A Dictionary of
FOOD & NUTRITION

J.L. Sharma
Silvano Caralli

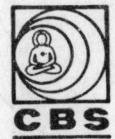

CBS

CBS PUBLISHERS & DISTRIBUTORS PVT. LTD.

New Delhi • Bengaluru • Chennai • Kochi • Mumbai • Pune

ISBN: 81-239-0628-5

First Edition: 1998
Reprint: 2002, 2004, 2005, 2011, 2015

Published by:
Satish Kumar Jain for CBS Publishers & Distributors Pvt. Ltd.,
CBS Plaza, 4819/XI Prahlad Street, 24 Ansari Road,
Daryaganj, New Delhi – 110002, India
delhi@cbspd.com, cbspubs@airtelmail.in • www.cbspd.com
Ph.: 23289259, 23266861, 23266867 • Fax: 011-23243014

Branches:
• *Bengaluru:* Seema House, 2975, 17th Cross, K.R. Road,
 Bansankari 2nd Stage, Bengaluru - 560070
 Ph: +91-80-26771678/79 • Fax: +91-80-26771680
 E-mail: cbsbng@gmail.com, bangalore@cbspd.com
• *Chennai:* No. 7, Subbaraya Street, Shenoy Nagar, Chennai - 600030
 Ph: +91-44-26681266, 26680620 • Fax: +91-44-42032115
 E-mail: chennai@cbspd.com
• *Kochi:* 36/14, Kalluvilakam, Lissie Hospital Road, Kochi - 682018
 Ph: +91-484-4059061-65 • Fax: +91-484-4059065
 E-mail: cochin@cbspd.com
• *Mumbai:* 83-C, Dr. E. Moses Road, Worli, Mumbai - 400018
 Ph: +91-9833017933, 022-24902340/41 • E-mail: mumbai@cbspd.com
• *Pune:* Bhuruk Prestige, Sr. No. 52/12/2+1+3/2,
 Narhe, Haveli (Near Katraj-Dehu Road Bypass), Pune - 411041
 Ph: +91-20-64704058/59, 32342277 • E-mail: pune@cbspd.com

Printed at :
J.S. Offset Printers, Delhi

Preface

The dictionary of food and nutrition, has been compiled as a clear, convenient, and immediately accessible reference book. Every aspect of its conception and layout has been planned to help the reader to find the scientific information he needs with minimum difficulty. Most of the terms come from a wide range of disciplines- such as biology, botany, chemistry, biochemistry, microbiology, and engineering. While compiling this dictionary, emphasis has been placed on the composition of food items, their chemical composition and uses; and the basic scientific principles, phenomena and processes. Entries include the descriptions of the plants and their useful parts such as roots, leaves, or fruits; essential oils and herbs; showing their botanical identities, medicinal values, where they grow, how they are used, their history and folklore, and the examples of the foodstuffs in which they are constituents. Animal ingredients are similarly described, together with the principal chemical and synthetic materials now employed. In this dictionary, the energy content of the foods is mostly expressed in joules, and the vitamins are expressed, where appropriate, in both micrograms and in International units. Restraint must prevail, particularly in a dictionary such as this of modest proportions; the terms included have been selected in a somewhat pragmatic manner, partly on the basis of those most frequently encountered within the context of food and nutrition in daily life.

Comments by the users which might be useful in considering the later revisions of, and additions to, this dictionary will be welcomed and appreciated.

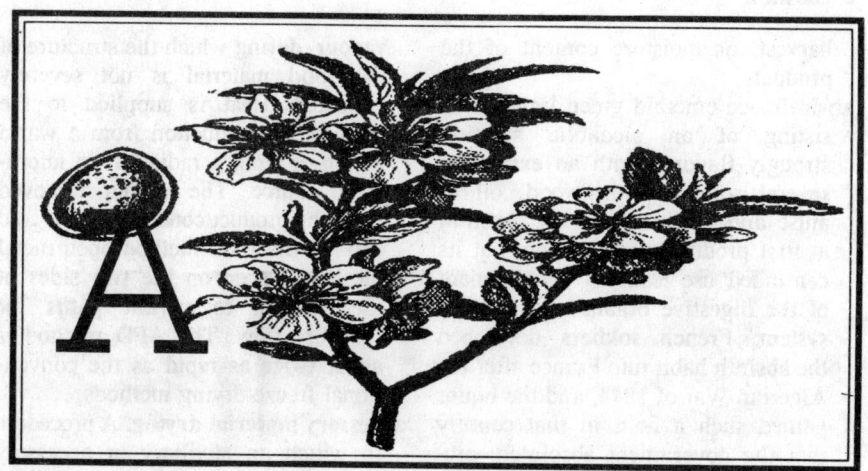

A24 protein. The protein complex resulting from the conjugation of ubiquitin to histone H2A. The amount of H2A histone that is in the form of A24 varies in different cells. Some evidences exist to suggest that chromatin, which includes the actively transcribed DNA sequences is enriched in 24 protein.

abalone drying. See ablone.

abalone. A shellfish, gastropod mollusc of the genus *Haliotis;* found in the water round Japan, California, Channel Islands and France. The abalone is an ear-shaped shell marine animal containing edible meat; commonly harvested on the Pacific Coast. It is dried in the sun after removing the shell, washing, and boiling.

abernethy. A variety of hard biscuit flavoured with caraway seed.

ablimation. The process of condensation of vapour directly to ice without going through the liquid phase. Ablimation is a process which occurs in a direction opposite to sublimation, as commonly defined.

ABO blood group system. The major human blood typing system the reflects the presence or absence of the A and B antigens in erythrocyte plasma membranes. It is the most important in blood transfusion serology because natural antibodies against ABO blood group antigens occur in serum. Humans belong to one of four groups: A, B, AB and O; the red cells of each group carry respectively the A antigen, the B antigen, both A and B antigens, or neither antigen. The antibodies in serum are specific for those ABO antigens not present on the red cells of the bearer, *e.g.,* persons of group A have serum antibodies to B antigen.

abrin. A protein present in the seeds of *Abrus precatorius,* that is toxic and has antitumor activity; interferes with binding of aminoacyl t-RNA to ribosomes.

abscission. The separation of a body part, such as seeds, fruits, and leaves, from the plant either naturally or artificially. A special layer of cells weakens and dies is a result of natural aging, or through the use of a chemical to induce aging or death. Plants may be treated to cause abscission before drying so as to control growth of plant, timing of harvest, or moisture content of the product.

absinth. An emerald green liquor consisting of an alcoholic solution strongly flavored with an extract of several sorts of wormwood, oil of anise and other substances. Absinth at first produces exhilaration, but its continued use leads to derangement of the digestive organs and nervous system. French soldiers developed the absinth habit into France after the Algerian War of 1844, and the liquor gained such a hold in that country that the government absolutely prohibited its use in 1915. Previously its use had been barred in the army and navy. Also spelled as absinthe.

absinthe. *See* absinth.

absolute pressure controller. An instrument used in the operation of a vacuum pan or evaporator to control the vacuum on the product. The absolute pressure is independent of the atmospheric pressure. Absolute pressure measuring elements use a bellows or U-tube and do not have to be compensated for atmospheric conditions because these units measure from zero absolute pressure. These units are preferred for evaporator control because the boiling temperature depends on absolute pressure.

absolute specificity. The extreme selectively of an enzyme that allows it to catalyze only the reaction with a single substrate in case of a monomolecular reaction, or the reaction with a single pair of substrates in the case of a bimolecular reaction. Also known as absolute group specificity.

Ac'cent. Trade name for monosodium glutamate.

accelerated freeze-drying. In freeze-drying heat is added to a product, usually food or pharmaceutical, such that the moisture is removed as a vapour, during which the structure of the solid material is not severely damaged. Heat is supplied to the product by conduction from a warm platen or from a radiation or microwave source. The vapour removed from the product condenses on a cold coil. In the AFD method open metal mesh is placed on the two sides of the product to permit paths for moisture flow. The AFD method is about twice as rapid as the conventional freeze-drying methods.

accessory material drying. A procedure in which an auxiliary or accessory material is added to the material being dried. The material is used to hasten the speed of heating and/or to absorb moisture to increase the rate of drying. An accessory material such as filter paper when used with sand increases the drying rate, whereas filter paper with a hygroscopic material, such as potatoes or carrots, increases the first part of the drying rate then decreases the remainder of the drying rate. The decrease in drying rate is caused by a decrease in heat and mass transfer. Accessory materials can also be used for heating a material to be dried, such as the use of heated sand, which has been used for drying cereal grains. For drying with accessory materials, conduction heating predominates in contrast to convection heating for many drying operations.

Acesulfame K. Trade name for the potassium salt of 6-methyl-1,2,3-oxathiazine-4(3H)-one-2,2-dioxide; used in several food products. It is believed to be on the market in the form of tabletop sweeteners, chewing gum, instant coffee and tea, and dry bases for beverages, gelatins, puddings, pudding desserts, and dairy product analogs. There is an intent to releasing carbon dioxide and the sulphydral form of acyl carrier protein. It exists at least in two isoform differing in amino acid sequence. These are required for fatty acid synthetase activity.

acyl carrier protein transacylase. A rate limiting enzyme encountered in fatty acid synthetase system It catalyzes the formation of medium chain fatty acids products by transferring acetyl-CoA to ACP-SH, forming acetyl-S-ACP and CoA.

acyl lipids. The lipids forming a major component of plant membrane. These are water insoluble containing a long hydrocarbons chains. Mostly glycerol is backbone in their structure.

acyl thiokinase. An enzyme which catalyzes the esterification of free fatty acids with extramitochondrial-CoA using adenosine triphosphate and producing high energy fatty acyl-CoA. It is localized in glyoxysomes.

acyl transferase. An enzyme which catalyzes the transfer of the palmityl moiety of palmityl-ACP to a suitable acceptor e.g., 1-monoacylglycerol-P during ACP-chain termination.

acyl-CoA dehydrogenase. An enzyme which catalyzes the removal of hydrogen from fatty acid giving β-unsaturated acyl derivatives of CoA, FAD acts as prosthetic group. This enzyme is of four different types and their specificities depend upon the chain length of fatty acid.

acyl-CoA oxidase. An enzyme which catalyzes the formation of acyl-CoA from propionyl-CoA during oxidation of odd number carbon atoms containing fatty acids.

adaly. Coix lachryma-jobi. A tall grass that grows wild in parts of Asia and Africa. It is used as a cereal to eke out rice suppliers in parts of India, China, Siam and Philippines. It belongs to the same family (Tripsaceae) as maize. The average composition per 100 g is: protein 14%, fat 4%, food energy 1.52 MJ, Ca 20 mg, Fe 5 mg, vitamin B_1 0.2 mg, B_2 0.2 mg, nicotinic acid 3 mg. Also known as Job's tears.

additives. Any material deliberately added to food to help manufacture and preserve food, improve palatability and eye-appeal; such as emulsifiers, flavours, thickeners, curing agents, humectants, colours, vitamins, minerals, and mould, yeast and bacterial inhibitors. Most of these are controlled by law in all countries.

adenosine diphosphate. ADP. Nucleotide composed of adenine, ribose and two phosphate groups. It is an important coenzyme and can undergo further phosphorylation to yield adenosine triphosphate (ATP), which is the prime energy-rich intermediate in cellular metabolism. The phosphorylation of adenosine diphosphate (ADP) to adenosine triphosphate (ATP) occurs within mitochondria, and ADP/ATP ratios and levels within the cell help to determine rates or anabolism and catabolism.

adenosine monophosphate. AMP. Nucleotide consisting of adenine linked to ribose and a single phosphate group.

adenosine triphosphate. ATP. A nucleotide that is of fundamental importance as a carrier of chemical energy in all living organism. It consists of adenine linked to D-ribose (i.e., adenosine); the D-ribose component bears three phosphate groups, linearly linked by covalent bonds. Adenosine triphosphate drives most of an organism's energy-requiring reactions by yielding the high free-energy of its phosphate-phosphate (pyrophosphate) bonds. It is formed in the mitochondria of cells under aerobic conditions by the oxidative phosphorylation of adenosine diphosphate (adenosine diphosphate), and also by transfer of phosphate to adenosine diphosphate from other energy-rich molecules, for example phosphoenolpyruvate; this latter is the only means of energy generation under anaerobic conditions. Of the three phosphate groups in adenosine triphosphate, two are attached by pyrophosphate bonds, and hydrolysis of these bonds results in a substantial release of free energy. This energy release on hydrolysis of adenosine triphosphate is used widely in biological systems to drive energy-requiring processes. Adenosine triphosphate is derived from adenosine diphosphate during photosynthesis, using solar energy, and during oxidative phosphorylation in which energy from carbohydrate catabolism is used.

adenosine. Combination of the base, adenine, with the sugar, ribose. Of special importance, as adenosine triphosphate plays a central part in the energy release in muscle.

adenyl cyclase. The enzyme that catalyzes the formation of cyclic adenosine monophosphate from adenosine triphosphate by the splitting out of pyrophosphate. This enzyme is involved in many cellular processes and particularly in the action of polypeptide hormones attach to the plasma membrane of a cell they stimulate adenyl cyclase to produce cyclic adenosine monophosphate. This is the initial step in the second messenger system, which enables these hormones to effect the gene expression of cells to which they bind.

adenylic acid. Nucleotide found in RNA consisting of the purine base adenine, a pentose sugar and a phosphoric acid group.

adenylosuccinate lyase. An enzyme which catalyzes removal of fumaric acid from 4-N-succinocarboxamide-5-aminoimidazole ribotide to form 4-carboxamide 5-aminoimidazole ribotide.

adenylosuccinate synthetase. An enzyme which catalyzes the combination of inosine-5'-monophosphate with aspartic acid in presence of ATP. Thus adenylosuccinic acid is formed.

adhesive hardening. The process of hardening of an adhesive is variously called curing, drying, hardening, and setting. Curing is generally used to represent the process when chemical polymerization is involved. Drying is generally used with starch adhesives. Setting is the term commonly used for emulsion and gelatin glues.

ADI. Abbreviation for *A*cceptable *D*aily *I*ntake; refers to chemical additives used in food processing.

adipose tissue. Groups of cells that sore and mobilize fat; constitutes a fifth to a quarter of the total body mass, and more in fatty people; composed of 82-88% fat, 2-2.6% protein and 10-14% water and contains 8-9 kcal (34-38 kJ) per gram.

adjuvant. A material added to an antigen to increase its immunogenicity. Some of the common examples include alum, killed *Bordetella pertussis*, and an oil emulsion of the antigen, either alone or with killed mycobacteria.

A DNA. Form of double helical DNA which, like the common B form, is a right-handed double helix of antiparallel strands, but differing slightly in helical pitch and base pair orientation from the B form. It may be noted that only very localized regions of DNA occur as A-form molecules, but the A-form helix is the most stable configuration for double-stranded RNA.

adoptive immunity. The immunity acquired by an animal organism when it is injected with lymphocytes from another organism.

adoptive tolerance. The immunological tolerance acquired by an animal organism when it in injected with lymphocytes from another organism.

adrenaline. Hormone secreted by the medulla of the adrenal glands; the first hormone to be discovered. It is secreted under conditions of emotional stress and causes an increase in blood pressure, blood sugar levels and metabolic rate, thus mobilizing the body's reserves of energy.

adrenocorticotropic hormone. Hormone extracted from the anterior part of the pituitary gland of animals and used in the treatment of rheumatoid arthritis. Acts by stimulating the adrenal gland to secrete corticosteroids.

adsorbent carbon. *See* activated carbon.

adsorptionally bound water. A monomolecular layer of water on the internal and external surfaces of a capillary-porous body, represented by equilibrium moisture content curves or similar relationships.

adulterated milk. *See* milk, adulterated.

adzuki bean. Family: *Leguminosae*. Genus: *Phaseolus*. Species. *Phaseolus angularis*. In macrobiotics these beans are used to help kidney complaints.

aequm. Amount of food necessary to maintain body weight under normal or specified conditions of activity.

aeration. 1. The process of forcing air or gas, usually carbon dioxide, under pressure into a liquid. 2. Exposure of milk to the atmosphere, i.e., while heating to pasteurization temperature (not during holding period) to minimize feed flavour if present. Milk is commonly aerated over surface coolers after milking to help remove undesirable gases and odours. Introduction of air into a substance such as soil or a liquid.

aerobes. The microorganisms that need oxygen for growth. Obligate aerobes cannot survive in absence of oxygen.

aerobic sporeforming bacilli. Members of the genus *Bacillus* are widely dispersed in soil, plant matter, and air. These bacteria are aerobic or facultative anaerobic, Gram-positive, motile rods that grow readily on laboratory media. Under adverse conditions *Bacillus* spp. form true endospores that are extremely resistant to heat, desiccation, ultraviolet light, and chemical treatment. Subgroups of the *Bacillus* genus have been constructed based on endospore shape (oval, spherical), position of spore in the cell (central, terminal), and the species' ability to ferment sugars. Many species of *Bacillus* can be isolated from soil by planting a pasteurized soil suspension on a selective medium. The spores survive this heat treatment and grow into colonies on aerobic agar plates. These bacteria grow on a wide range of organic compounds including amino acids, organic acids, and sugars. Most *Bacillus* spp. are mesophilic; however *Bacillus stearothermophilus* is a thermophile that grows at 338K.

aesculin. A glycoside (dihydroxycoumarin glycoside) found in chestnuts, with vitamin P activity.

aflatoxicosis. *See* aflatoxin poisoning.

aflatoxins. Toxic metabolites of the mould *Aspergillus flavus*. Eight forms have been isolated; chemically it is related to furocoumarins; carcinogenic to several animal species. Also formed by other strains of *Aspergillus* and *Panicillum puberulum*. *See also* aflatoxin poisoning.

aflatoxin poisoning. The etiologic agents of this food-borne illness are Aflatoxin B_1, B_2, G_1, and G_2 from Aspergillus flavus-oryzae group. These fungi are found worldwide and grow on practically any substrate. They are carcinogenic to rats, ducks, and trout and some authorities implicate them in involvement with human cancers. These toxins are heat-stable. Suspect food sources include cottonseed meal, Brazil nuts, palm, kernels, groundnuts (peanuts), corn (maize), other cereals, and animal feeds. Preventing measures include control of moisture during storage of aforementioned materials, preventing of damage during harvesting, insect control, fungicidal mold control, and physical removal of contaminated products, such as groundnuts. Also known as aflatoxicosis.

ageusia. Lack or impairment of sensitivity to taste stimuli.

agglomeration. The process of gathering fine particles together into larger particles to form coarser particles. The process is used to join small particles into agglomerates of food particles to form instantized dry products. The agglomerated products are more readily soluble in water when reconstituted than the fine particles.

agglutination. A term used to refer to a form of aggregation occurring in antigen-antibody reactions in which proteinaceous particles, such as bacteria, blood cells, etc., form clumps or clusters. The action is quite specific to the proteins involved. Agglutination may occur in transfusion if blood of the wrong group is given. The surfaces of the donor's red blood cells contain antigen molecules that are attached by antibody molecules in the serum of recipient, which causes the red cells to clump together. These clumps may block capillaries, causing fatal damage to the heart or brain. Agglutination of bacteria by antibodies causes them to disintegrate. *See also* antibody; blood groups.

agglutinin. One of a class of substances found in blood to which certain foreign substances or organisms have been added or admixed. As the name indicates, agglutinins have the characteristic property of causing agglutination, especially of foreign substances or organisms responsible for their formation.

aggregate fruit. A fruit which is formed form numerous carpels of one flower. The fruit, therefore, consists of a cluster of small, individual fruitlets. Examples are blackberry, raspberry, and strawberry. The fruitlets of the blackberry and raspberry, and strawberry. The fruitlets of the blackberry and raspberry are actually small drupes. In the strawberry, the seedlike achenes are fruitlets, embedded in a fleshy, edible floral receptacle.

aggressin. A substance that is produced by a microorganism and that, though not necessarily toxic by itself, promotes the invectiveness of the microorganism in the host; the enzymes hyaluronidase and collagenase are two examples.

aging. 1. A term applied to treatment of flour with oxidising agents, i.e. aging agents. When freshly milled flour is stored for several weeks it undergoes an aging effect and produces a stronger and more resilient dough and a bolder loaf, and the flour slowly bleaches. Chemical agents can produce these effects immediately. Oxidising agents, such as ammonium persulphate used (160 mg/kg) and potassium bromate (20 mg/kg), are improvers but do not bleach. Nitrogen peroxide (5 mg/kg) and benzoyl peroxide (20-40 mg/kg) bleach but do not improve. Nitrogen trichloride (60 mg/kg) and chlorine dioxide (30 mg/kg) bleach and improve. The use of only one bleaching agent, that is benzoyl peroxide at concentration not exceeding 50 mg/kg, has been recommended. No specific limit is set on maturing agents such as ascorbic acid. potassium bromate, ammonium and potassium persulphate, chlorine dioxide, chlorine (cake flour only) sulphur dioxide (brown flour only).

2. In reference to wine "aging" refers to the development of bouquet and smooth mellow flavour, and disappearance of harsh and yeasty taste-due to slow oxidation and formation of esters. *See also* wine.

agnelloto. Envelope of pasta stuffed with minced meat or vegetables; cut in half-moon shape, so differing from ravioli, which is cut in squares.

air brush. A method by which is dried product is separated from the air in a spray dryer. Air from outside of the dryer, either at room temperature or conditioned to a lower temperature, is used to direct a jet of air to move the product from the bottom of the dryer.

air dehumidification. The process of removing a water vapour from a mixture of air and water vapour in which the humidity is reduced. Dehumidification is carried out by condensing the moisture on a surface at a temperature below the dew-point, by spray dehumidifiers, with a chemical such as an acid in an absorption tower, or with chemical dehydrating agents such as calcium chloride.

air dry lumber. Lumber dried by exposure to air outdoors or under an unheated shed for any length of time. The range of the final moisture content is from 6% (in the southwest) to 24% (in winter in the northwest), but usually in the range from 12-15% moisture content.

air humidification. The process of evaporating a liquid such as water into air and the diffusion and convection of the moisture throughout the air. The humidity of the air is increased as a result of humidification. Humidification may be done to increase the moisture content of a product or to condition a product for subsequent processing.

air lock. A chamber with valves located between two other chambers at different pressures or between a chamber at a vacuum or pressure and the outside air. The air lock is operated in a procedure similar to the lock in a canal to move a ship from one level to another. The purpose of the air lock is to permit moving a product from one pressure chamber to another without losing the pressure (or vacuum) of the chamber, such as with a vacuum freeze-dryer and for moving grain into and out of a dryer.

air moving device. AMD. A revolving, wheel type, mechanical device, driven by a power source, used to move air for drying or aeration. For the ASAE standard, an AMD includes the wheel or blade assembly, mounting structure and casing, and may or may not include a power source.

air oven. A nearly closed container, with or without air circulation, usually heated with electricity, having a carefully controlled temperature, with or without vacuum, used to dry weighed samples of product to determine the moisture content. The time and temperature of dehydration have been standardized for most commercial products.

air separator. A mechanical device for separating liquid and/or solid contents from air. The most common principle used is centrifugal force. Also known as dust collector; centrifugal separator; cyclone collector; and cyclone separator.

air trunking. The ducts, tunnels, or

channels which direct air to storages, silos, or drying chambers. The velocity of air flow normally should not exceed 7.6-10 m/s to prevent excessive pressure drop. Trunking is constructed from sheet metal, wood, plywood, chipboard, etc. It is a general term for an air distribution system.

air-lift dryer. The name may be applied generally to a fluidized bed or pneumatic dryer. A more precise use of the term is for a dryer which was used to partially dry potato granules during World War II. The dryer consisted of a vertical feed chamber into which the product was fed by a vibrator into a hot air stream at a venturi section. The product was carried vertically while being dried in the hot air stream. The vertical chamber had an enlarged cross-section as the exit was approached, thus decreasing the velocity and therefore the carrying capacity of the air. The product hit a deflector and was dropped to a collector and removed. The moist air exited vertically after passing around deflector.

air-straightening-vanes. The mechanical channels, guides, etc., placed in airflow ducts to assure a more uniform distribution of the air at bends or elbows and throughout pipes, tubes, or ducts.

Ajinomoto. Trade name for range of flavour enhancers such as - Ajinomoto IMP, disodium inosinate; Ajinomoto GMP, disodium guanylate; Ajinomoto, monosodium glutamate.

ajwan oil. A yellow essential oil distilled from ajwan seed of the herbaceous plant *Carum copticum,* or *Ptychotis ajowan,* of India. The seed yields 3 to 4% oil containing up to 50% thymol and some cymene, most of the thymol separating out on distillation. Thymol is known as ajwan ka phul,

meaning flowers of ajwan in Hindi, and the latter part of the name is Anglicized to thymol. Ajwan oil has a specific gravity of 0.900 to 0.930. It is used in pharmaceuticals. Thymol, $(CH_3)_2 CHC_6H_3(CH_3)OH$, is a white crystalline solid with a strong thyme odour, soluble in alcohol, and melting at 50°C. It is used in antiseptics and as a deodorant for leather. Thymol is also obtained from horse-mint oil and from eucalyptus oil, or can be made synthetically from *m*-cresol. It was originally distilled from the thyme plant, *Thymus vulgaris,* of the Mediterranean countries, the dried leaves of which are used as a condiment. Cymene is used as a scent in soaps, and has high solvent properties. It is also obtained from spruce turpentine. Also called ptychotis oil.

akee. *Blighia sapida.* The fruit of West African origin, grown in West Indies; unripe fruits are toxic.

Alaska pollack. *Theragra chalcogramma.* A kind of fish is not to be confused with the pollock. The Alaska pollack has the same distribution as the Pacific cod, but is less dependent on being near the coast and may be found at depths as great as 300 m. This species is found in open, warmer (as compared with Pacific cod) water. Its diet consists of plankton and small fish. In the western Pacific Ocean, isolated populations have developed difference in growth and the spawning season. In recent years, the Alaska pollack has become quite important commercially.

albedo. White pith of the inner peel of citrus fruits, also known as the mesocarp; 20-60% of the whole fruit. It consists of sugars, cellulose and pectins; used as a source of pectin for commercial manufacture.

albumin index. A measure of the quality

of an egg; the ratio of height of the albumin to the width when broken on to a flat surface. As the egg deteriorates the albumin index decreases, i.e. the egg white spreads.

albumin/globulin ratio. Ratio of the blood albumin to the globulins; in normal human serum 1.82. Change in the A/G ratio is of diagnostic value.

albuminoid ammonia. Ammonia obtained by decomposition of albuminous material. The quantity present is utilized in water analysis to determine the percentage of organic nitrogen in the sample.

albuminoids. Fibrous proteins that have supporting or protective function in the animal (in plants cellulose fulfils this function). The three types are:
(a) collagens in skin, tendons and bones, resistant to pepsin and trypsin, converted to water-soluble gelatin by boiling with water;
(b) elastins in tendons and arteries, not converted to gelatin;
(c) keratins, proteins insoluble in dilute acids and alkalis, not attacked by any animal digestive enzymes, comprise horns, hoofs, feathers, scales, nails.

albumins. A mixture of water-miscible globular proteins occurring in the tissues and fluids of the body. It crystallizes on drying but can be reconstituted with water. It is heat-sensitive and coagulates irreversibly at about 353K. Albumin is the chief component of egg white in the form of ovalbumin and conalbumin, it also occurs in lower percentages in egg yolk, milk, and blood serum. It is produced for commercial use in food products and for photographic emulsions. The molecular mass of the albumins is about 50,000. Humans serum albumin is a simple protein carrying a negative charge at neutral

pH. By maintaining the colloidal osmotic pressure of blood plasma, it plays an important role in osmoregulation. Ovalbumin, found in the water-soluble part of bird egg white, is a protein that contains a carbohydrate prosthetic group.

alcaptonuria. A rare inborn error of metabolism of the two amino acids phenylalanine and tyrosine. Their metabolism ceases at homogentisic acid, which is excreted in the urine. Homogentisic acid oxidizes to black melanoid pigments, hence the urine of alcaptonurics slowly turns black. The defect appears to be harmless.

alcohol test for milk. A test used to indicate stability or acidity of milk which is to be subjected to high temperatures as in evaporation or sterilization. The test consists of mixing in a test tube 2 ml each of milk and ethyl alcohol of a definite percentage (68-75% alcohol by volume) and noting whether or not coagulation occurs. White particles of coagulated casein on the inner walls of the test tube indicate an acidity of at least 0.21%; the coarser the particles, the greater the acidity. The alcohol test is said to be more useful than an acidity determination in predicting the stability of milk destined to be evaporated and sterilize by heat. In genera, milks not precipitated by 70% alcohol are stable enough for this purpose.

alcohol, denatured. Alcohol to which unpleasant materials have been added to make it unfit for drinking, e.g., methylated spirits contains 10% methyl alcohol, a blue dye and unpleasant-smelling pyridine. Denatured alcohol is used for industrial purposes.

alcoholic beverages. Yeast fermentation of sugar or starchy materials yields a solution of approximately 10-15% alcohol, (wine) at which strength the alcohol kills off the yeast. If sweet wines are required the fermentation is stopped at an earlier stage when there is still some sugar left. If stronger wines are needed, such as port, they are fortified by the addition of brandy. The strong spirit are made by distilling the alcohol from wine. Alcohol content of some of the alcoholic beverages are (per cent by volume):

Spirits- gin, whisky, brandy, rum- 25 under proof, 43% alcohol; 35 under proof, 37%.

Wines- Port, Sherry, Madeira 20%; Burgundy, 14%; Champagne, Charet, Hock, 10%; Cider, 4.3%; Ale 3.1 to 6.6%; Sout, 3.9 to 5.3%; Porter 4.0%.

Liqueurs- Curacao, 55%; Benedictine, 52%; Absinthe, 59%; Anisette, 42%; Chartreuse, 43%; Kummel, 34%.

See also ale, brandy, Champagne, rum, whisky and wine.

alcoholic fermentation. The anaerobic process of hexose decomposition, such as that of glucose to ethanol and carbon dioxide, caused by the zymase produced by yeasts, *e.g.,*

$$C_6H_{12}O_6 = 2C_2H_5OH + 2CO_2.$$

It occurs in many yeasts. The same enzymatic pathway of glycolysis is followed except the two last steps. *See also* fermentation.

ale. A type of wine in which the process of fermentation has been stopped before all the sugar is changed to other compounds. This sugar is changed by later fermentation in the barrel into alcohol and carbonic acid, and this change makes ale stronger and more harmful than beer. The strength of ale depends upon the time given it in which to cure; for mild ale, this is one week; for pale ale, from two to four months, and for strong ale, from ten to fifteen months.

Alemtejo cheese. A kind of cylindrical shaped, soft cheese made in the province of Alemtejo, Portugal. For the most part, sheep's milk is used although goat's milk is often added. It is ripened for several weeks.

aleurone layer. Single layer of large cells under the bran coat and outside the endosperm of cereal grains; about 3% by weight of the grain, rich in protein. Botanically, it is part of the endosperm but during milling remains attached to the inner layer of bran. It contains about 20% of the thiamine, 30% of the riboflavin and 50% of the riboflavin and 50% of the nicotinic acid of the grain.

alewife. A food fish found abundantly along the eastern coast of North America. It is not large fish, weighing at most not over 1 kg, but it makes up in numbers what it lacks in size. The alewife somewhat resembles the shad in colour and shape, and is related to that fish and to the herring.

alfalfa. *Medicago sativa.* A perennial herb commonly found on the edges of fields, in low valleys and is widely cultivated by farmers for livestock feed. An erect, smooth stem grows from an elongated taproot to a height of a foot or more. Flowers are blue-to-purple during the summer months, finally producing the characteristic spirally coiled speed pods. The plant is remarkable for the depth to which its roots penetrate the soil, ten to twenty feet being common. For this reason it thrives in dry regions where many forge plants could not exist. Above ground alfalfa attains a height of 30-60 cm. It bears leaves in three parts, purplish flowers resembling those of the pea, and small seed pods curiously twisted into spirals. As it is a rapid grower, producing a crop about every forty days during the season of growth, from three to seven crops a year may be harvested. The readiness with which alfalfa adapts itself to different soils and climates is one of its most striking characteristics. The latter are injurious in the their shorter roots take nourishment from the upper soil layers. Since alfalfa, like other pod-bearing plants, adds nitrogen to the soil through the bacteria that form on the nodules of its roots, fertilizers containing nitrogen are not necessary for its growth. Artificial liming, however, must sometimes be resorted to, a ton of unslaked lime to the acre being applied one year before the crop is sown. Bacteria do not usually develop spontaneously on the roots of the plant when it is first sown, and for this reason alfalfa growers sprinkle the new field with soil taken from an old field. This practice is called artificial inoculation. In the preparation of the seed bed the ground is plowed six weeks before sowing time. For hay it is customary to make the first cutting when the plants are just coming into bloom, and thereafter every forty days or so, as long as the season lasts. The plant is utilized as pasture grass, and as hay and silage, and is fed to dairy cows, beef cattle, poultry, sheep, horses and hogs. As bees eagerly visit the blossoms, an alfalfa field contributes to the production of honey.

Alfalfa or Lucerne was used by the Persians to feed their horses to make them look sleeker and feel stronger. The Arabs designed this common hay feed for livestock, "The Father of All Foods." Some modern herbalists have gone even further than this, characterizing alfalfa as being the Big Daddy in terms of nutritional value, considering that the plant is so rich in calcium that the ashes of its leaves are almost 99% pure calcium. Powered alfalfa contains vitamins A, B-6, B-12, C, E and K-1, niacin, pantothenic acid, biotin, folic acid, etc., as well as many essential and nonessential amino acids. Additionally, it contains 15-25% proteins, major minerals and trace elements like calcium, phosphorus, manganese, iron, zinc and copper, together with many naturally occurring sugars (sucrose, fructose, etc.)

alfalfa dehydrating. Dehydrated alfalfa is a metal product resulting from the rapid drying of alfalfa by artificial means at temperatures above 100°C. Because alfalfa meal is used in chicken rations, cattle feed, hog rations, sheep feed, turkey mash, and other formula feeds, it is important that the protein content, growth and reproductive factors, pigmenting xanthophylls, and vitamin content be altered or reduced as little as possible during the dehydration process. Standing alfalfa is mowed and chopped in the field and transported by truck to a dehydrating plant, which is usually located within about 16 kilometres of the field. The truck dumps the chopped alfalfa (wet chops) onto a feeder, which carries it into a direct-fired, rotary drum. Within the drum, the wet chops are dried from an initial moisture content of from 60% to 80% (weight to about 8% to 16%. Typical combustion gas temperatures (oil or gas is used) within the drums range from 980° to 1092°C at the inlet to 250°-300°C at the inlet to 120°-150°C at the outlet. From the drying drum, the dry chops are pneumatically conveyed into a primary cyclone that separates them from the high-moisture, high-temperature exhaust steam. From the primary cyclone, the chops are fed into a hammer-mill which grinds the dry chops into a metal. The meal is pneumatically conveyed from the hammer-mill into a meal collector cyclone in which the meal is separated from the air steam and discharged into a holding bin. Meal is then fed into a pellet mill where it is steam-conditioned and extruded into pellets. From the pellet mill, the pellets are either pneumatically or mechanically conveyed to a cooler, through which air is drawn to cool the pellets and, in some cases, remove fines. Fines removal is more commonly accomplished in shaker screens following or ahead of the cooler, with the fines being conveyed back into the meal collector cyclone, meal bin, or pellet mill. Cyclone separators may be used to separate entrained fines in the cooler exhaust and to collect pellets when the pellets are pneumatically conveyed from the pellet mill to the cooler. Following cooling and screening, the pellets are transferred to bulk stored. Dehydrated alfalfa is most often stored and shipped in pellet form. In some instances, pellets may be ground in a hammer-mill and shipped in meal form. When the finished pellets or ground pellets are pneumatically transferred to storage or load-out, additional cyclones may be used for product air-steam separation at these locations. Particulate matter is the primary pollutant of concern from alfalfa dehydrating plants, although some odours arise from the organic volatiles driven off drying. Particulate emissions can be reduced if the feeder discharge rates are uniform, if the dryer furnace is operated efficiently, if proper airflows are used in the cyclone collectors, and if the hammer-mill is well maintained and not overloaded.

algae. Sub-group, mainly aquatic, of the division of plants called *Thallophyta* which show no differentiation into root, stem and leaf. Includes seaweeds, such as Dulse and Irish Moss, which have long been eaten by man. Unicellular varieties such as *Chlorella, Scenedesmus* and *Spirulina* are being grown experimentally in tanks as a potential source of food. They require only carbon dioxide and mineral salts since they obtain their energy by photosynthesis. Protein content on dry weight basis: Spirulina 60-70%, Scenedesmus and Chlorella 50-60%; fat, spirulina 2%, Chlorella 8-20% depending on growing conditions; nutritional value of the proteins is similar to that of casein, i.e. NPU 50-70, per 2.2 - 2.5.

Green algae, most resembling the genus Chlorella, are found in many freshwater protozoa, sponges, hydra, and some flatworms. Most of these algae reproduce by simple cell division and are found within the host cell's vacuoles, which divide when the alga divides. Another green alga, Platymonas convolutae, is found mostly in the subepidermal cells of the marine flatworm. Within the flatworm, Platymonas has no cell wall and an irregular shape; its plasma membrane, greatly increased in surface area by fingerlike projections, is more or less in direct contact with the vacuole membrane of the host cell. When removed from the flatworm and cultured, Platymonas has a cell wall, four flagella and an eyespot, all lacking when it is symbiotic. The most direct relationship between green algae and invertebrates involves certain nudibranchs, which are marine molluscs, and the chloroplasts of some siphonaceous green algae, such as Codium. The chloroplasts, which are presumably acquired when nudibranchs eat the algae, are found in cells that line their entire respiratory chamber. In the presence of light these chloroplasts carry on photosynthesis so efficiently that individuals of the nudibranch Placobranchus ocellatus are reported to evolve oxygen more rapidly than it its consumed. Certain dinoflagellates (division Pyrrophyta), which resemble the nonflagellated cells of Chlorella when they occur as symbionts, inhabit the cells of various marine sponges, coelenterates, molluscs, flatworms, and protozoa. In the giant clams of the family. Tridachnidae, the dorsal surface of the inner lobes of the mantle may appears chocolate-brown as a result of the presence of symbiotic algae of this group, which are found in the blood sinuses and probably occur mainly within amoeboid blood cells. Dinoflagellates are also important symbionts in reef-building corals. Coral tissues may contain as many as 30,000 microscopic algae per cubic millimetre. The exact role of these algal symbionts in the coral economy is not known, but tracer studies using radioactive carbon have shown that organic substances pass from algae to the coral, and it has also been shown that the reef grows much more rapidly when the algae are present. Even though the coral animals are heterotrophic, the reef as a whole is autotrophic.

People of various parts of the world, especially in the far east, eat both red and brown algae. One of the red algae, Porphyra (nori), which is eaten by many of the inhabitants of the north Pacific Basin, has been cultivated in Japan and China for centuries. Various other red algae are eaten on the islands of the Pacific and the shores of north Atlantic.

Seaweeds are generally not of high nutritive value, because humans, like most other animals, lack the necessary enzymes to break down the seaweed carbohydrates. Seaweeds do, however, provide necessary salts as well as a number of important vitamins and trace elements and so are valuable supplementary foods. In many north temperate regions, kelp has been harvested for its ash, which is rich in soda and potash and is therefore valuable for industrial processes. Iodine is also produced commercially from kelp. Algae are often harvested and used directly for fertilizer. Alginates, derived from beds of kelps such as Macrocystis, are widely used as thickening agents and colloid stabilizers in the food, textile, cosmetic, pharmaceutical, paper, and welding industries. Off the west coast of the United States, Macrocystis beds can be cropped just below the surface several times a year. One of the most useful direct commercial applications of any alga is the preparation of agar, which is made from a mucilaginous material extracted from the cell walls of a number of genera of red algae. Agar is used to make the capsules that hold vitamins and other drugs, as a dental-impression material, as a base for cosmetics, and as a culture medium for bacteria and other microorganisms. It is also employed as an antidrying agent in bakery goods, in the preparation of rapid-setting jellies and desserts, and as a temporary preservative for meat and fish in tropical regions. Agar is produced in many parts of the world, but Japan is the principal source.

alginates. Salts of alginic acid found as the free acid and calcium salt in many seaweeds. Alginic acid is a polysaccharide complex built from mannuronic acid units. Salts such as iron, magnesium and ammonium alginates form viscous solutions. They hold large amounts of water and are useful as thickeners, stabilisers and gelling, binding and emulsifying agents in ice-cream, synthetic cream. The propyl glycol ester is used under the trade name of "mannucol ester".

Aliment de severage. Trade name for a protein-rich baby food, 20% protein. Algerian version made from wheat, chick peas, lentils, skim milk powder and sugar with added vitamin D. Senegal version made from millet flour, peanut flour, skim milk powder and sugar with vitamins A and D and calcium.

alimentary pastes. Shaped dried doughs made from semolina or wheat flour with water, and sometimes egg and milk. The dough is partly dried in hot air, then more slowly. Macaroni. tubular-shaped, about 10 mm diameter; at 20 mm it is called fovantini or maccaroncelli; at 12 mm, zitoni. Spaghetti is solid rod; vermicelli is a third of the thickness of spaghetti. Noodles are shaped into sheets or ribbons. *Farfals* are ground, granulated or shredded.

alizarin test for milk. A test for acidity, depending on the colour changes observed in a neutral alcohol solution of alizarin dye (deoxy-anthraquinone) when 2-3 ml are added to an equal amount of milk in a test tube and shaken. Coagulation changes may also be observed. With fresh normal milk of 0.16% acidity, colour is lilac-red. As acidity increases, the colour becomes brownish, then yellowish, until, with milk of 0.36% acidity or more than colour is yellow. There is no coagulation of milk in this test until the milk is over 0.18% in acidity. At this stage, coagulation takes place and size of the flakes increases with acidity to maximum size at an acidity of 0.36%. If milk has a normal acidity

of 0.16-0.18% but coagulates in very large flakes, the colour being dark brick-red, it is evidence of the presence of rennet-forming bacteria and the milk is considered to be of doubtful value as market milk. If milk turns violet and coagulates in fine flakes, the milk is alkaline, probably from a diseased udder, and is regarded as unfit for making cheese or any other edible milk product.

alkaloids. One of a group of organic compounds found in plants, that are poisonous, insoluble crystalline compounds. They contain nitrogen and usually occur as salts of acids such as citric, malic, and succinic acids. Their function in plants remains obscure, but it is suggested that they may be nitrogenous end-products of metabolism, or they may have a protective function against herbivores. Important examples are quinine, nicotine, atropine, opium, morphine, codeine, and strychnine.

alkalosis. Decrease in the acid base ratio in the blood plasma, or an increase in its buffering power. Causes may be excessive loss of carbon dioxide, excessive intake of base as in antacid drugs, loss of gastric secretion by vomiting, high intake of sodium or potassium salts of weak organic acids.

alkanet. Colouring obtained from root of *Anchusa tinctoria (Alkanna tinctoria)*; legally permitted in food in most countries; colouring principle is alkannin. It is insoluble in water but soluble in alcohol and ether; blue in alkalies, blue with lead, crimson with tin, violet with iron; used for colouring fats, cheese, essences (and inferior port wine). The colouring principal is alkannin, which can be recovered by extraction with petroleum ether. Alkannin (or orcanella) is a naphthaquinone derivative and is dark reddish-brown, somewhat coppery crystalline powder. It is insoluble in water, but soluble in ethanol (95%) and fixed oils to give a bright red solution. In alkaline solution, the colour changes to a deep blue.

All Bran. Trade name for breakfast cereal derived from wheat bran. The average composition per 100 g of the product is: 14 g protein, 2 g fat, 65 g soluble carbohydrate, 6.3 g fibre, food energy 1.4 MJ, 11 mg iron, 0.6 mg vitamin B_1, 2.5 mg vitamin B_2, 32 mg nicotinic acid.

allergen. Any Antigen or hapten that induces an allergic reaction, particularly through the production of antibodies of immunoglobulin IgE. The allergen and antibody combine to form a histamine-like substance, which in turn weakens the blood vessels sufficiently to release fluids. This causes the commonly experienced edema, sneezing, and swelling well-known to hay fever sufferers. Only those who are predisposed to certain allergens are capable of forming such antibodies. Severe allergens can cause extremely serious conditions which have been known to be quite fatal. Protein-containing substances are the most common allergens (wool, hair, pollen, etc.), but allergic reactions may be experienced by a few individuals from exposure to almost any substance.

allicin. A sulphur containing compound responsible for the flavour of garlic.

alligator pear. The fruit of an evergreen tree. It resembles a large pear, is one to two pounds in weight, and has a firm, marrow-like pulp of a delicate flavor. It is called also avocado pear or vegetable butter. The plant is a native of tropical regions.

Allinson bread. A whole wheat bread named after Allinson who advocated its use in England at the end of the nineteenth century, as did Graham in the United States (thus Graham bread).

allosteric enzyme. Any of several regulatory enzymes whose catalytic activity is modulated by the non-covalent binding of a specific metabolite at a site other than the catalytic site. These enzymes show end product inhibition. The first enzyme in such multienzyme system is known as allosteric enzyme. The classical Michaelis-Menten relationship is generally not confirmed. These enzymes show two types of control;
(a) heterotrophic, and
(b) homotrophic.

allosteric inhibitors. The low molecular mass compounds, though not resembling with substrate, which bind on the inhibitor sites of a regulatory enzyme. Thus the inhibitors could either decrease the affinity for the substrate at the catalytic site, or affect the catalytic efficiency of the enzyme, or do both.

allosteric modified enzyme. Enzymes modification due to binding of one or more metabolites to the catalytic sites of a regulatory enzymes.

alloxan. Pyrimidine derivative that can induce diabetes when given orally or by injection, by damaging the Islets of Langerhans (that part of the pancreas which secretes insulin).

allspice. Dried fruits of the evergreen *Pimenta officinalis,* also known as pimento or Jamaican pepper (differs from pimiento). The whole spice comes in the form of a reddish-brown seed with a fairly smooth surface. The predominant flavor of allspice is that of cloves and is due to the presence of eugenol. Most allspice is produced in Jamaica, but alternative sources include Guatemala, Honduras, and

Mexico. Jamaican allspice is considered by many to be the best because it has a more rounded flavor, higher oil content, and cleaner appearance. In the spice trade this material is often called pimento. The name comes from the fact that allspice is thought to resemble in flavor a mixture of cinnamon, nutmegs and cloves. The fruit is also called Jamaica pepper. It is employed in cooking, and in medicine as an agreeable aromatic, and it forms the basis of a distilled water and an essential oil. The volatile oil content of the dried material will run from about 2.5% to 3.5% and the moisture content will be 9% to 12%. Allspice has been used in some cakes, especially dark fruit cake types, and in mince meat.

allura red AC. Red. No. 40. FD&C Red 40. A dark red powder, which is very soluble in water. It was added to the permitted list of food colours in the US in 1971. Red No. 40, with the addition of various shading colours, can be used satisfactorily to replace amaranth in most food products. It is most effective in opaque and translucent products, but does not give the right shade of red in transparent products.

almond oil, bitter. Essential oil from seeds of almond tree (*Prunus amygdalus*) or apricot tree (*Prunus armeniaca*); mostly manufactured from the apricot; contains 95% benzaldehyde, with hydrocyanic acid and benzaldehyde cyanhydrin. When feed from hydrocyanic acid is used as flavour, in perfumes and in cosmetics.

almond. Family: *Rosaceae*. Genus: *Prunus*. Species: *Prunus amygdalus.* The fruit of the almond, a tree which grows usually to the height of 7-8 metres, and is akin to the peach and nectarine. It has beautiful pinkish flowers that appear before the leaves, which are oval, pointed and delicately serrated. It has a downy outer coat which covers the flatfish, wrinkled stone that encloses the seed. There are two varieties, one sweet and the other bitter.

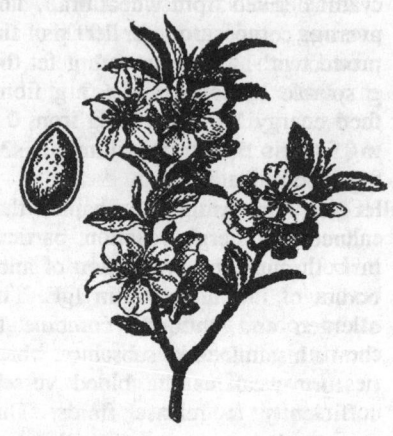

Sweet almonds are a delicious food and furnish an oil used in flavoring. Bitter almonds contain prussic acid, a highly poisonous substance. Almonds are extremely nourishing and have been valued as a good muscle- and body-building substance. They are high in fat, carbohydrate and protein and their calcium content is particularly valuable for building children's teeth and bones. Almond meal contains almost twice the vitamin B content of the same weight of roasted almonds.

almond flavouring. Some food processors find it more convenient to use almond flavouring rather than almonds *per se* in various products. Bitter almond oil is a principal source of almond flavouring. Bitter almond oil is obtained by cold expressing the fixed oils from previously ground bitter almond (*Prunus amygdalus*), apricot (*P. armeniaca*), and peach (*P. persica*). The kernels of these fruits contain the glucoside amygdalin, which when hydrolyzed by enzymes, will yield benzaldehyde and hydrogen cyanide. Distilled bitter almond oil for use as a flavouring must be distilled to render it fully free of hydrogen cyanide (HCN; prussic acid). After pressing, the ground kernels are mixed with water to complete the enzymatic hydrolysis. The mixture is then steam distilled to yield from 0.5 to 0.7% essential oil. Oil intended for food use is further treated to remove HCN by precipitation as an insoluble calcium ferrocyanide. The oil is used in both nonalcoholic and alcoholic beverages, in ice creams, candies, baked goods, gelatins and puddings, chewing gums, and marschino cherries. Levels of usage in these products ranging from about 30 parts per million up to about 340 parts per million. Most countries generally regard the oil as safe (GRAS) if it is free from prussic acid.

aloe. *Aloe vera.* A perennial succulent native to East and South Africa, but also cultivated in the West Indies and other tropical countries. The strong, fibrous root produces a rosette of fleshy basal leaves. They have fleshy leaves, which are thick and more or less armed with spines at the edges or ends. The flowers have a tubular corolla. The fibrous parts of the leaves of some species are made into cordage, fishing nets, lines and cloth; the juice of several species is used in medicine as a bitter drug; under the name of aloes. The principal drug-producing species are the Socotrine aloe, the Barbados aloe and the Cape aloe. A beautiful violet colour is afforded by the leaves of the Socotrine alone. The so-called American aloe is

a different plant altogether, as are also the aloes or lignaloes of Scripture.

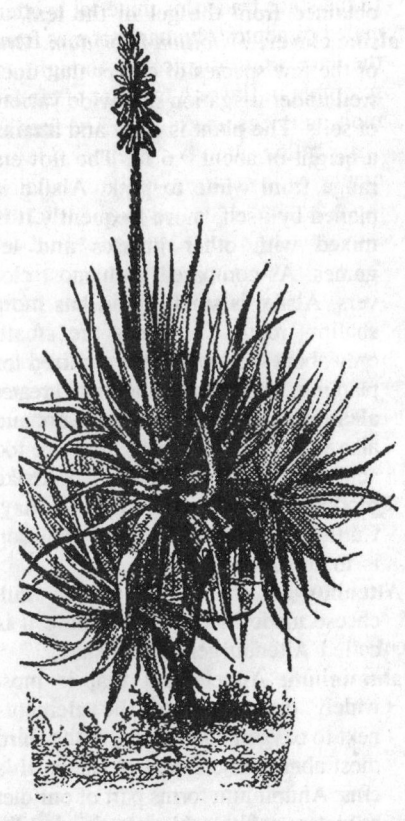

The tissue in the centre of the leaf contains a mucilaginous gel which yields aloe gel or aloe vera gel. Aloe vera contains 96% water, which provides water to injured tissue without closing off the air necessary for tissue repair. The remaining 4% of the pulp contains complex carbohydrate molecules, believed essential to aloe's natural value as a moisturizer. Substances present include enzymes, trace sugars, a protein containing 18 amino acids; vitamins; minerals like sulphur, silicon, iron, calcium, copper, sodium, potassium, manganese and more. The mixture of active ingredients in aloe is called aloin, and is obtained from the gel in the leaf.

alsike clover. *Trifolium hybridum.* One of the few species of clover that does well under irrigation in a wide variety of soils. The plant is erect and attains a height of about 0.6 m. The flowers range from white to pink. Alsike is planed by itself, more frequently it is mixed with other grasses and legumes. As compared with most clovers, Alsike is smaller and has more shallow roots. The seeds are small, only about 4.5 kg/hectare required for planting. The plant will tolerate greater alkalinity than most other clovers and also will do well in soils that are too acid for red clover. Usually, Alsike produces only one crop of hay. Cuttings usually done when the crop is in full blood.

Altenburger cheese. A goat's milk cheese made in Germany where it is called Altenburger Zingenkase.

aluminium. An element that is most widely distributed of the elements next to oxygen and silicon, is the third most abundant element in the earth's crus. Aluminium forms part of our diet as instant coffee, table salt, dried milk, some food additives and in tea bags. The mineral is also a component of many stomach medicines, including antacid tablets, that can increase the levels of aluminium excreted in the urine by 8 times. Aluminium hydroxide in stomach medicines also binds to phosphates and means they cannot be taken up by the body. This can lead to inadequate levels of phosphorus in the body. Several vaccines for diseases also contain aluminium.

Aluminium is released from the soil by the action of acid rain lowering the pH, and the mineral then enters the ground water and may be taken into supplies of drinking water. Concentrations of aluminium in drinking water in many developed countries seem to correlate to the prevalence of Alzheimer's disease. It has been proposed that the disease results from the deposition of aluminium in the brain cells, which would impair their functioning. Aluminium is an extremely reactive chemical, and it is inclined to bind to other substances. Since aluminium ions (Al^{3+}) are similar to ferric iron ions (Fe^{3+}), aluminium can change places with iron in proteins such as ferritin and so enter the cells. When in the body, aluminium causes demineralization of the bones, changes the metabolism of calcium and allows cross-linkages to form in collagen. The mineral also brings about zinc loss, and this may play a part in the development of dementia. Dyslexic people often have high level of aluminium and low levels of zinc in the body. When zinc is lacking, aluminium can bind to proteins that carry zinc, and supplementation with zinc is necessary to reverse the deficiency, correct the protein structures and restore normal function to many enzyme complexes. Patients who are drip-fed or who need dialysis treatment absorb much more aluminium than normal people, and this can cause damage to bones and brain damage. This is why dialysis fluids are normally purified and the aluminium removed because aluminium poisoning can be fatal.

alveographe. Measures stretching quality of dough as index of protein quality for baking. A standard disc of dough is blown into a bubble and the pressure curve and bursting pressure measured; gives the ability, extensibility and strength.

amaranth. Class: *Dicotyledon*. Group: *Thalamiflorae*. Order: *Caryophyllales*. Family: *Amaranthaceae*. Genus: *Amaranthus*. Amaranth seeds were an important food for some of the American Indian tribes as early as 4,000 BC. Not a true cereal, but rather a fruit, it belongs to the same family (chenopodium) as the edible weed, lamb's-quarter. Looking like a sesame seed, it has a pleasant, nutty flavour and can be popped like corn or steamed and flattened into a flake. It requires very little water and fertilizer, growing almost anywhere the common weeds do. It is thought that amaranth was brought to this hemisphere by those first migrants from the Tower of Babel, who travelled eastward across China and launched their barges on the Pacific, eventually reaching what is now western Mexico around 2000 BC. The Mayas were probably among the first to cultivate the plant, and it was also extensively cropped by both the Aztecs and the Incas. Estimates place total production by the Aztecs at about 15 to 20 thousand tons per year prior to the Spanish Conquest, at which time it was the third ranking crop, following corn and beans. Leaves of this plant were also used as food, and it is said that even today the leaves are favored much more than the grain. In most countries outside Central America, amaranth is regarded as a weed. There are over 60 accepted genera of Amaranthaceae and over 50 species of Amaranthus. About 35% of the total protein is found in the endosperm, the remaining 65% being distributed in the germ and seed coat. Using milling processes which separate germ and hulls from the endosperm, the former fraction had a protein content of 4.2.0% while the endosperm contained 7.7%. Proximate composition of amaranth seeds (dry basis) was 7.5% fat, 15.5% protein, 64.5% starch, 3.2% ash, 0.06% tannins, and 17.7% total dietary fiber. Calculated energy content per gram was 3.66 kcal, while the observed value was 4.76. The starch content is slightly higher than for most wheat samples, but lower than for corn. The starch granules are about 1 to 2 microns in diameter (which is extremely small compared to cereal starches) and may contain either waxy or nonwaxy types of starch. The fat content of amaranth seeds is about 7.6%, which is much higher than the normal fat content of wheat, rice, or corn kernels. The fatty acid distribution is about 77% unsaturated, and there is a relatively large ratio of linolenic acid. Lipid classes are 81% triglycerides, 5.4% steryl esters, 1.8% galactosyl diglycerides, and 3.6% phosphatidyl esters. The oil also contains a significant amount of squalene, an isoprenoid which is a precursor of sterols such as cholesterol. The yellow oil they obtained is similar in appearance and composition to corn oil, but comparison with previously published analyses revealed a considerable variation in the content of the principal fatty acids (palmitic, oleic, and linoleic) although the squalene content of 5 to 8% was in the expected range. Representative fatty acid composition of the oil is 19% palmitic, 4% stearic, 25% oleic, 50% linoleic, and 1% linolenic, with a total unsaturated of 77%. Typical vitamin content (as mg per 100 gm) is: 0.10 thiamin, 0.21 riboflavin, and 1.31 niacin. Mineral contents on the same basis are 187 calcium, 10 iron, 455 phosphorus, 288 magnesium, 3.8 zinc,

0.9 copper, 32 sodium, and 420 potassium. The phytate content was reported as 0.56%. Notable differences, as compared to wheat, brown rice, and oats are much lower content of thiamin, about double the content of riboflavin, and considerably lower content of niacin in the amaranth. Also much higher content of sodium, calcium and magnesium, higher content of iron and copper, and lower content of phytate.

Amaranth colour. FD&C Red 2. Trisodium salt of 1-(4-sulpho-1-naphthylazo)-2-naphthol-3,6-disulphonic acid. It is a reddish-brown powder, soluble in water (20% at 25°C) to yield a magenta-red to bluish-red solution. It is readily soluble in glycerol (18% at 25°C), but poorly soluble in glycols and ethanol (95% ethanol: 5% water). Amaranth is moderately light-stable and is very stable in acid media. It has not been permitted for food use in the US since it was delisted in 1976, but may be returned to use since there has been no demonstrated safety problem with it.

ambergris. Morbid concretion obtained from the intestine of the sperm whale. Contains cholesterol, ambrein, benzoic acid. Appears as a mottled or striped grey-brown or black wax. It is used in drugs and perfume.

AMD. *See* air moving device.

American process cocoa. Cocoa prepared in the usual manner without treatment with alkalies. Sometime called acid cocoa. It is used to a considerable extent, in the manufacture of chocolate-flavoured dairy products, but not so desirable under most conditions as Dutch Process Cocoa.

amino acid profile. Amino acid composition of a protein.

amino acid, limiting. That essential amino acid present in the protein in question in least amount (relative to the dietary needs). The ratio of the amount of the limiting amino acid to the requirements serves as a chemical estimation of the nutritive value of the protein. Most cereal proteins are limited by lysine and most animal and vegetable proteins by the sulphur amino acids (methionine plus cystine). In complete diets it is the sulphur containing amino acids that are usually limiting.

amino acid. Any of a group of water-soluble organic compounds that possess both an amino ($-NH_2$) and a carboxyl (-COOH) group attached to the a-carbon atom. Amino acids have the general formula $R-CH-(NH_2)COOH$, where R may be hydrogen or an organic group with an alkyl, aryl, or heterocyclic structure, and determines the properties of the particular amino acid. Amino acids occur both as free molecules and, when linked together by peptide bonds, as structural units of peptides, polypeptides, and proteins. Since amino group is basic and carboxyl group is acidic, amino acids are amphoteric; in water solution they forms zwitterions, *i.e.*, ions having a positive electric charge at one end and a negative charge at the other.

All amino acids except glycine are optically active, *i.e.*, they contain one or more asymmetric carbon atoms; most have the left-handed (L) configuration. Amino acids can be obtained by the hydrolysis of proteins (which occurs in the digestive process), though many are now prepare synthetically. In earlier century, amino acids were prepared in the laboratory by passing an electric discharge through a mixture of ammonia, methane, and water vapour. It is believed that a similar reaction may have accounted for the origin of amino acids, and hence of life on earth.

8 amino acids are regarded as essential in diet, since they cannot be synthesized within body; 12 others are considered to be nonessential. Over 80 amino acids have been identified in the free or uncombined state; of these, 22 are known to be the constituents of proteins. Amino acids in proteins are L-isomers, but short peptides of microbial origin (e.g., certain antibiotics) contain D-isomers as well as certain amino acids not found in proteins.

Amino acids combine in chains of great complexity and form proteins. The critical importance of their arrangement and sequence in these chains has been established. Amino acids in excess of the amount required for protein synthesis are used for energy generation or other processes, since there is no mechanism for protein storage in animals.

The metabolism of amino acids by transamination and deamination liberates ammonia; this is converted to urea in mammals by the urea cycle. In birds and terrestrial reptiles, uric acid is the end-product of amino acid metabolism. The non-nitrogenous 'carbon skeleton' of the various amino acids is metabolized by the Krebs cycle and other pathways. Those amino acids whose skeletons can give rise to glucose are termed glucogenic; others, especially those with aliphatic alkyl groups, yield acetyl-CoA and so can be converted to fat or ketone bodies; hence they are sometimes termed ketogenic.

amino acids, antiketogenic. Those which are metabolized to glucose. They are glycine, alanine, serine, cystine, aspartic acid, glutamic acid, arginine, proline and hydroxyproline.

amino acids, ketogenic. Those which are metabolized to acetoacetic acid (ketone bodies). They are leucine, isoleucine, phenylaline and tyrosine.

amino sugars. The monosaccharides in which a nonglycosidic hydroxyl group is replaced by an amino or substituted amino group, e.g., D-glucosamine, (from glucose) occurs in many polysaccharides of vertebrates and is a major component of chitin. Galactosamine or chondrosamine (from galactose) is major component of the cartilage and the glycolipids. Amino sugars are important components of the bacterial cell walls.

aminogram. Amino acid composition of a protein.

aminopeptidase. Enzyme of the pancreatic juice that splits polypeptides to dipeptides. Removes the terminal unit of the polypeptide chain at the end at which the amino radical is free, hence is an exopeptidase.

aminopterin. Aminopteroylglutamic acid, specific antagonist to folic acid.

amydon. Starchy material made by steeping wheat flour in water and drying the starch sediment in the sun; used for many centuries for thickening broths.

amygdalin. Glucoside in almonds, apricot and cherry stones, hydrolyzed by the enzyme, emulsin, to glucose, hydrocyanic acid and benzaldehyde. The benzaldehyde gives the characteristic odour.

amylases. The enzymes which act on starch and starch-containing plant materials. Enzymes have been used to hydrolyze starches into sugars. The amylases may be applied to starch liquification as well. This requires gelantinization of the starch. Inasmuch as the viscosity of such gelatinized preparations makes them unwieldy at concentrations greater than 20%, amylases may be added to

liquefy the gelatinous structure and permit higher concentrations of starch to be processed. The principal reaction catalyze by α-amylase is the hydrolysis of α-1,4-glucan bonds in polysaccharides (starch, glycogen, etc.) yielding dextrins and oligo- and monosaccharides. The main reaction catalyzed by β-amylase is the similar hydrolysis of α-1,4-glucan bonds in polysaccharides, yielding beta limit dextrins. Some authorities place the amylases into three categories:
(a) glucoamylases;
(b) bacterial amylases; and
(c) fungal amylases.

Some glucoamylases are prepared from *Aspergillus niger*. Glucoamylase (Amyloglucosidase) hydrolyzes α-1,3- and α-1,6-glucan bonds in polysaccharides, yielding glucose. Some bacterial amylases are derived from *Bacillus licheneformis* of *Bacillus subtilis*. Several commercial fungal amylases are derived from *Aspergillis oryzae*, sometimes by fermentation of wheat bran cultures.

amyloamylose. Old name for amylose, as distinct from erythroamylose, old name for amylopectin.

amylopectin. Starch consists of 20-25% amylose and the remainder amylopectin. Amylose consists of 1,4 alpha-linked glucose units and gives a pure blue with iodine. Amylopectin is a branched structure built up of 20-24 glucoside units linked 1,4 and gives a purplish colour with iodine.

amylopsin. Pancreatic amylase.

anabolism. The assimilation of nutrient material by the living organism to build or restore its tissues and other living matter. It is phase of intermediary metabolism concerned with the energy requiring biosynthesis of cell components from smaller precursor molecules. Starch, glycogen, fats and proteins are products of anabolic pathways. Anabolic reactions generally require energy provided by ATP produced by catabolism.

anaerobic respiration. Respiration, found in yeasts, bacteria, and occasionally in muscles tissue, in which oxygen is not involved. The organic substrate is not completely oxidized and the energy yield is low. In the absence of oxygen in animal muscle tissue, glucose is degraded to pyruvate by glycolysis, with the production of a small amount of energy and also lactic acid, which may be oxidized later when oxygen becomes available (*see* oxygen debt). Fermentation is an example of anaerobic respiration, in which certain yeasts produce ethanol and carbon dioxide as end products. Only two molecules of ATP are produced by this process.

anchovy. *Engraulis encrasicholus.* A small fish of the herring family. Fifteen genera have been identified with a total of some 100 species in the tropical and temperate regions of the northern and southern hemispheres. Distribution is chiefly in the Indian and Pacific Oceans. Due to the great masses in which they occur, the family has large commercial importance to several countries for the production of fish meal and oil. Seven species in the main genus *Engraulis* have been identified from the Pacific and Atlantic Oceans. The common anchovy, esteemed for its rich and peculiar flavour, is not larger than the middle finger. It is caught in vast numbers in the Mediterranean and frequently on the coast of France, Holland and the south of England. A similar species is found on both the Atlantic and Pacific coasts of America. Anchovies feed on small plankton, chiefly on crustaceans of various families. Fish eggs have also been found in their stomachs. The anchovies are prey to many predatory fishes and marine birds. It is usually prepared semipreserved with 10-12% salt and sometimes benzoic acid, and is extensively used in the preparation of sauces.

ancillary equipment. Equipment added to a primary piece of equipment to assist in meeting the functional requirements of the system. The operation of a dryer is influenced by ancillary equipment, used preceding, following, surrounding, or associated with the dryer. Ancillary equipment for dryers include: mechanical dewaterers, grinders, choppers, lacerators, pulverizers, mixers, pelleters, materials handling devices, heating equipment, dust collectors, exhaust systems, and ventilation (external) equipment.

aneurine. Obsolete name for vitamin B_1.

angelica. Family: *Umbelliferae*. Genus: *Angelica*. Species: *Angelica archangelica*. A giant member of the parsley family, angelica grows up to 1.5 m high, with a spread a spread of about 90 cm. It is native both to northern Europe and to Syria, and grows wild in many parts of the world, decorating the countryside with its bright green shoots of treelike proportions. The fleshy steams are candied as cake decorations and sweetmeat. The young shoots may be blanched, chopped, and added to salads, and the leaves used to flavour *court bouillon* for fish, stewed fruits (rhubarb, in particular), and preserves. Oil from the seeds is used as a flavouring in several aperitifs and other alcoholic drinks, including absinthe and gin. It is also used as an aromatic ingredient in pot pourri. Medicinally, the dried roots may be used as an aid to flatulence, and the leaves, shoots, and seeds to help relive coughs, colds, and other respiratory disorders. The seeds may also be used as an appetite stimulant and an aid of digestion. Angelica contains a volatile oil and derivatives of coumarin, which helps to stimulate gastric secretions, controls peristalsis and increases appetite. It also contains bitter principles, sugar, valeric and angelic acids and a resin called Anglican. Angelica is used to improve the circulation and warm the body. It is one of the best herbs to use against the cold in winter, particularly during convalescence. when the coldness one feels is subjective. Because of its warming properties, it will relieve spasms of the stomach and intestines and dispel gas. It is said that its prolonged and regular use will create a distaste for alcoholic drinks. However, it is a strong emmenagogue and should not be used by pregnant women. Neither should it be used by diabetics as it tends to increase the level of sugar in the blood. It can be used externally as a poultice for rheumatism. It is of great benefit in the treatment of colds, coughs, pleurisy and all lung diseases. It improves the mucous membrane of the bronchial tubes and tones up the heart muscle. The fresh leaves were used to heal wounds in the old days and athletes used to bathe in decoctions of the root to ease over-strained muscles. However, be aware that angelica can irritate the skin, and should not come into contact with the eyes. If using the seeds, use only freshly harvested ones, since they lose their vitality very quickly. Medicinally, decoction of the root can be prepared by using 2.5 g to 600 ml water and taken 3 tablespoons three times a day.

angostura. Essential oil distilled from the bark at *Galipea cusparia*. Contains galipol, cadinene, galipene and pinene; used in preparation of bitters and liquors.

angular somatitis. An affection of the skin at the angles of the mouth, characterized by heaping up of epithelium into ridges, giving the appearance of fissures; a symptom of riboflavin deficiency but also a symptom of other diseases.

anhydrous milk fat. Dry fat which according to the US standards must contain not less than 99.8% butterfat and not more than 0.1% moisture or curd. This fat is made only from high quality fresh milk or fresh sweet cream and is not to be confused with butter oil which may be made from butter or sour cream and does not meet rigid specifications of anhydrous milk fat.

aroma. A distinctive, pleasant odour of certain plants and other substances; as the aroma of the flavouring materials in dairy products.

anhydrovitamin A. Form of retinol in which the -OH group has been removed by treatment with hydrochloric acid, with a corresponding shift in the double bonds. Once incorrectly called cyclized or spurious vitamin A. it has very slight biological activity. When fed in large doses to rats, a more active material called rehydro-vitamin A is obtained.

animal protein factor. Name given to certain growth factor or factors which were found to be present in animal but not vegetable proteins. Vitamin B_{12} was identified as one of these.

aniseed. The dried fruit of *Pimpinella anisum* (parsley family). Chief component of the volatile oil is anethole (methoxypropenyl benzene). The seed is used to flavour backed goods, meat products and drinks.

Anjou pear. A variety of pear, the Anjou is the principal winter pear, usually making up about 75% of the winter total. Full name of variety is Beurre d'Anjou, but French origin has not been authenticated. There is some evidence that the variety originated with Vans Mons at Louvain, Belgium in about 1819 and appeared in the Van Mons catalog in 1823 under the name of Nec Plus Meuris. Fruit is medium size to somewhat large, with short stem; oval to globular shape with sides slightly unequal; short, obscure, thick neck; yellowish-green skin, occasionally sprinkled with russet, sometimes shaded to dull crimson. Flesh is yellowish-white, fairly fine, buttery, juicy, some grit cells at center. The fruit is aromatic, spicy, and of sweet flavor. The variety stores well. Tree is vigorous, upright, spreading, but somewhat temperamental as to production. Moderately susceptible to blight.

annatto. The fruit of a shrub, *Bixa orellana* L., which is cultivated in South America, the southern United States, India and East Africa. The principal colouring matter is recovered by pulping the pericarp of the fruits with water, allowing the mass to ferment and filtering out the insoluble annatto which is then sun-dried into cakes. These contain 6-12 % of the colouring principal, bixin. Bixin is a carotenoid and chemically is the monomethyl ester of norbixin, a symmetrical dicarboxylic acid. It is insoluble in water and only slightly soluble in ethanol (95%) but readily soluble in organic solvents and fixed oils to give a brownish-yellow solution. Alkalies saponify bixin giving a clear reddish-brown aqueous soluble solution.

Annatto is marketed as a light-yellow to deep orange spray-dried powder (15 % bixin), as a solution in vegetable oil (0.25-0.5 % bixin), or as a water-soluble form. This latter product is normally in potassium hydroxide/propylene glycol solution with a pH in excess of 8. Some products may contain polysorbate (Tween 80) and this is stated in the specification. Most water-soluble annatto products contain 1.5-2.5 % bixin or are standardized on a colour value. Annatto is listed in the US as a colour additive for use in foods and is widely employed in the manufacture of butter, margarine, cheese and related products. The colour from seedpods of *Bixa orellana;* used for colouring butter and cheese (not margarine); it is legally permitted, and contains orellin, of minor importance, soluble in water, and bixin, the major colour, insoluble in water. Also known as bixin; butter colour.

annexin. A family of at least eight distinct group of calcium dependent, phospholipid binding proteins which have some roles in membrane-cytoskeletal linkage, membrane fusion events in exocytosis and regulation of cell surface receptors. They have conserved internal repeat sequences of about 70 amino acids which occur at least four times in the primary structure. In pea annexin like proteins of 35 KD have been purified.

anorexia nervosa. Psychological disturbance resulting in a refusal to eat; sensations of hunger usually non felt. These may be a restriction of the diet to particular foods. The result is great weight loss, atrophy of tissue and fall in basal metabolic rate.

anorexigenic drugs. Drugs that depress the appetite and are used as an aid to weight reduction; e.g. amphetamine (or dextroamphetamine or dexedrine) preludin (phenmetrazine hydrochloride) "Tenuate" (diethylpropion).

anta-acids. *See* antacids.

antacids. Mild bases or buffers that neutralize acid; used generally in relation to the partial neutralization of stomach acidity. Substances such as magnesium carbonate, sodium bicarbonate, magnesium hydroxide, glycine, etc., are used as antacids. Also spelled as anta-acids.

anthelminthics. Chemicals used to destroy intestinal worms.

anthocyanins. Violet, red and blue water-soluble colouring matter of many fruits, flowers and leaves. Consists of glucose pus anthocyanidins (these consists of two 6-membered carbon rings containing one oxygen atom). Examples are delphinin, pelargonidin, cyanidin. The colour hue and light stability characteristics are dependent on the hydroxyl and methyl groups as well as the nature of the glycoside linkages involved. The glycoside moiety comprises one or more molecules of glucose, galactose, rhamnose or arabinose. Some anthocyanins are acylated with *p*-coumaric, cafferic or ferrulic acids at the 3'-hydroxy group of the sugar. The colour of anthocyanins is dependent on several factors. The removal of the 3'-hydroxy group shifts the colour toward yellow; methylation results in a reddening effect. As the anthocyanins are ionic, they are pH-sensitive; solutions at low pH are bright red, those at high pH are bright blue and intermediate shades result as the pH alters. High concentrations of anthocyanins, such as occur in the skins of many fruits, result in a deep purplish to almost black appearance. Anthocyanins are traditionally recovered from suitable plant material by extraction with methanol, acidified with a mineral acid or a fruit acid such as tartaric, followed by removal of the solvent under vacuum and purification by ion-exchange chromatography. The acid remains in the final product; hence, the use of tartaric acid makes the product more widely acceptable for use in foods where a red colour is desired. Anthocyanins are widely permitted throughout the world for use as a food colorant. In the US, they may be used only in the form of grape skin extract and grape colouring. Grape skin extract is made from the aqueous extraction (steeping) of fresh deseeded marc remaining after grapes have been pressed either for juice or wine. Grape colouring is an aqueous solution of grape pigments made from Concord grapes or a dehydrated powder prepared from the aqueous solution. The aqueous solution is prepared by extracting the pigments from precipitated less produced during the storage of Concord grape juice. The anthocyanins can attack iron and tin and thus may cause trouble in canned foods.

anthoxanthins. Alternative name for flavonoids.

antibiotics. The microbial products which in low concentrations, are capable of inhibiting or killing susceptible microorganisms. Natural antibiotics are produced by microorganisms living in the soil or aquatic environments. Techniques have been developed for screening soil and water samples around the world for antibiotic producing microorganisms. These microorganisms are limited to a few genera of bacteria and fungi. Penicillin is produced by species of *Penicillium*, and the prototype of the cephalosporins is produced by another fungus, *Cephalosporium*. Members of the genus *Streptomyces* are by far the most important bacterial producers of antibiotics. Clinically important antibiotics produced by a *Streptomyces* species include streptomycin, tetracyclines, vancomycin, kanamycin, rifampin, and chloramphenicol. Each antibiotic is active against a limited number of genera and species of bacteria. Broad-spectrum antibiotics inhibit a wide range of Gram-negative and Gram-positive bacteria. Narrow-spectrum antibiotics act against only a few groups of bacteria. Each antibiotic has its special mode of action which can be broadly characterized as inhibiting protein synthesis, nucleic acid synthesis, cell wall synthesis, or interfering with membrane function.

antibody. A protein molecule formed within the body of an animal in order to neutralize the effect of a foreign invading protein (called an antigen). These serum proteins (immunoglobulins) are produced by certain cells of the lymphocyte series in response to the presence of antigens. Antibodies bind specifically to molecules of the eliciting antigen but not to other antigens. Antibodies are produced by lymphocytes in response to the presence of antigens. Each antibody has a molecular structure that exactly fits the structure of one particular antigen molecule, like a lock and key. Antibody molecules attach themselves to invading antigen molecules (on or from bacteria, transfused red blood cells, or grafted tissue of another animal) and so render them inactive. It may also assist in the ingestion of antigenic matter by phagocytes (opsonization) and also activate complement. Immunoglobulin molecules each comprise two parallel heavy chains (of high molecular mass) and two light chains, all united by disulphide bonds. The amino acid sequence in certain regions of both heavy and light chains is highly variable. These variable regions contribute to the three-dimensional structure of the two antigen-binding sites on each molecule, and confer specificity on the antibody.

There are several classes of antibodies, according to the nature of the invariable regions of their heavy chains. IgM antibodies have mu (μ) heavy chains; they are a polymerized form of the antibody secreted during the early response to antigens. IgG antibodies, with gamma (γ) heavy chains, appear later in the immune response and are most abundant immunoglobulin class in normal blood serum. IgA antibodies, with α-heavy chains, are secreted at mucous surfaces, especially in the alimentary and respiratory tracts. IgE, with epsilon heavy chains, has a special role in relation to mast cells and in the mediation of Type I hypersensitivity. Maternal IgG antibody passes to the fetus across the placenta before the birth in primates and rodents.

In most herbivores mammals, antibody transfer takes place in the first two days of life of newborn, which absorbs the IgG and IgA antibodies in colostrum across the gut mucosa. Antibody can the detected and estimated by means of the *in vitro* reactions with antigens. They are also used in a wide range of assays and tests to label specific antigenic components.

anticaking agents. Some food products, particularly those that contain one or more hygroscopic substances, required the addition of an anticaking agent to inhibit formation of aggregates and lumps and thus retain the free-flowing characteristic of the products. Calcium phosphate, for example, is commonly used in instant breakfast drinks and lemonade and other soft drink mixes. The term drying agent is also sometimes applied to such substances, but the term also applies to substances used to dry air in processing and for use in packages and containers that hold food substances that tend to be hygroscopic or deliquescent. Many anticaking agents, including silica gel, also act as dispersants for powdered products. Many food products, when stirred into water, tend to form lumps which are difficult to disperse or dissolve. The agent not only improves flow properties of the dry powder but also increases speed of dispersion by keeping the food particles separated and permitting the water to wet them individually instead of forming lumps.

A number of commonly used anticaking additives include calcium carbonate, magnesium stearate, calcium phosphate, myristates, calcium silicate, palmitates, calcium stearate, phosphates (calcium tribasic, magnesium tribasic, microcrystalline, cellulose, powdered, kaolin, silicon dioxide, magnesium carbonate, sodium ferrocyanide, magnesium hydroxide sodium silicoaluminate magnesium oxide, starches, magnesium silicate. The uses for microcrystalline cellulose include incorporation in imitation mozzarella cheese. The general function of an anticaking agent can be described by using silica gel as an example. Generally, these substances are available from manufacturers as very small particles (ranging from 2 to 9 mm) average size with surface areas ranging 310-675 m^2/g. Average pore diameters range from 200 to 2000 nm. They have a bulk density ranging from 80.1 to 464.6 kg/m^3. Depending upon manufacturer's formulation, the *p*H of 5% (weight) solutions will range from 4.3 to 7.2. A typical application for a silica gel formulation is admixture with orange-juice crystals to assure a free-flowing product, avoiding formation of crystal cakes and hard lumps, as may result from high temperature, humidity, or pressure. The very high adsorption properties of the anticaking substance removes moisture that can cause fusion. The billions of extremely fine, inert particles coat and separate each grain of powder (product) to keep it in a free-flowing state.

anticoagulants. With reference to blood, substances that prevent clotting by interfering with the mechanisms. Oxalate and citrate are anticoagulants as they combine with the calcium which is needed; dicoumarin and heparin inhibit the formation of prothrombin, needed to release fibrin from fibrinogen; hirudin inactivates the thrombin.

antienzymes. Substances that specifically inhibit enzymes: produced by the lining of the digestive tract to prevent attack by the digestive enzymes, by intestinal parasites, and as antibodies in the blood stream.

antifoaming agents. Octanol (capryl alcohol), sulphonated oils, silicones; reduce foaming often caused by the presence of dissolved protein or other stabilizer.

antigalactic. Substances that suppress the secretion of milk.

antigen. An agent that stimulates the animal to synthesize antibodies that can specifically react with that antigen. Antigens are usually complex macromolecules that are foreign to the animal, that is, self recognizes self and does not make antibodies against its own complex molecules.

Some substances such as large foreign polysaccharides and proteins are excellent antigens, whereas other foreign substances do not stimulate antibody formation. As a rule, substances that are degraded by metabolic activities are good antigens, whereas nondegradable organic polymers are poor antigens.

antihistamine. One of about 40 synthetic organic compounds developed in recent years to inhibit the irritant and sometimes toxic effects of histamine. The latter substance is a degradation product of the amino acid histidine; it is a pharmacologically active compound formed in body tissues as a result of an external stimulus (allergen) in a manner similar to that of an antibody. The allergic effect is usually in the nasal tissues, and it is for this that antihistamines are generally used, though they are also effective in more severe disorders involving an allergic response to penicillin and other drugs. Chemically, they are complex aromatic amines. Since some have undesirable side effects, antihistamines must be used after proper investigations.

antimycotics. Substances that inhibit mould growth, such as sodium and calcium propionate, methyl hydroxybenzoate, quaternary ammonium chloride, sodium benzoate, sorbic acid.

antioxidants. These food additive chemicals may be defined as substances that oppose oxidation, or inhibit or retard reactions promoted by oxygen (or peroxides) and, therefore, its effects. Antioxidants are substances that retard atmospheric oxidation and the degradative effects of oxidation, thus extending the useful storage period (shelf-life) of the substrate when they are added in very low concentrations-usually on the order of a small fraction of 1% of their full strength. Composition of the substrate, processing conditions, impurities, and desired shelf-life are among the most important factors in selecting the best antioxidant system for a given food product. The desirable features of antioxidants may be summarized as:

(a) effectiveness at low concentrations;

(b) compatability with the substrate;

(c) nontoxic to consumers;

(d) stability in terms of conditions encountered in processing and storage, including temperature, radiation, pH, etc.;

(e) nonvolatility and nonextract-ability under the conditions of use;

(f) ease and safety in handling;

(g) freedom from off-flavours, off-odours, and off-colours that might be imparted to the food product; and, of course, they must be cost effective.

It could appear that inasmuch as oxidative degradation occurs in a variety of organic materials that are dissimilar in appearance and have entirely different applications and different properties, with degradation producing different effects, the oxidation mechanism itself might be different. Current knowledge indicates, however, that the mechanism of oxidative degradation is the same for all organic substances. They appear to degrade by the same free-radical mechanism. Common examples of food oxidative degradation include products that contain oils and fats. For example, some antioxidants have made it possible to store groundnuts (peanuts) and other nuts, maize (corn) products, and bakery and cereal products on the shelf for periods well

in excess of the 4 months that was considered the traditional limiting period prior to the appearance of such additives. Other examples of food products that tend to become rancid by way of oxidation include various meat-flavour stuffing mixes, cake mixes, unbaked cheesecake mix, and essentially all foods that incorporate lipids. The stability of natural fats and oils present in raw materials varies over a wide range and hence the amount of antioxidant required must be tailored to each product situation. Enzymatic "browning" is another example of oxidative degradation. The enzymes in fruits and vegetables cause apples, apricots, bananas, cherries, peaches, pears, and potatoes, among others, to darken when they are exposed to air after being cut, bruised, or allowed to overmature. Some antioxidants can prevent or delay enzymatic browning much in the same manner as dipping fresh-cut fruits in lemon, orange, or pineapple juice. Limonene and ascorbic acid naturally present in these juices serve as antioxidants. Oxidative changes may affect carbohydrate, protein, and fat substances, the primary building blocks of foodstuffs, but generally, the oxidative rancidity problems results mainly from autoxidative degradation of fatty (glyceridic) components. *Mechanism of Oxidation and Inhibition.* Some authorities describe oxidation as a free-radical, chain-type reaction. At usual processing temperatures and more slowly at room temperature, organic free radicals (R.) are formed. These react with oxygen to form peroxy radicals (ROO.), which can abstract a hydrogen atom from the affected substance to form a hydroperoxide (ROOH) and another organic free radical. The cycle repeats itself with the addition of oxygen to the new free radical. The unstable hydroperoxides left along with the substance are the major source of degradation. Under the influence of heat, light (and any metals if present), the hydroperoxides decompose to form carbonyl groups. When this happens, the organic molecule breaks and splits off another organic free radical. Ultimately, this type of degradation can lead to rancidity and color deterioration in oils and fats. An antioxidant ties up the peroxy radicals so that they are incapable of propagating the reaction chain or to decompose the hydroperoxides in such a manner that carbonyl groups and additional free radicals are not formed. The former, which are called chain-breaking antioxidants, free-radical scavengers, or inhibitors, are usually hindered phenols or amines. The latter, called peroxide decomposers, are generally sulphur compounds or organophosphites. A number of antioxidants useful in rubber and plastics, for example, are not suited to food products because of their toxicity. By using two or more different types of antioxidants, the resistance to oxidation or deterioration may be improved to a greater extent than would be predicted on the basis of strict additivity. The two additives are then said to show a synergisitic effect toward one another. Probably the most generally effective mixtures of antioxidants are those in which one compound functions as a decomposer of peroxides (sulphides, thiodipropionates) and the other as an inhibitor of free radicals (hinders phenols, amines). Although the latter retards the formation of reaction chains, some hydroperoxide is nevertheless formed. If this hydroperoxide then reacts with a decom-

poser of peroxides, instead of decomposing into free radicals, the two antioxidants act together to complement each other. Moreover, the peroxide decomposer may itself be subject to oxidation by peroxy radicals, and its efficiency will therefore be increased in the presence of an inhibitor of free radicals. In case of phenol-sulphide mixtures, the sulphide (peroxide decomposer) also continuously regenerates the phenol (radical scavenger) to accentuate synergistic nature of the mixture. Metal chelators or deactivators, such as citric and phosphoric acids, ultraviolet light absorbers (carbon black, substitute benzophenones, benzotriazoles, and salicylates), and antiozoants (substituted phenylenediamines) also develop synergistic effects along with antioxidants.

anti-spattering agents. The substances added to fats used in frying, such as lecithin, sucrose esters (laurates and stearates), and sodium sulphoacetate derivatives of mono- and diglycerides. They function by preventing the coalescence of water droplets.

anti-staling agents. Substances that retard the staling of backed products, and also soften the crumb, such as sucrose stearate, polyoxyethylene monostearate, glyceryl monostearate, stearoyl tartarate.

antisticking agent. An additive used primarily in certain finely divided food products that tend to be hygroscopic to prevent or inhibit agglomeration and thus maintain a free-flowing condition. Such substances as starch, calcium metasilicate, magnesium carbonate, and magnesium stearate, among several others, are used for this purpose in table salt, flours, sugar, coffee whiteners, and similar products. Anticaking agents provide a nonadhering (some-times slippery or friction-free) boundary between substances, such as salt crystals. In the case of common salt, the sticky and clammy condition of the crystals poses an inconvenience to the consumer. In the case of the food processor, non-freeflowing salts and powders that tend to bridge over in hoppers and to clog conveyances, chutes, etc., are a serious problem, contributing to inefficiency Anticaking agents usually are relatively water-absorbent in themselves, but do not become sticky within their moisture-holding limitations. Insoluble phosphates often play this role. Surfactants are also effective.

anti-toxin. Antibody that, by its specificity for a particular toxin antigen, can neutralize the toxin. Antitoxins are produced by the organisms following the injection of, or the elaboration of, toxin, derived from pathogenic bacteria in to the blood. These substances appear to combine with and neutralize the corresponding toxin and so immunize the organism against it, but they are inactive toward other toxins. This has been considered as due to an asymmetric configuration so that only those antitoxins which are constituted similarly to a certain toxin can unite with it.

antizymotic. A substance that prevents, inhibits, or retards fermentation, and is frequently used for that purpose in medicine, in food products, etc. Antizymotic agent reduces fermentation and gas formation in the gastrointestinal tract or reduces the stability of foam and allows the release of gas. Antizymotics that reduce the number of gas-producing organisms in the digestive tract include oil of turpentine, linseed oil, formalin, and antibiotics.

apocarotenal. A purplish-black crystalline substance which imparts a light-orange to orange-red coloration to oil solutions, and from an orange to tomato-red coloration to aqueous dispersions. Solubility of the substance in fats and oils ranges between 0.7-15 g/L; in water, it is essentially insoluble. The vitamin A value (biological activity) is rated at about 1200 international units/mg. Apocarotenal (sometimes blended with β-carotene) finds application for color enhancement in cheese (natural and processed) and in a number of simulated food products.

apoenzyme. The protein part of an enzyme that has a nonprotein component; polypeptide moiety of a conjugated enzyme after removal of its prosthetic group. As the activity of conjugated enzymes depends on their prosthetic groups an apoenzyme is inactive, but its presence can sometimes be demonstrated by binding of specific antibodies raised against the whole enzyme (holoenzyme).

apoferritin. The protein part of ferritin, the iron storage complex in the intestinal mucosal cells.

apollinaris water. Popular name for a kind of alkaline, highly aerated, natural water, containing sodium chloride and calcium, sodium and magnesium carbonates; obtained from a spring in the valley of the Ahr (Prussia).

aporinosis. A term used in food science for any disease due to deficiency of an element in diet.

aporrhegma. Ptomaine or other toxic substance split off from an amino acid during the bacterial decomposition of a protein.

aposia. A term used in food science for the absence of feeling of thirst.

apositia. A term used in food science for the aversion for food.

Appenzeller cheese. A variety of cheese which is similar to Emmentaler made of cow's milk (skim or whole) in the Canton of Appenzell, Switzerland.

appertization. A term applied by the French to the process of destroying all the microorganism of significance in food, i.e., commercial sterility; it has been found that a few organisms remain alive but are quiescent.

apple butter. Apple that has been boiled in an open kettle to a thick consistency. It appears to be similar to the apple sauce but is darker in colour due to the prolonged boiling.

apple drying. Apples are peeled and usually sliced, ringed, or diced before drying. Drying or dehydrating with heated air is usually done in a tunnel, kiln, or belt dryer. In the tunnel dryer, apples at 85% moisture content are loaded on trays, and moved through the tunnels where the temperature is about 74°C. Using counter-current flow technique, about 8 hours are required to dry apple slices to about 20%. With two stage drying, temperature of 85°C in the first stage and 74°C in the second stage are used. As per US standards, the dry apples possess 24% moisture and dehydrated apples possess about 2.5% or less moisture. Sulphuring of the peeled fruit is done to reduce discolouration, either before drying or after the first stage of drying. It has been found that 100 kg of apples produces approximately 10 kg of dried apple pieces.

apple jack. American name for apple brandy; distilled cider. Also known as Calvados.

apple, liquid. A preparation of apple juice plus pulverized apple pulp in suspension.

apple nuggets. Crisp granules of apple of low moisture content, Dehydrated apples of 24% moisture content are cut into small cubes and dried down to 2% moisture; used to make applesauce.

apple powder. Drum-dried apple powder is a product used in cake mixes and in baked pastries. The dried product rehydrates readily and may reasonably be termed "instant apple sauce." Considerable amounts of drum-dried apple powder are now being produces by processors in the Pacific Northwest. It may be prepared by grinding low-moisture dried apples, or preferably by drum-drying apple puree. Apples are peeled, cored, cooked in clean steam, and dried on a double drum dryer of the type once used for drying milk. The puree is applied to the drum by a travelling spray feeder which distributes product uniformly on the upper surface of the drum.

apple tea. *See* apple.

apple. Family: *Rosaceae.* Genus: *Malus pumila.* The tree which bears this popular fruit can be grown in many parts of the world. The blossoms are very susceptible to injury from frost, but they appear much later than peach or apricot blossoms and so avoid the late frost which would be fatal to fruit bearing. Apple trees reach a moderate height and have spreading branches. The leaves are nearly oval, and the pinkish-white flowers are produces from very short shoots or spurs, which are usually of two years' growth. It is true in general that the apples of the cold northern climates are smaller and harder than those of the hot summer climates. By placing winter apples in cold storage or even in cool cellars, the fruit can be kept in good condition through out the year and until the earliest varieties which are raised in the warmer regions are on the market, so that it is possible to have apples the entire year. New varieties are obtained by planting the seed, but a desirable variety is seldom secured in this way, because the seeds do not reproduce the fruit from which they were taken; therefore orchard trees are prepared by grafting. In setting trees, the ground should be carefully prepared.

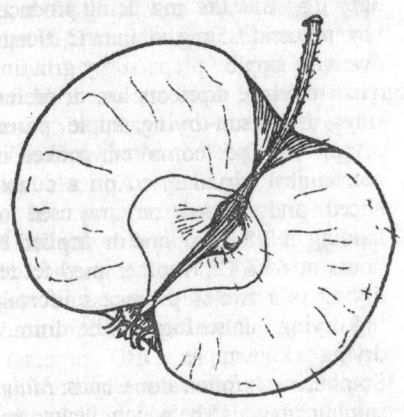

Pyrus malus, the apple or crab apple grows throughout Europe and as far as Central Asia, where it seems to have originated. The people of Asia Minor took no notice of it for a long time, but the Greeks had already cultivated it. In Rome at the time of the Emperor Augusts there were no less than 30 different varieties recorded. It is by far the most generally cultivated of any grown in the temperate regions, and it is also one of the most appreciated. The person who does not enjoy eating apples is a rarity. All of the numerous varieties have been derived from two species, the wild crab and the common apple. The fruit is a rather hard juicy pulp that is formed around a core, which consists of five cells bearing two seeds each. The pulp is white or slightly pinkish. Most apples are nearly round, though some are elongated. In colour there are nearly as many shades as there are varieties, though these shades are limited to red, green and yellow. Several thousand varieties of cultivated apples are known, though of this number not more than 100 are profitable, and not over twenty varieties are successful in any one locality. The numerous varieties are adapted to the soil and climate of widely different sections, and if removed from their native locality will seldom succeed.

Apples contain vitamins, easily assailable sugars, and enzymes that are indispensable for the digestion. They also contain essential acids, such as malic acid, and minerals like potassium, sodium, calcium, magnesium and phosphorus. The skin is richest in these but modern pesticides and insecticides sometimes contaminate apples, so they should be meticulously washed.

Traditionally, the apple is thought to be very healthy, hence the old saying, 'An apple a day keeps the doctor away.' However, they actually have a relatively low vitamin C content and food value. The processing of apples further reduces their nutritional value. An apple loses half its vitamin C content when peeled, and frozen apples lose most of their vitamin A and potassium. Since apples are about 84% water and most of their goodness is found in their fruit sugar, dried apples naturally have a higher food value (weight for weight) than fresh apples. Apples are said to stimulate body secretion and can be taken as a health tonic medicine and bowel regulator. The malic and tartaric acid in them prevents disturbances of the liver and activity aids digestion. Unsweetened apple cider is said to prevent the formation of kidney stones. The low acidity of apples stimulates saliva flow and removes debris from the teeth. However, cheese is probably better for this purposes because it is not so acidic.

Eating several apples daily is believed to help arthritis, and lung and asthma complaints, and there was a time when apples were said to prevent emotional upsets and tension headaches. The pectin in apple peel certainly helps to remove noxious substances from the body by supplying galacturonic acid. The pectin helps to prevent protein matter in the intestines from spoiling. Apples are recommended for obesity, poor complexions, bladder inflammations, gonorrhea, anemia, tuberculosis, neuritis, insomnia, catarrh, worms and halitosis, and chewing unpeeled apples will strengthen bleeding gums.

Apple tea, which comes in easy-to-use powdered form, is said to cleanse the urinary tract and prevent diseases of the reproductive system. It is made from the peel, which is dried in ovens. Processed apples and apple products have far less vitamin C and A than raw apples. Unsweetened apple sauce and artificially sweetened apple sauce have fewer calories than apples of equivalent weight and less of the vitamins and minerals.

Apple butter, not surprisingly, has three times the number of calories, as well as more carbohydrate and phosphorus and twice the calcium, iron, sodium and potassium, of its fresh cousin, but it has no vitamin A.

The average composition for the fruit per 100 g is: water 84%, protein 0.3%, fat 0.3%, sugar 9%, kcal 49 (210 kJ), Ca 5 mg, Fe 0.3 mg, vitamin A 23 μg, B_1 0.03 mg, nicotinic acid 0.2 mg, vitamin C, 4 mg. It contains 0.7% malic acid, 3% pectin and the aromatic constituents are largely amyl ester of formic, caproic and caprylic acids and geraniol.

apples, dried. The average composition (per 100 g) of the dried apple is: protein 3.1%, fat 0.6%, kcal 280 (1.2 MJ), Ca 54 mg, Fe 2.3 mg, vitamin A 300 μg, B_1 0.06 mg B_2 0.12 mg, nicotinic acid 1.5 mg, vitamin C 10 mg. See also apple.

apricot drying. Apricots are dried on trays using sun or heated air. Sun drying for 3-5 hours may precede mechanical drying. Apricots are sliced and placed on trays at a loading of 9.8 kg/m² and drying for 8 hours at 65.6°C. Another method of drying is a two-step process involving drying, blanching, and continued drying (known as DBD process). Sulphuring is often done by burning sulphur may also be accomplished by dipping the apricots in a bisulphite solution before drying.

apricot. Fruit of *Prunus armeniaca*, closely resembling the peach in appearance. It was first grown in Armenia and other parts of Asia, and also in Africa. The apricot is a low tree of rather crooked growth, with somewhat heart-shaped leaves. The fruit is sweet, more or less juicy, of a yellowish colour, about two-thirds the size of the peach and resembling it in delicacy of flavor. It is one of the most highly esteemed fruits of the temperate climates. Botanists have characterized this sweet-sour fruit as more of a plum, although it does belong to the same family as peaches and almond nuts. This brass- or copper-coloured fruit originated in earlier days in Central Asia. It is said that when the first body of emigrants to leave the Tower of Babel in central

Iraq crossed over the Caucasus Mountains then turned westward towards the Caspian Sea, they brought with them young apricot tree seedlings, some of which were planted along the way.

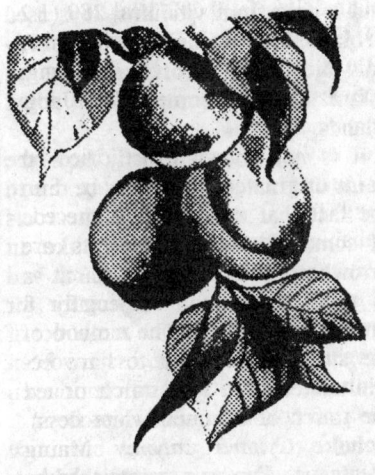

The average composition per 100 g of apricot is: raw-protein 0.6%, fat trace, carbohydrate 7%, kcal 28 (120kJ), Fe 0.2 mg, vitamin A 830 μg, vitamin B_1 0.04 mg, vitamin B_2 0.05 mg, nicotinic acid 0.6 mg, vitamin C 7 mg. Apricot kernel sometimes used (plus oil of almonds) in place of almond to make marzipan substitute.

arachin. One of the globulin protein from the peanut. Precipitated by 40% saturated ammonium sulphate from a salt extract of peanut. Conarachin can be precipitated from the residue by 85% saturated ammonium sulphate.

Araka. An intoxicating brandy-like liquor obtained from the distillation of koumiss - a fermented milk drink. Also known as rack or racky.

archidonic acid. Straight-chain fatty acid containing 20 carbon atoms and four double bonds (a tetrene). Found only in animal fats, e.g. brain, liver, egg yolk,

areca. A genus of lofty palms which have feather-shaped leaves, and bear a one-sided berry or nut enclosed in a fibrous rind. One species of the Malabar coasts is the common areca palm, which yields areca or betel nuts, and the astringent juice catechu.

arginase. Enzyme that hydrolyze arginine to urea and ornithine, the last stage of urea synthesis from the amino groups of the amino acids. Present in most animal cells.

argol. Crust of crude cream of tartar (potassium acid tartrate) that forms on the sides of wine vats (also called Wine Stone). White argol from white grapes, red argol from red. 50-85% potassium hydrogen tartrate and 6-12% calcium tartrate. It is used in vinegar fermentation, as mordant in dyeing, and in the manufacture of tartaric acid.

ariboflavinosis. Name given to set of symptoms caused by deficiency of riboflavin (vitamin B_2). Characterized by swollen, cracked, bright red lips (cheilosis), enlarged tender, magenta-red tongue (glossitis), cracking at the corners of the mouth (angular stomatitis), congestion of the blood vessels of the conjunctiva.

Arlac. Protein-rich baby food (42% protein), made in Nigeria by, from peanut flour and skim milk powder with added vitamins B_1, B_2 B_{12} and D and minerals.

Armenian bole. Ferric oxide; occurs naturally as hematite or prepared by heating ferrous sulphate, etc.; used in metallurgy, polishing compounds, paint pigment and as a food colour.

arnica. A genus of plants, consisting of about twelve species, one of which is found in Central Europe. It has a perennial root, a stem about two feet high, bearing on the summit heads of a dark golden yellow. In every part of the plant there is an acrid resin and a volatile oil, and in the flowers an acrid bitter principle called arnicin. The root contains also a considerable quantity of tannin. A tincture of arnica is employed as an external application to wounds and bruises, as it drives away the blood that collects around the injury.

Arogel. Trade name, Arogel 909 P for a potato starch preparation used as thickener in gravies, sauces and canned foods; it is stable to heat.

arrowleaf clovers. The three varieties of arrowleaf clovers (Amclo, Meechee, and Yuchi) are well adapted to the south-eastern US. The varieties are similar, but with differences in date of maturity. Amclo is the earliest, maturing 2 to 4 weeks later than crimson clover. Yuchi matures about 2 weeks later than Amclo. Meechee matures 2 to 4 weeks later than Yuchi. Arrowleaf clovers usually produce less fall growth than does crimson clover. However, late winter, spring, and early summer growth is greater than crimson clover. Forage quality of arrowleaf clovers and been good even in the bloom stage of growth. The clovers can be used for both hay and grazing. However, when an accumulated growth sufficient for hay is cut, little regrowth or reseeding occurs. Arrowleaf clovers can be overseeded on a Bermuda grass sod or seeded in a mixture of small grains and rye grass. Arrowleaf clover seeds have a very hard seed-coat. This seems to delay germination of volunteer seed in late summer and provides a good supply of seed for fall germination. Arrowleaf clover germinates at lower temperatures better than does crimson clover. These clover require a specific types of inoculant. Commercial type O inoculant is usually used.

arrowroot. Tuber of the West Indian plant, *Maranta arundinacea*, mainly used to prepare arrowroot starch, the most refined of all feculas. The starch contains only a trace of protein (0.2%) and is free from vitamins. It is used in bland, low-salt and protein-restrictedly diets and, unfortunately, as an infant food in some West Indian islands.

It is not known exactly how the name originated, but it may be due to the fact that the scales on the roots of some plants are shaped like an arrowhead. It is a delicate starch and is used as a food, especially for invalids and infants. The arrowroot of the stores is very apt to have been adulterated with rice starch or even the starch of common white flour.

artichoke. *Cynara scolymus.* Maurice Messegue, Europe's greatest herbalist, says that the part of the artichoke we are in the habit of eating is the least active, while all the rest of it, which is unbelievably bitter, is actually the most nutritious and therapeutic for you. Two vegetables are called artichokes, but have absolutely no relation to each other. We distinguish them as the globe artichoke and the Jerusalem artichoke. The former is a green vegetable somewhat like a tiny cabbage, except that its leaves are smaller and thicker. While the latter isn't even an artichoke, nor has anything to do with Jerusalem. It came here from South America, and first was called "girasole" from its likeness to the sunflower. Later this was corrupted into "Jerusalem." The tubers are pleasant enough to consume, but have no medical value.

artificial food. Chemically or mechanically prepared food, for humans or animals; examples of animal foods are oil cakes and bone meal.

asadero, oaxaca. A white whole milk Mexican cheese. The curd is heated and the hot curd is cut or braided into different sizes.

asafoetida. Gum asafoetida is an oleo-gum-resin exudate from the fleshy rhizomes and stems of *Ferula asafoetida. L., F. foetida, F. rubricaulis Boiss.*, and probably others of the 60 or so species of Ferula, members of the Umbelliferae that grow in Afghanistan, northwest India, Iraq and Turkey. It has a strong, persistent, peculiar odour with a warm sweet balsamic undertone and a characteristic bitter back-note, which is not disagreeable in dilution but in its natural form is objectionably strong. Some commercial samples, often in the form of a paste, may consist of gum mixed with various diluents such as gypsum, cereal flours, etc. The genuine material should contain 40-64% resin consisting of asoresinotannol both free and combined with ferulic acid, 25 % of gums, and 6-19% of essential oil The volatile oil obtained by distilling gum asafoetida is of little commercial value, although small lots are available. Very little work has been carried out to establish the chemical composition of oil of asafoetida. The presence of the following compounds has been reported in asafoetida: pinene, 2-butyl propenyl disulphide (about 40%), several disulphides with boiling points between 92-127°C (about 20%) said to be responsible for the disagreeable odour, diallyl disulphide and about 20% of an unidentified component. Presence of three major disulphides, viz. 2-butylpropenyl disulphide, 2-butyl-3-methylthioallyl disulphide, and 1-(1-methylthiopropyl) 1-propenyl di-

sulphides has also been reported. Dimethyl trisulphide, 2-butyl methyl disulphide, 2-butyl methyl trisulphide, di-2-butyl disulphide, di-2-butyl trisulphide, di-2-butyl tetrasulphide and di-1-butyl trisulphide have also been found. Some effort has focused on terpenes and numerous have been identified to date.

ascomycetes. The Ascomycetes comprise about 30,000 described species, including a number of familiar and economically important kinds. Most of the blue-green, red, and brown molds that cause food spoilage are Ascomycetes, including the salmon-coloured bread mold Neurospora, which has played such a notable role in the history of modern genetics. Ascomytcetes are the cause of a number of serious plant diseases, including the powdery mildews that attack fruits, the chestnut blight (due to the fungus *Endothia parasitica*, accidentally introduced from northern China), and Dutch elm disease (caused by *Ceratocystis ulmi*, a European fungus). Yeasts are also Ascomycetes, as are the delicious morels and truffles. Ascomycetes, like most fungi, are filamentous when they are growing. In general, their hyphae are septate (divided by crosswalls) instead of the aseptate hyphae characteristic of the Oomycetes and most Zygomycetes. The crosswalls are perforated, however, and cytoplasm with its included nuclei can move freely through them. The hyphal cells of the vegetative mycelium may be either uninucleate or multinucleate. Some species of Ascomycetes are homothallic, other are heterothallic. Asexual reproduction in the majority of Ascomycetes is by formation of specialized spores, called *conidia* (from the Greek meaning "fine dust"), which are cut off at the tips of the modified hyphae known as *conidiophores* (spore bearers). No flagellated cell appears at any point in the life cycle of these fungi. Sexual reproduction in Ascomycetes always involves the formation of an *ascus* (little sac), a structure that is characteristic of the group and distinguishes the Ascomycetes from all other fungi. Ascus formation usually takes place within a complex structure composed of tightly interwoven hyphae, the *ascocarp*. Many ascocarps are macroscopic, and they have been used extensively in the classification of the Ascomycetes.

ascorbic acid. $C_6H_8O_6$. A water soluble vitamin (Vitamin C). Both ascorbic acid and its first oxidation product, dehydroascorbic acid function as the vitamin. Milk as secreted contains about 20 mg of ascorbic acid per litre but it is rapidly oxidized to the dehydroascorbic acid by air. The latter is destroyed by heating so that pasteurized milk may have little vitamin C, unless added after pasteurization.

Ascorbic acid is found abundantly in citrus fruits, tomatoes, cabbage and other raw green leafy vegetables and forage plants. It is also artificially produced as a crystalline colourless compound with mild citric acid taste, which oxidizes easily especially in the presence of moist heat. It is essential in the formation of collagen. Connective tissues and tissues of the walls of the capillary blood vessels are weakened by a lack of ascorbic acid. Severe deficiency results in scurvy, capillary bleeding into skin and muscle tissue and bloody diarrhoea.

ascorbin stearate. Ester of ascorbic acid and stearic acid; a fat-soluble form of the vitamin which is used as an antioxidant at 0.1% concentration.

ascorbyl palmitate. Ester of ascorbic acid and palmitic acid used as an anti-staling agent in bakery products. Amounts of 0.1-0.4% by weight of the flour retard staling for 2-4 days.

aseptic filling. A term used in connection with the filling of sterilized sweet milk and with the filling of sterilized sweet milk and sweet cream cans or bottles. The entire machine is sterilized under pressure and the sealing is accomplished by means of a cap sealer to bottles or cans in an atmosphere of steam. When food, solid or liquid, is sterilized in the can it is subjected to heat treatment that can affect that quality of the food. Instead it can be sterilized in thin films or in narrow tubes by shorter treatment that inflicts less damage, and must then be filled into cans under strictly aseptic conditions.

aseptic. The condition of a surface, substance, or air in which microorganisms are either not present, or are killed and are not able to multiply. Most often the term 'aseptic' refers to the absence of pathogenic organisms in contrast to sterile which refers to absence of all organisms. Substances used to provide aseptic conditions are known as antiseptics.

ash. The residue left behind after all the organic matter has been burned off. It serves as a measure of the inorganic salts that were present in the original material.

asparagine. Amide of the amino acid, aspartic acid; serves in plants as a store of ammonia. During the growth of seedlings ketonic acids are formed during photosynthesis, and these are aminated to amino acids at the expense of ammonia in asparagine.

asparagus. Family: *Liliaceae.* Genus: *Asparagus.* Species: *Asparagus* *officinalis.* Asparagus was cultivated in ancient times by the Romans. The vegetable is a member of the Lilly family, and grows like weeds. Cattle and horses graze on it with delight. The plants should be allowed to grow three years from the seed before they are cut; after that, for ten or twelve years, they will continue to afford a regular annual supply. The beds are protected by straw or litter in winter. The full-grown plant has a beautiful feathery top, shaped like a miniature trees, and it bears small flowers and bright red fruits. Some varieties are cultivated for ornament and are incorrectly known as ferns.

Boiled, drained asparagus offers good amounts of protein, fat and vitamin A, B_2, C and E. Minerals include calcium, copper, magnesium, iron phosphorus, sulphur and traces of sodium. Canned asparagus is very salty although diet canned asparagus has very little salt. Otherwise it has the same food value as cooked fresh asparagus except that it has less vitamin B_6. Frozen asparagus has the same nutritional value as fresh cooked, except that it has slightly less vitamin A and less B_6 than fresh cooked asparagus.

Asparagus is an excellent diuretic and is often recommended for patients who enjoy it on bladder cleanses at the beginning of the summer. The urine they produce as the result of a fast on asparagus smells like motor oil, and looks about the same colour, but it is a wonderful kidney cleanser. Asparagus is also a good diaphoretic, and a laxative (due to its high fibre content). It is said to calm people under stress and it contains an amino-acid which is essential for the growth, division and regeneration of the body's cells. The juice of asparagus helps to break up oxalic acid present in the kidneys and the whole muscular system, so relieving rheumatism, uritis and arthritis.

The average composition per 100 g asparagus is: protein 1.5%, fat 0.1%, Ca 15 mg, Fe 0.5 mg, food energy 65 kJ, vitamin A 220 µg, vitamin B_1 0.11 mg, vitamin B_2 0.13 mg, nicotinic acid 1 mg, vitamin C 22 mg.

aspartame. A synthetic compound which does have significant caloric content, but the energy value it adds to finished products is negligible in most applications. Aspartame is the methyl ester of 1-aspartyl-1-phenylanine and it is prepared by chemical synthesis, as is saccharin. The substances is said to taste about 180 times as sweet as sucrose, but its sweetening power depends on the conditions under which the two materials are compared. Although aspartame is only about a half to a third as sweet as saccharin, and is much more expensive, aspartame does not contribute the bitter and metallic notes frequently observed when foods and beverages containing saccharin are ingested. Aspartame tends to slowly hydrolyze and become ineffective as a sweetener under certain rigorous conditions. The reaction is accelerated by high temperatures and high pH.

aspartic acid. A nonessential amino acid; amino succinic acid (dibasic). Its amide its asparagine.

aspic jelly. A jelly flavoured with lemon, tarragon vinegar, sherry, peppercorns and vegetables; used as a garnish.

aspiration psychrometer. An instrument used to measure the relative humidity of air, in which the air is moved over a thermometer sensing element (bulb) to evaporate moisture using an aspirator to propel the air.

astaxanthin. A carotenoid pigment; the

pink colour of salmon musçle.

atherosclerosis. The deposition of a fatty material, called atheroma, on the inner lining of the arteries. If atheroma is laid down in the coronary arteries the formation of the thrombus or clot may be encouraged, it is called coronary thrombosis. Several dietary factors have been implicated in causation of atherosclerosis.

atmospheric double drum dryer. Two hollow drums into which steam is fed for heating, with the two drums rotating towards each other, with the product placed above and between the two rolls, evaporation with the product placed above and between the two rolls, evaporation taking place at atmospheric pressure, and the dried product removed after 3/4-7/8 revolution of the drum. Devices are available to hold the knife off the drum for more than one revolution. The product is in contact with the drum for drying about 3 seconds or less. The spacing between the drum may be varied. Condensed product, or products at 30-70% moisture, are usually placed on the dryer and dried to 2-8% moisture content.

atmospheric dryer. A device for removing moisture from products using atmospheric air forced through or over product at atmospheric pressure.

atmospheric evaporator. A steam jacketed cylinder inside of which a moving blade moves the liquid product over the heating surface, with evaporation at atmospheric pressure and at a temperature only slightly above 100°C. Vapour is removed and discharged into the atmosphere. Also known as atmospheric concentrator.

atmospheric tray dryer. Trays containing materials to be dried are placed in one or more compartments at atmospheric pressure. These dryers are operated as batch or continuous units. Hot air is blown over the trays, around the trays, or through the product and trays, some having screened or perforated bottoms. The atmospheric tray dryer can be used for drying paste-like as well as other conventional materials.

atomization. The process of breaking or dividing a liquid into very small drops or droplets. Atomizers are used for fuels and for drying or dehydration of liquid products in spray dryers. The total surface area of a unit volume available for heat and mass transfer is greatly increased as the size of drop is decreased. During spray drying the temperature of the atomized particles approaches the wet-bulb temperature of the drying air.

atomizer. A device for producing droplets from a liquid, such as for atomization of fuels for a burner and for atomization of liquid products for spray drying. The atomized fuel is burned in a combustion chamber. The atomized product for drying is introduced in the drying chamber where heated air evaporates moisture from the atomized product and carries the moisture out of the dryer. Atomization of products for drying is accomplished by a high pressure nozzle, a two-fluid (air or steam) atomizing nozzle, or a centrifugal disc (disk).

Atwater factors. Factors used to calculated the energy content of foods in kilojoules after allowing for losses indigestion and urinary nitrogen: Protein 4, fat 9, carbohydrates 4, derived by Atwater from the heats of combustion, namely, protein 5.7, fat 9.4, carbohydrates 4.1

aubergine. Family: *Solanaceae.* Genus: *Solanum.* Species: *Solanum melongena;* native of Southeast Asia. It is 10-15 cm in diameter and up to 30 cm long, purple in colour. Aubergines are valuable for their vitamin B content, particularly B_1, B_2 and B_3 and for vitamin C, and they contain a little iron, calcium and carbohydrate. They are low in calories, but remember that they absorb enormous quantities of fat. They are helpful for constipation, colitis, stomach ulcers and nervous conditions. The average composition per 100 g aubergine is: carbohydrate 6%, protein 1.4%, vitamin B_1 0.06 mg, vitamin B_2 0.05 mg, nicotinic acid 0.8 mg, vitamin C 5 mg. Also known as egg plant.

Aufait. A molded ice cream and fruit combination consisting of two or more layers of ice cream with pectinized fruit spread between the layers. For example, to make Strawberry Aufait, fill a brick mold half full with vanilla ice cream; harden; spread over this a layer of pectinized strawberries (not too thick since it is difficult to cut through the fruit layer when it hardens); harden; and finish filling the mold with vanilla or strawberry ice cream. Many variations both as to number of layers and combinations of fruits are possible. Aufaits are also made in bulk by gently stirring the pectinized fruit into the ice cream as it comes from the freezer. The fruit should be heavy enough and cold enough so that it will make a more or less continuous line in the ice cream, giving a marbled effect.

aurantiamarin. Glucoside present in the albedo of the bitter orange; partly responsible for the flavour.

Aurore grape. A French-American hybrid variety of grape, parentage of which includes *Vitis linecumii, V. rupestris,* and *V. vinifera.* Although identification of flavour components from many studies on grape juices and wines from California and Europe have appeared, very little information is available on volatile components of native North American species and hybrids.

autoclave. A vessel in which high high pressure and temperatures can be reached. The domestic pressure cooker is an example. Autoclaves have two major use is in sterilization. Bacteria are destroyed more readily at these elevated temperatures, and autoclaves are used to sterilize food, for example in cans, and for sterilizing instruments and dressings in surgery.

autolysins. Enzymes that partially digest peptidoglycan in growing bacteria so that the peptidoglycan can be enlarged.

autolytic enzyme. A bacterial enzyme, located in the cell wall that causes disintegration of the cell following injury or death.

automation of dry kiln. The automation of kiln operation which consists of:
(a) the automatic determination of the moisture content; and
(b) the automatic changing of drying conditions to meet needs of the process.

The moisture content is determined by automatic continuous weighing of a part of the kiln load from which the moisture content is determined. Drying times can be reduced about 20% with an automated system.

auxins. Plant hormones produced in the growing buds, embryos and young leaves of plants, as well as many fungi and bacteria. They are manly organic acids, such as indole acetic acid, indole butyric acid and naphthalenic acetic acid. Auxns are used to stimulate root formation and control growth.

available nutrients. In some foodstuffs nutrients shown to be present by chemical tests may not be available, or only partly available, to the animal. For example, the calcium combined in phytin, and lysine that is combined with sugar in the Milliard complex, are not available they cannot be liberated by the digestive enzymes.

avenin. The glutelin protein present in oats.

avermectin. Any of a group of macrocyclic lactones, first isolated from the actinomycete bacterium Streptomyces avermitilis, with activity against helminth parasites. They include the commercially available anthelmintic ivermectin.

Avicel. Trade name for microcrystalline alpha-cellulose-natural cellulose partly hydrolyzed with acid and reduced to a fine powder. It disperses in water and has the properties of a gum; used to make oily foods such as cheese peanut butter, as well as syrups and honey, into dry granular powders; also used in sauces and dressings.

avidin. Protein in white of which combines with vitamin H (biotin), and renders it unavailable to the body. It is inactivated in cooked eggs.

avidity. A term used to describe the total affinity of an antibody for its specific antigen as a summation of all possible binding sites.

avitaminosis. A term used to describe the absence of vitamin; may be used specifically, avitaminosis A.

avocado. Family: *Lauraceae.* Genus: *Persea.* Species: *Persea Americana.* The avocado tree, which is related to the laurel, grows in semitropical climates. Orchards occur from Santa Barbara, California all the way to Lima, Peru. Giant prehistoric ground sloths feasted on ripe avocados, rapidly packing masses of oily flesh into their mouths, and later defecating seeds with hardly a sense of their passing. Avocados are always eaten raw and are best combined with a sharp taste as a good foil for their creamy blandness. The nutritional value varies according to their geographic origin but they are extremely rich in protein, vitamins A and B, potassium, and folic acid, and have some vitamin C. They contain a rare digestible oil which is not found in other fruits. The high fat and caloric content of avocado make it unsuitable for people trying to slim. Avocados are, on other hand, excellent for the malnourished, and are often recommend to patients who have stomach ulcers or ulcerative colitis. Their richness make them good for male impotency, constipation, insomnia and nervousness. Unusual as a fruit in high fat content.

The average composition per 100 g of avocado is: carbohydrate 5%, protein 2.1%, fat 16-25%; iron 1 mg, vitamin A 70 µg, vitamin B_1 0.12 mg, vitamin B_2 0.15 mg, nicotinic acid 1.1 mg, vitamin C 16 mg. Also known as alligator pears.

avocado oil. An oil obtained from the ripe, green-coloured, pear-shaped fruit of the avocado. *Persea americana,* a small tree of which more than 500 varieties grow profusely in US and many other parts of the world. The avocado oil is extracted from the fruit pulp, the dehydrated pulp yielding 70% oil. In Central America the oil is extracted by pressing in bags, and the oil has been used by the Mayans since ancient times for treating burns and as a pomade. It contains 77% oleic acid, 10.8 linoleic, 6.9 palmitic, and 0.7 stearic, with a small amount of myristic and a trace of arachidic acid. It is also rich in lecithin, contains phytostearin, and valued for cosmetics because it is penetrating like lanolin. It also contains mannoketoheptose, a highly nonfermentable sugar. The oil has good keeping qualities and is easily emulsified. The oil-soluble vitamins are absorbed through the skin, and the oil for cosmetics is not wintered in order to retain the sterols. The specific gravity is 0.9132. The oil is also called alligator pear oil.

Avocet. A trade name for a sterilized cream of 20-30% fat content. The fat emulsion is stabilized with an alginate and some corn product is also added. The combined amount of these two added products does not exceed 0.3%.

avoparcin. A glycopeptide antibiotic produced by a strain of the bacterium Streptomyces candidus. It is active against Gram-positive bacteria and is used in feed for pigs, cattle, and poultry as a growth promoter. Absorption from the gastrointestinal tract is extremely low and most of drug is excreted unchanged in faeces. Development of resistance by bacteria is not widespread and there is not cross-resistance with other antibiotics.

axial-flow fan. A mechanical device consisting of a power driven blade or propeller which moves air or gas parallel to the axis of rotation of the fan blade. Axial flow fans are characterized by operating at high air flows and low static pressures. Axial flow fans consists of propeller fans or other axial flow fans with an impeller or propeller fans with an enlarged hub, known as a disc fan. The other major classification of fans is the radial flow fan.

azaserine. An antibiotic, either produced by a species of Streptomyces or prepared synthetically, that inhibits the purine biosynthesis and leads to chromosomal aberrations.

azeotropic drying. The removal of moisture from a product (such as wood) in a heated chemical mixture which has a constant boiling point. The process may be carried out in a vacuum. An azeotrope is a given mixture of liquids which has a constant boiling point, for which the composition of the liquid does not change as it is converted to vapour.

Azlon. A popular name given to textile fibres produced from proteins, such as casein, zein.

azoprotein. A modified protein in which a tyrosine residue has been coupled to an aromatic diazo compound. Diazotization is often employed to form protein-heptan conjugates.

azotobacter. Genus of bacteria of family *Azotobacteriaceae* which can use atmospheric nitrogen and synthesize nitrogenous tissue from it. The cells are plump rods or cocci, surrounded by slime. A multilayered wall may be synthesized around the cell to produce a microcyst resistant to desiccation.

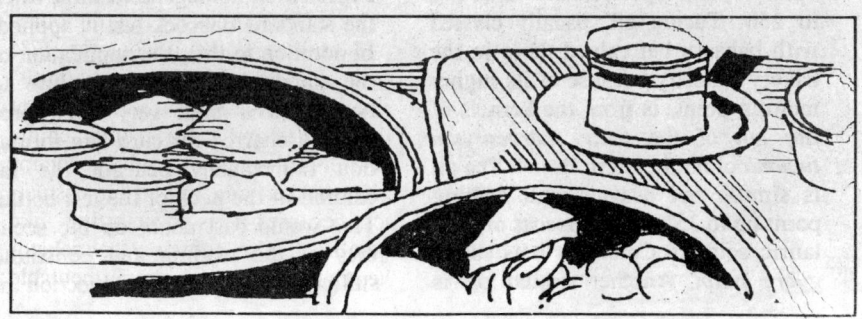

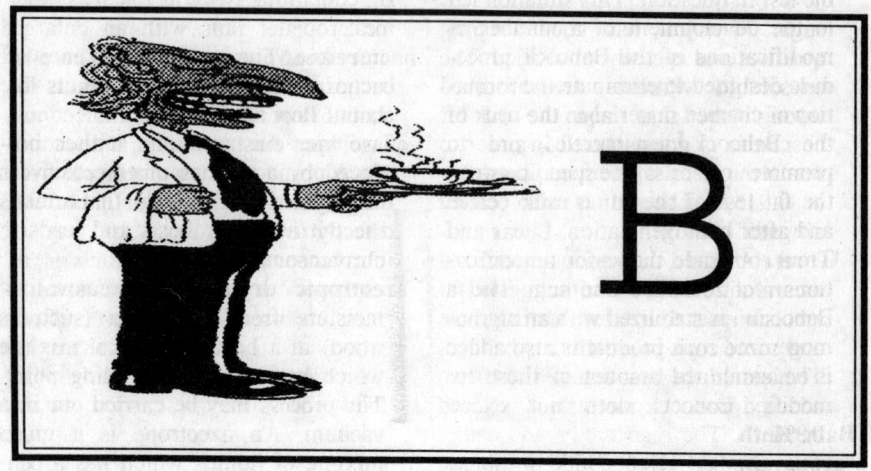

babassu oil. An edible oil from the Brazilian palm nut; similar to coconut oil and used in food, soap and cosmetics. It is obtained from the kernels of the nut of the palm tree *Attalea orbignya* which grows in vast quantities in north-eastern Brazil. There are two to five long kernels in each nut, the kernel being only 9% of the hearty-shelled nut, and these kernels contain 65% oil. A bunch of the fruits contains 200-600 nuts. The oil contains as much as 45% lauric acid, and is a direct substitute for coconut oil for soaps, as an edible oil, and as a source of lauric, capric, and myristic acids. The melting point of the oil is 22-26°C, specific gravity 0.868, iodine value 15, and saponification value 246 to 250. Tucum oil, usually classed with babassu but valued more in the bakery industry because of its higher melting point, is from the kernels of the nut of the palm *Astrocaryum tucuma* of northeastern Brazil. The oil is similar but heavier with melting point up to 35°C, and consists of 49% lauric acid. In Colombia it is called *guere palm.* Another similar oil is

murumuru oil, from the kernels of the nut of the palm *A. murumuru,* of Brazil. The name is a corruption of the two Carib words maru and moru, meaning bread to eat. The oil contains as much as 40% lauric acid, with 35% myristic acid, and some palmitic, stearic, linoleic, and oleic acids. It is usually marketed as babassu oil.

Babcock test for fat in homogenized milk. It has long been recognized that the standard Babcock test procedure for fat in non-homogenized milk does not yield comparable results when applied to homogenized milk. General experience has indicated that somewhat lower fat tests (usually not more than 0.10% lower) may be expected on homogenized milk when the standard Babcock test is applied. In addition to this, the application of the standard Babcock procedure to homogenized milk very often produces a charred for curd-like formation immediately beneath the fat column in the neck of the test bottle. This would cast doubt on the accuracy of the reading and constitute sufficient cause for the rejection of the test in question. This situation led to the development of a number of modifications of the Babcock procedure designed to eliminate the formation of charred material in the neck of the Babcock test bottle, and to promote closer agreement between the fat test of the same milk before and after homogenization. Lucas and Trout compared the various modifications recommended and suggested a Babcock procedure for testing homogenized milk in which they believe is embodied the best features of these modified Babcock methods.

Babe Ruth. The registered trade name of a product similar to chocolate covered ice cream bars, except that it is in the form of a base ball and is poured into molds instead of being cut out of bricks.

baby beef. A young beef animal that has been rapidly fattened while still in the rapid growth period. Such animals generally go to market for slaughter at the age of 12-20 months and weigh from 700-1200 kg live. Aberdeen Angus and Herefords are the most popular breeds for this trade. Also, the trade name for this type of meat.

bacalao. South American name for klipfish.

bacitracin. Antibiotic isolated from a organism of the *B. subtilis* group; a polypeptide.

bacon. Cured and smoked flesh of pigs raised with less subcutaneous fat than pigs for pork and with long backs. Streaky, fried. The average composition is: protein 24%, fat 45%, food energy 2.1 MJ, vitamin B_1 0.6 mg, vitamin B_2 0.24 mg, nicotinic acid 2 mg. The average composition per 100 g of gammon, fried is: protein 31%, fat 33%, food energy 1.8 MJ, vitamin B_1 0.6 mg, vitamin B_2 0.24 mg, nicotinic acid 2 mg. Pig meat is rich in vitamin B_1, containing twice as much as other meat.

bacteremia. The transient presence of bacteria in the blood. It accounts for about 6% of all nosocomial infections. Two types exist: primary, and secondary. A primary bacteremia results from the accidental introduction of bacteria directly into the body by way of intravenous infusion, transducers, respiratory devices, prostheses, catheters, endo-scopes, or parenteral nutrition. A secondary bacteremia results from an infection at another body site such as urinary tract, respiratory tract, or surgical wounds. The organisms most responsible for bacteremia are Gram-negative bacilli. Bacteremia occur primarily in neonates and the elderly, whose natural defense mechanisms are compromised.

bacteria. A large and diverse group of organisms, which, in terms of numbers and variety of habitats, includes the most successful life forms. In nature, bacteria are important in the nitrogen and carbon cycles, and some are useful to man in various industrial processes, especially in the food industry. However, there are also many harmful parasitic bacteria that cause diseases such as botulism and tetanus. Bacterial cells are simpler than those of animals and plants and do not contain complex organelles such as chloroplasts and mitochondria. They may divide every 20 minutes and can thus reproduce very rapidly. They also form resistant spores. Bacteria are resident in the digestive tracts of most animals, including humans, where they aid in the digestion of food. They live in nodules on the roots of some plants, especially the legumes, assisting them in the take up of nitrogen from the air and the soil. Some are able to decompose environmentally dangerous compounds such as petrochemicals. A few bacteria obtain their food by means of photosynthesis, some are saprophytes, and others are parasites, causing disease in man, animals, plants, and other microorganisms. It has been estimated that the weight of all living bacteria, taken together, equals or exceeds the weight of all other organisms on the earth. Bacteria include all prokaryotic organisms except the blue-green algae, from which they can be distinguished by the latter's ability to photosynthesize aerobically. They include the *eubacteria, actinomycete, spirochetes, rickettsiae*, slime bacteria, iron bacteria, and sulphur bacteria. Bacteria can be classified into five major divisions based upon their requirements for gaseous oxygen or air:

(a) Obligate aerobes, that have an absolute requirement for oxygen as they metabolize sugars; members of this group include the genera *Bacillus* and *Pseudomonas*.

(b) Obligate anaerobes, that cannot multiply if oxygen is present. Some members are killed by even traces of oxygen because they cannot modify the toxic forms of oxygen produced in metabolism. The best known members of this group are in the genus *Clostridium*.

(c) Facultative anaerobes, which can utilize oxygen in metabolic processes if it is available but can also grow in its absence. Growth is generally rapid, if oxygen is present, since more ATP, the readily utilizable storage form of energy, is generated by metabolic pathways that require oxygen. *Escherichia coli* and *Saccharomyces* are common examples of facultative anaerobes.

(d) Microaerophilic organisms, the microorganisms require small amount of oxygen (2-10%) but the higher concentrations are toxic. Few disease-causing organisms such as *Helicobacter pylori*, are included in this group.

(e) Aerotolerant organisms, which can grow in the presence or absence of oxygen, but unlike facultative anaerobes, they derive no benefit from oxygen. Many aerotolerant organisms grow better in containers used for anaerobic cultures because they contain higher levels of carbon dioxide and water vapours than found in air. *Streptococcus pyogenes*, the cause of strep throat, is aerotolerant bacterium.

bacterial disease. The disease caused by the bacteria. Many of the bacterial diseases remain major cause of death in underdeveloped countries. Bacterial disease may be acquired through different routes, including:

(a) the respiratory tract,

(b) the alimentary tract,

(c) sexual transmission,

(d) congenital transfer, and

(e) the skin and mucosa (including the bite of insect vectors).

Immunity to bacterial diseases involves both the humoral and cell-mediated responses of the host. The bacterial surface is composed of a number of antigens, which vary considerably from species to species and between various strains within a species. Many of these antigens induce the formation of specific protective antibodies in the host, which accounts for the resistance to future infection as well as recovery from primary infections. Those surface antigens that do not elicit a protective antibody response often belong to agents that cause chronic infections such as tuberculosis and brucellosis.

bacterial transposon. Any one of a number of different DNA sequences found in some strains and species of bacterial cells that are characterized by their mobility in the genome, since they can move from one site to another within the circular chromosome. They owe their mobility to the existence of short insertion elements at each end of the transposon, and they may carry bacterial coding sequences within the transposon itself. Transposons betray their presence in bacteria by the movements of a coding sequence within a transposon (as revealed by mapping the gene sequence through an interrupted mating experiment) or by the altered expression or mutation rate of other bacterial genes adjacent to the site of insertion of transferable sequence.

bacteriochlorophyll. A modified Chlorophyll that serves as the primary light trapping pigment in purple and green photosynthetic bacteria. It is structurally similar to chlorophyll.

bacteriocins. The substances produced by bacterial strains that inhibit or kill other closely related strains. Bacteriocins are composed of proteins and in some cases are coded for by plasmids. Bacteriocins are named in accordance with the species of organism that produce them. Thus, in *E. coli* have colicins, coded by Col plasmids, *Bacillus subtilis* produces subtilisin, and so on.

bacteriophage. A substance of biological origin which has a lytic (dissolving) action on bacteria and thus destroys them. Little is known of the nature of bacteriophages; they are ultramicroscopic and pass through filters readily.

bacteriostat. A substance that prevents the growth and multiplication of bacteria but does not kill them. The use of such agents to treat infections depends on a competent host immune system to kill the organisms. Also, it is essential to maintain an effective concentration of the bacteriostat during the course of treatment or the organisms may recover and resume reproduction.

bacteroids. A genus of Gram-negative anaerobic bacteria, commonly found as saprophytes in the gastrointestinal tract. *B. nodosus*, however, is an important cause of foot rot in sheep and possibly also in goats and cattle, usually in association with *Fusobacterium necrophorum*. Morphologically, *B. nodosus* appears as a large curved or straight rod, both ends of which are enlarged. The organism survives better during prolonged wet and warm conditions.

bactofugation. A Belgian process for removing bacteria from milk by high-speed centrifuging.

bagasse. The cellulosic residue of sugar-cane after it has been disintegrated to extract the sugar. It is converted by high-temperature compression into a heavy board of high thermal insulating value which is useful for heat- and soundproofing in building construction. Paper can be made from bagasse on a commericial basis; also applicable in the manufacture of furfural; and used an an extender in animal feeds.

bag dryer. A unit especially designed to remove moisture from seed or grain in bags or sacks by forced air. A unit consists of a fan and air distribution system upon which sacks of seeds or grain are placed over 25 cm X 60 cm openings with each opening provided with a door.

bagasse. Mill residues from sugar cane

consisting of the crushed stalks from which the juice has been expressed; 50% cellulose, 25% hemicelluloses, 25% lignin. Sometimes also applied to residues from other plants such as beet. It is used as fuel, cattle feed, preparation of paper and fibre board, and in the manufacture of furfural, and for boiler fuel having a heating value of 18,500-21,000 kJ/kg (8000-9000 Btu/lb) of dry matter.

bagozzo cheese. A Parmesan type cheese similar to Reggiano and Parmigiano. The red coated cheese has a hard yellow body and a sharp flavour. Also known as grana bagozzo.

bakers' cheese. A skim-milk cheese that is softer, more homogenous, and contains more acid than the cottage cheese. Bakers' cheese usually is used commercially in making such bakery products as cheese cake, pie, and pastries. It may be creamed and eaten like cottage cheese. The milk is pasteurized, cooled to a temperature of 32.2°C and inoculated with lactic starter and rennet. After 4-6 hours the sour coagulated mixture is stirred, or broken without cooking or washing. It is drained or pumped into special draining bags, which are tied and piled to allow whey drainage. The bags are piled several times to form a drier cheese. Crushed ice may be placed between the bags to retard acid development during overnight drainage. The salted or unsalted curd may be packed in polyethylene bag-lined cans for stored. It will keep for several months if stored frozen at a temperature below -17.8°C, but preferably it is kept at 0°C. Weight of cheese yielded about 15 to 20% weight of skim milk used. Bakers' cheese may be made from spray-dried nonfat milk solids. Reconstituted milk, containing 11% solids, is warmed to 32.2°C 3.6 kg of lactic starter and 0.2 mg of rennet (which has to be diluted in water) are added. In 4-6 hours of coagulated curd is bagged and drained by the same method as described above for regular skim milk. The yield is 8.6-10 kg of cheese. Continuous centrifuges have been used successfully to recover the cheese solids instead of the bag method. The centrifuged curd is cooled under pressure and packaged directly into a polyethylene-lined tin can. Control of the acid development is maintained and the keeping quality is extended considerably.

baking additives. The materials added to baked products to improve their appearance, performace and taste. For example in bread-making yeast-stimulating preparations may be used, and bleaching and improving agents (ascorbic acid, potassium bromate, ammonium persulphate, chlorine dioxide, benzoyl peroxide). Cakes may contain added sodium lactate to improve the texture of the sponge and biscuits may contain the same substance to prevent 'checking'.

baking powder. A mixture capable of liberating carbon dioxide when moistened or heated. Sodium bicarbonate is the source of carbon dioxide and an acidic substance is required, such as tartaric acid or acid salt, calcium acid phosphate, sodium pyrophosphate or sodium aluminium sulphate. Quick-acting powders contain tartrate and liberate carbon dioxide in the dough before heating; slow-acting contain phosphate and liberate most of the carbon dioxide during heating. Legally baking powders must contain not less than 8% available, and not more than 1.5% residual, carbon dioxide. Golden raising powder (similar but coloured yellowed; called egg substitute) must contain not less than 6% available, and not more than 1.5% carbon dioxide.

Bal-Ahar. Protein-rich baby food (22-26% protein) made in India from wheat flour, oil-seed flour and vegetables with added vitamins and calcium.

balance. With reference to diet means equilibrium between intake and output, e.g., nitrogen balance, calcium balance, etc. Negative and positive balance respectively refer to net loss from or gain to the body.

ball clover. *Trifolium nigrescens.* A variety of clover that is a winter annual reseeding legume for pastures. Ball clover has long, succulent branching stems growing prostrate to partially upright. It has white to yellowish-white flower heads. Ball clover makes major growth about one month later in the spring than does crimson clover. In comparative tests, ball clover has not produced as much total forage as crimson clover. This type of clover is favoured in some areas of the southern states.

bambarra groundnut. *Voandzeia subterranea.* Resembles true groundnut but seeds are low in oil content. Seeds are hard and need soaking or pounding before cooking. The average composition per 100 g is: 18 g protein; 6 g fat; 60 g carbohydrates; food energy 1.5 kJ; 65 mg calcium; 6-7 mg iron; 0.3 mg vitamin B_1; 0.1 mg vitamin B_2, and 2 mg nicotinic acid.

bamboo shoots. Thick pointed shoots of *Bambusa vulgaris* and *Phyllostachys pubescens* eaten in many parts of eastern Asia. The average composition per 100 g is: 2.5 g protein; 0.2 g fat; 6 g carbohydrates; food energy 0.15 MJ; 0.15 mg vitamin B_1, 0.07 mg vitamin B_2; 0.6-0.7 mg nicotinic acid; and 4 mg vitamin C.

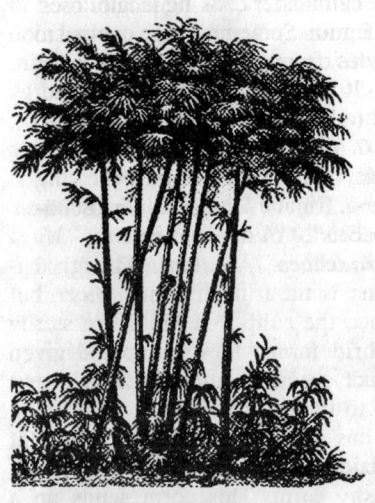

banana drying. Bananas may be dried in many forms using one of several different methods. Sun-dried bananas are used for flour or powder. Diced or sliced peeled bananas are dried on trays in a heated air chamber or tunnel. Air heated to not more than 93°C initially and 65.5°C finally is used to dry bananas to 20% moisture content. The bananas can be pulped in a disintegrator or homogenizer and dried on a double drum atmospheric dryer. Flakes are produced on a drum dryer. The flakes may be pulverized to make a powder. The pulped material can be diluted with water and dried in a spray dryer. Discolouration can be reduced by sulphuring after peeling, before processing.

banana figs. Bananas are split longitudinally and sun-dried without treating with sulphur dioxide. The product is dark in colour and sticky.

banana, false. *Ensete ventricosum,* closely related to the banana; fruits are small and contain seeds (bananas are sterile and have no seeds); the rhizome and inner tissues of the stem are eaten after cooking (major food in S. Ethiopia). The average composition of rhizome per 100 g is: 1.5 g protein; 45-50 g carbohydrates; food energy 0.8 MJ; 5 mg iron; 0.02 mg vitamin B_1; 0.07 mg vitamin B_2; 0.3 mg nicotinic acid; and 0.5 mg vitamin C.

banana. Family: *Musaceae*. Genus: *Musa*. Species: *Musa sapientum; Musa paradisiaca (plantian)*. Though banana is the fruit of genus *Musa*, but since the cultivated kinds are sterily hybrid forms, they cannot be given exact species names. Banana grows up to the height of about 5-6 metres. It has a stout, cylindrical, succulent pseudostem arising from a large, fleshy corm. This corm sends up a series of suckers, forming clumps. Bananas are native, in various forms, from India and Burma through the Malay Archipelago to New Guinea, Australia, Samoa and tropical Africa. It's universally cultivated in tropical regions.

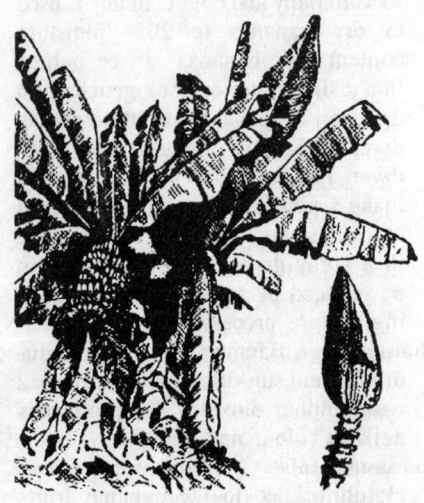

Bananas have high content of carbohydrates, potassium, folic acid and vitamin C. They contain a large amount of starch which changes to sugar as they ripen; unripe bananas are starchy and potato-like, and are indigestible. Contrary to popular belief, bananas are not particularly fattening. Desert bananas have a high sugar content (17-19%) and are eaten raw. The average composition per 100 g of banana is: 1 g protein; 0.3 g fat; 27 g carbohydrates; food energy 0.49 MJ; 0.5 mg iron; 30 mg vitamin A; 0.05 mg vitamin B_1; 0.05 mg vitamin B_2; 0.7 mg nicotinic acid; and 10 mg vitamin C. Sodium content is low, that is, about 1.2 mg/100 g; it is therefore recommended in low-sodium diets. An average banana contains 85-90 calories, which makes it lower in calories than a good-sized serving of cottage cheese, besides which the banana is not only easily digestible but helps the body to store protein. A banana a day gives one fifth of the recommended daily intake of vitamin C. Bananas are used naturopathically as a dietary method of controlling allergic-type reactions. Their protein content is of such a benign nature that allergy suffers adding a banana to their diet find it reduces the distressing symptoms of runny nose and puffy eyes. Calcium, phosphorus and iron are richly present in bananas. It has been found that there is more iron in banana than that found in apple. Under the skin of unripe bananas, there is an antibiotic-type substance, hence the custom of cooking them in their skins in the West Indies and the Pacific islands. Like apples, bananas contain pectin, which helps to digest other foods, and they are very useful for normalizing bowel function in patients with either chronic constipation or chronic diarrhoea. Banana actually helps to increase the quantity of bacteria in the intestine, particularly if it is mixed with plain yoghurt. Bananas have been recommended for colitis, intestinal ulcers and colic disease. They are also excellent for edema because kidneys that are under-functioning, sluggish or slow as a residual symptom of disease can be helped to function better as a result of the fruit's high potassium content. They are extremely nutritious when mashed and given ripe to babies, and have the added advantage of coming in a nice germ-proof, dirt-proof skin. Banana flour, made from the dried unripe fruit, is as nutritious as double the amount of wheat flour. Dried bananas have four times the nutritional value but less vitamin C than fresh bananas.

banbury. A soft, rich cheese popular in England in the early 19th century. It is a cylindrically shaped cheese about in inch thick.

band through-circulation dryer. A device for removing moisture in which the wet material is in particulate or granular form of nearly uniform size, such as pellets, placed on a perforated band or conveyor, and moved through a forced air stream in a drying chamber.

bannock. Flat round cake made of oat, rye or barley meal; baked on a hearth or griddle. Pitcaithly bannock is a type of almond short-bread containing caraway seeds are chopped peel.

Barbados rum. A variety of rum made in Barbados which is about medium boiled. The distillation of the fermented molasses is carried out with high rectification to over 90% alcohol. A strange mixture of lime, soda, vegetable roots and coconut shells is placed in the still with the fermentation liquid. An equally interesting mixture of Sherry, Madeira, spirits of nitre, bitter almonds and raisins are added to make this spirit into a nice drink. A little rum is made in Mexico, from simple sugarcane. This is a high-bodied drink and is not very popular. A limited quantity of rum is made in South America, Jamaica and US. Such rums acquire flavour during fermentation, but all the others have flavouring materials added to it. Jamaican rum is very popular in Canada and the US, and many other European countries.

Barberey cheese. A soft rennet cheese similar to Camembert, and deriving its name from the village of Barberey, near Troyes, France. In summer it is often sold without ripening. It is 10-15 cm in diameter and 3-4 cm thick.

barbiturates. A group of drugs that are derivatives of barbituric acid (malonyl urea), so called beause it was first prepared on St. Barbara's day in 1863. Barbituric acid itself is inactive. Many barbiturates are therapeutically useful and exert a depressant action on the central nervous system (such as phenobarbitone, amylobarbitone, thiopentone, methohexitone), but stimulant barbiturates have been synthesized. Depressant barbiturates exert sedative, hypnotic, antiepileptic and anaesthetic activity. Their uses as sedatives or hypnotics are now largely obsolete, but the long-acting ones (e.g., phenobarbitone) remain in use as anticonvulsant drugs in epilepsy, and the short-acting ones (e.g., sodium thiopentone and sodium methohexitone) are used as intravenous anaesthetics. Their main mechanism of action is probably exerted at GABA recepotrs, where they act to potentiate GABA. The problems with barbiturates that have led to a substantial reduction in their use as sedatives and hypnotics include serious tolerance and drug dependence, and enzyme induction.

barley. Family: *Gramineae.* Genus: *Hordenum.* Species: *Hordeum vulgare.* The edible grains which are rich in protein and have substantial amounts of calcium, iron, potassium and phosphorus. The same amount of pearl barley contains only about two-thirds of the protein and mineral content and half the amount of B vitamins. Barley is nutritious and easily digested and encourages healthy hair and nail growth. It will also soothe stomach ulcers. The grain of *Hordeum vulgare,* are of considerable importance as human and animal food and in brewing; one of the hardiest of cereals. The whole gain with only the outer husk removed is called *Pot, Scotch* or *Hulled Barley* (this requires several hours cooking).

Barley Meal is ground hulled barley; *barley flour* is ground pearl barley; *barley flakes* are the flattened grain. *Pearl Barley* is most of the bran and germ removed, ash reduced from 2.5-1%, vitamin B_1 to one tenth. The average composition per 100 g of barley is: protein 9%; fat 1.4%; calcium 20 mg; iron 0.7 mg; vitamin B_1 0.15 mg; vitamin B_2 0.08 mg; and nicotinic acid 2.5 mg.

barm. Another name for yeast or leaven, or the froth on fermenting malt liquor. Spon or virgin barm (short for spontaneous) is made by allowing wild yeast to fall into a sugar medium and multiply there.

Barmene. Trade name for yeast extract prepared from autolyzed brewer's yeast, plus vegetable juices, used for flavouring. The average composition per 100 g is: 38% protein; 13% carbohydrates; 6 mg thiamine; 6 mg riboflavin; 60 mg nicotinic acid; 3 mg pantothenic acid; 1.5 mg pyridoxine; and 1 mg folic acid.

barn drying. The process of completing the drying of hay, grass, or other forage in the now of the barn using forced air or forced heated air after wilting the forage in the field, drying a maximum of 50-15% moisture content, wet basis. Duct systems are provided for distributing air through the storage or mow. A centre main duct, a main duct with laterals, or a slatted floor is used to distribute the air through the forage. For heated air systems, temperatures up to 82.2°C are commonly used. For unheated air, airflows of 0.076-0.10 m³/m²s are used, and for heated forced air, airflows of 0.10-0.15 m³/m²s are used. Airflows are designated on the basis of 0.16 X 10^{-3} to 0.26 X 10^{-3} m³/kgs, with higher airflows for heated air systems. These systems will have a static pressure of 0.19 to 0.38 kPa. Also known as barn hay drying.

barn hay drying. *See* barn drying.

Barolo. An Italian red wine comparable to the French wines of the Rhone Valley. Regarded by some tasters as the best red wine of Italy. The wine takes its name from Barolo, a small village south of Turin. The Nebbiolo grape is used in its preparation. It requires considerable ageing, usually 3 years in wood and a year or so in the bottle prior to consumption.

Bartlett pear. The main variety of pear grown in Europe, US, and many other moderately colder regions of the world. The fruit is medium to large in size, oblong-obtuse-pyriform (bell-like), somewhat irregular. Skin is fairly thin, somewhat tender, clear yellow in color when ripe, occasionally blushed. The surface is somewhat uneven, with rather inconspicuous dots. Flesh is white, fine, quite free of grit, melting, juicy. It has sweet vinous flavour with traces of muskiness. It ripens early in season.

basal metabolic rate. BMR. The rate of energy metabolism required to maintain an animal at rest. It is measured in terms of heat production per unit time: it indicates the energy consumed in order to sustain such vital functions as heartbeat, breathing, nervous activity, active transport, and secretion. Different tissues have different metabolic rates (*e.g.,* the BMR of brain tissue is much greater than that of bone tissue) and therefore the tissue composition of an animal determines its overall BMR. For any comparable group of animals (such as mammals) BMR is proportional to body weight according to the allometric equation; small animals tend to have a higher metabolic rate per unit weight than large ones. The thyroid hormones are prime regulators of the BMR. When the body is at complete rest, free from draughts, at moderate room temperature and 12-14 hours after a meal, energy is being used as the basal rate-the basal metabolism. This energy is needed to maintain the heart beat and respiration, but largely to maintain body temperature and the tension of the muscles. BMR is therefore related to muscle mass and the surface area of the body. It is calculated from surface area, the output per square metre varies with age and sex. For male infants BMR is 50-70 kcal per m²/hour, falling steadily with age to 30-40 kcal at the age of 70, about 10% less for women. It is, under control of the thyroid gland, increased in fever and hyperthyroidism and by administration of thyroxine or dried thyroid, and reduced when the thyroid is underachieve.

base. A base is a substance that:

(a) liberates hydroxyl ions when dissolved in water;

(b) that liberates negative ions of various kinds in any solvent;

(c) that receives a hydrogen ion from a strong acid to form a weaker acid;

(d) that gives up two electrons to an acid, forming a covalent bond with the acid (Lewis).

Lewis bases are considered hard if they have high electronegativity and are difficult to oxidize and soft if they have low electronegativity and are easily oxidized. These properties relate to the presence or absence of vacant orbitals. Bases react with acids to form salts and water; when the proper proportions are used, neutralization occurs. All water-soluble bases give solutions having a *p*H of more than 7.0, the neutral point.

basic amino acids. Amino acids, such as lysine, arginine and histidine, that carry a positive charge on their sidechains, the prevalance of these amino acids in some proteins (*e.g.,* histones) renders these larger molecules basic also, especially since they are also depleted in the acidic amino acids glutamic acid and aspartic acid.

basic 7 foods plan. Division of foods into seven groups, with the recommendation that some food from each group should be eaten every day, so ensuring a well mixed diet.

Group 1. Green and yellow raw vegetables.

Group 2. Grapefruit, oranges, tomato, and raw salads.

Group 3. Potatoes and other vegetables and fruits.

Group 4. Milk and cheese.

Group 5. Meat, poultry, fish and eggs.

Group 6. Bread, flour, and cereals.

Group 7. Butter and margarine.

basic fondant. A mixture of sucrose, dextrose, levulose, maltose, lactose and/or dextrins or a combination of two or more such products and water, boiled to a predetermined temperature. The ratio of sugars used determines the final temperature. The ratio of sugars used determines the final physical characteristics of the basic fondant, i.e., short, medium, or chewy. Fondant finds major use in coated or dipped candies, such as bonbons, chocolate candies, candy bars, cast cream centres, among others. Nearly are kind of confectionery can be dipped in fondant. Sugar cream, or fondant, is a versatile class of candy that typifies the entire category of soft candies.

basil. Family: *Labiatae.* Genus: *Ocimum.* Species: *Ocimum basilicum.* Basil contains an essential oil, comprising mainly estragol, which is also present in French and Russian tarragons. *Ocimum basilicum* is Cultivated worldwide as an annual plant. Many varieties have different compositions and flavouring characteristics. The herb is strongly affected by environmental factors like temperature, geographic location, soil and amount of rainfall. Its thin branching root produces bushy stems growing 30-60 cm high and bearing leaves of a purple hue, and two-lipped flowers, varying in colour from white to red, sometimes with a purple tinge. It sometimes (depending on the variety) contains thymol and it also contains basil camphor which gives it its specific fragrance and taste. Basil is used as an anti-spasmodic and carminative in treating gastrointestinal problems like stomach cramp, and vomiting constipation and enteritis. It is also used to treat whooping cough, head colds, headaches and warts. Its weak -sedative action is sometimes used in the treatment of nervous headaches or anxiety.

batch dryer. A device in which the product to be dried is placed in batches for drying, the complete drying or drying and cooling operations performed, and them removed. Usually the unit is self-contained comprising of a drying compartment, either horizontal or vertical, through which heated air is forced or drawn from a central portion usually called a plenum chamber. A large range of heated air temperatures is used. Cooling is usually carried out in the same manner. Integral conveying equipment provides for loading and unloading the dryer. Also included as part of the dryer are the air moving device, burner, and control system. Batch dryers are often portable, but may be stationary. The following are included in the category of batch dryers: tray dryer, agitated batch dryer, and rotary dryer, all of which may be for either atmospheric or vacuum operation.

batch-in-bin dryer. A drying unit in which wet grain in shallow depths of about 1.25 m or less, is placed in a bin with a false floor and is dried with forced heated air, 50 to 70°C, at flow rates of 0.1-0.25 m^3/m^3s. The system for batch-in-bin drying is characterized by:

(a) all of the floor on which grain is placed is exposed to the air plenum;

(b) improved equipment has made loading and unloading the grain, and in-bin materials handling, workable;

(c) possibility of a large variation in moisture throughout the bed; and

(d) cooling grain with fan but without the heater.

Battlemat cheese. A variety of cheese made in Canton of Tessin, Switzerland, western Austria, and northern Italy. It ripens faster than Emmentaler, being ready for consumption in about 4-5 months.

Bauden cheese. A sour milk¯ cheese made in herder's huts in the Bohemian and Silesian mountains. Locally it is known as Koppen. It is made in two forms, one conical with a diameter and a height of 10 cm, and the other cylindrical with a diameter of 12.5 cm and a height of 7.5 cm.

bay laurel. *Laurus nobilis.* A small evergreen shrub or tree native to the Mediterranean region and Asia Minor. Bay leaves are among the most versatile of herbs, and the plants, if regularly clipped, rank among the most decorative of shrubs. The glossy and sweetly scented leaves are indispensable in both French and Mediterranean cooking, a traditional ingredient in bouquet garni, and a 'must' in marinades, *court bouillon,* stocks, and pickles. Bay leaves are used in all types of cookery, such as in soups, stews, casseroles, stocks, syrups, sweet and savoury sauces, and as a garnish. An infusion of the leaves may be taken for flatulence, and the dried leaves are crumbled into pot pourri. To dry the leaves, they are simply hanged in bunches in a warm and dry place. It has been admired for its beauty and aromatic leaves since the Greek and Roman times. The leaves are leathery, lanceloate, pointed and experience maximum oil content increases, during early and midsummer only. Several botanicals are known by the name of 'bay', *i.e.,* West Indian bay (*Pimenta racemosa*) and California bay (*Umbellularia californica*). Hence, the term 'bay' in the existing herb literature can mean any one of these botanicals, among others. Also known as sweet bay.

bayberry bark. *Myrica cerifera.* Wax myrtle or bayberry is an evergreen shrub native to the eastern US and also grows in the Bahamas, West Indies and Bermuda. The fruit is a greyish-white, round drupe-like nut covered with a waxy crust. The medicinal properties of bayberry bark are similar to those of wild Oregon grape root or barberry (*Berberis vulgaris*).

Baycovin. Trade name for diethyl pyrocarbonate.

B-complex. A group of growth-promoting compounds produced by living cells. Each member of B-complex is essential, and no member can be substituted for any other member. Their physiological effect is additive, throughout each is a distinct compound which has specific functions in metabolism. The complex may be thought of as a role, each strand of which is represented by an individual and unique substance. The complex occurs in all the cells of all organisms, both plant and animal, and among its components are thiamine; riboflavin, niacin, biotin, pyridoxine, folic acid, and cyanocobalamin.

Bdellovibrio. The small vibroid organisms having the unusual property of preying on other bacteria, using as nutrients the cytoplasmic constituents of their hosts. Phylogenetically, Bdellovibrio fall into the delta group of purple bacteria. These bacterial predators are small, motile cells, which stick to the surface of their prey cells. Because of the latter property, they have been given the name Bdellovibrio. A wide variety of Gram-negative bacteria can be attacked by a single Bdellovibrio, but the Gram-positive cells are not attacked.

Bdellovibrio obtain its energy from the oxidation of amino acids and acetate (*via* citric acid cycle). It apparently is unable to utilize sugars as electron donors.

bean drying. Edible beans, such as pea, yellow eye, kidney, pinto, great northern, and lima beans or soybeans, are often harvested when too wet (above 18% moisture) to store, so must be dried. Drying is done with forced air or heated air. If dried too slowly, spoilage may occur. If dried too rapidly, the seed coat and bean may crack and/or split, reducing the market quality. Continuous heated air drying can be done at 36°C or less. Cracking is prevalent when more than 3-4% moisture is removed rapidly. Following at 4-6 hours holding period, drying may be continued. Beans handled by conventional means when cold, below 1.7°C, or too dry (less than 12% moisture) may cause intensive damage.

beans, baked. Usually mature haricot beans *phaseolus vulgaris*; cooked by autoclaving.

beans, broad. *Vicia faba.* The edible beans of average composition after cooking, whole beans without pod: water 84%; protein 4-5%; carbohydrate 6.8%; food energy 175 kJ; Fe 1 mg; nicotinic acid 3 mg; and vitamin C 15 mg. Also known as horse bean.

beans, butter. *Phaseolus lunatus.* A variety of edible beans. The average composition of this kind of beans per 100 g, after cooking, is: water 70%; protein 7%; carbohydrates 17-18%; food energy 390 kJ; Fe 1.6 mg. Also known as lima beans, curry beans, Madagascar beans and sugar beans.

beans, French. *Phaseolus vulgaris.* A variety of beans eaten unripe in the pod. The average composition per 100 g is: water 95%; protein 0.9%; carbo-

hydrates 1.2%; food energy 30 kJ, Fe 0.6 mg; carotene 800 i.u., and vitamin C 5 mg.

beans, haricot. Ripe seeds of *Phaseolus vulgaris* (unripe seed is the French bean). The average composition per 100 g of the cooked beans is: water 70%; protein 6.5%; carbohydrates 16.7%; food energy 370 kJ, Ca 66 mg; and Fe 2.6 mg. Also known as Navy beans; pinto beans; snap beans.

beans, runner. *Phaseolus multiflorus.* A variety of beans eaten unripe with pod. The average composition per 100 g after cooking is: water 93.5%; protein 0.8%; carbohydrates 0.99%; food energy 30 kJ; carotene 500 i.u., nicotinic acid 0.5 mg; and vitamin C 4-5 mg.

beans. A general term having several meanings in food science:
(a) the seed of certain plants or, in numerous cases, the pod and the seeds;
(b) a plant, commonly leguminous, that bears seed pods which generally are called beans when they are marketed;
(c) food substances that may have the shape of a bean.

This term is concerned here with bean plants and their edible parts. Most commercially important beans are of the family Leguminosea (pea family) and, like the other members of this very large family, have the distinct advantage of obtaining nitrogen from the air and transferring the nitrogen to the soil, thus enriching the soil. This is an advantage not only because of the soil-nitrogen restorative powers, but also because bean plants will produce nutritious food substances from soils where many other plants do not prosper well without extensive nitrogen feeding.

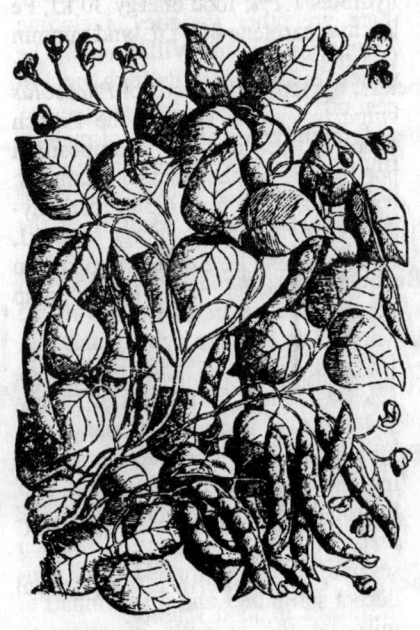

Several kinds of bean plants are used as forage for livestock. Beans of various genera, types, and varieties are closely related to peas. There is no sharp demarcation in the use of the words bean and pea. In some countries, certain kinds of beans may be called peas and vice-versa. The majority of plants and their pods and seeds that are classified as beans are of the genus Phaseolus, and those called peas are of the genus Pisum, but this is not an exclusive differentiation. A wide variety of leguminous seeds are rich in protein (20-30%) and moderate sources of iron (2-10 mg per 100 g) and of vitamins B_1, B_2 and nicotinic acid. When soaked in water and allowed to germinate they become a good source of vitamin C. Many beans have different names in different countries, e.g., Lima bean (US), butter bean (UK), curry bean, Madagascar bean, sugar bean (*Phaseolus lunatus*). Navy, pinto, or snap bean (US), haricot (UK), kidney, French- the pods sometimes called string beans (*Phaseolus vulgaris*). Broad bean, horse bean (*Vicia faba*). Scarlet runner bean (*Phaseolus multiflorus*). Mung bean, black gram, woolly pyrol (*Phaseolus mungo*). Field bean, hyacinth bean, Egyptian kidney bean, tonga bean (*Dolichos lablab*). The different types of beans used commonly as food iinclude:

Black beans. These are small, oval beans with a tender texture and a mushroom-flavoured, somewhat earthy taste to them.

Black-eyed peas. These oval, medium sized beans have a nutty crunchiness to them and posses a fine-flavoured taste reminiscent of a meatless vegetable stew.

Chick-peas. These round beans have a distinctive nutty flavour and chewy fieriness to them.

Fava beans. Such beans are large, flat and oval with a firm texture and a dainty taste. They are very popular in Europe, especially in UK.

Kidney beans (Dark Red, Light Red and White). All three colours of beans are oval-shaped with a somewhat soft, bland taste to them. The dark red ones are mostly sold in cans and used in salads, while the light red are sold dry and made into chilli, refried beans and Creole dishes.

Lentils. These small, disk-shaped beans disk-shaped beans have a subtle mildness characterized with a distinctive flavour and rather firm texture.

Lima beans. These large, white oval beans date from 7000-5000 BC in Peru and yield a mild taste and a soft texture when cooked. Quite often, though, they are dried, canned and marketed under the names of wax or butter beans. Three principal types are:

(a) large lima bean (large and flat);
(b) Dreer lima bean, the seeds of which are smaller than the large lima, rounded, and rather closely crowded in the pod. Along with the sieva bean, the Dreer lima bean is sometimes referred to as a dwarf lima bean or dwarf butter bean.
(c) Small lima or sieve bean (Phaseolus lunatus), described later in this list. The plant is quite widely used as forage for livestock.

Mung beans. They are highly esteemed for their tiny seeds, which becomes rather sticky on cooking, but are accounted both wholesome and nourishing. These are dried and boiled whole or split, or else parched and ground into flour. In China they are added to green noodles and used for bean sprouts, a use to which they are also put here in America. Also known as green or golden gram in India.

Navy, white and great northern beans. All three of them are firm, mild beans in varying sizes, ranging from small to medium and large.

Pinto beans. These are small, oval beans with a mild flavour and texture to them.

Split and Whole peas (Yellow and Green). Both varieties are small and possess a soft, grainy texture marked with a certain distinctive flavour.

Soybeans (*Glycine* or *Soja max*). These firm, round, bland-tasting beans are not of the genus *Phaseolus* as the others happen to be.

Bearss lemon. A variety of lemon which is categorized as Sicilian type and considered to be within the Lisbon group. In Europe and US, the Bearss is one of the most widely grown variety of this category, although there are other varieties, including Avon, Harney, and Villafranco. The variety is known for its high yield of peel oil.

beauty mandarin. A variety of mandarin; a Dancy-type mandarin believed to have originated in Australia (near Brisbane) as nuclear seedling of the Dancy.

Beche-de-mer. *Stichopus japonicus.* An occasional food in most parts of the world. The average composition per 100 g is: protein 22%; carbohydrates 1%; Ca 120 mg; Fe 1.4%; food energy 394 kJ. Also known as trepang.

Bedouin test. A colour reaction involving the addition of cane sugar and hydrochloric acid to a fat. The test is used to detect sesame oil. When sesame oil cakes are fed, they produce a soft butter and often impart to milk fat the property of giving a Baudouin oil test.

beech family. *Fragaceae.* A nut fruit partially enclosed in basal bracts (acorn, beech nut, chestnut) is the most familiar characteristic of this family of 6 genera, which are deciduous or ever-green trees and shrubs. The simple leaves have lobed, toothed, or entire margins and deciduous stipules. The flower are usually unisexual and wind-pollinated. The male flower occurs in catkins or singly and has 4-7 sepals, 4-40 stamens and a vestigial pistil. The female flower can be single in a cup of bracts or in a cluster of 2-3 flower, which may have bracts. Fused sepals of the female flower have 4-6 lobes. The pistil has an inferior ovary of 3-6 carpels, chambers, and styles. Two ovules in axil placentation develop in each chamber, where one develops and the other aborts. The family include: *Castanea* spp. (chestnuts), *Fagus* spp. (beeches), *Quercus* spp. (oaks; in the US, oaks are the second most important source of lumber after conifers); *Castanea* spp. (chestnuts), *Lithocarpus* (tanoak), *Quercus* spp. (oaks); *Castanea dentata* (American chestnut).

bee wine. A kind of wine produced by the usual alcoholic fermentation of sugar, but using yeast in the form of a clump of yeast and lactic bacteria. The clumb rises and falls with bubbles of carbon dioxide produced, hence the "bee".

beef fats. A product obtained from edible fatty tissues of cattle. Its physical properties are variable and depend on the feeding history and genetic constitution of the cattle from which the fat is taken. It is normally a hard plastic fat having a melting point of about 40-45°C. Because of its hardness, it may be subjected to further processing rather than used in its native form. Beef fats rendered by special methods can be separated by fractional crystallization into oleo oil (the low melting fractions) and oleostearin (the high melting fractions). Its short plastic range and relatively low melting range make oleo oil a fair substitute for coconut oil in some applications. Minimally refined beef fats retain a slight meaty flavor that has been found valuable in, for example, French frying potatoes.

beef tea. An extract of stewing beef prepared by stammering for 2-3 hours.

beef, carcass. Prime grade beef carcasses and wholesale cuts are blocky and compact and very thickly fleshed throughout. Loins and ribs are thick and full. The rounds are plump and the plumpness extends well down towards the hocks. The protrusion of well down toward the hocks. The protrusion of fat between the chine bones is liberal and the overflow of fat over the inside of the ribs is abundant and fairly evenly distributed. It has abundant marbling and the marbling is extensive especially in the heavier carcasses. Carcasses must also be symmetrical and uniform in contour and the rib eye muscle must be fine in texture. A carcass must have certain evidences of quality to be eligible for the Prime grade. Slightly abundant marbling must be evident in the rib eye muscle of carcasses with soft, red chine bones terminating in soft pearly white cartilage. Progressively more marbling is required in carcasses with evidences of more advanced maturity. Only beef produced from steers and heifers will quality for the Prime grade. Choice grade beef carcasses and wholesale cuts are moderately blocky and compact and moderately thick-fleshed throughout. Loins and ribs are moderately thick and full and the rounds are moderately plump. The fat covering of beef within the grade will vary within moderate limits depending on evidences of the maturity attained by the animal from which it was produced. Interior and exterior fats are fairly firm and brittle. In carcasses whose chine bones are tinged with white and which terminate in cartilage in which some ossification is evident, the rib eye has moderately abundant marbling and is usually moderately firm and fine in texture. The colour of the muscle usually ranges from a light red to slightly dark red. It is usually uniform and bright in colour but any be slightly two-toned or slightly shady. Carcasses showing evidences of maximum maturity permitted in the Choice grade have chine bones which are tinged with white and cartilage on the end of the chine bones which are partially ossified. However, the carcasses must also be at least moderately symmetrical and uniform in contour and the rib eye muscle must be fine in texture. The minimum marbling permitted will vary from a small amount in very red-boned, lightweight carcasses to a moderate amount in carcasses approaching the maximum maturity permitted.

Carcasses which are slightly compact and blocky and with slightly pump rounds and slightly thick fleshing may meet the minimum requirements for the grade provided they have finish and evidences of quality equivalent to the midpoint of the Choice grade. Beef produced from steers, heifers, and young cows may qualify for the Choice grade. Good grade beef carcasses and wholesale cuts are slightly compact and blocky in conformation and the fleshing tends to be slightly thick throughout. Loins and ribs are slightly full and the rounds are only slightly pump. Chucks are slightly thick and full and the neck and fore shanks tend to be slightly long and thin. The fat may be somewhat soft or slightly oily. Characteristic of the cut surface of the rib eye muscle will vary depending on evidences of maturity attained by the animal from which it was produced. Carcasses showing evidence of maximum maturity permitted in the Good grade may have chine bones tinged with white and the cartilage on the end of the chine bones may be moderately ossified.

Carcasses must also be at least moderately symmetrical and uniform in contour and the rib eye muscle must be at least moderately fine in texture. Beef qualifying for the Commercial grade is quite variable in conformation, finish, and quality and

in the evidences of maturity attained by the animal from which it was produced. Young, red-boned carcasses are ragy, angular, and slightly thin-fleshed throughout. Loins and ribs tend to be flat and are slightly thin-fleshed. The fat is moderately soft or oily. Carcasses from mature animals with conformation and evidences of quality which only slightly exceed the minimum requirements of the grade are not eligible for the Commercial grade if they are excessively patchy or uneven in distribution of external fat.

beef. The composition of beef varies with the breed of the animal and amount of fat present; usually classified as fat, medium and lean with following average composition per 100 g:

Fat: 22 g fat; 14.2 g protein; food energy 1.1 MJ; 1.7 mg iron; 1.2 mg vitamin A; 0.05 mg vitamin B_1; 0.13 mg vitamin B_2; and 3 mg nicotinic acid.

·*Medium:* 17 g fat; 14.9 g protein; food energy 0.9 MJ; 1.8 mg iron; 9 mg vitamin A; 0.05 mg vitamin B_1; 0.13 mg vitamin B_2; and 3.1 mg nicotinic acid.

Lean: 10 g fat; 1.54 g protein; food energy 0.66 MJ; 1.8 mg iron; 6 mg vitamin A; 0.05 mg vitamin B_1; 0.14 mg vitamin B_2; and 3.2 mg nicotinic acid.

beer. Alcoholic beverage produced be fermentation of cereals. Beer is an ale beverage made by fermentation of farinaceous extract which is obtained from the carbohydrate-rich material, barley (used in the form of malt). Barley differs from the other common cereals in that, the husk adheres to the kernel of the threshing as it does in spelt. It renders the process of malting and subsequent extraction of the fermentable products much easier than with wheat or other grains. Beer can be broadly classified into two categories:

Lager Beer: These beers are so named because they are stored or lagered after fermentation in cold store houses for clarification and flavour purposes. They are also called 'bottom fermented' beers because the yeast settles to the bottom during fermentation and is removed by sedimentation. It is rich in extract and aged after fermentation.

Ales: These are 'top fermented' beers wherein the yeast floats to the top during fermentation and is removed either by skimming or suction. The first step in manufacture is malting of the barley. It is allowed to sprout when the enzyme amylase develops and hydrolyses the starch to dextrins and maltose. The sprouted barley is dried and extracted with hot water (the process is called mashing) to produce wort. After the addition of hops for flavour the wort is allowed to ferment. Ale is a light-coloured beer made by top fermentation and containing more alcohol and hops. Porter is made from partially charred malt and is darker in colour; it is also a top fermentation. Stout is similar to porter but contains more extract and a higher alcohol content. Most beers, ale and stout contain 3-7% alcohol and 30-60 kcal of food energy per 100 ml of the beer.

Beerenauslese. Trade name for a very high quality, rare, costly, somewhat sweet German white wine produced only in the good or best seasons. The grape berries are individually selected and picked only when they are over-ripe. Some authorities consider these wines among the most remarkable of the world's white wines. The white Riesling or Sylvander (Silvaner) grape is used for making this wine.

beet (red) drying. Red beets are used for coloring, flavoring, and food. Beets are sliced, diced, or cut into strips prior to drying. Beets are dried to 5% moisture content, or below, often in two steps. Blanched diced beets are dried at 93.3°C on conveyor or in tunnel dryers with final drying which may take place in a bin dryer.

beet powder. Beet or red beet (*Beta vulgaris* L.) contains up to 0.15 % water-soluble colouring principals known as betalains. These comprise the red betacyanins and the yellow betaxanthins. The major betacyanin of red beet is betanine, which accounts for 75-95 % of the total betacyanins present and far exceeds the betaxanthins present. The natural colorants derived from red beets are readily available commercially and are comprised of concentrated syrupy liquid beet juice (40-60% total solids and 0.5-1% betanine) or spray-dried powder (40% betanine or diluted to a stated figure). Many of these products contain ascorbic acid as a colour stabilizer and may also contain a permitted preservative whose nature must be stated in the specification. In view of the diversity of the products available, reference should be made to the manufacturer for advice on colouring power and use levels. The colour of betanine is not affected by *p*H within the range 3-7, but in alkaline media above *p*H 7 the colour intensity is reduced and the hue changes from red to violet. The colour is relatively heat-stable.

beet pulp drying. Beet pulp is the wet material leaving the diffusers following the removal of sugar from sugar beets. The beet pulp is dewatered in a press. It may be fed, stored, or processed. One process of preparing an animal feed consists of mixing the pulp with molasses followed by drying.

beet sugar. Sucrose extracted from the

sugar beet. It is identical with sucrose extracted from any other source.

beet, common red. Root of *Beta vulgaris*.

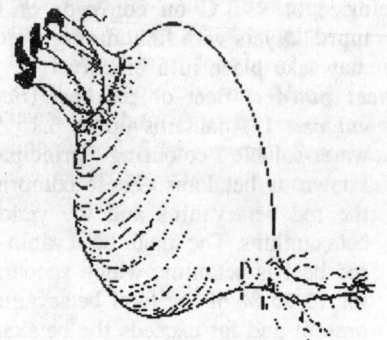

The average composition per 100 g of the boiled beet is: water 83%; protein 1.8%; carbohydrate 10%; food energy 185 kJ; Fe 0.7 mg; Ca 30 mg; vitamin A traces, vitamin B_1 0.02 mg; vitamin B_2 0.04 mg; nicotinic acid 0.06 mg; and vitamin C 5.2 mg. Edible beet roots are related to the sugar beets (*Beta vulgaris saccharifera*), grown for the making of sugar, the extraction of which began in the 18th century. The edible roots of beets are of two basic colours, red and yellow. The English pioneered the red variety, but elsewhere in Europe the yellow-rooted kind was once much preferred because of its sweeter taste and greater suitability for pickling. There is also a white-rooted beet which is cultivated chiefly for its leaves and stalks. The tops are used in place of spinach and the ribs are like asparagus in some ways. In the Middle Ages, no meal was considered complete without a soup made from the leaves of this Swiss chard, as it is often called.

beeturia. Red pigmented urine after eating beet-root; occurs only in one person in eight and not consistently.

The colour is due to the presence of pigment betanin.

Beggiatoa. The organisms of this genus are morphologically similar to filamentous cyanobacteria. The filaments of *Beggiatoa* are usually quite large in diameter and long, consisting of many short cells attached end-to-end. In addition to movement by gliding, that can flex and twist so that many filaments may become interwined to form a complex tuft. *Beggiatoa* is found in nature primarily in habitats rich in hydrogen sulphide, such as sulphur springs, decaying seaweed beds, mud layers of lakes, and waters polluted with sewage. In these habitats the filaments of *Beggitoa* are usually filled with sulphur granules. An interesting habitat of *Beggitoa* is the rhizosphere of plants (rice, cattails, and other swamp plants) living in flooded, and hence anaerobic soils. Such plants pump oxygen down into their roots, so that a sharply defined boundary develops at the root surface between oxygen on the root and hydrogen sulphide in the soil. *Beggitoa* (and probably other sulphur bacteria) develop at this boundary, and it has been suggested that *Beggitoa* plays a beneficial role for the plant by oxidizing and thus detoxifying hydrogen sulphide. It has been suggested that the plant promotes the growth of Beggitoa in its rhizosphere via catalase production, thus leading to the development of mutualistic relationship between plant and the bacterium.

bel paese cheese. A popular uncooked soft, sweet, fast-ripened Italian table cheese. About 0.25% starter is added to milk at 38-40° C. Rennet is added and the coagulated curd is cut in cubes. After firming, the whey is removed and the cheese is placed in hoops.

Beledi orange. A variety of sweet, nonbloody, seedy orange having thin skin. It grows throughout Mediterranean region including Egypt, Greece (Koines), Iran, Iraq (Mohali), Italy (Biondo Comune), Lebanon (Mawardi Beledi), Spain (Comuna), and Syria. In Italy, this variety accounts for about one-third of the country's orange production. In Lebanon, the Mawardi Beledi is native and is sometimes grown from seedlings.

Belgian cooked cheese. A variety of cheese. The skim milk is curdled and the curd is heated to 60-65° C, placed in a cloth, and allowed to drain. When dry it is thoroughly kneaded and allowed to ferment. This takes from 6-8 days in summer and about 10-14 days in winter. When the fermentation is complete, salt and cream are added, and the mixture is slowly heated and stirred until it is homogenous. It is then put into molds and allowed to ripen 8 days. Lager is made by bottom fermentation, is low in alcohol content, rich in extract and aged after fermentation.

Belladonna orange. A variety of sweet orange, (of nonblood colour), having very few or no seeds; matures in early midseason. The fruit is of medium-size, oblong to oval in shape at maturity. The fruit holds well on tree after maturing. It is produced in Italy for many years, and is of unknown origin, and ranks second only to Ovale Calabrese in Italian orange production.

Bellelay cheese. A soft variety of rennet cheese made from sweet, whole milk. It originated with the monks in the Canton of Bern, Switzerland. The milk is set at 35°C with rennet enough to coagulate it in 20-30 minutes. The curd is cut rather fine and is stirred while being heated slowly to a temperature of 40°C, being cooked much firmer than Limburger cheese but not so firm as Emmentaler. When cooked the curd is dipped into wooden hoops lined with cloth. After being pressed, the cheeses are wrapped in bark for two weeks and are cured in a cool, moist cellar, as eyes should not develop. It takes about a year to ripen and will keep well for 3 to 4 years. It is soft and buttery and may be used as cheese spread. Also known as Monk's head; Tete de Moine.

belt dryer. A unit used in food processing for continuously drying granular, aggregated, lump, pelleted, and similar products on a belt passing through a moving heated air stream. The product usually does not exceed 10 cm depth. The belt may be an open mesh type, such that air will pass through while retaining the product. The unit may be provided with a heating section, primarily for drying, and a cooling section in which temperature of product is reduced and additional drying takes place. The unit may operate under vacuum or atmospheric conditions. Examples of products dried on belt dryers are fruits and vegetables, particularly apples, beets, carrots, onions, and potatoes.

belt-trough dryer. A type of continuous dryer used in the food processing in which the granular material being dried flows through the unit on a slowly overturning bed in the path of heated air forced through the bed.

Bemax. Trade name of a wheat germ preparation. The average composition per 100 g is:, protein 27.8%; fat 9.3%; carbohydrates 44.5%; Ca 55 mg; Fe 7.8 mg; food energy 1.55 MJ; vitamin B_1 1.6 mg; vitamin B_2 0.7 mg; and nicotinic acid 6.8 mg.

Bence-Jones protein. An abnormal immunoglobulin that consists only of light chains, generally in the form of dimers, and that is produced by individuals suffering from plasma cell tumors. Each complete immunoglobulin is made up of two pairs of polypeptide chains; a pair of light (short) and a pair of heavy (long) chains. The Bence-Jones protein is identical to the light chain of immunoglobulin. All light chains are divided in to a region of variable amino acid sequence and a region of constant sequence. The variable region occupies the $-NH_2$ terminal half of the light chain (about 110 amino acid residues) and the constant sequence region occupies the half, and is essentially identical in all human light chains. Heavy chains are also divided in to VH regions and CH regions. The VH region is smaller in size to the light chains, but the CH region is about three times as long. Bence-Jones protein has unusual thermostability properties.

Benson model. The model of a biological membrane according to which the proteins are largely globular and are located in the interior of the membrane, and the lipids are intercalated into the folds of the protein chains, with the polar portions of the lipid molecules at the exterior surfaces of the membrane.

benzoic acid. C_6H_5COOH. An aromatic carboxylic acid prepared by the oxidation of toluene. The free acid and the sodium and potassium salts are effective preservatives, but in UK, its use is permitted only in limited foodstuffs such as coffee extracts, pickles, sauces and soft drinks. It has antimicrobial activity, especially in acid solution (little effective at pH above 5), and is almost half as effective as sulphur dioxide. Its permitted level in concentrated soft drinks is 600 mg/L. One view is that benzoic acid appears to be harmless as it is excreted in the urine in combination with glycine as hippuric acid; up to 4 g per day can be consumed and excreted in this way. Esters of the acid are more potent preservatives than the salts.

bergamot. *Monarda didyma.* The plant has a pleasant smell of oranges and, with its red, pinky-red, or purple flowers, is an attractive addition to any border. It is strongly attractive to bees. Besides the most common red bergamot, there is wild bergamot (*M. fistulosa*), and lemon bergamot (*M. citriodora*), which too, has a strong citrus aroma. Fresh leaves may be used sparingly in salads, fruit salad, and fruit drinks, and fresh or dried leaves made into a refreshing and relaxing tea that is said to be soporific. The dried leaves impart a pleasantly citrus aroma to pot pouri blends; and used for extraction of the peel oil for perfumery.

bergamot orange. A variety of sour orange grown principally for its rind oil. It is considered to be sour orange hybrid. Its main variety is Castagnaro whose production is limited to Province of Calabria in Italy. Bergamot oil is used as base of cologne water and other perfumery. In Calabria, sometimes the peel of the fruit is separated from the flesh to form 2 half-spheres. These are allowed to dry on a mold. After drying, the 2 halves make up the vase and lid of small boxes for jewel cases, delicately scented and sometimes grace with antwork. In Turkey, Bergamot fruit and/or the rind is processed into a jam.

Bergkase cheese. The name given to Alpine cheese of the Swiss type. This may include: Battlematt, Piora, Gruyere,

Fontina, Walliser and Vacherin.

Bergquara cheese. A kind of Swedish cheese resembling Gouda.

Berna lemon. A variety of lemon. It is estimated that about 90% of lemon trees grown in Spain's Murcia region consists of the mid season Berna variety. The fruit closely resembles the Lisbon lemon planted in California. The lemon trees in Murcia are heavily pruned and are described by some authorities as very precocious. Fruits of the early blooming (early March). They are distinguished by very smooth skins and locally are called Mesero.

Bernarde cheese. An Italian cheese prepared mainly from cow's milk, which is coloured with saffron. The cheese is dry, salted and is cured for about 2 months.

berries, golden. The berries of the Cape Gooseberry or Chinese Lantern, (*Physalis peruviana*). The average composition per 100 g is: water 85%; fat 0.5%; protein 2%; fibre 2.8%; carbohydrates 10%; food energy 0.2 MJ; Fe 1.5 mg; vitamin A 600 μg; vitamin B_1 0.1 mg; vitamin B_2 0.04 mg; nicotinic acid 2.7 mg; and vitamin C 28 mg.

berries. Botanical name for fruits in which seeds are embedded in pulpy tissue, e.g., strawberry, currant, tomato. The selected varieties of berries known for both their nutritional as well as medicinal values include:

Blackberry. *Rubus villousu.* They are known by their deep purple-black fruits.

Boysenberry. *Rubus* species. A huge blackberry-like fruit with a raspberry-like flavour.

Cranberry. *Vaccinium macrocarpum.* A low, creeping shrub common to boggy areas. It is distinguished by its bright red berry. Most commonly used around holidays like Thanksgiving and Christmas.

Currants (black, red). *Ribes nigrum, R. rubrum.* Small red, black and even white berries closely related to gooseberries, which a tart flavour.

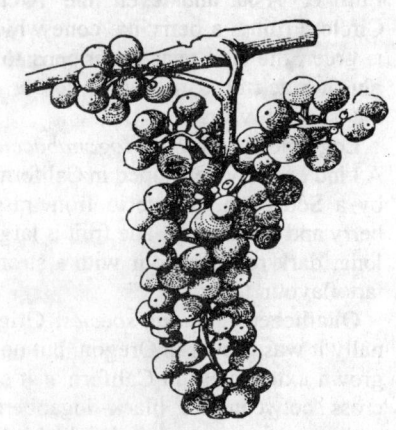

Dewberries. *Rubus canadensis.* Part of the blackberry family and regarded as one of the tastiest of the entire *Rubis* species. The hybrid youngberry was developed from it.

Elderberry (sweet, black, red). *Sambucus canadensis, S. nigrum, S. racemosa.* A small shrub or tree yielding red-brown to shiny black berries.

Gooseberry (Garden). *Ribes grossularia.* The small fruit looks like a little green basketball with a stem because its skin has striated lines that appear to divide the berry into uneven sections.

Hawthorn berry. *Crataegus oxyacantha.* Many species of Hawthorn berry are found around the world. Some are tastier than others. Berries can be red, purple or nearly black, depending on the species, and are found on either trees or large bushes.

Huckleberry. *Vaccinium myrtillus.* It is almost same as the blueberry, only more noted for its medicinal uses. Fruit can be either blue-black or red. Both kinds of blueberries are more closely related to the cranberry.

Juniper berry. *Juniperus connumis.* An evergreen shrub found in dry, rocky soil throughout North America, Europe, Asia and even the Arctic Circle. Fruit is a berrylike cone which is green the first year and ripens to a bluish-black or dark purple colour in the second year.

Loganberry. *Rubus loganobaccus.* A kind of berry developed in California by a Scotsman. A hybrid from raspberry and blackberry. The fruit is large, long, dark red in colour with a strong tart flavour to it.

Ollallieberry. *Rubus species.* Originally it was grown in Oregon, but now grown extensively in California; it's a cross between the black loganberry and youngberry, and is bright black, medium size, firm and sweeter than loganberry is.

Mulberry. *Morus alba, M. rubra, M. microphila.* The white mulberry occurs throughout New England, the red in the Appalachias and the Texas variety, with many hybrids as well. Tart, but juicy and tasty.

Rose hips. *Rosa species.* Over 100 kinds of Rosa hips are found in the world. Fruit resembles a berry, but is actually a ripened hypanthium (an enlargement of the torus below the calyx). Noted for its strong vitamin C content.

Salmonberry. *Rubus spetabilis.* Its name comes from its yellow colour. Common to the north-western U.S. Has a strong, sour taste. Better cooked than raw.

Strawberry (cultivated, wild). *Frangaria ananassa, F. vesca.*

Thimbleberry. *Rubus paraviforus* or *R. nutkanus.* It is common throughout the Pacific Northwest, its raspberry-red berries are shaped like a thimble, hence the name. It has an especially soft texture like juicy velvet that almost seems to literally melt in your mouth.

See also bilberry; raspberry.

berseem clover. *Trifolium alexandrinum.* A variety of clover that looks something like alfalfa. However, in the Mediterranean region, including the Nile Valley of Egypt, berseem clover is the main forage crop. It does well in many regions that are humid and frost-free. Of all true clovers, berseem is least tolerant to cool temperatures.

betaine. Trimethyl glycine. Occurs in beet-root and cottonseed; also known as lysine and oxyneuine (obsolete names). Related to choline; possesses labile methyl groups.

betel. Leaf of the creeper *Piper betel* or *betle,* which is chewed in some parts of the world for its stimulating effect (due to the presence of the alkaloids arecoline and guvacoline).

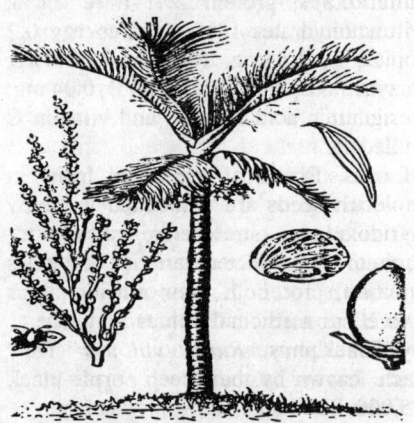

The leaves are chewed with nuts of the areca palm, *Areca catechu,* which is therefore often called the betel palm and the nut is called the betel nut.

bezoar. A hard ball of undigested food that forms in the stomach and is capable of causing intestinal obstruction. Foods with a high content of indigestible pectin such as orange pith can form bezoars if swallowed without chewing.

Bgug-cheese. A variety of Armenian cheese prepared from sheep's milk, partly or entirely skimmed. Rennet is used to coagulate the milk, the curd drained, after which it is broken up and salt and herbs added. After being pressed again, the cheese is put into a salt bath for at least two days. Also known as Daralag cheese.

biffins. Apples that have been peeled, partly baked, then pressed and dried.

bifidus factor. Name given to factor present in human milk, now known to be lactulose, that stimulates growth of *Lactobacillus bifidus* and makes faeces of breast-fed infants slightly more acid than those of babies fed on cow's milk.

bifunctional oligomeric enzymes. The bifunctional enzymes such as tryptophan synthetase of *E. coli*. This enzyme consists of two proteins designated A and B. Protein A has a molecular mass of 29,500 and consists of one subunit, a. Protein B has a molecular mass of 90,000 and has two pyridoxal phosphate binding sites per mole of B. In the presence of 4M urea solution, protein B dissociates in to two b subunits, each containing one pyridoxal phosphate binding site and each having a molecular mass of 45,000. The complete tryptophan synthetase consists of two A proteins and one B protein designated as a_2b_2. The association of the subunits to form fully active and associated synthetase is greatly increased by the presence of both pyridoxal phosphate and the substrate L-serine.

bigflower clover. *Trifolium michelianum.* A variety of clover probably native to Turkey. Generally, bigflower clover resembles Alsike clover. The plant is adapted for both pasture and hay in many parts of the world.

bilberry. Berry of shrub of the species *Vaccinium,* which is not cultivated but grows wild. The average composition per 100 g of bilberry is: water 76.5-88%; protein 0.7%; free acids 1.1-1.7%; sugar 3.8-6.9; pentosans, etc., 0.5-1.5%; fibre 3.7-12%; ash 0.3-1.0%. Also known as whortleberry; blaeberry (Iceland) windberry; huckleberry

bile acids. The acids (or their sodium or potassium salts) that are present in bile and play an important role in fat digestion in the small intestine. They are based on cholic acid and chenodeoxycholic (chenic) acid, which are synthesized in the liver from cholesterol and are conjugated with glycine or taurine to form bile acids, that is, glycocholic, taurocholic, glycochenic, and taurochenic acids. These conjugated forms are less susceptible to precipitation and more slowly absorbed from the proximal small intestine. Thus increasing their effectiveness. A high proportion of both forms in reabsorbed and recycled to the liver for resecretion in the bile. The bile acids are effective emulsifying agents and assist stabilization of fats. The conjugated acids also reduce the pH optimum of pancreatic lipase thereby rendering it more effective in the small intestine, where it acts to hydrolyze fats. Bile acids form multimolecular aggregates (micelles) with the monoglycerides and fatty acids, thereby maintaining them in a soluble form and accelerating their diffusion towards the intestinal mucosa. The micelles split up at the intestinal surface and fatty acids and bile acids are absorbed separately.

bile pigments. A mixture of pigments bilirubin and biliverdin, which are present in bile and and impart yellow, green, or brown colour to it, depending on their relative proportions; they are excretory products of degradation of haemoglobin and other haem-containing proteins. When haemoglobin is destroyed in the body the protein portion, globin, is degraded to amino acids, while the porphyrin or haem portion gives rise to the bile pigments. The green pigments biliverdin is the first of the bile pigments; it is easily reduced to the red-brown pigment bilirubin. Bilirubin is the major pigments in human bile, there being only slight traces of biliverdin, which is the chief pigment in the bile of birds. A specific enzyme, biliverdin reductase, catalyzes the reduction of biliverdin to bilirubin. The formation of biliverdin and bilirubin from haem takes place in reticuloendothelial cells of the liver, spleen, and bone marrow. The pigments are then transported to the liver where they are excreted in bile into the duodenum. In the intestine, bilirubin undergoes further chemical modification and is secreted in the faeces.

bilin. A coloured bile pigment, such as urobilin or stercobilin, formed by the oxidation of bilinogen pigment.

bilirubin. One of the bile pigments; formed by the degradation of haemoglobin. Since haemoglobin is the most abundant haem-containing protein, most bilirubin results from the normal process of erythrocyte destruction. In the normal physiology of the body, bilirubin is absorbed by the liver form circulation and excreted into the bile; its clinical accumulation in tissues and plasma results in the yellow colour of jaundice.

biliverdin. One of the bile pigments; formed during the degradation of haemoglobin.

Biltong. Popular name given to the dried meat strips in South Africa. The meat is cut in 5 cm strips, 60-90 cm long, along the muscle fibres, which are salted, spiced and dried in air for 10-15 days. The average composition per 100 g of Biltong is: 11.6 g water; 1.8 g fat; 12.5 g ash; 66 g protein; and 1.3 MJ food energy.

bin drying. A procedure commonly used to complete the dehydration or drying of vegetables, nuts, grain, or forage by holding a batch in a deep bin or container with slow movement of heated or unheated air.

binning. A term used to describe laying away bottled wine for aging. Always with table and sparkling wines, the bottle should be stored on their side so that the wine is in constant contact with the cork. The wine should be stored at cool temperature. The relationship of size with time of aging also applies to final container sizes. A half-bottle will be ready earlier than a full bottle. Because of the adverse affects of light upon aging, the coloured bottles (brown or green) are used. It has been claimed that about three-fourths of the wines produced is as good when about 2 years old as it is likely to be and deterioration is likely to start after 3 years. the avrieties of wine recommended for consumption within 3-5 years include: Vin Rose (California, France, etc.); most prepared from Chardonnay, Chenin Blanc, Pinot Blanc, Sauvignon Blanc, and Johannesberg Riesling; most white Burgundies, with exception of those from the excellent vineyards in good vintage years; nearly all Italian wines, except a few selected red wines.

bioassay approach. Analytical method used to determine the measure of biomass in a certain water environment. A sample of water is filtered through fibres, and inoculated with a culture to test algae. Subsequently the inoculated sample is incubated for about ten days. The amount of growth during that period is a measure of the biomass in test region from which the sample were obtained.

bioassay. Determination of the potency and activity of drugs of derivatively, the amount of active ingredient they contain, by observing their effect upon animals. Also known as biological assay.

biochemical oxygen demand. See biological oxygen demand.

biocytin. One of the bound forms of biotin that occurs naturally, the lysine derivative; not fully utilized by all organisms until it has been hydrolyzed to free biotin.

biodegradability. The susceptibility of an organic material to decomposition as a result of attack by microorganisms. The term is applied especially to detergents and insecticides, which vary widely in this respect. For ecological reasons, a high degree of biodegradation is desirable to minimize the adverse environmental effect of such materials. The process of decay or decomposition of organic matter accomplished by bacteria or by secretions and chemicals involving these bacteria, fungi and other microorganisms. Any organic matter that can be broken down by bacteria is called biodegradable matter because it undergoes biodegradation, an abbreviated description of biological degradation. Biodegradable materials such as plastic bags have been developed to reduce the solid waste disposal problem.

bioflavonoids. Alternative name for flavonoids.

biologic transmission. A type of vector-borne transmission in which an infectious organism goes through some morphological or physiological change within the vector.

biological control. The use of one or more organism (such as bacterium) to control the growth of another organism (such as insect). It has been found that some microorganisms can interact with plants in highly beneficial ways and even act as insecticides in certain cases. For example, the leaf-inhibiting bacterium *Pseudomonas syringae* produces a protein that brings about the formation of ice crystals on the leaves of plants at temperatures higher than would otherwise be case, leading to premature frost damage. Because of great agricultural significance of frost damage, it is desirable to prevent this frost-inducing action of *P. syringae*. A number of bacilli, most notably *B. larvae*, *B. popillae*, and *B. thringiensis*, function as biological control agents by serving as insect larvicides.

biological degradation. The biochemical process of the breakdown of complex, large organic molecules into small, simple molecules. See biodegradability.

biological oxygen demand. BOD. Microorganisms consume oxygen for their respiration and the uptake of oxygen by a contaminated material, *e.g.*, sewage, water, milk, etc., is a measure of microbial activity. Also termed biochemical oxygen demand.

biological value. A quantitative measure of the nutritive value of a protein food carried out under conditions where quality of the protein is the limiting factor. It is defined as the amount of absorbed protein that is retained in the body (expressed as a ratio), *i.e.*, digestibility is not taken into account. If digestibility is included, *i.e.*, the amount retained is expressed as a fraction of the amount in the diet, the measure is net protein utilization.

NPU = BV X Digestibility.

Previously, it was expressed as a percentage scale, now as a ratio; thus the perfect protein has BV = 1.0 (100% retained). Examples are egg and human milk protein, 0.9-1.0; meat, fish and cow's milk, 0.75-0.8; wheat bread, 0.5; peanut, 0.4-0.45.

Biondo comune orange. A variety of the Beledi orange grown in Italy. It matures in mid-season. The fruit is medium-large and round. The peel is yellowish-orange at maturity. The fruit is not highly regarded as a fresh fruit. About 40% of the crop is processed, although processing quality is also pour because of low juice and soluble solids content, as well as high limonin content. In Italy, concentrated juice of the fruit is added to mineral water to make an orange drink called Aranciata, containing about 12% juice.

bioregulators. Biologically active low molecular mass compounds, either naturally occurring or synthesized, which regulate biosynthetic and/or metabolic system and thus affect the expression of biological responses in living tissue.

biosterol. Obsolete name for vitamin A.

biotin. $C_{10}H_{16}O_3N_2S$. A water soluble vitamin present in milk to the extent of about 50 mg/L. Formerly, it was known as Vitamin H or Factor H of the B complex. It is one of the most recently discovered vitamins known to be essential in human nutrition. Deficiency of biotin in the diet of rats produced egg white injury, a condition characterized by severe dermatitis, skin hemorrhages, edema, nervous disturbance, anemia, and complete loss of hair. In humans, somewhat similar condition (except loss of hair) have been reported, which were cured by addition of biotin. Important sources of biotin include eggs, liver, kidney, yeast, fresh vegetables, some fruits, and milk.

biotoprotein. A soluble biotin protein complex that occurs naturally.

birch beer. Non-alcoholic carbonated beverage flavoured with oil of wintergreen or oil of sweet birch and oil of sassafras.

Birch family. *Betulaceae.* The flowers of the deciduous trees and shrubs in this family are borne in catkin-like clusters of cymules. Many cymules make up a cyme (cluster of clusters). Each cymule has 2-3 flowers and several bracts. The clusters of male and female flowers occur on the same tree (monoecious). The male flower may have 4 tepals with 2-20 stamens per cyme. The female flower has 1 pistil with an inferior ovary, 2 styles, and 2 stigmas. These spring flowers utilize wind for pollination and produce a nutlet or a winged samara fruit. Leaves are alternate and simple and have saw-tooth (serrate) margins. Stipules are present at petiole bases. The bark is prominently marked by lenticles (openings for gas exchange). The family includes: *Betula* (birch), *Ostrya* (hophornbeam); *Alnus* (alder), *Betula;* Corylus (hazel nut, filbert); *Betula papyrifera* (paper birch, white birch), *B. pendula* (European white birch). White birch grows to about 20 metres in height and is found mainly in the northern U.S., Canada and northern Europe. It has white bark and bright green leaves that are minutely hairy. Black birch averages 20-25 metres in height. The bark is brown when the tree is young, dark grey later and is horizontally striped. On older trees the bark is more irregularly broken. The leaves are ovate, pointed and alternate in pairs on the tree.

biscuit check. The development of splitting and cracks in biscuits immediately after baking.

biscuit. Essentially bakery confectionery dried down to low moisture content, name derived from Latin for twice-cooked. Made from soft flour-mostly rice in fat and sugar and consequently of high energy content 450-550 kcal, per 100 g. Termed cookie in the United States, where the word biscuit means a small cake-like bun.

bisquit tortoni. A Neapolitan ice cream to which is added, when partly frozen, heavy or medium heavy sweet cream. A further modification of this speciality is the addition of meringue and macaroons just before drawing from the freezer.

bitter cress. It designates the genus *Cardamine* and includes the cuckooflower (*Cardamine partensis*), which grows in wet places and bogs in the northern US. Rock cress is a term that designates plants of the genus *Arabis*. Indian cress, a species of *Tropabolum*, is the popular garden flower, nasturtium, the foliage of which also can be used in salads.

bitters. Gentian, quassia and calumba, and, in small doses, quinine and strychnine; used to stimulate gustatory nerves in the mouth and thus stimulate appetite.

Bitto cheese. A cheese of the Emmentaler group that is made in Italy. It may be eaten fresh or ripened or as long as 2 years, at which time it is very hard and has small eyes.

Biuret test. A test reaction for proteins (actually for peptide bonds). Violet colour is developed when a drop of copper sulphate solution is added to a solution of protein is caustic soda.

bixin. A carotenoid pigment found in the seeds of the tropical plant *Bixa orellana*, the crude extract is the colouring agent annatto.

black (green) tea. *Camellia sinensis.* Tea drinking in some Asian countries has evolved into quite a delicate art, much as wine sampling or tasting has done in France. There are connoisseurs of finely brewed tea, who can tell what type of water was used, what kind of utensils were involved and the approximate conditions under which a particular tea is prepared. In China, some varieties of tea are so strong to the palate that they are served in (literally) thimble-sized cups.

black (white) pepper. *Piper nigrum.* Black pepper is the dried full-grown but unripe fruit, while the white kind is the dried ripe fruit with the outer part of the pericarp removed by soaking in water and then rubbing it off. It is less aromatic than black, but has a more delicate flavour. Major producers of both kinds include India, Indonesia, Malaysia and China. They should not be confused with red or cayenne pepper which comes from the *Capsicum* species.

black cohosh. *Cimicifuga racemosa.* A perennial plant native to North America; occurs frequently on hillsides and in woodlands at higher elevations. The plant has a large, creeping, knotty rootstock which is often scarred with the remains of old growth. It produces a stem up to 3 m in height and has flowers yielding an offensive, stinking smell.

black diamond watermelon. A standard shipping variety of watermelon. A high-yielding variety, but somewhat inferior in texture, flavor, and flesh color. It weighs from 15-18 kg, but may sometimes reach 22 kg. Its shape is nearly round. The outer layer is very dark green, slightly ribbed, thick, tough, and hard, factors contributing to its excellent shipping quality. Flesh is red, rather coarse-grained, sweet, and crisp. Seeds are brownish-black. In some strains, it is relatively free from whiteheart. It is resistant to anthracnose and tolerant to Fusarium wilt. Vines are vigorous and prolific. From planting to maturity, it takes about 90 days.

black PN. Food colour, tetra-sodium salt of 8-acetamide-2-(7-sulpho-4-p-sulphophenylazo-1-naphthlazo)-1-naphthol-3:5-disulphonic acid. Also called Brilliant black BN.

black tongue. A symptom of nicotinic acid deficiency in dogs that was used in the isolation of the vitamin.

blackberry. Berry of bramble, *Rubus fruticosus*. The average composition per 100 g is: protein 1.2%; fat 1.0; Fe 1.0 mg; vitamin A 50 μg; B_1 0.03 mg; B_2 0.05 mg; nicotinic acid 0.4 mg; vitamin C 24 mg; food energy 0.24 MJ.

blackcurrant. Fruit of the bush, *Ribes nigra*. Of special interest as a fruit because of its high vitamin C content. The average composition per 100 g is: protein 0.9%; carbohydrates 6.6%; water 77%; Fe 1.3 mg; vitamin A 90 μg; B_1 0.03 mg; B_2 0.06 mg; nicotinic acid 0.25 mg; vitamin C 200 mg; and food energy 0.12 MJ.

black-eyed pea. Family: *Leguminousae*. Genus: *Vigna*. Species: *Vigna unguiculata*. Like the other members of the bean family; they are valuable source of protein and contain a variety of vitamins and minerals.

blackfish oil. A pale-yellow oil extracted from the pilot whale, porpoise, or blackfish, *Globicephala melas*, found along the North Atlantic Coast. The blackfish averages 4.6-5.5 m in length, with a weight of about 450 kg. The oil has a saponification value of 290, iodine value 27, and specific gravity 0.929. The dolphin oil, of the common dolphin, *Delphinus delphis*, of all seas, is also classed as blackfish oil, as is also the oil of the killer whale, *Grampus orca*, of all seas. The oil is used as a lubricant for fine mechanisms, in cutting oils, and for treating leather. The product from the head and jaw is of the best quality, and is known as jaw oil, although the best grade of sperm oil is also called jaw oil. The jaw oil from blackfish does not oxidize easily, and is free-flowing at low temperatures, having a pour point of -29°C. It consists of about 70% mixed acids, of which 85% is valeric acid, $C_2H_5(CH_3)CHCOOH$, and 14% oleic and palmitic acids. The normal valeric acid is methyl ethyl acetic acid, and can be made by the oxidation of amyl alcohol. It is produced in the human system by the action of enzymes on amino acids.

blackstrap. A term referring to the molasses which remains after all the economically recoverable sugar has been removed from cane or beet syrup. It can be used as a source of alcohol and other fermentation products and as an animal feed base.

blanching. A term used in the food industry to describe the mild heating of fruits and vegetable at 93-100°C primarily to inactivate enzymes that would cause deterioration or loss of flavor. This process usually precedes canning, dehydration, freezing, and other preservation methods. Notwithstanding the name, it has little effect on colour. Fruits and vegetables are blanched before canning, dehydrating, or freezing, for a variety of reasons: softening of texture, shrinkage, removal of air, destruction of enzymes, removal of undesirable flavours. Also done to remove excess salt from preserved meat and to aid removal of skin, *e.g.*, from almonds. It can result in losses of 10-20% of sugars, salts, and protein, some of the vitamins B_1, B_2 and nicotinic acid, and up to one-third of the vitamin C. The procedure is sometimes called "scalding." If vegetables such as sweet potatoes, carrots, and spinach are blanched before dehydration, there may be less loss of carotene during dehydration.

blanching, infra-red. Superior to steam blanching for apples, celery, peas and potatoes as it reduces the amount of water left in the product, does not leach out flavour and nutrients, and improves the texture, flavour and appearance. In potatoes the process reduces fat absorption during frying.

blancmange powders. Usually a cornflour base with added flavour and colour.

bland diet. One that contains the minimum of crude fibre or roughage and is therefore non-irritating and soothing to the intestine.

bleeding bread. Bacterial infection with *B. prodigiosus* that stains the bread bright red. Under optimal conditions of warmth and damp the infection can appear overnight and contamination of shewbread with this organisms in churches has led to accusations and riots against religious minorities over the centuries.

blessed thistle. *Cnicus benedictus.* A plant widely used during medieval times. This particular herb had religious connotations surrounding it, hence other common names for it like holy thistle or Holy Ghost herb are also popular. Blessed Thistle apparently helped to relieve pain and

inflammation of the heart in the 16th and 17th centuries. The herb is found in moist areas, waste places, meadows and pastures.

bleu. A roquefort type cheese (blue-veined) made outside the Roquefort area. Also known as fromage bleu.

blind. A cheese that has no "eyes" or gasholes.

block (of milk). A product, tablet-like in appearance, made from condensed or dried milk or milk products. Agglomerated nonfat dry milk is compressed with 1300-4100 kPa presses to a density of 450-600 kg/m³ to make milk blocks or tablets. Another procedure is to concentrate milk in an evaporator to one-third the original volume, add sugar, homogenize, dry in a scraped surface heat exchanger-dryer, and solidify in molds to form blocks or cakes. Cream tablets are made from a high fat product (30 to 55% fat) by compressing a spray-dried product.

blood (human). A heterogeneous suspension, considered to be liquid tissue, containing the followings:

(a) red cells, or erythrocytes, which contain hemoglobin, an iron-protein complex; they are not actually living cells, but rather are aggregates of haemoglobin, liquids, and water.

(b) white cells, or leukocytes, which are true biological cells, and contain nucleoproteins and liquids and function as a protective mechanism against infections.

(c) platelets, made up of cephalin and other proteins, which play a part in blood clotting. Besides these major components, blood contains many proteins, sugars, cholesterol, fatty acids, and in organic substances in ionized form.

Blood acts in the body as a transport agent for nutrients and for oxygen and carbon dioxide. It is strongly buffered system and maintains pH of about 7.3-7.5. The coagulation mechanism involves protein fibrinogen; serum is the fraction remaining after coagulation. The blood is the vehicle for metabolic communication between the organs of the body. It transports nutrients from the small intestine to the liver and other organs and transports waste products to the kidneys for excretion. The blood is also the vehicle for transport of oxygen from lungs to the tissues and for the transport of carbon dioxide generated during the respiratory metabolism of the tissues to the lungs for excretion. Moreover, the hormones are transported from the endocrine glands via the blood to their specific target organs, in their function as chemical messengers. The blood in the vascular system of an adult human has a volume of about 5-6 litres. Almost half of its volume is occupied by cells, which consists largely of red blood cells (erythrocytes), much smaller number of white blood cells (leukocytes), and blood platelets. The liquid portion is the blood plasma, which is about 90% water and 10% dissolved matter. Over 70% of the plasma solids is constituted by plasma proteins. About 20% consists of organic metabolites, which are passing between various organs, and the waste products urea and uric acid, which passes to the kidneys to be excreted into the urine. The remaining 10% of plasma solids consists of inorganic compounds. Some of the blood components normally vary in concentration, depending upon the nature of the nutritional intake. The blood glucose level, for example reaches a maximum just after the meal, especially if it is rich in sugar, and then may decline below the mean level after several hours. Similarly, the concentration of chylomicrons in the blood varies during the period between the meals. The concentrations of the various components of blood plasma are maintained at characteristic levels by certain regulatory systems.

blood cells. Cells of the blood, consisting of red blood cells and their various precursors, erythroblasts and reticulocytes- white blood cells (see leukocytes) of many kinds, such as plasma cells, lymphocytes, granulocytes and macrophages, and in some diseased states, earlier precursor cells normally found only in bone marrow or other erythropoietic sites. Also known as blood corpuscles.

blood clotting. Process in which fibrinogen, a protein present in blood plasma, is acted upon by the enzyme thrombin and, by the removal of a terminal peptide, is modified to form fibrin. This protein is capable of rapid polymerization to form clot. Thrombin is not normally freely available in blood, but becomes so by the conversion of prothrombin, a process requiring calcium ions a lipoprotein factor released from broken platelets and an anti-hemophilic globulin molecule. Also known as blood coagulation.

blood coagulation. *See* blood clotting.

blood corpuscles. *See* blood cells.

blood drying. Animal blood can be dried with a spray dryer using an entering drying air temperature of 166°C and an exit temperature of 71.1°C for the incoming product at 65% moisture, wet basis. Freeze drying is also used for moisture removal so there will be minimal thermal effect on the product while drying. Two general approaches are used for drying blood for food and feed purposes:

(a) Blood is collected from the animal and held in a cool place and clotted or coagulated. The coagulated material is placed on screen-bottom trays, and the serum is drained and dried in pans or trays in a cabinet dryer.

(b) Blood is collected and treated with an anticoagulant (such as sodium citrate and sodium chloride solution). The blood is screened and centrifuged. The blood is separated into 40% hemoglobin (28-30% solids) and 60% plasma (9% solids). The fibrin is removed from the plasma, leaving serum. The serum is condensed to 25% solids. The serum and the hemoglobin are spray-dried separately to 8% moisture. In one procedure, the blood is coagulated with steam before drying. Disagreeable odors may be minimized by injecting an aerosol mist (propylene glycol base) into the stack discharge of the dryer.

blood group substance. A genetically determined particulate isoantigen that is attached to surface of red blood cells ad that may be attached to the surface of other cells; the related blood group substances represent the alternative antigens, specified by the allelic genes.

blood serum. Blood plasma from which clotting factors, such as blood platelets, have been removed by centrifugation.

blood sugar. The glucose, normally present (before breakfast) at 80-100 mg/100 ml. The level rises after a meal (to around 150 mg/100 ml) but rapidly returns to normal as glucose is taken up by the tissues (except in cases of diabetes mellitus).

blood, citrated. Blood that has been prevented from clotting by the addition of citrate, which combines with the calcium. 600 mg of sodium citrate prevents coagulation of 100 ml blood.

blood, defibrinated. Blood clots rapidly after it has been shed when the soluble protein fibrinogen is converted into insoluble fibrin. If the blood is stirred with a rod the fibrin can be removed as it forms and the blood, still containing the cells, will remain fluid. This is called defibrinated blood.

blood, oxalated. Blood sample that has been prevented from clotting by the addition of oxalate, which combines with the calcium. 160 mg of sodium oxalate has been found to be sufficient to prevent clotting of 100 ml of the blood.

bloody milk. A popular term for the milk appearing red in colour, especially near the bottom of the bottle or container. This is usually due to the presence of blood which comes into the milk from a ruptured blood vessel in the udder of the animal. Bloody milk is also indicated when on separation, the separator slime is pink or red, inasmuch as the red cells are thrown out due to centrifugal force. The same is true on clarification.

bloom gelometer. Instrument used for measuring the strength of jellies, and also for any test of firmness, *e.g.*, staleness of bread. For jelly strength the jelly is prepared at 6.66% concentration and chilled at 10°C for 16-18 hours. The instrument measures the load in grams needed to produce a 4 mm depression in the gel with 12 mm diameter plunger. Gelatin at 250 bloom grams is used in jellied meat, 200 in marshmallows.

bloom. Fat bloom is the whitish appearance on the surface of chocolate that sometimes occurs on storage. It is due to a change in the form of the fat at the surface or to the fat diffusing outward and being deposited on the surface.

blueberry. Highbush blueberry (*Vaccinium corymbosum*) and lowbush (*V. augustifolium*) grown in North America. The cultivated kind of a blue-black colour used principally for its food value.

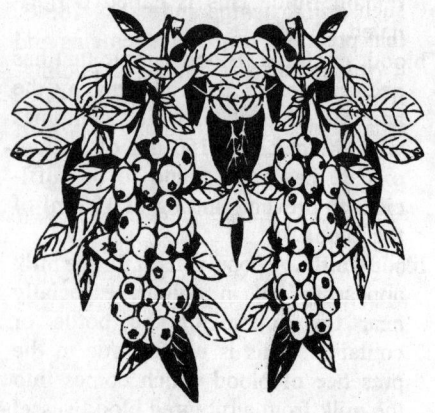

blue milk. A very uncommon condition of milk caused by a bacterium, *Bacillus cyanogenes.* The blue colour develops when milk is allowed to stand. Immediate pasterization of the milk will prevent this condition from developing.

blue mold. A term often used for Roquefort or Roquefort-type cheese, especially that made in the United States. A cheese made outside the Roquefort area of France, with Penicillium roquerforti.

blue value. 1. Referring to vitamin A, it denotes the transient blue colour produced by reaction with antimony trichloride, the intensity of colour being proportional to the amount of the vitamin present. 2. Referring to starch, it is an index of free soluble starch, i.e., the amylose, in food, *e.g.*, potatoes.

blue VRS. A blue coloured dye; the sodium salt of 4,4'-di-(diethylamino)-4",6"-disulphotriphenyl-methanolan-hydride.

blueing process. Development of blue mold on Stilton cheese is somewhat similar to that used for blue mold cheese. The blue mold grows best in rooms containing much carbon dioxide and little oxygen.

BOD. *See* biological oxygen demand.

body-building food. A term indiscriminately used, usually refers to proteins. The code of practice suggests that no claim should be made for the body building properties of a food unless a reasonable amount of protein (not specified) is present in a normal proportion.

bodying agents. The body of a food substance is generally associated with the textural qualities of a food substance, notably with mouth-feel or chewiness. Much effort is required by the food technologists as regards the sorting out of properties and their terminology in this presently very active area of technology. The term `body' refers to a number of essentially unprocessed foods that, by their fundamental nature, possess desirable mouth-feel or chewiness. For maximum consumer appearance, these qualities must fall within those parameters which have been established by tradition for a given food substance (not too chewy, thick, or tough and thus difficult to eat; but also not too thin, watery, pasty, mucilaginous, etc.). In the case of tough meats, a key target in texture investigations, excessive chewiness is reduced by various processing operations and the use of certain chemical substances which act enzymatically on muscle and connecting tissue. Such additives, while affecting texture, normally are not considered bodying agents, but fall into a special classification of tenderizers.

More often, the term bodying agent is associated with semiliquid food substances. Their use may increase the consistency and otherwise alter rheological properties to achieve a sensation of "thickness" or an apparent increase in viscosity that imparts mouth-feel sensations, some resistance to flow, creaminess, stiffness, etc., as contrasted with the sensations of a watery, thin substance. Some products, particularly those of a fabricated nature, may possess a full complement of desirable consumer appeals (taste, odour, colour, nutritive value, etc.) and yet lack the desirable texture quality of body. Thus, soups, gravies, sauces, cheese foods and spreads, dressings, snack dips and spreads, margarines, among others, can be improved through the addition of bodying agents. For example, formulations for frozen desserts can be improved by the addition of low levels of microcrystalline cellulose (about 0.25% weight), in combination with soluble hydrocolloids, such as guar, locust bean gum, alginates, or carrageenans. Microcrystalline cellulose achieves about the same degree of body and substance in frozen desserts that is normally obtained only in well-emulsified products with a 2-4% higher fat contents. This is the result of the ability of microcrystalline cellulose, like carrageenan, to stabilize the serum solids. Microcrystalline cellulose imparts body and smoothness to ice cream and ice milk, and tends to make them feel less cold. There are no off-flavours associated with the substance, and frozen desserts melt to smooth, creamy consistencies.

bog-butter. Norsemen, Finns, Scots and Irish used to burry firkins of butter in bogs to ripen it for the strong flavour that developed. This old Irish custom, not now in practice, dates back to the 15th and 16th centuries. Reports indicate that the butter was either packed in firkins or wrapped in skins before it was buried in the peat bogs.

boiled sweets. Sugar and water boiled at such a high temperature, 149-166°C, that practically no water remains and a vitreous mass is formed on cooling. It may be regarded as a supersaturated solution of sugar, to which other ingradients are added to modify its colour and taste.

boiling(stewing). For meat of second quality, *i.e.*, containing much connective tissue, boiling or stewing is the preferred method of cooking since it slowly breaks down the connective tissue to water-soluble gelatin and improves the tenderness. The meat extractives expressed into the water through shrinkage, are not lost since the water is normally used. Destruction of vitamin B_1 approx. 75%, B_2 30%, and nicotinic acid 50%. It has been estimated that fish loses about 20% B_1 on boiling.

bone broth. The product obtained by prolonged boiling of chopped bones. Of little nutritive value, consisting of 2-4% gelatin, with very little calcium.

bone charcoal. Bones degreased, broken to required size and heated in closed retorts. The organic matter is carbonized leaving about 10% carbon deposited on a framework of calcium phosphate. It is mainly used to clarify solutions by virtue of its properties of absorbing colouring matter and impurities.

bone. The organic matrix of collagen, osseoalbumoid and osseomucoid with an inorganic mixture of about 85% calcium phosphate, 10% calcium phosphate, 10% calcium phosphate, 10% calcium carbonate and 1.5% magnesium phosphate. The inorganic mixture has the crystal structure of the mineral hydroxyapatite which is composed of one molecule of calcium hydroxide and three of calcium phosphate. Fluoride and sulphate are also present in bone.

bone meal. The product obtained from degreased animal bones; in high purity state, it is used as supplement for both, animal feed as well as human food, as a source of calcium and phosphate. it is also used as plant fertilizer as a source of phosphate.

Bontrae. Trade name for textured vegetable protein preparation made by spinning or extrusion.

borage. *Borago officinalis*. The bright blue, star-shaped flowers of borage make it one of the prettiest of herb plants, though the leaves, dark green, downy, and with no fragrance, are unremarkable. It is a hardy annual plant, a native of northern Europe, and grows well in temperate regions of North America. Borage flowers and leaves are the traditional decoration for gin-based summer cocktails, and may be set in ice cubes to garnish other drinks. The flowers may be used to garnish salads and cake decoration. Borage tisane, an infusion of the leaves, may be taken to ease coughs, and the leaves may be used as a poultice to alleviate muscular strains.

Bosc pear. *Beurre Bosc*. A variety of pear, which is second to Anjou pear in terms of volume as a winter pear, making up about 20% of the winter crop in US. Fruit is uniquely shaped and colored. It has a long tapering neck, skin is dark yellow, overlaid with cinnamon-russet, which varies in intensity, depending upon climatic and cultural conditions. The fruit is medium to large in size, and the flesh is yellowish-white, some grit at centre,

buttery, but not melting, very juicy. It has rich vinous, aromatic flavour and rates high as a dessert fruit. The tree is vigorous, upright, spreading, productive, difficult to shape during formative years. but well shaped and stately at maturity. It has been found to be quite susceptible to blight.

Boston brown bread. In the US, name given to a spiced pudding steamed in the can.

bottom yeast. The yeast used in beer production that tends to settle at the bottom of the fermentation vessel.

botulism. A form of food poisoning caused by neurotoxin (botulin) produced by the Gram-positive, spore-forming *Clostridium botulinum*; sometimes found in improperly canned or preserved foodstuffs. The spores can germinate and an exotoxin is produced during vegetative growth. If the food is then consumed without adequate cooking, the toxin remains active and the disease results. The toxin binds to the synapses of the motor neurons and appears to prevent the release of acetylcholine. As a consequence the muscles do not contract in response to motor neuron activity, and flaccid paralysis results. The various characteristics of the disease and the organism are:

(a) The disease is an intoxication and not an infection.

(b) The organisms releasing the toxin grow only under anaerobic conditions.

(c) The toxin can be inactivated if it is subjected to boiling for more than 5 minutes.

(d) The toxin is resistant to digestive enzymes.

(e) In the smoking process of meats if the salt concentration is high enough, the organism causing botulism cannot multiply. Wound botulism is characterized by spore germination in the wound and release of toxin to the systemic circulation. The symptoms of the disease are the same as for food-borne botulism. Ingestion of the spores, contaminating such foods as honey, vegetables, or fruits, is apparent cause of infant botulism. The spores germinate in the intestinal tract and the toxin is released.

Boudanne cheese. A variety of French cheese made from cow's milk, either whole or skim. The milk is heated to about 28°C, enough rennet added to coagulate it in an hour, and the curd cut to the size of peas, stirred, and heated to at least 37°C. After standing for 10-15 minutes, the curd is pressed into molds. They are drained, turned often and ripened for about 3 months.

Bouillabaisse. The popular name for fish stew common in Southern France, made from several kinds of fish and shellfish, cooked with oil, spices and herbs. It is so named because it is repeatedly boiled.

bouillon. Popular name for plain, unclarified beef or veal broth.

bound auxins. Indole-3-acetic acid or any other auxin, present in the bonded form with various metabolites. In this form higher level of free auxins is reduced and kept at physiological concentration. Free auxins are released from bound auxins by hydrolysis either enzymatically or autolysis e.g., Ascorbigen, glucobrassicin and auxin peptides etc.

bound water. In reference to the cheese, the water which is tied up with the protein of cheese. The amount of bound water has been reported to be 200-350 g/ kg of cheese. This bound water has been measured by the freezing point depression technique based on the assumption that part of the water molecules appear to be unable to act as solvent for substances which cause a freezing point depression. Bound water cannot be determined accurately by any known method. The amount of bound water in cheese is affected by amounts of fat, solids and sodium chloride and also by the pH of the cheese.

Bournvita. Trade name for preparation of cocoa, malt, milk, sugar, eggs and flavouring agents, for consumption as a beverage when added to milk. The average composition per 100 g is: protein 11.4%; fat 7.5%; carbohydrate 67.6%; Ca 89 mg; Fe 3 mg; food energy 1.6 MJ.

Bovril. Trade name for a preparation of meat extract, hydrolyzed beef, powder and yeast extract used as a beverage, breadspread and flavouring agent. The average composition per 100 g is: protein 28%; vitamin B_2 3.5 mg; nicotinic acid 24 mg; Fe 12 mg.

Bra cheese. A kind of cheese made first by the Nomads in the region of Bra in Piedmont, Italy It is a hard rennet cheese about 30 cm in diameter, 8 cm high, and weighs about 5 kg.

bradycardia. An abnormal condition characterized by unusually slow heartbeat; a symptom, among other causes, of certain vitamin deficiencies.

braising. The process of brief frying in shallow fat followed by stewing. Proteins coagulate very rapidly during frying and may become tougher. During braising, the loss of vitamin B_1 may be up to 50%, B_2 25%, and nicotinic acid 35%.

bran. Wheat bran. *Triticum aestivum.* Sorghum bran. *Sorghum vulgarie.* Bran is a relatively inexpensive and abundant source of dietary fibre, being the coarse outer coat or hull of the grain of wheat, separated from the meal or flour by sifti ig or bolting.

Diabetics and those with a tendency towards poor blood sugar tolerance, like hypoglycemics, may also benefit from bran, particularly from oat bran, because these types of fibre slow down the emptying of the stomach during digestion, so reducing the rise of sugar as food is turned into available energy in the blood stream. The only problems with bran as far as medical treatment is concerned are the it can cause a lot of flatulence and with very tender and inflamed colons can actually scour them and make the situation worse, besides which it is now recognized as inhibiting the absorption of iron in certain people. Bran from wheat is rich in protein, carbohydrate, fibre, phosphorus iron, sodium, potassium, vitamins B_2, B_3 and B_6 and folic acid. Sorghum bran, on the other hand, comes from sorghum, a major cereal crop in many third world and developing nations. In fact, it's the world's third largest cereals food grain. Sorghum is a coarse kind of grass with a stalk very similar to that of corn.

Bran plus. Trade name for a cereal food containing untreated wheat bran. The average composition per 100 g is: 13.7 g protein; 57.4 g carbohydrates; 13 g water; 3.6 g fat; 4.5 g ash; 7.8 g fibre.

Brand cheese. A variety of German hand cheese weighing about 150 g, made from sour milk curd that is cooked at a slightly higher temperature than is usual. The curd is salted and allowed to ferment one day. Then it is mixed with butter, pressed into shaped, dried, and placed in kegs to ripen, during which time is occasionally moistened with beer.

brandy. A spirit distilled from wine, The name 'Brandy' was originally called Brandwine or Brandewine derived form the Dutch 'Brandewijn', that is burnt or distilled wine. In the British Pharmacopoeia brandy is defined as a spirituous liquid distilled from wine and matured by age, and containing not less than 36.5% by weight or 43.5% by volume of ethyl alcohol. There are two major types:

(a) of high alcohol content, 80-94.5%, used to fortify dessert wines; and

(b) beverage brandies of 50% alcohol. The age of brandies used to designated by stars (*) (one for 3 years, two for 4 years, three for 5 years). Brandies are also designated by initials such as V.S.O. (very special old, 12-17 years (V.S.O.P. (very special old pale, 18-25 years), V.V.S.O.P. (very, very, special old pale, up to 40 years old) but these designations have largely lost their meaning through indiscriminate use.

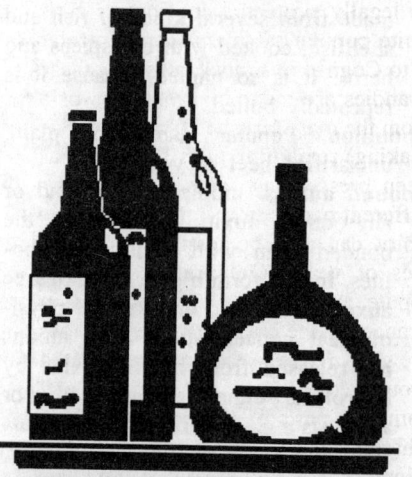

Like whisky, 'Brandy' is one of the distilled liquors of commerce known all over the world, and may be safely branded as "the king of spirits". Indeed, the French do think of it as a basic necessity and in many places it is known '*Eau-de-vie*' or water of life'. It is obtained by the distillation of fermented saccharine liquids and contains, beside alcohol, certain congeneric substances produced during fermentation and storage, which are responsible for their characteristic flavour and bouquet. Brandy is most often distilled from grape-wine, but there are many other types known as Fruit Brandies are also made from many fruits such as plums, cherries etc., and are obtained from fruit wines.

Of Brandy, fundamentally a fresh spirit, there are subdivisions. The best quality of brandy is Cognac made only in France. Although this is often referred to as brandy, the French do not agree and consider it illegal. Armagnac is also of good quality though it is not a patch on Cognac from an outsider's point of view. Its quality is high and its name is legally protected in France. It is quite popular, as many people prefer it to Cognac in France. Besides, these brandies are made all over the world from the marc (crushed grapes in wine making) remaining after the wine has been pressed out. This is known by different names in different countries. Spirit can also be distilled from the lees of yeast. The brandies of best repute are distilled and matured in France in the districts where grapes are grown. These districts are situated around the town of Cognac and comprise parts of the departments of Charente and Charente Maritime. For a long time the vines of this and other districts of France suffered greatly from the attack of the phylloxera, but increased scientific knowledge, leading to a system of replanting and hybridizing has enabled the vinegrowers to cope with the disease. After the distillate has been prepared

from the wine, it is stored in casks of oak-wood, which imparts a brown colour to the spirit. Brandy used to be described as a straw coloured liquid but the colour is invariably deeper, a certain intensity of tint being obtained at by the addition of caramel or burnt sugar colouring to the spirit. The maturing requires several years in the case of the finest brandies, but too long a period is disadvantageous, as the evaporation of the liquid may result in too great a weakening of the spirit.

Brandy is seldom bottled straight. Most palates are suited by a blend of different vintages. The blending is carried out in vats shortly before bottling and it is the proper carrying out of this process which determines the quality associated with particular names. Some proprietary brands obtain a distinct flavour by means of flavouring essences. Brandy has a sweet, smooth ethereal flavour and fine bouquet. The flavour is due to the presence of capric ester and other volatile constituents of wine. The constituents present include esters of acetic, butyric, and valeric acids, volatile oils, tannin, fixed acids and colouring materials.

Brandy is the form in which alcohol is usually administered as a medicine, as its stimulating properties are quickly exercised. It is used as a stimulant in cases of suspended animation or exhaustion. Imitation brandies are made by 'cutting' strongly flavoured brandy with diluted rectified grain alcohol, colouring and sweetening with caramel and cane sugar syrup, and 'dosing' with Lees' oil or an extract of oak wood chips. Extract of cedar wood chips, bitter almonds, stored plums, and walnut shells are often added to give aged characteristic and herb-like flavour. Sometimes orris root, coumarin, cinnamon, pekoe tea or vanilla are added.

brawn. A product made from meat, ears and tongue of the pig; boiled with peppercorns and herbs, minced and pressed into a mould. Mock brawn differs in that other meat by-products are used.

Brazil nut. Family: *Lecythidaceae.* Genus: *Bertholletia.* Species: *Bertholletia excelsa.* Brazil nuts are high in calories and fat and are a rich source of protein, containing many vitamins and minerals.

bread. The generic term for breads containing enough bran and other non-endosperm fractions of the grain to give a distinctive colour and texture to the baked product. These varieties are not to be confused with whole wheat bread, which should in theory, contain all the fractions of wheat in the same proportions as they exist in the unmilled grain.

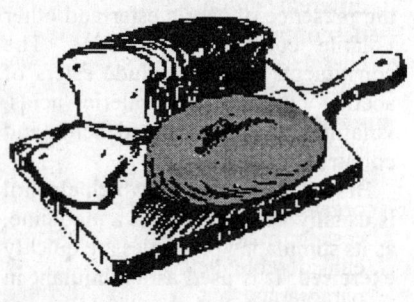

Whole wheat bread is by its very nature a coarse, dark, chewy, and rather highly flavoured product, but wheat bread can be very close to standard white bread in density, texture, crust appearance, colour, and flavour. It appeals to consumers who believe there are some health problems with white bread but who have not yet been converted to the view that the worse a product tastes the better it is for you. There is no specified standard for the identify of wheat bread; but any product purporting to be `whole wheat bread,' Graham bread, entire wheat bread, whole wheat rolls, Graham rolls, entire wheat rolls, whole wheat buns, Graham buns, or entire wheat buns, must conform to certain Standards laid down by the department of food. They must be made from whole wheat flour, brominated whole wheat flour, or a combination of these. White flour can not be used for making any kind of bread. Wheat bread is formulated and processed similarly to regular white bread. Because it contains structurally inert ingredients in the form of bran, germ, etc., supplementation by strong flour or even by vital wheat gluten is sometimes necessary in order to get volume and grain that will be accepted by the consumer.

One slice of either pumpernickel, rye or wheat bread would be about equal to 8 slices of white bread for increasing stool output. The best way to increase intake of fibre-rich food is to increase bread consumption, making sure that white bread is replaced by bread made from flour that is as near as possible to wholemeal. Whole wheat bread has three times the amount of dietary fibre compared to white bread. Composition depends on extraction rate of flour and on enrichment with vitamins and minerals; may also be enriched with milk powder, fish protein concentration or other sources of protein. The average composition of white bread (enriched with iron, calcium, thiamine and nicotinic acid) per 100 g is: 38 g water; 53 g starch; 8 g protein; 1.4 g fat; 0.18 mg B_1; 0.04 mg B_2; 1.7 mg nicotinic acid; 1.8 mg iron; 90 mg calcium; and 1.0 MJ food energy.

bread, aerated. A variety of dough that is made with water saturated with carbon dioxide under pressure. The object is to produce an aerated loaf without the loss of carbohydrate involved in a yeast fermentation (7% of the total ingredients).

bread, Allison's. Trade name for a wholemeal cereal loaf. The avergae composition per 100 g is: protein 8.2%; fat 2%; carbohydrate 47.1%; Ca 26 mg; Fe 3 mg; food energy 0.97 MJ.

bread, black. Coarse wholemeal wheat or rye bread leavened with saurteig, which is a mixture of fermenting microorganisms. These include :

(a) peptonizing bacteria that turn the dough to a more plastic state,

(b) yeast, and

(c) lactic or acetic bacteria that produce the sour flavour.

bread, brown. A loaf may not legally be described as brown (or wholemeal) unless it contains not less than 0.6% fibre (on dry weight), *i.e.*, a high rate of extraction.

bread,Cornell. Loaf of increased nutritional value by addition of 6% soya flour and 8% skim milk solids.

bread, gluten. Loaf with added wheat gluten to increase the protein content. The name may legally be applied only to loaves containing not less than 16% protein (calculated on dry weight). When the protein level is not less than 22% the loaf may be designated protein bread.

bread, malt. A loaf containing 6-13% ground malt or malt extract which produces a sweeter, stickier and darker loaf.

bread, milk. A loaf cannot legally be described as milk bread unless it contains not less than 6% whole milk solids or skim milk solids.

bread, protein. Loaf containing not less than 22% protein (calculated on dry weight). High protein bread is an alternative designation.

bread, salt-rising. A specialty product having some superficial resemblance to white bread. It has an unusual texture and a pungent aroma, which it gets from a combined yeast and bacterial fermentation. It was formerly prepared by using a natural sour or starter made by encouraging the proliferation of salt-tolerant organisms present in the environment and/ or the ingredients. Some bakers still use this method for developing starters, but practically all commercial salt-rising bread being made (and there is not much) is based on a proprietary dry yeast preparation. The salt-rising bread exhibits a dichotomous distribution of acceptance. Some people find it appetizing while others dislike it. There is wide variation in texture and flavour of the samples made by different producers, but a frequent description of odour is that it is like cheese. The specific volume is about 70-75% of the white bread.

bread, San Francisco sourdough. A highly specific sourdough preparation that gives a product of unique organoleptic characteristics. A process for making it will be described in considerable detail in the following paragraphs, but it should be understood that other procedures may also achieve similar results. It is necessary to have a starter sponge containing the specific organisms required for this bread. Without the correct microflora, it is useless to try any formula or procedure. The starter sponge is made up of 100 parts of the previous sponge, 100 parts of high gluten flour, and 46-52 parts of water. This mixture begins with a pH of 4,.4 and, after about eight hours of fermentation, levels off a pH of about 3.9-4.0. The starter sponge is rebuilt in the same manner about three times a day, seven days a week. The bread dough is formulated with about 20 parts of starter sponge, 100 parts of patent flour, 60 parts of water, and 2 parts of salt. After about one hour of floor time, the bread is made up, and the dough pieces proofed for five to seven hours. During pan proof, the pH drops from about 5.3-3.9. The dough surface is cut immediately before baking, and these cuts are said to be necessary to the development of the typical eating quality of this loaf. Baking is done for 45 to 50 minutes, the exact time depending on the oven conditions, piece size, etc. Low pressure steam is injected into the oven during the first half of the baking cycle or until the crust begins to colour. The dough pieces are placed directly on the hearth. The pH of the crumb does not change must as a result of baking,, so the final bread has pH of 3.9-4.0. Pure cultures of *L. sanfrancisco* bacteria are primarily responsible for the unique flavour of this bread, are available in freeze-dried or frozen form.

bread, scones. A common type of quickbread prepared in the kitchens and retail bakeries of the UK. It is usually made from a considerably richer dough that used for baking powder biscuits, they sometimes include currants, and they are occasionally made in a pie-wedge shape.

bread, soda. Any of the various kinds of bread leavened with sodium bicarbonate and an acidic substance instead of yeast, although legally it may contain yeast as well. Most soda breads are similar to hearth loaves of yeast-leavened bread in shape, size, and usage, but are make from chemically leavened doughs. Their texture and flavour are considerably different from their yeast-leavened counterparts. Irish soda bread is a typical example of this group. These does not seem to be much demand for such products, but their novelty appeals to some consumers. For best result, a moderately strong flour is required, and the dough is developed much like the dough for yeast-leavened bread and rolls. Soda breads are often baked as hearth breads, usually in round (hemispherical) shape with a cross slashed in the top to promote oven spring. Some loaves described as "soda breads' are made from batter-like mixtures deposited in loaf pans.

bread, starch-reduced. Legally the term starch-reduced bread may be applied only to bread containing less than 50% carbohydrate and the wording claiming its value as a slimming aid is legally controlled. Bread generally contains 9-10% protein and about 50% starch; if the starch is reduced either by washing some part of it out of the dough or by adding extra protein, the bread is referred to as starch-reduced and is often claimed of value in slimming and diabetic diets.

breadfruit. The starchy fruit of the tree *Artocarpus communis* or *incisa;* seasonal food of the West Indies; eaten roasted whole when ripe or boiled in pieces whole when ripe or boiled in pieces when green. Not only is the tree attractive and excellent for shade, but it is also an important source of staple food. When ripe, the fruit ranges from 10-15 cm in diameter and weighs up to 13.5 kg and is used in a variety of foods, including puddings. The large ovoid fruits usually have a rough surface, but may be smooth in some varieties. Each fruit is composed of many achenes, each surrounded by a fleshy perianth and growing on a fleshy receptacle. Usually yellowish-brown when ripe, the fruit is roasted or boiled before serving. Some improved varieties are seedless. However, the seeds also can be boiled and eaten. Whereas the fruit of the mulberry tree (also of *Moraceae*) contains sugar, the breadfruit is rich in starch. The large leaves, from 0.3-0.6 m in length, are deeply cut into pinnate lobes. Condensation dripping from the deeply lobed leaves aids in keeping the soil under the tree moist during dry periods. There are over 40 species of breadfruit. The breadfruit is valued in west Africa, as well as in the Pacific islands, because it is well suited to the west African climate.

Propagation of the breadfruit is by root cuttings. The trees grow quite tall, about 9-12 m. They are planted at a spacing of 10.5 by 10.5 m. The fruits do not appear to be damaged to any appreciable extent by insects or fungi. The breadfruit tree shows a definite preference for moist soils, and trees are usually planted in valley soils where water is plentiful. The average composition per 100 g of the fruit is: water 72%; carbohydrate 25%; protein 1.5%; fat 0.4%; Fe 1.2 mg; vitamin B_1 0.1 mg; B_2 0.05 mg; nicotinic acid 1.2 mg; vitamin C 20 mg; and food energy 0.47 MJ.

Breadsoy. Trade name for unheated (enzyme-active) full-fat soya flour.

breakfast food, cereal. Legally defined as any food obtained by the swelling, roasting, grinding, rolling or flaking of any cereal.

Brewers' grains. Cereal residue from brewing, contains about 25% protein; used as animal feed and also a source of unidentified growth factors.

Brewers' pounds. Before specific gravity was used in breweries the strength of wort was expressed as the difference between the weight of a barrel of wort and that of a barrel of water (360 lb.). The excess weight over 360 lb. is denoted by Brewers' pounds.

brewing. The production of beer and ale by enzymatic conversion of the starches contained in barley malt to wort, or malt extract. This is then hydrolyzed to sugars and proteins by a process known as mushing, followed by boiling with hops and fermentation with yeast. These processes (all of which are of the batch type) involves complex reactions induced by enzymes and require extremely close control and careful selection of ingredients. Barley is the grain chiefly used a source of malt; its enzymes are activated by controlled cycles of water absorption and aerating, white induce partial germination of the barley. Beer and ale also contain colloidal proteins which cause foaming; they are clarified by filtration through adsorptive clays or diatomite.

brick cheese. A soft, smear-ripened, high moisture cheese which was developed in America and is largely made in Wisconsin. The body is softer than Cheddar and has a flavour between Cheddar and Limburger. It derives its name from the fact that is made in bricks.

brickbat cheese. A rennet cheese made in Wiltshire, England as early as 1700. It is made from fresh milk to which a small amount to cream has been added. It is supposed to be fit for consumption even one year after being made.

brick tea. A kind of tea made from coarser leaves of the tea plant and may include some pruning. These materials are gathered and heated and steamed while under suitable covers. After some time, a black fungus spreads through the mass. The materials are further processed, including mixing with a glutinous rice paste. After moderate steaming, the mass is molded into bricks (dry weight = 2 kg). This product also is made in smaller tablet form.

bright-leaf tobacco drying. The curing of bright-leaf tobacco with natural air or with a heat supply and a method of obtaining full or partial recirculation of the air in a tightly-built barn. Natural draft ventilation is often used with an adjustable ridge ventilator at the top of the storage building. The desirable temperature and humidity at various stages of the curing. The initial curing process consists of yellowing the tobacco leaves during which large quantities of starch are converted to sugar and the tobacco leaf is maintained in a physical condition which permits the moisture to be removed quickly from the cells. As soon as the proper colour is reached the leaf cells are killed by using a high temperature. The water must be removed from the leaves as rapidly as possible when the desired colour has been obtained. The heating system for drying is larger than required for yellowing only. Drying can progress vary rapidly as long as scorching of the leaves is avoided. After the tobacco is dried it is ordered, meaning that it absorbs moisture from the atmosphere and becomes pliable.

brilliant black PN. The tetrasodium salt of 2-4-(p-sulpho-phenylazo)-7-sulpho-1-naphthylazo-8-acetamino-1-naphthol-3,5-disulphonic acid. It is a dense black powder, which is readily soluble in water and glycerol but only slightly soluble in 95% ethanol. Brilliant black has excellent light fastness and is stable in acid media and under heat treatment. Although a general purpose food colour, it is used mostly in blends. It is not permitted for use in foods in the U.S.

brilliant blue FCF. FD&C blue 1. A triarylmethane dye having a structural formula similar to that of Fast Green. It is the disodium salt of 4-{4-N-ethyl-p-sulphobenzylamino-phenyl)-(2-sulphonium-phenyl)-methylene}-[1-(N-ethyl-N-p-sulphobenzyl)-δ-2,5-cyclohexadienimine]. It is bright blue powder, which is very soluble in water, glycerol and the glycols (all at 20 % at 25°C) and is slightly soluble in ethanol (95 %). This colour is lightfast, and has good stability in a wide range of pH and in the presence of sulphur dioxide and sodium benzoate.

brislings. Popular name for young sparts, *Clupea sprattus.* Canned brislings contain 1,000 i.u. vitamin A and 1-2,000 i.u. vitamin D per 100 g.

brix. A table of Specific Gravity based on the Balling tables calculated in grams of cane sugar in 100 g solution at 20°C, i.e., degree Brix = per cent sugar. It is used to refer to concentration of sugar syrups used in canned fruits.

broad bean. Family: *Leguminosae.* Genus: *Vicia.* Species: *Faba Vicia faba.* Broad beans are a good source of protein and contain calcium and iron together with some vitamins.

broad-spectrum drugs. Chemotherapeutic agents that are effective against many kind of pathogens.

broad-spectrum pesticide. A pesticide such as DDT or Lindane, which kills a wide variety of living organisms. The 'shotgun approach' that the broad-spectrum pesticides represent is now discredited as a pest-management tool due to the indiscriminate killing of non-target species (including bees, ladybugs, and other beneficial insects) following their use.

broccoli. *Family: Cruciferae. Genus: Brassica. Species: Brassica oleracea var. italica.* Cooked frozen broccoli is similar to fresh but has slightly less vitamin C (73 mg to 100 g of the vegetable). It is a good source of fibre, potassium, vitamin A, B_2 and C, calcium, iron and potassium, and is low in calories unless of course you cheat and lavish it with sauces. Broccoli is good for constipation, toxemia, neuritis, hypertension, and to brighten up the sluggish digestive system. People with underactive thyroids should avoid it, as it exacerbates the problem.

Brodie's solution. A solution of specific gravity of 1.033 so that 10,000 mm equals 1 atmospheric pressure. It contains 23 g sodium chloride and 5 g bile salts dissolved in 500 ml water, coloured with crystal violet or gentian violet, and preserved with thymol. It is used in the Warburg manometer.

broiler. Name given to the chicken that are about 10-12 weeks old and weighing about 1.2 kg. Alternative definition is: chicken 70-76 days old weighing 0.9-1.2 kg of a rapidly growing strain. At this stage the chicken is at its most rapid, and therefore economically most profitable, growth.

bromatology. Science of food (derived from the Greek word *Broma-* food).

bromelain. A protein-digesting and milk-clotting enzyme found in pineapple fruit juice and stem tissues; *Ananas comosus* (L.) Merr. Enzymes from fruit juice and stem tissue are distinguished as fruit bromelain and stem bromelain. From pineapple juice the enzyme is obtained by precipitation with acetone and also with ammonium sulphate. It is white to light-tan in colour and available as an amorphous powder. Bromelain is soluble in water (the solution being colorless to light-yellow and somewhat opalescent) but practically insoluble in alcohol, chloroform, and ether. Bromelain has molecular mass of about 33,000 and is probably the first proteolytic enzyme of plant origin to be established as a glycoprotein. Typical applications include chill-proofing of beer, as a meat tenderizer, in the preparation of precooked cereals, and the production of protein hydrolysates. Its major function performed is the hydrolysis of polypeptides, amides, and esters (especially at bonds involving basic amino acids, or leucine or glycine), yielding peptides of lower molecular mass. Fungal bromelain is a mixture of proteases from pineapple, capable of hydrolyzing both plant and animal proteins to peptides and amino acids. Depending upon conditions, the material can hydrolyze protein substrates to large or small peptides. The substance is used in meat tenderizers. In processing of proteins, it is claimed that the substance can reduce viscosity of protein solutions used in the manufacture of protein hydrosylates.

brominated oils. Brominated olive, peach, apricot kernel, soya oils, etc., used to help to stabilize emulsions of flavouring substances in soft drinks; also described as weighting oils.

brose. A Scottish dish made by pouring boiling water on oatmeal or barley meal; fish, meat or vegetables may be added.

broth. A soup made from meat or bone extractives, with vegetables, meat, farinaceous material, spices, and herbs. Legally, in the case of canned soups, the "meat nitrogen" content must be equivalent is not less than 1% protein.

brown colours. Some of the brown colours used in food industry are:

Brown FK. A mixture of the disodium salt of 1,3-diamino-4,6-di-(*p*-sulphophenylazo)benzene and the sodium salt of 2,4-diamino-5-(*p*-sulpho-phenylazo)toluene. Also known as Skipper brown.

Chocolate brown FB. The product obtained by coupling diazotized naphthionic acid with a mixture of moraine and maclurin.

Chocolate brown HT. Disodium salt of 2,4-dihydroxy - 3,5-di-(4-sulpho-1-naph-thylazo) benzyl alcohol. Chocolate brown FB and Chocolate brown HT are also known as baking browns.

brown fat. A type of adipose tissue containing small fat cells with multiple small fat droplets in their cytoplasm. Brown fat tissue is particularly abundant in rodents and in new born and hibernating animals, occurring in various parts of the body, including the axillary and neck regions. Compared to normal white fat, deposits of brown fat are more richly supplied with blood vessels and have a higher proportion of unsaturated fatty acids. They can also be more rapidly converted to heat energy, especially during arousal from hibernation and during cold stress in young animals. Since the deposits are strategically placed near major blood vessels, the heat they generate warms the blood returning to the heart. It is also postulated that brown fat turnover may be used to dispose of excess fat intake in the food, rather than increasing the white fat deposits.

brown sugar. A general term for the sugar crystals coated with molasses. They are composed of small crystals covered with a film of highly refined, dark-colored, cane-flavored syrup. On a solids basis, these sugars are always slightly more expensive than ordinary granulated sugar. They contribute characteristic colors and flavors that are considered desirable in several kinds of bakery foods.

At one time, sugar refiners produced 15 grades of brown sugars, ranging from No. 1, with a slight creamy tint, to the very dark brown No. 15. Moisture contents range from about 2% in the lightest colored type to about 4% in the darkest type. The total sugar content varies from about 95% in No. 6 to 91 in No. 13 From 1% to 5% of the sugar is present as invert. Brown sugars remain soft and easy to measure and dispense as long as their moisture content remains constant. If the sugar is exposed for weeks to atmospheres of low relative humidity, much of the water will evaporate and the sugar crystals will become cemented together. It is this familiar change that creates numerous difficulties in the commercial use of brown sugar. A bag of brown sugar that has become cemented into a solid block is very difficult to handle in the plant. To circumvent this problem, suppliers offer brown sugar syrup, brown sugar flavors (to be used with granulated sugar), and granulated brown sugar. Another expedient is to use a good grade of cane molasses in combination with granulated sucrose as a substitute for an equal quantity of brown sugar. Because of the differences in the way beet sugar is refined, molasses prepared from beets is not considered suitable for human consumption and, therefore, brown sugars can not be made from beet sugar by withdrawing partially purified sugar crystals during the refining process. The solubles found in feet extract are different, and less acceptable, than those in sugar cane juice. Some of the processing aids used in the initial stages are also different from those added in cane sugar refining. As a result of these differences, molasses obtained during beet sugar processing is not a food ingredient. Large quantities are, however, used as fermentation substrates and in animal feeds. Brown sugar can be made from beet sugar by coating the beet sugar crystals with a type of molasses made from cane.

browntop millet. *Panicum remosum.* The name given to a plant that was introduced into the US from India in 1915. There are relatively limited plantings in the southeastern states for hay and pasture. As a dividend, the seed supports wild birds (quail, doves, etc.). The plant is self-seeding, a disadvantage for use in rotation with other crops. At one time, the plant was known as German hay grass. The plant is not to be confused with browntop panicum (*Panicum culatum*), who is a native of Central and South America.

Brown-Duvel method. A method of moisture determination in food products, in which the moisture is removed from the product by heating a weighed sample, usually 0.1 kg, in oil. The moisture content is determined on the basis of the moisture removed when collected as condensed vapor or from loss of weight of sample. It is one of earliest standard methods for determining the moisture content of grain. The original method required about 1 hour to obtain the moisture content. The modified Brown-Duvel utilizes more rapid heating of sample using a higher oil temperature for heating and stirring of the oil. The oil is heated to 145°C for forages and 190°C for grains.

Brussels sprout. Family: *Cruciferae.* Genus: *Brassica.* Species: *Brassica oleracea* var. *gemmifera.* There is so little difference between cooked fresh Brussels sprouts and frozen ones that they can be regarded as nutritionally identical. They are rich in vitamins A, B and C, calcium, potassium, and also a good source of fibre; they possess a fine nutty flavour. Recommended for catarrh, obesity, constipation and pyorrhoea, Brussels sprouts are said to be good general tonic. The average composition per 100 g is: protein 3.5%; fat 0.4%; Ca 25 mg; Fe 1.0 mg; vitamin A 90μg; B_1 0.05 mg; B_2 0.12 mg; nicotinic acid 0.6 mg; vitamin C 71 mg; and food energy 0.15 MJ.

Bryophyta. A division of simple plants possessing no vascular tissue and rudimentary rootlike organs. It contains the classes Musci (mosses), and Hepaticae (liverworts). Bryophytes grow in a variety of damp habitats, such as from freshwaters to even rocky surfaces. They show a marked alteration of generations between gamete-bearing forms (gametophytes) and spore-bearing forms (sporophytes), the later being dependent on the form of water and the nutrients. The leaves, stems, and roots of the gametophyte generation are not equivalent to those of higher (vascular) plants since the whole structure is haploid.

buckeye. Genus: *Aesculus.* Family: *Hippocastanaceae* (horse chestnut family). The fruits of several species of buckeye and horse chestnut trees. The species range from shrubs to trees, they are deciduous with compound leaves. The meat of the nut is tempting, but must be leached several times before it is edible. The American Indians used the nutmeats as a starch in their diet, but records to not indicate buckeyes being used as a serious foodstuff since that time.

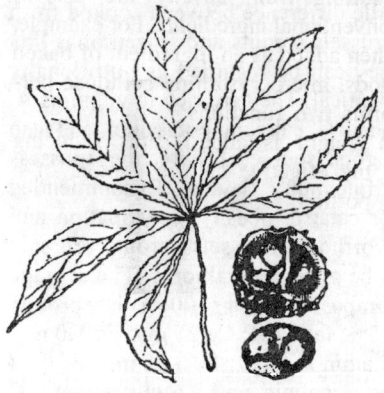

The name buckeye comes from the seed pod which has a light-brown scar resembling the partly opened eye of a buck or deer. Also known as horse chestnuts.

Buckwheat family: *Polygonaceae.* On these plants, the stem nodes have a sheathing membrane consisting of 2 fused stipules, called an ocrea. While mainly herbs, there are also a few shrubs, trees, and vines in this family. Small, wind-pollinated flowers are borne in clusters or in heads. Usually the flower is bisexual and with a variable number of parts of 3-6 sepals and petals that look alike (tepals), 6-9 stamens, and 1 pistil. The superior ovary of fused carpels has 1 chamber with 1 ovule which develops into an achene fruit. The family include: *Fagopyrum* (buckwheat), *Rheum* (rhubarb); *Antigonon* (mountain-rose vine), *Coccoloba uvifera* (sea grape), *Polygonum aubertii* (silver-lace vine), *P. sachalinene* (sacaline); *Polygonum* spp. (knotweeds, smartweeds, wild buckwheat). *Fagopyrum esculentum* is a cereal, unsuitable for bread-making, eaten as the cooked grain, porridge or pancakes. The average composition per 100 g is: protein 11%; fat 2%; carbohydrates 70%; Fe 3 mg; vitamin B_1 0.3 mg; vitamin B_2 0.3 mg; nicotinic acid 3 mg; and food energy 1.5 MJ. Also known as Saracen corn, when cooked, as Kasha (Russian).

buddeizing. A method to prolong the keeping quality of milk and to render milk safe by means other than heat. It consists of adding 12 ml of hydrogen peroxide to 1 quart of milk and keeping the mixture at 52°C. for several hours. The majority of bacteria are destroyed, but a small excess of hydrogen peroxide imparts a disagreeable bitter taste to the milk. This can be overcome by adding a catalase. The method is too complicated to be of practical value.

budding yeast. A kind of yeast that can reproduce by budding as well as by sexual means. The common budding yeast used for baking and brewing is *Saccharomyces cerevisiae.*

buffer. An acid-base balancing or control reaction by which the pH of a solution is protected from major change when acid or bases are added to it. The protection is afforded by the presence in the solution of a weak acid and related salt; for example, acetic acid and sodium acetate (acidic buffer); or ammonium chloride and ammonia (basic buffer), which maintain the equilibrium by means of the ion transfer and neutralization. The same effect can be obtained by use of a blend of two acid salts such as phosphates, carbonates, and ammonium salts; which are common buffering agents.

The ability to prevent large changes in pH is an important property of most intact biological organisms. The cytoplasmic fluid which contain dissolved proteins, organic substrates, and inorganic salts resist excessive changes in pH. The blood plasma is a highly effective buffer solution almost ideally designed to keep the range of pH of the blood between 7.2-7.3. In animals a complex and vital buffer system is found in the circulating blood. The components of this system are CO_2-HCO_3^-; Na_2HPO_4; the oxygenated and nonoxygenated forms of haemoglobin, and the plasma proteins.

bulgar. Family: *Gramineae*. Genus: *Triticum*. Species: *Triticum vulgare*. Prepared, precooked wheat originating in the Near East. Wheat is soaked, cooked and dried; it is lightly milled to remove the outer bran and cracked. Eaten with soups, cooked with meat, etc. Bulgur is the oldest processed food known. Bulgar wheat retains much of original nutritional content of the whole-wheat grain. It is easy to digest and therefore invaluable for young children and invalids. It is a good source of iron and phosphorus and contains trace of the B vitamins. Also called ala; American rice; when cooked with meat, it is called Kibbe.

Bulgarian buttermilk. A type of buttermilk, similar in its method of manufacture to *Acidophilus* buttermilk, this product is made with a culture of *Lactobacillus bulgaricus*. It has been shown that *L. bulgaricus* is not readily implanted in the intestine as claimed for *L. acidophilus*. Although the bacteria can produce a milk with a titrable acidity up to 4%, any drink containing more than 1.25% titrable acidity is less than palatable.

bulkhead. A partition of wood, concrete, or metal, usually at the end of a container used for drying or storage, to retain the products.

bulking agents. These substances are added to semiliquid and solid food products to add bulk to the end product over and beyond the bulk resulting from strictly the use of conventional ingredients. For example, when added as an ingredient of baked foods, microcrystalline cellulose performs two functions:

(a) Weight is added, thus reducing the effective caloric content of a portion; and

(b) water is tied up so that considerably more liquid can be incorporated into the formulation.

However, it should be stressed that microcrystalline cellulose can only partially substitute for fat, which is needed for air entrapment, or flour which provides the elastic gluten structure. As an additional advantage, crude fibre content of the product is increased. In the manufacture of low-calorie foods, a bulking agent essentially can be considered as a diluent even though it may play other important roles. Thus, the diet-conscious consumer can eat cookies, doughnuts, or portions of cake of traditional size, and yet consume considerably fewer calories.

The important factor in selecting a bulking agent for low-calories foods is that of finding a substance that combines noncaloric qualities with other functional capabilities so that lower amounts of relatively high-calorie ingredients can be reduced or replaced without detracting drastically from the consumer appeals of the finished product. Commonly used bodying and bulking agents include cellulose (microcrystalline); glycerine, methylcellulose; sodium carboxymethylcellulose; PVP (polyvinylpyrrolidone; povidone; and poly[1-(2-oxo-1-pyrrolidinyl)-ethylene].

bulk temperature. The average temperature of the mass of a product, usually as would occur in a bin dryer, bulk storage, or flowing mass. To determine the temperatures, thermocouples may be placed at appropriate locations in the mass such that average readings will represent the bulk temperature. The bulk temperature in the free stream is the weighted mean of the temperature of a cross-section of fluid.

bulk ventilation dryer. A unit for removing moisture from grain, forage, or aggregates in which the air is directed by ducts or an open (slotted, perforated, mesh) floor through the product, usually in large batches, usually without moving the product during or after drying.

burdock. *Arctium lappa.* There are basically two kinds of burdock. Common burdock (*A. minus*) is the kind more commonly found intercropped with corn and wheat in the Midwest. On the other hand, greater burdock is the one primarily harvested for its root as an important source of food for the Japanese. They use it there as we use carrots here. This variety of burdock has big, round, brown bristle burrs, hence common name of cocklebur.

burghu. Alternative name for bulgur.

Burgundy wines. A range of red and white wines made in the Burgundy region of France, south-east of Paris. Because of tight governmental regulations, not all wines grown in the region may carry the name Burgundy. A Burgundy wine is made from specified superior varieties of grapes and in specific townships of the district. Red Burgundies are made from the Pinot Noir grape and white Burgundies from the Chardonnay grape. Juice of Pinot Noir is colourless, the colour of the red Burgundy wine resulting from fermentation taking place in the presence of the skins. One stretch of hillside vineyards extends from close to Dijon southward and past Beaune and is known as the Golden Slope. The wines from these vineyards were responsible decades ago for generating the high international regard enjoyed by Burgundy wines. Over the past several years, wine production in Burgundy has declined and obtained exceptionally fine Burgundy wines has become increasingly difficult. Outside France, as its the case in the United States, the term Burgundy essentially has become a generic reference for any red wine, regardless of grape used, characteristics, or location of vineyard. For example, sweet red wines from New York State and the Midwest have been called Burgundies. The California wines labelled Burgundy, however, are usually prepared from varieties of European grapes. It has been observed that Burgundy and Claret have been bottled out of the same tank. Closer to the characteristics of the French Burgundies are wines designated as Chardonny, Pinot Blanc, Pinot Noir, and Gamay-Beaujolais.

Burri method. A method for estimating the number of bacteria in milk. It consists essentially in using a loop for measuring the milk and smearing the contents of the loop on dry agar slants. After incubation at the temperature desired, the colonies on the slants are counted. In as much as 0.001 ml of milk is used as the original inoculum, the number of colonies found on the slant is multiplied by 1,000 to give the total count per ml of milk being examined.

Burton. A bitter ale made at Burton-on-Trent out of water having a great deal of permanent hardness. Many breweries try to imitate Burton beers by the artificial addition of salts to the normal water supply. The 'Burtonization' of water is usually accomplished by the addition of calcium sulphate to the hot liquor tanks along with small quantities of sodium chloride. In view of the difficulties in dissolving the calcium sulphate completely resulting in variation in the salt content in the liquor, some breweries prefer to 'Burtonize' their beer by adding calcium chloride and sodium sulphate to the brewer liquor.

busa. A fermented milk beverage of Turkey produced by the growth of lactobacilli (*L. bulgaricus*), yeasts, and streptococci (*S. lactis*) in the milk. The sour, flavoured product is similar to Yoghurt, Kefir, Koumiss, Leben.

butter bean. Common designation in the US for the lima bean, although it is sometimes used to identify any garden bean of a yellow color. In particular, the name applies to the baby lima bean.

butter colour. A material used in artificially colouring butter when the colour naturally present is insufficient to satisfy the trade. The colouring principle in butter colours is of either vegetable or mineral origin. The former is derived from the seed pod of the annatto plant while the latter is derived from harmless oil-soluble coal tar dyes. The medium carrying the colouring principle is a neutral oil such as corn oil or cotton-seed oil. Only two coal tar colours are used for tinting butter. They are FDC#3 (1-Phenylazo-2-naphthylamine), and FDC #4 (1-*o*-Tolyazo-2-naphthylamine), both certified as harmless and suitable for use as food colouring by the Federal Food and Drug Administration of United States.

butter defects. Some of the principal defects associated with the properties of butter are:

Brittle Texture. (Crumbly Texture). A defect of butter characterized by crumbliness of the butter which makes it difficult to cut. It is believed to be caused by the abnormal firmness and short grain characteristic of winter butter and by processing and storing at low temperatures.

Briny flavour. A flavour defect of butter characterized by a salty taste resulting from failure to incorporate salt and water satisfactorily.

Carton flavour. A flavour defect of butter sold in cartons or parchment wraps heavily inked. A disagreeable oily flavour caused by the linseed oil in the ink used for printing and absorbed by the butter. Danger of carton flavour might be completely eliminated by drying all cartons before applying paraffin.

Cheddar cheese flavour. A butter defect caused by sour curdy cream, or by over-ripened cream (thin cream especially), or by the use of an over-ripe curd starter. Prevention lies mainly in improving the quality of the cream and the starter. The flavour is not volatilizable and cannot be removed after it has once appeared.

Cheesy flavour. A defect of butter caused by excessive bacterial action in cream or starter, especially during the hot summer months. The presence of excessive amounts of buttermilk may also lead to this defect. Large numbers of yeasts and molds often cause distinct flavours resembling Limburger cheese and Roquefort cheese. The common cheesy flavour resembles cheddar cheese.

Cloudy brine. A serious defect of butter evident from the appearance of milky water droplets on the trier. This defect is usually caused by over-churning which prevents proper washing of the buttermilk from the butter.

Coarse flavour. A term to indicate butter that lacks the delicate flavour and aroma of good butter, and yet has no specific off-flavour. Coarse flavour is usually caused by a high acid cream, over-ripened cream, over-ripened starter excessive salt, or butter in which the salt was not properly incorporated.

Colour specks. A defect caused by the particles of colour not evenly distributed in the butter.

Cooked flavour. A butter defect generally thought of as a custard flavour. It is caused by pasteurizing cream at a very high temperature. This flavour is most commonly noticed in freshly churned butter which has been made from pasteurized cream. It is not considered objectionable and is permitted in butter scored as high, i.e., 93. This flavour usually disappears when butter has been in storage for a little while. *Fishiness,*

Fishy flavour. A flavour defect of dairy products, particularly butter. It very closely resembles salted mackerel. The compound, trimethylamine, responsible for this flavour is a colourless liquefiable gas of the fishy, ammoniacal odour, soluble in water, alcohol, and ether. It results from the hydrolysis of the lecithin in the butter or other milk product and the oxidation of the liberated choline. The presence of salt, acid, copper and iron accelerates this defect.

Gasoline flavour. A rather uncommon off-flavour in butter. Its presence is easily detected, especially when the sample is heated. The flavour is due to the presence of gasoline or kerosene in the cream from which the butter was made.

Greasy texture. A body defect of butter. When a sample is taken into the mouth it leaves a greasy sensation. Due quite often to overworking soft butter.

Gritty salt. A kind of butter defect caused by the presence of undissolved particles of salt, resulting from improperly working the salt into the butter, the addition of dry salt to soft butter before working, use of salt of slow solubility.

Gummy bodied butter. A kind of butter defect indicated by the tendency to stick to the roof of the mouth and it gives a gum-like impression. It is due to abnormally firm condition of the butterfat. It is more prevalent in sections where cottonseed products are fed as the protein supplement in the dairy ration. This defect is not too serious but it does interfere somewhat with the spreading ability of the product.

Leaky body. A kind of butter defect indicated by a wet appearance and, when bored, shows large breads of water on the plug and a wet trier. Leaky butter generally originates from cream not held long enough at churning temperature followed by improper methods of washing and working.

Mealy texture. A body defect of butter characterized by a grainy, corn meal type character, noticeable when tasting. Mealiness in butter is usually the result of one of two conditions: ether a hardened condition of the casein particles brought about by improper neutralization with lime, or oiling off due to freezing of the cream and subsequent melting in too hot water, or inadequate agitation during pasteurization and holding.

butter extender. A product which when blended with one pound of butter will make up to two one pound of butter will make up to two pounds of butter spread, depending on amount used. The extender is composed of gelatinized starch, certified colour, rennet, powdered buttermilk and salt. This is mixed with lukewarm milk then blended with the butter and cooled. Not much used and generally confined to home blending.

butter flavour. The various flavours of associated with butter and related dairy products are:

Metallic flavour. Indicative of the flavour of metal. It gives a slightly puckery feeling to the mouth. This flavour may be detected as soon as the butter is placed in the mouth but the flavour becomes more intense as the sample is melted on the palate. Metallic flavour is generally attributed to the holding of sour cream in copper or iron lined salts. It is thought that the butter. Quite often this flavour is traced to old, rusty cans or cans from which the tin has been worn off. The flavour is rather objectionable.

Mottled butter. Butter which is streaked and uneven in colour. This condition appears as the result of an uneven distribution of water droplets in salted butter because of insufficient or uneven working. Large droplets from in the presence of salt giving a deeper translucent colour.

Musty flavour. A kind of flavour defect of butter and often of other dairy products, characterized by lack of freshness. This kind of flavour resembles the odour of poorly ventilated area. Usually the flavour is most noticeable when the sample has been expectorated.

Neutralizer flavour. A flavour defect of butter and other dairy products wherein the standardization of the acid present has been improperly done. The presence of a soapy or washing powder flavour suggests the use of soda types, while a bitter taste remains on the tongue when calcium and magnesium neutralizers are used.

Oily flavour. A term used to designate a flavour defect in butter brought about by oxidation of the butterfat.

Old cream flavour. A common defect of butter brought about by the use of cream of poor quality. It may later develop into more serious off-flavours.

Onion or garlic flavour. Detected by the distinctive flavour of onion that becomes more intense after holding the sample in the mouth. It is very objectionable in butter and are score is cut as much as 15 points in flavour when this defect is present.

Rancid flavour. Hydrolysis splits butyrin into butyric acid and glycerin causing the strong pungent flavour and odour in butter which is typical of butyric acid. Commonly caused by improper pasteurization or recontamination with raw cream containing the enzyme lipase and other fat splitting substances.

Salvy texture. A body defect of butter. It is characterized by a lack of grain or texture. The bore fails to show a sharp, even edge, but rather like one cut with a dull knife. Such butter often has a smeary feel to the palate.

Short-grained texture. Butter in which the fat globules are small and firm so that they do not pack and cohere readily. Short-grained butter is of brittle or crumbly texture, which is more common in butter made in winter than in summer, due to the predominance of high melting point fat in winter feeds and the relatively small globules in the advanced periods of lactation. Freezing and subsequent improper thawing may be contributing causes also, due to the loss of colloidal binding properties in frozen casein, and the oiling off of fat. Exposure of butter to low temperatures near the freezing point is another factor. Linseed meal, gluten feed, and other feeds containing low melting point fats, if fed to the cows, will help to correct the defect as will succulent roughage. Brittleness may be avoided by churning, washing and working the butter at temperatures high enough to secure a fairly soft butter that binds and is readily compacted. Avoiding excessively low temperatures during holding and cooling is important.

Sticky texture. A texture defect of butter characterized by the product's sticking to the knife rather than cutting clean. Stickiness is caused primarily by the predominance of hard fats and is most common during the winter months. Lack of succulent feeds, and in areas where alfalfa hay is a major roughage, stickiness often develops. Avoiding holding cream at low temperatures and churning immediately after pasteurization is quite helpful.

Storage flavour. A common off-flavour of dairy products which are frequently held in storage for a long time develop the characteristic flavour. There is a lack of freshness. The flavour seems to be retarded and is observed generally during the latter part of the tasting routine. Many people compare this to a woody taste.

Surface taint. A flavour defect of butter characterized by an offensive, putrid odour and taste. This defect begins on the surface of butter and is often classed as a cheesy flavour. Proper pasteurization, sanitation and a clean water supply are necessary precautions.

Tallowiness. The taste and odour of spoiled tallow in butter, a defect which renders butter unfit for the market. A bleached colour accompanies this flavour development. Tallowiness is due to a decomposition of the butterfat but, unlike rancidity which is due to hydrolysis of the fats, tallowiness is due to oxidation. It may be caused by:

(a) exposure to air, light, or heat;
(b) metals and metallic salts;
(c) excess lactose; and
(d) excess neutralizer.

It may be prevented by:

(i) not exposing the butter either in the process of being made or in storage to air, light, and heat.
(ii) using bright, non-rusty cans for cream and using only wrappers which are free from metallic rusts.
(iii) making butter under the proper conditions with a normal amount of acidity.
(iv) careful standardization of the entire operation of neutralizing to prevent over-neutralization. Also, the butter should be protected against contact with alkalies.

Unclean or "dish-ratty" flavour. This flavour manifests itself by an unpleasant odour which becomes rather intensified as the sample is melted. Some describe this odour as somewhat similar to the one gets from poorly washed cans with the lid closed tight. Sometimes the odour is spoken of as utensil flavour. In most cases it strongly indicates poor sanitary care of utensils, cans or milk machine equipment with which the milk, cream or butter has come in contact.

Wavy butter. A colour defect of butter indicating the incomplete mixing of two butters having a different shade of colour or uneven working of the butter.

Weak body. In butter this often yields an imperfect plug, there being a tendency for the butter to stick to the trier and it is difficult to break the plug clear. It also has a greasy appearance. Weak body is thought to be due to incomplete fat crystallization which results in an excess of liquid fat in the butter. It may also be due to incomplete cooling of the cream after pasteurization or to too large a percentage of low-melting glycerides in the butterfat.

Woody flavour. A flavour defect of butter. The flavour may resemble the fragrant, sometimes piney, odour of a new churn. It may have the freshness of new hardwood or may have somewhat musty odour of decayed wood.

Yeasty flavour. In butter this is easily observed particularly in the early stages of development because it gives a typical fruity, slightly fragrant aroma particularly noticeable when the sample is first taken into the mouth. More careful tasting gives a rather distinctive yeasty flavour. Yeasty flavour is most often encountered in butter made in hot summer months and is due to the by-products formed by yeast growing in the cream, inasmuch as the cream from which the butter was made had undergone decomposition.

buttercup family. *Ranunculaceae.* The plants in this primitive family are mostly herbs with a few woody vines. They prefer moist habitats. The leaves are usually alternate and palmately compound and, typically, the flower is bisexual with spirally arranged parts. There are usually 5 sepals (may be 3 to many) and 5 petals or varying numbers or none. The petals sometimes serve as nectaries. The ovary is superior with 1 to many carpels and 1 to many ovules in parietal placentation. Fruit types are follicles, achenes, berries, and capsules. The family includes: *Aconitum* (monkshood, extremely poisonous), *Anemone* (windflower), *Anemonella* (rue aneumone), *Aquilegia* (columbine), *Caltha* (marsh marigold), *Clematis, Cimicifuga* (bugbane), *Delphinium* (larkspur),

Helleborus (Christmas rose), *Helpatica, Hydrastis* (golden seal), *Paeonia, Ranunculus* (buttercup), *Thalictrum* (meadow rue).

butter granules. Small particles of butter which form in the churn toward the end of the churning process and are indicative of the completion of the churning. The churn is usually stopped when these granules are the size of wheat or corn kernels.

butterhead lettuce. A variety of lettuce characterized by soft pliable leaves, which barely overlap to form a head. The butterhead cultivars are smaller and softer than the crisphead type. The veins, midribs, and stem are smaller and less prominent than those of crisphead-type lettuce. It is difficult to ship butterhead-type lettuce long distances without losses due to mechanical damage and breakdown of the delicate leaf tissue. For this reason, this lettuce is usually grown in market garden areas close to cities. The main butterhead lettuce cultivars are White Boston; Big Boston; Bibb; and Buttercrunch.

buttermilk cheese. The cheese is made from the curd of buttermilk and is somewhat finer grained than cottage cheese, which it closely resembles. Buttermilk with an acidity of 0.5-0.6% is run into a steam-heated vat or starter can, or into a pail which can be heated in a tub of hot water. The buttermilk is stirred, heated to a temperature of 23.9-25.6°C, covered, and left for 1.5-2 hours. The temperature is then raised to 60°C, and in about an hour the curd settles to the bottom. The whey is removed and the curd is transferred to a cloth to drain for about 10 hours. It should be stirred occasionally while draining. When dry, the curd is salted, and wrapped in parchment paper. In an attempt to utilize sweet buttermilk in cheese-making, sometimes about 10% of the sweet buttermilk is added to milk used in making cheese by the Cheddar method. Cheese made in this way is said to ripen faster than Cheddar cheese. It is illegal to add buttermilk to Cheddar cheese milk in many countries.

butter oil (north process). A patented process by which butter oil is extracted directly from cream without the necessity of first churning the cream into butter. The undesirable curd material is eliminated by running the nearly churned cream into hot water, thus causing precipitation and settling of the curd. The oil is purified by centrifugation method.

butter oil with bland flavour. A form of dehydrated butter much used in the confectionery industry. The proteins and other constituents are first removed by coagulation and staining; the oil then is heated not higher than 110°C to prevent any cooked taste. The natural antioxidants normally in the butter are transferred to the oil to give it a bland, uncooked flavour.

butter scores. *93 Score Butter.* This type of butter shall posses fine flavour. It may possess a very slightly normal feed or slightly cooked flavour. It is made from cream to which a culture (starter) may or may not have been added. The total permitted defects in body, colour, and salt are limited to a rating of one-half.

92 Score Butter. This type of butter shall possess a pleasing flavour. It may possess a slightly normal feed, slightly storage, slightly heated cream (summer defect), slightly flat, slightly coarse-acid, or a definitely cooked flavour. The total permitted defects in body, colour, and salt are limited to a rating of one-half unless the flavour rating is sufficiently high to permit the total ratings for defects in these factors to exceed one-half; provided, however, that the total ratings for defects in body, colour, and salt do not exceed one in 92 score butter regardless of the flavour rating.

91 Score Butter. This type of butter shall possess a fairly pleasing flavour. It may possess any of the following flavours if present only to a slight degree: acidity, utensil, scorched, neutralizer, aged (butter), greasy, woody, bitter, and old-cream. It may possess any of the following flavours even when present to definite degree: storage, normal feed, heated cream (summer defect), flat, coarse-acid, and smothered. The total permitted defects in body, colour and salt are limited to a rating of one-half unless the flavour rating is sufficiently high to permit the total ratings of defects in the factors to exceed one-half.

90 Score Butter. This type of butter may possess a fairly pleasing flavour. It may possess any of the following flavours if present only to a slight degree: cabbage, turnip, potato, rape, weedy (ordinary-common), and musty. It may possess any of the following flavours even when present to definite degree: acidity, utensils, scorched, neutralizer, aged (butter), greasy, woody, bitter, old-cream, The total permitted defects in body, colour, and salt are limited to a ratings for defects in these factors to exceed one-half.

89 Score Butter. Such butter may possess any of the following flavours if present only to a slight degree: Fruity, yeasty, cheesy, oily, metallic, and barny. It may possess any of the following flavours even when present to a definite degree: Sour, sorched-neutralizer, scorched-old cream, alkaline, cabbage, turnip, potato, rape, weedy (ordinary-common), musty, and sale-cream. The total permitted defects in body, colour, and salt are limited to a rating of the one unless the flavour rating is sufficiently high to permit the total ratings for defects in these factors to exceed one.

88 Score Buttery. This type of butter may possess a slightly obnoxious weed flavour or any of the following flavours even when present to a definite degree: Fruity, yeasty, cheesy, oily, metallic, cabbage, turnip, potato, rape, and barny. It may possess any of the following flavours even when present to a pronounced degree: Alkaline, musty, and stale-cream. The total permitted defects in body, colour, and salt are limited to a rating of one unless the flavour rating is sufficiently high to permit the total ratings for defects in these factors to exceed one.

87 Score Butter. This type of butter may possess a fishy, onion and garlic flavour if present only to a slight degree. It may posses an obnoxious weed and barny flavour even when present to a definite degree. It may also possess a yeasty and cheesy flavour when present to pronounced degree, and a stale-cream flavour when present to a very pronounced degree. The total permitted defects in body, colour, and salt are limited to a rating of two unless the flavour rating is sufficiently high to permit the total ratings for defects in these factors to exceed two.

86 Score Butter. This type of butter may possess any of the following flavours: Definitely fishy, definitely onion or garlic, and pronominally obnoxious weeds. The total permitted defects in body, colour, and salt are limited to a rating of two unless the flavour rating is sufficiently high to permit the total ratings for defects in these factors to exceed two.

85 Score Butter. This type of butter may possess a pronominally obnoxious weed, onion, and garlic flavour. The total permitted defects in body, colour, and salt are limited to a rating of three unless the flavour rating is sufficiently high to permit the total ratings for defects in these factors to exceed three."

butter spreads. Butter mixed with other food products in a way as to increase the quantity of resulting product.

butter yellow. *p*-dimethyl-aminoazobenzene; a food colour. According to the U.S. Food and Drug Administration, this dye should not be used as a food colour and may not be certified for such use. Only those coal tar dyes which are certified by the Food and Drug Administration as suitable for use in foods may legally be added to foodstuffs.

butter, dehydrated. Butter which has had its water content removed in order to prevent rancidity. The butter is first melted, then the fat is floated off the water and serum; the oil is then centrifuged to remove curd and water. Final drying to remove last traces of water, oxygen and other gasses is done in vacuum, under agitation. The oil flows into containers. The head space is filled with nitrogen and the container is sealed. This butter can easily be reconstituted by the addition of skim milk, water and salt. The New Zealand process is as described below:

The unsalted whey butter is melted over a jet of steam. The melted fat and condensed steam are run into cylinder which automatically separates the water that settles out by gravity from the butter-fat-water mixture. The fat is then run through cream separators, and finally goes through vacreator for final dehydration.

butter, dry. A term generally used to indicate the condition of butter which has been correctly worked in the churn until it appears "dry", that is, until no water droplets can be pressed from a lump of butter between two paddles. A product prepared thus far only experimentally. To produce butter, only water need be added to the dry material and the ingredients stirred and chilled.

butter, black. Butter that has been browned by heating then vinegar, salt, pepper or other seasoning added, and used as a sauce.

butter, renovated. Butter that has been melted and rechurned with the addition of milk, cream or water.

butter, whey. Made from the small amount of fat left in whey. It has a fatty acid composition slightly different from that of ordinary butter. Also known as serum butter.

butter. The product obtained from cream by souring it naturally or with bacterial culture (starter) and churning. Legally in UK must contain not less than 80% fat (may be 78% if salt added), not more than 2% other milk solids and not more than 16% water; usually contains 1% protein, 0.4% lactose, 1.5-4.5% salt and coloured with annatto. The vitamin A content varies between 500 μg per 100 g in winter and 1350 μg in summer; the vitamin D content is up to 1 mg. Butter has mainly two basic forms:

(a) Sweet cream butter, which is manufactured without the addition of a selected bacterial culture; and

(b) a cultured butter product. When lactic cultures are used in butter manufacture, they enhance the basically bland flavor of sweet cream butter.

buttermilk powder. Buttermilk from which most of the water has been removed by heat or vacuum process. It is used by bakers; also for livestock feeding. The approximately composition is: water 1.9%; protein 38.7%; fat 5.8%; lactose 39.9%; mineral matter 7.7%; lactic Acid 5.9%. Also known as dry buttermilk.

buttermilk, condensed. Creamery buttermilk which has been ripened to an acidity of 1-1.8% and then condensed at a ratio of approximately 3-3.5 kg of buttermilk to one kg of the condensed product. Condensed buttermilk is a valuable feed for hogs and poultry. It contains approximately 28% total solids. The average composition is: water 65-70%; protein 10.4-14%; fat 0.3-2.0%; lactose 15-18%; mineral matter 2.1-2.8%; lactic acid 4.5-6.0

buttermilk, cultured. It is prepared by pasteurizing milk at a temperature of approximately 65°C for 30 minutes and then adding a starter (a mixture of bacteria that will produce the desired flavour and quantity of lactic acid). The milk is held at approximately 25°C until sufficient acid has developed, then stirred to break up the curd. Generally a small amount of cream is added. Approximately between 1-2% of fat. This greatly improves the flavour. To more closely imitate natural buttermilk some makers add a small amount of melted butter which is sometimes sprayed into the product. Some prefer to add a small amount of milk or cream that has been churned until small butter particles appear. Buttermilk or "cultured buttermilk" drinks are very popular in many parts of the world.

buttermilk, semi-solid. Buttermilk which has been ripened to an acidity to about 1.6% to 2.0%, then heated and condensed in vacuum pans until it reaches a concentration of from 3:1 to 4:1. It is packed in barrels and sold as hog and chicken feed. A smaller proportion is sold to bakeries, confectioneries, and various food manufacturers. The ingredients of product are: water 65-70%; fat 0.3-2.0%; protein 10.5-14.0%; milk sugar 15-18%; acid 4.5-6.0; mineral matter 2.1-2.8%.

buttermilk cheese. A cottage cheese made from raw, sour cream buttermilk, or from sweet cream buttermilk to which a starter has been added. It may also be made from sour, pasteurized cream buttermilk, in which case the curd formed is chalky and must be recovered from the whey by means of a centrifuge; or the curd may be recovered by first dissolving with lye the fine curds formed by pasteurization, and then precipitating the curd again with hydrochloric acid. The flavour may be sharp and acid.

buttermilk. Residue left after churning butter, 0.1-2.0% fat, with the other milk constituents proportionately increased. It has a slightly acid flavour together with a distinctive flavour due to diacetyl and related substances.

butylated hydroxyanisole. An antioxidant, used for fats and fatty foods, derived chemically from phenol, not destroyed by heat and therefore useful in baked products: active at concentration of 0.01-0.1%.

butyric acid bacteria, test for. Approximately 10 ml of milk is placed in each of three test tubes. These samples are heated for 20 minutes at about 75° C for two days. If butyric acid is present the samples will have a noted pinkish colour at the surface and there will also be a characteristic smell of butyric acid. The test is not very sensitive but if two of the three tubes show no characteristic colour or smell, it may be concluded that the milk is fairly free from bacteria producing excessive amounts of butyric acid.

butyric fermentation. Type of oxidative fermentation of hexoses, such as that of glucose, caused by *Bacillus butylicus*, leading to decomposition of carbohydrate with formation, of *n*-butanol, butyric acid, ethanol, formic acid, acetic acid, lactic acid and carbon dioxide.

bynin. Name given to an alcohol soluble protein of malt; later shown to be identical with the alcohol-soluble protein of barley and the name was abandoned.

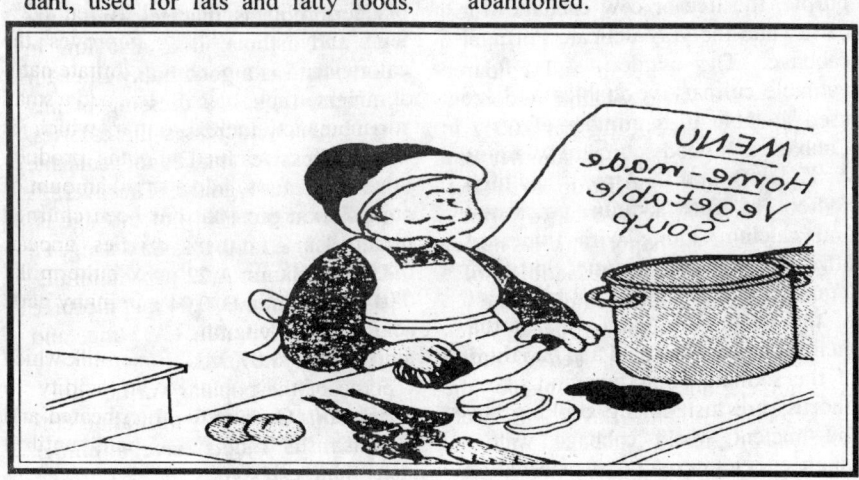

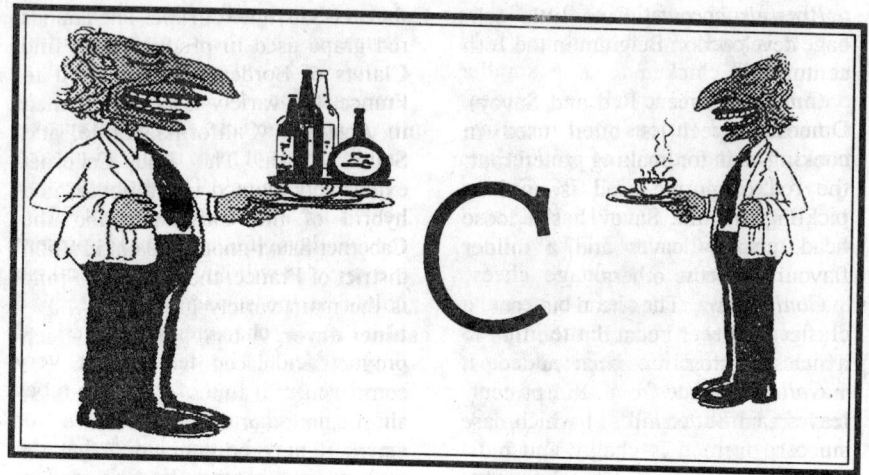

cabbage. Family: *Cruciferae*. Genus: *Brassica*. Species: *Brassica oleracea*. A common garden vegetable cultivated for its edible leaves, which in the common varieties are crowded together in dense heads. The kinds most cultivated are the common cabbage, the savoy, the broccoli and the cauliflower. The common cabbage forms its leaves into heads or bolls, the inner leaves being nearly white. Its varieties are the white, the red or purple, the tree or cow cabbage, for cattle, and the very delicate Portugal cabbage. The garden sorts form valuable culinary vegetables and are used at table in a number of ways. Cabbage is a good source of vitamins A, C, B_2, B_3 and D. Also, it has high content of iron, sodium, potassium and calcium, along with traces of other elements such as zinc. However, a quarter of the original calories, half of the vitamin B and C, all of the vitamin B_6 and folic acid and one third of the sodium, potassium and phosphorus, are lost during cooking. In the ancient world cabbage water, taken either internally or externally,

was considered a panacea capable of alleviating everything from freckles to drunkenness, and some even went so far as to say the mere act of slicing it made one feel better. Nowadays we acknowledge its muscle-building and blood-purifying properties and fresh raw cabbage juice is an excellent treatment for gastric ulcers and anaemia. The chlorine and sulphur in it cleanse the internal mucosa and so it is also helpful for kidney and bladder problems, diabetes, skin problems and asthma. It is also low in calories and is a good bulky filler for slimmers, though a dressing of any sort obviously increases the calories. Very excessive intakes of cabbage juice can cause goitre. The average composition per 100 g of cabbage is: protein 1.2%; fat 0.1%; Ca 34 mg; Fe 0.35 mg; vitamin A 22 μg; vitamin B_1 0.04 mg; vitamin B_2 0.04 mg; nicotinic acid 0.2 mg; vitamin C 35 mg; and food energy 0.07 MJ.

Some of the popular varities are:

Broccoli. Originally an Italian ethnic dish. Its shoots have a milder taste than cabbage.

Brussels sprouts. Cute little cabbage developed in Belgium in the 16th century.

Cabbage (Green, Red and Savoy). Domestic green is often used in cooking and for making sauerkraut; the red or purple kind is used in pickling and the Savoy has a loose head, crinkly leaves and a milder flavour than the others.

Cauliflower. The head is not a cluster of flower buds, but the tips of a mass of closely compacted stems.

Collards and kale. Kale has curly leaves, while collards have broad, smooth ones.

Kohlrabi. A vegetable from outer space, some say, due to its pale-green bulb with gangly tentacle-like stems sprouting from all sides.

cabbage drying. A method of .drying cabbage. Cabbage is shredded and placed on trays and dried in a two-stage tunnel dryer, with the first stage at 82.2°C with parallel air and product flow, and the second stage at 62.8°C with counter-current air and product flow with the product dried from 95 to 8% in six hours. Bin drying follows using heated air at 48.9°C to dry to 4% in 7-10 hr.

cabbage palm. A name given to various species of palm trees, because the terminal bud, which is of great size, is edible and resembles a cabbage. It is a species of the areca palm. The palmetto is a variety of cabbage palm found in the West Indies and Southern United States.

cabbage rose. A species of rose of many varieties, supposed to have been cultivated from ancient times, and eminently fitted, because of its fragrance, for the manufacture of rose water and attar. The name Provence rose is sometimes given this species.

Cabernet-Sauvignon grape. The famous red grape used in production of fine Clarets of Bordeaux. In addition to France, the variety is also cultivated in Australia, California, Chile, and South Africa. The Rub Cabernet extensively planted in California is a hybrid of the Carignane and the Cabernet-Sauvi-gnon. In Saint Emilion district of France, the Cabernet Franc is the main variety grown.

cabinet dryer. A batch dryer in which products are placed in closed box-like compartments, equipped with heated air circulation or thermal radiation for drying. The products are placed on trays or racks. Natural air circulation can be used but usually forced ventilation is used.

cacao. *See* cocao.

cachexia. An extreme state of general ill-health, with a malnutrition, wasting, anaemia, and circulatory and muscular weakness.

Cacio fiore cheese. A soft yellowish cheese with a delicate buttery flavour similar to that of Bel Paese. The whole milk is coloured with saffron and coagulated with a vegetable rennet (artichoke family). It is cut, drained on straw mats and is cured for 10 days. Also known as Caciotta cheese.

Caciocavallo Siciliano cheese. A pasta filata cheese like the Italian Provalone and Caciocavallo, essentially a pressed Provolene. It is used as a table cheese and for grating.

Caciocavallo cheese. A hard, rennet-curd, bacteria-ripened Italian cheese. it is ripened several months and is characterized by a hard sharp flavour. It is molded in the form of a ten-pin. A pasta filata type cheese identical to Provolone, except for the shape, a slightly lower fat content. and the fact that it is not smoked.

Caciotta cheese. *See* Cacio fiore.

cadmium. An element considered to be of no biological interest until the recent isolation of metal lothionein from horse kidney cortex. This is a protein complex including 2.9% cadmium and 0.6% zinc per gram of protein. Cadmium is highly toxic and three have been many cases reported of poisoning arising from cadmium derived from cadmium plated vessels. In 1858, probably the first reported cases of cadmium poisoning was described. Three servants, polishing silverware with cadmium carbonate, apparently inhaled great quantities of cadmium dust and developed respiratory and gastrointestinal problems. During the early 1900s cadmium salts were used sporadically in treating human syphilis and tuberculosis.

Cadmium is a good inhibitor of sulphhydryl enzymes. It also has affinity for other ligands in cells, such as hydroxyl, carboxyl, phosphatyl, cysteinyl and histidyl side chains of proteins, purines and porphyrin. It can disrupt pathways of oxidative phosphorylation. Cadmium interacts or competes with other metals. For example, in animal studies high dietary levels of this element have been shown to depress copper uptake and to change the distribution of tissue copper. Reduced weight gains, induced in mice and rats by excess cadmium in the diet, are largely overcome by zinc and copper supplements. It was found that rabbits fed cadmium developed hyperplastic bone marrow and a hypochromic microcytic anaemia similar to that induced by iron deficiency. The development of anaemia in other animal studies has been demonstrated also. The mechanism of this cadmium effect is not known. High intakes of cadmium, as well as zinc, copper and manganese, interfere with iron absorption possibly through competition for protein binding sites in the intestinal mucosa. In the studies with Japanese quail, an increase in plasma transferrin was noted to occur concurrently with the severe anaemia. Cadmium interference with the release of iron by transferrin has been suggested as a possible mechanism.

Cadmium has been shown to aggravate zinc deficiencies in various animals. A partial replacement of zinc by cadmium in various tissues has been reported by scientists. The investigations, wherein it was demonstrated that the sum of zinc and cadmium bound to renal metallothionein remains constant while the concentrations of the individual metals vary, suggest that these elements compete for protein-binding sites. It has been postulated that metallothionein acts as the transport protein for cadmium. industrial exposures to cadmium occur via the respiratory tract, though bad hygienic practices may result in some gastrointestinal absorption.

Inhalation of fumes or dusts containing cadmium and its compounds primarily affects the respiratory tract, but there are subsequent systemic effects as well. Some hours after exposure a dryness of the throat, a sense of constriction, a difficulty in breathing are experienced. There may be headache, vomiting, muscle cramps. Because of the delayed onset of symptoms following even massive exposures, workmen have been known to inhale fatal concentrations without experiencing much discomfort. In fatal cases, a pulmonary edema, acute inflammatory changes in the kidney, and fatty degeneration of the liver have been noted. The symptomatology of chronic cadmium poisoning was recognized only in recent years. Friberg reported that the main findings in workmen employed at an accumulator factory for over 20 years were: emphysema of the lungs, mild liver damage, anaemia, proteinuria, renal tubular damage, some dental changes, and impairment of the sense of smell (anosmia).

Ingestion of cadmium compounds produces symptoms suggestive of food poisoning of microbial origin. Nausea, salivation, vomiting, followed by diarrhoea with abdominal discomfort and pain may appear. While some cases of poisoning due to ingestion of cadmium have occurred in industry because of improper hygienic practices, most instances result from common household items. When cadmium-plated cooking utensils, ice cube trays, and coffee urns were in use, outbreaks of 'food poisoning' due to cadmium occurred with frequency. Acidic foods and beverages solubilized the cadmium plating. Cadmium-based paints can be as hazardous in the environment of a child as their lead counterparts.

Poisoning due to cadmium has been misdiagnosed as lead poisoning, primarily because of physicians' unawareness. One such case is as follows: Many years ago, a two-year-old white male, febrile, with an encephalopathy, and unconsciousness was admitted to a hospital. X-ray examination revealed the presence of radiopaque material in the abdomen. Blood and urine lead levels were not significant, being 50 μg and 250 μg 1-1, respectively. The blood cadmium was 25μg and the urinary excretion 1000 μg 1-1. History revealed that the child's parents, quite cognisant of the dangers of leaded paint, had painted his crib with a red, lead-free paint containing 0.5% cadmium. The child had chewed off most of the paint. Furthermore, he liked to lick white shoes, amply dusted with cadmium sulphate. In addition, his sisters cooked food for him in their cadmium-plated toy pans and dishes.

Cadmium is present only in minute amounts in tissues at birth, but concentrations increase as a function of age. Apart from industrial exposures, the increase in the body's cadmium burden stems from the environment. All foods, seafood, meat, milk, grains, and water contain the element. The major hazard arises when cadmium coated substances are heated, soldered, welded, or burnt and the fumes are given off. Acute poisoning due to inhalation of fumes may result in tightness of chest, dry and uncontrollable cough, headache and shivering, and in some cases even death. Chronic poisoning due to cadmium may cause shortness of breath, impaired sense of smell, loss of weight and apatite, and golden-yellow staining of teeth.

Cadmium is present in tobacco; one cigarette generally contains about 1-2 mg of cadmium. Because it is volatile at elevated temperatures, some of the metal will be inhaled during smoking. Estimates have been made of the contribution made by various types of tobacco in different countries. Typically, about 2-4 mg of cadmium per 20 cigarettes is inhaled; out of which probably 50% is deposited in the lungs.

Occupational exposure to cadmium is defined as any work involving handling, storage, use of cadmium at a concentration above the action level. In industries, the exposure to cadmium should be controlled in such a manner so that no employee is exposed to cadmium at a concentration greater than 40 mg/m^3 of air, determined as a time-weighted average (TWA) concentration limit for up to a 10-hour work shift in a 40-hour workweek, over a working lifetime. The ambient water quality criterion for cadmium is recommended to be identical to that of drinking water standard which has been set at 10 mg/L.

caeruloplasmin. A blue copper protein complex present in traces in the blood.

caffeine. An alkaloid drug (trimethylxanthine) found in coffee and tea. It raises blood pressure, stimulates kidneys and averts fatigue temporarily. Coffee beans contain about 1% caffeine, hence the beverage contains about 18 mg per cup; tea contains 1.5-2.5% caffeine, about 12-15 mg/100 ml of beverage: cola drinks contain 3-4.5 mg/100ml. It has been suggested that caffeine stimulates the expenditure of energy and the burning of fats. It has a thermogenic effect (*i.e.*, raises body heat) when taken in moderate doses on a daily basis. When caffeine is taken together with physical activity, the thermogenic effect is enhanced. The mechanism by which caffeine exerts this fat burning effect is thought to be associated with the thermogenic Cori cycle. This is where glycogen and glucose are converted to lactate in fat and muscle tissues. Lactate then triggers thermogenic processes in the liver.

caffeol. Volatile oil giving characteristic flavour and aroma to coffee.

cajeput oil. A greenish essential oil obtained by distilling the leaves of the tree *Melaleuca leucadendron*. It has camphor-like odour. It is used in medicine as an antiseptic and counterirritant, and in perfumes. Naouli oil is a similar oil from the leaves of the tree *M. viridi* of New Caledonia. Cajeput bark, from the same tree, is used as an insulating material in place of cork.

cake, sponge. A part of a recipe continuum that starts with the original formula for pound cake and continues through sponge cake and chiffon cakes to layer cakes. Some bakers call any kind of cake made with whole egg foams a sponge cake, and there is a certain logical justification and tradition behind this nomenclature, but the classification followed in this chapter is though to be more information. It is very common to find baking powder or soda plus some acidic ingredient in sponge formulas, and the shortening content is less than in a pound cake (sometimes none). A formula for sponge cake that does not contain shortening or baking powder is:

32.1% granulated sugar, 20.0% liquid whole eggs, 26.5% cake flour, 21% liquid whole or skim milk, and 0.4% salt. For maximum volume, the eggs can be beaten separately, the sugar, milk, and salt mixed in, and then the flour folded in with minimum agitation. If baking powder is to be obtained with a one-stage mixing procedure, employing the wire whip at high speed to aerate the batter. An emulsifier must be added obtain proper volume development. Flavour varieties are the same as those suggested for pound cake. Sponge cakes perform very well as the basis for jelly rolls, lady fingers, tortes, berry shells, and the like.

caking. The mixing of powdered, ground, or crushed material into a larger solid mass. The formation of cakes by applying pressure may be carried out, such as for blocks, pellets, and tablets. When it is desired to maintain the powdered dry state, caking is undesirable. Hot bagging or storing of moist or dried materials, such as sugar and dry milk powder, will increase caking and may lead to deterioration of the food product.

calabar bean. The seeds of an African plant, nearly allied to the kidney bean. It is such a powerful narcotic poison that six beans are sufficient to cause death. The calabar bean is the famous ordeal bean of Africa, administered to persons suspected of witchcraft. If the accused vomits the bean and recovers, it is a sign of innocence. It is employed in medicine, chiefly as an

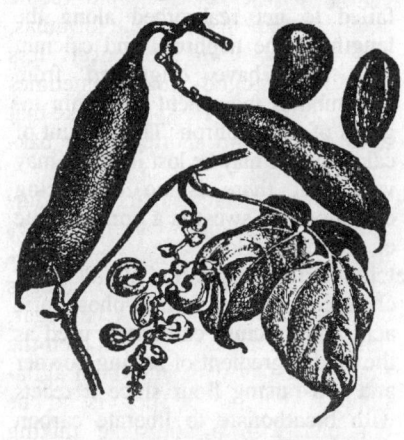

agent for producing contraction of pupil of the eye, and in the treatment of neuralgia, lockjaw and rheumatism.

calamint. A genus of plants, some species of which are known respectively by the names of mountain balm, catmint, basil balm and wild basi. The first, also termed common calamint, has aromatic leaves, employed to make herb tea.

calamondin. A citrus fruit resembling a small tangerine, with a delicate pulp and a lime-like flavour.

calciferol. Old name for ergocalciferol or vitamin D_2, made by irradiation of ergosterol.

calcium. An essential element for animal and plant growth. It is present between plant cell walls as pectate, and is found in the bones and teeth of animals. In most animals including humans, calcium absorption occurs mainly in the upper portion of the small intestine. The amount of calcium absorbed from the gut are function of intake, age, nutritional status, and health. Generally, the fraction absorbed decreases with age and intake and as nutritional status improves. The absolute amount absorbed increases with intake and may or may not decrease with age. The mechanisms by which calcium is absorbed are not well understood. Active transport of the ion against an electrochemical gradient seems to be involved, but not all of the calcium appears to be absorbed by this process, because calcium absorption continues with conditions when active transport is severely depressed, as in vitamin D deficiency. Calcium absorption can be enhanced by administration of large doses of vitamin D and is depressed in vitamin D deficiency. There is uncertainty regarding effect on calcium absorption of the parathyroid hormone, the major endocrine control of the blood calcium level. Patients with hyperparathyroidism have been shown to have higher than normal absorption and patients with hypoparathyroidism to have lower than normal absorption. Similar effects have been observed in acute animal experiments, but in most of these instances a possible indirect effect has not been excluded.

Calcium ions, Ca^{2+}, are important in triggering muscle contraction where their rapid release from the cisternae of sacroplasmic reticulum is thought to set off the reaction between ATP and the myofilaments. Calcium is important in resting muscles in maintaining the relative impermeability of the cell membranes. If calcium concentration falls, the potential difference across the membrane also falls so that muscles may spontaneously contract without activation by acetylcholine, giving twitching and spasms. The concentration of calcium ions is also important in influencing the breakdown of glycogen in muscles. Calcium is important in the clotting of blood in the conversion of prothrombin to thrombin. In mammalian stomach it is also important in precipitating casein from milk. Calcium is a dietary essential needed for the formation of bones and teeth, which are composed largely of calcium phosphate. It is present in the body in larger amounts than any other mineral (1.0-1.5 kg). The small amount circulating in the blood (9-11 mg/100 ml) and in the soft tissues plays a vital part in the metabolic processes, controls the heart beat and the excitability of muscle and nerve, plays a part in blood clotting and in the maintenance of acid-base equilibrium. A fall in the level of blood calcium results in increased sensitivity of the motor nerves to stimuli, i.e., tetany. Its absorption from food is aided by vitamin D and protein and hindered by excess fat, phosphate, oxalate and phytate; the result is that only 15-35% of dietary calcium is absorbed. Daily requirements (0.4-0.5 g) increased to 0.4-0.7 g in growing children, and 1.0-1.2 g in pregnancy and lactation. Richest sources are milk and cheese; calcium is added to flour as *creta praeparala*; eggs and vegetables are moderate sources. The chemical form in which calcium is added to foods for enrichment does not appear to be important, e.g., carbonate, phosphate, chloride, etc., appear to be equally well absorbed.

The principal routes of excretion for calcium are stool and urine. Calcium in the stool may be considered as made up of unabsorbed food calcium and nonreabsorbed digestive juice calcium. The latter is termed the faecal endogenous calcium. The proportion of fetal endogenous calcium to urinary calcium varies in different species. It is about 1:1 in human and 10:1 in the rat and in cattle. Calcium in urine may have a dual origin-calcium that was filtered at the glomerulus and failed to get reabsorbed along the length of the nephron, and calcium that may have originated from transtubular movement in certain regions of the nephron. The amount of calcium that may be lost in sweat may vary, but there is no convincing evidence that sweat is a normal route of significant loss.

calcium acid phosphate. $Ca(H_2PO_4)_2$. A chemical obtained from o-phosphoric acid and calcium carbonate, used as the acid ingredient of baking powder and self-raising flour since it reacts with bicarbonate to liberate carbon dioxide. Chemically, it is similar to superphosphate fertilizer but is much purer. Also known as monocalcium phosphate; acid calcium phosphate.

calcium gluconate. Water-soluble salt of calcium and gluconic acid useful for intravenous administration (e.g., in the relief of tetany).

calcium ionophores. Low molecular weight lipophilic compounds which are able to translocate Ca^{2+} from an aqueous phase across the intact bilayer mambrane into another aqueous compartments. Artificial Ca^{2+} ionophore is A 23187 or calimycin derived from *Streptomyces chartrensensis*. Oxidised polyunsaturated fatty acids and phosphatidic acid are endogenous Ca^{2+} ionophores, whose action increase during senescence leading to leakiness of the membranes.

calcium-phosphorus ratio. It has been suggested that a high ratio of phosphate to calcium in the diet hindered the absorption of calcium from the intestine into the blood stream and gave rise to rickets. It was thought that a Ca:P ratio of between 1:2 and 2:1 was essential for maximum absorption but this belief has been discarded.

calendula. *Calendula officinalis.* A plant having bright yellow to orange flower heads. It is prolific in numerous waste places and gardens as a hardy weed of sorts. An old folk belief says that if its flower heads should close up after 7:00 a.m., it will rain for sure the next day. Its greatest value in either salve or dilute tincture form is for any kind of external skin, muscle or blood vessel problems, wounds, sores, varicose veins, pulled muscles, boils, bruises, sprains, athlete's foot, burns, frostbite, etc.

Calfos. Trade name for a prepared bone meal, *i.e.*, calcium phosphate used as a source of calcium and of phosphate in foods.

calibration chart. A graphical representation of the value read from an instrument, usually placed on the abscissa, and the true value of the variable, usually located on the ordinate. Calibration consists of comparing an instrument to a known standard for measuring values. The instrument should be calibrated at a sufficient number of points on the scale to assure the proper relationship between measured value and indicated value. A calibration chart may be furnished with the instrument by the manufacture, or may be developed by the user after calibration.

callose. An insoluble polysaccharide which is a β-1,3-linked polymer of glucose and found in plants, particularly enveloping the connecting strands in sieve areas and sieve plates of sieve elements and around tetrads of microspores during pollen development in angiosperms. As the sieve tube ages the callose layers become thicker, eventually blocking the sieve element. Such blocking may be seasonal or permanent.

calmodiulin. A widely distributed intracellular protein that binds calcium ion with high affinity and specificity. It exists as a monomer of molecular weight 17000 daltons. It resembles, but is not identical with, the troponin C of skeletal and cardiac muscle. Binding of Ca^{2+} results in a conformational change which causes the calcium ion-calmodiulin complex to activate a number of cellular enzymes and so modulate a range of cellular functions including secretion, motility, mitosis, cyclic nucleotide metabolism and glycogen metabolism.

calorie. A unit of heat defined as the heat required to raise the temperature of one gram of water from 14.5 degree Celsius to 15.5 degree Celsius (the 15 degree calorie). Another artificial calorie, used in engineering steam tables is the International Table calorie;

1 I.T. calorie = 1/860 international watt-hour

= 0.00116298 absolute watt-hour.

The conversion of its value to other energy units gives:

1 cal. = 0.00396573 B.T.U.

1 cal. = 0.0412917 litre-atmosphere

1 cal. = 0.999346 I.T. calorie.

calorie, 15 degree. cal$_{15}$. An obsolete unit of thermal energy; in SI system, 1 cal$_{15}$ = 4.1855 J.

calories, empty. Refers to foods that supply only energy with little, if any, of the nutrients.

calorimetry. Measurement of the quantity of heat involved in various processes, such as chemical reactions, changes of state, and formation of solutions, or in determination of the heat capacities of substances. Calorimetric measurements are useful in determining important thermodynamic properties of substances, for example, heat capacity, entropy, and free energy.

calpain-1. A protease enzyme that uniquely catalyses the degradation of fodrin. Calpain may play a part in memory storage. Repeated synaptic activity at certain cortical synapses facilitates the enty of large amounts of calcium into the dendritic cytoplasm of the postsynaptic cell. Consequent activation of calpain and breakdown of fodrin cause a permanent change in the synaptic connection and expose an increased number of glutamate receptors.

Calymmatobacterium granulomatis. Encapsulated, pleomorphic, Gram-negative rods with rounded ends that occur in clusters and singly; will not grow on most bacteriological media but have been reported to grow on an egg yolk medium. It is responsible for granuloma inguinale, a chronic, indolent ulcerogra-nulomatous disease of skin and mucous membranes usually involving genitalia. In stained smears of lesions, the organisms lie intracellularly in phagocytes.

Camden process. The preservation of food by addition of sodium bisulphite which liberates sulphur dioxide. Also known as cold preservation since it replaces heat sterilization.

Camden tablets. Trade name for the tablets of sodium bisulphite; used as cheap food preservative.

camellia. A genus of plants, with showy flowers and dark green, shining, laurel-like leaves, nearly allied to the plants which yield tea. The camellia of Japan and China is a lofty tree of beautiful proportions, which is the origin of many double varieties of our gardens. Besides this species, one with small, white, scentless flowers, and another with large, peony-like flowers, are cultivated in America.

Camembert cheese. A soft rennet cheese of French origin made from cow's milk testing 3.5% fat or less. After setting and draining, the cheese is salted and mold-ripened at 20-25° C in a room with a high humidity. The ripening period is generally 4-6 weeks. The interior is yellow and waxy or creamy. the mold used in *Penicillium camemberti.*

campanula. A genus of herbs with bell-shaped flowers, usually of a blue or white color. It includes several American species which are known to all lovers of wild flowers. The harebell, also known as the bluebell of Scotland, is found on damp rocks and rocky hillsides, and is an exceedingly pretty and delicate plant. The Canterbury bell is a European species, with large tubular flowers, formerly popular in gardens.

Campbell's process. A method of drying milk by first concentrating by blowing hot air through, followed by drum-drying.

camphor. $C_{10}H_{16}O$. A whitish translucent gum with a bitterish, aromatic taste and a strong stinging odour. It is derived from the bark and wood of *Cinnamomum camphora,* belonging to the laurel family, found in various parts of the Far East. In food industry, it is used for flavouring many drinks. Camphor is used in great quantities in pharmaceuticals, disinfectants, and in the manufacture of pyroxylin, an explosive constituent. It is also used for hardening nitrocellulose plastics.

Campylobacter. A Gram-negative, curved rod which grows as a micro-aerophile. Two major species have been recognized, *C. jejuni* and *C. fetus*, and together these species are thought to account for the majority of cases of bacterial diarrhea in children. *Campylobacter* is transmitted to the humans via contaminated food, most frequently in poultry, pork, raw clams, and other shellfish, or by water route in surface waters that have not been subjected to chlorination. *Campylobacter* species also infect domestic animals such as dogs.

camu-camu. A Peruvian fruit from the bush *Myrciaria paraensis;* Burgundy red in colour. It contains about 3,000 mg vitamin C per 100 g pulp.

canapes. Small open sandwiches.

Canberra oil. Oil extracted from genetically selected variety of rapeseed with not more than 2% erucic acid.

Candida albicans. An oval, budding yeast that forms smooth, creamy colonies when grown at around room temperature, on enriched media. Under less favorable conditions, such as less nutritious medium at room temperature, pseudohyphae are formed along with the budding yeast cells. These pseudohyphae consist of very elongated budding cells in chains, resembling hyphae in a mycelium. Frequently, round, thickened spores form at the ends of its pseudohyphae. These morphological characteristics along with characteristic carbohydrate fermentation patterns are used to distinguish *C. albicans* from other yeasts. In addition, this organism produces tubelike projections called germ tubes in human serum. No other mycotic pathogen produces as diverse spectrum of disease in humans as does *C. albicans*. Most infections involve the skin or mucous membrane. It occurs because *C. albicans* is strict aerobe and finds such surfaces very suitable for growth. Cutaneous involvement usually occurs when the skin becomes overtly moist or damaged.

candied peel. A material used in confectionery; prepared by softening peel, often of citrus fruits, and boiling for prolonged periods with sugar syrup.

candle plug. A desirable plug removed from a Cheddar cheese by means of a trier, free from holes and which exhibits is slight translucence similar to a candle, hence candle plug.

candlefish. A sea fish of the salmon family, of about the size of the smelt, frequenting the northwestern shores of America. It is converted by the Indians of Alaska into a candle, simply by passing the pith of a rush or a strip of the bark of the cypress tree through it as a wick, when its extreme oiliness keeps the wick blazing. The oil is sometimes extracted and used as a substitute for cod-liver oil. Though the fish is very oily its flesh has an aggreeable flavor, and the oil itself is not unpleasant.

candy. A term used in US for sugar confectionery.

candytuft. A group of plants related to the mustard, three species of which are commonly grown in gardens. Purple candytuft is so called because of its purplish flowers, which are borne in flat-topped clustres. There are four petals to a blossom. Like other members of the group, purple candytuft has petals of irregular formation, as the two inner are shorter than the outer ones. Bitter candytuft is notable for the medicinal properties of its root, stem, leaves and seeds. Its profuse growth of pure white flowers is the distinctive characteristic of the evergreen candytuft, which is a native of warm regions.

cane sugar. Sucrose extracted from the sugar cane; identical with sucrose prepared from any other source, such as sugar beet.

canned butter. Butter packed into non-absorbent, hermetically sealed tin cans. The butter is packed in tins to prevent leakage of water and oil, and to preserve the keeping quality of the butter by exclusion of air. Canned butter is used in tropical regions.

canner's alkali. Mixture of sodium hydroxide and sodium carbonate used to remove skin from fruit before canning (sodium hydroxide alone more frequently used).

canning. A method of food preservation in which the food is placed in metal containers, hermetically sealed, and heated to 380-385K for intervals ranging from 25 to over 100 minutes, to destroy the pathogens and spoilage microorganisms. The precise time and temperature depend on the nature of the food. After heat treatment, the cans are cooled as rapidly as possible, usually with cold water.

During aseptic canning the foodstuffs are presterilised at very high temperatures for a few seconds and then sealed into cans under aseptic conditions. The flavour, colour and vitamin retention are superior with this short time-high temperature process compared with conventional canning. The rate of bacterial spore destruction is approximately multiplied tenfold for every 10°C rise in temperature while the chemical reactions responsible for loss of quality are doubled for every 10°C rise in temperature.

canthaxanthin. 4,4'-diketo-β-carotene. A brown-violet crystalline substance which imparts a red-orange to red coloration to oil solutions and aqueous dispersions. Its solubility in fats and oils ranges from 0.05-8 g/L; essentially insoluble in water. It is a red carotenoid pigment, chemically related to β-carotene but without any vitamin-A activity. It has been approved for use in foods since 1969. It has been suggested to add this compound to the diet of broiler chickens to impart a pigmented skin and shanks, and to the diet of trout to produce the bright colours of wild trout; these colours are normally derived from natural foodstuffs which may be variables in short supply. It is also widely used in the colouring of simulated meats. It has a more orange colour than β-carotene and has an unusually high tinctorial power. This makes it a good colorant for tomato products. It is commercially sold as water-dispersible formulation containing 10% canthaxanthin or as a spray-dried powder (2.5-10% canthaxanthin) in the gelatine/carbohydrate base. These products give clear aqueous solutions.

capelin. *Mallotus villosus*. A cold-water pelagic fish occurring extensively in the north Atlantic and north Pacific and adjoining regions of the Arctic. It is a soft-rayed fish and, together with the smelts, comprises the family *Osmeridae*. In the eastern Atlantic, the caplein occurs abundantly from the Trondheim Fjord region of northwestern Norway northwest to Jan Mayen, Spitzbergen, and Novaya Zemyla at the eastern extremity of the Barents Sea. Growth is greatest dur-.

ing the initial 2 years of life, after which it decreases until in the fifth year the size increment is negligible. During the first year, both male and female are the same size, but during the second year a differential growth rate sets in, favouring the male, which is from 1 to 2.5 cm larger than female at sexual maturity.

capers. Buds of unopened flowers of *Capparis* which grows from the crevices of rocks and walls and among rubbish, in the countries bordering on the Mediterranean. The buds are pickled in vinegar and used in making sauces for meats. The flower buds of the marsh marigold and nasturtium are frequently pickled and eaten as a substitute for capers.

capillary fragility. Refers to the resistance to rupture of the walls of a blood vessels, which would result in the leakage of red blood cells into the tissue spaces. There is some evidence that the flavonoids increase the resistance to rupture and this has given rise to unverified suggestions that this group of compounds will protect against the common cold by increasing the resistance of the capillaries to infection.

Capnocytophaga canimorsus. A slow growing, gliding, Gram-negative rod showing growth enhancement in carbon dioxide. It is present in saliva of normal dogs, and causes septicemia in patients with alcoholism, cancer, and other chronic conditions.

capon. Castrated cockerel; slightly increased growth with more tender flesh than the cockerel. Surgery mostly replaced by "chemical caponization", implantation of pellets of female sex hormone.

capric acid. $C_9H_{19}COOH$. One of the fatty acids occurring as triglyceride in coconut, goat and cow butter, and in the fat of the spice bush.

caproic acid. $C_5H_{11}COOH$. One of the fatty acids occurring as triglyceride in goat and cow butter and coconut fat.

caprylic acid. $C_7H_{15}COOH$. One of the fatty acids Occurring as triglyceride in goat and cow butter, coconut oil and human fat.

capsicum. A genus of annual, shrubby plants, with a wheel-shaped corolla, projecting and converging stamens and a many-seeded berry. They are chiefly natives of the East and West Indies, China, Brazil and Egypt, but they have spread to various other tropical or subtropical countries, being cultivated for their fruit, which at times reaches the size of an orange, is fleshy and variously coloured and very sharp to the taste.

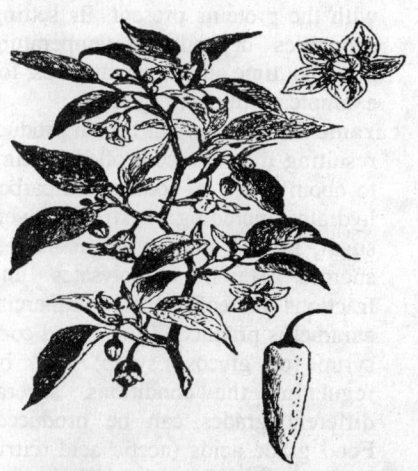

The fruit or pod is used for pickles and sauces, and also is valuable medicinally. Dried or powdered, the pods are used in making a gargle for sore throat, and they are also employed in the treatment of neuralgia and rheumatism. Cayenne pepper and chili, the favorite condiment of the

Mexicans, is prepared from a species of capsicum.

capsomer. The morphological unit, one or more of which constitute the viral capsid. The capsomer, in turn, consists of one or more structural units, or monomers. A capsomer that consists of five structural units if known as a pentagonal capsomer, or pentamer, and a capsomer that consists of six structural units is known as a hexagonal capsomer, or hexamer.

carageenan. Extract of red seaweed, *Chondrus crispus* (Irish Moss) and *Gigartina stellata;* the name is also given to extracts of other red seaweeds (*Eucheuma* and *Iridea* varieties). It is used in low-calorie jams and jellies, chocolate milk drinks, ice-cream, instant milk puddings, oil emulsions, toothpastes and processed cheese. It increases viscosity, binds water and emulsifies and stabilises by reacting with the proteins present. Its setting properties depend on temperature only, not time and temperature as, for example, with pectin gels.

caramel. An amorphous brown product resulting from the controlled heating to about 190°C of food grade carbohydrates including: dextrose, invert sugar, lactose, malt syrup, molasses, sucrose, starch hydrolysates and fractions thereof. Most commercial caramel is produced from liquid corn syrup (or glucose syrup) and, by regulating the conditions, several different grades can be produced. Food grade acids (acetic acid, citric acid, phosphoric acid sulphuric acid and sulphurous acid), alkalis (ammonium hydroxide, calcium hydroxide, potassium hydroxide and sodium hydroxide) and salts (ammonium, sodium, or potassium carbonate, bicarbonate, phosphate, sulphate or sulphite) may be employed to assist carmeliation in amounts consistent with good manufacturing. The preferred catalyst is ammonium sulphite. The chemistry of the reaction that takes place is complex, and depends not only on the starting material and its concentration but on the nature of any catalysts used and the temperature and pH of the system. There is considerable art in the manufacture of food grade caramels. Although chemical reactions are not well understood, two main types are thought to occur:

(a) Maillard reaction; and

(b) pure caramelizing reactions.

These reactions produce aldehydes and dicarbonyls of high molecular mass. All caramels are aqueous, colloidal in nature and are characterized by the electrical charges that bind the particles together. Depending on the method of manufacture, these may be either positive or negative. It is the isoelectric point, or pH at which the ionic charge is electrically neutral, which determines the most suitable end use of the product. At a pH above the isoelectric point the caramel is negatively charged, and below this pH it is positively charged.

Caramel is purchased not only by type, but by tinctorial power. This is determined either by empirical tinctometer, comparative methods or spectrophotometrically. It is now a common practice to quote the tinctorial power in terms of EBC (European Brewers Convention) units. The following grades of caramel are generally available, but in many countries caramel is manufactured for specific end uses.

Acid proof. Isoelectric point below 2.0 Single-strength, double strength, foaming and powdered (spray-dried or drum dried).

Bakers. Isoelectric point 4.0 or higher. Regular, positive-type chocolate brown, burnt sugar flavour, powdered. Caramel has been evaluated toxicologically by the Joint FAO/WHO‐Expert Committee on Food Additives and those products not made by the ammonia process are listed with an unlimited ADI, whereas caramel made by the ammonia process has been given an ADI of 100 mg/kg be based on a product having a colour intensity of 20,000 EBC units and containing not more than 200 mg/kg of 4-methyl imidazole. Being viscous, it is usual to dilute caramel products before use to facilitate handling and incorporation into product mixes. Such dilutions are readily fermentable and must be used as soon as possible after preparation. It is preferable to dilute only as much as required at the time. Brown colour prepared by heating sugar above its melting point; permitted additive to foods. It is used in cooking as a coloring and flavoring ingredient and in giving a brown colour to spirits and other liquids. The name is also applied to a certain preparation of candy. If only caramel colour is desired, without the flavour, caramelized sugar can be dissolved in a small amount of water and then alcohol added. Most of the sugar will thus precipitate out and the colour will be then be concentrated by evaporation and the colour can be added in suitable proportions to produce the light brown colour generally used in caramel ice cream or as a suitable colour for maple ice cream. Caramel colour and flavour can be brought from most of the ice cream supply houses. Also known as black Jack.

caramelization. The brown colour produced when sugars are heated or treated with acid. Sweetened fruit juices turn brown on storing at higher temperatures through carmelization. The effect is distinct from the Maillard reaction between sugar and proteins which also occurs on storage.

Carignane grape. A productive wine grape used for ordinary red table wines. Cultivated in Algeria, California, France, Israel, Italy, and Spain.

carmine. Alkaline salt of the aluminium lake of carminic acid, prepared directly from cochineal and containing not less than 50 % of carminic acid. It is a bright red pigment, which is insoluble in cold water, partially soluble in hot water and readily soluble in alkalis. The colour of the solution is dependent on the *p*H. Commercially, carmine is available as a deep red powder or as a solution in a mixture of ammonia and propylene glycol (about 0.3% carminic acid). Carmine is almost universally accepted for use as a natural food colorant consistent with good manufacturing practice.

caraway. Family: *Umbelliferae.* Genus: *Carum.* Species: *Carum carvi.* A common biennial plant, with a tapering fleshy root, a furrowed stem and white or pinkish flowers. It produces a well-known seed used by confectioners and bakers and in medicine. Caraway seeds are characterized by a spicy fragrance and an aromatic taste. Hollow, furrowed, angular, branched stem commences to grow in the second year from a white, carrot-shaped root. The leaves are bi-or tripinnate and deeply incised, the upper ones on a sheath-like petiole. The small white or yellow flowers make their appearance in the late spring. The seeds are dark brown, flat and oblong in shape. Caraway is a two-in-one plant. The bright green, feathery leaves have a mild flavour, somewhere between that of parsley and dill, while the seeds, a spice, have a strong aroma and pungent taste. The plant is grown commercially for its seed in northern Europe, the US, and North Africa. A flavouring for use in baked goods and sweets is made from the essential oil distilled from the dry, ripe seed. The leaves may be used in salads and soups, the seeds in baked goods, in dumplings, cream cheese, and meat dishes such as goulash and pork casserole. The roots can be boiled as a vegetable and served with a white sauce. The leaves, seeds, and roots can be used as an aid to digestion. Main component of the volatile oil is carvone, with smaller amounts of limonene. Caraway grown in northern climates contains noticeably less oil than that grown further south. It also contains fibre, limonene, minerals, protein and wax. The volatile oils promote digestion and prevent flatulence. For this reason, caraway is an excellent aid to digestion. It is taken for indigestion, gas, colic and nervous conditions. Simply infuse 25 g of the crushed seeds in a pint of freshly boiled water and steep for 20 minutes. Take the tea in frequent doses of 2 teaspoonfuls until relief is obtained. This is particularly useful to prevent griping in babies. Caraway is also useful for congestive bronchitis and colds in the chest. Chew 2 grams of the dried seeds, three times daily. It has in the past been used to promote the onset of menstruation, relieve uterine cramps and increase lactation.

carbohydrase. *Aspergillus niger var.* The material produced by the controlled fermentation of *Aspergillis niger* var. and is an off-white to tan amorphous powder, or a tan to dark-brown liquid. The substance is prac-

tically insoluble in alcohol, chloroform, and ether. The major active components are:
(a) α-amylase;
(b) pectinase (usually a mixture and
(c) glucoamylase (amyloglucosi-dase).
Typical applications include the preparation of starch syrups juices, chocolate syrup, bakery products, liquid coffee, wine, dextrose, and dairy products.

carbohydrase *Rhizopusoryzae var.* This is a group of enzyme preparations produced by the controlled fermentation of Rhizopus *oryzae var.*, taking the form of powders or liquids. Major active principles are :
(a) α-amylase;
(b) pectinase; and
(c) glucoamylase (amyloglucosidase).
Typical applications include the preparation of starch syrups and fruit juices, as well as the manufacture of various cheeses.

carbohydrase *Saccharomyces spp.* The purified enzyme produced by the controlled fermentation of a number of species of *Saccharomyces* traditionally used in the manufacture of various foods. The substance is a white to light brown coloured amorphous powder, which is soluble in water (the solutions usually are light in color), but practically insoluble in alcohol, chloroform, and ether. The major active principles are:
(a) invertase, and
(b) lactase.
Typical applications include the manufacture of candy and ice cream, and modification of dairy products.

carbohydrate metabolism. Breakdown of simple sugars, particularly glucose, is one of principal sources of energy for living organisms. The dissimilation may be anaerobic, as in fermentation, or aerobic, that is respiratory. In the both types of metabolism, the breakdown is accompanied by evolution of energy rich bonds, mainly the pyrophosphate bond of the coenzyme adenosine triphosphate (ATP); which serves as a coupling agent between different metabolic processes. In the higher animals, glucose is the main carbohydrate constituent of blood, which carries it to the tissue of the body. In higher plants, disaccharide sucrose if often stored and transported by the tissues. Certain polysaccharides, especially starch and glycogen, are stored as endogenous food reserves in the cells of the plants, animals, and microorganisms. Others, such as cellulose, chitin, and bacterial polysaccharides, serves as structural components of cell walls. As constituents of animals and plant tissues, various carbohydrates become available to those organisms for their source of nutrients. Hence, the naturally occurring carbohydrates can be dissimilated by some animals and/or microorganisms. Starch and other digestible carbohydrates are converted into monosaccharides by a series of hydrolytic enzyme. Salivary amylase (Ptyalin) is the enzyme present in saliva. It acts upon starch to hydrolyze it to maltose because the food is swallowed rapidly not much hydrolysis occurs in the mouth. However, the activity of the enzyme continues until the low pH of gastric juice inactivate it. About 40% hydrolysis occurs before inactivation by gastric acidity. Pancreatic amylase (Amylopsin) splits starch and dextrin to maltose. Pancreatic maltase catalyzes the hydrolysis of maltose to glucose. The intestinal lactase hydrolyses lactose to glucose and galactose. Intestinal maltase hydrolyses maltose to two molecules of glucose. Intestinal sucrase hydrolyses sucrose to glucose and fructose. Only monosaccharides are absorbed and can be utilized by the body at different rate into the blood stream. After absorption they are carried by the portal circulation to the liver. In the liver, monosaccharides other than glucose are converted to glucose. This glucose may pass into general circulation or may be carried to tissues or may be converted to glycogen. This glycogen is the storage form of glucose. Glucose in tissue can be converted to muscle glycogen, which serves as a available source of energy for muscle. Lactic acid which results from glycogen breakdown is carried to liver where it is converted to liver glycogen.

carbohydrate productivity. Amount of carbohydrate produced per square metre of the area on which light is falling. It is equal to carbohydrate assimilation rate into duration of full light interception.

carbohydrates, unavailable. The term includes pentosans, pectins, hemicellulose, cellulose, lignin and gums which are not digested and gums which are not digested and therefore unavailable to monogastric animals, but some are available to ruminants.

carbohydrates. A class of compounds which are main components of plants of all types; they collectively constitute most abundant group of natural organic substance. They include both simple compounds (sugars) and polymers of these (starches and cellulose), the latter being called polysaccharides. Their molecular formula correspond to the hydrates of carbon having general formula $C_n(H_2O)_x$. These polyhydroxy aldehydes or ketones have at least one asymmetric carbon. The atoms are so arranged that each molecule contains a hydroxyl group and a carbonyl group, a structure known as a saccharose unit. Carbohydrates are a widely distributed group of natural compounds which constitute one of the three major classes of our food. Sugars, starches, and cellulose are probably the best known members of this group. Carbohydrate moieties are also found in a variety of complex substances such as glycosides, mucoproteins, and nucleic acids. Low molecular mass carbohydrates are called sugars or saccharides. They are classified as tetroses, pentoses, or hexoses, according to the number of carbon atoms present in their molecules. The aldehyde or ketone-like of most sugars leads to their further classification as aldoses or ketoses, depending up on the location of the carbonyl group in the carbon skeleton. Carbohydrates composed of chains of pentose or hexose units bonded together by ether linkages are referred to as disaccharides, trisaccharides, and in the case of large polymers as polysaccharides. Polysaccharides are also called glycans, and are polymeric substances composed of many hundreds or thousands of monosaccharide units bound together by glycoside linkages. Some of these compounds provide structural rigidity and strength to plants, where as others serve as reserve food supplies. They form the major part of the diet of man in the form of starch and sucrose in particular, and provide energy at the rate of 4 kcal or 15 kJ per g. The loss of water in the formation of disaccharides and polysaccharides from the monosaccharides results in slight differences in energy content-monosaccharides 3.74 kcal or 15.6 kJ, disaccharides .395 kcal or 16.5 kJ, starch 4.18 kcal or 17.5 kJ and glycerol 4.32 kcal or 18.0 kJ per g.

In the analysis of foods it is difficult to determine the various carbohydrates and they are usually approximated by subtracting the measured protein plus ash plus fat from 100. The figure can be corrected by subtracting crude fibre which is non-available carbohydrate. Carbohydrate by difference is the sum of:

(a) unavailable carbohydrate pentosans, pectins, hemicelluloses and celluloses;

(b) available carbohydrate, that is, dextrins, starch and sugars;

(c) non-carbohydrates, such as organic acids and crude fibre.

carboligase. The enzyme that catalyzes the formation of acetoin from acetaldehyde and active acetaldehyde.

carbon black. A finely divided form of carbon made by the incomplete combustion of hydrocarbons. That most widely accepted for use in food is of vegetable origin. Depending on the source material and the method of manufacture, they are normally fine, bulky, black powders insoluble in water and may contain a considerable quantity of ash.

Channel black is a special grade made by the impingement of a luminous flame of natural gas against an iron plate from which the carbon is removed at regular intervals. Channel black is characterized by having a very small particle size, but may also be somewhat aromatic. Its use is permitted in certain countries but not universally. Liquid dispersions of carbon black are commercially available and these are much easier and cleaner to use than the powdered form. They are normally oil-based and may contain added emulsifiers to stabilise the product. Carbon black is an effective colo ng or use in the manufacture of licorice paste.

carbonic anhydrase. An enzyme which helps in release and transport of carbon dioxide by catalyzing the synthesis, and the dehydration, of carbonic acid from, and to, carbon dioxide and water.

carboxylase. An enzyme that catalyzes the decarboxylation of ketonic acids and transfer of carbon dioxide from one molecule to another. Carboxylase are usually found in yeasts, bacteria, plants, and animal tissues. Pyruvic carboxylase brings about decarboxylation of pyruvic acid wiliest oxaloacetic carboxylase helps the breakdown of oxaloacetic acid into pyruvic acid and carbon dioxide. Carboxylases are thus involved in the transfer of carbon dioxide in respiration.

carboxyl transferase. An enzyme which catalyzes the transfer of carbon dioxide moiety of carboxybiotin to acetyl-CoA and thus malonyl-CoA is formed during palmitate synthesis. It is one of the active components of acetyl-CoA carboxylase complex.

carboxymethylcellulose. A compound repared from pure cellulose of cotton or wood. It absorbs up to 50 times its weight of water to form a stable colloidal mass and used (in combination with stabilisers) as a whipping agent, in ice-cream, confectionery, jellies, etc., and as an inert food filler in slimming aids.

Methyl cellulose is another cellulose derivative but differs from the above (and other gums) since its viscosity increases with rise in temperature instead of decreasing, hence it is soluble in cold water and gels on heating. It is used as thickener, emulsifier, in foods low in gluten, etc. Other cellulose derivatives with similar properties are ethyl methyl cellulose, and hydroxyethyl-cellulose.

carboxypeptidase. The exopeptidase enzyme that catalyzes the hydrolysis of peptide at the end of a molecule containing the free carboxyl group. Carboxypeptidase-A catalyzes the hydrolysis of most amino acids and leads to sequential degradation of the polypeptide chain from the C-terminal; carboxypeptidase-B catalyzes only the hydrolysis of C-terminal lysine and C-terminal arginine.

carboxysome. Polyhedral inclusion bodies that contain the carbon dioxide fixation enzyme ribulose 1,5-biphosphate carboxylase; found in cyanobacteria, nitrifying bacteria, and thiobacilli.

carcinogenic index. A measure of the activity of a carcinogen; equal to $100A/B$, where A is the number of animals bearing a tumour divided by the number of animals living on the day of appearance of the first tumor, and B is the mean time is days of the appearance of tumors.

cardamom. *Elettaria cardamomum.* The dried fruits and seeds of different species of plants called cardamoms.

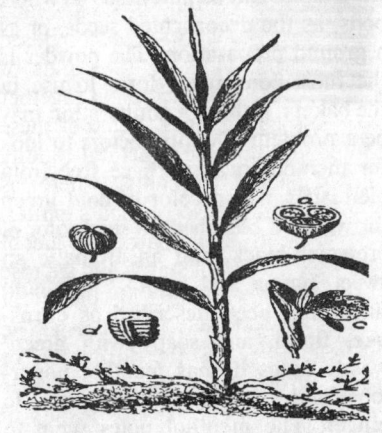

The volatile oil contains cineol and terpineol. It is used as flavouring agent in a large number of sausages, bakery goods and in curry powder and used in whole, mixed pickling spice. They have a sharp, aromatic taste, and are used to make curries, sauces and cordials, as well as for the relief of colic. Cardamom spice is reputed to be an essential ingredient in Indian curries. Those recognized in Europe as true or official cardamoms and known in commerce as Malabar cardamoms, are the produce of a plant of the mountains of Malabar, in British India, from which country they are imported. Cardamom is a perennial found throughout southern India, but is also cultivated quite extensively in the tropics as well. Indian Malabar cardamom is supposed to be the best. The Indian Mysore variety has a slightly harsh flavor. The simple, erect stems reach an average height of about 2.5 metres. The leaves are lanceolate, dark green and glamorous above, lighter and silky-like beneath. The small, yellowish flowers grow in loose racemes on prostrate flower stems. The fruit is a three-celled capsule holding up to 18 seeds. Cardamom can be purchased as whole pods, as the decorticated seeds, or as a ground preparation. The powder is the most convenient form to use in the bakery, although adulteration may be a problem. Quality factors to look for include an appearance free from blemishes, a pod color of bold green (or white, if bleached), a seed color of brownish-black, and an aromatic an sweet flavor and odor. Cardamom flavor has been described as citrus-like, floral, and soapy with green/woody notes. It has menthol undertone and has some similarities to ginger. The menthol notes seem to predominate in some preparations. The spice contains 2% to 3% volatile oil, of which the principal flavouring component is 1,8-cineole. The chemical composition of cardamom oil has been the subject of numerous studies. More than 70 compounds have been identified in it; most of them are monoterpenoids.

carmelization. The excessive heat treatment of the sugar may cause a darkening of the product, such as of lactose during drying of milk, and others sugars in many products. Carmelization usually produces an undesirable effect, but for some foods, such as candies, carmelization may be desirable.

carmine. A beautiful red dye derived from the dried bodies of a class of insects found in Mexico and Central America. This coloring matter is used in silk dyeing, in minature painting and in manufacturing of artificial flowers, rouge, red ink and water colors.

carmine-fibrin. Chopped blood fibrin that has been soaked in ammonical càrmine solution. It is used as a test for proteolytic activity, since, when digestion takes place, the liberation of the carmine into the solution acts an indicator.

carmoisine. The disodium salt of 2-(4-sulpho-10-naphthylazo)-1-naphthol-4-sulphonic acid. It is a red powder, which is soluble in water (4 % at 25°C) to give a bright magenta solution. It is only moderately light-stable, is very stable in acid media, but only poorly so in alkaline media. It has good stablity in the presence of both benzoic acid and sulphur dioxide. Carmoisine was not permitted for use in foods in the United States till 1990, but is undergoing toxicological testing as a possible replacement for amaranth. Also known as azorubine.

carnitine barrier. The limited ability of long chain fatty acids to cross the inner mitochondrial membrane in the form of fatty acyl-CoA, as contrasted with their ability to cross the membrane in the form of fatty acyl carnitine.

carnitine. A vitamin-like compound, found in muscles, and responsible for the transport of fatty acids across mitochondrial membranes in fatty acid oxidation. Although higher animals can synthesize it; also it is a dietary requirement for some insect species. It functions in β-oxidation by transporting fatty acyl groups across the inner mitochondrial membrane. It plays a role in transferring the acetyl group from inside the mitochondrion to the outside where fat synthesis takes place. Carnitine occurs in animal muscle and is particularly rich in meat extract but is not a dietary essential for man and the higher animals. the only organisms that have been shown to require carnitine as dietary essential are the meal worm and a few related species; it was originally called vitamin B_T.

carnosine. β-alanylhistidine; a dipeptide of β-alanine and histidine occurring in vertebrate muscle; function unknown.

caroa. The fibre obtained from leaves of the plant *Neoglaziovia variegata* of north-eastern Brazil. It is more than twice as strong as jute and is lighter in colour and lighter in weight, but is too hard to be used alone for burlap. It is employed as a substitute for jute in burlap when mixed with softer fibres and also for rope, and in mixtures with cotton for heavy fabrics and suiting. Some suiting is made entirely of the finer caroa fibres. Fibrasil is a trade name in Brazil for fine white caroa fibres used for tropical clothing.

carob. Family: *Leguminosae*. Genus: *Ceratonia*. Species: *Ceratonia siliqua*.

An excellent, well-balanced food rich in vitamin A and the B-complex vitamins and it contains valuable minerals, particularly calcium and phosphorus, as well as iron, copper zinc, and magnesium. The flower is recommended for non-specific diarrhoea and is good for weak babies who can not keep food down. Carob pods grow on a dome-shaped evergreen tree with dark-green compound leaves consisting of 2-5 pairs of large, rounded glossy leaflets. The tree can reach a towering height of about 17-18 m and is native to south-western Europe and western Asia, but is also widely cultivated in the Mediterranean region. The pods are the so-called "locusts" consumed by John the Baptist during his wilderness residency, hence the other common name of "St. John's bread." Seeds were used in ancient times as weight units for gold from which the term "carat" is reportedly derived. It is a natural pectin and recent research has shown that this makes it useful for diarrhoea and stomach upsets. It has a distinct advantage over chocolate in as much as all cocoa-bean products contain caffeine and need to be artificially sweetened with sugar which carob does not.

carotenal. apo-8-carotenal. A modified form of beta-carotene found in the intestine and is possibly the first intermediate in the conversion of carotene to retinol. Also found in nettles, spinach and citrus fruits. When fed to laying chickens it is deposited in the egg yolk and so it is added to chick diets to produce deeply coloured yolks.

carotene. A chemical compound with yellowish-orange coloured pigment in leafy portions of many plants, such as alfalfa, carrots, sweet potatoes, and

It is changed to vitamin A in human and animal bodies. Pure carotene is oxidized when exposed to air, causing deterioration. The oxidation is accelerated by heat and sunlight. The carotene loss is greatly reduced if alfalfa, for example, is dried by hot air as contrasted to field drying for several days in the sunlight. Carotene loss in vegetables during drying may be reduced by blanching preceding drying, particularly for spinach, sweet potatoes, and carrots. About one-third of the vitamin A of western diets is supplied as carotene. Present to only a limited extent in animal tissues, for example there is some caretone as well as retinol in milk. Before the preparation of pure retinol, b-carotene was used as the vitamin A standard, 0.6 mm of b-carotene = 1 i.u. of vitamin A. a and g-carotenes have only half the vitamin A potency of betacarotene. Carotene itself occurs in nature in four isomeric forms: a, b, g and k, which differ only in the position of the double bonds.

Since carotene is poorly absorbed from foods (about 33%) and the efficiency of conversion to vitamin A the body is one-half of the available β-carotene, the utilisation efficiency is taken as one-sixth. Thus 1 μm of β-carotene in the diet is equivalent to 0.167 microgram retinol. It is used as a colouring material in foods and as a source of vitamin A in vegetarian and kosher margarine. A wide variety of food products and colouring extracts owe their distinctive yellow to reddish-yellow colour to the presence of carotenoids. These include annatto, apricots, butter, egg yolks, paprika, safffron, salmon, tomatoes, yellow corn, etc. In food products that are coloured with carotenoids, the observed shade is more directly related to the concentrated and physical form of the colorant than to its precise chemical structure.

carotenoids. A class of oil-soluble, yellow to violet-red isoprenoid lipochrome pigments. They are present in plant and animal tissues, either in solution in the fats, as colloidal dispersions, or in combination with proteins in the aqueous phase. Some 200 carotenois have been characterized in nature representing aliphatic or aliphatic alicyclic structures and a further 200 carotenoid molecules have been synthesized in the laboratory. The basic chemical structure of the carotenoids consists of two rings and an extended system of conjugated double bonds. Most have a C_{40} carbon skeleton comprising a C_{18} central chain of 7 double bonds with 4 side chain methyl groups. The characteristic absorption spectra of these compounds is due to the conjugated double bond system, as the chain lengthens, the colour changes toward red and as it shortens the change is toward yellow. In nature, carotenoids are primarily all *trans* isomers but *cis* isomers do exist. Modifications in the structure of the carotenoid molecule account for the characteristic colour shades associated with many plants. Only β-apo-8'-carotenal, β-carotene, and canthaxanthin are marketed for food applications in the US β-carotene produces a bright yellow color and has been recommended as a replacement for FD&C Yellow No. 5. Apocarotenal gives an orange-yellow color similar to that obtain from FD&C Yellow No. 6. Both beta-carotene and apocarotenal have provitamin A activity, with the former compound equivalent to 1,667 IU of vitamin A per milligram, and the latter equivalent to 1,200 IU per mg.

These substances are insoluble in water and slightly soluble in fats and oils. They are somewhat unstable inn air because oxidative reactions occur, and light increases the rate of oxidation. In their marketed forms, beta-carotene and apocarotenal are either suspended or dissolved in an oil or are emulsified into a water-soluble matrix that can be converted into beadlets or spray-dried powders. Beta-carotene is used in such bakery products as sweet doughs, cakes, and rich yeast breads. A suspension of 30% beta-carotene in vegetable oil has been recommended for production systems where it is convenient and practical to color the fat phase. This is also the most economical version of the colorant. If a water dispersible form is needed, the usual choice is a beadlet which includes surfactants and other dispersing agents in addition to about 2.4% of the β-carotene.

There are several biochemical functions of carotenoids. These include carotenoid in photosynthetic apparatus of green plants, algae, and photosynthetic bacteria, where carotenoids function as blue light harvesting pigment (antenna or accessory pigment for photosynthesis. Thus carotenoids make it possible for photosynthetic organisms to utilize solar energy in the visible spectral region. The other important function of carotenoids is to protect biological systems as the photosynthetic apparatus from photodynamic damage. The most widespread is β-carotene. This is the orange pigment of carrots whose molecule is split into two identical portions yield vitamin A during digestion in vertebrates. Xanthophylls resemble carotenes but contain oxygen.

carotenols. Carotenoid pigments carrying the hydroxyl group. The term xanthophylls is often used collectively for these hydroxylated carotenoids, apart from the substance xanthophyll itself.

carotin. Obsolete spelling of carotene.

caroto-albumin. Carotene-protein complex in the blood serum, presumed to be the mode of transport of carotene in the body.

carp. A family of fresh-water fishes native to South-western Asia, but now acclimated in all parts of the world. Carp is a favorite food fish of Europe, but because of the coarseness of its flesh it is not so well liked in the US. It thrives and multiplies rapidly in ponds and sluggish streams. The leather carps have no scales. Many species are brilliantly colored, while some are dull.

carrot. Family: *Umbelliferae*. Genus: *Daucus*. Species: *Daucus carota*. A plant whose slender, tapering root is widely used as a table and stock food. Carrots are grown from seed and belong to the biennial group; that is, their period of growth lasts through two seasons. They can be easily grown in a soil containing sand and clay, and they do not require much attention. The roots are white, reddish or yellow, but those cultivated for the table are smaller and of a finer grain than those intended for stock. Carrots around the world grow in all shapes and colours. Westerners would mistake the Asian types, with their bulbous purplish red roots, for beets. Other colours are pale and deep yellow, red and white. The roots range from spherical to cylindrical. One variety in the Far East grows up to a yard long. As a table food they compare favourably with other vegetables, as they are nine per cent sugar. If cooked whole or cut into large pieces, carrots will lose less of their sugar content in boiling than otherwise. Carrots are immensely rich in carotene (provitamin A) and contain significant amounts of vitamins B_3, C and E, and sodium, calcium phosphorus, potassium, fibre and folic acid. They are very high in sugar. Carrots are best scrubbed not peeled as most of the nutrients are stored close to the surface.

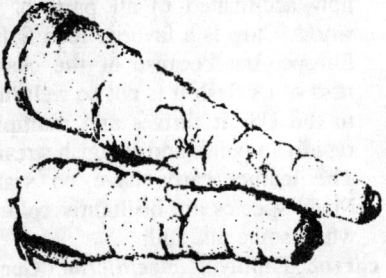

The cooked carrots lose some of their nutrients including one third of their potassium. The ordinary canned carrots are far too high in salt, but diet canned carrots have less salt than fresh ones. The average composition per 100 g of the carrot is: protein 1.0%; fat 0.2%; Ca 30 mg; Fe 0.6 mg; food energy 0.16 MJ; vitamin A 500 mg; vitamin B_1 0.05 mg; vitamin B_2 0.05 mg; nicotinic acid 0.6 mg; and vitamin C 6 mg.

Carr-Price reaction. A test for vitamin A which gives a blue colour with a solution of antimony trichloride in chloroform (the Carr-Price reagent).

Carter's spread. Trade name for a kind of breadspread containing a mixture of butter (68%), hydrogenated oils (12.4%) common salt, preservative and lecithin.

cartilate. A product consisting mainly collagen, chondromucoid (protein plus chondroitin sulphuric acid) and chondroalbumoid (a protein similar to elastin). New bone growth consists of cartilage on which calcium salts are depo-sited as a later stage to form the bone.

Cartose. Trade name for a steam hydrolysate of maize starch; used as a carbohydrate modifier in milk preparations for infant feeding. It consists of a mixture of dextrin, maltose and glucose.

Casaba melon. A large variety of muskmelon, so called because it came originally from Casaba, in Asia Minor.

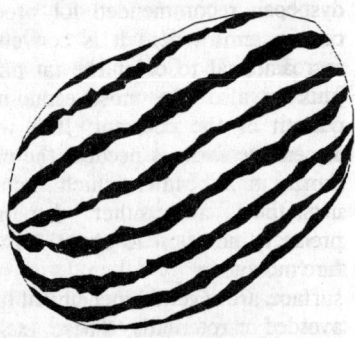

Its flesh is yellow and of a very agreeable flavor. On the outside the Casaba melon has lengthwise grooves, as have other muskmelons, but it lacks the network of lines seen on the ordinary varieties.

cascara extract. A fluid extract of the cascara buckthorn, or California buckthorn. It is employed with other laxatives by physicians for the relief of constipation. It is nearly always one of the ingredients of so-called liver pills.

cascara sagrada. *Rhammus purshiana.* The tree from which the valuable reddish-brown bark is obtained, is a small to medium-sized deciduous with hairy twigs, capable of reaching a height of about 20 metres. The tree is native to the Pacific Coast states and provinces of the US and Canada. The bark is removed is removed from trees with trunk diameters of about 1.2 metres or more. It's then permitted to dry and aged for 1 year before use, as the fresh bark has an emetic principle which is destroyed on prolonged storage or by heating.

cascarilla. A term applied to several to several different medicinal barks, but used most often to designate the bark of a small shrub found on the Bahama Islands. From this bark is prepared a medicine used in some cases of dyspepsia, chronic bronchitis and certain fevers. It has the effect of increasing the flow of the digestive juice, but if taken in too large quantities it is nauseating.

case hardening. In dehydration, or during rapid heating of some products, the formation of a layer in the product that resists passage of moisture movement from the interior to the surface. Case hardening of lumber is avoided or reduced by periodic steaming of approximately 2 hours throught the drying process. Case hardening of fruits, cereal grains, and beans may be reduced by steaming, using saturated exhaust air from the drying process to heat and wet incoming products. Case hardening of some products is avoided by using an initial high temperature of drying and in other products is avoided by using a low temperature.

casein. A group of at least three milk proteins, two of which are phosphoproteins. Casein comprises up to 3% of normal cow's milk. It occurs in milk in combination with calcium, magnesium and phosphate as complex colloidal particles. It is the chief constituent of cheese, being coagulated for cheesemaking by acid or rennet. It may also be precipitated from milk by saturation with sodium chloride. Casein is prepared in a more or less pure state for industrial uses as paper sizing agent, and in the manufacture of glue, paint, and plastics. Casein is precipitated under acid conditions, while the other two are not, thus cheese contains the casein, and the lactalbumin and lactoglobulin are left in the why. Casein is one of the most easily prepared proteins and is therefore used as a dietary supplement. Its biological value is 70. Casein may be precipitate by acid or by rennet. Acid casein contains 2% ash, 0.1% calcium, and is used a binder for Chinese clay in coating paper, for glue and in casein-bound water paints as well as for food. Rennet casein contains 8% ash, 3.5% calcium and is used in plastics.

α-casein. A protein of the casein fraction of milk. It is characterized by a phosphorus content of about 1.00%. α-casein constitutes about 75% of casein.

β-casein. A protein of the casein fraction of milk. It is characterised by a phosphorus content of about 0.6%. Casein contains about 22% β-casein.

V-casein. A protein of the casein fraction of milk. It is characterized by its solubility in 50% aqueous alcohol and by its freedom from phosphorus. It constitutes 3.4% of casein. Also known as free casein.

casein, acid. Casein exists in milk as a colloidal suspension. Calcium and tricalcium phosphate are associated with the protein molecule. Casein precipitated near the iso-electric point by acid results in the removal of most of the calcium and phosphorus. This term distinguishes between calcium and phosphorus free casein, and the more complex parent substance existing in milk and the casein formed by the action of rennet which still contains a large portion of the calcium and phosphorus.

casein, dried. A commercial casein product usually obtained from skim milk by dilute sulphuric acid precipitation. The curd is washed, drained, placed in trays, and dried in a heated chamber. When the moisture has been reduced to 2.3%, the curd is ground fine. It is then packed and shipped to be refined and made into glue, paints, plastics, etc.

casein, iodinated. When iodine is introduced into the casein molecule it has thyroactive properties similar to those of the thyroid hormone, but without some of the hypermetabolic effects of, for example, thyroxine.

casein/fat ratio. The proportions of case in and fat in milk are often stated in terms of kg of casein per kg of fat. This ratio is used to predict fairly accurately the proportions of casein and fat in the finished cheese. A casein/fat ratio of 7 produces approximately 52% fat in the dry matter of the cheese.

casein lactate. A chemical compound formed by the action of lactic acid on the casein of milk. Casein may be precipitated as mono-calcium caseinate as well as base-free or uncombined casein. A common belief was that in the natural souring of milk the lactic acid formed by microorganisms dissolved the calcium from the calcium caseinate and re-placed it, forming casein lactate.

casein number. The ratio of the casein nitrogen to the total nitrogen in milk. This index has been suggested as a method of diagnosis of mastitis.

caseinogen. According to older nomenclature, caseinogen is the form present in milk, and when precipitated with rennin it becomes casein. In American nomenclature the two forms are casein

and paraceasein, which is now the accepted usage.

cashew nut. Family: *Anacardiaceae*. Genus: *Anacardium*. Species: *Anacardium occidentale*. The cashew tree grows best in the tropical summer rainfall regions with 500-3500 mm rainfall. It is very drought tolerant, and on dry sloping sites is often the only cultivated plant grown as cash crop. After the development of an industrial roasting procedure for the separation of the shell oil, the nuts are obtained as the main product. The separation of the shells and seed coats from the kernels was carried out by hand in earlier days, but now there are fully mechanized plants, which make the processing possible with less efforts and time.

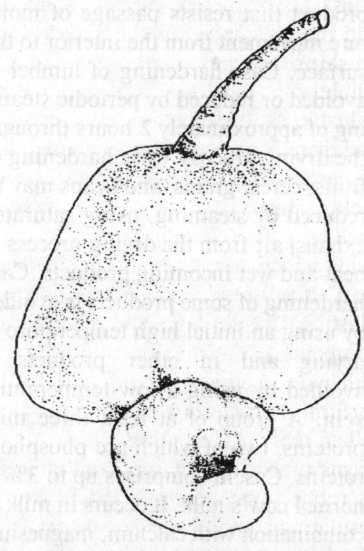

Cashew-nuts are good body-builders and easily digested when raw (having first been deprived of their acrid fluid) and so help in cases of emaciation and in building good teeth. Boiling them in oil or salting them makes them harder to digest, so they are best eaten in their natural state. They go best with acid fruit and non-starchy vegetables rather than sweet fruit and heavy starch. Like all nuts cashews contain a great deal of unsaturated fatty acid, mostly in the form of oleic acid.

cashew shell oil. An amber-coloured, poisonous, viscous oil obtained by extraction from the by-product shells of the cashew-nut industry of India and Brazil. The cashew nut grows on the distal end of the fruit of the tree *Anacardium occidentale*. The thin-skinned, yellow, pear-shaped fruit may be eaten or used in preserves. It is also distilled into a spirit in India. The kernel of the seed nut, known as the cashew nut, is roasted and widely used as an edible nut or in confections. The kernel is crescent-shaped, and the nuts are graded by sizes. On crushing, the nuts produce 45% of an edible oil, but the nuts are more valuable as a confection than for oil, and there is no commercial production of cashew-nut oil. One kg of shells yields about 0.3 kg of cashew-nut shell oil, which contains 90% anacardic acid, which causes blistering to the skin. It is used in the production of plastics, drying oils, and insulating compounds. The oil reacts with form-aldehyde to give a drying oil. With furfural it produces a molding plastic. When reacted with other chemicals it forms rubber-like masses, and is used as rubber extenders and in electrical insulating compounds. The other 10% of cashew-nut shell oil is cardol.

Casilan. Trade name for a casein preparation containing 90% protein, 1.8% fats, 3.8% mineral salts, and calcium.

cassareep. The juice of the bitter cassava or manioc. It is boiled to a thick syrup and used as a base for sauces.

cassava. Tuber of the plant *Manihot utilissima;* the plant of humid tropics, which grows upto 3 m in height, and bears broad, shining, hand-shaped leaves, and beautiful white and rose-colored flowers. The stems are very woody, with swollen nodes.

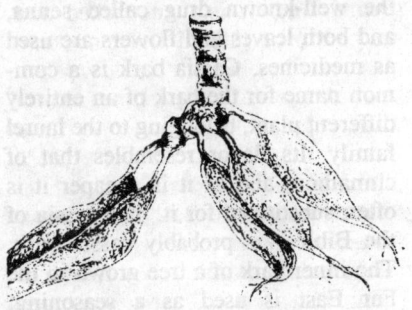

The roots contain bitter tasting glycoside linamarin, from which hy-drocyanic acid is released by the action of enzyme linamarase. There are two species of cassava, bitter and sweet, but roots of both are valuable. In the tuberous roots, the linamarin content is higher in the rind than in the pith; in the sweet cultivars there are less than 50 mg/kg in the pith, for the bitter cultivars, the corresponding value is over 100 mg/kg. From bitter cassava is obtained a juice used in making a sauce called casareep. In South America it is known as manioc and yuca. It is a staple article of diet in many tropical countries although an extremely poor source of protein. The average composition per 100 g is: protein 0.9%; fat 0.2%; Ca 25 mg; Fe 0.5 mg; vitamin B_1 0.04 mg; vitamin B_2 0.02 mg; nicotinic acid 0.4 mg; vitamin C 27 mg, and food energy 0.46 MJ. The juice from the roots is Cassareep, used in sauces and fermented with molasses. The leaves are eaten as a vegetable. The tuber is a source of Tapioca.

cassia. A large genus of plants belonging to the pea family and found in the tropical parts of the world. The cassia consist of trees, shrubs or herbs. The leaves, which are compound, usually bear glands on their stalks. The leaflets of several species constitute the well-known drug called senna, and both leaves and flowers are used as medicines. Cassia bark is a common name for the bark of an entirely different plant, belonging to the laurel family. Its flavor resembles that of cinnamon, and as it is cheaper it is often substituted for it. The cassia of the Bible was probably cassia bark. The inner bark of a tree grown in the Far East is used as a seasoning; similar in appearance and flavour to cinnamon.

cassina. Beverage (tea substitute) made from cured leaves of a holly bush, *Ilex cassine;* contains 1-1.6% caffeine and 8% tannin.

castor oil. The oil obtained from the seeds of bean, *Ricinus communis* L. It is native of India, but is distributed over all the warmer regions of the globe. The tree can attain height up to 10 m. This plant is often cultivated in gardens for ornament. The oil is obtained from the seeds by bruising and pressing.The sees contains 42-56% oil. Before pressing or extraction, the seed is usually shelled; the seed coats form 17-20% of the weight. The castor oil of commerce, which is used as a purgative, is chiefly imported from India. The taste of castor oil is very disagreeable, and can be swallowed without a feeling of nausea only when it is enclosed in capsular piece of fruits. The oil contains about 91-95% ricinoleic acid, which is chemically more reactiv than any other fatty

acid due the presence of a double bond on the 9th carbon atom and hydroxyl group on the 12th carbon atom. The oil itself is non-irritating, but in the small intestine is hydrolysed by lipase to liberate ricinoleic acid which is an irritant to the gastro-intestinal mucosa and therefore acts as a purgative.

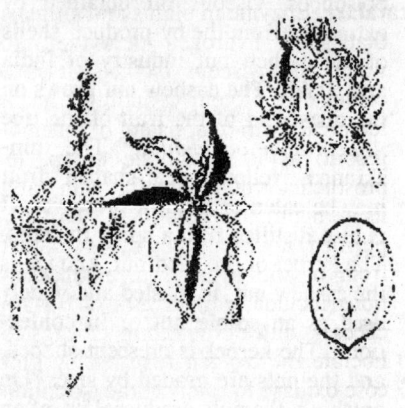

The castor oil itself retains its viscosity at high temperatures, and is therefore used as a lubricant. It is also used as plasticizer. Due to its ability to dissolve certain colours, it finds applications in lipsticks and other cosmetics.

catabolite repression. Effect of glucose in preventing the induction of enzymes required for the catabolism of sugars (*e.g.,* lactose, arabinose and galactose) and certain amino acids (*e.g.,* tryptophan) in *E. coli* and related bacteria. Glucose, or a breakdown product (a catabolite), prevents expression of the genes for the catabolizing enzymes by regulating the intracellular concentration of cyclic amp (cAMP). In glucose-grown bacteria the concentration of cAMP is low, cAMP is required to bind to and activate a catabolite activating protein, which in turn binds to a site on the DNA close to the promoter of a glucose-regulated gene and facilitates transcription initiation by RNA polymerase. The catabolite repression ensures that the glucose is used in preference to inferior carbon substrates (*e.g.*, lactose) which support slower growth. Also known as glucose effect.

catalase. Enzyme in plants and animals that splits hydrogen peroxide into water and gaseous oxygen. It is a conjugated protein containing haem identical with the haem of haemoglobin) as its prosthetic group. Its prosthetic group contains iron, and its pH optimum is 6.5-7.0. It is partially purified liquid or powdered extract from bovine liver. Typical applications include manufacture of certain cheeses, and desugarging of eggs to liberate the oxygen required by glucose oxidase to catalyze the oxidation of glucose to gluconic acid.

catchup. Alternative spelling of catsup or ketchup.

catechu. A resinlike substance obtained from the wood of certain species of acacia found in India. It is employed in tanning and dyeing, and is used medicinally as an astringent. In the East the natives chew it. Catechu is extracted from the heartwood, small chips of which are boiled in water until the extract is nearly as thick as tar. The mass is then allowed to harden and is formed into balls. These are wrapped in leaves and thus placed on the market. Cutch is a familiar commercial name of this product.

catenase. A collective term for an enzyme of either the endo- or the exo-type that catalyzes the cleavage of a polymeric chain; ribonuclease, lysozyme, and carboxypeptidase are examples.

catfish. A large family of fishes inhabiting both fresh and salt water. All species are characterized by their smooth skin and the sharp spines, or thorns, at each side of the head, which, when the fish is frightened or attacked, are erected at right angles to the body. Their names refers to their habit of making a peculiar purring sound when taken out of the water. The fresh-water species in North America are often known as horned pout and bullhead. Specimens weighing 70 kg have been reported, but the average weight is about 15-20 kg. The flesh has a sweet flavor and is highly nutritious.

cathepsins. Group of intracellular proteolytic enzymes in animal tissues. Probably function in the normal breakdown and resynthesis of tissues proteins. They are responsible for the autolytic softening of the flesh. There are four enzymes in the group, cathepsins I, II, III and IV, respectively similar to pepsin, trypsin, aminopeptidase and carboxypeptidase.

catmint. *See* catnip.

catnip. A plant of the mint family, widely found throughout North America and Europe. It has whorls of rose-tinged, whitish flowers, and stalked, downy, heart-shaped leaves. It has much the same fascination for cats as valerian root. In some sections a tea brewed from the leaves is used as a home remedy for colic and as a tonic. Its erect, square, branching stem is hairy and grow from 1-2 metres high. The oblong or cordate, pointed leaves have scalloped edges and grey or whitish hairs on the lower side. The flowers are white with purple spots and grow in spikes. Also known as catmint.

cauliflower. Family: *Cruciferae*. Genus: *Brassica*. Species: *Brassica oleracea* var. *botrytis*. A garden variety of cabbage, in which cultivation has caused the flowers to assume, when young, the form of a compact, fleshy head, which is highly esteemed as a table vegetable. It has a more delicate flavour than cabbage and is not quite so rich in vitamins and minerals as some of its relative varities but contains phosphorus, sulphur, calcium, sodium, zinc, and vitamin A and C. In fact an average helping of cauliflower supplies half the daily recommended vitamin C requirement (though the amount recommended is far too low in my opinion). The tender pale green leaves that encase the head are rich in minerals. Cauliflower has a high sulphur content which may cause indigestion and poor and assimilation, so do not combine it with other sulphur-rich foods like onions. Cooked frozen cauliflower retains two-thirds of its calories, half its protein, to-thirds of its carbohydrate and loses one third of its vitamins. Cauliflower is a good blood purifier and helps asthma, kidney and bladder disorders, hypertension, gout, constipation and biliousness. Eaten raw it will strengthen bleeding gums. The average composition per 100 g is: protein 1.2%; fat 0.1%; Ca 14 mg; Fe 0.5 mg; food energy 0.05 MJ; vitamin A 15 μg; vitamin B_1 0.05 mg; vitamin B_2 0.06 mg; nicotinic acid 0.025 mg; and vitamin C 35 mg.

caustic. A term which has the general meaning of corrosive and is applied to the water-soluble hydroxides of the light metals to distinguish them from their carbonates. It is also used in medicine to designate substance that destroy body tissues; thus lunar caustic is silver nitrate.

caviar. A food prepared from the sturgeon. Caviar is made by freeing the eggs from the tissue which holds them together, then washing them and rubbing them with salt, after which they are dried and packed in kegs. It is considered a great delicacy, especially among the Russians, in whose country it is manufactured in large quantities. It is not a general article of diet because of its high cost; the piquant flavor is agreeable only to a cultivated taste. Also spelled as caviare. The average composition per 100 g is: 30% protein; 20% fat; and food energy 1.42 KJ.

cayenne, bell peppers, and paprika. *Capsicum frutescens, C. Annuum.* The capsicum species are divided into two groups: The sweet or mild-flavoured varieties primarily used as vegetables; and the hot peppers, often referred to as chillies, that are used for spiking sauces and seasonings. The bell pepper is the sweetest and largest variety. It's typically sold green, but later in the season one can usually get red, yellow and purple varities as well. The bright-coloured ones have merely been allowed to ripen longer on the vine and are sweeter. Then there's the fiery kind, often measured in BTU's according to their individual hotness. Cayenne pepper is a perennial in its native tropical America, but is annual when cultivated outside of the tropical zones. Growing to a height of 1 m or more, its glabrous stem is woody at the bottom and branched near the top. The leaves are ovate to lanceolate, entire and petioled. The drooping, white to yellow flowers grow alone or in pairs of three. The ripe fruit or pepper, is a many-seeded pod with a leathery outside in various shades of red or yellow.

Celacol. Trade name for derivatives of cellulose, methyl hydroxyethyl, etc.

celeriac. *See* celery.

celery. Family: *Umbilliferae.* Genus: *Apium.* Species: *Apium graveolens.* A plant of the parsley family, native to the temperate parts of Europe, but extensively cultivated in other regions of the world, where it is highly popular as a salad vegetable. Celery is one of the oldest vegetables ever used in recorded history. The ancient Egyptians were known to gather wild celery from marshy seaside areas for food. It is a plant of many uses and little waste: the leaves and dried seeds make good seasoning; the outer ribs are best cooked and the inner ribs may be consumed raw as they are good for the heart. The variety most commonly available is the light-green to medium-green Pascal celery. In its natural state it is bitter and tough, but the crisp, tender stalks of the cultivated varieties have a delightful flavor. Celery is grown from seed, which is placed in a hotbed for an early crop, and in the open for a late crop. If the plants are desired for summer or fall use, boards are placed about the stalks to shut out the light. By this means the coloring matter in the tissues is destroyed and the stalk are whitened, or blanched. Celery grown for winter use is blanched by having earth heaped up about the stalks. On the approach of winter the plants are taken up and set in pits or in a cool cellar. Moist earth is packed around the roots and the blanching process continues. Another method consists in making rows from 15-30 cm apart, whereby the plants are self-blanched, only the outside rows needing artificial darkening. Celery needs moisture and a fertile soil. The ancient Greeks on the Isthmus of Corinth around 450 BC regularly crowned their winning athletes with crowns of celery stems and leaves.

Celery was once widely recommended for the treatment of rheumatic patients. It is excellent for those trying to lose weight, through it is also good for stimulating the appetite. The fresh juice is strong diuretic and is good for nephritis. Celery is also helpful for high blood pressure, catarrh, diarrhoea, diabetes and acidosis as it eats the acid in the body and raises the alkali levels, thereby clearing the complexion. It is one of the best sources of organic calcium and so is useful for strengthening the nervous system and helping insomniacs. A decoction made of the celery leaves was once used as a footbath to help chilblains, and in the past it had reputation as an aphrodisiac. The average composition per 100 g is: protein 0.75%; fat 0.1%; Ca 30 mg; Fe 0.25 mg; vitamin B_1 0.04 mg; vitamin B_2 0.02 mg; nicotinic acid 0.2 mg; vitamin C 5 mg; and food energy about 0.05 MJ.

Cellofas. Trade name for derivatives of cellulose, e.g., Cellofas A, methyl ethyl, Cellofas B, sodium carboxymethyl.

celluflour. Powdered cellulose; used in experimental diets to provide indigestible bulk.

cellular slime molds. *Class: Acrasiomycetes.* Slime molds with a vegetative phase consisting of amoeboid cells that aggregate to form a multicellular pseudoplasmodium. The cellular slime molds, like the Myxomycetes, exist for part of their life cycle as amoeba-like organisms but differ from the plasmodial slime molds in that the amoebas, on swarming together, retain their identify as individual cells. The cellular slime molds comprise approximately 26 species, grouped into seven genera. One of the example of the cellular slime molds is *Dictyostelium discoideum,* which begins life as a group of individual amoeba that are smaller than common *Amoeba proteus* but not strikingly different in appearance. These amoebas grow and divide repeatedly, increasing in number; then quite suddenly they stop growing, swarm together, and adhere to form a many-celled sluglike mobile mass that is capable of moving several cm. Movement toward light, especially green light, is characteristic. The aggregation stage begins when all of the amoebas begin to emit pulses of cyclic adenosine monophosphate at intervals of approximately 5 minutes. An amoeba that receives a signal pulse of cyclic AMP evidently moves toward it, pauses, and then lets off a pulse of its own. The consequence of this is that each amoeba is attracted to its nearest neighbour, because its own signal is automatically delayed until a certain its own signal is automatically delayed until a certain time after the one it has just received. The amoebas form streams, all flowing toward the centre of growing aggregate in a series of waves and sticking together. The amoeba at the centre, the pacemaker, is the one that emits pulses of AMP at the fastest rate. After a period of migration, the cells in the mass begin to differentiate, those in the anterior third of the sluglike mass forming stalk cells, and the remainder forming spores. Evidently the higher concentrations of cyclic AMP at the front of the mass determine the fate of the cells, as isolated amoebas subjected to high concentrations of cyclic AMP differentiate into stalk cells. The gradient in cyclic AMP seems to develop as the sluglike mass migrates and will arise even if one mass is divided into two, or four, if the resulting masses migrate for a sufficient length of time. As the stalk grows, it is strengthened with fibrils of cellulose, and the mass of amoebas quite abruptly rise up in a fruiting body on the pinnacle of which is a droplet containing hundreds, or, in some instances, thousands of spores. These spores are dispersed, and if they fall on warm damp ground, they germinate. Each releases one small, quite ordinary-looking amoeba, and the entire cycle begins again.

cellulase. Enzyme that attacks cellulose; present in the digestive juices of various snails, wood-boring insects, and microorganisms. The cellulase present in the intestinal microorganisms of ruminants is responsible for the ability of these animals to obtain energy from straw, for their own digestive juices do not contain cellulase. Many animals, including herbivores, lack cellulases implying either that they are unable to digest cellulose or that they can only do so by harboring, in the gut, bacteria or protozoa which themselves produce cellulase. It is only within the last few years that the chemistry of cellulose and of cellulases (enzymes that act on cellulose) has been well established. Presently, cellulases are used widely for the recovery and utilization of previously unavailable plant materials. For some processes, cellulases substantially increases yields. The principal reaction catalyzed by cellulase is hydrolysis of β-1,4-glucan bonds in such polysaccharides as cellulose, yielding β-dextrins. A variety of cellulase-containing preparations are commercially available. For example, there is a fungal cellulase system that is primarily active on soluble forms of cellulose with minor activity on highly-ordered forms. The hemicellulase component of the system rapidly reduces the viscosity of several plant gums, such as locust bean, guar, soybean, and coffee. Application of this material to fruit juice manufacture has resulted in improving the extraction and clarification of juice from citrus fruits. Other applications of cellulase preparations include increasing sucrose yield from beet and cane sources, dextrose production, improved recovery and processing of fruits and vegetables, the recovery of vegetable extracts, etheric oils, flavors from cellulose- and hemicellulose-containing materials and the manufacture of various foods in solid form.

cellulobiose. Two molecules of glucose joined together in the 1,4'-β position (as distinct from the 1,4'-α bond in maltose). Cellobiose is the basic structural unit of cellulose and does not exist in the free state in nature.

cellulose synthetase. An enzyme which catalyzes the polymerization of glucose to cellulose by β-1,4-glucan bonding. Its activity is mainly confined to microfibrils which are situated near cell membranes.

cellulose. Polysaccharide that forms the supporting cell structure in plants, does not occur in animals. It consists of long chain of glucose units. Is not digested in man or other monogastric animals, but serves a useful purpose in providing bulk for intestinal functioning. It is digested by the bacteria in the rumen of ruminating animals, which can therefore subsist on grass and hay. Paper and wood are essentially cellulose. Commercial sources are cotton and woe pulp. It is one of the most abundant organic compound

in nature, and has general formula as $(C_6H_{10}O_5)_n$, in which n stands for an under-terminated number of carbohydrate units. It is a straight-chain molecule comprised of glucose units connected by oxygen atoms and can be converted to simpler forms (starches, etc.) by hydrolysis. It is composed of a linear array of β-D-glucose molecules. In the plant cell wall, microfibrils of cellulose form crystalline latices known as micelles, linked by groups of more randomly arranged cellulose fibrils. Cellulose is present in plant cell walls and its synthesis resembles those of starch and glycogen except that the nucleoside of the NDP-glucose is in this case guanosine. Moreover, the final glycosyl transferase reaction results in the formation of β-glucoside linkages, for unlike starch and glycogen, cellulose comprises β-glucoside residues. In leaves, the synthesis of starch, sucrose and cellulose may at certain times be going on simultaneously, but the NDP-glucose compound is different in each case (ADP-glucose for starch, UDP-glucose for sucrose, and GDP-glucose for cellulose. In contrast to starch, the β-1,4 linkages of cellulose are highly resistant to acid hydrolysis; strong mineral acid is needed to produce D-glucose; partial hydrolysis yields the reducing disaccharide, cellobiose. β-1,4 linkages of cellulose are not hydrolyzed by glycosidases found in the digestive tracts of humans or other higher animals.

central metabolic pathway. The metabolic pathway composed of the reactions of the citric acid cycle and some of the reactions of glycolysis. The pathway occupies a central position in metabolism, since it can be used either catabolically for the oxidation of metabolites to carbon dioxide and water, or anabolically for synthesis and inter-conversion of metabolites.

central nervous system stimulants. The drugs capable of producing generalized stimulation of the brain or spinal cord which may lead to convulsion. They are of limited therapeutic value because of their convulsant activities. There are, however, some that are used as respiratory stimulants. A few central nervous system stimulants exhibit predominant central stimulant action, *e.g.*, strychnine, nikethamide, leptazol, etc., others produce multiple side effects. In ususal practice, the central nerveous system stimulants find their use in emergencies for prompt and short-term excitation of central nervous system, because a prolonged stimulation may be followed by depression. Also known as CNS stimulants.

centrifugal fan. A centrifugal fan or radial flow fan consists of a wheel with appropriate blades which is rotated in a spiral housing. The air pressure at the centre of the rotating wheel is less than the surrounding air pressure. Air pressure is increased in the spiral housing as the wheel rotates. The air flows axially into the wheel and is moved from centre to the periphery of the fan by the centrifugal force of rotating wheel. It is possible to get higher pressure on a centrifugal fan by increasing the length of the blades because greater centrifugal force exerted. These fans may be further classified into forward-curved, backward-curved, and straight-bladed. The highest mechanical efficiency obtained with these fans is 80%.

centrifuging. A separation technique based upon the application of centrifugal force to a mixture or suspension of materials of closely similar densities. The smaller the difference in density, the greater is the force required. The equipment used (centrifuge) is a chamber revolving at high speed to impart a force up to 17,000 times that of gravity (much higher in the ultracentrifuge). The materials of higher density are thrown toward the outer portion of the chamber, while whose of lower density are concentrated at or near the inner portion. A common cream separator is a type of centrifuge in which flow is continuous. The centrifugal force throws the heavier milk into a different chamber from the lighter cream. This technique is used effectively in the production of numerous food products and thus can be classified as one of the unit food processing operations. For example, important applications occur in the separation of milk components. In food research laboratories where proteins, polymers, and other substances with high molecular weights are investigated, the ultracentrifuge is widely used. The sedimentation of large molecules in a strong centrifugal field enables the distribution of molecular weights in certain systems. When a solution containing polymer or other large molecules is centrifuged at forces up to 250,000 times gravity, the molecules begin to settle, leaving pure solvent above a boundary which progressively moves toward the bottom of the cell. This boundary is a rather sharp gradient of concentrations for molecules of uniform size, such as globular proteins. For polydisperse systems, the boundary is diffuse, the lowest molecular masses lagging behind the larger molecules. An optical system can be provided for viewing this boundary, and a study as a function of the time of centrifuging yields the rate of sedimentation for the single component, or for each of many components of a polydisperse system. The sedimentation rates may then be related to the corresponding molecular weights of the species present after the diffusion coefficients for each species are determined by independent experiments. Both sedimentation and diffusion rates are affected by interactions between molecules, so that each must be studied as a function of concentration and extrapolated to infinite dilution, as is done for the colligative properties. Extrapolation of diffusion coefficients to infinite dilution is difficult for high-molecular-mass linear polymers, and so alternate means are used to relate sedimentation constant to molecular masses in these important applications.

cephalins. Alternative spelling to kephalins.

Ceplapro. Protein-rich baby food (18-20% protein) made in granular form from degerminated maize flour, wheat, defatted soya and skim milk powder with added calcium and vitamins.

cereal coffee. Coffee prepared from roasted cereal grains.

cereal cream. A very light commercial sweet cream usually testing about 10% to 12% butterfat. It is more commonly known under the name of cereal milk but is sold in a number of markets as "Half in Half."

cereal grain drying. Cereal grains, often harvested at moisture contents which are too high for storage, are dried before storage. For safe storage, the moisture contents should be in the range of 11-14%, wet basis, depending on the type of grain, storage conditions, microorganisms associated with the grain, and temperature. Field losses from shattering and weather are reduced by early harvest

when the grain is wet. Maximum production is secured when the seed is in the range of 30-40% moisture. Mechanical drying can be done by forced air or heated forced air in a bin with appropriate ducts with grain 5 metres or less over the ducts, using 0.013-0.134 m³/m³s of air. Continuous drying can be done in a vertical column or on a horizontal belt in which the grain thickness if 10-45.7 cm, air temperature 71-121°C, and airflow of 0.65 to 3.9 m³/m³s. To avoid decreasing germination the grain temperature should be kept below 52°C; to avoid damaging baking quality, below 60°C; and to avoid causing reduction in feeding quality for animals, below 82.2°C. With appropriate control the air temperature for drying may exceed the grain temperature.

cereals. Any grain or edible fruit of the grass family that may be used as food. Include wheat, rice, oats, rye, barley, maize and millet. Provide the largest single type of foodstuffs.

cerebrosides. Part of the structural matter of brain and the myelin sheath of nerves. Contain phrenosin, kerasin, fatty acid, sphingosine and galactose. This is the only structure of the body that contains the sugar galactose.

cerelose. Commercial glucose with about 9% water.

ceroid. A lipid granule that may be formed in an animal, particularly in the liver, as a result of either the injection of oils rich in unsaturated fatty acids or the ingestion of various experimental diets.

Cerophyl. A patented preparation in concentrated form made from selected young wheat, oats, barley, and rye grasses, dried and tableted. It is a natural food supplement. The vitamin content per 100 grams is: carotene 70000 I.U.; thiamin; 0.9 mg; ascorbic acid 350 mg; riboflavin 2.5 mg; vitamin K 15 mg; chlorophyll (a non-vitamin factor) 750 mg. It is a source of the entire vitamin B complex.

Cetavlon. Trade name for detergent and bacteriostat, cetyltrimethylammonium bromide.

cetyl alcohol. A solid, waxy, straight chain alcohol of sixteen carbon atoms, found in spermaceti (from the sperm whale) and waxes. It can be spread as a thin film on the surface of water in reservoirs where it reduces evaporation of water.

Chablis. A French white wine prepared from the Chardonany grape, which some authorities feel is only matched in quality, by white Riesling grape.

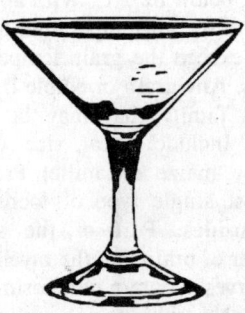

The wine derives its name from a small town, Chablis, located Southeast of Paris and in the north-western portion of Burgundy wine-producing district. Some ordinary white wines in various parts of the world masquerade under the name Chablis. French Chablis wines are divided into four grades: Grand Cru, Premier Cru, Chablis, and Petit Chablis.

chalones. Substances that act as growth regulators but, unlike hormones, they are effective against the tissue that produce them. They therefore constitute a mechanism of inhibition of growth by positive feedback. They are postulated to be glycoproteins, although some doubt continues to surround claims for their activity. Many different tissues such as epithelial tissue, liver parenchyma and erythrocytes are said to have effective chalones, which prevent the growth of these tissues beyond certain limits. They are assumed to be released into circulation and to act as mitotic inhibotors on the target tissue. They are tissue specific, but not species-specific, in their actions. They act, reversibly, to inhibit mitosis and thereby cell multiplicatio. Chalones may play a role in determining the shape and size of organs, and deficiency may be involved in the aetiology of cancer, and in wound-healing. An obsolete meaning of chalone is a substance that inhibits the action of a hormone.

chamber dryer. A unit used for removing moisture from brick or clay products heated by steam or hot air, in which the air from a partially dried chamber of products can be directed to a chamber with wet products. Four or five chambers may be used with appropriate controls to direct and mix the air for drying.

chamomile. Any of the two herbs, *Anthemis nobilis* and *Matricaria recutica*. Essential oil used for flavouring liqueurs; chamomile tea made by infusing dried flower heads, used as old-fashioned tonic; whole herb used to make herb beers. Apple-scented chamomile, a perennial plant of the composite family, is one of the daintiest of herbs. A low-growing type known as Roman chamomile can be grown as an effective ground cover to form a green and white daisy-flowered lawn. A tisane of the flowers is taken for dyspepsia, flatulence, and other stomach ailments, and used as a mild antiseptic. It can also be taken as an appetite restorer. An infusion of the dried flowers is used as a rinse for fair hair, as a skin cleanser, and a skin tonic. One species, *A. tinctoria,* is sued as an orange-brown dye. Roman chamomile is a strongly fragrant, hairy, half-spreading and much branched perennial with white ray-like flower heads and can grow to a foot in height

Champagne. A French wine, white or red, which is made chiefly in the department of Marne, in the former province Champagne. It is generally characterized by its property of frothing, or effervescing, when poured from the bottle, though there are also still Champagne wines. The creaming or slightly sparkling Champagne wines are more highly valued and command greater prices than the full-frothing wines, in which the smaller quantity of alcohol they contain escapes from the froth as it rises to the surface, carrying with it the aroma and leaving the liquor nearly tasteless. The property of creaming, or frothing, possessed by these wines is due to the fact that they are partly fermented in the bottle, carbonic acid being thereby produced.

Wine of a similar kind is made elsewhere; some of the German champagnes are very much like the French. Champagne, the best known of the sparkling wines, has an air of high society of dissipation about it. It is a white wine, but part of the grapes used in making it are black grapes. In some vineyards the proportion is as high as four black to one white. The fire Burgundy grapes used to prepare Champagne are the 'Pinot Noir' and the 'Pinot Balnc'. A sparkling wine is one which after the normal fermentation is over, is cleared of bottled, and then a second fermentation is carried

out in the bottle by adding extra sugar and yeast. In growing the grapes and making the wine which to become Champagne, greater care is taken than usual. If the black grapes are allowed to become too ripe, it will be almost impossible to prevent a little colour getting into the wine. In the gathering unusual care is taken to prevent bruising, for bruising leads to premature fermentation which may result finally in spoiling the delicate taste of Champagne. The pressing of the grapes is carried out with equal care. Only the first part of the expressed 'must' is used for Champagne. This amounts to a little over half the juice which could be extracted. The rest of the juice goes for inferior wines.

Fermentation of the first juices (450 gallons) proceeds for about 2-3 days, a process that is carried out in glass-lined or concrete vats in the modern winery, whereas in traditional wineries, the must is racked off into oak casks that contain a little less than 50 gallons. Although the initial fermentation lasts but a few days, the fermentation at a slower rate keeps on persisting for about 2 months. The appearance of a clear wine is an indication to wine-maker that fermentation has virtually ceased. Although it would be the desire of the wine-maker that all batches be of the very highest of quality, there is not absolute uniformity in dealing with a naturally derived product. Thus, at this juncture in processing, there is blending. The blended wines are called the wine-making firm's Cuvee. The blend is tested for residual sugar. If low, a predetermined amount of liqueur de triage (pure cane sugar dissolved in Champagne wine) will be added. This is a critical operation because too much sugar will cause the bottle to burst and too little will detract from the sparkling qualities of the product. Bottles are filled and corked, using a strong steel clamp to hold the cork in place. A second fermentation occurs in the bottle, producing carbonic acid gas and building up a pressure of 6 atmosphere or slightly less. The length of time the wine is retained in this configuration varies from one maker to the next and may range from about 1.5-5 years. At the end of this period, the bottles are removed and shaken. After which they are placed in titled racks known as pupitres. It is necessary to remove the deposit of sediment resulting from the second fermentation caused by adding the liqueur de tirage. This sediment removal is called remuage in French. Usually the bottle is shaken and turned in its rack by just a few degrees each day (up to 24 such shakings and turnings). This results in a relatively uniform deposition of sediment against the cork, a condition important prior to disgorging. In California, remuage is sometimes called *riddling*. Removal of the deposit is called disgorgement. In modern facilities, a freezing machine is used. Bottles, in an upside-down configuration, are exposed to a low temperature to a distance of about 5 cm along the neck to form an ice plug perhaps 12-13 mm thick. Within this plug will be embedded the sediment which it is desired to remove. In disgorging the plug, an operator will loosen the clamp and open the bottle in essentially the usual fashion, pointing it upward and at an angle. Once the plug is blown out, it is necessary to allow some of the wine to flow out, but not too much. After the bottle is inspected for traces of deposits, it is then ready for dosage. Cane suga. dissolved in mature wine or old brand (*liqueur d'expedition*) is added to the bottle. It is at this time that the final sweetness of the Champagne is determined, ranging from *Brut* (considered drier than extra dry and not containing over a 2% dosage); to *Demi-Sac* (half-dry, a term no longer used very much). Usually the dosage is comprised of 3 parts cane sugar and 2 parts of old wine. Rock candy is sometimes used and in some cases a small amount of special brand (espirit de Cognac, double-distilled, 140 proof) is added in the dosage. The final cork is then placed in the neck of the bottle and clamped. The bottle is then shaken thoroughly to mix the wine with its dosage, after which the Champagne is again stored. Vintage champagne continues to improve for about 10 years, after which it loses its equality, including sparkle. The wine produced thus undergoes a supplementary fermentation 'in the bottle'. Especially thick strong bottles are used, free from flaws, and the wine is filled into them together with some sugar and a pure yeast culture. The yeast is a specially cultured one which acts vigorously, but is not sensitive to high concentration of carbon dioxide. A little tannin is usually added at the same time. The bottles are stored at 20°C and inside them the yeasts display their normal activity on the pure sugar. The bottles contain a dry wine with a high pressure of carbon dioxide. At one time, before the bottle manufactures became expert, a considerable proportion of breakage took place and to work in a champagne cellar was a dangerous occupation. When the fermentation was almost complete the temperature of the cellar was lowered to about 15°C. At this stage, the bottles contain good Champagne, as well as dead yeast cells. The major difficulty is to get these yeast cells out without releasing the pressure. It is a very tedious process and is carried out by an expert.

chaparral. *Larrea divericata.* One of the most amazing herbs ever found in the plant kingdom. It thrives on nutritionally bankrupt soil and settles in where even the hardiest of cacti fear to tread. Chaparral secretes a powerful anti-growth substance that keeps all other vegetative intruders away. Nothing grows around the immediate perimeter of shrub - not even other chaparral!

chapati. Flat, pancake-like baked product usually made from wheat flour, commonly eaten in India, Nepal, and Pakistan. The standard chapti is made from wheat flour and water only; other types are leavened or may be made with white flour (Nan), gram, barley or maize flour; and/or may have added oils and fats, milk, common salt, sugar, and baking powder.

chard. A form of garden beet cultivated for its leaves, which are eaten as greens, but particularly for the center rib of the leaf. The latter is cooked about the same way as asparagus. Chard is grown in the same way as the garden beet, from which it differs in having small, woody roots.

Chardonnary grape. A variety of renowned white grape used in production of superb white Burgundies (Chablis, Montrachet, Pouilly-Fuisse, etc.) in France. It is also the white grape used in production of Champagnes. The grape is also cultivated in Alsace and California. Although the term Pinot is sometimes used in connection with this variety, such as Pinot Chardonnay (considered by some authorities as the best American white table wine), botanists have not established a true relationship between the Pinot Noir and Pinot Blanc, among others. In recent years a French hybrid of the Chardonnay has been cultivated in Canada.

charge pan dryer. A unit for removing moisture consisting of shallow cylinder-shaped. The containers are top-loaded and bottom-emptied with an agitator in each container. Heat is supplied through the walls of the containers. The unit may be operated under vacuum or atmosphere.

Charleston grey watermelon. A variety of melon that is long and blocky, mostly weighing 12.6-15.8 kg. The rind is light grayish-green with darker green veins. The flesh is bright red, crisp, sweet, of superior quality and flavor. Seeds are black. Very resistant to anthracnose (Race 1), and, to some degree, to Fusarium wilt. The rind is thin, hard, and resistant to Sunburn. Keeping and shipping qualities are excellent. From planting to maturity, about 87 days.

charqui. Dried meat of Brazil, chiefly from beef but also from sheep, llama and alpaca in Peru. Strips of meat cut lengthways and pressed after salting then air dried; finished form is in flat, thin sheets, rather flaky, so differing from the long strips of biltong.

Chartreuse. Liqueur made by monks of Chartreux, using, it is said, more than 200 ingredients. There are three varieties: green, 96% of proof spirit; yellow, 74.5%; and white, 52.5%.

Chasselas grape. A white and sometimes pink grape cultivated in Alsace, Australia, France, Germany, and Switzerland. It is known as the Gutadel in Germany. In Europe, it is also a table grape. It produces wines of medium quality.

checking. As applied to lumber drying, the small cracks which develop during drying as a result of closing of the pores by the hardening of the albumen and resins in the sap before the water constituents have been abstracted. The hardened constituents expand with increasing temperature and cause cracks in the timber. Also applied to grains, particularly corn and beans, in which the seedcoats or seed may check as a result of rapid drying, excessive heating, or rough handling.

cheddar cheese. A kind of cheese named after the village of Cheddar in Somerset-shire, England where it was first made. The first Cheddar cheese factory was established by Jesse Williams near Rome, Oneida country, N.Y. in 1851. This hard, rennet cheese, ranging in colour from white to orange, is usually made from pasteurized whole milk. The milk is cooled to the setting temperature, 30°C, run into the cheese vat and starter (lactic acid bacteria) added and milk stirred as it ripens for approximately an hour. Rennet and colour are added and stirring is stopped. The curd sets in about 30 minutes and is then cut with curd knives into very small cubes to allow the whey to drain doff. The stirring process is continued either by hand or by use of curd rakes until the whey is drained. Then the curd is heated gradually to about 37°C and maintained until the curd is ready to be removed from the whey. When the desired firmness of the curd and degree of acidity of the whey is reached, the whey is drained (dipping process) from the vat. When the curd is firm enough to be turned without breaking it is cheddared, and piled and cut into strips. Next, the curd is run into a curd mill and spread evenly over the bottom of the vat and stirred; salt is added and curd is pilled at either side of the vat to allow whey to drain. After the salt has completely dissolved, the curd is removed to cloth lined metal hoops and pressed. When pressing process is complete the curd is dried for 3-4 days at a temperature of 20-22°C, then dipped in paraffin or cheese wax and boxed for shipment to be cured. Curing temperatures range usually from 20-22°C, sometimes as low as 15°C and as high as 25°C. Curing time usually is 3-6 months, but may extend to one year. Also known as American cheese.

cheddaring. The process of piling, matting or packing of the cheese curd and cutting into strips 10-15 cm wide at right angles to the vat, when repelling until it is firm enough to be piled in layers. The purpose of the cheddaring process is to control moisture content by regulating the removal of whey, and to form the characteristic body and texture in the curd. In the manufacture of cheese, after coagulation of the milk, heating of the curd and draining, the curds are piled along the floor of the vat when, in the case of Cheddar cheese, they consolidate to a rubbery sheet of curd. This stage is the Cheddaring process. (In the case of Cheshire cheese it is not allowed to settle so densely and has a more crumbly texture.) Also known as matting.

cheese. A concentrated dairy food product made from the coagulated portion (curd) of milk, cream, skim milk, whey or buttermilk; and consisting chiefly of casein, fat and moisture. It is made by coagulating the casein thereof with rennet or lactic acid, with or without the addition of ripening ferments and seasoning, and contains, in the water-free substance, not less than 50% of milk fat. Switzerland is famous for this so-called King of Cheeses, and a large part of the milk produced in Switzerland is used in its production. It was first made, probably about the middle of the 15th century, in the Canton of Bern in the Emmental Valley (which accounts for its native name Emmentaler). The industry was well developed and cheese was being exported by the middle of the 17th century. Only the best cheese is exported, and it is commonly called Switzerland cheese. Swiss cheese is made in many other countries besides Switzerland, including France, Denmark, Germany, Bavaria, Italy, Austria, Finland, Russia, Argentina, and the United States. Emmentaler, Bellunese, Formaggio Dolce, Fontina, Fontine d'Aosta, and Traanen are local names for similar cheese made in Switzerland and nearby countries. Gruyere, made mostly in France, is similar to Swiss but is smaller and cures somewhat differently. Danish Swiss is called Samso. Swiss cheese is one of the most difficult kinds of cheese to make. Natural cheese is that made directly from milk or whey, as opposed to processed cheese which is usually made from a blend or combination of several kinds of natural or hard cheese. It is made by coagulating or curdling milk, heating and stirring the curd and eventually draining off the whey and accumulating and pressing the curd.

In general, three species of bacteria are used as starters: *Streptococcus thermophilus*, called the *coccus* culture; a lactobacillus, *Lactobacillus bulgaricus* or *L. lactis*, called the rod culture; and *Propionibacterium shermanii* (a propionic-acid-forming microorganism), called the eye former.

The lactobacillus and streptococcus produce lactic acid, which acids in expelling the whey, and they probably contribute to the breakdown of the curd during ripening. The propionic-acid bacteria are largely responsible for the characteristic flavor and eye formation. Flavours and texture requirements are usually obtained by curing the cheese during the holding period at specific temperatures and humidity.

Milk is coagulated either by the addition of rennet or by the lactic acid produced by the addition of starter. A portion of the water is removed by cooking, stirring or draining the curd or by the application of pressure. The cheese may or may not be ripened, the ripening period varying from a few days to many months, depending upon the type of cheese. A true organic cheese should come from a cow which is not rattling with chemicals and emerge at about 38.6°C. It is then immediately chilled to 10°C or less or held at that temperature to prevent the multiplication of bacteria until it is dumped into the cheese vat. Then it is heated to 31-32°C to active the starter and the temperature is increased to 37-39°C to separate the whey from the curd and so produce the proper moisture levels. Since certain amino acids are destroyed at 40°C, milk should not be heated to above 39.7°C). Edam cheese may also contain colourings.

The processed cheese and cheese spreads or cheese-flavoured spreads are made by heating cheese from various sources and blending them together to obtain a consistent result. Emulsifying agents, lactic and acetic acid, salt and flavourings are added. The cheese is then heat-fixed so that it cannot mature any further and the flavour will not change. Many hard varities of cheese are flavoured with added ingredients such as beer, coffee, garlic, onions, and spices.

The different varities of cheese vary enormously nutritionally, but as a group they can be considered as a very potent food. Cheddar, the most common type of cheese in the West, on the whole appears nutritionally in the middle of the range of cheeses. Cheddar cheese is 25% protein, and cream cheese with 8% protein contains much less. It is very fatty, 32% fat, which is slightly more than most of the other hard cheese. Edam cheese contains less than 25% fat. Cream cheese is nearly 38% fat while cottage cheese contains only 0.3%. Cottage cheese emerges with the most favourable ratio of protein to fat but it really does need to be tarted up to taste anything like palatable. Protein and calcium are the chief nutritional features of cheese, and many cheeses contain significant amounts of vitamins A, B_2 and D. Milk is the most common of all food allergies and cheese may cause more allergic reactions than the milk. Symptoms of cheese and milk intolerance are excess of mucus, susceptibility to colds and sinus problems, and indigestion accompanied by flatulence. Solutions to the problems include boiled milk, yoghurt or butter-milk, or better still no milk at all. Milk and cheese are undeniably rich nutritional sources, but the many alternatives to both should be considered by people who experience allergies to them.

Cheese other than cottage or cream are cured by being left to mature with salt, under various conditions that produce the characteristic flavour of the particular type of cheese. The average composition (hard cheese) per 100 g is: protein 25-30%; fat 31%; Ca 750 mg; Fe 1 mg; vitamin A 410 mg; vitamin B_1 0.01 mg; vitamin B_2 0.5 mg; nicotinic acid 0.1 mg; and food energy 1.62 MJ. Most of the lactose of the milk is lost with the whey. Legally must contain not less than 40% fat on a dry weight basis and fat must be milk fat.

cheese, blue. Cheese that contains an internal growth of the mould, *Penicillium roqueforti;* e.g., Blue Vinney, Stilton and Roquefort.

cheese, cottage. A kind of soft, uncured white cheese made from pasteurised skim milk (or milk powder) by lactic acid starter (with or without added rennet) heated, washed and drained (salt may be added). It contains more than 80% water. The baker's cheese or hoop cheese is like cottage cheese but is not washed and is drained in bags so giving a finer grain and contains more water and acid than cottage cheese. Also known as pot cheese; Dutch cheese; Schmierkase cheese.

cheese, processed. Natural cheese passes its peak of flavour rapidly and processing temporarily arrests deterioration, while the processed cheese is loaf cheese, melted, pasteurized, flavourings added (pimento, caraway, etc.), plus emulsifiers, and repacked. Its nutritive value is identical with the original cheese.

cheese, whey. A kind of cheese made from whey by heat-coagulation of the proteins (lactalbumin and lactoglobulin).

cheese body. This characteristic of cheese usually associated with the moisture content is composed of several elements such as firmness, springiness, crumbliness and smoothness. Body is usually measured organoleptically as the resistance to pressure when manipulated between the thumb and the first two fingers.

cheese colour. A colour or dye material commonly added to milk for cheese-making in order to bring and colour of the cheese to the desired shade. It is also used in the artificial colouring of ice cream. The colouring material is either water soluble extract or annatto or coal tar dyes and is carried in an alkaline water solution. These materials add colour to both casein and fat in contrast to butter colour which is an oil solution and mixes only with the fat.

cheese curd. The coagulated or thickened part of milk as distinguished from whey or watery part. The composition of curd made from whole milk is approximately as follows: fat 34%; casein 23%; water 37%; milk sugar and mineral matter 6%.

cheese food (pasteurized process). A food prepared by mixing with the aid of heat one or more of the following; cheese, part skim cheese, an emulsifying agent, an acidifying agent, water, salt, colouring, spices or flavouring. Other optional ingredients are cream, milk, skim milky, cheese whey, or a mixture of two or more of these, or any of the foregoing from which part of the water has been removed, and albumin from cheese whey. The moisture content of this product is not more than 44% and the fat content is not less than 23%. the product must be pasteurized for not less than 30 seconds at 65° C.

cheese insects. Insects which affect the appearance and quality of cheese. There are two particularly injurious species. The cheese hopper, or cheese skipper, is a small black fly white deposits its eggs deep in the cracks of cheese, ham and beef. The maggot has two horny, claw-shaped mandibles, with which it digs into the cheese and moves about, as it has no legs. By bringing the two ends of its body together and separating them by jerk, it can throw itself 20-30 times its own length. The other cheese pest is the cheesemite, a minute creature which leaves upon the cheese a brown, powdery mass of skins. Scrupulous cleanliness in places where cheese is kept is the best defense against these pests.

cheese mite. A small insect scarcely visible to the naked eye. It affects flavour and body of cheese during ripening but does not prevent proper ripening.

cheese paraffining. The act of dipping or coating cheese with wax or paraffin or a mixture of these. The amount of paraffin adhering to the surface depends upon temperature (higher the temperature, thinner the coating) and number of times the cheese is dipped. The cheese is paraffined to protect the surface and to prevent moisture shrinkage.

cheese reaction. A popular term that refers to potentiation by monoamine oxidase inhibitors of the pressor actions of indirectly acting sympathomatic amines, notably tyramine, in certain foods, including some cheeses. The antidepressant action monoamine oxidase inhibitors is predominantly associated with inhibition of MAO-A. Selective inhibitors of MAO-A might therefore have some advantage, in the MAO-B would be left intact, especially in the gut where it represents the first line of defence against ingested tyramine.

cheese spread. Pasteurized process cheese spread with fruits, vegetables or meat conforms to the definitions and standards of identity of pasteurized process cheese spread except that it contains a mixture of one or more of the following : cooked, canned or dried fruit; cooked canned or dried vegetables; cooked or can meat. In general, cheese spreads are food products, usually of a buttery consistency, which contain cheese and other ingredients such as milk or whey solids, emulsifying agents, seasonings, condiments and colouring matter. The difference between spreads and processed and pasteurized cheese is that the spreads are soft and may contain substance other than cheese and emulsifying agents. Because the manufacturing processes are similar, cheese spreads may be considered as modified processed cheeses. There are three principal types of spreads available in the market:

(a) cream cheese with pickles, pimentos, olives, etc.;

(b) processed cheese of sufficient moisture content to be buttery in consistency;

(c) processed cheese to which concentrated whey or skim milk has been added, and which contains sufficient moisture and fat so that it spreads easily.

Cheddar, Swiss, Roquefort and Neufchetel are the varieties of cheese used principally in cheese spreads, but most other varieties may be used. Condensed and dried whey and skim milk are produced for use in cheese spreads. Federal Regulations now specify minimum amount of butterfat and maximum amount of water that they may contain.

chemical ice. Ice containing chemicals used as preservative, *e.g.*, a solution of antibiotics or other chemicals frozen and used to preserve fish.

chemical indicators. Dyestuffs that have one colour in acid solutions and a different colour in basic or alkaline solutions. They are used to indicate the relative acidity of chemical solution, as the different materials have different ranges of action on the acidity scale. The materials are mostly weak acids, but some are weak bases. The best known is litmus, which is red below a pH of 4.5 and blue above a pH of 8.3, and is used to test strong acids or alkalies. It is natural dye prepared from several varieties of lichen, *Variolaria,* chiefly *Rocella tinctoria,* by allowing them to ferment in the presence of ammonia and potassium carbonate. When fermented, the mass has a blue colour and is mixed with chalk and made into tablets of papers. It is used also as a textile dye, wood stain, and as a food colorant. Azolitmin, $C_7H_7O_4N$, is the colouring matter of litmus, and is a reddish-brown powder. Orchil, or cudbear, is a red dye from another species.

Alkanet, also called orcanette, anchusa, or alkanna, is made from the root of the plant *Alkanna tinctoria*. The colouring ingredient, alkannin, is soluble in alcohol, benzene, ether, and oils, and is produced in dry extract as a dark red, amorphous, slightly acid powder. It is also used for colouring fats and oils in pharmacy and in cosmetics, for imparting red colour to wines, and for colouring wax. Alkannin paper, also called Boettger's paper, is a white paper impregnated with an alcohol solution of alkanet. The paper is red, but it is turned to shades from green to blue by alkalies. Some coal-tar base indicators are: malachite green, which is yellow below a pH of 0.5 and green above 1.5; phenolphthalein, which is colourless below 8.3 and magenta above 10; and methyl red, which is red below 4.4 and yellow above 6.

A universal indicator is a mixture of a number of indicators that gives the whole range of colour changes, thereby indicating the entire *p*H range. But such indicators must be compared with a standard to determine the *p*H value. The change in colour is caused by a slight rearrangement of the atoms of the molecule. Some indicators, such as thymol blue, exhibit two colour changes at different acidity ranges because of the presence of more than one chromophore arrangement of atoms. These can thus be used to indicate two separate ranges on the *p*H scale. Curcurmin, a crystalline powder obtained by percolating hot acetone through turmeric, changes from yellow to red over the *p*H range of 7.5-8.5, and from red to orange over the range of 10.2-11.8. Test papers are strips of absorbent paper that have been saturated with an indicator and dried. They are used for testing for acidic or basic solutions, and not for accurate determination of acidity range or hydrogen-ion concentration such as is possible with direct use of the indicators. Litmus paper is used for testing the acidity. Starch-iodide paper is paper dipped in starch paste containing potassium iodide. It is used to test for the presence of halogens and oxidizing agents such as hydrogen peroxide.

chemical score. A chemical method of defining the nutritional value of proteins. It is based on a comparison of its amino acid composition with that of egg, which has a nearly ideal balance of essential amino acids. The amount of each amino acid in the protein is expressed as a percent of the amount of the same amino acid in egg; the lowest value, or score, is given by the essential amino acid that is limiting for growth and is a measure of the nutritionally quality of the protein. A later modification is Protein Score, in which a standard amino acid reference mixture is used instead of egg protein.

Chenin-Blanc grape. A variety of white grape highly regarded for its quality, and sometimes referred to as the Pineau de la Loire. In addition to France, the variety is successfully cultivated in northern California. White wines made from this variety are the predominant wines in several of the French provinces where it is grown. The variety is sometimes referred to as the Pinot Blanc.

cherry, west Indian. Fruit of a small bushy tree native to tropical and semi-tropical regions of America, *Malpighia punicifolia*. It is one of the richest known source of vitamin C; the edible portion of the fruit contains 1000 mg of vitamin C per 100 g when ripe, and the green fruit 3000 mg. Also known as *Barbados cherry* and *Acerola* (Spanish), and Antilles cherry.

cherry. Fruit of *Prunus avium* species. Since the caveman era, wild cherries have existed in the temperate parts of Asia, Europe and North America. The hundreds of varieties on the market today may be classified in terms of sweetness and colour. The Bing and Royal Ann varities of cherry are sweet, but Bings have deeply coloured juice, whereas the juice of the other variety is colourless. Sour cherries are most favoured for pies, tarts and turnovers, are similarly divided. The very popular tart cherry, Montmorency, is light to dark red with red juice. The average composition per 100 g of cherries is: protein 1.0%; fat 0.42%; Fe 0.4 mg; vitamin A 170 µg; vitamin B_1 0.06 mg; vitamin B_2 0.04 mg; nicotinic acid 0.5 mg; vitamin C 6 mg; and food energy 0.24 MJ.

chervil. Family: *Umbilliferae.* Genus: *Anthriscus.* Species: *Anthriscus cerefolium.* A herb used in the fresh green state for flavouring salads and soups, and as a granish. Chervil comes from a Greek word meaning leaf of rejoicing or cheer-leaf. Chervil is East European origin and is to be found growing wild in Southeast Russia and most of Iran. This annual plant has a round, finely grooved, branched stem which grows 30-65 cm high from a thin, whitish root. The leaves are opposite, light green and bipinnate, the lower leaves petioled, the upper sessile on stem sheaths. Chervil, together with chives, parsley, and tarragon, is one of the *fines herbes* mixture used in French cookery, particularly to flavour omelettes. It is also one of the herbs used in ravigote sauces, and is often blended with tarragon to flavour béchamel and other creamy sauces. It is a hardy annual, one that is easy to grow but that quickly goes to seed. The leaves quickly lose their flavour and are best added fresh to a dish just before serving. They can be chopped into softened butter to serve with grilled meats or poultry; added as an aromatic garnish to creamy soups; and stirred into egg and cheese dishes. The leaves are also used to flavour white wine vinegar, and may be infused in water as skin freshener. Chervil contains a volatile oil which stimulates the metabolism. The fresh roots are antiseptic and used to be prescribed by herbalists for girls during puberty. However, there is some division on this because some herbalists now feel that the root itself is poisonous. The distilled water of chervil is a diuretic and acts on the kidneys. A warm poultice applied locally will ease painful joints. It was popular for soothing gout at one time.

Cheshire cheese. A hard, rennet cheese first made in England, from sweet whole cows' milk. The cheese is very highly coloured, cylindrical in shape. It is one of the oldest and most popular of the English varieties of cheese. It is crumbly or flaky in body and mild in flavour.

Cheshire-stilton cheese. A combination of the characteristics of Cheshire and Stilton varieties of cheese. The manufacturing procedure, size and shape are similar to Cheshire cheese but the mold of Stilton is used.

chestnug, water. *Trapa natans,* also known as *Caltrops* and *Singharanut.* Seed is eaten raw or roasted. The average composition per 100 g is: 3 g protein; 15 g carbohydrate; 0.8 mg iron; vitamin B_1 0.05 mg; nicotinic acid 0.06 mg; 16 mg C; and food energy 0.32 MJ.

chestnut. Family: *Fagacea.* Genus: *Castanea.* Species: *Castanea dentata* (American); *Castanea sativa* (European). Chestnuts which are raw should be approached with caution because of their high tannic-acid content. They make good body-building material and are helpful for strengthening gums.

chewing gums. The confections prepared from various masticatory substances. In the chewing gum manufacture, selected gum or combination of gum bases is finely chopped, dried, and then cooked, usually under vacuum. When fully mastic, various flavouring ingredients (sugar and/or artificial sweeteners, etc.) are added to the batch, after which they are mixed to form a kind of dough. After kneading, the material is rolled into sheets for cutting or extruded into final forms. The cut pieces are then dried, dusted to avoid sticking, and packed. Although chewing gum is consumed in several parts of the world, it is mainly an American product.

Chianti. A common red wine in Italy. The quality of Chianti varies considerably from one manufacturer to the other. Some varieties of good quality Chianti have built an international appreciation for its characteristics, which by habit or other reason, seem to blend exceptionally well with various Italian foods. More than hundred million gallons of Chianti is produced in Italy during an year, a considerable portion of this being of modest to poor quality. Some observers · have noted that common California red wines are better than a number of the Chianti imported. Such observers also hasten to add that the classical Chianti, prepared from San Gioveto and Cannaiolo grapes and with other touches provided by the producer, can be a superior wine. A special method of vinification is used in the Chianti country of Italy and is locally referred to as *Voverno*. For the high-quality wines, about one-tenth of the grapes harvested (some of the more exotic varieties, such as Cannai-olo, Mammolo, and Colorino) are put aside to raisin after they are pressed. Fermentation of these berries is delayed until late fall. Once their fermentation has commenced, they are added to the principal batch of wine. This results in early spring. The somewhat prickling sensation produced by some varieties of Chianti is considered by some experts to arise from this "hint of sparking."

chick anti-pellagra factor. Obsolete name for pantothenic acid.

chicken. The average composition per 100 g of a young and healthy chicken is: protein 12.5%; fat 7.9; Ca 7-8 mg; Fe 1 mg; vitamin A 75 µg; vitamin B$_1$ 0.06 mg; vitamin B$_2$ 0.1 mg; nicotinic acid 4.9 mg; and food energy 0.5 MJ.

chick-pea. Family: *Leguminosae*. Genus: *Cicer*. Species: *Cicer arietinum*. Chick-peas are rich in iron, calcium and vitamins, especially vitamin C, and have been used to treat deficiency diseases in children.

chickweed. *Stellaria media*. This apparently feeble member of the pink group is actually a lusty annual with matted to upright green stems that take over many areas. It vigorously thrives through the sleet and snowstorms of winter, even in the far north, survives most weed killers, beginning to bloom while the snow is often still on the ground, and many times it finishes its seed production in the springtime.

chicle. The partially evaporated latex of the evergreen sapodilla tree (*Achras zapota*). It is used mainly as base for chewing gum, sometimes diluted with gutta gums. For chewing it is compounded with polyvinyl acetate, microcrystalline wax, and flavours. The crude chicle is in reddish-brown pieces, and may have up to 40% impurities. The purified and neutralized gum is an amorphous white to pinkish powder insoluble in water, which forms a sticky mass when heated. It contains about 40% resin, 17 rubber, and about 17 sugars and starches. Under the name of txixtle, the coagulated latex was mixed with asphalt and used as chewing gum by the Aztec Indians, and this custom of chewing gum has been widely adopted in the United States.

chicory, endive and escarole. *Cichorium intybus, C. endiva-latifolia.* The plant native of Europe and Asia, but long since naturalized in other parts of the world. It has a fleshy root, spreading branches, coarse leaves and bright bue flowers. The leaves are sometimes blanched, to be used as salad. But the most important part of the plant is its long, fleshy and milky root, which, when dried, roasted ground, is now extensively used for adulterating coffee. The presence of chicory in coffee must be stated on the label of the package, in accordance with recent pure food laws. Its presence may easily be detected by putting a spoonful of the mixture into a glass to clear, cold water, when the coffee will float on the surface and the choice will separate and discolor the water as it subsides. The plant has stick-like stems; open, widely spaced foliage and milky sap. The striking thing about chicory, however, is its bright, almost iridescent blue flowers that bloom incongruously on the stems as if stapled to the wrong plant. The rootstock is light yellow outside, white inside and contains a bitter milky juice too. In US the name endive usually refers to the small, pale, cigar-shaped plant, while escarole refers to the broad, bushy head with waxy leaves. Endives have a slightly bitter taste. All three salad plants in the family, endive, chicory and escarole, were believed to have some bitter herbs consumed by the Children of Israel during the Passover before their hasty exodus from Egypt. Chicory root is frequently used in natural coffee substitutes and added to regular coffee to give it a richer flavour and reduce its caffeine content somewhat. The leaves are eaten as a salad and the root, dried and partly caramelised is often added to coffee as a diluent to cheapen the product. The leaves are grown in the dark to prevent the development of the bitter flavour and so are very pale in colour. Also called succory

and (in Belgium). The French call chicory "Endive Belge" and endive is called "Chicoree". Chicory is rich in inulin, like dandelion root, and contains minerals salts and vitamins B, C, K and P. It is a weak tonic, a diuretic and a laxative and was once used to help jaundice. It was also believed to protect the liver from the effect of too much coffee drinking, and certainly it makes a much more effective enema than coffee, opening up the haemorrhoidal portal vein so that waste products can be dumped from liver. It increases glandular secretion slightly. Average composition of leaf and stem per 100 g is: water 96%; protein 0.8%; carbohydrate 1.5% (some of which is inulin); Fe 0.7 mg.

Chiffon cakes. The cakes similar to Angel food cakes in the leavening occurs mainly as the result of whipping the egg whites to a low density foam. In addition to egg whites, flour, and sugar-as found in angel food batters-chiffon cakes contain egg yolks and added fat, the latter characteristically in the form of vegetable oil rather than plastic shortening. Ingredients comprising the batter (shortening, flour, etc.) are mixed separately from the foam ingredients, then these two parts are combined by folding the batter into the foam. Sometimes the foam is folded into the batter, depending on the type of results the formulator wishes to obtain. "Chiffon" was the name given by the originators to the completed mixture before baking, but it is now applied to the cakes as well. Baking powder is often used to improve the oven spring in chiffon cakes, but the structure and volume are primarily due to the foamed egg ingredient. A typical formula, expressed in percent of batch weight, is: 10.7% egg yolks,

10.7% salad oil, 32.0% egg whites, 0.4% salt, 16.0% granulated sugar, 14.0% cake flour, 1.0% powdered sugar, and 0.2% cream of tartar. The egg whites, cream of tartar, and salt are whipped until a soft foam is developed, then the sugar is added and beating is continued until a soft peak is obtained. The egg yolks are whipped in separate equipment until they are thoroughly blended and aerated. The egg yolk and oil mixture is carefully folded into the meringue using minimal agitation. The sugar and flour are sifted, together and then folded into the eggs. If baking powder is to be added it goes in with the flour. Although chiffon cakes may be used in many of the same combinations suggested for pound and sponge cakes, the greater difficulty of making them and their somewhat coarser and less resilient structure reduces their utility in these items. Flavoring preferences are similar to those for sponge cakes, although orange and lemon chiffon cakes seem to be the most common varieties. Chocolate-flavored chiffon cakes are also well accepted.

chili sauce. Sauce made from tomatoes with species onions, garlic, sugar, vinegar, and salt-similar to tomato catsup but containing more cayenne, onions and garlic.

chillproofing. A term used in reference to beer; treatment to prevent appearance of haze when the beer is chilled. Chillproofs include tannic acid to precipitate proteins, materials such as bentonic to adsorb them, and proteolytic enzymes to hydrolyse them.

chimche. Basic Korean dish (in addition to fish and rice) consisting of fermented cabbage with garlic, red peppers and pimientos. Vitamin C content 126 mg per 100 g, led to the suggestion that the Koreans have the highest intake of vitamin C.

Chinese cabbage. Family: *Cruciferae* (mustard family). Genus: *Brassica.* Chinese cabbage is more closely related to mustard than to cabbage. It is sometimes called celery cabbage even though it is unrelated to celery. Other names, such as crispy choy, chihili, michili, and wong bok, refer to different varieties of the plant. Generally, the flavour of the leaves and stalks of these plants is quite similar to lettuce. Its use in salads is popular, but the plant parts also may be cooked and served as a vegetable or incorporated into other dishes, such as casseroles and Chinese recipes. There are two principal species of this cool-weather plant. *Brassica chinensis,* of which crispy choy is variety, achieves a height of 30-46 cm and furnishes an edible stalk that is of greenish-white color. The leaves are ustered loosely about the stalk. More commonly cultivated in the US is *B. pekinensis,* of which michili, is a variety. This plant achieves a height 46 to 51 cm and features a core of tender, lightly compressed green leaves. The silhouette of the growing plant, when the outer leaves are intact, has an unlike appearance.

Chinese eggs. A Chinese dish prepared by covering fresh duck eggs with a mixture of caustic soda, burnt straw ash, salt and slaked lime, and storing for several months. The white and yolk of the egg coagulate and become discoloured with partial decomposition of the protein and phospholipids. Also known as Pidan, Houeidan and Dsaoudan, according to variations in the method of preparation.

chitin. A nitrogen-containing heterosaccharide having a basic structure similar to that of cellulose but also containing amino (nitrogen) groups. It is homo-polymer of N-acetyl-D-glucosamine. This structural polysaccharide constitutes the shell of crustaceans and scales of insects. It forms hard layers or accretions and is found in integuments of shellfish. It is found in some animals and the cell walls of most fungi. The outer covering of arthropod, the cuticle, is impregnated in its outer layers with chitin, which makes the exoskeleton more rigid. It is associated with protein to give a uniquely tough yet flexible and light skeleton, which also has the advantage of being waterproof. The chitinous plates are thinner for bending and flexibility or thicker for stiffness as required. The plates cannot grow once laid down and are digested at each moult. Chitin is also found in the hard parts of several other groups of animals. It consists of many glucose units, in each of which one of the hydroxyl groups has been replaced by acetylamine group ($-CH_3CONH_2$).

chitinase. An externally secreted digestive enzyme produced by certain microorganisms and invertebrates that hydrolyzes chitin.

chitterlings. Intestine of ox, calf or pig.

chives. Family: *Amaryllidaceae*. Genus: *Allium*. Species: *Allium schoenoprasum*. It belongs to the same *Allium* species that garlic and onions belong to, and is seldom found in the wild anymore, this hardy perennial is cultivated all over the world, from Corsica, Greece and Sweden to Siberia and throughout North America. The bulbs grow quite close together in dense clusters and are of an elongated form, with white, rather firm sheaths. They also thrive in temperate regions of North America. The leaves have a delicate, onion-like flavour and are widely used in cooking, particularly in egg and cheese dishes, in salads, and as a garnish. If protected, they can be harvested for about nine months of the year. Chives are included in the *fines herbs* mixture used in French cookery. Snipped chives, for it is easier to cut them with scissors than chop them with a knife, give a hint of onion flavour in many dishes, from scrambled egg to cheese soufflé. They are good sprinkled on green and tomato salads, on soups, in cream cheese sandwiches, and on jacket potatoes with soured cream dressing. Chive butter, made by beating snipped chives and lemon juice into softened butter, is good with grilled chops and steak. Chives contain very similar health-giving properties to garlic but they are altogether milder. They are rich in vitamin C and sulphur. They are a digestive and have antiseptic properties. Chives (usually referred to in the plural) are the smallest, though one of the finest-flavored of the onion tribe. Since the leaves are slightly antiseptic, and were used to relieve rheumatism. Chives are used to season omelettes, cottage cheese, baked or mashed potatoes, sour cream sauces or dips, salad greens as well as salad dressings. Chives used in food as a flavouring and as a garnish are the hollow thin green stems of the alliaceous bulb, *Allium schoenoprasum* L. The plant grows wild throughout northern Europe, Canada and northern United States, but is most widely cultivated as a pot herb. It has a pleasantly delicate onion-like flavour, which is strongest in the young, freshly chopped leaves. The flavour is lost on dehydration, but can be retained for several months under frozen storage.

chlorella. A nonmotile unicell, which

was the first alga to be isolated in axenic (pure) culture and has been widely used for experimental studies of photosynthesis. In nature, Chlorella is widespread in both fresh and salt water and in soil. Each Chlorella cell contains a single cup-shaped chloroplast, with or without a pyrenoid, and a single minute nucleus. The only known method of reproduction in Chlorella is asexual, each haploid cell dividing mitotically two or three times to give rise to either four or either nonmotile cells. Chlorella is currently under investigation as a potential food source for humans. Pilot farms have been established in the United States, Germany, Japan, and Israel. The Japanese have processed Chlorella as a tasteless white powder, rich in vitamins and protein, that can be mixed with flour.

chlorine. An element that is found in biological tissues as chloride ion. The body contains about 100 g of chloride and the average diet contains 6-7 g, mainly as sodium chloride. Free chlorine is used as a sterilising agent e.g., in drinking water. Acute poisoning due to chlorine causes severe coughing, difficulty in breathing, burning sensation to the nose, throat, and eyes, and skin irritation. Occupational exposure to chlorine gas should be controlled in such a manner so that no employee is exposed to gaseous chlorine at a concentration greater than 0.5 mg/m^3 of air, for any 15 minute sampling period.

chlorine demand. The amount of chlorine required by any given volume of sewage or polluted water, to kill all pathogenic bacteria therein.

chlorine dioxide. A highly reactive, hazardous compound of chlorine; used for bleaching and as disinfectant. The occupational exposure to chlorine dioxide is defined as exposure to airborne concentration of this compound at or above one-half of the recommended workplace environmental limit. Occupational exposure to chlorine dioxide should be controlled so that no employee is exposed to chlorine dioxide at a concentration greater than 0.3 mg/m^3 of air (0.1 ppm), for any 15 minute sampling period. The recommended standard is designed to protect the health and safety of workers for up to a 10-hour workshift, 40-hour work week over a working lifetime.

chlorocruorin. The copper-containing protein that carries oxygen in the bloodstream of the Annelid worms, analogous to haemoglobin in mammals.

chlorophylls. The green colouring matter of leaves by which they carry out pohtosynthesis. The chlorophylls in plants is somewhat analogous to hemoglobin in blood and their structural formulas are very similar. Chlorophylls are magnesium complexes having a porphyrin structure and contain two hydroxy groups; one is esterified with phytyl alcohol and the other with methyl alcohol. In nature, the molecular complex is bound with a protein moiety. Commercially, chlorophyll is recovered from various grasses by alcohol or acetone extraction of the finely powdered dehydrated grass-meal with the subsequent removal of the solvent under vacuum. The initial dark, olive-colored, firm extract is a mixture of pigments including chlorophyll-α (about 60%), chlorophyll-β (about 25%) together with xanthophyll (about 10 %) and carotene (about 5%). This extract is soluble in fixed oils and organic solvents, and is used as the strting material for the manufacture of a range of oil, and water-soluble derivatives. Wilstater found that chlorophyll was an ester of chlorophyllin with phytol and that the compound could be saponified by alkalis to give a nitrogenous compound known as pheophytin and the free unsaturated alcohol, phytol. This reaction is the basis for the production of purified chlorophyll and chlorophyllins. The colour of chlorophyll depends on the nature of the coordinated element, which is normally magnesium. As a result of natural acids present during the extraction, this element is replaced by hydrogen. To produce a bright green colour, it is necessary to introduce copper into the molecule. This is done by treating the separated pheophytins with a calculated quantity of copper sulphate and removing all excess ionic copper. The total and ionic copper content of these products is determined in aqueous solution by atomic absorption spectrophotometry. Whether coopered or uncoopered, the chlorophylls are soluble in ethanol (95%), hydrocarbon solvents, fixed oils and fats. They are insoluble in diluted alcohol and water. Chlorophyll is almost universally accepted for use in foods, but the cooper complex is not (neither is accepted in US). In many countries, its use is limited to certain products (e.g., chewing gum). Before using the coppered chlorophyllins in any food product, reference should be made to the specific regulations. In the case of the water-soluble products, it should be remembered that these salts are not stable in acid solution as the pheophytin is precipitated. In neutral and alkaline media, these chlorophyllins are stable and light-fast.

chlorophyllide. The green colour found in the water after cooking certain vegetables. the fat-soluble chlorophyll is converted to water-soluble chlorophyllide by removal of the phytyl side-chain by alkali or enzyme.

chloroplast. Semiautonomous cell organelles enclosed by double membrane lipoproteinaceous envelope. Like a mitochondrion, a chloroplast has an outer membrane and a inner membrane with an intermembrane space. The inner membrane surrounds a stroma containing soluble enzymes and membranous structures called thylakoids, which are flattened sacs, where carbon dioxide is fixed. The lamellae are stacked to form thylakoid and these form the grana where photolysis of water, production of ATP and $NADPH_2$ are completed. Thus a chloroplast is an organelle with considerable autonomy. The inner membrane of a chloroplast, which contains translocators for a variety of compounds such as ATP and dicarboxylic acids, is the site of interaction between chloroplast and the rest of the cell. The outer membrane of the chloroplast, like that of a mitochondrion, is highly permeable to small molecules and ions.

chocolate (from cacao beans). *Theobroma cacao.* Chocolate is obtained from the ground, roasted beans of the cacao tree. This evergreen with leathery, oblong leaves reaches a height of about 10 m and a trunk width of about 15 cm. The leaves are typically evergreen, with whitish or yellowish flowers slightly tinted with orange and pink. The berries are borne directly on the trunk and the branches may be red, yellow, purple or brown in colour. Inside the thick ridged and furrowed fruit find, are a white or pinkish acid pulp enclosing 25-60 brown or purple, bitter and somewhat oily seeds. It is these seeds or cacao beans which are of prime economic importance and yield cocoa powder, cocoa butter and chocolate upon curing by fermentation and drying, followed next with roasting and finally by grinding while still very hot.

chocolate brown HT. CI Food brown 3. A diazo compound that is used for the colouring of vinegar. It is very soluble in water and has excellent stability in acid media.

chocolate liquor. The solid or plastic product obtained by grinding cocoa nibs. Chocolate liquor contains about 50% fat. Also known as liquor chocolate, plain chocolate, and chocolate. The cooled liquor may be molded and put up in large or small slabs or packages such as are sold in grocery stores as bitter cooking chocolate, or it may be further processed into cocoa.

chocolate. Chocolate nibs, refined and mixed with sugar, cocoa butter, lecithin, and, if milk chocolate, milk solids. The average composition (plain unsweetened) per 100 g is: protein 5-6%; fat 50-55%; Ca 100 mg; Fe 4.5 mg; vitamin A 20 μg; B$_1$ 0.06 mg; B$_2$ 0.25 mg; nicotinic acid mg; and food energy 2.2 MJ.

choking. The interruption of breathing by pressure, by an obstruction or breathing in polluted atmosphere. The blocking usually occurs in the larynx, or voicebox, which opens into the throat. The cause of choking may be illness, injury, a foreign body.

cholagogue. A substance that promotes the flow of bile from the gall bladder into the duodenum.

cholecystokinin. A hormone secreted by the mucosa of the duodenum and jejunum and carried in the blood of gall-bladder which is thus stimulated to contract and secrete bile.

choleretics. Substances that stimulate the secretion of bile; such as bile salts themselves taken by mouth, or cholic acid by intravenous injection.

cholesterol. An unsaturated polycyclic alcohol (sterol) having one hydroxyl group and one double bond. It is closely related to phenanthrene in structure and falls into the general classification of lipids. Cholesterol is a component of all eucaryotic plasma membranes, and is essential for the growth and viability of cells in higher organisms. However, too much of cholesterol can be lethal because of the atherosclerosis resulting from the deposition of plaques of cholesterol esters. Cholesterol is synthesized by all higher animals; its oxidation product in the body are bile acids and steroid hormones. In esterified form it is a component of the saturated fatty acids occurring in animal fats such as butter; it is thought by some workers to have an adverse effect on the circulatory system, but according to recent researches, this has not been proved. In vertebrates, cholesterol is the substrate for a complex of modifications of the side-chains and the ring system to form progesterone, androgens, estrogens, and corticosteroid.

choline. Essential dietary factor. trimethyl hydroxyethyklammonium hydroxide, usually classed as a vitamin, although the quantities involved are far from catalytic. It functions in the animal organism as a source of mobile methyl groups, and in a number of species as a lipotropic agent by aiding the conversion of neutral fats to phospholipides in the liver. Choline occur in the body as a constituent of lecithin or as acetyl choline. its classification as one of the vitamins of the Vitamin B-complex is not universally accepted. A deficiency of choline prevents normal functioning of liver and kidney. Liver is an excellent source of choline; good sources are meat, eggs, cereals and certain vegetables. Specific dietary deficiency does not occur; daily requirements not established but the daily intake is 0.25-0.5 g. Choline can be synthesized in body tissues from the essential amino acid methionine, and dietary requirements thus depend on the quantity of methionine and fat in the diet. Most foods are good sources of choline.

Without sufficient choline, animals develop fatty livers and hemorrhage kidneys. The absence of choline for long periods causes basic physiological changes in the animal that shorten life span. Perosis (slipped tendon) in poultry, can result from a deficiency of choline (or manganese). In pigs, a choline deficiency may result in spraddled hind legs in the newborn; fatty infiltration of liver; and poor reproduction and lactation in sows. Suggested choline level vary considerably. For example, for finishing swine, the suggested level ranges from as 100 g/ton to 1995 g /ton of complete feed. For poultry layers, the amounts of choline required vary with geography and traditional area feed substances. Level from 75-300 g/ton are suggested for the northeastern US, whereas the much higher levels of 300-500 g/ton are suggested for the Midwestern states. Choline occurs in fats and usually is an sufficient supply in feeds that contain fats with the exception of those that may be very limited in methionine.

cholinesterases. Enzymes that break down acetylcholine at the neuromuscular junctions, so permitting a return to the resting state prior to any further stimulation by acetylcholine release. The term usually refers to acetylcholinesterase, which breaks down the neurotransmitter acetylcholine into choline and acetic acid. It is found in all cholinergic nerve junctions, where it rapidly destroys the acetylcholine released during the transmission of a nerve impulse so that subsequent impulses may pass. Other cholinesterases are found in the blood and other tissues. Two types have been distinguished, true and pseudo. True cholinesterase is thought to be responsible for the destruction of acetylcholine at neuromuscular junction and is found in nerve tissue and in the red blood cells. Pseudocholinesterases are found in various tissues such as liver, heart muscle and intestine and it is this type which is present in plasma.

Cholla. Loaf of white bread made in twist form (or Biblical beehive coil) from one large and one small piece of dough plaited together. The dough is made from white flour, enriched with eggs and a pinch of saffron, and the loaf is decorated with maw or poppy seed. Mentioned in the Bible and translated as loaves; used for benediction on the Jewish Sab-bath and Festivals.

chondroitin. A polysaccharide containing galactosamine and glucuronic acid. The sulphuric acid ester, chondroitin sulphate, is found in cartilage and the organic matrix of bone. Classed as a mucopolysaccharide.

Chorleywood bread process. A method of preparing dough for bread-making in which the dough is submitted to intense mechanical working so that, together with the aid of oxidising agent, the need for bulk fermentation of the dough is eliminated. This is a "no-time" dough process and saves 1.5-2 hours. The process permits the use of an increased proportion (20-25) replacement of weaker flour, and produces a softer, finer bread which stales more slowly.

choux pastry. A light, airy pastry as used in eclairs and cream buns. The batter is pre-cooked in the saucepan, the baked. The name choux is the French for cabbage, the characteristic shape for cream puffs.

chowder. An American term for a seafood soup; often made with clams or shrimps.

Chromobacterium violaceum. Facultatively anaerobic, motile, oxidase-positive, Gram-negative rods that are found naturally in soil and water. It causes chromobacteriosis, a rare systemic infec-tion that occurs mostly in tropical and subtropical climates. Most strains produce a water-insoluble, violet pigment.

chromatography. The widely used analytical technique which is based on different rates of migration of components in a mixture in which one phase is immobile layer of developed surface and the other is a mobile stream of gas or liquid flowing through it. In general, chromatography involves passing a gaseous or liquid mixture known as mobile phase, through a column of porous material sometimes coated with a nonvolatile liquid, called the stationary phase. The components of the mixture are adsorbed selectively and pass through the porous material at different rates, emerging as distinct separation zones at the bottom of the column. A carrier gas or liquid is necessary to provide movement of the material through the adsorbent. When the components have been thus separated, the identity of each can be determined by an appropriate analytical method. The best known types of chromatography are gas, liquid, paper, ion-exchange, and thin layer, the name depending on the characteristic aspect of the method. This technique has been widely used for quantitative determination of carbohydrates, proteins, amino acids and a number of metals present in various foodstuffs.

chromium. A grayish-white, hard and brittle metal, which itself is not so toxic except in the form of fume, but some of its compounds are irritant and damaging to the skin, especially those involving hexavalent chromium. Its major uses are as an alloying agent in stainless steel and other alloys and for electroplated coatings on exposed metal parts. It can also be plated on plastics. Its isotope, chromium-51, is radioactive and is, obtained by neutron bombardment of chromium; it radiates gamma rays. Some of its compounds have been recognized to possess carcinogenic or cocarcinogenic potential.

Chromium occurs in a variety of foodstuffs in the form of a complex with nicotinic acid and possibly glycine, glutamic acid, and cysteine. Chromium in this complex, termed as glucose tolerance factor, is absorbed better than in an inorganic form. Animal protein is the best and most reliable source of chromium. The chromium content in all tissues decreases with age. It has been postulated that this decline in chromium may be involved in the etiology of disease states with ageing. The concentration of chromium in human blood is estimated to be 0.5-5 µg/L and in urine, 5-10 µg/L. The daily chromium intake by man ranges from 5-100 µg. The chromium levels in the hair of 33 normal children and of 19 juvenile diabetics have been composed. Normal children showed a mean chromium concentration of 0.85 µg/g (range of 0.36-1.87 µg/g (range 0.26-1.19 µg/g). The development of corneal lesions in squirrel monkeys maintained on a low chromium diet has been demonstrated.

In past, interest in chromium was confined to its toxic effects. However, the element is now considered essential. It has been demonstrated that the synthesis of cholesterol and fatty acids from acetate by rat liver was enchanced when chromium ions were present. In the rat experiments addition of chromium to a low-chromium diet suppressed serum cholesterol levels and inhibited the tendency of levels to increase with age. Scientists observed impaired glucose tolerance in rats fed various diets. The cause was traced to a chromium deficiency. Chromium is now considered essential for maintaining normal glucose metabolism. It was later hypothesized that Cr (III) acts as a cofactor with insulin at the cellular level through the formation of ternary complex between membrane sites, insulin, the chromium. Evidence has accumulated that chromium is involved in glucose tolerance in man. The rats fed diets deficient in protein and chromium exhibit impaired capacity to incorporate the amino acids, glycine, serine, methionine and α-aminobutyrate into the protein of their hearts. The slight improvement in incorporation achieved with insulin alone was significantly enhanced by supplementation with trivalent chromium. Subsequently, it was demonstrated that raising rats in plastic cages on a low protein, low chromium diet resulted in moderate depression of growth that could be alleviated by chromium supplements.

The oxidizing agent chromic acid and the dichromate salts are irritating to mucous membranes, skin, and conjunctiva. Allergies and dermatitis are induced through exposure to these compounds. The penetrating ulcers which occur around the fingernails, the surface of exposed fingerjoints, eyelids, and occasionally forearms, are not painful and do little if any permanent damage. The lesions on nasal mucosa are more troublesome. In some instances the septum is perforated, and breathing through the nose makes a whistling sound. A higher rate of bronchitis among chromate workers has been reported. 'Chronic chromate lung' has also been described. Alkali bichromates can be absorbed through skin lesions in sufficient quantity to cause renal damage. For many years it was not realized that chromium compounds could be carcinogenic. However, certain epidemiological studies seem to have established a significant increase in pulmonary malignancy in workers exposed to chromium and all its compounds. Hypersensitivity to chromium is not restricted to industrial workers. Chromium present in detergents has been implicated as the cause of dermatitis in housewives in Europe and Israel.

It has been shown that noncarcinogenic compounds of chromium (VI) are chromates and dichromates of lithium, sodium, potassium, rubidium, and ammonium, while most of the other compounds of chromium (VI) have been found to possess carcinogenic activity. The occupational exposure to carcinogenic chromium (VI) is defined as exposure to airborne concentration of carcinogenic chromium (VI) at or above one-half of recommended workplace environmental limit; while occupational exposure to noncarcinogenic chromium (VI) is defined as exposure to airborne concentration of the noncarcinogenic chromium (VI) at or above one-half of the recommended workplace environmental limit. Occupational exposure to noncarcinogenic chromium (VI) should be controlled in such a manner so that no person is exposed to noncarcinogenic chromium (VI) at concentrations greater than 25 mg/m^{-3} of air, determined as the timeweighted average (TWA) concentration limit for up to a 10-hour workday in a 40-hour workweek, over a working lifetime.

For total recoverable chromium (VI), the criterion to protect freshwater aquatic life as 0.29 mg/L as a 24-hour average and the concentration should not exceed 21 mg/l at any time. The available data for chromium (VI) indicate that chronic toxicity to freshwater aquatic life occurs at concentrations as low as 44 mg/L, and would occur at even lower concentrations among the species that are more sensitive than those tested. For the protection of human health from the toxic effects of chromium (III) ingested through water and contaminated aquatic organisms, the ambient water criterion to be 170 mg/L; while for the protection of human health from the toxic properties of chromium (III) ingested through contaminated aquatic organisms alone, the ambient water criterion has been determined to be 3433 mg/L. The ambient water quality criterion for total chromium (VI) has been recommended to be identical to the existing drinking water standard, which is 50 mg/L.

chromogen. A colourless substrate that is acted on by an enzyme to produce a colored end product.

chromoproteins. A class of proteins conjugated with a metal-containing prosthetic group, *e.g.*, vertebrate haemoglobins contain iron, invertebrate haemocyanins contain copper, chlorophyll contains magnesium, and are characterized by being colored. The prosthetic group is a coloured compound in such cases.

chromosomes. The protein-nucleic acid complex formed from chromatin in the nucleus of the biological cell; it is made up of DNA, the genetic code carrier, and various other nucleoproteins. Chromosomes are unit structures formed during cell division from standards of the parent complex, chromatin, the number of chromosomes in a given cell being characteristic of a particular plant or animal species. They contain the genes, which are the specific agents of hereditary transmission.

chuck. A part of a side of dressed beef, including some of the neck and the parts about the shoulder blade, also including the meat on the first three ribs.

churn. A vessel used for making butter. An early and simple pattern was shaped like the lower part of a cone. A plunger operated through a hole in the cover stirred the cream within until the butter was separated from the buttermilk. The modified forms of churns are now in general used and these secure the desired result by rotary motion. In creameries large churns operated by power are in use.

chutney. A sweet-sour, moist condiment originating in India and the Orient. It is commonly consumed with curries. The principal ingredients of chutney include the ripe fruits of mango and tamarind, combined with raisins, various herbs, chillies or cayenne, vinegar or lemon juice. Numerous spices, in varying quantities and combinations, that may be added include fenugreek seed, ginger, and turmeric. Bottled and preserved chutney is usually available at restaurants and gourmet departmental stores.

chyle. The digested alkaline fluid resulting from the action of the biliary and pancreatic juice upon the chyme which is thus prepared for absorption by the lacteals of the intestines. It passes mixed with the blood into the veins by the thoracic duct.

chylomicrons. Droplets of unhydrolysed fat in the lymph or bloodstream.

chymase. An enzyme usually obtained from the inner lining of the fourth stomach of young calves and lambs although it is widely distributed in other animals and in extracts from various plants. The chymase of mammals is usually called rennin. The extract containing the enzyme is known as rennet and is used in the manufacture of cheese.

chyme. The partially digested food as it exists in the stomach. A thick grayish-white substance formed by the action of gastric juice on food in stomach. The walls of the stomach contract in such a way as to churn the masticated food and mix it thoroughly with the gastric juice, and the resulting chyme passes into the small intestine to be changed into a fluid called chyle.

chymosin. Obsolete name for rennin, also chymase.

chymotrypsin. Proteolytic enzyme of the pancreatic juice; it attacks parts of the protein molecule different from those attacked by pepsin and by trypsin. It is secreted as the inactive precursor, chymotrypsinogen, and activated by trypsin.

CI acid blue 3. patent blue. A calcium salt of *m*-hydroxy-tetraethyldiaminotriphenyl carbinyldisulphonic acid. It is a bright blue powder, which is soluble in water (15% at 25°C), glycerol and ethanol (95%). It is very light-fast and is heat stable, but acquires a greener shade in acid media and in the presence of sulphur dioxide and sodium benzoate.

cider. An alcoholic beverage made by fermenting apple juice; contains 5-6% alcohol (by volume) and 0.7-2.0% sugar. In US, cider or fresh cider are names given to fresh (unfermented) apple juice, and the fermented materials is called hard or fermented cider. The apples are ground and crushed until they are reduced to a pulp; the juice is allowed to run into casks, where it is freely exposed to the air until partial fermentation takes place, when a clear liquor of a pale brown or amber colour is the result. Unfermented cider is extensively used as a beverage, and it is also boiled to the consistency of sirup and used in cooking. Also known as cyder.

ciguatera. Poisoning from eating fish feeding in the region of coral reefs in the Caribbean sea and the Indian and Pacific Oceans. The species of fish are normally edible and appear to derive the toxins, ciguatoxins, from their diet.

Ciliophora. The phylum *Ciliophora* is the largest of seven protozoan phyla. There are about 8,000 species of these unicellular, heterotrophic protists that range from about 10-3,000 mm long.

cinchona. An important genus of plants belonging to the *madder* family. They are trees, shrubs or herbaceous plants, with simple, opposite leaves. The fruit is dry. The plants are found in tropical regions, and many species are of great medicinal value. For example, quinine is produced from one of them. The bark is taken off in strips, longitudinally; it is in time renewed by naturl growth. Cinchona plants have been taken from Peru, their native home, and they are now cultivated in large plantations in Ceylon, India, Jawa and other tropical countries.

cinnamon. *Cinnamomum zeylanicum.*

The bark, of various species of the genus *Cinnamomum*; it is split off the shoots, cured and dried. or Chinese cinnamon comes from Burma, while true cinnamon is a native of Ceylon. Cassia is more pungent, while true cinnamon is more light and delicate; it's also more expensive than cassia is. During drying the bark shrinks and curls into a cylinder or "quill". Ceylon or true cinnamon differs from other types (*Cinnamomum zeylanicum*) and the oil contains mostly cinnamic aldehyde, together with some eugenol. Saigon cinnamon contains also cineol; Chinese cinnamon has no eugenol. In its native state, it is the bark of the under branches of a species of laurel, which is chiefly found in Ceylon, but grows also in other parts of the East Indies. The tree attains the height of twenty or thirty feet, has oval leaves, pale yellow flowers and acorn-shaped fruit. The Ceylonese bark curls up into rolls or quills in the process of drying and the smaller quills are introduced into rolls or quills in the process of drying and the smaller quills are introduced into the larger ones for shipment. These are later assorted according th quality by tasters and are made into bundles. The leaves, the fruit and the root of the cinnamon plant all yield oil of cinnamon, a drug of considerable value. Cinnamon is a peasing condiment, popular with cooks for certain pastries and confections. It is also used as flavour in meat products.

cissa. Unnatural desire for foods, alternative words cittosis, allotriophagy and pica.

citral. $C_{10}H_{16}O$. An important constituent of many essential oils, especially lemon. It occurs in β- and α- form (*cis*- and *trans*- isomers); it is used as the starting material for the synthesis of ionone (the synthetic perfume with the odour of violets), a stage in the synthesis of retinol.

Citrange orange. A variety of orange which is hybrid between the common orange and the hardy trifoliate orange (*Poncirus trifoliata*). The trees are resistant to cold weather and can withstand temperatures as low as -9.4° or -12.2°C with minimal if any injury. The fruits are similar to those of the common orange and range in size from 1.5-10 cm. in diameter. This hybrid is flavored for gardens in regions of the southern US that are too cold for growing the common orange.

citric acid. A tribasic acid, which occurs widely in nature in fruits, especially citrus fruits. Is a normal metabolite in the body, therefore when consumed, it is completely metabolised. It is widely used as flavouring in beverages and confectionery. Commercially, it is produced by moulds or extracted from lemons.

citric acid cycle. The oxidation stage in the metabolism of food-stuffs. Carbohydrates and fats are broken down to acetate (active acetate or acetyl coenzyme A) and the first step in the cycle is the combination of the acetyl with oxaloacetate to form citrate. This passes through a series of reactions in which energy is released and carbon dioxide and water produced; the end-product is oxaloacetate. Since many of the amino acids can be converted into substances that lie on this pathway, the citric acid cycle is the common metabolic pathway for all three major foodstuffs. Also known as the Kerb's cycle.

citric acid fermentation. A type of oxidative fermentation of hexoses, such as of glucose, caused by *Citromicetes, Aspergilla and Penicilla*. resulting in the decomposition of carbohydrates to citric acid.

citrin. A mixture of two flavanones found in citrus pith, namely hesperidin and eriodictin (demethylated hesperidin). It is prepared from Hungarian red pepper, and from orange and lemon peel. It is said to be distinct from ascorbic acid, and useful in the treatment of obstinate capillary bleeding which did not yield to treatment with large doses of ascorbic acid. It is also called hesperidin.

citron. *Citrus medica.* First of the citrus fruits of become known to Europeans. Very sensitive to cold and can be grown only in warm regions.

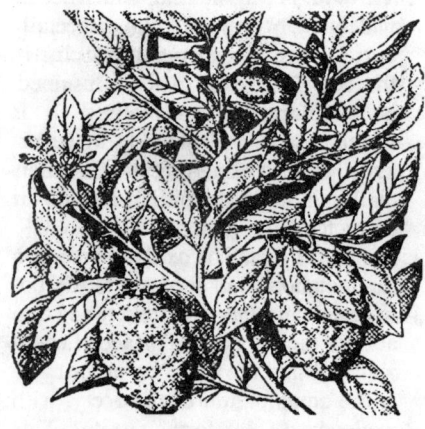

Very thick peel, solid, sweet and acid-free pulp with practically no juice; used for preparing candied peel. The citron tree is small, and has been a favorite since the days of ancient Rome. The name citron is also given to a small, hard watermelon that is used for pickles and preserves almost everywhere.

citronin. Flavanone glycoside from the peel of immature Ponderosa lemons - methoxy dihydroxy rhamnoglucoside.

citrovorum factor. Name given to a growth factor for the organism *Leuconostoc citrovorum.* Now known to be tetrahydro formyl pteroyl glutamic acid, which is believed to be the active form of the vitamin, folic acid.

citroxanthin. Yellow carotenoid pigment in orange peel; has vitamin A activity. Also known as mutachrome.

Citroze. Trade name for a lemon flavoured glucose drink.

citrulline. Amino acid formed as an intermediate in the metabolism of urea in the body; not of nutritional importance since it is not found in food proteins.

citrus. Genus including *C. limonum* (lemon), *C. aurantifolia* (lime), *C. aurantium* (sour orange), *C. sinensis* (sweet orange), *C. medica* (citron), *C. nobolis* (tangerine), *C. maxima* (grapefruit), *C. bergamia* (bergamot), and *C. grandis* (pomelo). The citrus plants have rather long, pointed leaves or leaflets, united by a distinct joint to the leaflike stalk; their stamens are united by their filaments into several irregular bundles, and they have pulpy fruits with spongy rinds. Grapefruit (*citrus paradisi*) is not a hybrid, but a distinct plant species in itself.

Kumquat (*citrus japonica*). It is the smallest of all citrus fruits and have been cultivated in China and Japan for thousands of years. They are usually eaten skin and all, their rinds being quite sweet while the pulps are tart and juicy.

Lemon (*citrus limon*) and lime (*citrus aurantifolia*) originate from small evergreens with sharp and stiff thorns, they originated in Asia a long time ago. Lemons were known to the ancient Romans, while British seamen acquired their famous nickname "limeys" in the 19th century, after limes were added to their daily rum rations to prevent scurvy.

Both kinds of oranges (bitter and sweet) (*citrus aurantium* and *citrus sinensis*) are native to China and India. The bitter orange tree is hardier and more resistant to plant infections than the sweet orange tree. Like lemons, oranges were brought to the Mediterranean lands by the Moors, where their cultivation flourished.

Tangerine (*citrus reticulata*) is named after the city of Tangier in North Africa, this small, loose skinned citrus fruit is actually a variety of Mandarin orange-the most important variety. The juicy segments, which separate readily, are dark orange, with a sweet, delicate flavour. The skin ripens to a deep orange-red and is popular in Chinese folk medicine.

citrus juice drying. Orange, lemon, grapefruit, and other citrus juices are dried to produce a product having 2-4% moisture content. If the dried products are to be stored for 6 months or more, a moisture content of 1% or less is preferred. If dried to 1%, dehumidifying air in the final stage or in-package desiccation is required. Drying is carried out using procedures to assure that the product can be readily reconstituted in cold water. The dehydrated juice products are usually made from concentrated juice. Atomization is done by pressure or centrifugal device, which is used if suspended particles are present in the concentrate. Belt or tray dryers using puff drying or foam-mats, are other methods of drying. The modified drum dryers are also used in some cases. The essential oils may be removed from juices in the evaporation process, which is of benefit in minimizing the development of off-flavors. Various procedures may be used to return flavour to the juice.

citrus red 2. The colour additive is principally 1-(2,5-dimethoxyphenylazo-2-naphthol. Citrus Red No. 2. is used only for colouring skins of oranges that are not intended for processing.

Clapp favorite pear. A variety of pear fruit resembles Bartlett in size and form, but is somewhat smother and frequently has a clubbed stem. Its skin is greenish-yellow, and is quite free of blemish; often blushed, attractive. The flesh of Clapp favorite pear is fairly fine and juicy, with some grit at centre. It is sweet with pleasing, aromatic flavour, and is rated among the best of early pears in dessert quality. Clapp favorite pear is somewhat soft to withstand commercial handling, and is therefore highly susceptibile to core breakdown if left on trees for too long. It is very susceptible to blight.

claret. A general term to describe a light red wine. Regardless of origin or character, any American red table wine may be called a "claret". The English have always adopted a much narrower meaning for the word, claret signifying a red wine from the Bordeaux district of France. It is interesting to note, however, that these Bordeaux wines and not identified as clarets. The word Medoc, a district of Bordeaux, is regarded by discriminating English wine consumers as almost synonymous with claret. Since and word is so ill-defined and loosely used, the appearance of the word "claret" on a label really has little meaning.

clarification. The removal of colloidally dispersed solids from a liquid either by coalescence and sedimentation or by adsorption on active material surfaces. For example, aluminium sulphate causes flocculation and settling of solid particle in purification of potable water; finely divided clays, carbon and certain proteins effect clarification of vegetable oils, sugar solutions, beverages. The operation is sometimes called decolorization.

clarifixation. A method of homogenising milk in which the cream is separated, homogenised and re-mixed with the milk in one machine - the clarifixator.

clary. *Salvia sclarea.* A native of southern Europe; it is in close relation of sage and a decorative biennial that is usually treated as an annual. The strongly aromatic leaves can be added sparingly in the preparation of soups, casseroles, home-made wines and beer, or made into fritters. Medicinally, they may be used to make a gargle or mouthwash, as an antiseptic, and a skin cleanser. Clary's derived name, clear eye, suggests it was also used to concoct an eye bath.

Clementine mandarin. A variety of mandarin of deep orange-red colour, with smooth and glossy surface, and having globose-to elliptical shape, sometimes irregularly shaped. A medium size clementine will have a diameter about 5-6 cm. The base evenly rounded to slightly necked. The most common strain is self-incompatible and is seedless in the absence of cross-pollination. Another strain, the Monreal, is self-compatible, is always very seedy and bears regular crops. *Clementine de Nules* (*Clemenules*) is a Spanish Monreal clone and is believed to have originated in Ules (near Castellon). The fruit of the Moroccan Clementine is thin-skinned, juicy, with qualities that surpass the Clementines grown in other Mediterranean countries. The Clementines produced in US are sometimes called Algerian tangerines.

clostridia. Genus of bacteria of family *Bacillaceae;* sporeformers. *Clostri-*

dium botulinum is the most heat-resistant of the food-poisoning organisms; its destruction is generally accepted as the minimum standard of processing for low-acid and medium-acid canned foods, although other clostridia are more heat-resistant.

Clostridium perfringens. Gram-positive rods known to cause food intoxications. These microorganisms, which produce exotoxins, must grow to the levels of approximately one million bacteria per gram or higher in food to cause disease. They are common inhabitants of soil, water, food, spices, and intestinal tract. Upon ingestion, the cells sporulate in the intestine and produce enterotoxin. This is a spore-specific protein and is produced during the sporulation process. Enterotoxin can be detected in the feces of affected individuals.

cloudberry. *Rumus chamaemorus.* Golden-fruited berry growing in northern latitudes; used in similar fashion to blackberries. Extremely rich in natural benzoic acid and the soft fruit will keep for long periods.

clove. *Caryophyllus aromaticus or Syzygium aromaticum.* Cloves are one of the most famous of all spices.

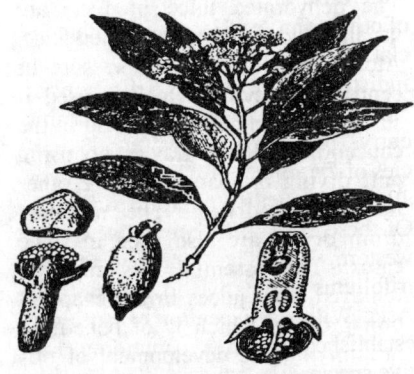

The 10 m long trees stand like neat

evergreen sentinels with their clustres of crimson flowers and seem to flourish best near the sea. That's probably why the island of Zanzibar today is the most renowned clove-growing country all. The dried flower buds of a tree which was first found in the Molucca Islands, but which is now grown in various warm countries, including, to some extinct, the West Indies. These buds, in powdered form, are used as a favorite condiment in cookery, and the oil of cloves has its place in medicine. The odour of cloves is fragrant; the taste sharp, warm and bitter. The tree is a handsome overgreen, from fifteen to thirty feet high, with large elliptic, smooth leaves and numerous purplish flowers on jointed stalks. Dried flower buds of *Caryophyllus aromaticus;* mother of clove is the ripened fruit, inferior in flavour. Contains 10% fixed oil and a volatile oil mostly eugenol, with small amounts of caryophyllene, vanillin and other substances.

clover. True clover plants are of the family *Leguminoseae* (pea or bean family), subfamily *Papilionoiceae*, genus *Trifolium* (trifoliate leaves). There are several clover like plants which also are called clovers, but which are of other genera and even of other families. Because the nomenclature is somewhat complex and indistinct, a list of short definitions of clover plants is given later in this entry. There are about 400-500 species of *Trifolium*, of which only about 10-15% are native to North America. Of these, a majority are native to the western US. The majority of the trifoliums are native to Europe and Asia. With the exception of naturally established pastures containing native species, the majority of important clovers species in Europe and US are of food production significance. With the exception of naturally established pastures containing native species, the majority of important clover species in the US have been introduced from other parts of the world. Clover performs a number of agricultural functions:

(a) as a pasture crop, either plain or mixed with some other grass or legume;
(b) for hay, plain or mixed;
(c) for soil-enrichment;
(d) as a cover crop, particularly desirable in some orchards;
(e) for silage; and
(f) for green manuring.

Several of these functions are interrelated. Clover is also an excellent honey crop. Several species of clover, including white and Alsike clover, must depend upon insect pollination. In the case of red clover, the normal honeybee is incapable of reaching the deeply located nectar, leaving this task to the bumblebee. Claims over the years also have been made for the medicinal characteristics of certain clover plants, potions usually being prepared as a tea by boiling leaves and flowers in water.

club cheese. A variety of cheese made from well ripened American cheddar by grinding to a smooth paste and mixing in a certain amount of butter, with or without other flavouring materials. It is often flavoured with pepper, and when coloured green and having a peppery taste it is called Chilli cheese. Formerly known as potted cheese.

clumping. The forming of aggregates or clumps of fat globules in cold milk. The fat globules coming in contact with one another have a tendency to adhere or form bunches. The degree to which this clumping takes place tin milk on cream depends upon temperature, age, heat treatment, fat content and its degree of dispersion, the degree of agitation, and the degree of fluidity of the milk and cream. Fat globule clumping is a pre-requisite of creaming. It is now thought to be due to the presence of an agglutinin (euglobulin) in the milk serum which is destroyed at temperatures above those used for normal pasteurization. Fat globule clumping also occurs as a result of homogenization when the fat content is over 8-10% or when the SNF/Fat ratio is less than 1.0. It is the cause of homogenized cream feathering in coffee.

Co I and Co II. The abbreviations for coenzymes I and II, officially named nicotinamide adenine dinucleotide and nicotinamide adenine dinucleotide phosphate, respectively.

coacervation. Heat-reversible aggregation of amylopectin-suggested as one explanation of the staling of bread.

coagulation, blood. The final stage is the precipitation of fibrils of insoluble fibrin from the soluble plasma protein, fibrinogen. The mechanism involves the conversion of prothrombin in the plasma by thromboplastin (released from blood platelets and damaged tissues) to thrombin, in the presence of calcium. The thrombin then reacts with the fibrinogen to form the fibrin clot. Hence the addition of oxalate or citrate, which combine with the calcium, will prevent clotting as effectively as heparin, hirudin and coumarin, which interfere with the prothrombin.

coagulation factors. A collection of soluble substances (chiefly proteins) that are present in blood plasma and, under certain circumstances, act together in a predetermined sequence to cause blood coagulation (blood clotting). Although each factor has a name, they are also referred to by the Roman numerals. Four of the factors (II, VII, IX, and X) are dependent upon vitamin K for their full expression in the liver; four (factors I, V, VIII, and XIII) are thrombin-dependent; four (factors XI, XII, XIV, and XV) are known as contact factors and are involved with the initiation reactions following injury. Factors III and IV are not proteins but are included because of their crucial roles in the clotting process. Bleeding disorders may be caused by the lack of a particular factor (inherited or acquired), the presence of an inhibitor (*e.g.*, heparin), or the synthesis of an abnormal molecule that is non-functional. Also known as clotting factors.

coating agents. Substances that are used to protect the surface (and penetration through the surface) of food materials that are being processed or final products, including fresh produce that requires very little processing per se. Wax-coated cheese is the simplest example of a coating application. Depending upon the materials involved, coating agents may be dusted or sprayed onto the substrate, or the latter may be dipped into a solution of the protective material.

Coating agents serve a number of functions. For example, some fruits may be dipped in 1-2% citric acid prior to freezing. This removes any residual lye from the peeling process and the further destruction of ascorbate is prevented. However, citric acid alone is not always sufficient to prevent deteriorative effects during freezing and thus a sequestrant/antioxidant may be added. For example, a solution of 0.5% citric acid along with 0.02% D-erythroascorbic acid may be used to prevent browning of some fruits during freezing and defrosting. The procedure is also useful with some vegetables. Dried fruits, such as raisins, prunes, and figs, require a residual moisture content because most consumers do not like a thoroughly dry or crispy product in this category. Residual moisture, of course, encourages mold and yeast growth. Protection can be gained by dipping the fruit in solutions of 2-7% potassium sorbate, this leaving a fine coating of antimicrobial agent on the fruit pieces. Acetostearin products (di- and triglycerides) solidify into wax-like solids and are used in some protective coatings for food products. It has been shown that these products are effective against moisture penetration, as well as against atmospheric gases. The coating is applied by dipping, or in the case of nuts, by spraying.

For table-like confections, coating techniques from the pharmaceutical industry have been used. One of the most common coating material used is sucrose, but number of transparent or opaque materials also make excellent film coatings. These include various gums and resins. Some products may be multi-coated and through the use of approved colorants, interesting shades and colouring effects can be obtained.

The film-type coatings generally use an organic solvent containing a gum or resin plus plasticizers. The film-forming characteristics of starch have been known and exploited by the food industry for may years. Numerous foods can be protective and decoratively coated with starch. Starch can be added to sugar solutions used for coatings, providing a less brittle and moisture-sensitive surface. Starch coatings also have the advantage of being oil and grease resistant. Methylcellulose when incorporated into sweet dough products performs a number of functions, one of which is improving glaze adherence.

Red meats, poultry, and fish can be coated with a protective film prior to freezing by dipping into successive solutions of 10-15% sodium alginate, 3-5% calcium chloride, and 10-20% glycerol, the latter used as a plasticizer. This coating procedure improves retention of juices on freezing and thawing. Sodium alginate coating for sausages, alone or with ethylcellulose, prevents salt rust and increases storage stability. The effectiveness of carrageenan as a way to prevent oxidative rancidity after freezing, has also been investigated.

cobalamin. Vitamin B_{12}.

cobalt. An element discovered in 1735, is a grey, hard, magnetic, ductile, somewhat malleable transition metal. Compounds of cobalt are highly coloured and are used as pigments. The chloride is blue; cobaltous arsenite, pink to blood red; the bromide, bright green; cobalt carbonate, pale red; the chromate, brilliant green; cobalt hydroxide, blue green; the nitrate, red; the oxalate, pink; cobalt oxide, olive green to red; the phosphate, pink to lavender; the sulphate, pink to red; and the thiocyanate, yellow brown. Cobalt blue, or zaffree, was known and used prior to 1540. The metal cobalt itself its used is the manufacture of alloys and in nuclear technology. Cobalt-60 is used in medicine as a source of radiation in treating malignancies. Salt of cobalt have appellations other than their use in pigments. Radioactive cobalt is manufactured from the chloride salt.

The acetate, carbonate, and chloride were used as foam stabilizers in the brewing of malt beverages. Cobalt carbonate and chloride are utilized in trace element supplement preparations for ruminants. The oxide is used in grinding wheels.

Inhalation of cobalt-containing dusts may cause pulmonary symptoms. Skin contact with powders or effluents in various industrial processes can cause dermatitis. Ingestion of soluble cobalt salts induces nausea and vomiting because of local irritation of the gastric mucosa. Scientists have determined cobalt, zinc, magnesium, and manganese contents of the heart tissue of patients dying from 'beer drinkers' myocardiopathy, by both neutron activation analysis and atomic absorption spectroscopy. The mean cobalt content of heart muscle was found to be 0.69 $\mu g/g$ wet weight as compared to 0.04 $\mu g/g$ for control cardiac tissue. Manganese, magnesium, and zinc in the former were all decreased compared to levels found in controls. The relationship between these changes is as yet uncertain.

Cobalt is believed to be a dietary essential in trace amounts although a simple cobalt deficiency has never been observed in man. It is part of the molecule of vitamin B_{12} but no other function is clearly known. It is acts as a growth factor for chicks, turkeys, pigs and rats, although large doses are toxic. Mechanisms of myocardial toxicity induced by cobalt salts have been investigated in rats. Scientists induced lesion in the pericardium, myocardium, and endocardium of guinea pigs by feeding 20 mg of cobalt per kg body weight/day. The lesion observed were strikingly similar to those seen in Quebec beer drinkers' cardiomyopathy. Addition of ethanol to the cobalt salt regimen failed to modify the incidence or severity of disease in the animals. After investigating some experimental aspects of cobalt cardiomyopathy concluded that the damage observed possibly reflects an enzymatic block of the oxidative decarboxylation at the pyruvate and ketoglutarate levels. The occurrence of cobalt intoxication in patients with uremic myocardiopathy has been described. Using neutron activation analysis, scientists studied blood and tissue cobalt concentrations in normal subjects and in patients with terminal renal failure. Patients on maintenance dialysis given cobalt chloride in an attempt to treat the existing anaemia showed a rise in blood cobalt from 3.5-138 $\mu g/L$. However, the maximum rise observed in hemoglobin levels was only 1 μg. The myocardial cobalt content of renal failure patients treated with the salt rose to 165 μg. Cobalt levels in the myocardial tissue of renal failure patients (non-cobalt treated) and in the tissue of cobalt-treated subjects without renal failure were 5 and 6 μg respectively.

Cobalt has been reported to cause a hyperlipemia in rabbits. The effect of cobalt chloride on blood lipids in man has not yet been investigated. The first evidence that cobalt was a dietary essential was obtained more than 50 years ago as the result of researches regarding the cause of two debilitating diseases of sheep and cattle known as 'coast disease' and 'wasting disease', or 'bush sickness'. In 1948, it was discovered that the antipernicious anaemia factor in liver is a compound containing 4% of cobalt. The compound is now known as vitamin B12.

coboglobin. An artificially prepared hemoglobin or myoglobin molecule in which the iron atom has been replaced by a cobalt atom.

coca leaves. From the S. American plant, *Erythroxylon coca;* contain cocaine, and chewed by the natives of Peru as a stimulant.

cocarboxylase. Coenzyme that assists the enzyme carboxylase to remove carbon dioxide from various compounds, *i.e.*, decarboxylation. Cocarboxylase is the diphosphate of vitamin B_1, alternatively known as thiamin pyrophosphate or *diphosphothiamin.* In deficiency of vitamin B_1 the body is unable to oxidize pyruvic acid, an intermediate stage in carbohydrate metabolism, which therefore accumulates in the blood.

cochineal Red A. Trade name for: *Ponceau 4R. 16255.* The trisodium salt of 1-(4-sulpho-1-naphthylazo)-2-naphthol-6, 8-disulphonic acid. It is a red powder, soluble in water (5 % at 25°C) to give a scarlet red solution. It has good light resistance and is stable in both acid and alkaline media. It has only a fair resistance to sulphur dioxide.

Red 2G. A monoazo compound. It is a red powder, which is soluble in water (6 % at 25°C) to give a bright red solution with a slight bluish tinge. It is fairly soluble in glycerol, but only very slightly so in ethanol (95 %). Red 2 G has excellent light-fastness and is table in both acid and alkaline media. This colour is not permitted for use in food in the U.S.

cochineal. A naturally derived red colorant from the female insect of *Coccus cacti.* It is sometimes used in foodstuffs as well as certain medicinals. Prior to the appearance of synthetic colours during the last century, cochineal was an important commercial colorant. Cochineal is the name of the female insect of *Coccus cacti*, a wingless insect that feeds on various species of cactus found in Central American countries, including Mexico. A different species of cochineal insect feeds on the leaves of the tamarisk tree (*Tamarix manifera*), found in the Canary Islands and párts of South America. During the egg-laying season, the cochineal insects are brushed from the leaves, killed in boiling water, and subsequently dried. The insects are dark reddish-brown in colour. About 20% of the insect eggs contains carbonic acid. Carmine red colour is obtained by boiling with mineral acid. A brilliant-red pigment is prepared by precipitating a mixture of cochineal and alum. Although cost prohibitive for many applications, carmine is sometimes used for specific food products to produce a pink colour in coatings and in retorted protein produces where other colours may be unstable. Many countries permit the use of cochineal colouring in foods in amounts consistent with good manufacturing practice.

cock-a-leekie. Scottish soup made from leeks and chicken.

cockle. Of the family Carbide, the cockles are worldwide in distribution and contain about 200 species. The common edible cockle (*Cardium edule*), also known as *Cerastoderma edule*, attains a length of 3.5-5 cm. This is one of the most common and best-known bivalves in Europe. Shells of this form have been found in superabundance swept up on sandy beaches from Iceland to western Africa. The animals are characterized by whitish-yellow shells with regularly spaced ribs. There is an exhaling and inhalant siphon. The long foot is bent and tapers to a point. It enables this bivalve to move in a peculiar way.

The animal extends the foot as far out of the shell as possible, up to nearly 5 cm and gropes for resistance from any object. When the bent portion of the foot is suddenly jerked into a straight position, which results in a push, the bivalve flings itself a distance of over 50 cm.

cocoa. The product prepared from the cocoa bean, *Theobroma cacao*. The bean is left to ferment before roasting; it is then cracked and the shell removed. The remainder constitutes the nib, which, when ground, is cocoa: 54% fat, 11% protein, 9% carbohydrate, 2% water, together with alkaloids, fibre, tannins, organic acids.

In the manufacture of cocoa and chocolate, the beans are cleaned and sorted to remove foreign bodies of all kinds and are also graded into sizes to secure uniformity in roasting. The roasting is done in rotating iron drums in which the beans are heated; the result is the peculiar aroma and the elimination of the bitter elements. The beans are dry and their shells are crisp. The beans are next crushed, the light shells removed and the beans left in the form of "cocoanibs" or kernels, occasionally seen in the shops. Cocoa-nibs may be prepared with hot water, in the same way that coffee or tea is, but for most people this beverage is too rich. The fat is usually extracted from the beans, which are then ground to a fine powder. It is then ready for use in the ordinary way.

In the preparation of chocolate the preliminary processes are followed as for cocoa, except that the fat is not extracted. Sugar and sometimes other materials are added to the ground paste, ttogether with vanilla or other suitable flavoring materials. The final result is a semi-liquid fluid which is molded into the familiar tablets or other forms in which chocolate comes on the market. Also spelled as cacao.

cocoa butter. A common name given to the oil which is prepared from the bean and is much used by confectioners in making candy. When the butter is used for table purposes, a little half-churned cream or butter colour is put in. When left white, cocoa butter is almost tasteless and odorless, and it is often used in the kitchen in place of cheap butter or lard.

cocoa, Dutch process. In Dutch process the cocoa beans are treated with certain alkalis at the time of roasting to break up the cell structure. This alkali treatment makes the cocoa more soluble and gives it the desired darker colour which distinguishes it from the Dutch process for natural cocoa. It also aids in bringing out the full fine chocolate flavour when the cocoa is used in the finished product. Because the alkalies counteract the puckery acid taste which is found in natural cocoa, the Dutch Process cocoa leaves no bitter taste when used a flavouring in ice cream.

cocoa, natural process. Cocoa made from chocolate liquor by subjecting the liquid to high pressure in hydraulic presses. This process removes a large amount of the cocoa (fat) butter, usually about 38–40% of the total, and leaves a hard, dry cake which normally contains about 22% fat, though some cocoas contain more and some less. It also contains nearly all the flavouring material from the cocoa bean. The fat is practically tasteless. This cocoa cake is then put through a number of processes known as milling which results in the finely sifted cocoa.

cocolait. A kind of coconut milk made by pressing coconut under high pressure and homogenising the oil and water emulsion along with coconut water (coconut milk) obtained. It is then bottled and used in place of cow's milk in some of the Asian countries.

coconut. Family: *Palmaceae.* Genus: *Cocos.* Species: *Cocos nucifera.* Coconut has less protein than other nuts and is unique in having a very high saturated fatty acid content, even more than milk. The saturated fatty acid in coconut meat contains a high proportion of lauric acid, which is liquid at room temperature. Because of this property it is used to make artificial milk and modified cow's milk products and this is another good reason for being a hawk-eyed label reader if you are on a diet low in saturated fats. Coconut is said to destroy tapeworms acquired through infected meat. It contains organic iodine and can prevent thyroid problems. It is also used to help with constipation, flatulence, dysentery and intestinal inflammation, as well as for body-building. In the tropics the milk is used to soothe sore throats and stomach ulcers.

coconut oil. The oil obtained from the thick kernel or meat adhering to the inside of the large nuts of the palm tree *Cocos nucifera* growing along the coasts of tropical countries. The tree requires salt air, and inland trees do not bear fruit unless supplied with salt. The name coco is the Carib word for palm. Copra is the dried meat of the coconut from which the oil is pressed, alkali refined, and bleached. The dried copra contains 60-65% oil. It is an excellent food oil, and is valued as a shortening for crackers, but its use for margarine has declined. It is also valued for soaps because of its high lathering qualities due to the large percentage of lauric and myristic acids, though these acids are irritating to some skins. It is also employed as a source of lauric acid, but lauryl alcohol is now made synthetically. Coconut oil has a melting point of 27-32°C, specific gravity 0.926, saponification value 251-263, and iodine value 8-9.6. It contains 45-48% lauric acid, 17-20% myristic, 10% capric, 5-7% palmitic, 5% stearic, and some oleic, caprylic, and caproic acids. During sun-drying coconut meat to make copra there is a loss of some of the sugars and other carbohydrates, and some proteins. The oil from copra contains more free fatty acid than that from fresh dried coconut and is rancid, requiring neutralization, decolorization, and deodorization. The meal and cake are also dirty and rancid but are useful for animal feed or fertilizer. Dehydrated coconut meat gives a better yield of oil and is not rancid. About 5,000 coconuts area required to produce a metric ton of copra, and the average yield of crude oil is 63%. The stearine separated from crude coconut oil by the process of wintering, to remove the more-liquid glycerides, is known as coconut butter. and is used in confectionery. Hydrogenated coconut oil is a soft solid with a melting point of 45°C. Desiccated coconut, produced by oven drying or dehydration of the fresh coconut meat, is used shredded as a food and also powdered in many bakery products as a food and stabilizer. It has high food value, containing not less than 60% oil, 15% carbohydrates, 15% cellulose, 6-7% protein, and various mineral salts and considerable vitamin B. It is easily digested and has antitubercular value, but its characteristic coconut flavour is not universally liked and its use is largely confined to confections.

Coconut oil is widely used as a skin lubricant and is commonly used in many countries on new-borns babies who are massaged daily with it for the first month or two of life. It is good for sunburn and for treating dry scalps as well as conditioning hair. The residue after oil extraction is used for animal feed. The hollow unripe nut contains a watery liquid known as coconut milk, which is gradually absorbed as the nut ripens.

The average composition of milk from the ripe nut is: 1.4% solids; 0.2% protein; and 3% carbohydrate (mainly sucrose). The composition of mature kernel per 100 g is: 40-80 g solids; 4 g protein; 35 g fat; 11 g carbohydrate; 4 g fibre; 2 mg iron; traces of vitamins B_1, B_2 and nicotinic acid; and food energy 1.57 MJ.

coddle. To cook slowly in water kept just below the boiling point.

codfish. Order: *Anacanthin*i. Family: *Gadidae*. All codfish are marine with exception of the burbot, *Lota lota*, a species with ranges from the polar regions southward in North America and Eurasia. The marine codfishes prefer cold or temperature water, as contrasted with tropical climes. The occurrence is much greater in the northern than in the southern hemisphere. Codfishes are among the greatest of world seafood sources. Included in the codfish family are the pollock, the haddock, and the whiting. Because of certain anatomical differences, some investigators do not consider hakes as members of the family *Gadidae*, but rather as belonging to a separate family, *Merlucciidae*. The Atlantic cod is the largest of about 150 species. It may attain a length 1.8 m, and weigh up to 95 kg. A 2-year-old cod will achieve a length

of about 38 cm. Normally, they are not capable of spawning until about 5 years old. The most noticeable external characteristics are its three dorsal and two anal fins, its protruding upper jaw, its almost square tail, and a pale line running along each side of the body from head to tail.

In the cod family there are two groups-the shore cod and the deep-sea variety. Millions are taken every year, but the supply remains constant, for cod are very prolific. The destruction of eggs and young, which are preyed upon by other fish for food, is enormous, but the number growing to maturity is always ample. Shore cod are confined to the temperate zones, but deep sea cod, which constitutes the well-known food fish, has a slightly flattened body which tapers abruptly to the tail. It reaches maturity in about three years, but it is of sufficient size to be marketable when two years old. The composition of all non-fatty fish, such as cod, hake, haddock, flatfish, is similar. The average composition per 100 g for cod fillet is: protein 16.4%; fat 0.5%; Ca 25 mg; Fe 0.7 mg; vitamin B_1 0.05 mg; vitamin B_2 0.08 mg; nicotinic acid 2.2 mg; and food energy 0.3 MJ. For cod round, the average composition per 100 g is: protein 7.4%; fat 0.2%; Ca 11 mg; Fe 0.3 mg; vitamin B_1 0.02 mg; vitamin B_2 0.04 mg; and nicotinic acid 1.0 mg.

There is a fleshy barbel under the lower jaw. In most fish, the upper part of the body is thickly speckled with small, round spots somewhat darker than the body color, which may range from reddish to brown, gray, or greenish. Cod can be found from shallow water near shore, down to 450 m. Its usual habitat is within a few fathoms of the bottom, but it also comes to the top of the water in pursuit of small fish or squid. It is most plentiful on the banks and in oceans of moderate depths. Cod live chiefly over rocky, pebbly ground, on sand or gravel, and seldom on soft mud. The movements on- and off-shore and from bank to bank are due chiefly to temperature influence, the presence or absence of food, and the search for proper spawning conditions. Cod prefer temperatures of 0°-5°C, but good catches can be made in waters up to 10°C. Cod feed on almost all types of sea life. The most important food is fish, especially herring, capelin, and sand lance, but mussels, crabs, and other bottom animals are also consumed. The common Atlantic cod is well known on both sides of the north Atlantic. On the American coast, it is found as far north as Greenland, Davis Strait, and Hudson Strait and south nearly to Cape Hatteras. The cod (*Gadus callarias*), is caught in large quantities by British fishermen and constitutes about one-third of the total tonnage taken in British fisheries. The whiting (*Gadus merlangus*) is essentially a near-water fish, and occurs in large quantities around the northern coast of Britain; it figures prominently in the landings at Scottish ports.

cod-liver oil. An oil extracted from the livers of different species of cod. It is a pale yellow oil, of very disagreeable odour and taste, and is obtained by pressing it from the livers in a cold state, or by heat. It is easily digested, and if not taken in too large quantities, is considered an extremely valuable remedy in all wasting diseases. On account of its disagreeable taste, it is administered in capsules and various otherforms. The milky mixture, known as emulsion, consists of a preparation of cod-liver oil with other remedies. The average sample contains 120-1,200 µg vitamin A and 1-10 µg vitamin D per gram. British Pharmacopoeia standard recommends minimum 180 µg vitamin A and 2 µg vitamin D per g.

coenzyme B-12. Coenzyme derived from cyanocobalamin. It contains a corrin ring having four pyrrole rings and a central cobalt atom. It is involved as a coenzyme in methylation reactions, as a methyl carrier and as a prosthetic group in rearrangement reactions such as the conversion of methylmalonyl coenzyme A to succinyl coenzyme A. It is also involved in the reduction of ribonucleotides to deoxyribonucleotides.

coenzyme Q. A group of substances that function in certain respiratory enzyme systems, found in the subcellular particles: identical with the ubiquinones. Also known as Q 275 and mitoquinone.

coenzyme Q_{10}. An electron-carrying coenzyme active in the electron-transport chain. Coenzyme Q_{10} serves as an acceptor of electrons not only from NADH dehydrogenase, but also from the flavin components of succinic dehydrogenase, glycerol phosphate dehydrogenase, and fatty acyl-CoA dehydrogenase.

coenzyme R. Obsolete names for biotin.

cofactor. A non-protein substance that helps an enzyme to carry out its activity. Cofactors may be cations or organic molecules, known as coenzymes. Unlike enzymes they are, in general, stable to heat. When a catalytically active enzyme forms a complex with a cofactor a holoenzyme is produced. An enzyme without its cofactors is termed an apoenzyme. Cofactors include metal ions, coenzymes and prosthetic groups. Prosthetic groups remain attached to the enzyme during the complete catalytic cycle, whereas coenzymes must be dissociated from the enzyme in order to function.

coferment. Any substance that increases or makes the action of an enzyme posible. The complex organic phosphates have been shown to increase the activity of the yeast ferment and blood does not clot in the absence of calcium salts, apparently because calcium salts are necessary for the conversion of the blood zymogen into thrombase, the clotting ferment.

coffee. Family: *Rubiaceae.* Genus: *Coffea.* Species: *Coffea arabica, coffea robista* and others. The seed or berry of an evergreen shrub, or small tree, which is cultivated in warm regions. The name also is given to a dark-brown, fragrant table beverage which is made from crushed coffee berries. The coffee tree, when wild grows from 5-10 metres high, but in cultivation it is seldom allowed to exceed 2 metres. The leaves are dark green and have a waxy appearance on the upper surface. The flowers are white and appear in the axils of the leaves. The fruit is an oval, dark red berry, resembling a cherry when ripe. Each berry contains two cells, and each cell has a single seed, which forms the coffee nib or bean. These parts of the plant are shown in the colour plate. Before roasting the seed is of a light green colour. The tree lives for about forty years and bears fruit from the time it is three years old When ripe, the fruit is gathered by placing canvas under the trees and shaking them. The berries are dried in the sun, then passed between rollers, which crush the dried pulp, but do not crush the seeds. The fragments of pulp are then removed from the seeds by winnowing. After being thoroughly dried, the seeds are packed in large sacks, in which they are shipped to market.

Among the volatile compounds contained in various varities of coffee are aldehydes, ketones, alcohols, esters, pyridine, sulphur compounds, mercaptans, hydrogen sulphide, carbon disulphide, and hydrocarbons. Acetaldehyde, which occurs in fruits, has a pungent, fruity aroma. Usually, its presence is only noticed in very freshly roasted and ground coffee. The acetaldehyde is retained in spray-dried powders and is more pronounced than in roast ground coffees, suggesting that acetaldehyde may result from the hydrolysis of roast coffee. Other aldehydes present, each of which contributes in a small way to characteristic aroma, are propionaldehyde, butyraldehyde, and valeraldehyde. Furfural, which imparts a haystack odour, is present in some coffees and may occur in soluble coffee up to 200 parts per million, believed to result from the hydrolysis of coffee solubles. Acetone is present in some varities of coffee up to a concentration of 60 parts per million. The odour is sweet and pungent (fingernail polish or solvent odour), and, when not present in excessive amounts, tends to contribute to the sweetness and smoothness of the coffee aromat. Diacetyl provides a definitely rich note to coffee aroma and may be present up to about 20 parts per million in roast coffee. The esters, such as methyl formate, ethyl formate, and methyl acetate, occur in coffees up to a concentration of 20 parts per million. Of these, methyl acetate contributes most to coffee essence. Pyridine, which can occur in a concentration of about 200 parts per million in coffee, has a most undesirable odour, accompanied by a sharp taste. The compound results from the decomposition of trigonelline during roasting. Highly roasted coffee tend to be heavy with pyridine. It is believed that the disagreeable odour of stale coffee is the result of the predominance of pyridine, which does not disappear (voltalize) with time as do other essence ingredients which tend to overcome pyridine in freshly roasted coffee. Trigonelline (white crystalline solid) occurs in coffee to the extent of about 1.3% in green coffee and somewhat smaller portions in roasted coffee. The taste is bitter (something like, but not so strong as caffeine). During roasting, nicotinic acid or niacin are developed to the extent of about 100 parts per million in light roasts and up to 400 parts per million in very dark roasts. A cup of coffee contains about 10% of minimum daily requirements of this particular vitamin. Dimethhyl sulphide and methyl mercaptan, as sulphur compounds, have disagreeable odour. However, as a very small part of the total coffee essence, they can contribute to a pleasant sensation. Hydrogen sulphide occurs in some coffees, but is not a problem when present in concentrations of less than 1 part per million. It has been noted that when this compound is present in coffee solubles at this low level, a popcorn-type odour may be detected. Also present in some coffees at low level is carbon disulphide, which by itself smells like bad cabbage.

The brown appearance of the coffee found in retail stores is due to the roasting. Since the aroma developed by the roasting evaporates rapidly, coffee should not be roasted until it is desired for use.

The different varieties, such as Moha, Java and others, may be due to the locality from which the coffee is obtained, the real Mocha coming from Arabia, but they are all liable to be produced from the seeds of the same orchard, the name Mocha usually being given to the small beans, and Java to the larger ones. Mixtures of these produce other varieties. Three types differing in shape and size Moka, Bourbon and Martinique. The average composition after roasting is: moisture 8%, protein 8.5%, fat 10.1%, carbohydrate 50%, fibre 18%, caffeine 1.3%, together with coffeol oil which supplies the flavour, caffeic acid, chlorogenic acid and trigonelline. The hot water extract from 100 g of coffee contains about 27 mg nicotinic acid, 1 mg Fe, 30 mg Ca, 8 g protein.

Different types of coffee are preferred in various parts of the world. Arabic coffee is produced mostly in South and Central America, particularly Brazil, Colombia, Mexico and Guatemala, while robust coffee is produced mainly by African countries such as the Ivory Coast, Uganda, Angola and so forth. In the US, Colombian and Central American coffees are preferred over Brazilian and African coffee. A breakfast-sized cup of fresh coffee contains 100 mg of caffeine, and the same amount of instant 80 mg.

Caffeine stimulates the central nervous system and brain. It panics the adrenal glands into releasing stored sugar into the bloodstream. Drinking coffee does release fats into the bloodstream, which is why many Marathon runners drink black coffee before and even during a race. It raises the pulse rate and may in certain sensitive people cause irregular heart rhythm or palpitations. Its tannic acid content can inhibit the proper digestion of protein and the absorption of iron. Decaffeinated coffee may still affect the digestive process because of the amount of tannic acid present. Alternative coffee substitutes include roasted dandelion and chicory roots (either separately or mixed) which are actively beneficial and various grain coffees made from roasted rye, oats, millet, barley, wheat, figs and molasses. The longer a bean is roasted the more niacin (vitamin B_3) it contains. A dark-roasted been will contain three or four times the amount found in a 'regular' roasted one. The longer a coffee is brewed the stronger the brew. If brewed for 10 minutes, it will grain 2 more calories per cup. Instant black coffee contains very few nutrients. Black coffee may be invaluable in certain cases of narcotic poisoning and in acute cases it can be introduced into the body by means of an enema.

coffee essence. Must contain not less than 0.5% w/v caffeine derived from coffee. Coffee and chicory extract must contain not less than 0.25% caffeine. *See* coffee.

coffee extract drying. Instant dry coffee is made from coffee extract or liquid coffee. The liquid coffee is made from blended, roasted, and ground coffee beans from which soluble solids are removed by percolators. A vacuum drum dryer may be used to dehydrate the coffee extract. A vertical tower spary dryer using a pressure nozzle at 208-3450 kPa with concurrent flow of extract 10-20% solids and heated air at 276°C to produce powder with particles of size 60-100 µm diameter at 3-4% moisture content.

coffee, decaffeinated. The coffee from which caffeine is removed by treating the aqueous extract of the coffee with boiling ethylene dichloride or methylene dichloride, and then drying.

coffee, soluble. Although the objectives of producing soluble coffee (instant) powders is essentially that of reproducing a cup of freshly brewed coffee simply by adding hot water to a soluble powder, this is not really what happens. Only a very small portion of the natural coffee flavour is actually present in the cup of instant coffee. Very similar, but substitute aroma and taste constituents are generated in the instant coffee and serve to make the instant coffee taste like freshly brewed coffee. Thus, the process of selecting green coffee for preparing instant coffee requires new precursors of the final characteristics of the instant coffee after its long process of percolation, freeze- or spray-drying, and finally dissolving in the hot water.

The substitute flavour and aroma constituents arise from the solubilization of normally insoluble carbohydrates and proteins at the higher temperatures, longer processing times, and stronger concentrations that occur in preparing the extract as compared with freshly brewing coffee from the same grind. Nearly all of the original volatile aromas and flavours of the ordinarily brewed coffee are removed during the drying of the soluble powder. But, in substitution, hydrolysis forms more and different acids than the natural acids lost in processing to provide the cup of instant coffee with its characteristically pleasing aroma and taste of instant coffee. A number of soluble coffee products are combined with soluble milk. The spray dryers first used for making soluble coffee products were an adaptation of milk powder dryers. However, these are found lacking in preserving much of the coffee flavour.

Pure coffee product (with no milk) has been introduced which dissolved well and fast. The flavour of this type of products is richer, the colour is darker and, from the standpoint of both manufacturer and consumer, the flowability of the product seems to be good.

Cognac. A kind of brandy produced in a limited area of France, from special varities of grape grown on shallow soil and claimed to be distilled only input not continuous stills.

coiled coil. Structure found in proteins such as keratin, myosin and fibrin in which the a-helix is itself further coiled, usually by interwining of two or more individual a-helices. Nucleic acids can also adopt a coiled coil configuration.

cola drinks. Carbonated drinks containing extract of cola bean, the seed of the cola tree. The seed contains caffeine. The drinks contain 3-4.5 mg caffeine per fl. oz.

cola nut. The seed of a tree (genus Col) of the family *Sterculiaceae* that is native to the coastal zone of west Africa. Cola trees have purple flowers and large brownish-yellow fruits which contain the cola seeds. The tree is most productive in its tenth year, yielding about 54 kg of nuts per year. There are two species of Cola that are of commercial interest: (a) *C. nitada*, the seeds of which are called large cola nuts; and (b) *C. acuminata*, of which the seeds are called small cola nuts. *C. nitada* grows wild in the forests of the Ivory Coast and is also cultivated. There is also some cultivation of this tree in the West Indies and in South America, where the tree has been naturalized for many years.

C. acuminata also is found growing wild in the same region. It also is cultivated. The seeds of these trees are used as the basis of tincture as well as the basis of fluid, soft, and dried extracts, which may be processed to make them tannin-free. These bitter substances (when concentrated) provide what has become known as a cola flavor. The substances are used as flavoring agents for various beverages (aperitifs, bitters, carbonated cola-type beverages (up to 120 ppm), as well as in ice creams, candies, and baked goods.

Cola nuts contain nearly all of the constituents that are present in coffee, tea, and cocoa-caffeine, theobromine, theophylline, xanthine, and tannin. Natives have been using cola nuts as stimulants and medicinally for centuries. With exception of cystine, the cola nuts have a reasonably good balance of amino acids, being particularly high in aspartic acid, glutamic acid, arginine, lysine, and alanine. Also spelled as kola nuts.

Colby cheese. A kind of cheese which is similar to Cheddar cheese. It may be made from either raw or pasteurised milk. It is made in the same way as Cheddar except that (as in granular or stirred-cured cheese) the curd is not matted and milled. However, in making granular or stirred-cured cheese, water is not added to the curd to cool it as is done in making Colby. After the curd has been cut, stirred and heated (as in the Cheddar process) the whey is drained to the level of the curd. Then the vat gate is closed and rather cool water (about 15.6°C) is added with continuous stirring until the temperature of the curd has been reduced to about 26.7°C. Stirring is continued for 10-20 minutes, then the curd is pushed to the sides of the vat and stirred enough to prevent matting as the whey drains. About an hour after the whey is drained, salt is added to the curd in 2-3 applications, each application being mixed thoroughly with the curd. The curd is again pushed to the sides of the vat to drain while the salt is dissolving, which requires at least 20 minutes. Then the curd is hooped and pressed. The cheese is cured for a somewhat longer period than washed-curd cheese, but not so long as Cheddar cheese. If it is made from raw milk, it must be cured for least 60 days unless it is to be used for manufacturing. Colby cheese has a softer body and more open texture than Cheddar cheese, and it contains more moisture. For these reasons, it does not keep as well as Cheddar. The average composition of Colby cheese is: moisture, not more than 40% (usually 36%); fat in the solids, not less than 50%; and salt, 1.5-1.8%.

colchicine. An alkaloid isolated from the meadow saffron, or Autumn crocus (*Colchicum*). It is an old remedy for gout. It inhibits cell division and is used in experimental horticulture to produce plants with abnormal numbers of genes.

cold packed fruits. Fruits which have been stored at freezing temperatures after the addition of sugar, generally at the rate of one kg of sugar to four to six parts of fruit (depending on the type of fruit). The fruit-sugar mixture is packed in sealed containers, quickly froze and held at freezing temperatures until ready for use. Cold packed strawberries and raspberries are widely used in the ice cream industry. Their flavour is generally considered to be equal, or in some cases superior, to that to fresh fruits.

Coleman diet. High calorie, largely liquid diet introduced by Coleman for the treatment of typhoid fever.

coliform. A Gram-negative, nonsporing, facultative rod that ferments lactose with gas formation within 48 hours at 308K.

collagen. A protein occurring in the connective tissue of the body, having a fibrous polypeptide chain comprised of many amino acids; possesses the unique property of shrinking in hot water within a specific temperature range from 62-65°C. This behaviour is a critical factor in leather tannage. For leather, shrinkage temperature increases within the extent of tannage. In addition to leather, it is use to some extent in the manufacture of animals glues and in many medical applications such as dialysis membranes, sutures, etc. Collagen is converted into gelatin by hydrolysis, after purification it is used as a protective colloid and gel-former in food products, for sausage casings, and for coating photographic film. Collagen is synthesized, primarily by fibroblasts, as tropocollagen.

collagenases. A group of enzymes that cleave peptide bonds located in the helical regions of collagen, which are otherwise very resistant to enzymatic attack. Some are endogenous in vertebrate tissue and are important in wound healing and development (*e.g.,* resorption of the tail of a tadpole). One type is formed by certain microorganisms. *Clostridium histolyticum*, a bacterium that causes gas gangrene, secretes a collagenase that splits each polypeptide chain of collagen at more than two hundred sites. This enzyme contributes to the invasion of this highly pathogenic clostridium by destroying the connective tissue barriers of the host. The bacteria are unaffected by the enzyme because they contain no collagen. The other type have been found in the amphibian and mammalian tissues undergoing growth or remodeling.

colloid. Fine particles (the disperse phase) suspended in another medium (the dispersion medium); can be solid, liquid or gas suspended in solid, liquid or gas. The examples of gas-in-liquid colloidal systems include beaten egg white, whipped cream; liquid-liquid colloids: emulsions such as milk, salad cream.

colloid, lyophillic. Colloids in which there is a high affinity between the particles of the disperse phase and the dispersion medium. Include proteins and higher carbohydrates, very viscous, electrically charged, require large amounts of electrolytes for precipitation which is reversible. Also known as emulsoids.

colloid, lyophobic. Colloids in which there is no affinity between the particles of the disperse phase and the dispersion medium. The particles carry an electric charge and are flocculated irreversibly by electrolytes. Also called suspensoids.

colony. A cluster or assemblage of microorganisms growing on a solid surface such as the surface of an agar culture medium; the assemblage is often directly visible through a microscope.

colony counts. A bacteriological term used to assess the general bacterial content of water. This term does not refer to the total number of microorganisms present in water, but simply those that are able to form visible colonies in nutrient media under specified culture conditions.

colostrum. The thin milky fluid secreted by the mammary gland a few days before or after parturition. It is yellowish in colour; contains a higher concentration of solids than does the later milk, especially the globulin fraction. It contains protective antibodies, hence colostrum is of special importance to young mammals. In farming practice where animals are weaned as early as possible on to artificial mixtures, weaning takes place only after all the colostrum has been given to the young animal. Colostrum is thick and yellow, has a strong odour, a bitter taste, and contains a very high percentage of globulin. Colostrum has a laxative effect and is two to ten days colostrum milk usually changes to normal milk. Colostrum is believed to be especially rich in antibodies which protect the calf from diseases to which it would otherwise offer little or no resistance.

colour fermentation. An abnormal fermentation produced in milk or cream resulting in colour changes. Many organisms commonly found in milk produce coloured bacterial colonies, especially yellow, orange or red, on agar and various other solid media.

colours. As used in food science context, colours fall into three groups; natural pigments derived mostly from plant materials, inorganic pigments and lakes (combination of organic colouring matters with metals), and synthetic coal-tar dyes. Most of those in the first two groups are legally permitted in most countries, but only specifically named coal-tar dyes are allowed. Greece and Iceland do not permit any synthetic dyes in foods with specific exceptions; the list of permitted colours varies so much from one country to another that there is not a single dye that is permitted in every country.

coltsfoot. *Tussilago Farfara.* One of the quirky creations of nature. Very early in the Spring, coltsfoot develops flat orange flower heads, but only after they eventually wither do the broad, hoof-shaped, sea-green leaves develop. It is fairly common and is not picky about the soil it grows in.

Columbard grape. A white wine grape of wood quality, cultivated principally in France (Cognac district). Also cultivated in California, where it is sometimes called French Columbard. Wine from the Columbard is sometimes blended with other California wines, such as Chablis and in some California Champagne. The grape is also well suited for distillation.

column dryer. A unit for removing moisture in which the product being dried moves by gravity through a vertical column, with the heated drying air moving through the column at right angles to the heated drying air moving through the column at right angles to the flow of grain. The vertical column dryer is usually a continuous flow crossflow dryer. The speed of discharge of products and temperature and flow of the drying air are regulated or controlled to provide proper drying of the product.

Comice pear. A variety of pear *Doyenne du Comice*. Fruit is medium to large in size, sometimes very large. Shape is obovate-obtuse-pyriform. Its skin is fairly thick, granular, susceptible to blemishes, sometimes russeted; greenish-yellow color, often blushed. The flesh of comice pear is very fine, melting, extremely juicy, quite free of grit. It is sweet and possesses rich, aromatic, vinous flavour, and is considered by many as among the very best of desert pears. Fruit is inclined to bruise easily in the ripe stage. The treeof comice pear is large, stately, girorous, but slow in coming into bearing. Its demands for soil and climate more exacting than for most pear trees.

compaction. The process of packing fine particles or aggregates as is purposely done for pelleting, cubing, or wafering; or the packing of products in a drying bin, which may change the air flow-static pressure relationships; or increasing the density of dried food products, such as dry milk or hay, which may be compacted into tablets, blocks, cakes, or pellets following drying to decrease space, improve handling, and reduce oxidation.

compartment dryer. A batch dryer or quasi-continuous convection heated air dryer which is equivalent to two or more cabinet dryers operating in series.

compartment kiln. A building or holding unit which is filled with a product, usually lumber or clay products; the doors are closed, and the drying proceeds, all done in one operation. The product remains stationary. The temperature and relative humidity in the kiln are controlled according to a drying schedule which depends on the nature of the product. The design of the compartment kiln is a contrast to the tunnel kiln or progressive kiln, in which the product is moved. Also known as box kiln; charge kiln.

Complan. Trade name for a mixture of dried skim milk, arachis oil, casein, maltodextrins, sugar, salts and vitamins. Its average composition per 100 g is: protein 30%; fat 17%; carbohydrate 45%; Ca 825 mg; Fe 8 mg; and supplemented with proper amounts of vitamins A, B_1, B_2, nicotinic acid, B_{12}, C, D, E, K, pantothenic acid and folic acid.

complement. A series of proteins in the blood that plays a major role in the body's immunological defence, by promoting the phagocytosis of invading cells and other antigens, and by undertaking the lysis of certain bacteria. Complement is also involved in inflammation, and may be responsible for some of the damage that occurs in autoimmune disease and in hypersensitivity. The series comprises nine dis-tinct protein components, which interact sequentially in a so-called 'cascade' effect: this means that a small triggering event sufficient to activate one of the components generates an amplified effect. In the classical pathway of complement activation, the first step is the binding of IgG or IgM antibodies to specific antigen. The binding action leads to a conformational change in the antibody, which permits the activation of first complement component, C-. Activated C-1 is then able to activate components C-2 and C-4, which at jointly as a proteolytic enzyme to cleave component C-3 into C-3a and C-3b. These are thus released in the vicinity of antigen-antibody complexes or at the surface of cells that have bound antibody. C-3b. stimulates the influx, binding, and phagocytic activities of macrophages and neutrophils, and the release of inflammatory substances by platelets. C-3a acts to release histamine from base cells; in this role C-3a is known as an anaphylotoxin. C-3 can also be cleaved by an alternative pathway, which bypasses C-1, C-2, and C-4. The pathway is activated by many substances, including bacterial lipopolysaccharide, thrombin and plasmin, zymosan from yeast, and various factors in cobra venom and helminth parasites. Once produced C-3b in conjunction with further proteins-B, D, and P (properdin), has the property of stimulating further breakdown of C-3. In order to prevent overproduction of C-3b, normal serum contains C-3b. inactivator, the absence of which may result in spontaneous exhaustion of C-3, C-3b, whether generated by the classical or the alternative pathway, has the additional property of being able to activate C-5, which is clea-ved to produce C-5a, another anaphylotoxin. The remainder C-5. molecule complexes with C-6 and C-7, and in this form acquires the power further to attract neutrophils. The activated complex of C-5,6,7 is finally able to fix components C-8. and C-9, which thus acquire the power to lyse certain bacteria and other foreign cells.

complementary bases. Bases that normally pair up when DNA or RNA adopts a double-stranded configuration. Guanine pairs with cytosine, and adenine with either thymine or uracil (depending on whether DNA or RNA is involved), the former pair having three hydrogen bonds between the bases, and the latter two pairs having only two hydrogen bonds between the bases.

complementary DNA. cDNA. A DNA that is usually made by the reverse transcriptase and is complementary to a given messenger RNA. It is used in DNA cloning. It is synthesized *in vitro* using RNA as a template and the RNA-dependent DNA polymerase. The reac-tion requires a primer, usually a synthe-tic oligonucleotide capable of base pairing to the RNA, and generates a DNA molecule complementary in sequence to the RNA template. Complementary DNA can be made highly radioactive for use as a probe in nucleic acid hybridization studies, or rendered double-stranded by a further round of polymerization and then cloned into a bacteriophage or plasmid vector.

complex hapten. A high-molecular mass

hapten that constitutes a separate part of a complete antigen and that gives a visible precipitin reaction with the appropriate antibody.

complex I. One of the four complexes derived from electron transport particles that, by itself, can catalyze the oxidation of NADH by coenzyme Q.

complex II. One of the four complexes derived from electron transport particles that, by itself, can catalyze oxidation of reduced coenzyme Q by cytochrome c.

complex III. One of the four complexes derived from electron transport particles that, by itself, can catalyze oxidation of reduced coenzyme Q by cytochrome c.

complex IV. One of the four complexes derived from electron transport particles that, by itself, can catalyze the oxidation of reduced cytochrome c by molecular oxygen.

complex medium. Culture medium that contains some ingredients of unknown chemical composition.

conalbumin. One of the proteins of egg-white comprising 12% of the total solids. It has the property of binding iron in an iron-protein complex that is pink. Accounts for the pinkish colour resulting when eggs are stored in rusty containers.

concentrated liquid milk. Milk from which water has been evaporated to the extent that it is reduced in weight about 3 to 1. It is generally homogenized and pasteurized after condensation and then bottled and marketed in a manner similar to fluid bottled milk. It has good keeping qualities; takes up less space; is more economical to handle due to reduced water content; and can be reconstituted to any desired degree as per requirement of the user. It is identical with plain condensed whole milk except for its

method of packaging.

Concord grape. A blue-black grape native to North America and used primarily in making Kosher-type wines, unfermented grape juice, and jellies. The wine is also used in New-York State Burgundies and Ports. The concord is also grown in Canada. The grape is of *Vitis labrusca*. This grape is of much current interest as a source of food colorant.

concurrent dryer. The arrangement of a unit for moisture removal in which the hot air for drying and the wet material to be dried enter at the same end of the dryer and travel through the dryer in the same direction. Higher air temperatures, up to 200°C, may be used for certain cereal grains. Also called cocurrent and parallel flow dryer.

condiment. A seasoning added to the flavoured foods, such as salt, mustard, ginger, curry, pepper, etc. Although some of these are relatively rich in nutrients they are generally used in such small quantities that they make a negligible contribution to the diet.

conditioning. Using processes to change the physical properties of a batch or of some components of a batch to improve the stae of the product for further processing, storage or packaging. Conditioning may be done by wetting with water or steam, by adding a chemical, by drying with forced unheated or heated air, or by equalizing and maintaining a uniform temperature of the product.

conduction solid-band dryer. An apparatus employed for the removal of moisture with a conveyor or solid band holding the product to be dried is moved over a hot surface, such as a steam heated chest. The conveyor and the product are heated by conduction. Drying is often done under vacuum.

congies. The water from cooking rice which contains much of the thiamine and nicotinic acid from the rice; used as a drink.

conidendrin. A substance isolated from a number of coniferous woods whose derivatives, *nor-conidendrin* and alpha and beta conidendrol, are antioxidants. Chemically similar to the phenolic substance, nordihydroguaiaretic acid.

conjugated proteins. Name given to the proteins consisting of a polypeptide chain to which a non-protein or prosthetic group is attached. The prosthetic group may be a flavin nucleotide (flavoprotein), a polysaccharide (glycoprotein), a lipid (lipoprotein) or a nucleic acid (nucleoprotein). Conjugated proteins include:

(a) Nucleoproteins; the prosthetic group of these conjugated proteins is a nucleic acid.

(b) Lipoproteins; the lipid prosthetic group in these proteins is variable, but usually contains glyceride, phospha-tide, and cholesterol.

(c) Mucoproteins; those substances having a carbohydrate prosthetic group, which almost always contain some hexosamine.

(d) Chromoproteins; the prosthetic groups of this class are not easily classified except for their colour, *e.g.*, haemoglobin.

consomme. A clear soup made from meat or meat extract.

constant rate drying. An initial phase in the drying of solids during which the rate of evaporation per unit of surface area remains constant. While drying wetted sand, most of the drying occurs at constant rate. When drying hygroscopic materials, such as grain, very little if any drying occurs during the constant rate period, depending on the initial moisture content of the product. The rate of drying during the constant rate period is dependent on the humidity of the drying air, coefficient of mass transfer, - and the velocity of the drying air.

constitutive enzymes. A set of enzymes present through out the life cycle of a plant, although operating at different rates at various phases *e.g.*, carbon reducing enzymes of photosynthesis and respiratory enzymes.

continuous band dryer. An apparatus used for the removal of moisture, in which the material moves continuously, usually in a horizontal position in a band or on a tray, through a heated chamber. The product may be dried by convection heating, or may be moved over a heated surface, in which case the product is heated by conduction, and/or the product may be moved under a radiation heat source, either on a conveyor or in trays on a conveyor. Conveyors may be perforated, permitting air flow, or of a solid-band dryer. Continuous band dryers are used for precipitated inorganic colors, china clay, dyestuffs, molded articles, and some natural fiber textile materials. Dryers of this type consist of band through-circulation dryer; convection solid-band dryer; conduction solid-band dryer; continuous tray dryer; radiation solid band or conveyor dryer.

continuous circulation. A term referring to a dryer or evaporator in which the product is moved continuously during moisture the removal of its moisture. It generally forms a product which has uniform moisture content throughout the batch being dried, as compared with a unit in which no circulation takes place.

continuous flow dryer. An apparatus in

which the product being dried is in continuous movement in contrast to a batch operation. The main continuous flow dryers are spray, fluidized bed, continuous band, pneumatic, continuous rotary (direct and indirect), crossflow, concurrent flow, and continuous tray. Also known as continuous operation dryers.

continuous tray dryer. An apparatus used for the removal of moisture, in which the product to be dried is placed in trays. The product is heated by convection or conduction, usually with air moving through the product on deep trays of uniform materials of granules, pellets, etc., or over the product on shallow trays.

continuous web dryer. A setup for the removal of moisture, which moves wet products on a web conveyor in a horizontal direction (similar to a belt or open chain dryer) through heated air, often with counter-current flow. It is used for bulky materials, industrial parts, clay products, leafy and forage croups, and grains.

contractile proteins. Proteins, present in plant cells, involve in streaming of cytoplasm in several systems. When such proteins *e.g.*, actin and myosin, are pre-sent in sieve element due to peristaltic movement of these contractile proteins strand material may be transported.

convenience food. A catchall term for designating a food product that has been pre-processed and packed so that, with exception of heating (sometimes thawing and heating), the product is ready to be consumed, such as, cooked meats, canned foods, baked foods, break-fast preparations, frozen foods etc. Although some authors use this term traditionally for canned and frozen foods, the common connotation of the term is the substitution of factory pre-processing for routine processing in the kitchen at the point of consumption. In terms of home use, the advantage is essentially convenience (normally for a higher price); but for larger consumtion, such as parties, hospitals, schools, and other institutions, convenience can be quickly translated into terms of labour savings at the point of consumption. When professionally pre-processed and effectively handled at the consuming end, convenience foods also have a number of other advantages, including greater uniformity, quality control, portion control, cleanliness, and flexibility to meet varying demand loads (easy storage provides a buffer).

cookie. An American term for biscuit.

cooking. The process of making food more palatable and more digestible. There is breakdown of the connective tissue in meat and softening of the cellulose in plant tissues. Some of the common methods of cooking are:

Broiling, cooking by direct heat over flame.

Pan broiling, cooking through hot dry metal over direct heat.

Sautéing, cooking with small amount of fat.

Simmering, cooking in water slightly below boiling point.

Stewing, the process of prolonged simmering.

Fricassee, combination of sauteining and stewing. Devilled, Grilled or fried after coating with condiments or bread crumbs.

Steaming, cooking by heat conveyed by steam either directly or through steam jacket as in double boiler. Steaming is also carried out above 100°C by means of pressure cookers. In general the water-soluble vitamins and minerals are leached into the cooking water, the fat-soluble vitamins are unaffected except at frying temperatures, and the proteins are not damaged except under extreme conditions.

Vegetables lose much of their vitamin C, mostly by leaching into the water, but also by oxidation during heating. The losses can be minimised by steaming or greatly reducing the volume of the cooking water, and maximised by storing hot after cooking. The vitamins show some destruction, B_1 being more sensitive, on heating, and the loss depends on temperature and time. For example, frying destroys 10% B_1, 10% B_2 and 15% nocotinic acid, while braising destroys 55%, 25% and 35% respectively and stewing destroys 75%, 30%, and 50% respectively.

coon. A cheddar cheese, originally produced in northern New York State, shelf-cured and coated with black wax. Cheese of 36% moisture content is cured at 2.5°C and 85-90% relative humidity whereas cheese with a moisture content of 40% is cured at 25°C and 75-80% relative humidity.

copper. A transition metal; one of the earliest known metals, is lustrous, ductile, malleable, and a good conductor of heat. It may have been the first metal worked by ancient man 8000 years ago. Copper is an essential element. It is present in all organisms, land and marine. Copper is part of the enzyme tyrosinase (and in plants, laccase and ascorbic acid oxidase) and is needed to assist the incorporation of iron into haemoglobin. It is therefore thought to be a dietary essential in amounts of about 2 mg per day, but there is no evidence that a dietary deficiency ever occurs in man. Traces of copper are normally present in the blood in combination with an α-globulin as caeruloplasmin. Its deficiency in cattle gives rise to "swayback." The traces of copper are also essential for plant growth. It has been found to be toxic in high concentrations and there is a legal limit to the amount permitted in foodstuffs.

The early literature is rich with accounts of investigations concerning the presence of copper in different life forms. Some of the earliest observations were made upon marine organisms. Copper was shown to be combined with the blood proteins of snails. The essential role of copper became established when its importance was observed in diets for rats, and demonstrated that copper, in addition to iron, was necessary for blood formation. The reports began to appear from various regions that certain disorders of grazing sheep and cattle were due to deficiencies of copper and had responded to copper supplements. The copper containing enzymes include tyrosinase, ascorbic acid oxidase, cytochrome oxidase, monamine oxidase, uricase, and the δ-aminolevulinic acid dehydratase. Several manifestations of copper deficiency in animals appear to be related to decreased tissue concentrations of certain of these enzymes. Various aspects as copper metabolism and transport in man and animals have been studied in depth in both health and in disease states. Copper occurs in all bodily tissues. The distribution varies with age, species and diet. Liver, heart, brain, kidney and hair contain high concentrations compared to other tissues. Glandular tissues, such as, pituitary, thyroid and prostrate, contain low levels. Tissues containing intermediate concentrations include bones, skin, muscles, pancreas and spleen. Brain copper increases with age while levels in the liver, spleen and lung decrease. Abnormally high copper levels in liver are characteristic of certain diseases. Wilson's disease, or hepatolenticular degeneration comes to mind first of all. Other conditions which manifest increased copper content in liver include thalassemia, hemachromatosis, cirrhosis, yellow atrophy of liver, tuberculosis and carcinomas. Blood copper levels of healthy animals vary rather widely, but for the higher mammals are of a similar magnitude. According to Beck, most values lie between 80 and 120 µg. Other investigators report similar blood copper levels. The mean copper levels for normal human females is somewhat higher than for males; there may be some hormonal involvement. Increases in serum or plasma copper levels of women taking oral contraceptives containing an estrogen have been reported. Copper levels ranging around 280 µg have been reported in women pregnancy. Scientists observed changes in plasma and hair zinc and copper concentration during pregnancy. By sixteen weeks, copper had increased to 162 µg from a 107 µg level; zinc decreased from 88 to 68 µg. After thirty-eight weeks, plasma zinc fell to 56 µg and copper rose to 192 µg. At delivery copper levels in maternal sera are four to five times those found in newborns. Levels in the latter range between 45-70 µg. Elevated serum copper levels in humans are manifest in certain other disease processes also, for example, infections, leukemias, Hodgkin's disease, hemochromatosis, and hyperthyroidism. Increased serum copper levels have also been reported in artherosclerosis. Serum zinc is significantly decreased and copper and iron levels markedly increased in thalassemia; copper levels were also found in epilepsy. A summary of serum and urine copper concentrations found in health and disease states. Comparable hypocupremia also occurs in cystic fibrosis and kwashiorkor, diseases with a coexisting protein deficiency. Copper deficiencies have also been observed following long-term parental nutrition. A rather rare case of an infant on parental therapy for eight and a half months did respond to copper supplementation. Hepatolenticular degeneration, or Wilson's disease, is characterized by the progressive development of neurological disturbances as manifest by widespread tremor and rigidity and, at times, dementia. Liver cirrhosis is also present. Copper metabolism is abnormal, and there are indications that other metals may be involved. Amino acid excretion is increased. Most cases of the disease become manifest between age 11 and 40 yeras. Often in the past this treatable disease was misdiagnosed. Many cases were reported subsequently. A rather interesting anomaly seen in some cases is a zone or ring of pigmentation in the cornea, referred to as a Kayser-Fleischer ring. Early investigators suggested that the greenish granules in the ring consisted of silver, melanin, malarial pigment, etc. The granules were identified to be copper containing, using both chemical and spectroscopic methods. Wilson's disease is treatable within limits. D-Penicillamine is the agent of choice. Copper stores from tissues are mobilized and urinary copper excretion increased. With adequate treatment there will be neurological improvement and arrest of the liver damage.

Penicillamine, incidentally, also induces a cupriuria in normal subjects and patients with active liver disease. Urinary copper levels in controls were reported to increase from levels of 16 to 140 µg per day to levels of 832-1325 µg per day after a dose of penicillamine. Excretion levels in active liver disease patients increased to 1390 µg per day. Following penicillamine, patients with Wilson's disease excreted between 1800 and 7000 µg per day. In 1962, researchers first described the 'kinky hair syndrome', a sex-linked recessive disorder with retardation of growth, peculiar hair, and local cerebral degeneration. noting the similarity between this syndrome and copper deficiency in sheep, they demonstrated that serum copper and copper oxidase (ceruloplasmin) were extremely law in all infants with kinky hair disease. Subsequently it was reported that the brain in this condition is smaller than that in the normal newborn. While the grey matter is apparently of normal quantity, there is a significant decrease in the white matter. Both the substantial nigra and locus coerulus are depigmented. Copper contents in the brain were found to be half the concentration in similar tissue of a normal infant suffering to a trauma. Liver, kidney and spleen copper contents in the control were approximately twice that found in the kinky hair syndrome. Copper levels in the duodenal tissue of the latter, however, were more than twice those of the controls. Some scientists are of the opinion that this generalized disorder of copper metabolism is already manifest in the developing fetus and can be demonstrated in amniotic fluid, liver and skin fibroblasts.

The toxic signs of copper intake have been known for centuries. A rather unusual incident is that reported in 1968 wherein 30 workmen suffered acute copper poisoning after drinking more tea made with water from an unserviced gas water heater. The copper concentration of the water in the brew pan was 3 mg per 100 ml. Salts of copper have found limited application as germicides, fungicides, insecticides and astringents. At one time, these were also used as emetics. Salts are used as pigments in ceramics and in the textile industry. During a limited interval a few years ago when it was the fashion for inner-city women to spray metallic streaks on their hair, a number of children were admitted as emergencies with a syndrome resembling metal fume fever. Symptoms included a pulmonary edema and transitory fever. These subjects had inhaled a spray known as 'Nestle's Copper Streak', a preparation consisting of fine particles of metallic copper, about 10-50 µm in size. Serum copper levels and urinary copper excretions were elevated for approximately three days. Children apparently recovered within a week. 'Copper streak' and similar metallic sprays were eventually withdrawn from the cosmetic market. A condition named 'vineyard sprayer's lung' has been reported in vineyard workers who sprayed Bordeaux mixture (1-25% copper sulphate solution neutralized with hydrated lime) on grape vines to prevent mildew. Patients exhibited diffuse pulmonary pathology suggestive of a pulmonary infection. Presenting symptoms included weakness, malaise, loss of appetite, and weight loss, and occasionally cough. Vineyard workers are also reported to show a high incidence of lung carcinoma. Recently, liver pathology with inclusion of copper was recognized in rural workers with 'vineyard sprayer's lung'. Morphologically, the hepatic lesions resemble those previously reported in workers exposed to inorganic arsenic and vinyl chloride. Abundant deposits of copper were demonstrated in hepatic and pulmonary lesions by the histochemical techniques.

Copper was also identified in the lymphatic system, spleen and kidney. A number of cases, some lethal, of copper poisoning following dialysis have been described. Copper was leached from the tubing in the dialysis bath. Serum copper levels rose above 2 mg per 100 ml in some instances. Copper sulphate is said to be a fairly common agent for suicide or homicide in many countries. Certain sections in India had reported that one third of all acute hospital admissions were due to copper poisonings. Copper salts are more usually the weapon of women.

Exposure to copper dusts and fumes generated during various industrial processes is manifested by respiratory and dermatological problems. Copper salts have been known to induce a conjunctivitis and edema of the eyelids. Copper in the soluble form, has been shown to be an inhibitor of δ-aminolevalinic acid dehydratse. Zinc activates ALAD. Chronic copper toxicity in animals can be ameliorated by feeding ammonium molybdate. The use of molybdenum has been suggested for the prevention of nutritional copper poisoning in house sheep. On the other hand, copper deficiencies in animals seem aggravated by feeding molybdenum. Both metals are components of enzymes that mediate the oxidation and reduction of iron and are therefore involved in its utilization. Manganese may increase retention of copper in the body. Serum copper is elevated and zinc decreased in leukemic states. As therapy becomes effective, levels of both elements approach normal. Effects of copper and lead upon ALAD are additive, presumably. Both elements together effect greater inhibition than either singly

copra. The dried kernel of the coconut, which yield an oil used in the manufacture of soap and candles. Copra is obtained in large quantities from the islands of the Pacific, and is an important article of commerce. The cocoanut meat is dried in the sun or in a kiln, and also by hot air, the latter method producing a higher percentage of oil. One gallon is the average yield of thirty coconuts. The cake remaining after the oil is extracted is utilized as fodder and manure.

core enzyme. 1. The portion of the enzyme RNA polymerase that consists of an aggregate of five subunits and that possesses catalytic activity, but that requires the attachment of the sigma factor before it can recognize an initiation site of transcription. 2. The smallest aggregate of DNA-dependent DNA polymerase having enzymatic activity.

Cori cycle. The sequence of reactions through which the liver converts lactic acid back to glycogen, namely liver glycogen-blood glucose-muscle glycogen-blood lactate-liver glycogen.

Cori ester. Name given to glucose-1-phosphate, one of the inter-mediates of glucose metabolism.

coriander. Family: *Umbelliferae*. Genus: *Coriandrum*. Species: *Coriandrum sativum*. A small annual plant that has been cultivated for several millenniums and is still grown in North and

South America, Europe and the Mediterranean countries. The round, finely grooved stem grows almost 50 cm tall from a thin, spindly-shaped root. The leaves are pinnately decompound while the flowers appear in flat, compound umbels that may be either white or red in appearance. The brownish, globose seeds have a disagreeable smell until they ripen, at which time they acquire a distinctly spicy aroma. The whole plant has an unpleasant smell, but the fruit, improperly called seed is very aggreeable and aromatic when dry. It is used in medicine as a remedy for dyspepsia, and as an ingredient in cookery and confectionery. Both the green feathery leaves and the spherical seeds of coriander are indispensable in the kitchen, especially to anyone who is fond of curries. Bunches of coriander, which looks like-fat-leafed parsley, are sold in many markets, especially where there is an Asian or Green community. The seed is sold both whole or ground, and is a major ingredient in curry powder. It has a sweet taste reminiscent of orange peel. The leaves do not dry well, but may be frozen. They are used in curries; ground to a paste with olive oil and the ground seed as covering for roast lamb in mariandes; sparingly, as they are rather bitter, in salads; and mixed with coconut and green chillies in a classic Indian chutney. The seeds, which may be roasted to bring out the full flavour, are widely used in curries and casseroles, in sausages, with fish and all *ala Grecque* dishes. They are also included in mixed pickling spice. Medicinally, the herb has been tried as a digestive and for the treatment of colic. The dried ripe fruit of *Coriandrum sativum* contains 20% fixed oil and 1% essential oil -

largely linool or coriandrol (an isomer of geraniol).

Coriander contains volatile oil (about 1 per cent) as well as fats, starch, sugar, protein, tannin, flavonoids, glycosides, vitamins, including niacin, riboflavin and thiamin, and minerals, particularly potassium and calcium. The leaves are higher in protein than the seeds but contain less oil. Coriander is usually used to stop griping caused by seena or rhubarb, which will mask the unpleasant taste of other medicines. Chewing the seeds stimulates the secretion of gastric juices. The brusied seed can be applied externally as a poultice between pieces of gauze to relieve painful joints in rheumatism. In China, ripe coriander seeds are sun-dried and then used to stop bleeding, to bread up phlegm and to eliminate odours. There is a Cantonese folk remedy for treating bad breath, foul urine and female genital odour which and female genital odour which requires fresh coriander herb to be used in soup. Its main use is for the treatment of haemorrhoids, dysentery, measles, indigestion, constipation and analprolapse. A decoction is sometimes used as a mouthwash to relieve toothache and also for gargling. It is also used as flavour in meat products, bakery goods, tobacco, gin and in curry powder.

corm. Thickened, underground base of stem of plants, often called bulbs as, for example, taro and onion.

corn, flour. A variety of maize with large, soft grains and very friable endosperm, making it easy to grind the grain to flour.

corn. In UK, a generic term for cereals. In US, it refers to maize.

corn steep liquor. The first stage in the preparation of starch from maize is to soak the maize in water containing sulphur dioxide for 24 hours. The liquor is termed corn steep liquor. It was found to be an excellent medium for growing mould to produce penicillin; the yield was greatly enhanced beyond that obtained with synthetic media since the liquor contained a "biochemical precursor" of penicillin.

corn sugar. *See* glucose.

corned beef. In UK it is a relatively cheap canned product made from lower quality beef; the chopped meat is partially cooked in boiling water when the water-soluble fraction is partly removed to produce, after evaporation, *meat extract.* The scalded meat is cured in brine, together with sugar and preservatives, and canned. The name is derived from grains or corns of salt. In the US, it is called *salt beef.* The average composition per 100 g is: 25 g protein; 15 g fat; 3 mg iron; 11 µg vitamin A; 0.4 mg vitamin B_1, 00.2 mg vitamin B_2, 3.5 mg nicotinic acid; and food energy 1 MJ.

cornflakes. Breakfast cereal made from maize grain. The average composition per 100 g is: protein 6.6%; fat 0.8%; carbohydrate 88%; Ca 7 mg; Fe 3 mg. Phytic acid phosphorus 25% of the total P (58 mg/100 g).

cornflour. Purified starch from maize; in US called corn starch; used in custard, balancmange and baking powders. The average composition is: protein 0.5%, fat 0.3%, carbohydrate 87%, fibre 0.2%, no vitamins present.

cornhusker cheese. A colby type cheese having numerous openings, a higher moisture content, and a more rapid making procedure than Colby cheese.

corn oil. Pale yellow in colour, it is very high in caloric value, furnishing more than 8.9 calories per gram). Because the oil is not assimilated as quickly as carbohydrates or proteins, its complete digestion provides energy over an extended period of time. Refined corn oil is widely used as a cooking and salad oil.

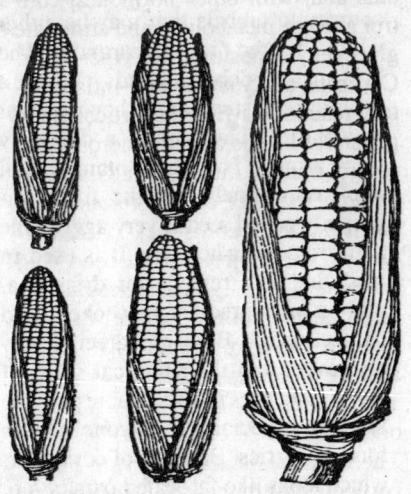

Refined corn oil is widely used in deep frying and for shortening because it does not smoke until it reaches a temperature above 232°C, withstands continued heating, is slow to oxidize, and provides a crisp crust with freedom from greasiness. In addition to providing energy some nutritionists feel that polyunsaturated fatty acids, such as those in corn oil, when properly used in diets, contributed to the reduction of blood serum cholesterol. Refined corn oil also finds wide application as a base for mayonnaise and salad dressings because the oil does not mask essential flavors and resists rancidity. Refined corn oil is also widely used in the production of margarine.

corticosteroids. The steroid hormones synthesized and secreted by adrenal cortex, or any related synthetic steroid. There are two main categories of corticosteroids-glucocorticoids and mineralocorticoids. Glucocorticoids are generally 17-hydroxylated corticosteroids and, with other hormones, control glucose metabolism and stimulate glycogen deposition in the liver. Cortisone also induces anti-inflammatory reactions. Mineralocorticoids are generally 17-deoxycorticosteroids and control mineral metabolism. Glucocorticoids include corticosterone and cortisol (hydrocortisone). Aldosterone is the major mineralocorticoid hormone. The glucocorticoids are essential for the utilization of carbohydrate, fat, and protein by the body and for a normal response to stress. The mineralocorticoids (e.g., aldosterone) regulate salt and water balance. The major naturally occurring glucocorticoid hormones are hydrocortisone (cortisol) and corticosterone. Their secretion is controlled by adenohypophysis via adrenocorticotrophic hormone, and there is a diurnal pattern of secretion, with a peak in the morning in most species (the peak occurs in the evening in nocturnal animals, e.g., cats). Secretion increases during periods of stress. The corticosteroids are distributed throughout tissues, are metabolized in liver, and excreted conjugated to glucuronide in the urine (synthetic corticosteroids are metabolized more slowly and can be excreted unchanged in the urine). The effects of gluconeogenesis (causing increased blood glucose and liver glycogen), muscle catabolism, lipolysis with redistribution of body fat stores, decreased absorption and increased urinary excretion of calcium, reduced levels of growth hormone, decreased bone growth, increased blood haemoglobin, increased numbers of circulating polymorphonuclear cells, decreased circulating lymphoid cells and eosinophils, and suppression of cell-mediated immunity. The glucocorticoids have marked anti-inflammatory effect, with activity at all stages of inflammation. They produce a decrease in capillary permeability, reduced exudation and migration of inflammatory cells, stabiliza-tion of lysosomal membranes, a reduction in phagocytosis by macrophages, inhibition of the release of arachidonic' acid (the precursor of inflammatory mediators prostaglandins, leukotrienes, and thromboxanes), suppression of granulation tissue formation, and reductions in collagen formation and fibroblast proliferation thus increasing the time taken for wound healing. Most glucocorticoids have some mineralocorticoid activity, although this is more marked with natural hormones and the early synthetic corticosteroids. This mineralocorticoid activity mimics the action of aldosterone, causing sodium retention, hypokalaemia, and fluid retention. The more recent synthetic corticosteroids have much less mineralocorticoid and mainly glucocorticoid activity.

corticotrophin. A polypeptide hormone secreted by the anterior pituitary gland. It acts on adrenal cortex, stimulating the secretion of corticosteroid hormones. Its release is controlled by the hypothalamus and by circulating corticosteroids, whose production it stimulates its secretion. It is used in the diagnosis of disorders of anterior pituitary gland and adrenal cortex and may be used therapeutically, for example to stimulate corticosteroid production in children.

cortisone. A steroid hormone, closely related biochemically to hydrocortisone and corticosterone; it is found in extracts of adrenal tissue, and is one of the first adrenal steroids to be isolated and synthesized, it has potent glucocorticoid activity and some mineralocorticoid action; it acts after being converted to hydrocortisone in the body.

coryneform bacteria. Gram-positive, aerobic, nonmotile, rod-shaped organisms that have the characteristic of forming irregular-shaped, club-shaped, or V-shaped cell arrangements during normal growth. The main genera of coryneform bacteria are *Corynebacterium* and *Arthrobacter*. The genus *Corynebacterium* consists of an extremely diverse group of bacteria, including animal and plant pathogens as well as saprophytes. The genus *Arthrobacter*, consisting primarily of soil organisms, is distinguished from *Corynebacterium* on the basis of cycle of development in *Arthrobacter* involving conversion from rod to sphere and back to rod again.

cos lettuce. A kind of cultivar which is easily recognized by the upright growth of the plant, long loaf-shaped head, and the long, relatively narrow spatulate leaves. The most common cos types are self-closing, that is, the leaves curl inwards at the tips and the inner leaves become blanched. The leaves are coarse with a ribby appearance, but are tender and sweet. Because of their shape and tenderness, they are damage easily. Thus, this type of lettuce usually is grown near the marketplace. Also known as romaine lettuce. The man cos cultivars are White Paris; and Dark Green.

cossettes. Thin chips of sugar beet into which it is shredded for hot-water extraction of the sugar.

costmary. A garden herb, the fresh or dried leaves of which may be used as a flavouring for salads, ale, and aromatic drinks. This perennial plant (*Chrysanthemum balsamita*) can be propagated from seeds or by dividing. Native to Italy, the plant was introduced into England as early as 1568. In America, the plant has become naturalized and is found growing wild in a region extending from Nova Scotia southward and westward through Ohio. The plant is easily recognized by its numerous small flowers and sweetly scented leaves. Also known as mint geranium.

cotherstone cheese. A rennet cow's milk cheese made in Yorkshire, UK. It resembles Stilton cheese. It is chiefly a local product manufactured on a small scale. Also known as Yorkshire-Stilton.

cottage cheese. A soft cheese made from sour skim milk, reconstituted concentrated skim milk or nonfat dry milk, curdled either with starter alone or with starter plus rennet, also known as Pot, Dutch or Schimierkase cheese. The large grained, low-acid variety is called sweet-curd, flake-type and low-acid rennet type Cottage cheese. Because the large particles of curd resemble popcorn it is also called Popcorn cheese. The small grained variety is known as country style or farm style cheese. When the cheese contains 4% or more fat, it is known as creamed cottage. Cottage cheese is perishable and should be stored at low temperatures. It has many uses and provides a convenient way of using surplus milk. Large quantities are consumed as table cheese and in salads. The approximate percentage analysis is: water 71.4-79.9%, proteins, amides, etc. 12.6-21.1%, fat 4-1.9% and ash 2-1.1%.

cottonseed products. The most important of the products derived from the seed of the cotton plant is a yellow oil. This is extracted by pressure after the seeds have been freed of fibres, pits of lint and hulls. The oil is employed in the manufacture of cottolene, which is used for lard; it is also a substitute for olive oil, and has a place in the manufacture of soaps. A hard, dry cake remains after the oil has been pressed from a mass of seeds, and when ground this cake forms cottonseed meal. It is an excellent stock food, and when mixed with acid phosphate it has value as a fertilizer. The hulls of the seeds are also used as stock food, and the fine pieces of lint (linters), which cling to the seeds in the ginning processes, are used in the manufacture of low-priced yarns, upholstering, wadding, etc. Another by-product is sludge, wich settles at the bottom of oil tanks. It is used in the manufacture of soap.

courgette. Family: *Cucurbitaceae.* Genus: *Cucurbita.* Species: *Cucurbita pepo.* Courgettes are high in vitamin C and contain a great deal of water, so are very low in calories unless boosted by oil or butter. Italian marrows, Italian Squash or Zucchini, a variety of gourd with small fruits.

courlose. Trade name for sodium carboxymethylcellulose.

covalently modified enzyme. A regulatory enzyme which is modified as a result of a chemical alteration of the enzyme, which in turn, is catalyzed by other enzymes. The inactive enzyme (zymogen) becomes active due to enzyme catalyzed activation *e.g.*, pepsin, trypsin and chymotrypsin. Such enzyme occurs in two forms *i.e.*, active and inactive and these are inter-converted by covalent modifications of their structures that are catalyzed by other enzymes.

cow manure factor. Vitamin B_{12}.

cozymase. An early designation of a heat-stable fraction-consisting chiefly of ATP, ADP, AMP, and NAD^+, that was isolated from yeast and participated in the reactions of alcoholic fermentation. Subsequently, cozymase I was used to denote NAD^+ and cozymase II was used to denote $NADP^+$.

crab apple. A tree which bears a small, tart fruit much used in making jellies and preserves. The name is somewhat loosely applied to any apple tree producing a sour, uncultivated fruit, but properly it refers to the wild varieties of the true apple, from which the latter is produced.

crabs. Shellfish of the suborder *Brachyura* of the Order *Decapoda.* Large spider crab, *Maina squinado*, occasionally used as food. The name given to nearly a thousand species of shellfish. Many of them are classed as food, but they contain slight nutriment, being really little more than a delicacy. Enough of the them are eaten to raise crab fishing to the plane of a profitable industry. The head and breast are united, and the whole is covered with a strong shell. The mouth has several pairs of strong jaws, in addition to which the stomach has its internal surface studded with hard projections for the purpose of grinding the food. The liver is the soft, rich, yellow substance usually called the fat of the crab. The young crabs throw off their covering at intervals as they increase in size, but after they are full-grown, three or four years at least may pass without a change of this character. The first pair of limbs are not used for locomotion, but are furnished with strong claws or pincers, and the right claw is generally larger than the left. The crab's eyes are compound and are placed upon stalks, which sometimes are over an inch in length. Edible crab, *Cancer pagurus,* found in shallow water among rocks; can grow up to 3-4 kg weight.

cranberry. The fruit of the cranberry (*Oxycoccus macrocarpus* L.) possesses a high colour value due to the presence of anthocyanins, principally peonidin, an enthocyanin. It is a small, red acid fruit, first found in Northern Asia and Central Europe, but now domesticated in nearly every temperate zone. Since it grows only on low, swampy land or on peat bogs it is called in some localities moss berry or moor berry. The berry when ripe, is globose and is a little more than a quarter of an inch in diameter. The American cranbery has larger berries than the European species. Commercially, this natural colorant is available as a concentrated juice (50° Brix) or as a spray-dried powder carried on maltodextrin. A techique has been developed for the recovery of anthocyanins from cranberry press cake as about 40% of the anthocyanins present in the fresh berries remain in the press cake after juice expression. These products are water-soluble and produce bright red solutions at *p*H 2.5 or lower. Unfortunately, cranberry juice is not a strong colorant and requires a relatively high use level; it also has a poor light-fastness.

cream. A soft, mild, rich uncured cheese made from cream or a mixture of cream and milk. Because of its soft consistency, its buttery, smooth texture, its pleasant aroma and its rich flavour, it is very popular as a spread for bread and in sandwiches or salads. Legally contains (in UK) not less than 18% fat; sterilised cream, 23%, double cream or thick cream, 48%, clotted cream, not less than 48% fat; whipping or whipped cream, not less than 35% fat.

creaming factor. An expression denoting the relation of volume of cream formed in milk upon standing to percentage butter-fat present. Also the relation between the fat content and the per cent of cream volume formed on milk. The normal relationship for raw milk is about 4.1 times and per cent of fat in the milk.

creaming quality. As applied to fats is the ability to adsorb air during mixing.

cream line index. The cream line or layer usually forms about 6% of total depth of the milk. The cream line index is the ratio of the percentage cream layer to the percentage fat in the milk. It is used as a test of the milk and in ordinary bulk pasteurised milk is about 1.7.

cream of tartar. Potassium hydrogen tartrate, used with sodium bicarbonate as baking powder because it acts more slowly than tartaric acid and gives a more prolonged evolution of carbon dioxide. This is tartrate baking powder; similarly phosphate baking powder contains calcium acid phosphate or sodium hydrogen pyrophosphate. Also used to "invert" sugar in making boiled sweets.

cream ripening. A term applied to the scientific fermentation of cream of butter-making. Ripening is accomplished by adding a starter culture to sweet cream which (preferably) has been pasteurized. this cream is then allowed to stand at a stated temperature for a definite period of time, to give the bacteria in the starter time to produce the required amount of acid in the cream.

cream separator. A machine by which cream is separated from milk. The various models now in use all conform to the same principle, that of centrifugal force. The separator consists of a revolving bowl, or drum, into which the milk flows. The bowl is made to whirl around at the rate of 5,000-8,000 revolutions/minute, and as it revolves the cream collects at the centre, while the heavier parts of the milk are thrown against the outer rim. There are separate tubes through which the cream and skim milk flow out. These machines are operated by hand, electric, steam, water and power.

cream, clotted. A kind of cream having high fat content even more than theat in double cream, which legally is 48% fat. Double cream is floated in a shallow layer on a layer of skim milk and scalded. The clotted cream at 63% fat is then skimmed off. This is Devonshire cream and contains 29.5% water, 4% protein, 2.8% lactose, 0.67% ash. Cornish cream is similar but is prepared by scalding the double cream alone, not floated on a layer of milk.

cream, plastic. A term used for a cream containing as much fat as butter (80-83%) but as a dispersal of fat in water, whereas butter is water in fat. Prepared by intense centrifugal treatment of cream; crumbly not greasy in texture; used for preparation of cream cheese and whipped cream.

cream, sleepy. Cream that will not churn to butter in the normal time.

cream, synthetic. Name given to:
(a) emulsion of vegetable oil, milk or milk powder, egg yolk and sugar, and to
(b) emulsion of water with methyl cellulose, monoglycerides, and other synthetic materials.

creatine. Methyl guanidine derivative of acetic acid. Essential part of the energy release system of muscle, as creatine phosphate, or phosphagen, possesses an energy-rich bond which is released when energy is required for muscular contraction. The anhydride of creatine is creatinine, in which form it is found in urine. Meat extract contains a mixture of the two, derived from the creatine that was present in the fresh muscle. Creatine plus creatinine is used as an index of quality of commercial meat extract, and as a measure of extract present in manufactured products, such as soups. Its phosphate, creatine phosphate (phosphocreatine, phosphagen), acts as a store of high-energy phosphate in muscle and serves to maintain adequate amounts of ATP (the source of energy for muscular contraction).

creatine phosphate. A compound that acts as a reservoir of high-transfer potential phosphoryl groups in vertebrate muscle; i.e., it is a phosphogen. When ATP is required for muscle contraction, creatine kinase catalyzes the transfer of phosphoryl groups from creatine phosphate to ADP. The same enzyme regenerates creatine phosphate from ATP and creatine when ATP is plentiful. Also known as phosphocreatine.

creatine test. A test for depth of flavour in starter, buttermilk, butter etc. It is dependent upon the development and depth of the red colour when concentrated sodium hydroxide is added to a small amount of sample containing creatine. The deeper the colour, the more is the flavour.

cress. The name of several species of plants, most of them of the mustard family. Water-cress makes a delicious salad, as its leaves have a moderately pungent, bitterish and salty taste. It grows in cool springs and rivulets.

creta praeparata. Official British

Pharmacopoeia name for prepared chalk, made by washing and drying naturally occurring calcium carbonate. The form in which calcium is added to flour (14 oz. per 280-lb sack).

creuse. A skim milk cheese made in the department of Creuse in France. The curd is produced either by rennet or by heating the sour milk. The curd is then put into perforated earthenware molds about 15 cm in diameter and 12-15 cm in height. After draining for several days the cheese is removed from the molds, salted and frequently turned. In time it becomes very dry and hard and may be preserved for a year or even longer. The cheese is also ripened by placing in tightly closed receptacles lined with straw, in which case it becomes yellow and soft and acquires a very pronounced taste.

crimson clover. *Trifolium incarnatum.* A true clover with red, pink, purple, or white flowers. The plant is erect, a hairy annual, and attains a height of from 0.2-1m. An excellent cover crop for orchards and for winter grazing. It is a winter annual that grows well on well-drained clay soils. It is often overseeded on Bermuda grass. For winter pasture, it is frequently used in mixtures of rye, oats, and ryegrass. Crimson clover is one of the more important forage crops in south-eastern Europe, the Near East, and in the south-eastern and west coast of the US. Records indicate that it has been cultivated in France, Hungary, Italy and Balkan countries since the 18th century. It was introduced into US in 1819. In US, crimson clover is grown as a winter annual, but in Maine, to a limited extent, it is regarded as a summer annual, where seedings occur in late spring.

Crimson sweet watermelon. A variety of melon which is large, round-oval in form, and blocky. The fruit has a fine texture, small dark seeds, and a high sugar content. The flesh is deep-red and sweet. Its rind is light-green with dark stripes and is tough and chin. It is resistant to anthracnose (Race 1) and Fusarium wilt. It takes about 87 days from planting to maturity,

crispbreads. Name given to a flour and water wafer originally Swedish and made from rye flour, but may be made from wheat flour. They have a much lower water content than bread and some brands are richer in protein because of added wheat gluten. Although popularly believed to be an aid in sliming they provide more energy than the same weight of ordinary bread since they contain less water.

crisphead lettuce. One of the most important type of lettuce grown commercially in the US. The cultivars of this type are distinguished by firm or hard heads, and by the texture of the leaf which is brittle or crisp. The leaves form a head by overlapping one another in a regular fashion. The heads are large, usually about 15 cm or more in diameter and normally weight 0.9 kg when packed for market. The midribs are prominent, the veins are coarse, and the stem is usually 2.5 to 5 cm in diameter before bolting. The leaves of crisphead-type lettuce cultivars are usually tough and firm enough to withstand rough treatment of harvesting, packing, and long-distance shipment without serious physical damage.

croutons. Small diced or shaped pieces of bread fried in fat.

crumpets. The food product customarily made from a yeast batter to which some soda is added just before they are cooked. Although similar in some respects to English muffins, crumpets will be discussed in this chapter because they seem to be allied to pancakes in method of preparation. The formula also has some similarities to that of pancake batter. Sales of crumpets in the US must be practically non-existent, but it is an interesting variant for the breakfast market that ought to be given some consideration as a new product, especially in view of the great success of English muffins. Crumpets have contours somewhat similar to English muffins, being round and thick, with straight sides. The batter is deposited in a ring or "hoop" placed on a greased baking surface. It is characteristic of crumpets that the top shows large, irregular holes and this coarse uneven structure extends throughout the piece. They tend to be moist and flexible instead of crumbly. It is said they are served in England at tea time, often together with muffins.

cryogenic freezing. A technique which has gained wide acceptance during recent years. Some of the advantages of this method over blast freezing are immediately obvious from the accompanying table. Because cryogenic freezing is very fast and accomplished at extremely low temperatures (down to -196°C), less dehydration occurs. Problems of cell damage, caused by sharp ice crystals formed during slower freezing processes, are largely overcome with short freezing times. Also, the sooner a product is deeply frozen, the sooner will be the halting of bacterial and enzyme degradation. For cryogenic freezing, nitrogen is used in several forms, as a shower of liquid droplets, as a liquid bath for direct immersion, or as a cold gas. Carbon dioxide is used as a liquid or in solid "snow" form. When used in a tunnel for IQF applications, liquid carbon dioxide can freeze product at a temperature from -62°C to -78°C. Fluorocarbons and halocarbons also have been used in conjunction with tunnel and spiral-type freezers that are used in IQF methods.

Cryovac. Trade name of rubber latex wrapping film. Can be heat shrunk on to foods to form a continuous film.

cryptoxanthin. Yellow colouring matter in certain vegetables such as yellow maize, and in the seed of *Physalis,* the Chinese Lantern. A hydroxy derivative of carotene; converted into retinol in the body.

crystallin. Protein of the lens of the eye.

CSM. Corn-soya-milk; protein-rich baby food (20% protein) made in US from 68% pre-cooked maize (corn), 25% defatted soya flour and 55 skim milk powder with added vitamins B_1, B_2 B_6, B_{12}, nicotinic acid, pantothenic acid, folic acid, A, D, and E and calcium carbonate.

Cuba rum. Cuba, which is the largest island in the Caribbean has more than half of the land ideal for agriculture. The soil is fertile and the climate is ideal for the growth of sugar-cane. About 80% of the exports are sugar and rum. In rum distilleries, molasses is mainly used. The rapid fermentation take three days and a special yeast culture is used. Distillation is usually carried out specially to a high alcohol content. Much of the flavouring material is removed by filtering through sand or charcoal. The product is then flavoured with sugar, wine, fruits, bay leaves and special ingredients. Cuba rum is mostly golden in colour and is known as 'white Cuban Rum'. There are two classes known as Ron Carta and a slightly heavier one called Ron Oro. Some of these rums are coloured with caramel. Daiquiri rum is a high class product with a special flavour (Ron is Spanish for rum).

cubebs. The fruit of species of plants belonging to the pepper family. The cubebs belonging to the pepper family. The cubebs of pharmacy are produced by a climing woody shrub, a native of the East Indies. It has round, ash-colored, smooth branches, each of which bears from forty to fifty small, globose fruits, about one-fifth of an inch in diameter. The odour of cubes is agreeable and aromatic; the taste, pungent, acrid and slightly bitterish. It is used by the natives for flavoring, but in other countries chiefly in medicine, and as astringent.

cubs. Trade name for a breakfast cereal made from wheat.

cucumber. Family: *Cucurbitaceae.* Genus: *Cucumis.* Species: *Cucumis sativus;* gherkins - *Cucumis auguria.*

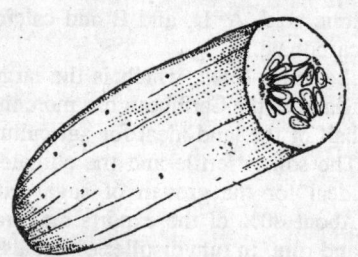

This familiar fruit is closely related to the muskmelon, and which was introduced to the world from the East Indies. In Southern Europe it is cooked before being used as an article of food, but in North America it is used principally as salad or pickle. The varieties are numerous, and each has its particular value. In a wild state in tropical Asia, the cucumber is very bitter and almost poisonous; even now it occasionally happens that a fruit is found that is bitter throughout, and almost always near the stem there is a bitter section.

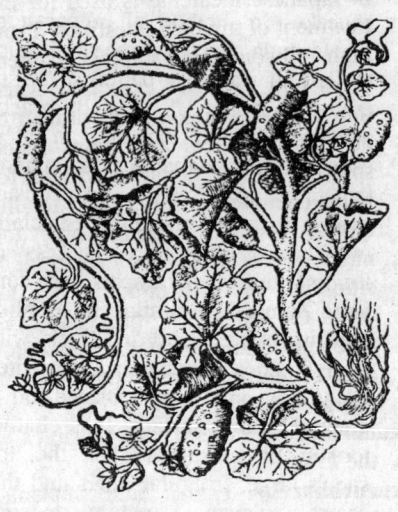

This ancient plant is a native of south-western Asia, where cultivated seeds almost 12,000 years old have been discovered. The cucumber is related to melons and, like them, has a high water content, which keeps its interior flesh cool in the hottest weather; hence, the expression "cool as a cucumber." Cukes are divided into three classes: the standard field-grown slicing kind; the smaller pickling kind, also field grown and the newer greenhouse varieties, some of which are seedless. A warm tea or cool vegetable drink is wonderful for eliminating excess fluid accumulations in body tissues, especially in chronic cases of gout and edema. Cucumber has few nutrients and no fat content or carbohydrates, which makes it ideal for slimmers. They are 95% water and once peeled lose all their vitamin A and the few trace minerals they have, but hang on to their vitamin C, folic acid and fibre. Cucumbers are an excellent diuretic and are high in potassium so do not strain the kidneys. Among the enzymes they contain is erepsin, an enzyme which helps digestion problems and which in Japanese medicine is used for the treatment of troubled intestines. Their high silicon and sulphur content helps hair to grow, especially when they are juiced and mixed with carrot or spinach juice, and helps mend splitting nails. Combined with carrot juice, cucumber juice is good for the type of rheumatism brought on by too much uric acid. The average composition per 100 g is: protein 0.6%; fat 0.1%; Ca 7 mg; Fe 0.2 mg; vitamin B_1 0.02 mg; vitamin B_2 0.03 mg; nicotinic acid 0.1 mg; vitamin C 6 mg; and food energy 0.04 MJ.

cucurbits. Term used for vegetables of the Cucurbitaceae.

cucurbitaceae. A small family of plants, largely restricted to tropical and warm climates. Most of its 650 species are climbing or trailing herbaceous plants which grow very rapidly. They are mostly annuals. Several members of this family are grown for food, as for example the cucumber, pumpkin, and squash. Some member also are used as the source of drugs. A botanical description of the plants of this family follows. The stems are hollow and, in most species, abundantly supplied with stiff bristly hairs. The large leaves are borne alternately on the stem, have a distinct, often long, petiole, and show a variety of shapes. The tendrils, which are a conspicuous feature of many members of the family, appear in the axils of the leaves and are interpreted as stems modified greatly. They are very sensitive organs, responding to the lightest touch of any solid substance, and often show a change in the direction of twining in the middle of a single tendril. In many species, the nutating or circling movement of the tendril is very rapid. The flowers are axillary, either borne singly or in various types of inflorescence, and are usually yellow or white coloured. The plants are either monoecious or dioecious. The calyx is adnate to the inferior ovary, the corolla is 5-lobed and inserted on the calyx. The stamens are typically 5, but show great variation in number through fusions. The inferior ovary is 1- to 3-celled and usually contains many flattened seeds. The latter lack endosperm. The fruit is variety of berry called a pepo, differing from a berry in that the receptacle enters into the formation of the rind or outer wall. The germination of the seeds of the commonly grown members of the family exhibits one rather striking peculiarity. When the arched hypocotyl emerges from the seedcoats, a small peg forms on its lower end. This peg prevents the seedcoats from sticking to the cotyledons, which are withdrawn and carried into the air by the straightening of the arched hypocotyl. Also known as cucurbits.

cultured half-and-half. This product, which contains a minimum of 11.5% milk fat, is manufactured much like cultured sour cream except that the starting material is a blend of milk and cream. Incubation of the product is halted when titrable acidity value of about 0.75% is attained.

cultured sour cream. A product, which contains a minimum of 18% milk fat, is made by adding lactic culture of pasteurized, homogenized cream. Because of adverse effects on viscosity, body, an texture of the final product, cream for cultured sour cream is pasteurized at a relatively low temperature 73.9°C for 30 minutes. This requires an excellent quality starting raw cream from bacteriological standpoint. Raw cream also can be pasteurized by the HTST process 85°C for 1 minute). When the pasteurized cream is cooled to a temperature of 21.1° to 22.23°C, a 1% lactic culture is added. The cream is incubated at this temperature until titrable acidity value of about 0.70% is attained.

cumin. *Cumin cyminum.* The stem of this small, annual herbaceous plant is slender and branched, rarely exceeding 30 cm in height and somewhat angular. The leaves are divided into long, narrow segments like fennel, but much smaller and are of a deep green colour, generally turned back at the ends. The upper leaves are almost without stalks, but the lower ones have longer leaf-stalks. The flowers are small, rose-colored or white, in stalked umbels with only 4-6 rays, each of which are only about 1cm in length. These bloom in the summer then eventually turn to the so-called seeds, which are oblong in shape, thicker in the middle and compressed laterally about 5 mm long. In some ways they resemble caraway seeds, but are lighter in colour and bristly instead of smooth, and almost straight instead of being curved. Their odour and taste is likewise reminiscent of caraway, but less agreeable to the senses than caraway is.

curacao. A liqueur made from the rind of Seville oranges and brandy or gin; 60% of proof spirit.

curd. 1. The coagulated portion of milk consisting almost wholly of casein and other proteins with some fat, lactose, and mineral matter, mechanically or chemically incorporated. Cheese is usually made from the curd, the coagulation being accomplished by the addition of starter or rennet or both. 2. In butter the curd is generally under stood to be the nitrogenous or protein substances present. However, in most cases the curd content is determined by subtracting the percentage of fat, moisture and salt from 100 and designating the difference as curd. Such a method for practical purposes considers not only the proteins but also the ash, lactose, and acid in the butter as curd.

curd, acid. The curd obtained by the action of acid (without rennet) as in some types of cheese-making. An acid curd is inelastic but is open and sticky as contrasted with a rennet curd. The calcium and phosphorus attached to the protein and phosphorus attached to the protein are converted into soluble salts and largely remain in the hey. Cottage cheese is largely an acid curd cheese. May also refer to normal cheese curd which has developed too much acid during the making process.

curd tension. A measure of the toughness of the curd formed from milk by the digestive enzymes and used as an index of the digestibility of the milk. The sample is coagulated with rennin and the force needed to pull a knife-blade through the curd is measured in grams under standardised conditions. Ideal score is zero, below 20 satisfactory; cow's milk 46, diluted with equal volume of water 20, reconstituted spray-dried milk 10, reconstituted roller-dried milk 5, evaporated milk 3, and human milk 1.

curd tension test. A test for determining the strength of gel produced by clotting the casein of milk with pepsin or rennin. The American Dairy Science Association has established a standard method in which the milk is clotted with a pepsin-HCl coagulant at 35° C and the strength of the curd measured after 10 minutes with a special automatically driven knife.

curdlan. A homopolysaccharide composed of β1-3 linked glucose units and is produced by *Alcaligenes faecalis*. It has been recommended for a number of applications including as gelling agent, thickener, and a stabilizer in foods. Because it is not degraded in the human body, it has been suggested as an ingredient in low-calorie food.

curing of meat. Aids colour, flavour and keeping properties. Saturated salt, sodium nitrate (and some nitrite) and sugar, preferably at 5.5°C. Only salt-tolerant bacteria develop, convert nitrate to nitrite which combines with muscle pigment, myoglobin, to give the red colour, nitrosomyoglobin.

currant. The name of two well-known shrubs cultivated in gardens for their fruit. The red current, which is used principally for jellies, is a native of Southern Europe, Asia and Americas. The dried currants of commerce are really raisins, a small variety of grape which originally came from Corinth and therefore received the name of currant. The average composition for per 100 g red currants is: protein 1.1%; carbohydrate 4.5%; water 84%; Fe 1.2 mg; vitamin C 40 mg; and food energy 0.9 MJ. For white currants, the average composition per 100 g is: protein 1.3%; carbohydrate 5.6%; water 83%; Fe 1 mg; vitamin C 40 mg; and food energy 0.1 MJ.

currants, dried. A product obtained by drying seedless black grape; usually dried in bunches on the vine or after removal from the vine on supports.

curry. Mixture of several spices such as turmeric, coriander, mustard, black pepper, caraway, ginger, cumin, cinnamon, cloves, mace, nutmeg, cayene and cardamom.

curry powders. The term is mainly associated with food preparations originally formulated in India and the Orient, for a number of curry mixes employed for different types of food preparations. In years past, curry powder has sometimes been referred to as the "salt of the Orient." The most common ingredients of curry powders and pastes are turmeric, fenugreek, and sago (a substance prepared from the pith of palm trees and related tropical plants). To the basic ingredients may be added varying amounts of caraway, coriander, ginger, black and Cayenne pepper. Frequently, the base of curry paste is tamarind (derived from the fruit of the tropical tree of the same name). The flavour of curry is characteristic and is described as piquant, strong, pungent, spicy, or aromatic. Food substances flavoured with curry sometimes include fish and sea-foods; beef; lamb; pork; veal; hamburger, meat-loaf; gravies and sauces; and certain vegetables such as beans, cabbage, carrots, potatoes, squash.

custard. A term that may refer to custard powder, or to egg custard. Egg custard is composed of milk and egg cooked together. *See also* custard powder.

custard apple. One of a number of species of tropical trees of the family Anonaceae; Sour sop, *Anona muricata*, white fibrous flesh, less sweet than the others, fruit may weigh up to 4 kg; sweet sop (*A. squamosa*) also known as 'true' custard apple, popular in West Indies; bullock's heart (*A. reticulata*) buff-coloured flesh. The average composition per 100 g is: 22 g carbohydrate; 1 g protein; 0.5 mg iron; 0.1 mg vitamin B_1; 0.08 mg vitamin B_2, 0.8 mg nicotinic acid, 30 mg C; and food energy 0.45 kJ.

custard powder. General term for maize starch, that is coloured and flavoured.

cutin. A plant material composed of a group of substances chemically related to fatty acids forming a continuous layer called the cuticle on the epidermis of plants, interrupted only by stomata or lenticels. Being fatty in nature, cutin is water-repellent, therefore helping to reduce transpiration. It is also protective, thus, preventing invasion by parasites.

cutlassfish. *Trichiuridae*. The edible fish which have an elongated, band-shaped body with a sharply tapered head. The fish is naked or covered with very tiny scales. The mouth opening is broad, and has several large teeth on the jaws and palate. The dorsal fin originates just behind the head and runs the length of the body; a finlet may be present. There are 100 to 160 vertebrae. Cutlassfish are divided into about 25 genera, most with very few species. They are known to have existed since the Lower Oligocene period, and teeth have been found in Eocene layers which resemble those of present-day *Trichirus* species. The cutlassfish (*Trichirus lepturus*) attains a length up to nearly 1.5 m and is one of the most widely distributed species. It is encountered in tropical and subtropical parts of the Atlantic, and in the Indian and western Pacific Oceans.

cuttlefish. The common name for certain mollusks, generally applied to the particular species from which sepia is prepared. A small shell or bone, sometimes called the pen, is inside the animal, and this is the cuttlefish bone placed in birdcages. When a cuttlefish is pursued and in danger of being captured, it throws out from a bag a black substance that sepia is obtained. All cuttlefish are marine animals, and in the tropics some very large specimens have been found.

cyanobacteria. A large group of photosynthetic bacteria with oxygenic photosynthesis and a photosynthetic system like that present in eucaryotic photosynthetic organisms; previously they were called blue-green algae. They are unicellular and non-motile, often coated with mucilaginous slime, and the photosynthetic membranes occur as thylakoids within the cell cytoplasm rather than being in a membrane-bounded chloroplast.

Cykelsoy. Trade name of a drying oil made by treating soybean oil with cyclopentadiene.

cyclosporin A. A cyclic polypeptide of 11 amino acids, one of which (has been given the name C_9-ene) is unique to the cyclosporins. Cyclosporins are obtained from the soil fungi *Trichoderma polysporum* and *Cylindrocarpon lucidium*. It acts by selectively inhibiting that part of the immune system that relies on T-lymphocyte proliferation, but it does not interfere with the myeloid system or the humoral system. Consequently, previously acquired immunity and immunity involving the myeloid and humoral systems are unimpaired.

Cymogran. Trade name for protein-rich food low in phenylalanine for feeding patients with phenyl ketonuria.

cysteine. One of the 20 common amino acids that contain -SH group, and is involved in oxidation reduction processes. Frequently used to protect enzyme against inactivation caused by oxidation of -SH group. Proteins rich in cysteine are often denatured by the rupture of disulphide bonds as in the action of hydrogen peroxide on the hair protein keratin. Cysteine is also a precursor of Co-A and of cystine. Sometimes used as a dough improver.

cytase. Any of several enzymes in the seeds of cereals and other plants, which hydrolyze the call-wall material.

cytochalasins. A class of more than 20 metabolites obtained from various moulds. The most widely studied is cytochalasin B, which was formerly called phomin because it was isolated from moulds of Phoma species. The actions include blockage of cytoplasmic cleavage in telophase so that the multinucleate cells are formed, inhibition of cell movement, induction of nuclear extrusion, inhibition of Na$^+$ independent glucose transport, inhibition of thyroid secretion and of growth hormone release, and inhibition of pha-gocytosis, of platelet aggregation and of clot retraction.

cytochrome a. A cytochrome in which the heme prosthetic group contains a formyl side chain; a cytochrome which contains heme A.

cytochrome b. A cytochrome that contains protoheme or a related heme (without formyl group) as its prosthetic group and in which the prosthetic group is not bound covalently to the protein.

cytochrome c. A cytochrome in which there are covalent linkages between the side chains of the heme and the protein. Cytochrome c is a ubiquitious protein found in all aerobic organisms. Its sole function is to transport an electron from a donor of lower reduction-oxidation potential to an acceptor of higher reduction-oxidation potential. The heme group in cytochrome c has a polypeptide chain of 104 amino acids attached and wrapped around it. All cytochromes have in their structure the sequence Cys$_{14}$-x-x-Cys$_{17}$-His$_{18}$ in which the two cysteine sulphydryl groups are co-valently linked to the heme by thioether bridges. In addition, the imidazole ring nitrogen atom of histidine-18 is coordinately bonded to one of the sides of heme iron as the fifth ligand. Cytochrome c therefore cannot react by simple coordination but must react indirectly by an electron-transfer mechanism. It can reduce the oxygen and transmit its oxidizing power toward the burning of food and release of energy in respiration. The cytochrome c of vertebrates possesses N-acetyl glycine as the terminal group, and 103 additional amino acids. Cytochrome c's of the two primates monkey and man are almost identical; they differ by an average of 10 amino acids from other mammals such as dog or whale, by about 15 residues from cold blooded vertebrates, by about 30 residues from insects, and by about 50 residues from plants and prokaryotes.

cytochrome d. A cytochrome with a tetrapyrolic chelate of iron as a prosthetic group in which the degree of double bonds is less than that is porphyrin; dihydroporphyrin is an example.

cytochrome oxidase. Cytochrome that is able to accept electrons from other cytochromes and to react with oxygen to produce water. It is thus the terminal member of an electron transport chain.

cytochrome P$_{450}$. The cytochrome component of an electron transport chain that is present in the endoplasmic reticulum of liver and some other cells. It is unique to the endoplasmic reticulum, being absent from the mitochondrial electron transport chain. The 450 denotes the fact that the reduced form of the cytochrome has an absorption band at 450 nm.

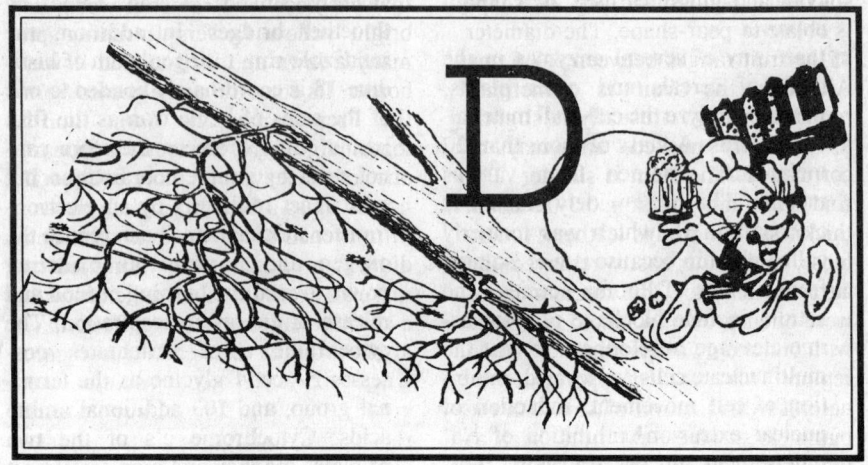

D-. A prefix attached to the chemical names, especially sugars and amino acids, indicating optical activity. When the first hydroxyl group of a sugar is on the same side as the alcohol group it is the D-form, on opposite sides it is the L-form. Both L- and D-glucose exist. In case of amino acids such as L-alanine is related to the sugar L-glyceraldehyde and follows the same nomenclature. The other amino acids follow alanine. All the naturally occurring amino acids are L-, synthetic are DL, few D- amino acids are found in nature. Capital L- and D- are not to be confused with *l*-, *d*- which are the old terms for (+) and (-).

d-. Obsolete prefix indicating dextrorotatory, now replaced by (+).

12D concept. One of the most important considerations in the commercial canning that ensures the destruction of *Clostridium botulinum* spores. This concept ensures that population of the most resistant spores is reduced to 10^{-12} of the original members. It has been shown that if 10^{12} botulinal spores per gram of food are heated at 394K, the time required for a 12 decimal reduction is 2.52 minutes. Also known as 12 decimal concept.

dahls. Indian term for split peas of various kinds, e.g., pigeon pea (*Cajanus indicus*), khesari (*Lathyrus sativus*), red dahl or Massur dahl the lentil (*Lens esculenta*). Also spelled as dal.

dal. *See* dahl.

Daltose. Trade name (of a carbohydrate preparation consisting of maltose, glucose and dextrin for infant feeding.

damson. Small dark-blue plum. The average composition per 100 g is: protein 0.45%; water 73%; carbohydrate 9%; Fe 0.5 mg; vitamin B_1 0.12 mg; nicotinic acid 0.25 mg; and food energy 0.15MJ.

Dancy mandarin. A variety of mandarin, familiarly known in much of the US as a tangerine. It is one of the best known of the tangerines produced in the US. The relatively small size of the fruit is sometimes considered a disadvantage, along with presence of seeds. However, is highly regarded for its high colour, flavour, and good quality. The fruit is of a deep red, sometimes scarlet coloration, with a smooth and glossy surface. Its shape is oblate to pear-shape. The diameter of the fruit ranges between 5-7.5 cm. Although the fruit is sometimes rounded evenly, it usually is slightly to distinctly necked, and may be corrugated. The stem is slender. The rind is thin ranging from 0.3-0.5 cm in thickness. The rind is leathery, tough, loose, and quite easily removed (an attractive feature). The kan mandarins were often grown in mixed plantings with pummelo varieties in the Canton region. This afforded opportunity for natural hybridization of kan with the pummelo to give new fruits, such as the unique sweet orange. Some of these may have been the Sekkan and Yinkan sweet oranges of China. Some authorities do not consider these sweet oranges to be progeny of the kan mandarins, but it is to be noted that the Chinese apply a "kan" ending to these tight-skinned sweet orange. The natural appearance of sweet oranges in China several centuries ago probably accounts for the lesser enthusiasm for these fruits than is evidenced by the western countries.

dandelion. Family: *Compositae*. Genus: *Taraxacum*. Species: *Taraxacum officinale*. A plant which carpets lawns and meadows with bright yellow in the spring summer and fall. The leaves are toothed, radiating from the crown of the very long root, and the name is from the French for tooth of a lion. The dandelion blooms profusely, bearing many slender stalks, each surmounted by one large, bright yellow head of many small flowers which mature into a beautiful white ball of feathered fruits. These are transported far and wide by the wind. The whole plant is full of a milky and bitter juice. Dandelion is native to Europe and Asia, and is herbaceous that has become a rampant weed, its bright yellow flowers intruding on many a lawn and well-tended flower border. Its common name comes from the French *dent de lion*, 'lion's tooth', signifying the toothed appearance of the leaves. Its more colloquial names - piss-a-beds in English *pis-en-lit* in French bear witness to its strong diuretic properties. The young leaves make an excellent salad, delicious with a slightly lemony dressing. They may also be lightly cooked like spinach, when they are good served with vinaigrette. The ground and roasted root is dried and used as a caffeine-free coffee substitute. The leaves and root are used to give a bitter flavour to country beers such as nettle and burdock, and a stout is made from the roots. Both the flowers and leaves are used, separately, to make wines.

Dandelion is valued as medicinal herb for all urinary troubles. The roots pro-duce a yellow or crimson dye, according to the mordant used. Some species have powerful medicinal properties, and the young leaves of all are often used for greens and salads. The leaves are particularly high in vitamins A and C and contain more iron than spinach, as well as potassium, potash and glutin. The raw leaves contain vitamin A to. There are also traces of vitamins B and D. The root contains tri-terpenes, sterols, choline and 25% inulin as well as sugars, pectin, phenolic acids, gums, and resins. The average composition per 100 g of the leaves is: protein 2.5%; fat 0.5%; Ca 135 mg; Fe 3 mg; vitamin A 3,000 mg; vitamin B_1 0.17 mg; vitamin B_2 0.13 mg; nicotinic acid 0.7 mg; vitamin C 25 mg; and food energy 0.17MJ.

Dandelion has a notable ability to clear obstructions and stimulate the liver to detoxify poisons. So dandelion acts as an excellent blood purifier and much of its beneficial action on the liver and the blood is as a result of its high content of easily assimilable minerals, especially in the root. Dandelion root is also supposed to clear obstructions of the spleen, pancreas, gallbladder, bladder and kidneys and is of tremendous benefit to the stomach and intestines. The root is a specific for hypoglycemia (the result of the high inulin content). Dandelion-root tea has been used to treat diabetes that has been acquired later in life. It is of benefit in helping to lower blood pressure. It has also been found to be useful for anemia, and is a great nutritive for the nerves and the blood. The raw roots made into a decoction are more effective medicinally than the roasted roots but a small amount of roasted roots, or some chicory (which has similar properties), can be added for flavour. In China, the powdered herb or fresh juice has been found to be most effective in treating upper respiratory tract infections, acute and chronic bronchitis, pneumonia, infectious hepatitis (serious cases can be cleared up within a week or two, when a diet is properly controlled), urinary tract infections, acute mastitis, acute pancreatitis, appendicitis and dermatitis, and for preventing postoperative infections. It has the advantage over modern antibiotics in such applications in that it causes fewer side-effects. Any side-effects there are, such as stomach upset and dizziness, disappear completely when the dandelion treatment is stopped.

dandelion greens. *See* dandelion.

dariworld. A semi-soft ripened cheese with a mild, pleasing flavour and a smooth slicing body.

dark adaptation. The change that takes place in the retina of the eye to assist vision in dim light. In dark adaptation a pigment, visual purple or rhodopsin, is formed from retinol (vitamin A aldehyde) and a protein. This is bleached in bright light. When body stores of retinol are inadequate poor dark adaptation, night blindness, results. This is the earliest indication of vitamin A deficiency.

dates. The fruit of the date palm, *Phoenix dactylifera*. The fruit is used extensively as an article of food by the natives of Northern Africa and of some countries of Asia. It consists of a fleshy coat, separable into three portions, and covering a hard, horny seed. Next to the cocoanut palm, the date is unquestionably the most interesting and useful of the palms.

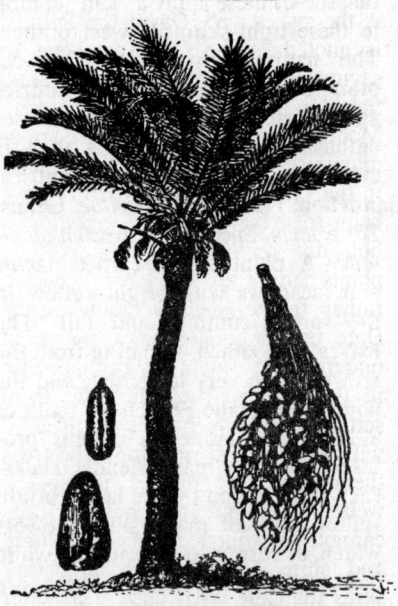

Its stem shoots up to the height of about 20 metres, without branch or division, and is of nearly the same thickness throughout its length. From the summit it throws out a magnificent crown of large, feather-shaped leaves, besides a number of stalks, each of which in the female plant bears a bunch of from 180 to 200 dates, each bunch weighing from twenty to twenty-five pounds. The fruit is eaten fresh or dried. Cakes of dates pounded and kneaded together are the food of the Arabs who traverse the deserts. A liquor resembling wine is made from dates by fermentation. There are hundreds of varieties classed as sweet, mild sweet and dry. The mild sweet are eaten fresh and the dry or camel date is pressed whole or grouped into flour and forms the staple diet of the Arabs. The variety normally found on the world markets is the sweet type. David the Palmist is quoted in the Old Testament as saying that "the righteous shall flourish like the (date) palm tree." Modern Arabs claim that there are as many uses for dates as there are days in the year. These sugary fruits are a boon to desert dwellers, growing in hot, dry regions where most food plants cannot yet they have their own rather temperamental requirements. Date palms must have a source of underground water, but any moisture in the air will keep the fruit from setting, and temperatures below 20°C will keep it from ripening. The trees themselves can survive in cooler, wetter areas, but their nutrias fruits cannot. Sun-ripened dates are plump and shiny, with lighter, smoother skins than the dried ones. The latter may contain added sweeteners and preservatives. Fresh dates are often described as either soft, semi-dry, or dry, depending of the softness of the ripe fruit. Covered and refrigerated,

they usually keep indefinitely. The average composition of dried date per 100 g is: water 20%; protein 2.4%; carbohydrate 70%; Fe 1.7 mg; vitamin A 30 mg; vitamin B_1 0.08 mg; vitamin B_2 0.05 mg; nicotinic acid 2.2 mg; and food energy 1.7 MJ.

David test for alcohol in essential oils. Extract the oil with a little water, and superimpose the water, on a solution of molybdic acid in concentrated sulphuric acid. A blue ring indicates the presence of alcohol. If the sample contains an aldehyde, it must be removed from the sample of oil with petroleum ether before performing the test.

deamination. Removal of amino groups ($-NH_2$) as, for example, the deamination of amino acids to ammonia and keto acids. This is an important process when an organism has more nitrogen in its food supply than it requires. Of genetic importance is the spontaneous deamination of cytosine to uracil that occurs in DNA at an estimated rate of 100 bases per day in every genome. Repair enzymes exist whose function is to replace the uracil produced by this accidental deamination. This repair is possible because uracil does not normally occur in DNA. A greater problem is caused by accidental deamination of 5-methylcytosine (relatively rare base in DNA) because the result is the normally occurring thymine that is therefore not repaired. L-Glutamic acid plays a key role in the metabolism of amino acids because of widespread occurrence of the enzyme glutamic dehydrogenase. This enzyme catalyzes the reversible oxidative deamination by NAD^+ of L-glutamate to form α-ketoglutaric acid, ammonia, and NADH. Oxidative deamination reactions are also catalyzed by a group of flavin enzymes known as amino acid oxidases. In contrast to the oxidative deamination, the non-oxidative deamination reactions also occur. One type of non-oxidative deamination is the reaction catalyzed by α-deaminases. Aspartase, which belongs to this group of enzymes, catalyzes conversion of L-aspartic acid in to fumaric acid. A somewhat different type of deamination is catalyzed by an enzyme in liver termed as serine dehydratase. The reaction, which is specific for L-serine, involves the loss of ammonia and rearrangement of the remaining atoms to yield pyruvate.

decarboxylation. The removal of carboxyl group, -COOH from a compound. This process is usually enzyme-catalyzed. For example, histidine is decarboxylated to histamine by histidine decarboxylase, and glutamic acid to GABA by glutamate decarboxylase. Some decarboxylations involve a concomitant oxidation (oxidative decarboxylation) (*e.g.*, the conversion of pyruvic acid to acetyl-coA by the pyruvate dehydrogenase complex). Many amino acids undergo decarboxylation reaction. In contrast to the deamination and transamination reactions which are involved in the catabolism of amino acids, the anabolic aspect of decarboxylation reactions is noteworthy. Some of the amines formed as a result of decarboxylation have important physiological effects. Thus, histidine decarboxylase, found in animal tissues, can produce histamine.

deciduous. A scientific term for the plants in which all the leaves are shed at the end of each growing season, usually the autumn in temperate regions or at the beginning of a dry season in the tropics. The seasonal leaf-fall help the plants to retain water that would otherwise be lost by transpiration from the leaves. The word deciduous is from the Latin, and means to fall down. A deciduous tree is one whose leaves fall off at a fairly regular time every autumn and are as regularly renewed in the spring. Nearly all forest trees are of this kind. While in most countries the loss of leaves is in the autumn, in some parts of the world the change from foliage to bareness is governed by arrival of the dry season. Such trees which are not deciduous are evergreen.

decimal reduction time. *D.* The time required to kill 90% of the microorganisms or spores in a sample at a specified temperature and pressure. Over the ranges of temperatures usually used in food sterilization, the relationship between D and temperature is essentially exponential, so that when the logarithm of D is plotted against temperature, a straight line is obtained. The slope of the line provides a quantitative measure of the sensitivity of the organism to heat under the conditions used, and the graph can be used in calculating process times for sterilization, such as in canning operations.

decolorizing agent. Any substance that removes color by a physical or chemical reaction. Charcoals, blacks, clays, earths, or other materials of highly adsorbent character are used to remove undesirable colours (and often odours) from sugar, vegetable and animal fats and oils, among other food substances. In a broad sense decolorizing agents also embrace bleaches which usually involve a chemical reaction for removing colour. The properties of representative adsorbents used for color removal are given in the accompanying table.

Activated carbon is one of the most widely used of the adsorbents. It is an amorphous from of carbon characterized by high adsorptivity. The carbon is obtained by the destructive distillation of wood, nut shells, animal bones, or other carbonaceous material. It is "activated" by heating to 800°-900°C, which results in a porous internal structure. The internal surface area of activated carbon averages about 929 m²/g. Numerous uses in the food industry include applications in the brewing and sugar refining industries. The diatomaceous earth also finds numerous adsorbent applications in food processing, in decolorizing, as well as a filter aid and clarifying agent. This is a soft, bulky solid material (88% silica) composed of skeletons of small prehistoric aquatic plants related to algae (diatoms). They have intricate geometric forms. Fuller's earth is also used as an adsorbent, it is a porous colloidal aluminium silicate (clay) which has a high natural adsorptive power. Silica gel is a regenerative adsorbent consisting of amorphous silica derived from sodium silicate and sulphuric acid. In addition to color adsorbent and bleaching powers, silica gel is used as a dehumidifying and dehydrating agent and as an anticaking agent in the food industry. Prior to crystallization in the refining of sugar, bleaching of the syrup is required. This is sometimes effected through treatment of the solution with calcium hypochlorite, usually in the presence of calcium phosphate which nerves as a buffer and aids in final precipitation of calcium from the bleached solution.

decomplementation. The removal of haemolytic activity of complement from serum by heat inactivation, cobra venom factors, zymosan, immune complexes, etc. or removal of complement activity from whole animals by treatment with such agents.

decomposer. An organism that breaks down complex materials into simpler ones, including the release of simple inorganic products. Such organisms obtain energy from the chemical breakdown of the dead organisms, animals or plant wastes. Organisms such as bacteria and fungi, participate in the decomposition of organic matter. Many decomposers (*e.g.*, nitrifying bacteria) are specialized to break down the organic materials that are difficult for the other organisms to digest. Decomposers perform a vital role in the ecosystem by returning the constituents of organic matter to the environment in inorganic form so that they can again be assimilated by plants.

decomposition. The breaking up of a compound into more simple parts. These parts may be either compounds or elements. In most cases decomposition separates one body into two or more bodies, but what is called double decomposition is a change or breaking up of two or more compounds into the same number of other compounds. Decomposition may be caused by such forces as heat, light, electricity and chemical reagents; or it may be due, as in the case of vegetable and animal matter, to very small animals or plants, called bacteria and ferments. *See also* decomposer.

decontamination factor. Ratio of amount of radioactive impurities present in substance before purification to that present after purification.

decontamination. In general, the removal of chemical, biological, or radiological contamination, from an area or a material. Specifically, this term refers to treatment of clothing, equipment, buildings, and the like to remove radioactive substances to which they have been exposed. Standard methods of decontamination include thorough washing with a soap/water solution with subsequent application of 5% sodium bisulphite solution. Sequestering agents such as ethylenediaminetetraacetic acid are also effective. The effectiveness of the decontamination can be checked with a radiation counter.

decontamination factor. Ratio of amount of impurities (biological, chemical, or radioactive) present in substance before purification to that present after purification.

decreasing rate drying. In deep bed drying, the rate of drying of the bed, bin, or batch decreases when the drying front reaches the top of the bed, when air is moving upward and out of the bed. This terminology refers to deep layer drying in contrast to the term falling rate drying for thin layer drying.

deep layer. When drying the products in beds, bins, or other containers in which a deep greater than the dimension of one particle of product is dried. It is usually possible to identify the following locations in deep layer drying: dried zone, drying zone, drying front, and damp undried zone. The initial period of drying in a deep layer, often after a heat-up period, is at the maximum drying rate period, which is followed by a decreasing rate drying period.

defecation. A term used chiefly in food technology to refer of the clarification or removal of impurities from sugarcane or beet juice by heating in the presence of lime to precipitate undesirable substance. The resulting mother liquor is then drained off and concentrated by evaporation and boiling. *See also* clarification.

deficiency disease. A disease caused by deficiency of a particular nutrient, usually with a characteristic set of symptoms. The essential elements for life are carbon, hydrogen, oxygen nitrogen, sulphur, phosphorus, potassium, magnesium, calcium, iron, and chlorine (macronutrients). Certain elements are commonly needed in trace amounts (called trace elements) like boron, manganese, zinc, copper, nickel and molybdenum. The latter are often part of the structure of enzymes or coenzymes. Heterotrophic organisms, namely animals and fungi, are not as competent at synthesizing their own organic requirements as autotrophic organisms like green plants. Thus whereas the latter are only likely to suffer mineral deficiency diseases, animals may suffer mineral, vitamin, protein etc. deficiency diseases.

defined medium. A culture medium made with components of the known composition.

definitive host. Host from which a pathogen cannot be transferred.

defloculation. The reverse process of flocculation, or the process of preventing flocculation, *i.e.,* the prcess of breaking up dispersing agglomerates to form a stable compound.

defoaming agents. The substances used to reduce foaming caused by proteins, gases, or nitrogenous materials, generally, which may interfere with processing. In certain food processes, the presence of foam severely limits the rate, if not the feasibility, of accomplishing certain kinds of operations, such as the production of sugar from beets and various fermentation processes where the progressive production of gases within a liquid phase cause excessive bubbling and foam production. Deforming agents, when used in small concentrations, are found to be quite effective.

The control of foam is of major importance in brewing operations, the advantages including:

(a) higher production through increased fermentation capacity, up to 10% more throughput;

(b) the lid of the fermentation tank can be left on, reducing oxidation and improving;

(c) lower oxidation rate, which gives a better physical and chemical stability to the beer as the denatured or partially denatured protein levels remain low, thus reducing turbidity; and

(d) less yeast build-up on the sides of the tank, thus reducing cleaning requirements.

Foam is a prime consideration in the quality of brewed products. The effective foam control during processing can later affect the "head" of the final product, providing for a stable, long-lived creamy foam. Thus, a defoaming agent must be insoluble in the beer and capable of removal so that it does not detract from the head of the finished product. Where a suitable chemical substance cannot be found, physical means are necessary which may be mechanical, electrical, or thermal in nature. The mechanical devices are fundamentally simple, frequently taking the form of rotating breaker bars. The presence of a hot surface near a foam tends to destroy the foam. Essentially, a portion of the foam is evaporated, causing the acceleration of its breakdown. It has also been established that electrical discharges tend to weaken or destroy films.

The chemical defoaming agents commonly used in the food processing include dimethylpolysiloxane, lauric acid, octanoic acid, decanoic acid, myristic acid, oleic acid, stearic acid, oxysterin, palmitic acid, petrolatum, mineral oil (white), petroleum wax (synthetic), silicon dioxide, and sorbitan mono-stearate.

The defoaming agents may be categorised as solubilized surfactants, as dispersions of hard particle, and as dispersions of soft particles. The classifications frequently overlap. In all cases, a liquid nonaqueous vehicle is present, even where the defoamer is represented as a solid formulation. Water may also be present, Particularly in emulsified silicone formulations. A common type of solubilized surfactant formulation is the fatty acid-fatty alcohol combination in oil. The spreading rate of such formulations is very rapid, which is largely responsible for their use. Either surfactant may be substituted by alkylene oxide adducts, mono-, di,- and triglycerides. The fatty acid or a derivative thereof by itself in oil is used. Mixtures of esters, waxes, alkyl phosphates, fats, et. al. have found application. Formulations of silicone and other polymers in oil are used, often in emulsion from. Soft-particle formulations may consist of paraffinic waxes or fatty amides among other components as the dispersed phase; a nonaqueous liquid serves as the vehicle. A fine particle size is generally desired, which is effected by grinding or chilling a hot solution rapidly.

In addition to the particulate components, members of the solubilized surfactant class are generally present. The hard-particle formulations most commonly consist of silica or a mineral coated with silicone which is dispersed in a vehicle. The optimal particle size may be as low as 0.02 μm.

A spreading agent, *i.e.*, a surfactant, is usually present. Dispersants may be added to promote stability since the rate of settling in such formulations is greater than for the soft-particle type.

Emulsifiers may be included in defoamer formulations to accelerate the dispersion of the defoamer throughout the foaming system. Such formulations are added to the foaming system neat or diluted with water. In addition to use of defoaming agents in food processing, foam inhibitors are used in minute quantities in certain products, such as containerized orange, pineapple, and other juices, to remove the "head" from the product.

defoliant. A chemical, sprayed on plants, that causes leaves to fall of prematurely.

degeneration. A term applied in biology to certain changes undergone by plant and animal life, whereby there is a falling off in size, productivity, vigor or other qualities. The causes of degeneration include lack of nourishment, disuse, and change of habit. The effect of long-continued disuse of a part or organ is shown in the uselessness of the small toe on the foot of man. Primitive man had flexible toes like those of the monkey, but as civilization caused changes of habit the toes, particularly the small one, degenerated, and the latter seems top be heading toward extinction. The vermiform appendix is an example of an organ which has lost whatever function it may originally have had. Not only do organisms degenerate, but whole classes, and this is true of the human race and of the lower animals. In the vegetable world the plants which are forced to grow for a succession of years in poor soil or

an unfavourable climate tend to become inferior. Mental and moral degeneration among civilized peoples is one of the vital questions with which eugenics, sociology and religion have to deal.

degradation. The breakdown of complex chemical structures to simpler compounds by the influence of bacteria, usually accelerated by the presence of oxygen and sunlight.

degumming agents. The substances used in refinishing of fats to remove mucilaginous matter consisting of gum, resin, proteins and phosphatides. They include hydrochloride and phosphoric acids, and phosphates.

dehisce. To open, split, or burst, usually during ripening of seed coats or capsules or vessels, naturally or during drying. Drying may be a natural process or an artificial process by forced air or heated air.

dehumidification. The process of decreasing the water vapour or the humidity of a body of air or gas such as through condensation on a cold surface, diffusion of vapour to a adsorbing agent, chemical action, and heating to reduce the humidity.

dehydratases. The enzymes catalyzing the reactions in which dehydration precedes deamination. For example, the α-amino groups of serine and threonine can be directly converted to NH_4^+ because each of these amino acids contains a hydroxyl group in its side chain. These direct deaminations are catalyzed by serine dehydratase and threonine dehydratase, in which pyridoxal phosphate is the prosthetic group.

dehydrated onion. The dehydration of onions to produce onion powder and pieces of various sizes is now a major activity in many countries. The onions are first flame peeled, washed to remove the burnt outer skin, and then mechanically sliced onto a perforated belt. The drying is carried out in a tunnel drier, the hot air circulating through the holes in the conveyor belt. Onions enter the system with a moisture content of about 80% and are dehydrated to about 4%. The dehydrated product may be sold as such, kibbled to various mesh sizes, or milled to a moderately fine powder. All of these products, particularly onion powder, absorb moisture and must be packed and retained in well-closed containers preferably having an impervious liner. Onions are dehydrated without blanching so that they retain their essential flavouring character. As a consequence, the products usually have a high microbiological count due to the presence of thermophilic spores that survive the drying temperature.

dehydrating press. A device used to squeeze moisture from pyrocellulose at 25% moisture, used for explosives, at about 17 atmospheres.

dehydration. Scientific term for drying, but tends to be used for factory-dried materials as distinct from wind-dried. 1. Removal of 95% or more of the water from a food product by intensive oven drying, spraying, or other means for the purpose of saving space, weight, and transportation cost. A number of common foods are available in dehydrated form (potatoes, fruit juices), requiring only addition of water to restore them to edible condition. The process called dehydrofreezing removes only about half the water content, after which the vegetable is frozen. 2. Elimination of water molecule from the molecule of a chemical compound.

dehydrator. A device used for dehydration of products for preservation. Some early literature uses the spelling dehydrator.

dehydroacetic acid. Also sodium salt (DHA-S). Active against moulds but not a permitted additive. Chemically can be regarded as the condensation product of acetic and acetoacetic acids, or 3-acetyl-6-methyl-1-pyran-2,4-dione.

dehydroascorbic acid. Oxidized form of vitamin C which can readily be reduced to the ordinary form, and is therefore biologically active.

dehydrobrining. The process of removing moisture and product preservation by partial drying (90-75% moisture content for vegetables) followed by sufficient salt to provide a saturated brine solution with the water remaining in the product after partial drying.

dehydrocanning. A process in which 50% of the water is removed from a food before canning. The advantages arc that the texture is retained by the partial dehydration and there is saving in bulk and weight.

dehydrofreezing. A method of moisture removal in which one-half to two-thirds of the moisture in a product to be frozen is first removed by conventional drying methods using heat, followed by freezing the product using standard or quick-freezing procedures. In some products, such as apples, from 20 to 50% of the moisture can be removed with little expense using normal heat drying, thus greatly reducing the amount of water which would need to be frozen. Considerable saving in shipping and storage of the product results. Product quality is not seriously damaged. Care must be taken to assure that the heating does not decrease the quality. It is employed for preservation of fruits and vegetables. The texture and flavour are claimed to be superior to either dehydration or freezing alone, and rehydration more rapid than with dehydrated products.

dehydrofrozen apple slices. The apple slices dried to atleast half of their original weight (*i.e.*, to atleast 70% moisture content), and then frozen. The slices are prepared by processors and are used by some of the large bakeries. Bakers utilize this product because it is easy to use and is free of drip when thawed. The dehydrofrozen apples may also be dried to one-third or one-quarter of the original weight before freezing.

dehydrogenases. Enzymes that carry out oxidation in the living cell by removing hydrogen from the substrate. They can only function by passing this hydrogen on to another substance, called the intermediate hydrogen acceptor. It is ultimately passed on to oxygen to form water. There are specific dehydrogenases for each substrate, *e.g.*, succinic dehydrogenase, lactic, malic, glucose etc. The oxidoreductase enzymes utilize a coenzyme, such as NAD or FAD, as a hydrogen acceptor in the oxidation of a metabolite. An example is lactate dehydrogenase, which catalyzes the reaction:

Lactate + NAD = pyruvate + NADH

Hydrogenases are usually called after the name of their substrate. Some dehydrogenases are highly specific, both with respect to their substrate and coenzyme, while others catalyze the oxidation of a wide range of substrates. Many require the presence of a coenzyme, which is often involved as a hydrogen acceptor. Dehydrogenases catalyze transfer of two hydrogen atoms from substances to NAD and NADP. They are transferases catalyzing the oxidation of one molecule with concomitant reduction of another, and hence fall into the wider group of enzymes known as oxidoreductases. A wide variety of molecules function as hydrogen acceptors for dehydrogenases, but when the acceptor is oxygen the enzymes are called oxidases. Cytosolic or soluble dehydrogenases (*e.g.*, glyceraldehyde-3-phosphate dehydrogenase and lactate dehydrogenase of the glycolytic pathway and glucose-6-phosphate pathway), usually have NAD^+ or $NADP^+$ as hydrogen-accepting coenzyme. Intrinsic membrane dehydrogenases forming parts of the electron transport chain in mitochondria, chloroplasts and bacteria are usually large complexes containing not only flavoproteins with FAD (succinate dehydrogenase) or FMN (NADH dehydrogenase) as a prosthetic group, but also iron-sulphur proteins. Quinones are typical hydrogen acceptors for this group of dehydrogenase. Another group of dehydrogenases found particularly in bacteria have pyrrolo-quinoline quinone as a prosthetic group (*e.g.*, glucose dehydrogenase and methanol dehydrogenase). Some of the common reactions involving dehydrogenases include:

(a) amino acid degradation;
(b) amino acid synthesis;
(c) citric acid cycle;
(d) fatty acid oxidation;
(e) fatty acid synthesis;
(f) glycolysis;
(g) oxidation of pyruvate;
(h) oxidative phosphorylation;
(i) photosynthesis; and
(j) pentose phosphate pathway.

dehydroretinol. The old name for Vitamin A_2; no longer in current usage.

Deinococcus. An unusual genus of Gram-positive cocci. Besides their unique phylogenetic stature species of *Deinococcus* differ from other Gram-positive cocci in a number of chemical and physiological properties. The cell walls of deinococci are structurally complex and consist of several layers, including an outer membrane layer normally only present in Gram-negative bacteria. However the outer membrane of *Deinococcus* is chemically unique and does not contain heptoses and lipid A typical of that of Gram-negative bacteria. Most dienococci are bright red or pink coloured because of the variety of carotenoids found in these organisms, and many strains are highly resistant to ultraviolet radiation and to desiccation. In addition to radiation resistance, *D. radiodurans* is resistant to mutagenic effects of many highly mutagenic chemicals.

de-lactosed milk. A patented product resembling sodium caseinate and sometimes used as a source of lactose-free serum solids in ice cream mix. Milk is coagulated with rennet, the whey siphoned off, and the curd then used in the mix. This product may also be used in certain instances when a sugar-free milk product is desired.

Delaware grape. A native North American pink grape that produces white juice. It is cultivated in New York States and Ohio as well as in Canada for making table wines. It is one of the most widely planted of the native North American varieties.

delmhorst. A commercial moisture detector or meter which measures the electrical resistance obtained by forcing an electric probe into the product. The moisture content of the wettest fibers in contact with the two electrodes near the end of the probe is measured. A device is provided for maintaining uniform pressure of the probe in the product.

Delshire cream. A very rich cream differing from ordinary cream only in the degree of its concentration. It contains about 65-75% butterfat. It is almost as rich in butterfat as is butter, which legally must contain not less than 80% butterfat. It is made by running milk warm from the cows, or cold milk heated to 37°C, thorough a cream separator having special parts for skimming heavy cream. It can be used as a spread, as cream or in place of other fats in cooking and baking. It is quite similar to the plastic cream.

Demerara rum. The molasses remaining after the brown Demerara sugars has crystallized out, is diluted with water and a little ammonium sulphate and sulphuric acid are added to stimulate the yeast and destroy the bacteria. Fermentation is completed in less than two days. Some of these rums have a fruity smell due to the addition of raisins, plums and spices. It is said that same distilleries add raw meat in the rum to remove impurities and to give it a characteristic flavour. A lot of caramel is added to give the particular colour. The rum is kept undisturbed for 3-4 days and is sold after ageing it.

demersal fish. A kind of fish that live on the sea bottom. Cod, haddock, whiting, hake, ling, saithe, halibut, sole, bream. It contains little fat. Also known as white fish.

denaturant. See denaturation.

denaturation. 1. With reference to ethyl alcohol, it means the addition of denaturants, such as methyl violet and pyridine (as in methylated spirits) to render it unpleasant and so prevent its consumption as a beverage and to make it tax-free. The qualities desired in a denaturant are that its boiling point should be so close to that of the alcohol that it is difficult to remove by ordinary distillation, and that is should be ill-tasting. Some of the denaturants are poisonous and cause death if the alcohol is taken internally. The usual denaturants are methyl alcohol, pyridine, benzene, kerosene, and pine oil. One or several of these may be employed, but denaturants must be approved by the government bodies. Completely denatured alcohol is a term used to designate alcohol containing poisonous denaturants, and these are employed only for antifreeze, fuels, and lacquers, but not in contact with the human body. Special denatured alcohol is alcohol containing denaturants authorised for special uses, such as pine oil for hair tonics.

Many legally permitted denaturants are marketed under different trade names. For example, Denol is a mixture of primary and secondary aliphatic higher alcohols. Agadite is a compounded petroleum product. Hydronol is a hydrogenated organic product. Denaturants are also used in imported oils that are permitted entry at lowered tax rates for industrial use so that they cannot be diverted for edible use. Rapeseed oil, for example, is denatured with brucine.

2. A reordering of the molecular structure of some proteins (globulins) induced by a number of external factors, such as heating to just below the boiling point, change of pH, or exposure to various radiation and detergents. It causes proteins to undergo unfolding of the characteristic structure of the peptide chain. The primary structure remains intact; no covalent bonds in the backbone of the protein chain are broken. Proteins vary in susceptibility to denaturation depending on their amino acid sequence; nucleic acids are less variable and generally need more extreme conditions than proteins before they denature. The denaturation of nucleic acids amounts to strand separation and is reversible, whereas denaturation of proteins is usually irreversible. A denatured protein consists of polypeptide chains randomly dispersed and not folded into the precise conformations necessary for biological activity. Denatured proteins only very occasionally renature spontaneously when returned to physiological conditions. The example of protein renaturation after prolonged boiling is ribonuclease.

dendritic salt. A form of ordinary table salt, sodium chloride, with the crystals branched or starlike (dendritic) instead of the normal cubes. The advantages claimed are the lower bulk density, rapid solution, and unusual capacity for absorbing moisture before becoming wet.

dent corn. *Zea indentata.* One of the principal type of corn. The name dent derives from the characteristic shape of the kernel. This dent is caused by shrinking of the soft starch in the crown at the time of ripening. Dent corn has large, long ears which are tapering, with white or yellow grains. Hundreds of varieties are known. In shoe-peg types, the dent is deep and narrow; in other types, the dent may be wide and shallow.

deodourization. In food technology, the term deodourization is generally applied to the removal of flavour (as in deodourized fish meal) but more specifically to the deodourization of fats during refining. Superheated steam is bubbled through the hot oil under vacuum, when most of the flavoured substances are distilled off. Substances such as activated charcoal or silica gel are also employed for this purpose.

deoxy sugar. A sugar in which oxygen has been lost by replacement of a hydroxyl group (-OH) with hydrogen (H). The most important example is deoxyribose, the sugar component of DNA.

deoxycorticosterone. 11-DOC. A steroid hormone, produced by the adrenal cortex, having mineralocorticoid activity. It is a metabolite in the biosynthesis of corticosterone. Small quantities are secreted by the adrenal gland. Synthetic 11-DOC has potent mineralocorticoid and slight glucocorticoid activity and can be used for the treatment of Addison's disease. Also known as deoxycortone.

deoxycortone. *See* deoxycorticosterone.

deoxyribonucleotide. Compound consisting of a purine or pyrimidine base attached to 2-deoxyribose which is in turn bonded to a phosphate group at either the 3'- or 5'- position. The ability of one phosphate group to form a phosphodiester link between two deoxyribose molecules is the basis for stringing nucleotides together in the polymer DNA. The ends of the polymer are thus characterized by whether the 3'- or the 5'-position is free. The four commonly occurring bases in deoxyribonucleotides are the purines adenine and guanine and pyrimidines cytosine and thymine.

deoxyribose. Sugar which, complexed to a phosphate group and to either a purine or pyrimidine base, goes to form the deoxynucleotides of the DNA molecule.

depectinization. Removal of pectins from fruit pulp to produce a clear thin juice instead of a viscous, cloudy liquid; achieved by the use of enzyme preparations.

derived protein. A product obtained by treatment of a protein with heat, acid, base, enzymes, or other agents. the primary derived proteins, such as proteins and metaproteins, are proteins that have been altered only slightly; secondary derived proteins, such as proteoses and peptones, are proteins that have been altered more extensively.

desaturases. The enzymes involved in biosynthesis of unsaturated fatty acid by introducing double bonds into previously synthesized saturated fatty acids *e.g.*, Acetyl-CoA desaturase and the stearyl-CoA desaturase etc.

desensitization. 1. The modification of a regulatory enzyme by either mutation or chemical means that results in an enzyme that has retained its catalytic activity but has lost the capacity to respond to effectors.
2. The attempt to minimize the response of an individual suffering from immediate-type hypersensitivity upon subsequent exposure to an allergen. Common methods include either the repeated injection of small doses of the allergen to form protective blocking antibodies, or depletion of the individual's tissue stores of histamine and serotonin.

desensitized enzyme. A regulatory enzyme that has been so altered by either mutation or chemical modifications that, while it is still catalytically active, it no longer responds to an effector.

desiccants. 1. Chemicals that kill leaves of plants, the leaves may either drop of or remain attached; Desiccants are used on many seed crops to hasten harvest.
2. Substance used to withdraw moisture from other materials. *Compare* desiccation.

desiccation. Removal of water vapour from a material by a hygroscopic substance, such as anhydrous calcium chloride, phosphorus pentoxide, or silica gel, placed in an airtight container with the material to be dried (often under vacuum). The term is conventionally restricted to laboratory control or chemical reagents, test samples, and the like and is not used for large scale drying or dehydrating operation.

desmolase. Any of a group of enzymes which catalyze rupture of atomic linkages that are not cleaved through hydrolysis, such as the bonds in the carbon chain of D-glucose.

detoxication. The enzymatic reactions in an organism whereby foreign compounds, produced within the organism or introduced in it, are converted to less harmful forms and to more readily excrete products; foreign compounds are either chemically altered or conjugated to normally occurring metabolites of the organism. In the body detoxication is effected by oxidation, reduction, hydrolysis, or by combination (conjugation) with glycine, glucuronic acid, glutamine, cysteine, or by methylation; e.g., the toxic substance benzoic acid is excreted in the urine as a complex with glycine, namely hippuric acid. Also known as detoxification.

detoxification. See detoxication.

dewberry. A large variety of blackberry, but different in flavour.

dextran. A polysaccharide composed of linked fructose units; unwelcome in the sugar factory but valuable clinically for blood transfusion (plasma extender). It is produced by the action of *Betacoccus arabinosaceous* on sugar.

dextrins. Mixture of soluble compounds formed by partial breakdown of starch by heat, acid or enzymes; (complete breakdown yields maltose). Formed when bread is toasted. Nutritionally equivalent to starch; industrially used as adhesives in the sizing of paper and textiles, and as gums.

dextrose equivalent value. D.E. A term used to indicate the degree of hydrolysis of starch into glucose syrup. It is defined as the total reducing sugar content, expressed as dextrose; calculated as a percentage of the dry solids content (i.e., the higher the D.E., more sugar and the less dextrins are present). Liquid glucose are commercially available ranging between 26-65 D.E. A complete acid hydrolysis converts all starch into glucose but produces bitter degradation products.

dextrose. A monosaccharide; dextrorotatory sugar, which occurs naturally in corn and grapes and is also found in blood. A member of the general class of carbohydrates, it is formed in plants by photosynthesis; it is Dextrose is an optical isomer of levulose (fructose), which is levorotatory. Dextrose polymers form amylose, a basic constituent of starch. As other stereochemical forms of glucose have no significance in biological systems the term glucose is often used interchangeably with dextrose. It is an alternative name for glucose. Commercially the term glucose is often used to mean corn syrup (a mixture of glucose, sugars and dextrins) and pure glucose is called dextrose.

diabetes mellitus. A metabolic disorder affecting mainly carbohydrate metabolism; an inability to metabolize glucose which therefore appears in the urine. Usually, it is due to a deficiency of insulin and is treated by insulin injections (also possibly due to increased destruction of insulin in the body, treated by oral drugs such as tolbutamide). Impaired glucose metabolism leads to excessive fat breakdown with the accumulation of the penultimate products of fatty acid oxidation, namely acetoacetic acid, β-hydroxybutyric acid and acetone (the so-called ketone bodies). These can cause diabetic coma.

diabetes, renal. The appearance of glucose in the urine without undue elevation of the blood sugar. It is due to a reduction of the renal threshold which allows the blood glucose to be excreted.

diabetic bread. In most of the breads, sugar is present in amounts too small to have much of an influence on the health of diabetics. Most of the carbohydrate in bread is in the form of starch. Some glucose and maltose is formed in the dough after water is added, provided amylases are present, but only a small quantity of sugar remains at the end of a normal fermentation. It is assumed that diabetics has received dietary guidance from their physician and this will include advice on whether or not to moderate or cease their consumption of bread and rolls. Of course, sweet baked goods (cakes, pies, pastries, etc.) will probably be unsuitable for the diet of diabetic person. In spite of all this, there appears to be a demand for sugar-free bread.

The term sugar-free can mean different things to different groups of consumers. Some health food buyers wish to avoid refined white sugar (sucrose, beet sugar, cane sugar), and would probably accept a product that contained honey, molasses, corn syrup, malt syrup, or even the so-called "raw" sugar. Few problems are encountered when one of these ingredients is substituted for the small amount of sugar usually added to bread dough. Even if sugar-free is interpreted to mean "does not contain added sucrose, glucose, or fructose," the demand can be met provided the baker is willing to make minor modifications in the standard bread formula. Sugar is usually added at the level of only a few percent in white bread and it is rapidly converted by yeast into glucose and fructose and then mostly metabolized, so the amount present is continually reduced as the dough ferments. Sugar does not play an important role in establishing the structure of dough, but it has an indirect influence on the physical properties of bread as a result of its effects on fermentation. As a source of preferred metabolities, its effect on fermentation is substantial but it can be replaced to some extent by the glucose and maltose generated by diastatic malt syrup or fungal amylases. Malt syrup does include quantities of glucose, maltose, and higher saccharides-these constituents should be taken into account when making labeling claims. Incidentally, corn syrup, honey, molasses, etc., must also be omitted from bread described as being "free of added sugar(s)." Milk products (except caseinates) include considerable lactose, a disaccharide sugar. It is obvious that bread from which all sugars have been omitted or consumed by yeast will be less sweet than regular white bread and, therefore, less palatable to most consumers. Also known as sugar-free bread.

diabetic ice cream. There is a great demand for ice cream which is low in carbohydrate and sugar content, for those who suffer from diabetes. The following formulation may help to meet such demand:

For a 5-gallon mix use: 3.25 gallons 30% cream, 1.75 gallons skim milk, 7 fresh eggs, 100 g gelatin, 50 g saccharin, 500 ml glycerine. The eggs, gelatin and saccharin are blended with the milk products, pasteurized and homogenized in the same manner as in making other ice cream mixes. The 500 ml glycerine is added at the freezer when the desired colour and flavour are added. It is imperative that the sugar content of the flavouring be held to the minimum; therefore vanilla, mint, and lemon are most satisfactory. Fruits such as pineapple, peaches, and apricots when well ripened can be used but are less satisfactory in this type of ice cream. Since the use of saccharin in ice cream is illegal in many states, special permission from health authorities must be precured.

diabetic milk. A modified milk suggested by Ringer to supply protein nourishment for diabetic patients. It is a solution of casein in a mixture of salts approximating those present in ordinary milk. Diabetic milk has been found to have the following composition: water 90.5%; milk sugar 0.12%; fat 2.4%; protein 2.44%; levulose 4.41%; ash 4.5%. Now it is not of much importance because of the easy availability of insulin.

diacetyl. $CH_3CO-CO-CH_3$. The flavour-aroma agent in butter formed during the ripening stage by the organism *Streptococcus lactis cremoris.* It is generally added as a synthetic compound to margarine as butter flavour.

dialysis. Separation of small molecules from larger in solution by virtue of their different rates of diffusion through a membrane. Membranes are natural, such as pig bladder, or artificial, such as cellulose derivatives or collodion. The solution is usually placed in a bag of the membrane and this immersed in water. The small molecules diffuse out into the water leaving the larger molecules inside the bag. This is a frequent method of separating proteins from solutions.

diaphorase. A flavoprotein enzyme in the cell respiratory system; function is to accept hydrogen from NADH. It catalyzes the reduction of artificial electron acceptor such as dye, ferricyanide, or a quinone, by either reduced nicotinamide adenine dinucleotide or by reduced nicotinamide adenine dinucleotide phosphate. Such enzymes were originally thought to function in the reduction of metabolites in electron transport system between NADH and the cytochromes, but this need not be the case. One preparation of diaphorase has been shown to be identical with lipoamide dehydrogenase.

diastase. An enzyme that hydrolyzes starch in barley grain to produce maltose during the malting process. It is a mixture containing amylolytic enzymes obtained from malt. Malt is obtained by artificially germinated barley grains, *Hordeum vulgare* (Fam. *Gramineae*). Barley is grown throughout the world in favorable climate. For preparing malt, wet barley grains in heaps are kept in warm room for germination until the caulicle protrudes. The grain is dried quickly to kill the embryo. The enzyme diastase in the moist warm grains converts starch to maltose which stimulates the embryo for germination. Dry malt contains maltose sugar (50-70%), dextrins (2-15%), proteins (8%), diastase and peptase enzyme. Malt extract is prepared by extracting the partially germinating grains of *H. vulgare.* It contains dextrin maltose, glucose and amylolytic enzymes. Diastase converts at least 50 times of its weight of potato starch into sugars (dextrin and maltose) in 30 minutes. Diastase is a yellowish white amorphous powder obtained from an infusion of malt. It is yellowish white, amorphous powder or translucent scales. It loses amylolytic power on storing; heating its solution at 85°C; or on adding excess of acid. It is soluble in water with some turbidity, and is almost insoluble in alcohol. It is used to manufacture starch, converting starch into sugar and to remove starch from fabrics. Also known as maltin.

diastatic activity of flour. A measure of its ability to produce sugar from its own starch under the influence of its own diastase. This sugar is needed for the growth of the yeast during the fermentation. It is measured as maltose figure.

diastatic malt. Diastatic malt products differ from their nondiastatic counterparts in possessing considerable enzymatic activity. The malted grain from which these products are, derived may be considered as a storehouse of enzymes. The two types that are of greatest interest to bakers are proteolytic enzymes and amylolytic enzymes. The latter group, comprising the diastase of older writers, contains at least two different enzymes, commonly designated α-enzyme (also known as dextrinizing enzyme) and the β-amylase (also known as the saccharifying enzyme). α-amylase splits the starch molecule at random points, forming smaller molecules of widely varying size. Two important effects of this action are the reduction of the viscosity of susceptibility starch suspensions and the production of relatively small amounts of fermentable sugars. End products of the reaction are chiefly dextrins (compounds containing several glucose residues) that cannot be used as substrates by bakers' yeast. It is doubtful if the amount of α-amylase normally encountered in sound wheat flour have any significant effect on its baking properties in the absence of native or added beta-amylase. The action of β-amylase on starch results in the production of maltose by the progressive release of terminal sugar residues from the starch molecule. β-amylase cannot attack the starch molecule inside the points at which it is branched, and so a residue of limit dextrin of high molecular mass remains after β-amylase has completed its action. These limit dextrins cannot be fermented, but they are customarily produced in smaller amounts than the dextrins resulting from the action of α-amylase.

dicoumarin. Toxic substance found in spoiled sweet clover; causes hemorrhage (hemorrhagic sweet clover disease) by interfering with the synthesis of prothrombin in the liver, *i.e.*, it has an anti-vitamin K action; it is used clinically to prevent the postoperative thrombosis.

dielectric drying. Moisture removal from substances, usually poor conductors of heat, by placing in the field of an alternating current. The alternating electrical field deforms the molecular field of the product, causing production of thermal energy. Heating is in proportion to the dielectric constant of the material, which for water is 80. The principle may also be used for moisture meters.

dietetic foods. Foods prepared to meet the particular nutritional needs of persons whose normal processes of assimilation or metabolism are modified, or for whom a particular effect is to be obtained by a controlled intake of foods or certain nutrients. They may be formulated for person suffering from physiological disorders or for healthy people with additional needs.

diethyl pyrocarbonate. Preservative that kills bacteria and yeasts (not moulds) and is hydrolyzed to ethyl alcohol and carbon dioxide; particularly suitable for beverages in the concentration range 50-300 mg/L; hydrolysis is complete after several days.

dietitian, dietician. One who applies the principles of nutrition to the feeding of individuals and groups; plans menus and special diets; supervises the preparation and serving of meals; instructs in the principles of nutrition as applied to the selection of foods.

digestibility. The proportion of a foodstuff absorbed from the digestive tract into the bloodstream, normally 90-95%. It is measured as the difference between intake and faecal output, making allowance for that part of the faeces which is not derived from undigested food residues (such as shed lining of the intestinal tract, bacteria, residues of digestive juices). Digestibility measured in this way is referred to as `true digestibility' as distinct from the approximately measure of `apparent digestibility' which is simply the difference between intake and output.

digestion of food. The digestion of food begins in the mouth and stomach, and the final stages of digestion of all major food components into the blood takes place in small intestine. During digestion in the gastrointestinal tract of mammals the three major nutrients (carbohydrates, lipids, and proteins) undergo enzymatic hydrolysis into their building block components. This necessary for their utilization, since the cells lining the intestine are able to absorb into the blood stream only relatively smaller molecules. For example, polysaccha-rides and even disaccharides must be completely hydrolyzed into monosaccharides by digestive enzymes before they can be absorbed. Similarly, proteins and lipids must also be hydrolyzed into their building block components. *See also* digestion.

digestion. 1. The breakdown of a complex into its constituent parts. Most frequently refers to the digestion of food which means the breakdown by the digestive enzymes of proteins to amino acids, starch to glucose, fats to glycerol and fatty acids - these simple breakdown products are then absorbed into the bloodstream. Digestion is also applied to the acid hydrolysis of a protein; the Kjeldahl digestion is the complete breakdown of a nitrogenous compound to ammonia by sulphuric acid.

2. The decomposition of solid or semisolid organic wastes such as garbage, cellulosics, sewage, etc., by the action of bacteria, either with or without the presence of air. Air is used in the activate sludges method of treating sewage wastes and in the composting of garbage and agricultural wastes. *See also* digestion of food.

dihydrofolate reductase. DHFR. The enzyme that catalyzes the NADPH-dependent reduction of folate to tetrahydrofo-late, an essential cofactor in the synthesis of glycine, purines and thymidine. It is target of the anticancer drug methotrexate. Cells resistant to this drug tend to have gene coding for DHFR amplified to high copy number.

dihydrolipoyl dehydrogenase. An enzyme with FAD prosthetic group; catalyzes the regeneration of the oxidized form of lipoamide.

dihydrolipoyl transacetylase. An enzyme which catalyzes the formation of di-hydrolipoate from the combination of acetylthioester of dihydrolipoate with coenzyme-A.

dihydroorotase. An enzyme which catalyzes the ring closure of N-carbamyl aspartic acid and leads to the formation of di-hydroorotic acid.

dilatation of fats. When fats change from solids to liquid at the same temperature there is an increase in volume. Measurement of this increase, dilatometry, may be used to estimate the amount of solid fat present in a mixture at any given temperature. The precise measure is the difference between the volumes of the solid and the liquid fat measured in microlitres per 25 g of fat.

dill. Family: *Umbelliferae*. Genus: *Anethum*. Species: *Anethum graveolens*. The plant originates from southern Europe and western Asia, and its use is recorded far back in time. As with so many umbellifers, this hardy annual yields two separate culinary components, its seeds and its feathery leaves, which are, somewhat ambiguously, known as dill weed. Dill is aromatic, somewhat like caraway is, but much milder and sweeter. The taste of dill resembles fennel in some ways, but is slightly more pungent and aggressive in flavour. The plant grows ordinarily from 60-75 cm high and looks a lot like fennel, although smaller but having the same feathery leaves, which stand on sheathing foot-stalks, with linear and pointed leaflets. But unlike fennel, it has seldom more than one stalk and its long, spindle-shaped root is only annual. It is of very upright growth, its stem smooth, shiny and hollow, and in midsummer bears flat terminal umbels with numerous yellow flowers, whose small petals are rolled inwards. The flat fruits or so-called seeds are produced in great quantities. The pickled cucumbers and beets would not be complete without dill seed. Nor would green apple pies, certain soups, beans, cabbage, cauliflower, peas, cottage cheese and some nut butters. The seeds produce an oil that is used to make dill water, or gripe water, used to alleviate colic in babies. The seeds are also said to act as a sedative and to ward off hunger.

Dill seed contains 2.5-4% volatile oil, composed mainly of carvone with lesser amounts of numerous other aromatic chemicals. It also contains coumarin, steroids, flavonoids, glucosides, phenolic acid, protein, fat, carbohydrates and minerals, particularly calcium and potassium, and vitamins, especially A and C. It stimulates poor appetite, soothes upset stomachs and helps with insomnia and flatulence. It is also used to promote lactation in nursing mothers. Oil from dill seed has been found, in animal experiments, to lower blood pressure, inhibit the growth of bacteria and relax spasms of the intestinal and uterine muscles. In China, dill seed is believed to benefit the spleen, kidney and stomach and is used mainly for treating gastrointestinal problems, including abdominal distension, colic, vomiting, lack of appetite and stomachache.

dinoflagellates. The *Pyrrhophyta* or dinoflagellates consist of more than 1,000 known species of unicellular, motile, photosynthetic protistan algae, responsible for the red tides that are poisonous to many forms of life. The majority of dinoflagellates are marine but some live in freshwater also. Along with the chrysophytes and diatoms, the dinoflagellates make up a large part of the freshwater and marine plankton and are at the base of many food chains. Most of the dinoflagellates have chlorophylls a and c, in addition to carotenoids and xanthophylls. As a result, they usually have a yellowish-green to brown colour. The biochemistry of their chloroplasts resembles that of brown algae and diatoms. The members of each of these groups probably acquired their chloroplasts as a result of independent symbiotic events. The energy-storage material is either starch or oil. Some dinoflagellates are capable of ingesting other cells; others are colourless and heterotrophic. A few occur as symbionts in many groups of jellyfish, sea anemones, mollusks, and corals. When dinoflagellates form symbiotic relationships, they lose their cellulose plates and flagella, become spherical golden-brown globules in the host cells, and are then termed zooxanthellae. Reproduction in dinoflagellates is primarily by longitudinal cell division, but sexual reproduction has been demonstrated in a few genera. Their nucleus very unusual. The DNA is complexed with histone-like proteins rather than normal histones, and their chromosomes remain condensed after mitosis. The nuclear envelope and nucleolus do not disappear during mitosis.

dinucleotide. Two nucleotides linked together through their phosphate groups. Two important dinucleotides are the coenzyme flavin adenine dinucleotide (FAD) and nicotinamide adenine dinucleotide (NAD⁺).

dipsa. Foods that cause thirst. Dipsetic -tending to produce thirst. Dipsosis means extreme thirst craving for abnormal kinds of drinks. Dipsomania refers to imperative morbid craving for alcoholic drink.

dipsogen. Thirst-provoking agent.

direct-fired dryer. A type of dryer in which the products of combustion for heating come into direct contact with the product being dried. Products which are not unfavorably affected by the products of combustion may be dried with a direct-fired unit. Direct-fired units have a thermal efficiency of 45 to 60%.

disaccharide intolerance. Impaired ability to digest maltose, sucrose or lactose, which may be inherited. Generalized lactose intolerance may be an adaptation to the absence of milk from the diet, and can be secondary to various inflammatory and degenerative diseases of the small intestine. Treatment is by omitting the offending sugar from the diet.

disaccharides. Sugars composed of two monosaccharide molecules combined, with the elimination of a molecule of water; e.g., glucose, $C_6H_{12}O_6$, plus fructose, $C_6H_{12}O_6$, produces sucrose, $C_{12}H_{22}O_{11}$. Conversely, when a disaccharide is hydrolyzed, either by acid or enzymatically, a molecule of water is added and two monosaccharides result.

disc fan. A type of air-moving device (AMD) or fan in which there is axial flow of air, parallel to the axis of rotation of the blade. It is essentially a propeller fan with an enlarged hub. The enlarged hub helps reduce the reverse airflow which may occur opposite the direction of major airflow through the fan. Reverse airflow may occur near the center of the fan wheel as the pressure is increased.

disc mill. One or more revolving circular plates between which substances, e.g., foodstuffs, are ground. The discs are separated by projecting tenth or pins; are ground. The discs are separated by projecting teeth or pins; used to grind grain, fruit, sugar,

chocolate, pastes, etc.
diseases of plants. A knowledge of plant diseases is of the greatest importance to the farmer. It is estimated that huge losses result every year from certain plant diseases. They are generally due to one of the following four causes; fungi, bacteria, insects or physiological cause. There are fungi which live wholly within the tissues of the plant, those that throw their spores in the air and those that live in the open air, fastening their rootlets to the plant and penetrating openings in the epidermis. When once the plant is attacked, the diseases progress with great rapidity. Familiar examples of diseases by fungi are rusts and smuts of corn, potato rot and mildews. In bacterial diseases insects visiting the plant introduce into the cells bacteria, which, when once they have gained entrance, seem to be beyond control of remedy and cause the injury or death of the plant without delay. It is impossible to cure plants when once infected by bacteria, but it is possible to prevent the spread of the disease to the other plants, by utterly destroying those which are diseased. The chief examples of these diseases are fire blight of apples and pears, black rot of cabbage, and celery disease, tomato disease and sweet corn disease. Certain insects, such as the eelworms or phylloxera, attack various plants. Phylloxera attack grapes and have been very injurious to whole vineyards in Europe. Orange trees, roses and cucumber plants are also subject to the attacks of these worms. It is said that lime is a good remedy, and in greenhouses it is possible to free the soil from infection by backing or freezing it. The physiological diseases are generally caused by unsanitary conditions, such as improper soil or lack or excess of light or water. The leaves generally turn yellow and drop, and the whole plant assumes an unhealthy appearance. Preventing of plant diseases requires careful study. If the seed is suspected, it should be treated before planting with some solution which will kill the spores. Fields in which the disease has appeared should have the old stubble burned over and be cleared of all shrubbery and other objects in which the spores may find refuge, before ploughing for the second crop.

dispersing agents. A term generally referring to surface-active agents, which are valuable for their dispersing action. A surfactant reduces energy levels between interfaces. Dispersions include emulsions (solubilization or macro emulsions, depending upon particle size involved), foams and aerosols, and suspensions. Effective dispersing agents employed n food industry include propylene glycol mono esters; glycerol mono esters; sorbitan esters; sucrose esters; polyglycerol esters; polysyethylene esters; polyoxyethylene sorbitan esters; and various complex esters, such as lactate, tartarate, among others. Phosphates also have a particular ability to effect dispersion and peptization of comparatively insoluble food constituents, for example, proteins in concentrated milk, pasteurised process cheese, and meat products. Phosphates (sodium or potassium di- and triphosphates) solubilize proteins and permit them to form protective film about fat globules and thus enhance their emulsification. Similarly, they stabilize milk proteins to prevent gelling during storage.

distilled liquors. Alcoholic liquors manufactured by the combined processes of fermentation and distillation. They may be made from raw material or directly from material which has been fermented, as in the manufacture of brandy by distilling wine. Most of the liquors, such as rum and whisky, are made directly from the raw material, corn, wheat and other grains being used. In some countries potatoes are used instead of grain. The grain is ground and soaked in warm water, preparing what is called the mash. Yeast is then added to this, and it is allowed to ferment, forming the wort. From this the spirit is distilled. The distilled spirit usually contains numerous substances that are not desirable, and these are removed by redistilling at different temperatures or by allowing the liquor to stand for a long time, when they are either absorbed or evaporated. The purification is generally known as the process of rectifying. Rum is made directly from fermented molasses.

diuresis. Loss of water from the body as urine.

diuretics. Substances that increase of secretion of urine; include organic mercury compounds, xanthines (therefore also coffee and tea) and substances that alter the alkaline reserve of the blood, such as urea, potassium nitrate, potassium chloride.

DNA gyrase. Enzyme that increases or introduces positive supercoiling in covalently positive supercoiling in covalently closed circular DNA molecules generated by DNA replication. This is achieved by breakage of at least one DNA strand followed by untwisting and subsequent resealing of the duplex. DNA gyrase is an alternative term for a type II topoisomerase. Also known as swivelase.

DNA helicase. An enzyme which binds ahead of the replicating fork in the discontinuous replication of DNA and it catalyzes the energy-dependent unwinding of the duplex. The enzyme has ATPase activity and hydrolyzes 2 molecules of ATP/DNA base pair broken.

DNA ligases. One of the enzymes involved in DNA replication in prokaryotes. The enzymes from *E.coli* and bacteriophage T4 have been characterized. The enzyme catalyzes the formation of phosphodiester bonds between adjacent 5'-phosphate and the free 3'-hydroxy groups in DNA duplexes. It is used in sealing restriction fragments together at Eco RI sticky ends generated, for example, by the restriction enzyme Eco RI.

DNA methylase. An enzyme which catalyzes the methylation of the bases in DNA; methylation occurs subsequent to, rather than prior, to the incorporation of the bases into the polynucleotide strand.

DNA polymerase I. A DNA-dependent DNA polymerase, originally thought to function in the replication of DNA but now it is believed to function in the repair-synthesis of DNA. It is a 109-kdal single polypeptide chain. It catalyzes the step-by-step addition of deoxyribonucleotide units to a DNA chain. DNA polymerase I adds deoxyribonucleotides to the 3'-hydroxyl terminus of a preexisting DNA (or RNA) strand. DNA polymerase I can also hydrolyze DNA starting from the 5' end of the chain. It can also add deoxyribonucleotides to a primary chain, but it cannot catalyze the joining of two DNA chains, or the closure of a single DNA chain.

DNA polymerase II. A DNA-dependent DNA polymerase that is sensitive to sulfhydryl reagents and that is believed to function in the replication of DNA. *See also* DNA polymerase III.

DNA polymerase III. A DNA-dependent DNA polymerase that is sensitive to sulfhydryl reagents and that is believed to function in the replication of DNA. Under certain conditions the enzyme behaves as a reverse transcriptase and utilizes polyriboadenylic acid preferentially. DNA polymerase II and III are like polymerase I in certain respects, such as:

(a) They catalyze a template-directed synthesis of DNA from deoxyribonucleoside triphosphate precursors.

(b) A primer with a free 3'-OH group is required.

(c) Synthesis is in the 5'-3' direction.

(d) They possess 3'-5' exonuclease activity. DNA polymerase III, but not II, also a 5'-3' exonuclease.

These polymerases differ in their template preferences. Polymerases II and III act optimally on double-stranded DNA templates that have short gaps. In contrast, extensive single-stranded regions near double helical regions are preferred templates for polymerase I.

DNA polymerases. Enzymes responsible for the synthesis of DNA form nucleotide precursors using single-stranded DNA as template. A number of different DNA polymerases can be recovered from eukaryotic cells, some of which are repair enzymes which polymerize short pieces of DNA where sections have been deleted from a sequence or help to substitute correct bases for incorrect bases. But at least one enzyme species (and probably more than one) is responsible for the polymerization of new DNA in the replication process.

DNA probe. A bit of DNA, labelled in some manner, which is used to identify the presence of similar DNA by hybridizing to it. DNA probes are usually labeled with either a radioactive isotope such as ^{32}P or a chemical such as biotin, that can be easily detected. Probes can be used to detect and:

(a) identify an organism that is extremely difficult to culture by common methods. In this case, the labeled probe is directed against the gene that is characteristic for a certain species, such as ribosomal RNA;

(b) quickly identify an organism if a reliable laboratory procedure is unavailable to culture the organism; and

(c) identify an organism when the organism is easy to culture but the toxin or product of interest that is characteristic of the organism is difficult to detect by standard methods.

DNA synaptase. An enzyme which catalyzes the fusion of double-stranded DNA molecules at a region of homology and that may play a role in genetic recombination.

DNA. Deoxyribonucleic acid. A nucleic acid, mainly found in the chromosomes, that contains the hereditary information of organisms. The molecule is made up of two helical polynucleotide chains coiled around each other to give a double helix. Phosphate molecules alternate with deoxyribose sugar molecules along both chains and each sugar molecule is also joined to a nitrogenous base, wither adenine, guanine, cytosine or thymine. The two chains are joined to each other by bonding between bases. The sequence of bases along the chain makes up a code- the genetic code- that determines the precise sequence of amino acids in proteins. Protein synthesis is achieved through the action of messenger

230 DNA-directed polymerase

RNA, which, (by transcription), relays the information in the genetic code to the protein-synthesizing sites (ribosomes), where it is translated into the amino acid sequence of the protein. The two purine bases (adenine and guanine) always bond with the pyrimidine bases (thymine and cytosine), and the pairing is quite specific: adenine with thymine and guanine with cytosine. DNA is the hereditary material of all organisms with the exception of RNA viruses. Together with RNA and histones it makes up the chromosomes of eukaryotic cells.

DNA-directed polymerase. An enzyme capable of forming an RNA polymer from ribonucleoside 5'-triphosphates, which has been isolated from bacterial extracts. It is similar in some ways to DNA polymerase. RNA polymerase requires all four ribonucleoside 5'-triphosphates (ATP, GTP, UTP, and CTP) as precursors of the nucleotide units of RNA, as well as Mg^{2+} ions. The purified enzyme also contains zinc as an essential part of its active group. In *E.coli* there is a single DNA-directed RNA polymerase that can make not only mRNAs but also tRNAs and rRNAs. It is a complex enzyme containing five polypeptide subunits. The first step in transcription is the binding of the holoenzyme to a specific site in the DNA, called promoter site. Once the RNA polymerase is positioned in the correct manner at the promoter site and has made a few phosphodiester bonds, the s subunit dissociates from the holoenzyme. The RNA is then elongated, step by step, by the remaining core enzyme. The end of the gene or genes being transcribed is signaled by a specific termination sequence in the DNA template. In order to terminate transcription and bring about release of RNA polymerase from the DNA, another specific protein is required.

DNA-like RNA. An RNA molecule that resembles DNA in its overall base composition and base ratios; the RNA is generally rich in adenine and uracil and has an adenine/uracil ratio of approximately 1.0.

DNase. Family of enzymes that degrade DNA, either by cutting the molecule one nucleotide at a time from the ends (exonuclease) or by cutting it internally, sometimes at specific sequences (an endonuclease). Enzymes that degrade both DNA and RNA are termed simply nucleases. Some DNases cut only single strands of DNA, even if the DNA is in duplex form; others cut both strands. An enzyme that is widely used to introduce nicks into DNA is the DNase I, a bivalent metal ion-requiring enzyme derived from boving pancreas. Enzymes referred to as DNase II, which may be derived form mammalian spleen or thymus, or form bacteria (now termed staphylococcal nuclease, previously referred to as micrococcal nuclease) have to metal requirement, but operate at a rather acid *p*H. They have been widely used for the digestion of chromatin to yield nucleosomes. The S1 nuclease is an endonuclease from Aspergillus that cuts single-stranded DNA selectively. Also known as deoxyribonuclease.

Doane-Buckley test. A method to determine the number of body cells in milk. It consists of concentrating the cells in milk by centrifuging and then counting the number in a definite volume of the concentrate by means of a blood cell counting apparatus.

Doblefina orange. A variety of sweet orange, blood-type. it is of unknown Spanish origin. The fruit was for many years the main blood-orange variety of Spain. Fruit is of medium of small size, shape is oval, fruit is seedless. It develops yellowish-orange coloration upon maturing and is more or less densely blushed. The flesh is firm, with blood flecks scattered densely blushed. The blood coloration is irregular; in some cases, the flesh has little coloration. Fruit drops rapidly from the tree. The Entrefina, a subvariety of Doblefina, is even smaller and less attractive.

dockage. Name given to foreign material in wheat which can be readily removed by a simple cleaning procedure.

dogfish. A name given to several species of small shark, common around the British Isles, so named from their habit of pursuing prey like dogs hunting. The rough skin of one of the species, the lesser spotted dogfish, is used in polishing various substances, particularly wood. This species is rarely three feet long. The greater dogfish is from three to five feet in length. It is black-brown in colour, marked with numbers small dark spots. Both species are very voracious and destructive. Their flesh is hard, dry and unpalatable. The common, or picked, dogfish is common in North American seas and is sometimes used as food. On the Pacific coast oil is made from the livers of the dogfish.

domiati cheese. A popular variety of Egyptian cheese made from partly skimmed cow's or buffalo's milk. It is soft, white, mild and salty with no openness. 5-15% salt is added to 2-3% of the milk before the addition of rennet, and the rest is heated to 60°C The portions are mixed and the rennet is added at 40° C If it is to be cured it is pickled in salt-whey or salt milk

brine. It is cured for 4-8 months.

Don joao orange. A variety of sweet orange, that is nonblood type. It was first identified in Portugal in 1943 in Don Joao orchard near Beja in Algarva region. The variety was traced back to a single very old tree, estimated to be at least 100 years old. Specifications of the Don Joao are essentially the same as for the Valencia. When Hodgson visited Portugal and compared Don Joao trees planted alongside Valencia trees, it was concluded that the 2 "varieties" are one and the same. This raised the question, "Is Valencia of Portuguese rather than Spanish origin?" But some authorities suggest the Valencia is of Chinese origin and was introduced into Portugal.

DOPA decarboxylase. A cytoplasmic enzyme present in kidney and liver cells and in adrenergic nerve fibres and chromaffin cells. It catalyzes the decarboxylation of DOPA with the formation of dopamine. It requires pyridoxal phosphate as a coenzyme. It also catalyzes the decarboxylation of other aromatic amino acids including m-tyrosine and 5-hydroxytryptophan. For this reason it is also called aromatic amino acid decarboxylase.

Dorscolene. Trade name of a drying oil made from fractionated and blended fish oils.

Dortmund. See Dortmunder.

Dortmunder. A variety of beer that required less hops than 'Pilsner' resulting in less bitter taste as well as head. The water used for making this beer is characterized by the presence of both carbonates and chlorides. The alcohol content is similar to Pilsners. Also known as Dortmund.

double-drum dryer. An apparatus consisting of two cylindrical, horizontal steam filled drums which turn toward each other, used for continuous drying. Commonly used to dry milk, juices, brewer's yeast, foods, and chemicals. The overall heat transfer coefficients range is 50-400 W/m²K.

dough cakes. Term includes crumpets, muffins and pikelets, all made from flour, water and milk; batter is raised with yeast and baked on a hot plate. Crumpets have sodium bicarbonate added to batter, muffins are thick and well aerated, less tough than crumpets, pikelets are made from crumpet batter that has been thinned down.

Doughe maker process. For continuous bread-making. Ingredients are automatically fed into continuous dough mixer, the yeast suspension being added in a very active state.

doum palm. A palm tree, remarkable for having repeatedly-branching stems. Each branch terminates in a tuft of large, fan-shaped leaves. The fruit is about the size of an apple. It has a fibrous, mealy rind, which tastes like gingerbread and is eaten by the poorer inhabitants of upper Egypt, where the doum palm grows.

dried cheese. Although not of major economic importance, procedures have been developed for making dried cheese from soft natural product. It is used in the manufactured food products, such as soup, salads, macaroni, and snack foods. A method of drying is by chemical treatment, such as addition of sodium citrate, followed by moisture removal on a drum dryer or in a spray dryer. The cheese may be dried in a vacuum at low temperature. Hard cheese, after curing, is grated, surface dried to 15% at a temperature of 24-27°C, followed by drying the pieces to 5% moisture content using air increased in temperature to 65°C. Throughout drying, special care must be given to physical properties of wey solids in soft natural cheese and the running of fat in hard cheese.

Drierite. Trade name of a dehydrating agent, consisting mainly anhydrous calcium sulphate; it is used for drying gases, liquids, and solids. The material may include a colour indicator to show the presence of moisture. The chemical may be regenerated by heating at 235 to 250°C.

Driocel. Trade name for a drying adsorbent made from activated bauxite (Al_2O_3) and regenerated by heating at 149-260°C.

drip dry. A textile product which dries rapidly using gravity for removal of surface moisture and heat in the normal ambient atmosphere for drying following laundering. Fibres are treated by covering the surface with resins to repel the water. The resins are primarily aminoplasts. Clothes made from drip dry fabrics are also called wash-and-wear. The usual ironing following washing of drip dry fabrics can be eliminated by hanging the fabrics to dry.

dripping. Unbleached and untreated fat from the fatty tissues or bones of sheep or oxen.

drum dryer. An apparatus in which drying is done continuously on the external surface of an internally steam heated rotating cylinder. A thin film is applied at one location and removed at another location, usually after less than one complete revolution of the cylinder. These dryers may be atmospheric or vacuum types and are classified as single drum; double drum, with two drums working together with a nip or sump fed from above; or twin drum, in which the two separate drums function almost as single drums. The single drum may have a dip, splash, or transfer roll feed; the double drum, usually has a nip feed; and twin drum, the dip or splash feed. Evaporation of moisture in an evaporator concentrating liquids from 2:1 to 3:1 often precedes drum dryer. Also known as roller dryer.

drupes. Botanical name for fruit that is a single seed, surrounded by stony and fleshy pericarp, e.g., apricot, cherry, plum.

dry-blanch-dry process. A method of drying fruit so as to retain the bright colour and flavour; it is faster than drying in the sun and preserves flavour and colour better than hot air drying. The material is dried to 50% water at about 82°C, balanced for a few minute then dried at 68°C over a period of 6-24 hours to 15-20% water content.

dry-cure. The process of curing by drying or moisture removal using a salt or brine.

dryer efficiency. The percentage of the total heat supplied by fuel used to evaporate water from a product. Dryer efficiency is the product of the efficiencies of the components and is normally 35 to 70%. Burner efficiency refers to the percentage of the heat in the fuel which through combustion leaves the burner and normally enters the heater. Overall thermal efficiency refers to the heat available in the fuel in relation to heat used to evaporate weather. Dryer efficiency may relate to the efficiency of heat utilization in the space where drying occurs.

dryer performance evaluation index. DPEI. The total energy required by a dryer to remove one kg of moisture from the product during drying under specified conditions. The total energy includes the energy to heat the drying air, the energy to move the drying and cooling air, and the energy to move the product. The specified conditions are ambient air conditions (tempera-

ture and humidity ratio), the inlet product moisture content, temperature, type and quality of product.

dryaeration. A modified drying process involving the portable batch or continuous-flow dryer. In this process, the product is dried with heated air to a moisture level of 16-18%, wet basis. The product is transferred immediately without cooling to a temporary storage (dryaeration) bin equipped for aeration. The product is allowed to set for some time to become tempered before aeration starts. Cooling is accomplished in about 12 hours with airflow rates of about $0.007 \text{ m}^3/\text{m}^3\text{s}$. At this low airflow rate, nearly all the heat in the product is utilized to further dry it. The moisture content may be further reduced 3-4% during the 12 hours of cooling.

dry farming. A term which does not mean the science of farming on dry soil; it relates to the production of crops on land favoured with only a slight rainfall. If less than 25 cm of rainfalls yearly upon any section of country that area is classed as an arid region, where agricultural effort is fruitless. Formerly it was believed that when rainfall did not exceed twenty inches in a year the prospects for agricultural returns were slight. It is still true that where there is less than fifteen inches of rain all effort is discouraging, but there has developed a principle embodying the conservation of moisture and its storage in the ground which makes good crops possible on millions of acres of land where there is from 30-35 cm of rain. The processes of this conservation and storage constitute dry forming. Dry farming is essentially a method of preparing the soil so that it will hold moisture as long as possible. The process of cultivation consists chiefly in deep, fall plough-ing, followed by harrowing. The disk harrow should be used before sowing and later as long as the growing crops permit. The deep ploughing and frequent harrowing form a mulch of fine soil upon the surface which prevents evaporation. The best crop for dry farming seems to be wheat. Corn is also profitable, and potatoes, sugar beets, alfalfa, and even peaches and other fruits have been success-fully cultivated.

dry fruits. The dry fruits are classified into dehiscent fruits, those which split open when ripe, and indehiscent fruits, which do not do so. Common dehiscent fruits are the legume, the follicle, and the capsule; dry indehis-cent fruits are the achene, the cary-opsis or grain, the samara, and the nut. A follicle is similar to legume, but splits along one side only. Milkweed pods are follicles. The fruits of the columbine and larkspur are also follicles. A capsule is a dehiscent fruit which develops from a compound ovary. The fruit of a lily or an iris is a capsule. The achene is a single seed indehiscent fruit which when mature has the seed from the ovary walls except at the point of attachment. Fruits of the buttercup are achenes; also the fruits of the strawberry, which are the small hard bodies borne on the surface of berry. The achene of the *Compositae* family differs from the others in having the calyx tube coalesced with the ovary wall. A caryopsis or grain is similar to an achene, but has seed coat fused with the pericarp so that the seed cannot be removed from the ovary wall. The fruits of all cereal grasses are cary-opses. The samara is an indehiscent fruit which has a wing. The fruits of the maple and elm tree are samaras.

dry frying. Frying without the use of fat by using an anti-sticking agents of silicone or a vegetable extract.

drying flowers. The procedure for drying fresh flowers is to use equal portions of powdered pumice and yellow cornmeal, or equal portions of borax and yellow cornmeal, with 3 tablespoons of uniodized salt to the above mixture. Place flowers in a pan (lined with oiled paper) with stems sticking up. Add small quanti-ties of the mixture to the bunch of flowers with a tablespoon into and around the petals and allow about 1 week to dry.

drying oils. Vegetable oils, the most common of which is linseed oil, which are easily oxidized in air which assist in producing a paint film. Nutritionally these oils are similar to edible fats, but when polymerized, are toxic. Drying oils have a high proportion of unsat-urated acids. The film develops by: (a) evaporation of solvent; and (b) oxidation of film, enhanced by driers.

The use of drying oils as the sole or main binder in alkyd coatings is steadily decreasing with the advent of water-based late paints. Currently, it is limited to solvent-thinned exterior house paints and some metal paints. The oils are also used in oleoresinous varnishes and in the manufacture of synthetic resins for coating binders, epoxy ester resins, and oil-modified urethane resins. Small amounts are used in printing inks linoleum, putty and caulking compounds, core oils, and hardboard. The best drying oils are those which contain the higher proportions of unsaturated acids, in which oxidation causes polymeriza-tion of the molecules. The drying of an oleoresinous varnish takes place in two stages. Initially, the reducer or solvent evaporates, leaving a continuous film composed of gums and drying oil. The drying oil is then oxidized by exposure, leaving a tough, hard skin. This oxidation is hastened by driers, but the drying oil itself is responsible for the film. The drying powder of oils is measured by their iodine value, as their power of absorbing oxygen from the air is directly proportional to their power of absorbing iodine. Drying oils have typical iodine values above 140, semidry oil above 120, and nondrying oils are below 120. Linseed oil is the most common of the drying oils, though tung oil and oticia oil are faster in drying action. Linseed oil alone will take about 7 days to dry, but can be quickened to a few hours by the addition of driers. Linseed oil and other oils may be altered chemically to increase the drying power.

Conjugated oils are oils that have been altered catalytically by nickel, platinum, palladium, or carbon to give conjugated double bonds in place of isolated double bonds in the molecules of the fatty acids. Conjulinol is a drying oil of this class made from linseed oil. The iodine value is 180, and the drying time is greatly reduced. Normally, soybean oil is not classed as a drying oil although it may be blended with drying oils for paint use. But by chemical alteration and, lately, by mixing with synthetic resins, it can be given good drying power.

Conjusoy is the trade name of a drying oil made by the conjugation of soybean oil. Its iodine value is 128, and the drying time is about one-half that of boiled linseed oil. Castor oil, which has poor drying properties, is dehydrated to form a good drying oil. Other methods are used to alter oils to increase the drying power, notably polymerization of the linoleic acid some other acids in the oils; or notably polymerization of the linoleic and some other acids in the oils; or oils may be fractionated and reblended to increase the percentage of acids that produce drying qualities.

drying potential. The unexpended or unused capacity of a body of air to hold water. The drying potential is represented by the distance from the saturation curve on the line of constant thermodynamic wet-bulb temperature on the psychrometric chart.

drying ratio. A dimensionless number representing the ratio of the weight of wet material entering a dryer to the weight of the same material as the material leaves the dryer at a lower moisture content. The number of pounds of fresh product (vegetable, fruit, or meat) prepared for drying required to produce one pound of acceptable dry product.

drying temperature. The temperature of a product during drying which is related to quality of dried product and rate of drying. Many biological products, pharmaceuticals, foods, seeds, fibers, etc., may be adversely affected by excessive heat treatment which involves a time-temperature exposure of heat, but the limit of exposure is often given by the maximum product temperature reached during drying period. During drying the evaporation of moisture may keep the product cooler than the drying air. The temperature of the product approaches the temperature of the drying air as the product dries.

dulcin. p-phenetylurea, or p-phenetolcarbamide. A sweetening agent which is about 250 times as sweet as sugar. It is used in the amnufacture of toothpastes and cheap candies, though its use is not permitted in foods. Also called sucrol and valzin.

dulcite. See dulcitol.

dulcitol. A six-carbon sugar-alcohol formed by reduction of galactose. It occurs in Madagascar manna (*melampyrum nemorosum*). Also known as dulcite; galacticol; melampyrin.

dulse. Purplish-red edible seaweed eaten raw or cooked.

dun. The brown discolouration caused by mould growth in salted fish.

dunst. Very fine semolina (i.e., starch from the endosperm of the wheat grain) approaching the wheat grain) approaching the fineness of flour. Also called break middlings (not to be confused with middlings which is the branny offal).

duodenum. The first part of the small intestine, between stomach and the jejunum. Pancreatic juice and bile are secreted into the intestine and major part of digestion takes place there.

durum. A grain that has been in existence for much longer than bread wheat, but it is now mostly used as a raw material of pasta. It is not a preferred ingredient for leavened bakery products, because durum flour will not make the extensible, elastic, cohesive doughs necessary for proper functioning of those formulas. Small amounts are used in flat breads mostly in the Middle Eastern countries, but that usage is largely based on economic and traditional considerations rather than on quality factors. The principal use of durum wheat is for the production of semolina to be used as a raw material in pasta, but durum can also be made into flour for bread and this was its major application for thousands of years. It is not nearly as satisfactory as hard or soft wheat for bread-making still accounts for about half for consumption of durum. The doughs will often consist of imported hard wheat flour mixed with a fairly large percentage of locally produced durum flour. Durum flour has a positive value in that it contributes a yellow color in the finished product. Leavening is by sourdough starters. A sponge is prepared by mixing soft wheat flour and hard wheat flour with water and allowing the dough to ferment until the following day. One part of sponge is then mixed with 0.7 parts of durum flour and 1.4 parts of water, and the new sponge is allowed to stand for two hours. To reduce acidity, another dough-up follows in which one part of the previous blend is mixed with 0.5 parts water and 0.9 parts durum flour. After four hours of fermentation, three parts of the final sponge are doughed up with 10 parts of flour, 0.3 part salt, 0.09 part compressed yeast, and eight parts of lukewarm water.

durian. *Durio zibethinus;* tropical fruit with disgusting odour; weighs 2-3 kg; its consumption is restricted largely to south-east Asia.

Duriff grape. A red wine grape grown mainly in France, which somewhat resembles the Syrah

durum wheat. See durum.

Dutch oven. A semi-circular metal shield which may be placed close to an open fire, and is fitted with shelves on which food is roasted. It may also be clamped to the fire bars.

Dyox. Trade name for chlorine dioxide used to treat flour.

dyspepsia. Any pain or discomfort associated with eating. Dyspepsia may be a symptom of gastritis, peptic ulcer, gallbladder disease, etc., or, if there is no structural change in the intestinal tract it is called functional dyspepsia.

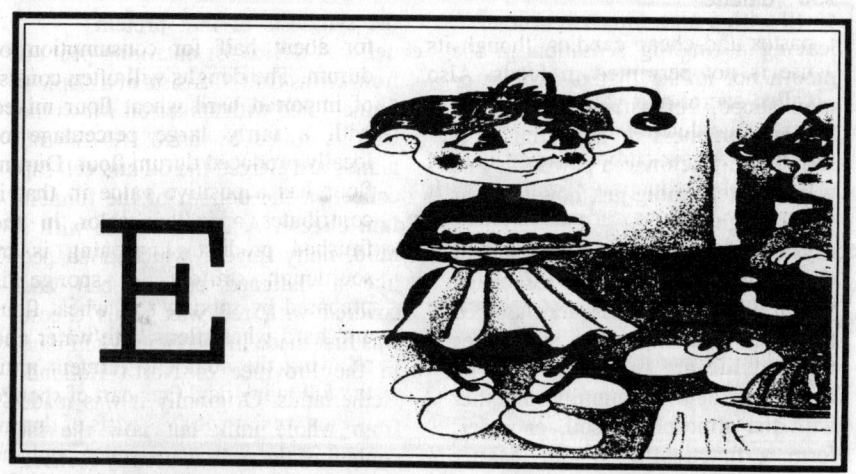

ear corn drying. A method of drying the ear corn involving natural air moving through the ears on piles or narrow open slotted cribs. Ear corn can be stored at a higher moisture content (25%) than shelled corn (13%) without spoilage unless forced air drying is used. Forced natural air and heated air drying of wet ear corn are used to reduced the moisture to a safe level in cribs exceeding 0.5-2 metres width in the major corn growing areas. Distances of air flow in ear corn of 4.5 m provide a static pressure drop of 0.1 to 0.2 pKa. An air flow of 0.065 to 0.13 m^3/m^3s heated to 43.3°C is used for ear corn drying. Moisture must move from the cob as well as the kernel.

Easter pear. A variety of pear *Easter Beurre*. The tree is moderately vigorous, upright, spreading in habit, reasonably productive, fairly susceptible to blight. Although many attempts have been made to grow the variety commercially, it has not received wide acceptance in the marketplace. The name Easter was adopted in England and America. Fruit is medium to large in size. Shape is ovate-pyriform with thick neck. Skin is thick and somewhat tough, deep green in colour, somewhat coarse, gritty, buttery, moderately juicy, fairly sweet, pleasing flavor when properly grown and handled. It usually fails to ripen unless held under refrigeration for several months.

Eau-de-Vie de Miel. Or honey brandy, made by distilling mead (which, in turn, is made by fermenting honey).

echinacea. *Echinacea augustifolia.* Echinacea is a native perennial growing from the prairie states northward to Pennsylvania, but also occurs in the cooler northern regions of some southern states as well. The stout, bristly stems bear hairy, linear-lanceolate leaves, tapering at both ends. Each of the distinctive rich purple flowers feature 12-20 large, spreading, dull-purple rays and a conical disk made up of numerous tubular florets. A weaker species (*E. purpurea*) is often substituted for *E. augustifolia* whenever the latter becomes scarce or too expensive for the herb industry's use. The plant has a faint aromatic smell with a nice, sweetish taste to it, leaving a tingling sensation in the mouth not unlike that of aconite or monkshood, but without the latter's lasting numbness or dangerous poison. Tasting echinacea powder is one way of determining just how fresh or old it might be.

ecosystem. A biological community and the physical environment associated with it. Living organisms are classified as biotic and inorganic substances that aid life are called abiotic. The organisms of a community, together with the atmosphere, soil, or water, form a functioning system. Matter and energy are taken up by the producer organisms from the physical surroundings, and passed from organism to organism through the food chain. Each ecosystem has an input of gases and mineral nutrients from the atmosphere, from the weathering of rocks and from other ecosystems, and input of energy as either light or organic matter or both. Also each ecosystem has an output of gases, and energy to the atmosphere, and often an output of nutrients and organic matters to the other ecosystems as well.

ectendomycorrhizal. A term referring to a mutualistic association between fungi and plant roots in which the fungus surrounds the plant root and also penetrates into the cortex to a limited extent, as found in orchids.

ectomorphy. Description given to a tall, thin individual, possibly with underdeveloped muscles.

ectomycorrhizal. A term referring to the mutualistic association between fungi and plant roots in which the fungus surrounds the root tip with a sheath.

ectopic protein. A protein produced by a neoplasm that is derived from a tissue that is not normally engaged in the synthesis of that protein.

ecuelle. A device for obtaining peel oil from citrus fruit. Consists of a shallow funnel lined with spikes on which the fruit is rolled by hand. As the oil glands are pierced the oil and cell sap collect in the bottom of the funnel.

Edam cheese. A Dutch cheese with a mild, nutty flavour which is shaped like a flattened cannon ball and covered with red wax. This cheese was first made in the vicinity of Edam in the Province of North Holland, Netherlands. Originally it was made from whole milk but now the fat content of the milk is usually reduced to about 2.5%. Pasteurized raw milk of 2.5% fat is normally used. About 1% starter is added to milk at 15°C and the milk is set with rennet. After 15 minutes the curd is cut into cubes and cooked to 25-30°C. The whey is removed until the curd is exposed. Water or weak brine may be added to the curd, which is then placed into hoops for draining and pressing. The cheese may be dry or brine salted. It is washed, dried and turned and usually coloured red. The average composition is: moisture 35-40%; fat 26-30%; salt 1.6-2%. Federal Standard recommends that the moisture should not be more than 45%, and fat should not be less than 40% in the solids.

edaphon. Collective name for the bacteria, fungi, and lower animals living in the soil. They play a vital role in biological decomposition.

eddo. W. Indian name for Taro.

edible oil. Any of the fatty oils obtained from vegetables, nuts, and seeds, commonly used in food products, either as a liquid or in hydrogenated form. They include corn, soybean, olive, safflower, cottonseed, coconut, peanut, and citrus seed oils. These oils are comprised largely of oleic, palmitic, linoleic, and many other fatty acids. Fish and shark liver oils are used as dietary supplements for their vitamin content, while castor oil finds numerous applications. They are also classed as edible oils. Flavoring oils derived from flowers, such as wintergreen, coriander, clove, and citrus peels, are of different chemical composition and are called essential oils, even though they are edible.

edible snail. *See* snail, edible.

Edifas. Trade name; Edifas A - methyl ethyl cellulose; Edifas B - sodium carboxymethylcellulose.

editing enzyme. Enzyme responsible for proof-reading the DNA and correcting errors in replication or following from mutation.

Edosol. Trade name for low-sodium milk substitute. The average composition per 100 g is: protein 30-3%; fat 26.4%; carbohydrates 37.9%; calcium 846 mg; iron 0.6 mg; sodium 43 mg; and food energy 2.1 KJ.

Edwardsiella **sp.** Three species of enterobacteria; one, *E. tarda*, can cause septicemia and possibly diarrhea; present in the intestines of a variety of mammals and reptiles.

effector. A metabolite that, when bound to an allosteric enzyme, alters the catalytic activity of the enzyme. The effector generally alters either the Michaelis constant of the enzyme or the maximum velocity of the reaction. An effector that functions as an activator and leads to an increase in the binding of the substrate and other effectors is known as a positive effector, while an effector that functions as an inhibitor and leads to a decrease in the binding of the substrate and other effectors is known as a negative effector. An effector may likewise bind to a nonenzymatic, allosteric protein and lead to a change in the properties of the protein.

effervescence. The formation of gas bubbles in a liquid as a result of chemical reaction. It occurs during fermentation, during the action of acids upon carbonates, etc. Boiling is not regarded as effervescence, nor is the frothing produced in such actions as that of concentrated sulphuric acid upon sugar.

egg. This term is usually thought of in connection with the eggs deposited by birds, from which the young are hatched, but zoologists apply the term to the reproductive cell from which all animals proceed, except those that are reproduced by cell division. The shell is composed almost of calcium carbonate and has for its purpose the protection of the parts which it encloses. Just within the shell is a thin, tough membrane, which forms the lining. Next to the lining, and surrounding the yolk, is the white, which is composed almost wholly of albumen. The yolk is also enclosed in a thin membrane and is spherical. It is composed of a variety of substances, some of which contain margarine and oleine; its colour is usually yellow. The germinal vesicle, or germ spot, is found within the yolk, and in the eggs of fowls it can be easily distinguished by its pearly-white appearance. It is from this that the young bird or chick is developed by incubation, the yolk and white serving for food during the process. In the large end of the egg there is a space between the lining and shell that is filled with air. As the egg grows old this increases in size. It is supposed by some that the air in this space is used by the chick while it is pecking out of the shell. The germ is developed by heat, which is supplied by the female's sitting on the nest.

The eggs of fowls and most birds require a temperature of 25°C for successful incubation. The period of incubation varies with the species. The number of eggs laid by different birds also varies with the species. Some birds lay only one during the year, and others, as the hen, lay a large number. The robin usually lays four, the swallow from four to six and the crow four, six or seven. In many instances the colour and shape of the egg are closely associated with the habits of nesting. Birds which lay their eggs on the ground without constructing any nest, lay an egg which is rounded at one end and nearly comes to a point at the other. It blown by the wind these eggs roll round in a circle, while if they were oval, like those laid in deep nests, they could easily be blown by the wind these eggs roll round in a circle, while if they were oval, like those laid in deep nests, they could easily be blown away. Eggs laid on the ground, or in nests built on the ground, usually take the colour of the pebbles or dead grass with which they are surrounded, while the bright colours belong to the eggs laid in well-constructed nests. Another peculiarity of the colouring is that the greatest variation is about the large end of the egg.

The economic use of eggs is well known, and the eggs of the hen, the guinea fowl, turkey and domestic duck constitute an important item in the world's supply of food. The eggs of hen are a rich source of the A and B vitamins and of highly assimilable minerals. Of particularly interest in eggs are the strong presence of inositol, choline and lecithin, all involved in cholesterol metabolism. The membrane mixed with the shell of the egg contains avidin, an enzyme which interferes with the biotin in the egg, which is essential for proper cholesterol metabolism. Avidin can be neutralized simply by cooking the egg in hot water 71°C for five minutes, after which it is possible to eat it raw. All the usual methods of cooking also neutralize avidin but the less the egg is cooked the more valuable it is nutritionally. Rubbery, extremely hard-boiled eggs not only make the protein difficult to assimilate but also destroy amino-acids.

All eggs of the same size and age have almost same food value, whether they are white or brown, and whether they have light or dark yolks. Stale eggs have the same nutritional value as fresh, except that the older the egg is the less vitamin B_{12} it contains. Half the folic acid is lost in cooking.

Hens' eggs are graded according to quality and size (European Economic Community). Quality A - fresh, A extra - packed less than 7 days ago, B - less fresh than A, preserved or refrigerated, C - fit for food manufacture only.

Sizes : Grade 1, 70 g and over, then grades 2 to 6 at 5 g intervals, with grade 7 under 45 g.

Microstructure of white and yolk. Yolk has been described as a system of a variety of different kinds of particles suspended in a protein solution. When yolk is separated by high-speed centrifugation, the granules sediment, leaving a clear fluid supernatant called plasma. The plasma constitutes about 78% of the yolk and contains about 49% water, 40% lipid, 1.1% ash, and about 9% other materials (mostly proteins). The granules contain about 44% water, 19% lipids, 34% protein, and 3% ash. Granules are said to be composed of

70% alpha- and beta-lipovitellins, 16% phosvitin (a phosphoprotein), and 12% low-density lipoprotein. Albumen has been described as a protein system of ovomucin fibers in an aqueous solution of numerous kinds of globular proteins. The relative proportions of these two categories of substances determine whether the albumen will be of the thick or thin type. Normally, the white as it exists in the intact egg can be seen to consist of an outer thin white, then proceeding inwardly, thick white, thin white, and chalaciferous layers (thick linear white). The relative proportions of these layers can vary greatly, depending upon numerous factors. The lipids of egg, all of which are located in yolk, are composed of glycerides and phospholipids in a ratio of approximately 2:1. About 30% of the fatty acids in the glycerides are saturated. The phospholipids, which are mainly responsible for the emulsifying properties of yolk, are made up about 60% lecithin, 25% cephalin, and 15% others. There is also a significant amounts of cholesterol in eggs yolk. Fat-soluble carotenoids in the lipid portion of lipoproteins are responsible for the yellow-orange color of yolk. These carotenoids are mostly xanthophylls, with minor amounts of carotenes. The intensity of yellow color in some egg-containing products-cakes, noodles, bread, etc., is regarded by many consumers as a token of richness or nutritional quality. Yolk color is not, however, a reliable measure of the nutrient content of an egg. Eggs with pale yellow yolks can have as high a content of vitamins, proteins, and minerals as eggs with intensely colored yolks. Most food manufacturers prefer to buy egg yolks and whole eggs with uniform color so that their finished products do not vary in appearance. On the other hand, egg noodle producers desire egg yolks and whole eggs with the highest possible color to improve the appearance of their product.

The colour of whole eggs and egg yolks depends to a very great extent on the plant pigments that are in the feed consumed by the chickens. Feed ingredients such as ground yellow corn, corn gluten meal, and alfalfa meal contain significant amounts of lutein, zeaxanthin, and cryptoxanthin, which are absorbed in the hen's digestive tract and then translocated to the ovary for deposition in the yolk as it is forming. The genetic capability of absorbing xanthophylls and depositing them in the yolk varies among individual hens. Also other feed components (particularly fats and antioxidants) and the hen's condition affect the efficiency of pigment translocation. Therefore, colour of the egg products may vary with the season, source, method of processing, and other factors. If the premium for dark yellow yolks is sufficiently high to justify and added cost, the egg producer may add feed supplements that contain large amounts of xanthophylls. Among these supplements are marigold petal meal and dried algae meal. About 0.4% to 0.5% glucose is present in egg albumen, and this represents virtually the entire amount of uncombined carbohydrate in eggs. There is about 0.5% of mannose and glucose (chemically combined with glycoprotein. Yolks may contain as much as 1% of carbohydrate, but this is mostly in combined form, with only 0.2% as free glucose. The small amount of glucose in dried egg white can lead to darkening and the development of off-flavors during storage as a result of the nonenzymatic browning (Maillard) reactions that occur between this reducing sugar and the amino groups of the proteins.

In the manufacture of dried albumen or dried whole egg, glucose is removed either by fermentation (using pure strains of yeast or bacterial) or by enzymatic oxidation using commercial preparation of enzymes. Albumen treated by these techniques is called stabilized. There is some glucose in liquid yolk (about half that in liquid white), but it is less of a storage problem in the dried yolk, as compared to dried white, perhaps because staling or spoilage usually occurs as a result of reactions other than nonenzymatic browning, and the odors, tastes, and colors resulting from these other reactions cover up changes involving glucose. Furthermore, because of the different percentage of solids in the liquid materials, dried yolk contains only about 0.4% glucose versus about 3.2% in dried unstabilized white. Stabilized yolks can be prepared by procedures similar to those used for stabilizing whites. Although egg white is low in vitamin content, except for riboflavin, yolk is a good source of many of these nutrients, particularly vitamins, A, D, E, folic acid, biotin, and choline.

The mineral content of albumen is quite variable, being influenced by the hen's diet and age, as well as environmental factors such as temperature, season, lighting, etc. The main influence, however, is the composition of the feed. Among the elements found are sulfur, potassium, sodium, phosphorus, calcium, magnesium, and iron.

egg drying. Eggs may be dried whole or separated into whites and yolks, which are dried. Whole eggs and yolks are dried in the same manner. Rehydrated eggs have 47% protein and 43% fat. Egg white drying includes:

(a) the removal of the free glucose by yeast, enzyme systems, or bacteria, to prevent the Maillard reaction;

(b) adjusting the pH with a food acid, such as lactic acid and citric acid; and

(c) spray-drying of the liquid egg white in a spray dryer, or tray-drying in a cabinet or tunnel system at 54.4°C.

Egg yolk drying consists of:

(a) pasteurization at 61.7°C for at least 3 minutes;

(b) storing after cooling to 4.4°C, or spray-drying immediately; and

(c) stabilization of yolks with a glucose-oxidase enzyme system.

Whole egg drying is similar to egg yolk drying. Carbohydrate products, such as sucrose and corn syrup solids are often added prior to spray drying to reduce foaming and to minimize emulsifying abilities of liquid eggs. Excessive heat, above 57.2°C, may have an adverse effect on the whipping properties of egg whites. An adverse effect from excessive heat is more likely to occur during tray drying than spray drying.

egg grading. Factors used in determining egg quality are shell, air cell, white and yolk. For eggs with dirty or broken shell, the standard of quality provide three additional qualities, namely, dirty, check, and leaker. Grade AA eggs "stand up" more than the Grade B eggs. The AA eggs are preferred for table use because of their appearance; the B eggs frequently are preferred for cooking. Eggs are labeled according to size and grade. Grade refers to interior quality and to the condition and appearance; the B eggs frequently are preferred for cooking. Eggs are labeled according to size and grade. Grade refers to interior quality and to the condition and appearance of the shell. Neither size nor color of the shell affect the egg quality. In the AA egg, the yolk stands up high and is surrounded by a large proportion of thick white with a very little thin white. Both AA and A eggs are ideal for all purposes, but are especially good for poaching and frying.

egg proteins. Ovalbumin, ovomucin, ovomucoid, ovoglobulin, conalbumin, and vitellin.

egg substitute. Name formerly used for golden raising powder.

egg, dehydrated. The average composition per 100 g is: protein 47%; fat 43%; Ca 186 mg; Fe 9.3 mg; vitamin A 100 μg; vitamin B_1 0.34 mg; vitamin B_2 1.08 mg; nicotinic acid 0.2 mg; and food energy 2.5 MJ.

egg products. Egg products are very susceptible to contamination by microorganisms, including some pathogenic species. These organisms can originate from the egg itself (especially from the egg exterior), from egg handlers, from equipment, from containers, from dispensing utensils, and from the air. If the liquid materials are held at room temperature, proliferation of bacteria or molds can occur very rapidly. Considerable progress has been made over the years in improving the microbiological quality of commercial egg products. Part of the impetus for this improvement has been the establishment of government regulations that require all egg products to be pasteurized or treated so they are rendered Salmonella negative. It is also necessary that all

egg products be inspected by the USDA. In spite of the generally good quality of commercial egg products, it is important to establish and enforce bacteriological standards for egg ingredients used in the bakery. Reasonable standards include maximums of 10,000 viable bacteria per gram in all frozen and dried products except for frozen whites where a limit of 50,000 per gram is more realistic. Yeasts, molds, and coliforms should be restricted to less than ten per gram. There has been much concern about contamination of egg products by Salmonella. This is an organism that can cause food poisoning, rarely fatal. Whole egg and egg yolk can be pasteurized in high temperature-short time equipment with little loss of nutrients, but treatment of albumen in a similar manner leads to deleterious changes in whipping quality. It was discovered that use of additives and modification in conditions of heat treatment greatly reduced the loss of foam-forming ability.

It is generally conceded, however, that treating egg whites to make them Salmonella-free causes some reduction in their response to whipping procedures. There are three general methods for pasteurizing egg products. One method is particularly applicable to whole eggs. It is based on the application of carefully controlled heat for a given time (minimum of 60°C for at least 3.5 minutes). A slight reduction in viscosity of treated product is frequently observed. The hydrogen peroxide-catalase method is more suitable for egg whites. A quantity of hydrogen peroxide solution is added to the egg white, the mixture is heated to within the range 5° to 54°C for 3.5 minutes, the cooled. When the mixture is cool, catalase is added to remove any residual hydrogen peroxide. A slight reduction in viscosity and some white clumps result. The third method is also suitable for egg whites. Aluminum sulfate and lactic acid are added, the eggs are heated at 60°C for at least 3.5 minutes and then cooled. There is a reduction in viscosity, some white clumps appear, and turbidity develops in the liquid phase. The rapidity with which egg white can be whipped to the desired volume, the maximum specific volume of the foam, and the stability of the foam can be improved by certain additives.

It has long been known that lowering the pH improves the functional properties of egg albumin. The type of acid used to accomplish this effect is a factor in the degree of improvement; that is, the anionic portion of the additive as well as the hydrogen ion concentration determines the effectiveness of the acid. Citric acid and lactic acid seem to be the preferred additives. When dry mixes are being formulated, phosphoric acid salts or tartaric acid salts are often used. Surface-active agents also influence whipping properties. Triethyl citrate and various anionic surface-active agents (*e.g.*, some common detergents) are effective. Apparently, these additives act to partially overcome the effects of the traces of yolk as well as to increase the speed of surface denaturation, thus permitting the more rapid formation of a stiff foam.

eggplant. *Solanum melongena.* A bushy vegetable belonging to the same family as the potato. Several varieties are cultivated. In some the fruit has a whitish peel and is the size of a hen's egg; in others it is a deep purple on the outside and attains a diameter of from 15-20 cm. This dark, satiny fruit was first imported from India by Arab merchant caravans centuries ago. The eggplant eventually was introduced to US by Thomas Jefferson, who experimented with seeds and cuttings of many foreign plants. Eggplants can be red, yellow or even white, but the most common kind is purple and pear-shaped. Other varieties include long, oval ones which Japanese refer to as nasubi; small egg-shaped varieties that may help to explain how this vegetable got its name.

egg rolls. The dough wrapped, fried, cylindrical items offered by virtually every Chinese restaurant as appetizers or main courses. The fillings can be combinations of everything that didn't sell as well as expected the day before, or traditional mixtures of shrimp, bean sprouts, etc. The dough is usually a thinly sheeted mixture of flour, water, salt, and perhaps egg white or whole egg. The dough is often bought ready-sheated from a specialty distributor rather than made in the restaurant. The dough mass is extruded into ribbon-like form, aged, then passed through calendering rolls to produce a continuous sheet of pastry material, commonly of 5 cm width. Because of the manner of forming, the grain extends longitudinally of the sheet. This strip is then cut into squares (18 cm each way), stacked with a powdering of cornstarch between, and allowed to age for some time.

egg-white. 87.8% water, 10.8% protein, 0.6% ash. It is composed of outer layer of thin white, layer of thick white, richer in ovomucin, and inner layer of thin white surrounding yolk. Eggs vary in ratio of thick to thin white, depending on the individual hen. Higher percentage of thick white desirable for frying and poaching helps the egg to coagulate into small firm mass instead of spreading); thin white produces larger volume of froth when beaten then does thick. Proteins are ovomucin, ovalbumin, ovomucoid, ovoglobulin and conalbumin.

einkorn. A type of wheat, the wild form of which, *Tricum boeoticum*, was probably one of the ancestors of all cultivated wheat. Still grown in some parts of the world, usually for animal feed. The name Einkorn, "one seed", derives from the single seed found in each spikelet.

elastin. A major component of elastic fibres which can stretch and recoil back to original size. It is also found in connective tissue, like collagen. It is present in the walls of large arteries and also in connective tissue of different tissues. Like collagen elastin synthesis also begins inside the fibroblasts and smooth muscle cells. There is only one genetic type of elastin. However different types can arise from alternative processing of the primary transcript. After peptide synthesis and post translational modifications the peptides are secreted as soluble elastin. Like collagen soluble elastin also has distinctive amino acid composition. It is rich in glycine (about one-third of the residues), proline and non-polar amino acids. However, there is no hydroxylation of proline and lysine unlike collagen. Elastin is very rich in nonpolar aliphatic residues. A single repeating unit -Gly-X-Y- was mentioned in the structure of collagen peptides. In the structure of elastin peptides repeating sequences of tetra (-Gly-Gly-Val-PrO), penta (-Pro-Gly-Val-Gly-Val-) and hexa (-Pro-Gly-Val-Gly-Val-Ala-) peptides have been found. Soluble elastin is secreted by the cells. Maturation occurs by assembly of soluble peptides, organization around microfibrillar proteins (also secreted by the cells which secrete soluble elastin), selective proteolysis, modification of some lysyl residues and cross linking. For cross linking some of the lysine residues under go oxidative deamination to yield a reactive aldehyde. The reaction is catalyzed by a copper dependent lysine oxidase. Aldol condensation and Schiff base reaction yield cross links. These cross links give elasticity to elastic fibres.

elder. *Sambucus nigra.* In springtime, the aroma of the umbrella-like trusses of creamy-white elder flowers scents the hedge rows and country lanes with a sweet aroma one longs to capture. The plant is common throughout Europe, western Asia, and North America, where a related species, *S. canadensis,* American elder, was used as a folk medicine by the American Indians. Elder flowers are traditionally used to flavour fruit compotes, salads, and jellies, and have a particular affinity with gooseberries. The berries - usually blended with apples - can be made into jam, jelly, and other preserves while both flowers and berries create excellent wines. The flowers, blended with lemon and sugar, are used to flavour summer drinks and cordials. Elderberry soup (again, mixed with apples) is a popular Scandinavian dish. Elderflower water is widely used, and sold commercially, as a skin toner and lightener.

elderberry. Family: *Caprifoliaceae.* Genus: *Sambucus.* Species: *Sambucus canadensis or Sambucus nigra.* The elderberries are good source of vitamin A and C, and rich in phosphorus. The fresh flower-heads made a sweet, rather pleasant honey-flavoured tea which is often combined with peppermint and yarrow as a cold cure. They act as a gentle circulatory stimulant with a strong diaphoretic effect and so are very helpful in fever, as an expectorant, and as a mouthwash and gargle for mouth and throat inflammation. When served cold, they make an excellent diuretic. Fresh and frozen flowers are far more effective than dried ones. The berries have been found to be useful for constipation and to dispel flatulence.

electro-analysis. Methods of chemical analysis based on phenomena occurring during electrode reactions and/or flow of current through electrolytic solutions. Many metals present in biological systems, after adequate matrix pretreatment, may be rapidly and accurately determined by depositing them on a weighed cathode and subsequently determining the difference in weight. Concentration may be determined by measuring potentials and conductivities, the end point of a galvanometer in place of an indicator, and concentration of hydrogen ions in acid and bases may be determined electrolytically.

electrocoagulation. The destructive coagulation of tissues by means of a high-frequency electric current concentrated at one point as it passes through them. The technique prevents or reduces haemorrhage and can be used as an alternative to crushing bleeding vessels with artery forceps or to legating such vessels.

electron transfer proteins. The proteins that serve as a donor and acceptor of either electrons or electrons and protons in oxidation-reduction reactions. Six types of electrons transfer proteins have been identified:
(a) flavoproteins,

(b) cytochromes,
(c) iron-sulphur proteins,
(d) cuproproteins,
(e) molybdoproteins, and
(f) proteins containing reducible disulphide groups.

electron transport chain. A sequence of biochemical of oxidation reduction reactions that forms the final stage of aerobic respiration. It results in transfer of electrons or hydrogen atoms derived from Krebs cycle to molecular oxygen, with the formation of water. At the same time it conserves energy in the form of ATP. Chain comprises a series of electron carriers that undergo reversible oxidation-reduction reactions, accepting electrons and the donating them to the next carrier in the chain. In the mitochondria, NADH and $FADH_2$, generated by the Krebs cycle, transfer their electrons to a chain comprising flavin mononucleotide (FMN), coenzyme-Q, and a series of cytochromes. This process is coupled to the formation of ATP at three sites along the chain. The ATP is then carried across the mitochondrial membrane in exchange for ADP. An electron transport chain also occurs in the light reaction of photosynthesis. In aerobic respiration the hydrogen is taken from the NADH formed in the Krebs cycle and transferred through a series of steps from one component to the next (respiratory chain). At these steps electron transfer occurs with oxidation-reduction of cytochromes. The electron transfer involves exchange of electrons between Fe^{2+} and Fe^{3+} in the haem part of the cytochrome. The energy released in these stages is conserved in the formation of ATP by oxidative phosphorylation. Final stage is transfer of electrons to molecular oxygen and reaction with hydrogen ions to form water. From succinate, two molecules of ATP are produced by the sequence. Malate and other acids yield three ATP molecules.

electrophoresis. The movement of electrically charged particles when current is passed through the solution. The electric charge on proteins is sufficient to make them migrate under the influence of current, the rate depending on the type of proteins. Electrophoresis is therefore a useful method for the analytical separation of proteins and can be applied to minute quantities in paper electrophoresis. It is valuable in examination of blood proteins for diagnostic purposes.

electropure process. A method of pasteurizing milk by passing a low-frequency, alternating current.

ELISA. *See* enzyme-linked immunosorbent assay.

Elm family : *Ulmaceae.* There are only about 15 genera in this family of trees and shrubs. Most of the genera have unisexual flowers. The alternate leaves usually have toothed margins, uneven blade bases, and deciduous stipules. Parts of the flower include fused sepals of 4-8 lobes, stamens the same number as sepal lobes, and 1 pistil. The flower has no nectaries and no petals, but does have abundant pollen, that is wind-carried to the pistil's plumose stigmas. A single ovule develops in a superior ovary consisting of 2 fused carpels. Fruit types are a winged samara, drupe, or nutlet. The family includes: *Ulmus* spp. (elms) *Planera abelica* (false sandalwood); *Ulmus glabra* (Scotch elm), *U. parvifolia* (Chinese elm); *U. pumila* (Siberian elm).

elongation cycle. The set of repetitive reactions that occur during the elongation stage of protein synthesis. These reactions are:

(a) attachment of the incoming amino-acyl-tRNA to the aminoacyl site on the ribosome;

(b) peptidyl transferase-catalyzed formation of a peptide bond between the incoming amino acid and the growing polypeptide chain; and

(c) translocase-catalyzed shifting of the peptidyl tRNA from the aminoacyl site to the peptidyl site on the ribosome with a simultaneous shift of the messenger RNA by one codon.

Elvira grape. A variety of grape used for production of white wines.

Embden-Meyerhof-Parnas scheme. The name given to the first series of steps in the breakdown of glucose in the tissues, as far as pyruvic acid, *i.e.*, the glycolytic part as distinct from the subsequent oxidation.

emblic. Berry of the southeast Asian malacca tree, *Emblica officinalis;* similar in appearance to the gooseberry. Also known as Indian gooseberry. It is quite rich source of vitamin C, containing about 600 mg/100 g.

EMIT. Acronym for *Enzyme Multiplied Immunoassay Technique.* A technique which does not involve the separation of bound fraction from free. The antigen is labelled with an enzyme in such a way that the enzyme retains its catalytic activity. When the antigen binds to the antibody the enzyme becomes inhibited, probably by an induced conformational change or by steric hindrance of the enzyme active site. This inhibition is reduced by the presence of free antigen in the test sample competing for the antibody binding sites. The greater is the amount of antigen present, higher is the activity retained, and more intense colour is obtained. Response of the unknown sample is compared with the standard dose of the antigen.

emmer. A variety of wheat known to be consumed more than 8,000 years ago; tetraploid (4 sets of 7 chromosomes). Wild emmer is *triticum dicocoides* and true emmer is *T. dicoccum.* Nowadays it is usually grown for animal feed.

Emprote. Trade name for a dried milk and cereal preparation consumed as beverage. 33% protein.

emulsifying agents. Substances which enable the creation of uniformly blended product (emulsions) from ingredients which, because of fundamental differences in their physical properties. Often cited as examples of two such incompatible substances are oil and water. Frequently mentioned as a successfully emulsified food product is salad dressing (oil and vinegar). The terms emulsifier and stabilizer derives from the fact that a stabilizer effectively assists in preserving an emulsion once created, with the practical result being a food product emulsion that enjoys a long shelf life. Substances such as gums, egg yolk, albumin, casein, soaps, agar, lecithin, glycerol monostearate, alginates, Irish moss, that aid the uniform dispersion of oil in water, i.e., form emulsions like margarine, ice-cream, salad cream etc. Stabilizers maintain these emulsions in a stable form. Emulsifying agents are also used in baking to aid the smooth incorporation of fat into the dough and to keep the crumb soft. Sodium citrate, sodium phosphates and sodium tartrate are used in the manufacture of milk powder, evaporated milk, sterilized cream and processed cheese. An emulsifying agent or stabilizer may perform:

(a) by supplying negatively charged ion for preferential adsorption on the globules;

(b) by surrounding each globule with adsorbed film, as of a protein; or

(c) by coating each globule with a mechanically strong layer of fine solid particles (so-called armor-plated emulsion).

Emulsions stabilized by electric charges on the surface of the globules occur almost exclusively with an aqueous continuous phase. Common examples include carbon black (lipophilic) which emulsifies water in oil; whereas silica (hydrophilic) emulsifies oil in water. Benzene can be emulsified in water by water-soluble sodium oleate; whereas water can be emulsified in benzene by oil-soluble magnesium oleate.

A surface-active emulsifying agent should be neither completely hydrophilic nor completely lipophilic. Some substances (such as sodium oleate) while soluble in water by virtue of its polar group, has in its molecule a large organic and lipophilic group with a high surface energy in an aqueous medium. Molecules arriving at an oil-water surface arrange themselves in a low-energy orientation, with the hydrophilic group in the water and the lipophilic group in the oil. Since molecules do arriving at an oil-water surface arrange themselves in a low-energy orientation, with the hydrophilic group in the water and the lipophilic group in the oil. Since molecules do not migrate spontaneously from low- to high-energy positions, this surface orientation is stable. Sodium oleate molecule acts as a bridge across the oil-water interface, reducing the interfacial energy, and the negative ions thus firmly attached to the surface cause mutual repulsion of the globules of oil. Even in the absence of an electric change, a judicious balance of the hydrophillipophil-balance (HLB) of a molecular structure has made commercially available a large number of effective nonionic emulsifying agents. These do not have harmful physiological effects of either anionic or the cation-active soaps and thus are suitable for use in foods and drugs. According to Bancroft's rule, an agent in which the hydrophilic character predominates will stabilize oil/water emulsions, and one in which the lipophilic character predominates will stabilize water/oil emulsions, an appropriate emulsifying agent can be selected in advance, on the basis of its HLB, for either type of emulsion.

Many emulsions are found in nature, as in the cases of milk, egg-yolk, and crude petroleum. Others are produced artificially, chiefly in the food, pharmaceutical, and cosmetic industries, by means of high-speed stirrers, colloid mills, or homogenizers. It has been found that the stability and other properties of an artificially prepared emulsion are affected by numerous, often apparently trivial, details of operating technique. For example, the order in which ingredients are added, the speed and duration of the process, intermittent or continuous operation of the stirrer or other machine.

Emulsions are sensitive to temperature and to small changes of concentration of the emulsifying agent. Instability can be determined microscopically by periodic measurement of the size-frequency distribution of the globules. An increase in average globules size, or decrease of interfacial area, shows coalescence of the disperse phase. Emulsion breaking is hastened by freezing, heating, aging, centrifuging, and the application of high-potential alternating current.

Generally, manufacturers of food additives have conducted extensive research, not only in the development of emulsifying agents (xanthan gum, for example) will be available in several formats and formulations for specific food product use. The physical and chemical properties of each formulation are adjusted to achieve as practically as possible the desired end viscosity, pseudoplasticity, and other qualities as may be required for puddings, pie fillings, salad dressings, canned potato salad, canned tomato aspic, freeze-thaw stable spoonable dressing, and a host of other products.

Of the over-600 food chemicals listed in the Food Chemicals Codex, emulsifiers, stabilizers, and thickeners are an important and extensive segment. Some of them include: acacia, acetylated monoglycerides, agar, alginic acid, ammonium alginate, calcium alginate, calcium stearate, calcium stearoly-2-lactylate, carrageenan, cholic acid, desoxychloic acid, diacetyl tartaric acid esters of mono- and diglycerides, dioctyl sodium sulphosuccinate, ethyloxylated mono- and diglycerides, gelatin, gibberellic acid and gibberellic plant growth hormones, guar gum, gums and mucilages, hydroxylated lecithin, hydroxypropyl cellulose, karaya gum, lactated mono- and diglycerides, lactylated fatty acid esters of glycerol and propylene glycol, lactylic esters of fatty acids, lecithin, locust bean gum, magnesium stearate, methycellulose, methyl ethylcellulose, mono- and diglycerides, pectins, polyglycerol esters of fatty acids, polysorbate 20, 60, 65, and 80, potassium alginate, tripotassium phosphate, potassium polymetaphosphate, potassium pyrophosphate, propylene glycol alginate, propylene glycol monosterate, sodium alginate, sodium aluminum phosphate, basic, sodium metaphosphate, sodium phosphate (dibasic), sodium phosphate (monobasic), trisodium phosphate, sodium pyrophosphate, sodium stearoyl-2-lactylate, sorbitan monostearate, starches, succinylated monoglycerides, tragacanth, xanthan gum, etc.

emulsin. Mixture of glycosidase enzymes in bitter almond that decompose the glucoside amygdalin, to benzaldehyde, glucose and hydrocyanic acid.

emulsion. An intimate mixture of two immiscible liquids, one being dispersed in the other in the form of fine droplets; e.g., oil and water. They will stay mixed only as long as they are stirred together unless an emulsifying agent is added to stabilize the emulsion.

encapsulated garlic flavors. These are generally spray-dried product containing garlic oil and/or garlic oleoresin or extract encapsulated either in gum acacia or a modified starch. The flavouring strength of these products depends on the manufacturer and range from equal to 10 times stronger than that of garlic powder.

encapsulated onion flavors. Onion oil encapsulated by spray drying in gum acacia or a modified starch is available as flavouring ingredient. The strength of these products depends on the manufacturer and may range from equal to ten times stronger than onion powder.

endive. Family: *Compositae*. Genus: *Cichorium*. Species: *Cichorium endivia*. A good source of vitamins A and C and contains iron, calcium, sodium and phosphorus as well. It is low in calories and have been used to help asthma tuberculosis, gout, diabetes,

hypertension, catarrh, liver ailments, neutritis, acidosis, stomach gas and biliousness. A tea made from the leaves was once drunk as a preventative measure against gallstones. The curly leaves are eaten as a salad; called chicory in US. The average composition per 100 g is: water 95%; protein 1.8%; vitamin A 1,000 µg; and vitamin C 12 mg.

endomorph. Description given to a stocky, fat individual.

endomycorrhizal. A term referring to the mutualistic association of fungi and plant roots in which the fungus penetrates into the root cells and arbuscules and vesicles are formed.

endonuclease. An enzyme that catalyzes the hydrolysis of a nucleic acid at an internal position on polynucleotide chain. Endonucleases may hydrolyze both DNA and RNA, but are more commonly specific (*i.e.*, endo DNase or endo RNase). Hydrolysis leads to the generation of 3'- or 5'-phosphate terminal, depending on the enzyme, and to the production of shorter oligonucleotides of varying lengths.

endopeptidases. Enzymes that split peptide bonds inside the protein molecule; *i.e.*, according to the older nomenclature, they are proteinases, like pepsin, trypsin and chrymotrypsin.

endorphin. One of a group of polypeptides, similar to encephalins, that have analgesic activity and are released in the body in response to injury or other stimuli. They act at the same receptors as the opiate drugs, causing depression of the central nervous system with analgesia and narcosis.

endosperm. The inner and greater part of cereal grains. In wheat comprises about 83% of the grain, mainly starch, and is the source of semolina. It contains about 10% of the thiamine, 35% of the riboflavin. 40% of the nicotinic acid 50% of the pyridoxine and pantothenic acid of the whole grain.

endotoxin estimation. One of the most accurate tests for endotoxins is the in vitro Limulus Amoebocyte Lysate (LAL) assay. The assay is based on the observation that when an endotoxin contacts the clot protein from circulating amoebocytes of Limulus, a gel-clot is formed. The assay kits available today contain calcium, pro-clotting enzyme, and pro-agulogen. The pro-clotting enzyme is activated by bacterial endotoxin and calcium to form active blood clotting enzyme. The active clotting enzyme then catalyzes the cleavage of procoagulogen into polypeptide subunits. The subunits join together by sulphide bonds to form a gel-clot. The protein precipitated by the lysate is determined spectrophotometrically.

endotoxins. The toxic substances formed inside the cells of Gram-negative bacteria, (e.g., *Salmonella*) and released on disintegration of the cell. They are heat stable polysaccharide-protein complexes causing nonspecific effects in their hosts. These are called endotoxins because they are generally cell bound and released in large amounts only when cells lyse. In most cases, endotoxins may be equated with lipopolysaccharide toxin. When injected into an animal, endotoxins cause a variety of physiological effects. Fever is an almost universal symptom, because endotoxin stimulates host cells to release proteins called pyrogens, which affect the temperature-controlling centre of the brain. Some of the main characteristics of the endotoxins are:
(a) heat stable;
(b) toxic only at high doses;
(c) weakly immunogenic; and

(d) usually capable of producing fever, shock, blood coagulation, diarrhea; weakness; and fibrinolysis.

Endotoxins initially activate Hageman factor (blood clotting factor XII), which in turn activates one to four humoral systems: coagulation, complement, fibrinolytic, and kininogen systems. *Compare* exotoxins.

Energen Rolls. Trade name for a light bread roll of wheat flour plus added wheat gluten. The average composition per 100 g is: protein 45%; fat 4%; carbohydrate 45.8%; calcium 46 mg; iron 4-5 mg; and food enrgy 1.63 MJ.

energy conversion factors. The amount of energy available in foodstuffs. When this was expressed in calories the factors were slightly different depending upon whether allowances were made for absorption. With the change to the joule it was recognized that conversion better values become available the following are used; protein 17 kJ/g, fat 37 kJ/g, carbohydrate (as monosaccharide) 16 kJ/g, ethyl alcohol 29 kJ/g.

energy converter. Any element or compound having ability to convert the radiant energy of sunlight into electrical, thermal or chemical energy. Prominent among them are silicon, and tellurium, as well as chlorophyll of plants in photosynthesis.

energy value. A measure of heat energy available by the complete combustion of a stated weight of the food; often expressed in joules per kilogram. It takes no account of the value of the food from any other point of view, or sometimes even of the suitability of the food for use by the human organism.

energy. The ability to do work. Exists in several forms such as chemical energy in fuels and food; kinetic, potential, light and heat energy. It is measured in joules. Total chemical energy in a food, as released in the bomb calorimeter, is gross energy. After allowance is made for the losses in the faeces the remainder is digestible energy. After allowance is made for loss in the urine (e.g., urea from dietary proteins the remainder is metabolisable energy. Finally after allowing for loss by specific dynamic action the remainder is net energy.

Energy expenditure of average adult man: basal 7.1 MJ per day; light work, total 9.7 MJ; medium work 12.6 MJ; heavy work 14.7 MJ.

enfleurage. Method of extracting essential oils from blossoms, by placing them on glass trays covered with purified lard or other fat, which eventually becomes saturated with the oil.

enhancer element. Eukaryotic promoter element that increases the transcriptional efficiency of nearby gene. The first enhancer element discovered was the 72-base pair tandem repeat of SV40 DNA. Deletion of this element, which is located upstream of the CAP site of early viral genes, reduces early gene expression by a factor of at least 100.

enocianina. Desugared grape extract used to colour fruit flavours. Prepared by acid extraction of skins of red grapes; bluish when neutralized, turns red on acidifying.

enolase. Enzyme that catalyses the conversion of 2-phosphoglyceric acid to phospho-enol-pyruvic acid, with the formation of an energy-rich phosphate bond. Important in the breakdown of glucose.

enrichment. A term applied to addition of nutrients of foods, such as addition of vitamins A and D to margarine, extra vitamin C to fruit juices, iodide to table salt, B vitamins to flour and

rice. The terms ennoblement and fortification are also applied to these procedures.

enteric bacteria. Members of the family *Enterobacteriaceae* (Gram-negative, peritrichous or nonmotile, facultatively anaerobic, straight rods with simple nutritional requirements); the term is also used for bacteria that live in the intestinal tract.

enterobiasis. An infection with the members of nematode genus *Enterobius*, usually with *E. Vermicularis.*

enterococci. Streptococci found in the intestinal tract of humans, a subgroup of the fecal steptococci, found in humans and other warm-blooded animals.

enterogastrone. Hormone found in the small intestine which inhibits both motor and secretary activity of the stomach. Its secretion is stimulated by fat, hence fat in the diet inhibits gastric activity.

enterokinase. An ingredient of intestinal juice that activates the trypsinogen and chymotrypsinogen of the pancreatic juice to form trypsin and chymotrypsin, the active enzymes.

enterotoxins. Exotoxin specifically affecting the cells of the intestinal mucosa, causing vomiting and diarrhea. Enterotoxins act on the small intestine, generally causing massive secretion of fluid into the intestinal lumen, leading to symptoms of diarrhea. Enterotoxins are produced by a variety of bacteria including the food-poisoning organisms such as *Staphylococcus aureus, Clostridium perfringens,* and *Bacillus cereus,* and the intestinal pathogens *Vibrio cholerae, Escherichia coli,* and *Salmonella enteritidis.*

entoleter. The machine used to disinfect cereals and other foods. The material is fed to the centre of a high-speed rotating disc carrying studs so that it is thrown against the studs and the impact kills any insects and destroys their eggs.

enzyme. A protein molecule that acts as a catalyst in' biochemical reactions. Each enzyme is specific to a particular reaction or group of similar reactions. Many require the association of certain nonprotein cofactors in order to function. The molecule undergoing reaction (substrate) binds to specific active site on the enzyme molecule to form a short-lived intermediate: this greatly increases (by a factors of up to 10^{20}) the rate at which the reaction proceeds to form the product. Many other molecules may compete for the active site, causing inhibition of the enzyme or even irreversible destruction of its catalytic properties. Enzyme production is governed by a cell's genes. Enzyme activity is further controlled by pH changes, alterations in concentrations of essential cofactors, feedback inhibition by the products of the reaction, and activation by another enzyme, either from a less active form or an inactive precursor (zymogen). Such changes may themselves be under control of hormones or the nervous system.

Enzymes are characterized by their specificity; each initiates a specific chemical reaction, but is of little significance for other reaction. There are four types:
(a) which effect removal of water;
(b) which aid transfer of electrons;
(c) which transfer radicals; and
(d) which act on a single carbon-carbon bond without removal or transfer of radicals.

All enzymes are proteins of high molecular mass ranging from about 10,000 to more than 1,000,000. An enzyme molecule may contain one or more polypeptide chains. Sequence of amino acids within the polypeptide chain is characteristic for each enzyme and is believed to determine the unique three-dimensional conformation in which the chains are folded. This conformation, which is necessary for the activity of the enzyme, is stabilized by interactions of amino acids in different parts of the peptide chains with each other and with the surrounding medium. These interactions are relatively weak and may be disrupted readily by temperature or pH variations, or changes in polarity unfolding of peptide chains and a concomitant loss of enzymatic activity, solubility and other properties characteristic of the native enzyme.

The names of most enzymes terminate in either -ase or -in, for example, rennin, diastase, amylase, phosphatase, cholinesterase, and epimerase. There are six classes of enzymes, namely:
(a) oxidoreductases, which catalyze oxidation-reduction reactions;
(b) transferases, which catalyze group transfer reactions;
(c) hydrolases, which catalyze bond cleavage by hydrolysis;
(d) lyases, which catalyze removal of a group, leaving a double bond;
(e) isomerases, which catalyzes the formation of isomers; and
(f) ligases, or synthetases, which catalyze the combination of two molecules with the concomitant hydrolysis of a high-energy bond (e.g., in ATP).

Enzymes are similar to proteins in their chemical nature and often are closely associated with them (coenzymes). An example is ribonuclease, composed of 124 amino acids arranged in a specific sequence and having four disulphide cross-links.

enzyme classification. The systematic arrangement and the naming of enzymes that is based on the 1972 recommendations of the Enzyme Commission of the International Union of Biochemistry. Each enzyme is denoted by a number composed four figures.

First figure denotes one of six main divisions: oxido-reductases, transferases, hydrolases, lyases, isomerases, ligases.

Second figure denotes the subclass and the third figure denotes the subsubclass.

The last figure denotes the serial number of the enzyme in its subsubclass.

enzyme I. A soluble bacterial enzyme that is part of the phosphotransferase system for the transport of sugars across the cell membrane. The enzyme catalyzes the reaction: P-enolpyruvate + HPr = pyruvate + P-HPr, where, HPr is a heat-stable, low molecular mass protein, and P designates phosphate.

enzyme II. A membrane-bound bacterial enzyme that is part of the phosphotransferase system for the transport of sugars across the cell membrane. The enzyme catalyzes the reaction: P-HPr + sugar = sugar-P + HPr; where HPr is heat-stable, low molecular mass protein, and P designates phosphate. The enzyme is responsible for the specificity of the transport with respect to the sugar and functions in some systems in conjunction with another protein (factor III).

enzyme induction. Synthesis of an enzyme by a bacterial cell in response to the presence of its substrate or some other inducing agent. This property of bacterial cells is engineered by a special gene regulatory mechanism, with a number of different enzymes often being coordinately produced in response to one inducer. Also known as adaptive enzyme synthesis.

enzyme inhibition. The prevention of an enzymic process as a result of the interaction of some substance with an enzyme so as to decrease the rate of the enzymic reaction. Enzyme inhibition are important as chemotherapeutic agents, as regulator in normal control of enzymic processes in living organisms, and as useful agents in the study of biochemistry.

enzyme labeling. A method for locating antigens or antibodies in tissues; based on binding the antigen or the antibody to an enzyme and then determining the location of the enzyme in the tissues by making use of the known properties of the enzyme.

enzyme-linked immunosorbent assay. ELISA. A very sensitive technique used to detect small quantities of specific proteins by antigenic means. A colorimetric reaction, often based on a peroxidase-conjugated antibody used to bind the protein, provides easy quantization of the results. The technique enables rapid analysis of multiple samples and is now used for the diagnosis of many animal diseases. Firstly, the antibody or antigen is absorbed onto a solid substrate, such as a plastic multi-wall plate. A solution of test material (*e.g.,* infected tissue or serum) is then allowed to interact with the adsorbed reagent. Any matching antigens and antibodies will form complexes, which adhere to the substrate; any uncomplexed material is washed away. An indicator is then put on the plate; this is either a second antibody to the antigen in the test material, or an antispecies antibody prepared against the antibody in the test material. the indicator has previously been conjugated to an enzyme; this causes a colour change in a fourth reagent, which is placed on the plate. The colour change is assessed either by eye or spectrophotometer, and its intensity indicates the presence and even concentration of antibody or antigen in the test material.

enzyme repression. The process where by synthesis of a repressible enzyme is decreased in response to either a repressor or a repressor-corepressor complex. The repressor or the repressor-corepressor complex binds to and blocks an operator and thereby prevents the transcription of the structural gene of the enzyme which is controlled by that operator.

enzyme unit. The amount of enzyme which, under specified conditions, will catalyze the transformation of one mole of substrate/minute, or, where more than one bond of each substrate molecule is attacked; one eq of the group concerned/minute.

epidemiology. The science concerned with the study of factors determining and influencing the frequency and distribution of disease, injury, and other health-related events and their causes in a defined human population for the purpose of establishing programs to prevent and control their development and spread.

epidermis. The outermost layer of cells on the primary plant body, and it constitutes the dermal tissue system of floral parts, fruits, and seeds, and of stems and roots until they undergo considerable secondary growth. Both functionally and structurally the epidermal cells are quite variable. In addition to the ordinary epidermal cells, which form the bulk of the epidermis, the epidermis may contain *stomata* many types of appendages, or *trichomes* and other kinds of cells

specialized for specific functions.

In most plants, the epidermis is only one layer of cells in thickness. However, in some plants, divisions in the protoderm of the leaf are parallel with the surface (periclinal divisions) and an epidermis with several layers (a multiple epidermis) is formed. Multiple epidermises are found in the leaves of such familiar house plants as the rubber plant and *Paperomia*. The multiple epidermis is believed to serve as a water-storage tissue. The main mass of epidermal cells is closely knit and affords considerable mechanical protection to the plant part. In order to minimize water loss, the walls of the epidermal cells of the aerial parts contain cutin and are covered with a cuticle. The cuticle may also be covered with wax, either in smooth sheets or as rods or filaments extending upward from the surface. It is this wax that is responsible for the whitish or bluish "bloom" on leaves. Interspersed among the flat, tightly packed epidermal cells are specialized cells filled with chloroplasts. These are the guard cells, which regulate the small openings, or stomata, in the leaf or young stem. (At one time the term stoma, the singular of stomata, was used to refer exclusively to the pore encompassed by a pair of guard cells. Today it is commonly used to refer to the entire stomatal apparatus: the guard cells plus pore between them). In order for photosynthesis to take place in the chloroplasts of the leaf or stem, carbon dioxide must be permitted to diffuse into the leaf or stem and oxygen must be allowed to pass out. But in the course of this exchange of gases, water is lost by evaporation from the moist interior surface of the leaf or stem. If the guard cells are turgid (bulging with water), they pull apart, permitting the stomata to open and gases to be exchanged freely. In responsible to a decrease in moisture, the guard cells relax, closing the stomata and conserving the plant's water supply. The ordinary epidermal cells of the leaf, like those of the stem, are compactly arranged and covered with a cuticle that reduces water loss. In leaves of hydrophytes that float on the surface of the water, stomata may occur in the upper epidermis only the immersed leaves usually lack stomata entirely. The leaves of xerophytes generally contain greater numbers of stomata there those of other plants. Presumably these numerous stomata permit a higher rate of gas exchange under conditions of favorable water supply.

In many xerophytes, the stomata are sunken in depressions on the lower surface of the leaf. The depression may also contain many epidermal hairs. Epidermal hairs, or trichomes, may occur on either or both surfaces of a leaf. Thick coats of epidermal hairs may retard water loss from leaves. In the leaves of dicotyledons, the stomata are scattered and randomly arranged, and their development is mixed-that is, mature and immature stomata occur side by side. In monocotyledons, the stomata are arranged in rows parallel with the long axis of the leaf. The development begins at the tips of the leaves and progresses downward.

epilithic microorganisms. The aquatic microorganisms which are associated with inanimate particulate materials in the water columns as well as on the surface of the water. This type of association is apparently more beneficial to bacteria than to other microbes. These bacteria are present at the interface between a particle and the water. The other major interface in the aquatic environment is between the water surface and the atmosphere. Organisms located at interfaces have a greater chance of survival, since the nutrient concentration is many times that found in the water column.

epiphytic bacteria. Bacteria that exist in association with plants or algae. Epiphytic bacteria have the subject of numerous studies designed to determine the exact relationships between these organisms. It is to the benefit of both the algae and the bacteria that such associations occur.

epizooic bacteria. The bacteria that exist in association with zooplankton or other aquatic animals. It is believed that in an association between bacteria and zoo-plankton the host derives the benefit of a convenient source of vitamins and other growth factors.

equilibrium humidity. See equiiibrium moisture.

equilibrium moisture. A condition or state of relationship of moisture in a product and its surroundings. A product is in moisture equilibrium with its environment when the rate of moisture loss from the product to the surrounding atmosphere is equal to the rate of gain of the product from the surrounding atmosphere. The atmospheric conditions are described by the temperature and relative humidity or absolute humidity. The moisture content of the product when the product is in equilibrium with the surrounding atmosphere is known as the equilibrium moisture content or hygroscopic equilibrium. The relative humidity of surrounding atmosphere at the same condition is the equilibrium relative humidity at particular temperature. Equilibrium moisture content values may be determined in an air stream and identified as dynamic equilibrium moisture content, or in a closed container and identified as static equilibrium moisture content. The graphical plots of equilibrium moisture and equilibrium moisture content are called isotherms.

eremosphaera. One of the largest group of unicellular green algae, large enough to be seen with the naked eye. It is found in acid water at the bottom of swamps and ponds. Each cell contains pyrenoid-bearing chloroplasts and a single large nucleus suspended in the centre of the cell by numerous radiating strands of cytoplasm. *Eremosphaera* reproduces by both asexual and sexual means. The former is similar to that in Chlorella. Sexual reproduction involves the union of biflagellated sperms with nonmotile cells that function as eggs. As in Chlamydomonas, meiosis is zygotic. Hydrodictyon, the water net, is an example of a nonmotile colony. Under favourable conditions it accumulates in massive aggregates in ponds, lakes, and gentle streams. Each colony consists of many cylindrical cells arranged in the form of a large hollow cylinder. Initially uninucleate, each cell eventually becomes multinucleate. At maturity the cell contains a large central vacuole and peripheral cytoplasm in which the nuclei and a large reticulate chloroplast with numerous pyrenoids are located. The hydrodictyon reproduces asexually through the formation of uninucleate, biflagellated zoospores. Eventually, the zoospores form groups of four to nine, typically six, within the cylindrical parent cell; lose their flagella; and form daughter colonies. Sexual reproduction in Hydrodictyon is isogamous, and its meiosis is zygotic.

erepsin. Name given to a mixture of enzymes contained in the intestinal juice, including amino-peptidases and dipeptidases.

ergot. Fungus that grows on grasses and cereal grains; the ergot of medical importance is *Claviceps purpurea* that grows on rye. The consumption of infected rye is harmful, causing the disease known as St. Anthony's fibre, and can be fatal. The active ingradients in ergot are alkaloids, ergotoxine, ergotamine, ergometrine, etc. Hydrolysis of all these forms lysergic acid, which is believed to be active components. Its effect is to increase tone and contraction of smooth muscle, particularly of the pregnant uterus. For this reason, ergot is used in obstetrics, but ergonovine maleate and ergotonine tartrate are preferable.

Although ergot seldom causes serious damage to the crop of rye, it is dangerous because a small amount mixed with rye grains is enough to cause severe illness among domestic animals or among the people who eat bread made with the flour. Ergotism, the toxic condition caused by eating grain infected with ergot, is often accompanied by gangrene, nervous spasms, psychotic delusions, and convulsions.

ergotism. See ergot.

Eriwani cheese. A kind of cheese made from sheep's milk in the Caucasus. Fresh milk is set at about 35°C, with enough rennet to coagulate it in 20 minutes. The curd is broken up and the whole is put in a sack, allowed to drain, and then pressed with stones until the whey stops running. The cheese is salted in brine.

erucic acid. Unsaturated fatty acid with one double bond at C_9 position, $C_{21}H_{41}COOH$, comprising 30-50% of various varieties of rapeseed oil; small amounts in other vegetable and marine oils. It has been found to cause the fatty infiltration of heart muscle of experimental animals and other changes. It is generally accepted that limited amounts of hardened rape seed oil may be tolerated in margarines.

erythropoiesis. Development of the red blood cells; takes place in the bone marrow.

erythroprotein. A protein hormone, produced by the kidney, that stimulates the production of additional red blood cells in response to low oxygen tension in the blood. Androgens also stimulate erythroprotein production.

erythrosine BS. Red colour permitted in foods in most countries. Disodium or potassium salt of 2,4,5,7-tetraiodofluorescein. It is used in preserved cherries, sausage and meat light and heat. In US, it is called Red No. 3.

erythrosine. FD&C Red #3. Disodium salt of 9-o-carboxyphenyl-6-hydroxy-2,4,5,7-tetraiodo-3-isoxanthone. It is a brown powder, which is soluble in water (9 % at 25°C) to give a cherry-red solution. It is readily soluble in glycols and glycerol (20% at 25°) and in ethanol (95%), giving a solution that has a slight fluorescence. Erythrosine is only fairly light-resistant. It is insoluble in acid media, hence its use is limited.

erythrotin. Obsolete name for vitamin B_{12}.

escalopes. Thin pieces of meat or fish.

Escherichia. Members of the genus *Escherichia* are almost universal inhabitants of the intestinal tract of the humans and warm-blooded animals, although they are by no means the dominant organisms in these habitats. *Escherichia* may play a nutritional role in the intestinal tract by synthesizing vitamins, particularly vitamin K. As a facultative aerobe, this organism probably also helps consume oxygen, thus rendering the large intestine anaerobic. The wild-type *Escherichia* strains rarely show any growth-factor requirements and are able to grow on a wide variety of carbon and energy sources such as sugars, amino acids, organic acids, and so on.

Some strains of *Escherichia* are pathogenic. The latter strains of *Escherichia* have been implicated in diarrhea in infants, occasionally occurring in epidemic proportions in children's nurseries or obstetric wards, and *Escherichia* may also cause urinary tract infections in older persons or in those whose resistance has been lowered by surgical treatment or by exposure to ionizing radiation. Entero-pathogenic strains of *E. coli* are becoming more frequently implicated in dysentery and generalized fevers.

essential amino acid. An amino acid that an organism is unable to synthesize in sufficient quantities. It must therefore be present in the diet. In man the essential amino acids are arginine, histidine, lysine, threonine, methionine, isoleucine, leucine, valine, phenylalanine, and tryptophan.

essential element. Any of a number of elements required by living organisms to ensure normal growth, development, and maintenance. Apart from the elements present in the organic compounds (C, H, N, O), the plants, animals, and microorganisms all require a range of elements in inorganic forms in varying amounts. The major elements, present in tissues in relatively large amounts (greater then 0.005%) are Ca, P, K, Na, Cl, S, and Mg. The trace elements occur at much lower concentrations, the most important of which are Fe, Mn, Zn, Cu, I, Co, Se, Mo, Cr, and Si.

essential enzyme. An enzyme without which a cell or an organism cannot grow or survive.

essential fatty acid. One of a group of long-chain fatty acid that must be supplied in the diet of all humans as well as animals. They contain two or more double bonds, and each double bond is separated by a single methylene group, *i.e.,* the double bonds are not conjugated. This confers important fluid properties on the membranes of animal cells. They are arachionic acid ($C_{19}H_{31}COOH$), linoleic acid ($C_{17}H_{31}COOH$) and linolenic acid ($C_{17}H_{29}COOH$). Only linoleic acid is actually required in the diet, since the other two can be synthesized form dietary precursors. All are crucial for fat metabolism and membrane structure since they are important constituents of glycerides and phospholipids. Deficiency in animals causes restriction of growth, abnormalities of skin and hair, damage to reproductive system, and abnormal composition of serum and tissue fatty acids. The need for EFA for man is not established (there are claims that babies suffer skin disorders in their absence). It has been claimed that a high dietary level of these unsaturated fatty acids lowers blood cholesterol levels and may therefore be beneficial in atherosclerosis. EFA are poorly distributed in animal fats and occur mainly in vegetable oils especially safflower, sunflower and corn oils, hence the use of these oils in diets sometimes recommended for the treatment of antherosclerosis.

essential oils. The volatile, odorous oils derived from plants. Most of these oils, chemically, are principally terpenes (hydrocarbons), but other types also occur. Essential oils, except for those containing esters, are not saponifiable. Some are almost pure compounds, for example, wintergreen oil (methyl salicylate). In cases of the type, the synthetic flavouring, depending upon quality control over purity, will be essentially identical with the natural flavouring. Many other essential oils, are mixtures of a number of chemical compounds, but generally in consistent proportional amounts so that, from a flavouring standpoint, the oil is a single substance. Most essential oils contain relatively sensitive organic components from a temperature standpoint. This thermal sensitivity, coupled with relatively high boiling points, makes separation of the oils from the plant raw materials somewhat difficult. Ordinary distillation cannot be used in majority of cases because of thermal sensitivity. High temperatures required for distillation degrade some and destroy other organic constituents that contribute to the various flavoring notes desired. Prior to distillation, the plant materials are dried in most cases, and some are subject to fermentation. Prior to separation procedures, the dried materials are ground so that a maximum of surface area is exposed.

ester. Any of the various compounds formed as a result of the chemical reaction between an organic acid and alcohol, *e.g.,* ethyl alcohol and acetic acid yield ethyl acetate, which is an ester. All esters have characteristic formula ArCOOR, or RCOOR, where R represents an alkyl group, and Ar an aryl group, that is, where R is a univalent straight-chain hydrocarbon having the formula C_nH_{2n+1}, and Ar is a univalent benzene ring C_6H_5.

The esters occur naturally in vegetable and animal oils and fats as combinations of acids with the alcohol glycerine. The natural fats are usually mixtures of esters of many acids, coconut oil having no less than 14 acids. Stearic, oleic, palmitic, and linoleic acid esters are the common bases for most vegetable and animal fats, and the esters of the other acids such as linolenic, capric, and arachidic give the peculiar characteristics of the particular fat, although the physical characteristics and melting points may be governed by the basic esters. Esters occur also in waxes, the vegetable waxes being usually found on the outside of leaves and fruits to protect them from loss of water. The waxes differ from the fats in that they are combinations of monacids with monohydric, or simple, alcohols, rather than with glycerine. They are harder than fats and have higher melting points. Esters of still lower molecular masses are also widely distributed in the essential oils of plants where they give the characteristic odours and tastes.

In the esters of low molecular mass which make the odours and flavours, the combination of different alcohols with the same acid yields oils of different flavour. Thus methyl acetate, CH_3COOCH_3 is known as peppermint oil; amyl acetate, $CH_3COOC_5H_{11}$ is known as banana oil; and isoamyl acetate, $CH_3COO(CH_2)_3(CH_3)_2$ is known as pear oil. Esters are used as solvents, flavours, perfumes, waxes, oils, fats, fatty acids, pharmaceuticals, and in the manufacture of soaps and many chemicals. Ester liquid lubricants have good heat and oxidation resistance at high temperatures and good fluidity at low temperatures.

esterases. Name given to a group of enzymes that attack simple esters rather than fats; they may be of low specificity as esterase itself, which attacks all simple esters, or of more specific nature e.g., choline esterase.

ethylene. $H_2C=CH_2$. A gas of much interest because of its use in assisting the ripening of fruits. For example, 0.4% ethylene accelerates ripening of pears; 0.5% will convert green lemons to yellow in one week at 30-40°C. In recent years, increasing attention has been paid to other natural substances that accelerate abscission. Ethylene is one such compound, that affects fruit ripening. It leaves, ethylene presumably triggers the enzymes that bring about the changes associated with abscission. Moreover, ethylene is produced when an unknown senescence factor, different from abscisic acid, is released from the cells of the leaf after protein synthesis in them is depressed by abscisic acid. Ripening in fruit involves a number of changes. In fleshy fruits, chlorophyll is degraded, and other pigments may form, changing the fruit color. Simultaneously, the fleshy part of the fruit softens. This is due to the enzymatic digestion of pectin, the principal component of the middle lamella is weakened, cells are able to slip past one another. During this same period, starches and organic acids or, as in the case of avocado, oils, are metabolized into sugars. As a consequence of these changes, fruits become conspicuous and palatable and thus attractive to animals that eat the fruit and so scatter the seed. During the time of ripening of many fruits, there is a larger increase in cellular respiration, evidence by an increased uptake of oxygen. This phase is known as the climacteric. The relationship between the climacteric and the other events of fruit ripening is not known, but the ripening of fruits can be suppressed by suppressing the intensity of the climacteric. For example, cold suppresses it, and in some fruits, cold stops the climacteric permanently. Fruits can be stored for very long periods in vacuum; under such conditions, amount of available oxygen is almost negligible, which suppresses respiration; and ethylene speeds the onset of the climacteric.. After the climacteric, senescence sets in, and the fruit becomes susceptible to invasions by fungi and other microorganisms.

Auxin, at certain concentrations, causes a burst of ethylene production in some parts of some plants. It is believed that some of the effects on fruits and flowers once attributed to auxin are related to auxin's effects on ethylene production. In addition to its effects on fruit ripening, ethylene causes leaves to abscise, chlorophyll to blanche, flowers to fade, and the petioles of seedlings to grow more rapidly on the upper side and therefore curve downward. This effect, which is known as epinasty, is so specific that it is used as a test for ethylene.

Ethylene is also responsible for a host of other effects that may or may not have anything to do with the growth of the plant under normal conditions. In some plants, ethylene has been shown to cause a lateral expansion (in contrast to the usual elongation) of the cell, apparently by changing the orientation of the microfibrils.

ethylenediamine tetra-acetic acid. EDTA. An organic compound which forms stable complexes with a number of metals, hence called sequestering agent or chelating agent. It has been suggested to use EDTA in foods to sequester traces of harmful metallic impurities that cause spoilage, and to inhibit certain bacteria; its use is not permitted in UK It inhibits the oxidation of vitamin C by trapping the copper that may be present (in acid solution); prevents off-flavours in canned fruits; prevents blackening of asparagus, cauliflowers and potatoes; aids prevention of struvite formation in canned seafood.

eubacteria. The large majority of bacteria that have cell wall peptidoglycan containing muramic acid (or are related to such bacteria) and membrane lipids with ester-linked straight chain fatty acids.

eucarytoic cells. The cells which have a membrane-delimited nucleus and differ in many other ways from prokaryotic cells; protists, algae, fungi, plants, and animals are eucaryotic. It appears that the eucaryotic cells arose from the prokaryotes about 1.4 million years ago.

euglobulin. The name given to that fraction of serum globulin which is precipitated by dialysis of blood serum against the distilled water. The name implies that this fraction is a typical globulin by reason of its insolubility in water.

Euler's yeast coenzyme. Nicotinamide adenine dinucleotide.

Eureka lemon. A juicy variety of lemon, whose tree tends to be medium in size, more open in growth habit, and more sparsely foliated than the Lisbon tree. Also, there are fewer and smaller thorns with some virtually thornless trees. In comparison to the Lisbon variety, the leaves are darker in colour and less sharply pointed. Leaf margins are somewhat more scalloped or crenated. In coastal areas, the Eureka tends to be more ever-bearing and to produce fruit in terminal clusters. Eureka lemon fruit is elliptical to oblong, sometimes egg-shaped, and commonly with a short neck. The blossom end or nipple is usually short, but sometimes long and often surrounded by an indentation or slight furrow. The medium-thick rind has a rugose (corrugated) texture, often slightly ridged longitudinally. The surface may be finely pitted with sunken oil glands. When mature, the fruit is a true lemon-yellow. Segments number about 10 and the seed count is variable, ranging commonly from a few to occasionally none. The quality of the juice is very acid, but with a good fresh lemon flavor. In desert locations, Eureka lemon is rougher in texture, with a more prominent ribbed surface and smaller flatter nipples. Eureka lemon comprises much of the lemon crop of Israel and the Eureka is planted in a number of other countries, including Argentina (near Tucuman) and Australia.

eutectic ice. The solid formed when a mixture of 76.7% water and 23.3% salt (by weight) is frozen. It melts at 21°C; 3 kg eutectic ice has the refrigeration effect equivalent to 1 kg solid carbon dioxide; particularly useful in icing fish and other sea foods.

evaporation. In the food technology, evaporation refers to the removal of solvent (usually water) from a solution or slurry. Compared with other related unit food processing operations, evaporation is the vaporization of a portion of a solvent (water) in which a solute or solid is present. Distillation is another form of evaporation in which the vaporization of one liquid from another liquid occurs. Sublimation is the vaporazition of a solid from other solids and its subsequent condensation, a situation that occurs during freeze-drying. Drying is the removal of a liquid from a solid generally by vaporization. All of these

processes are related because the common principles associated with vaporization must be present. Even with the entry of comparatively recent liquid food concentrating operations, such as freeze-concentrating, reverse osmosis, and ultrafiltration, as well as improvements in drying technology, evaporating remains the primary method for removing water from various food substances.

evaporation, flash. A short, rapid application of heat so that a small volume (about 1%) is quickly distilled off carrying with it the greater part of the volatiles. The flash distilled is collected separately from the later distillate and added back to the concentrate to restore the flavour; applied to products such as fruit juices.

evaporative efficiency. The amount of evaporation of water (liquid) which occurs in a direct dryer or evaporator compared to the amount of evaporation if the leaving air is saturated adiabatically.

evaporative limit. The maximum amount of moisture that can be evaporated adiabatically by a mass of moist air. The amount of moisture is proportional to the distance from the saturation curve along a line of thermodynamic wet-bulb temperature, which relates to the ability of air to dry and carry away moisture.

evaporator. A device for concentrating a solution or solid-liquid mixture by boiling. The temperature difference for evaporation is usually taken as the difference between the saturated temperature of the stream (neglecting superheating and sub-cooling) in the steam space and the temperature of the boiling liquid in equilibrium with vapor at the pressure of vapor-liquid. The evaporator usually refers to a vacuum pan or boiler for food or other heat sensitive products. Present literature, usually refers to the latter example as dehydrator or dryer. The evaporator is often used to remove bulk (50-80%) of the moisture in the product preceding dryer operation.

evian water. Non-gaseous, slightly mineralized; diuretic.

excretion. The process by which excess, waste, or harmful materials, resulting from the chemical reactions that occur within the cells of living organisms, are eliminated from the body. The main excretory products in animals are water, carbon dioxide, salts, and nitrogenous compounds: in unicellular or simple multicellular animals these substances are excreted by diffusion through the cell/body surface, but in more complex animals excretion occurs largely from special organs. In man and other vertebrates the main excretory organs are the kidneys: they eliminate excess water, salts, and nitrogenous compounds as urine. In addition, the lungs excrete carbon dioxide and water from respiration; the liver excretes bile pigments derived from the breakdown of hemoglobin, and small amounts of water, sodium chloride, and urea are lost from the skin in sweat. In invertebrates, the excretory organs include Malpighian tubules (of arthropod) and nephridia (of many invertebrates).

exhaust oven. A unique method of drying using the exhaust gases from a tractor engine. The unit consists of an open-ended cylinder which contains a sample and is dried with the exhaust gases. A scale is used to determine the weight of the sample before and after drying. The temperature of the sample is controlled at 140°C by adjusting the engine speed. The sample is turned about once each minute to prevent burning. About 6

minutes are needed to dry a sample of grass having 15% moisture and 10 minutes to dry a sample of oats at 27% moisture level.

exocellular enzyme. An enzyme that may readily be isolated from association with living cells, e.g., pepsin, maltase, zymase. Also known as extracellular enzyme.

exonuclease. Any enzyme which catalyzes the sequential hydrolysis of nucleotides from one end of the polynucleotide strand. The exonucleases may hydrolyze both DNA and RNA, but are more commonly specific (i.e., exoDNase or exoRNase). They usually lead to production of single nucleotides and are described as 3'-5' or 5'-3' depending on the direction of hydrolysis.

exopeptidase. An enzyme that catalyzes the sequential hydrolysis of amino acids from one end of the polypeptide chain.

exopeptidases. Enzymes the split peptide bonds near the terminal units, i.e., at the ends of the protein chain. According to the older nomenclature they were peptidases, such as aminopeptidase, carboxypeptidase and dipeptidases of the digestive juices.

exosome. A genetic fragment that is transferred to recipient cell in bacterial transformation and that is not readily integrated in recipient chromosome but can remain unintegarated and can replicate, be transcribed, and express biochemical function in this state.

exotoxins. A diverse set of extremely powerful poisons; as a group, they can affect a wide variety of different cellular structures and functions although each generally has a specific action. Exotoxins are heat-labile, toxic protein produced by bacteria as a result of their normal metabolism or because of the acquisition of plasmid

264 expeller cake

or prophage that redirects its metabolism. They usually released into the bacterium's surroundings. Generally, exotoxins are carried from the point of infection to other parts of the body where they can cause considerable damage. In case of botulism poisoning, ingestion of minute amounts of toxin is sufficient to cause paralysis that characterizes the disease.

expeller cake. The cake obtained after removal of most of the oil by pressing the oilseeds (cotton, coconut, groundnut, sunflower, sesame, etc.); it is a valuable source of protein.

extraction rate. A term referring to the yield of flour obtained from wheat in the milling process. 100% extraction (or straight-run flour) is whole-meal flour containing all of the grain; lower extraction rates are the whiter flours from which more of the bran and the germ are excluded, as low as 72% extraction which is the normal white flour of commerce. "Patent" flours are of lower extraction rate, 30-50%, and

so comprise mostly the endosperm of the grain. The average composition per 100 g for 72% extraction is: protein 8-12.5%; fibre 0.1-0.2%; vitamin B_1 0.1 mg; vitamin B_2 0.06 mg; nicotinic acid 0.8 mg; and iron 1.5 mg. For 80% extraction, the average composition per 100 g is: protein 9-12.5%; fibre 0.2-0.3%; vitamin B_1 0.25 mg; vitamin B_2 0.07 mg; nicotinic acid 1.6 mg; and iron 1.7 mg. For 100% extraction (wholemeal) the average composition per 100 g is: protein 10-14%; fibre 1.5-2.0%; vitamin B_1 0.4 mg; vitamin B_2 0.13 mg; nicotinic acid 5.5 mg; and iron 3.0 mg. 70-72 % extraction flour is now fortified to be equivalent to 80% flour and must contain not less than 0.24 mg vitamin B_1; 1.6 mg nicotinic acid; and 1.65 mg iron per 100 g flour. Sometimes it may be fortified with *creta praeparata* (chalk).

E-Z cheez. A kind of spray-dried bakers' cheese used in the preparation of cakes and other pastries. Aalso known as Whitson's cheese.

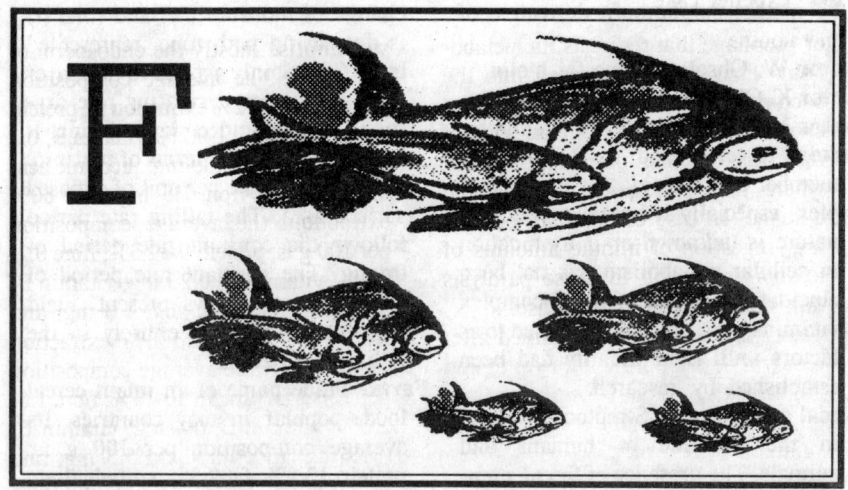

F factor. Fertility factor; a plasmid that carries the genes for bacterial conjugation and makes its *E. coli* host cell the gene donor during conjugation.

F.A.O. Abbreviation for Food and Agriculture Organisation of the United Nations.

fava beans. Large, flat and oval shaped beans with a firm texture and a dainty taste; very popular in Europe, especially in UK.

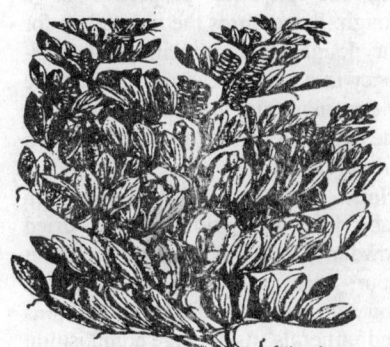

F₁ factors. The particles on inner mitochondrial membrane, which are site of ATP synthesis by oxidative phosphorylation.

F-actin. The polymerized, fibrous form of actin that consists of a double helix of G-actin monomers.

factor 3. An unknown agent present in wheat germ, wheat bran and whey, which protected rats against dietary necrosis of the liver; also protected against multiple sclerosis in mice, exudative diathesis in chicks and muscular dystrophy in mink. Since it was the third agent, the others being vitamin E and cystine, that was shown to be protective. Now, it is known to be an organic derivative of selenium, and the protective action of cystine is due to the presence of selenium contamination. Selenium compounds differ in their potency; selenate, selenite, selenium analogues of cystine, cystathione and methionine are effective at 2-3 micrograms per 100 g diet, Factor 3 is effective at 0.7 micrograms; one atom of selenium in this form is equivalent to 700-1000 molecules of vitamin E. Importance to man unknown.

factor I. Obsolete name for vitamin B₆.

factor U. Cabagin, antiulcer factor reported in cabbage leaves, believed to be methyl sulphonium derivative of methionine.

factor W. Obsolete name for biotin.

factor X. Obsolete name for vitamin B_{12}.

factor Y. Obsolete name for vitamin B_6.

factor. A term used to indicate any member of a biologically active complex, especially if its exact chemical nature is unknown or if its function in cellular metabolism has not been elucidated. Several of the B-complex vitamins were originally referred to as factors until their identity had been established by research.

faecal streptococci. Streptococci found in the intestine of humans and animals. The presence of faecal streptococci in water generally indicates fecal pollution. This term refers to those streptococci normally present in the faeces of man and animals. It includes S. fecalis, S. faecium. S. durans, S. bovis, and S. avium, as well as strains with properties intermediate between them. These organisms rarely multiply in polluted water and they may be slightly more resistant to disinfection than coliform organisms.

faeces. The matter composed of undigested food residues, remains of digestive secretions not reabsorbed, bacteria from the intestinal tract, cells and mucus from the intestinal lining, substances excreted into the intestinal tract. the main pigment present in faeces is stercobilin.

faggot. 1. Small bundle of parsley, thyme, marjoram and bay leaf tied together with cotton and added to the dish being cooked. Also known as Bouquet garni.

2. Name given to a dish prepared from liver, that is chopped, seasoned and baked.

falling rate drying. The period of drying in which the rate of drying, the change of moisture (M) and time (t) is decreasing with time, represented by dM/dt; mainly applied to thin layer drying, whereas decreasing rate drying is applied to deep layer drying. It is also expressed in terms of moisture loss per unit time per unit of exposed surface area. The falling rate period follows the constant rate period of drying. The constant rate period of drying is not always present. Field harvested grains dry entirely in the falling rate period.

Farex. Trade name of an infant cereal food; popular in may countries. Its average composition per 100 g is: protein 12.9%; fat 2.3%; carbohydrate 73%; calcium 885 mg; iron 24 mg; vitamin B_1 1.4 mg; vitamin B_2 1.6 mg; and food energy 1.45 MJ.

farina dolce. Italian name for the flour made from dried chestnuts.

farina. General term for starch. More specifically in UK, it refers to potato starch; in US, it is defined as the starch obtained from wheat other than durum wheat; starch from the latter is called semolina.

farinograph. An instrument for measuring the physical properties of a dough. It measures the time taken for the dough to attain standard consistency in a high-speed mixer, the time it can maintain this consistency and the extent to which the dough falls on further mixing.

Farlene. Trade name for a high protein baby food in the from of a dried powder. It contains protein-rich wheat flour, milk, peas, soya, wheat gluten and egg, and is fortified with vitamins and minerals. Its average composition per 100 g is: protein 25%; fat 5.5%; carbohydrate 61.5%; calcium 0.8 g; iron 12 mg; vitamin A 840 µg; vitamin B_1 0.8 mg; vitamin B_2 0.6 mg; nicotinic acid 15 mg; vitamin C 70 mg; vitamin

D 18 µg; and food energy 1.7 MJ.

fast green FCF. FD&C green no. 3. The disodium salt of 4-{[4-(N-ethyl-*p*-sulphobenzylamino)-phenyl]-(4-hydroxy-2-sulphoniumphenyl)-methylene}-1[(N-ethyl-N-p-sulfobenzyl)-δ-2,5-cyclohexadienimine]. It is a dull green powder, which is very soluble in water, glycerol and the glycols but almost insoluble in ethanol (95%). There is slightly fading of colour in acid media.

fat, blood. About 590 mg/100 ml plasma; 150 mg neutral fat, 160 mg cholesterol, 200 mg phospholipid.

fat, neutral. The triglyceride fats; used in distinction from other lipids, as, for example, in blood, where the subdivision is neutral fat, cholesterol and phospholipid.

fat-extenders. Substances that permit a reduction of fat content without much changing the texture; used in baked products, *e.g.*, glyceryl monosterate.

fat liquors. A mixture of neatsfoot oil and water, emulsified with a fatty acid or sulphonated oil; the neatsfoot oil is derived from water extraction of animal tendons; used in tanneries for treating tanned leather to lubricate the fibres, increase the flexibility, and improve the finish. Dyeing and fatliquoring are conducted in the same drum after tanned stock is aged, neutralized, and retained to impart special properties. There are two general type of fat-liquor emulsions: acid and alkaline. The acid group include sulfonated oils and some soluble-oil combinations. Alkaline types are emulsions of oils with soaps or alkalies. Leather may be treated first with an alkaline liquor and then with an acid, or borax or soda ash may be added to sulfonated oils to produce alkaline liquors. For suede and white leathers, egg-yolk emulsions may be used. The oils employed in emulsions may be sperm, cod, or castor oil, or a mixture of oils, and those that are neutral have a neatsfoot-oil base. The special kind of soaps are usually prepared for the tannery trade. Prepared fat liquors are marketed under trade names.

fats, high ratio. Shortenings with a greater proportion of the mono- and diglycerides, *i.e.*, superglycerinated. These shortenings disperse more readily into doughs, and allow the use of a higher ratio of sugar to flour than with ordinary shortening.

fats. The solid to semisolid glycerides of fatty acids of high nutritional value. Fats are chemically classified as lipids. Natural fats are produced by both plants and animals; the former are represented by coconut and cocoa butters, and the latter by lard, tallow, and milk-derived butter. Fats occur widely in plants and animals as a means of storing food energy, having twice the calorific value of carbohydrates. In mammals, fat is deposited in a layer beneath the skin (subcutaneous fat) and deep within body as a specialized adipose tissue. The insulating properties of fat are also important, especially in animals lacking fur and those inhabiting cold climates (*e.g.*, seals and whales). Fats derived from plants and fish generally have a greater proportion of unsaturated fatty acids than those from mammals. Chemically, such fats have the same composition as oils of the same origin.

Generally, fats are glycerides of stearic, palmitic, oleic, and similar fatty acids, varying only in the extent of their saturation, the animal fats being the more highly saturated. Thus, the only difference between a vegetable or animal fat and a similarly derived oil is that fats are solid and oils are liquid at room temperature. Some fats show traces of crystal formation of colin. Synthetic fats are made by catalytic hydrogenation of vegetable oils to a solid consistency, and are maily used for cooking. Some fish oils are also hydrogenated for use as dispersing agents. Fats can be hydrolyzed by reacting the glycerides with dilute alkali solutions/water at about 533 K to form glycerol and the salt of free fatty acids. Chemically,

(a) fats are substances which are insoluble in water but soluble in organic solvents such as ether, chloroform and benzene, and are actual or potential esters of fatty acids. The term includes triglycerides, phospholipids, waxes and sterols; also termed lipids;

(b) in the more general use the term fats refers to the neutral fats which are mixtures of esters of fatty acids with glycerol, *i.e.*, triglycerides.

fat-soluble vitamins. Vitamins A, D, E and K; occur in food in solution in the fats. Are stored in the body to a greater extent than the water-soluble. The distinction into fat-soluble and water-soluble is of historical interest and is convenient for chapter headings in text-books, but otherwise has no significance.

fatty acid activation. The conversion of a fatty acid to a fatty acyl coenzyme A ester which is the first step in the reactions of beta oxidation. The fatty acyl coenzyme A ester can be formed in a reaction catalyzed by a thiokinase or in a reaction catalyzed by a thiophorase.

fatty acid oxidation. Process by which acetyl coenzyme A oxidizes fatty acids in the mitochondria of animal and plant cells. Through this metabolic pathway neutral fat is utilized to release energy for the cell.

fatty acid synthesis. Fatty acids are synthesized in the cytosol by different pathway from that of β-oxidation. Synthesis starts with the carboxylation of acetyl CoA to malonyl CoA. This ATP driven reaction is catalyzed by the acetyl CoA carboxylase, a biotin enzyme. Citrate allosterically stimulates this step in fatty acid synthesis. The intermediates in fatty acid synthesis are linked to an acyl carrier protein (ACP), specifically to sulphydryl terminus of its phosphopantetheine prosthetic group. Acetyl-ACP is formed from acetyl-CoA, and malonyl-ACP is formed from malonyl CoA. Acetyl-ACP and malonyl-ACP condense to form acetoacetyl-ACP, a reaction driven by the release of carbon dioxide from the activated malonyl unit. This is followed by a reduction, a dehydration, and a second reduction. NADPH is the reductant in these steps. The butryl-ACP formed in this way is ready for a second round of elongation starting with the addition of a two-carbon unit from malonyl-ACP. Seven rounds of elongation yield palmitoyl-ACP, which is hydrolyzed to palmitate. The synthesis of palmitate requires eight molecules of acetyl-CoA, fourteen NADPH, and seven ATP. In higher organisms, the enzymes carrying out fatty acid synthesis, are organized in to a multienzyme complex. The two kinds of polypeptide chains in this complex contain several covalently linked enzymes. A reaction cycle based on the cleavage of citrate carries acetyl groups from mitochondria to the cytosol and generates some of the required NADPH. The rest is formed by the pentose phosphate pathway. Fatty acids are elongated and unsaturated by enzyme systems in the endoplasmic reticulum membrane. Mammals lack the enzymes to introduce double bonds distal to C-9, and so they require linoleate and linolenate in their diets.

fatty acid synthetase complex. A cytoplas-mic, multi-enzymic complex that catalyzes a cyclic set of reactions whereby a fatty acid is synthesized from one molecule of coenzyme A and successive molecules of malonyl coenzyme A; the complex consists of six enzymes and the acyl carrier protein.

fatty acid. 1. A general term for a group of monobasic organic acids derived from hydrocarbons by the equivalent of oxidation of a methyl group. They include both saturated and unsaturated fatty acids; for example, the simplest acid is formic acid, $HCOOH$; propionic acid, CH_3-CH_2-$COOH$; sorbic acid, CH_3- $CH=CH$-$CH=CH$-$COOH$. 2. Three members of the fatty acid series (those whose glyceryl esters compose the largest part of the most fats), palmitic acid, $C_{15}H_{31}COOH$; stearic acid, $C_{17}H_{35}COOH$; and oleic acid, $C_{17}H_{33}COOH$. Fatty acids are physiologically important both as components of phospholipids and glycolipids, and as fuel molecules. They are stored in adipose tissue as triacylglycerols (natural fat), which can be mobilized by the hydrolytic action of the lipases that are under hormonal control. Fatty acids are activated to acyl-CoA, transported across the inner mitochondrial membrane by carnitine, and degraded in the mitochon-drial matrix by a recurring sequence of four reactions:

(a) oxidation linked to FAD;

(b) hydration;

(c) oxidation linked to NAD^+; and

(d) thiolysis by CoA.

Fatty acid are in the general classification of lipids. Natural fats contain many unsaturated fatty acids having up to six double bonds along the chain (polyunsaturates), and many isomeric structures are possible. Saturated types occur in animal fats and some nut fats (coconut); unsaturated acids occur chiefly in such vegetable oils as castor, linseed, and safflower. Most fatty acids are mixtures of several types of glycerides. They are produced commercially by catalytic hydrolysis (splitting) of the fat or oil to separate the acid from it (Twitchell process), with glycerol as by-product. The best known saturated fatty acids are stearic, palmitic, butyric, and lauric; among the unsaturates are oleic, linolenic, linoleic, and ricinoleic.

Some fatty acids are synthesized within the animal and are thus called nonessential; others that are nutritionally necessary but are not formed within the organism and thus must be obtained from external sources and are hence called essential. These are arachidonic, linoleic; and linolenic acids. Fatty acids are used primarily as raw materials for soap manufacture, as dispersing and activating agents in the rubber industry, in synthetic detergents, and in candle making. Fatty acids are synthesized by cells from acetyl-CoA and malonyl-CoA in the presence of fatty acid synthetase complex, one molecule of acetyl-CoA (from mitochondria) being linked to two carbons from malonyl-CoA.

fatty acids, free. The free acids liberated from triglycerides when subjected to hydrolytic rancidity, therefore determination of FFA is an index of quality of fats.

fatty alcohol. An aliphatic alcohol containing from 8-20 carbon atoms in the chain; they are derived from natural sources by reduction, hydrolysis, or hydrogenation and may be saturated (ocetyl and stearyl or unsaturated (oleyl and linoleyl). Those having more than 12 carbons in the molecule are solids.

fatty oil. A nonvolatile oil of vegetable or animal origin, and consisting of glyceryl (and other) esters of fatty acids (sometimes other organic acids), often with some of the free acid present.

favism. Acute haemolytic anameia induced in sensitive animals by consuming broad beans (*Vicia faba*) or by contact with the pollen. It arises due to an inherited metabolic defect, namely a deficiency of the enzyme glucose-6-phosphate dehydrogenase in the red blood cells, causing a reduction in the glutathione level.

feathering. A defect associated with cream, indicating that it has not been properly processed. As a result, there is some coagulation of the cream in hot coffee. A condition in which the cream forms a flaky, feathery condition at the top of cup. Cream purchasers object to this "feathering" because of its abnormal appearance. However, consumers are in error in thinking that it invariably indicates sour cream. It usually does with unhomogenized cream but with homogenized cream it is almost always the result of using excess pressure in homogenizing.

feather meal. Hydrolyzed poultry feathers is the product resulting from the treatment under pressure of clean, undecomposed feathers from slaughtered poultry, free of additives and/or accelerators. The specifications require that not less than 75% of the crude protein of the meal shall consist of digestible protein (as determined by the pepsin digestibility method). Feathers are almost pure protein. Most of this is keratin protein, which in the raw or natural state is not readily digestible by animals. Processing with live steam to partially hydrolyze the protein breaks apart some of the chemical bonds that account for the peculiar structure of the feather fibers. The resulting feather meal is a free-flowing, palatable product that is easily digested by all classes of livestock and poultry. Processed feather meal is quite uniform because it is a single-source protein and such proteins have a relatively constant composition and amino acid pattern.

Feather meal is a rich source of cystine and thus conserves methionine which otherwise must be used to provide the required cystine. It has been demonstrated that amino acids in swine feeds, a 2:1 ratio of soybean meal and feather meal provides a protein supplement of good quality for growing pigs. As a protein source for ruminants, the comparative value of feather meal and the oilseed meals is roughly proportioned to their respective protein contents. It has been shown that feather meals serves as an effective ingredient in cattle concentrates that contain high urea levels. When high urea cattle concentrates contain about 7.5-10% feather meal, the power requirements for pelleting are reduced and handling properties of the pelleted-concentrate are improved. Some feather meal is now incorporated in pets foods-to the extent of 2-4%.

fecula. Name given to foods which are almost solely starch; prepared from roots and stems by grating, such as tapicoa, sago and arrowroot.

feed-grade animal fat. FGAF. The triglycerides, ranging from the more unsaturated poultry and pork fats (greases) to the more saturated beef tallow. Lower-melting fats with a higher level of unsaturated fatty acids are to some extent digested more efficiently and rapidly than saturated fats, such as hydrogenated oils and tallows. There are additional, indirect advantages of fat in animal feed: Improvement of overall nutrient efficiency and digestibility by lowering feed spoilage through reduced dustiness and improved physical acceptability. In feeds, small levels of added FGAF bind smaller, dustier particles of cereal starch into aggregates. A decreases in the incidence of pneumonia and respiratory difficulties among swine has been attributed to reducing the dust particle count. The colour, improved appearance, and palatibility tend to aid in appetite control and increase feed consumption and hence to improve feed consumption and growth rate.

The fats may be regarded as a means for improving the availability and absorption of fat-soluble vitamins, pigments, and amino acids. The so-called protein-sparing effect can lead to weight gain in excess of calculated caloric value, when protein or amino acids, such as lysine, are growth limiting. In feeds without added fats, the low content of preformed fatty acids will be almost entirely oxidized and utilized for energy production.

Animals need certain amounts and types of fatty acids for the synthesis of special body fats. The growing pig puts on about 500-800 g of liveweight every day. Of this a substantial amount (20-30%) is laid down as fat; this is because the genetic of the pig and its temperature threshold dictate a layer of insulating fat in addition to fat which is laid down between the muscles. Unless a minimum amount of preformed fatty acids is already provided in the feeds, they must be obtained from the metabolic breakdown of carbohydrates and/or proteins. From the economic point of view, the latter is an inefficient and wasteful process because such chemical transformations involve losses of energy. Consequently, the avoidance of such steps results in higher energy utilization, being proportional to the amounts of preformed fatty acids when are directly absorbed through the gut wall and moved to the side of deposition with less energy loss. Once this requirement is met, the value of fat riverts to its energy contribution.

Fehling's test. For reducing substances, mostly used to distinguish reducing from non-reducing sugars. Depends upon the reduction of blue cupric hydroxide to yellow cuprous oxide on heating the alkaline solution. Fehling's solution A is copper sulphate, and solution B is alkaline tartrate; mixed immediately before use to prevent deterioration.

Femminello ovale lemon. A variety of lemon which accounts for about 75% of Italy's lemon production. The fruit is medium-size, rounded at the base. It is ever-blooming, with the crop thus well distributed throughout the year. In Italy, about 25% of the crop is processed into single-strength juice. The variety is susceptible to the *mal secco* disease.

fennel seed. *Foeniculum vulgare.* A wild or cultivated biennial or perennial growing in the US, Europe, the Mediterranean and Asia Minor. It has a rather stiff, erect, branching stem, which bears deeply cut greyish-green flowers, followed by odd, toothed seed-vessels, filled with small somewhat compressed seeds, usually three-cornered, with two sides flat and one convex. These black or brown seeds yield a strong, agreeable, aromatic odour somewhat reminiscent of nutmegs and have spicy, pungent taste. **fennel.** Family: *Umbelliferae.* Genus: *Foeniculum.* Species: *Foeniculum vulgare.* Fennel seed contain about 2-6% volatile oil, 17-20% fat, and 16-20% protein, and is relatively high in vitamin E, with traces of other vitamins and calcium and potassium. For centuries fennel has been used in cooking with fish and used medicinally as a digestive. It is an antispasmodic, calminative, diuretic, expectorant and stimulant. It has also been shown to have antibacterial and insecticidal properties. The seeds are chewed as a breath freshener, particularly appropriate after eating curries. Sweet or Roman fennel, the herb, should not be confused with Florence fennel (*finocchio*), the vegetable grown for its creamy-white bulbous roots. The leaves are used with pork, veal and fish, in stock, sauces and stuffing, and in mayonnaise and salad dressings. The dried stalks are placed under grilled or barbecued fish to impart flavour. The seeds are used as a spice, particularly in breads, savoury scones, and biscuits. At the two-leaf (cotyledon) stage, the seedlings make a pungent salad, reminiscent of mustard. Medicinally, the leaves and dried seeds are used for flatulence and in gripe waters, which are still popular for babies; colic, while an infusion of the leaves may be used for eyestrain.

One of the more interesting uses of fennel seed is in the treatment of hernia of the small intestine. For this purpose, it has been suggested, tea using 15 g fennel seed is drunk while very hot. The patient then lies on his or her back with the legs together and knees half bent. If no response is noticed within half an hour the same dose can be repeated but generally the pain disappears about 30 minutes after treatment. Patients who do not respond 1 hour after this treatment are advised to undergo surgery. Hernias successfully treated in this way are generally those formed no more than three days before, hernias of longer duration do not respond so readily. Fennel and ginger make an excellent digestive tea and will help with griping colic and flatulence. Fennel oil inhaled in a steam bath can vaporise mucus loosening it and causing it degenerate so that the eliminatory process can remove it through the bloodstream far more easily than can be done by coughing, sneezing or blowing the nose. This process is aided by fennel's high mineral content. Also with its umbels of minute yellow flowers and dark green or bronze wispy leaves, fennel is a decorative addition to a herbaceous border, where, because of its size, it makes a good background plant.

fenugreek. *Trigoenella foenumogra-ecum.* The name comes from *foenum-graecum* meaning "Greek Hay," the plant being used in times past to scent inferior hay. The name of the genus, *Trigonella*, is derived from the old Greek name denoting "three-angled," from the form of the plant's corolla. It is an erect annual, growing about 60 cm high, similar in habit to lucerne hay. The seeds are brownish, about 10-15 mm long, oblong, with a deep furrow dividing them into unequal lobes. They are contained (10-20 together) in long, narrow, sickle-like pods. Fenugreek is an animal fodder crop grown around the Mediterranean region since ancient times. This leguminous plant is eaten as vegetable, and the seeds are used for flavouring. It is consumed by women in Orient to help gain weight. The sprouting seeds may also be eaten at the cotyledon stage as a spicy salad; the fully developed leaves, too bitter to cook as spinach, are served in the Indian way, as a curry; and the lightly roasted seeds are used as a spice, also principally in curries. The ground seeds, containing coumarin, are major ingredient in commercially prepared curry powders. The sprouted seeds are good as salad, tossed in vinaigrette dressing. The roasted seeds are used in Middle Eastern variations of *halva,* a rich sweetmeat, as well as in curries. Medicinally, an infusion of the seeds may be taken for flatulence. The seed produces a yellow dye. The Indian material is considered to be more uniform in colour and a have a better appearance than that from Morocco. Flavour of this spice is characterized as being maple-like, and its most important use is as an ingredient in artificial maple flavours. The average composition per 100 g of the seeds is: 29 g protein; 5 g fat; 50 g carbohydrate; 180 mg calcium; 22 mg iron; 0.4 mg vitamin B_1; 0.3 mg vitamin B_2; 1.5 mg nicotinic acid; and 1.45 MJ food energy.

ferguzade. Trade name for a glucose beverage.

ferment. A material which catalyzes certain organic reactions and consists of an enzyme in association with other substances produced by the living organism, or with the organism or cell itself.

fermentation test for milk. A test usually run in conjunction with the methylene-blue reduction method or reductase test. Milk is held in test tubes at 37°C until it coagulates so that the type of fermentation can be determined, furnishing an insight into the types of bacteria present. The results of the fermentation and reductase tests mean more when used together because the former indicates the type of bacteria and the latter the number. Detailed directions for the fermentation test are as follows:

A sample of milk is taken in a clean glass tube, placed in a warm box and kept at about 37°C for 20-24 hours. At the end of 20 hours the tubes are inspected and classed as:
(a) no gas or only a trace,
(b) moderately gassy,
(c) very gassy.

Gassy milk will have off flavours and is not desirable for market milk or for cheese-making.

fermentation, acetic. A fermentation which produces acetic acid, commonly in the dilute form (vinegar) from alcohol-containing solutions or substances.

fermentation, alcoholic. A fermentation which produces ethyl alcohol, commonly by the action of a yeast, such as *Saccharomycs cerevisiae,* on a sugar, or a sugar-containing solution.

fermentation, amylolytic. In general, this term means a fermentation of starch; specifically, it is an incomplete fermentation of starch that does not yield simple sugars.

fermentation, butyric. A fermentation reaction which produces butyric acid.

fermentation. The transformation or metabolism of compounds without the use of oxygen. The breakdown of sugar by yeast to carbon dioxide and alcohol is a fermentation, as also is the production by microorganisms of substances like lactic acid, citric acid, riboflavin. From the point of view of the organisms it is an anaerobic method of liberating energy. In mammalian muscle the first stage in glucose metabolism is anaerobic break-down to pyruvic acid, followed by oxidation. Fermentation is an energy-yielding process in which organic molecules serve as both electron donors and acceptors. It involves the breakdown of organic substances, particularly carbohydrates, under anaerobic conditions. It is a kind of anaerobic respiration and is seen in certain bacteria and in yeasts; it involves the production of chemical energy in the form of ATP through the degradation of carbohydrate and other organic molecules in a reaction that does not require molecular oxygen. In obligate anaerobic cells fermentation is the only energy-yielding process, but in facultative aerobes it will be followed by oxidation of the products of fermentation. Some yeast and bacterial cells use alcoholic fermentation in which ethanol appears as a fermentation product. Glycolysis is the most common form of fermentation in animal cells and involves lactic acid fermentation.

fermentograph. An instrument for measuring the gas-producing power of a dough. The fermentating dough is contained in a balloon immersed in water and as gas is produced the balloon expands and rises in the water, the rise being measured continuously.

ferredoxins. Non-haem iron-containing proteins isolated from a number of bac-teria and plants. They possess low redox potentials. Ferredoxins are involved in nitrogen fixation and photosynthesis. They are strong reducing agents (negative redox potentials) and function as electron carriers, for example in photosynthesis and nitrogen fixation. They are also called non-haem iron proteins to distinguish them from proteins in which the iron

is part of haem prosthetic group (*e.g.,* cytochromes). They contain clusters of iron-sulphur, which have equal numbers of iron and inorganic sulphur atoms complexed to the protein by way of four cysteine residues. Treatment with acid leads to the production of an acid-labile sulphide. Usually two (Fe_2S_2) or four (Fe_4S_4) iron and sulphide atoms are present, the iron being tetrahedrally coordinated to the sulphur atoms. Ferredoxins are usually small, water-soluble proteins which undergo single-electron oxidation/reduction reactions. The midpoint redox potentials of the ferredoxins are usually negative (ranging from -0.4 to -0.7V). They function in electron transport chains during respiration, photosynthesis and in mono-oxygenase systems. In anaerobic bacteria they function as the electron acceptor for pyruvate dehydrogenase During photosynthesis, ferredoxin reduces NADP.

ferrihaemoglobin. *See* methaemoglobin.

ferritin. A ferric-hydroxide-phosphate-protein complex (containing 23% iron) present in the cells of the intestinal mucosa, liver, spleen and bone marrow, as a storage form of iron. It is the major storage form of iron in the animal body, comprising a complex of the protein apoferritin and iron.

ferroprotoporphyrin. A protohaeme in which the iron is in the ferrous form: ferroprotoporphyrin IX is the prosthetic group of hemoglobin, myoglobin, catalase, peroxidase, and cytochrome b.

festoopen dryer. A device for removing moisture from paper materials in which the material is kept tension-free and is continuously fed in loops on supporting poles carried by conveyor chain, passed through forced warm air convection (air flow downward).

feverfew. *Chrysanthemum parthenium.* A plant with its bright lime green or yellow-green leaves that retain their colour through the winter, feverfew is a year-round decorative garden plant. It is low growing, bushy, a vigorous, quickly thickening up, spreading, and self-seeding. The white flowers, which may be like single or double daisies, are particularly pretty and dry well for flower arranging. The plant's bitter taste rules out culinary uses, but is worth tolerating for its medicinal properties. The fresh as well as dried leaves can be particularly effective (made into sandwiches) as a cure for migraine, and as a general tonic. The flowers are used in skin preparations.

fibre saturation point. Moisture content of wood and other cellulose products above which free moisture exists and below which the water is bound. For other materials this point is often called the critical moisture content. The fibre saturation point, depending on the species, is between 20-35% dry basis. Other parameters related to the fibre saturation point are electric conductivity, dielectric constant, elastic and strength properties. For wood, the fibre saturation point is the moisture content reached when all the fibers are completely swollen and saturated with colloidal water and no liquid or free water exists in the coarse capillary structure.

fibre. General term used for the indigestible parts of food. It is defined as the residue left after successive extraction with petroleum ether, boiling 1.25% sulphuric acid, and 1.25% caustic soda, minus ash. According to the earlier definition, crude fibre as the residue remaining after treatment with hot sulfuric acid, alkali and alcohol. It consists primarily of cellulose, lignin, and trace amounts of other polysaccharides. This definition appears somewhat narrow in terms of present views of the subject. Based upon writings of a number of investigators, fibre may be defined as that part of plant material in the diet which is resistant to digestion by the secretions of the human gastrointestinal tract-consisting of variable proportions of complex carbohydrates, such as celluloses, hemicelluloses, pentosans, and uronic acids, as well as linin. From an analytical point of view, because it is difficult to measure the undigested fractions (may be different from one person to the next), a definition of dietary fibre probably should be amended to include, "the residue remaining after an analytical procedure, such as the neutral Detergent Fibre method; or the Acid detergent fibre method. A definition of dietary fibre should include all the components of a food that are not broken down by enzymes in the human digestive tract to produce small molecular compounds which are then absorbed into the blood stream. Thus, dietary fibre includes hemicelluloses, pectic substances, gums, mucilages, as well as certain other carbohydrates in addition to lignin and cellulose. These chemical compounds are found largely in the cell walls of plant tissues.

The term crude fibre as traditionally used may represent as little as one-seventh of the total dietary fibre of a given food. It is possible that the term fibre may be somewhat misleading, inasmuch as not fibrous in the usual physical sense, while, inasmuch as all components of presently regarded dietary fibre are not fibrous in the usual physical sense, while, at the same time, some foods that contain recognizable fibres, such as muscle meats, do not yield undigestible residue.

Burkitt's definition of dietary fibre is mostly celluloses and lignin and lignin material, varying in different plants according to type and age. Basically, it passes through the small intestine undigested by our enzymes. Digestion of some components of dietary fibre, especially the hemicelluloses, takes place in the colon as a result of bacterial action. White flour, for example, is high in hemicellulose. The volatile fatty acids produced from this soluble fibre in the digestive process attract water from the surrounding tissues by osmosis, and thus may have a cathartic effect.

Some fibres, such as bagasse from sugarcane, are very sharp abrasives to intestinal tract; while others, such as lignin, may actually be constipating. There are such great differences in the physiological effects of various constituents of dietary fibre and some feel that it is essentially meaningless to consider higher-fibre diets in the abstract. They do not deny that needs may exist for components of dietary fiber with specific properties, but rather that these needs may vary with different physiological states. A wide variety of foods supply significant amounts of dietary fibre. Fundamental are those foods, such as fruits and vegetables, which provide significant quantities of fibre as the result of their naturally high fibre content. In many other instances, fibrous components (powdered cellulose; rice and soy hulls; soy, corn (maize), rice, wheat brans; coconut residues, citrus byproducts, ground almost skins, groundnut (peanut) hulls, etc.) can be added to processed foods, such as breads and, particularly to fabricated foods which provide excellent opportunities for improving the dietary aspects of many products in this latter category. A number of the fibre-containing components for addition to food products are not strange because for years past some of these materials have been considered additives, but for other purposes, such as thickening and bulking agents.

fibrin. The insoluble protein that forms fibres at the site of an injury and is the foundation of a blood clot. It is formed when thrombin acts upon fibrinogen. Conversion from soluble fibrinogen to insoluble fibrin is brought about by the enzyme thrombin. If fresh blood is rapidly whipped a stringy mass of fibrin is obtained. The fibrin polymerizes to form an unstable network, which, by the further action of activated Factor XIII, is strengthened into an insoluble clot by the introduction of covalent calcium cross-links between the fibrin molecules. Once a fibrin plug has served its purpose in wound healing it is digested by the fibri-nolytic enzyme plasmin. Fibrin is produced by the action of thrombin on plasma protein fibrinogen. Thrombin is normally produced only in blood that has escaped from circulation and is a product of an inactive precursor, present in normal plasma, called prothrombin.

fibrinase. The enzyme that catalyzes the cross-linking of fibrin molecules in blood clotting so that a hard clot is formed; the enzyme catalyzes joining of the g-carboxyl groups of glutamic acid residues to the ε-amino groups of lysine residues.

fibrinogen. One of the proteins of the blood plasma that is responsible for the clotting of blood. Under the influence of thrombin is converted to fibrin, which is deposited as strands that trap the red cells and form the ficin 277

clot. It is a major protein component of blood plasma; when activated by the enzyme thrombin at the onset of bleeding, the fibrinogen undergoes chemical modification to fibrin; this in turn triggers the protective agglutination or clotting of blood. Fibrinogen is water-soluble and has a fibrous structure; it is synthesized in the liver. Blood clotting is an involved series of reactions in which fibrinogen plays the vital role.

fibrinolysis. Process by which blood clots are dissolved and dispersed. This degradation involves the action of plasmin on the fibrin of the clot and is rather slow in normal circumstances, taking many hours to achieve complete dispersal of even small clots. Although the exact mechanism remains controversial it is generally regarded that physiological and pathological fibrinolysis are identical processes regulated by endogenous inhibitors and dependent upon a number of activators for initiation. These activators are present in all body tissues, including plasma, but not in the liver. High concentrations are found in vascular endothelium, which is the main source of plasma activator activity. Activators are also secreted by granulocytes in the blood and by some types of malignant neoplasm. This gives rise to pathological bleeding states induced by nonspecific lysis of clotting proteins other than fibrin.

fibrinopeptide. One of two peptides, denoted A and B, that are removed from fibrinogen during its conversion to fibrin by the action of thrombin.

fibroin. A protein which is the major component of silk, a material used by spiders to build webs, and by insects to construct larval nests and cocoons. Silk is produced only by specialized cells within the silk glands, and is composed of long chains of the amino acids glycine and alanine, with occasional serine residues.

fibronectin. The group of large proteins secreted by many type of cells, and which form fibrillar matrix linking cells to other extracellular proteins, such as collagen. It can interact with bacteria and mediate their nonspecific clearance from the body. Fibronectin is also involved in cell-cell interactions.

fibrous protein. One of the basic forms adopted by amino acid chains to construct proteins. Fibrous proteins consist most commonly of inter-linked chains of polypeptides forming a rope, as in the molecule of collagen, Packing of the amino acid chain into a relatively tight three-dimensional form is the chief alternative to fibrous protein: such molecules are known as globular proteins. Fibrous proteins are long, stringy molecules. Some typical fibrous proteins are α-keratin of hair and wool, and fibroin of silk. They may constitute about one-half or more of the total body protein in larger vertebrates, and provide external protection. Since, they are the major components of the outer layer of the skin, hair, feathers, nails, horns; they provide support, shape, and form because they are major components of connective tissues.

ficin. A concentrate prepared by filtering and drying the latex of *Ficus glabrata* (Fam. Moraceae) and a variety of tropical fig trees. They are white to off-white powders, which are completely soluble in water. Liquid-fig latex concentrates are light-brown to dark-brown in color. Typical applications include chill-proofing of beer, meat tenderizing, and dough conditioning in the baking industry.

The principal reaction catalyzed by

ficin is the hydrolysis of the polypeptides, amides, and esters (especially at bonds involving basic amino acids, or leucine or glycine), yielding peptides of lower molecular weight. One available ficin concentrate material is described as one of the most potent protease systems, exhibiting a faster initial reaction rate than other plant proteases. The substance has demonstrated a strong proteolytic action at temperatures of up to 50°C. It is a proteolytic enzyme of molecular mass ranging between 23,800-25,500, which requires a free sulphydryl group for activity and as such as a member of a group which includes papain and bromelain. Ficin has tissue, dissolving properties. Therefore, it must be handled with care.

Ficin is 10-20 times more active as papain in regard to milk clotting; 4-10 times as active in general. It is used as protein digestant in the brewing industry, and as a chill-proofing agent in beer; in the cheese industry it is used as a substitute for rennet for the coagulation of milk; in the meat industry, as a meat tenderizer and as an agent for removing castings from formed sausage. In the leather industry it is used for the bating of leather; in the textile industry for shrink proofing wool, for removing gelatin from sized thread, and mixed with amylases and maltases as spot remover. It is also employed in the preparation of peptones, for determining protein material in spent grains and in determination of Rh factor. It speeds 10 times the agglutination of human blood cells by the Rh factor when in contact with the anti-Rh serum. It has also been used as trichuricide. Also known as ficus proteinase; ficus protease.

field bean. Any of numerous varieties of beans that are produced on a large scale, as contrasted with garden beans, and which are not harvested until the pods are ripe and the leaves have fallen. Before threshing, vines are allowed to cure in the absence of moisture. Some of the field beans, such as dry edible beans, are produced for human consumption, while others are grown for animal feed.

fig. *Ficus carica.* Fresh figs have been a prized delicacy. They were grown in King Nebuchadnezzar's famous Hanging Gardens of Babylon, mentioned frequently throughout the Bible, and exported by the ancient seafaring Greeks and Phoenicians, who may have introduced them to Italy. In the 18th century, Jesuit priests planted figs at the first Catholic mission in San Diego, California. This so-called black Mission fig is still an important variety in that state.

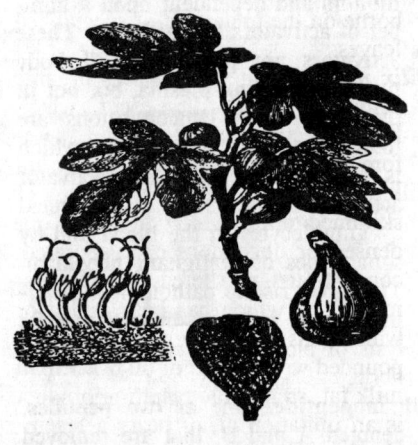

Fresh figs are usually pear-shaped, with either greenish-yellow, purple or black skins. When ripe, they are usually soft but not mushy. Ancient Roman gladiators ate a lot of figs prior to combat in the amphitheaters to give them extra physical strength and an advantage over their opponents. The average composition per 100 g of figs is: 1.3 g protein; 11 g carbohydrate; 1 mg iron; 24 mg vitamin A; 0.05 mg vitamin B_1; 0.05 mg vitamin B_2; 0.4 mg nicotinic acid; 2. mg vitamin C; and food energy 1.2 kJ. The average composition of the dried figs is: 4 g protein; 63 g carbohydrate; 269 kcal (1.1 KN), 200 mg calcium; 4 mg iron; 30 mg vitamin A; 0.1 mg B_1; 0.08 mg B_2; 1.7 mg nicotinic acid.

Filicinae. A class of terrestrial vascular plants, the ferns, belonging to the Pteropsida. Ferns are perennial plants bearing large conspicuous leaves (fronds) usually arising from either a rhizome or a short erect stem. Bracken is a common example. Only tree ferns have stems that reach an appreciable height. There is characteristic uncurling of the young leaves as they expand into the adult form. Spores are borne on the underside of specialized leaves.

filix mas. Male fern; contains organic acids, including filicic acid, which have selective action on, and therefore used in treatment, for tapeworm.

filled milk. Any kind of milk, cream, or skimmed milk, which may be condensed or uncondensed, evaporated, concentrated, powdered, dried or desiccated, to which has been added or which has been blended or compounded with any fat or oil other than milk fat, so that the resulting product is an imitation of, or bears a resemblance to milk, cream, or skimmed milk. The definition does not encompass any distinctive properties food compound not readily mistaken in taste for milk/cream or associated products, provided that such compound is prepared and designed for feeding infants and young children; is packed

in individual containers that bear a label in bold type that the content is to be used for specific purposes, etc. Any time materials are added to or subtracted from milk, excepting water, in the interest of formulating a new product, such product formulation should be carefully checked with regulatory bodies in the respective country or locate of manufacture and distribution.

filter pad butter test. A method for the detection of filth in the from of dirt, insects, and other extraneous materials in butter. To 100 g of butter in a beaker is added 120-200 ml of a solution of 40 g borax dissolved in 1 litre of water. The mixture is boiled and filtered through a Buchner suction funnel equipped with rapid flow filter paper. The paper is washed with gasoline to remove any remaining grease, and then with hot water. Very moldy butter may require as many as 10 separate filter papers. In this test the borax solution changes the curd into a soluble caseinate which passes readily through the filter paper. Mold, insects, and other extraneous material remain on the filter paper and may be removed with a needle, then placed in a drop of glycerine on a slide for examination under the microscope.

filter. Device used to remove components, usually undesirable, from gases and liquids. The size of the pores in a filter determines the size of particles retained. The air supply a controller is filtered so that particles will not cause malfunction. Fuel to the burner is filtered. Air entering the spray dryer for food drying may be filtered. Air for ventilation may be filtered. Absolute filters will remove 99.9% of 0.3µ particles and will remove microorganisms as well as larger particles. Filters are classified as roughing, medium efficiency, high efficiency, and ultra high or absolute. Coarser filters may be called strainers.

filth test. Name given to a test originated in USA for determining the contamination of a food with rodent hair sand insect fragments as an index of the hygienic handling of the food.

final moisture content. A representation of the moisture control of a product leaving a dryer or other process. The lowest moisture content of a product being dried is not necessarily the best moisture content. The optimum final moisture content depends on mechanical properties to avoid damage for handling (grain), excessive loss of leaves (forages), likelihood of rapid regain of moisture by some highly hydroscopic materials, crumbling of sheets or flakes (paper), splitting (lumber), and loss of stability (food products). Dehydrated food products appear to be most stable with minimum oxidation where there is a monomolecular layer of water internally (rather than a lower moisture content) which for milk and protein is 3.5%; potatoes, 6.5%; high sugar foods, near 0%; and nuts (walnuts), 3.0%

fines. Small diameter particles such as those which form from larger particles during handling and drying. The fines may be carried by the drying air. These fines may be removed by a filter, centrifugal separator, electronic precipitator, washing, etc., to avoid are pollution by the exhaust. Fines, often of high moisture content, may obstruct uniform flow and distribution of drying air. Fines may include dust, with sizes primarily in the range of 1-400 μm diameter, as well as particles much larger.

fines herbes. A mixture of chopped parsley, chervil, chives and tarragon.

finger millet. *Eleusine coracana.* A variety of millet grown in Africa and in south-east Asia (notably India in states of Mysore and Tamilnadu) for human consumption. The plant is hardy and tolerates poor soils. Unlike millets in general, finger millet is tolerant of moisture. In India it is frequently found near rice-growing areas. The plant does not do well, however, in frequent heavy rains. Moist mountainous slopes (the foothills of the Himalayas, for example) are particularly favorable to the plant. The annual plant achieves a height of between 0.9 to 1.2 meters with numerous branches. The inflorescence extends from a long peduncle from which 4 to 6 spikes or fingers radiate. Each finger contains 60 to 80 spikelets in 2 rows. The spikelets have from 4 to 5 florets, subtended by 2 glumes. Each floret incorporates a lemma, plea, ovary, and 3 stamens. The ovule develops into a globular seed. Nominally, finger millet is self-pollinating. The grain may be white or brown, depending upon variety. Frequently, finger millet may be intercropped with maize (corn). Seeding is done in irrigated beds in late spring and seedlings are transferred, commencing at the start of the rainy season. Finger millet is used in breads, cakes, and puddings. In some parts of India (Gujarat), unripe ears are eaten as a vegetable. This millet also can be used for making beer. also known as African millet, birdsfood millet, coracana millet, nagli, and ragi.

fining. A term used to describe traditional methods for bringing about clarification of wine. Fining agents include gelatin, casein, tannin, isinglass, and bentonite. Fining is most efficiently accomplished in relatively small vessels, including barrels. Because of so many variables involved, a careful laboratory examination of the wine is made prior to selection and determination of amount of fining agent to be used. Fining of white wines is sometimes accomplished by adding small amounts of gelatin and tannin, in solution form, using small amounts of wine as the carrier of the agents. Tannin is usually added first and then gelatin solution is added after atleast one day. In wine, gelatin has positive charge and thus tends to precipitate the negatively charged tannin. Commonly, the wine is left undisturbed for 3 weeks for settling to take place, after which the clear wine is drawn off and often given a polishing filtration. Overfining can cause a permanently cloudy wine. Egg albumen and enzymes also have been used as fining agents. In some countries (where permitted), potassium ferrocyanide is added to remove excessive copper, iron, manganese, and zinc from wines. This also helps to remove excessive proteins. Sometimes, magnesium phytate is used to remove excess iron. Centrifugation also has been considered for use in wine clarification. Centrifugation tends to reduce the amount of wine loss in the clarifying operation.

fining agent. A substance added to a liquid to clarify it by precipitating and carrying down suspended matter. Examples are the addition of certain colloids or other materials to fermented beverages to remove suspended matter. *See also* fining.

finish drying. The product leaving a particular dryer often is not at the desirable low moisture content desired. If the dryer were used to remove last 2-5% moisture, excessive heat effects (too long, or too high a temperature or both), there could be a deterioration in organoleptic properties. Finish drying is done to remove the final 2-5% moisture in a product, without destroying the physical structure, without producing undesirable chemical changes, and without permitting biolological contamination. Several procedures are used for finish drying :

(a) dehumidified air, at a low temperature moved slowly through the product,

(b) air forced through a deep bed (called finishing bins),

(c) intermittent heating, permitting moisture diffusion; and

(d) tumbling product through controlled air environment. Although it is applicable to many products, finish drying is more commonly used for wood particle drying.

finnan haddock. Smoke-cured haddock.

fire curing. The curing the tobacco in presence of the smoke from the burning or smoldering wood. The tobacco leaves remain in the barn for about three months until they are as brown as dark mahogany.

fire point. A term used with reference to frying oils; the temperature at which the fat will sustain combustion.

firkin. A quarter of a barrel of beer, *i.e.*, 9 imperial gallons; also 56 pounds of butter.

firming agents. The fresh fruits contain insoluble pectins as a firm gel around the fibrous tissues and keep the fruit firm. Breakdown of the cell structure allows conversion of pectin to pectic acid, with loss of firmness; while the addition of calcium compounds (such as chloride or carbonate) forms calcium pectate gel which protects the fruit against softening. Such compounds are known as firming agents. Alum is sometimes used to firm pickles.

Fischer (karl) method. A procedure for determining the moisture content of a product using chemicals often used as a standard. The material to be analysed for moisture is finely ground. Chemical solvents are used which penetrate the cells and provide rapid removal of moisture. Anhydrous methyl alcohol is used to extract the moisture. As compared to the oven method of moisture determination, a higher moisture content is indicated for hydroscopic materials because the procedure removes some of the water of hydration which might not otherwise be removed. As much as 2.5% higher moisture content may be obtained using this method as compared to thermal methods.

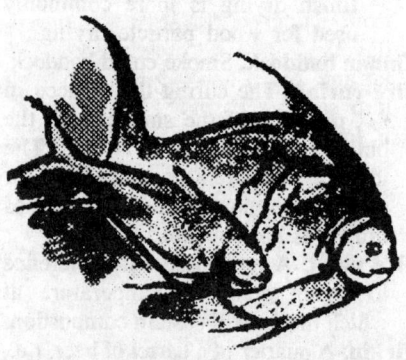

fish drying. The drying of fish may be carried out by several methods, of which salting is one, usually utilizing the fish available in excess of the fresh market needs. The gutted, fish, placed on screened or slotted shelves or trays, can be dried in a cabinet dryer with a current of heated air. Air temperatures should be kept low enough to avoid dripping of the fat. Pickle curing is another method in which 17 kg of salt are used per 100 kg of fish, the salt and fish are layered, with 1-1/2 weeks required.

Tunnel dryers, trays or belt roller dryers have been used, with forced air at 23.9°C, 40% relative humidity, to dry fish to 40%. Sun drying of shrimp is widely employed, following boiling in brine. A depth of 5-7 cm of shrimp is spread in the sun the turned every half hour, taking 3-4 days to dry. Freeze-drying cubes or strips of fish meat can be used as a method of moisture removal. Fish flour can be prepared by spray drying a wet slurry or by azeotropic drying, using dichloroethane solvent. Moisture contents of dried fish.

fish flour. A low-cost source of protein, and is used for enriching flours, baby foods, sauces, and prepared soups, and for adding proteins to breads, cakes, pastries, and other bakery products. It is prepared from fish meal by refining and deodorizing. It is an additive rather than a flour; it does not thiken soups, and in bakery products it does not have the elastic and extensible properties inherent in cereal flours. In the food industries it is called animal protein concentrate, and the high-protein grade contains 95% animal protein. It is also high in calcium and phosphorus, and contains thiamin, niacin, and riboflavin. An edible fish-protein concentrate may now be made directly from finely ground industrial fish. Oils, fats, fatty acids, and lipid-containing materials are extracted by a solvent such as isopropyl alcohol. About 20% by weight of raw fish is recovered as dry, odourless, tasteless powder which can be mixed with a variety of foods to upgrade human diet. Fish flour has almost negligible contents of carbohydrate, and does not contain more than 0.4% fat; but Viking egg white, an odourless grey powder made in Germany from whitefish, is a soluble albumin used as a substitute for egg white in bakery goods.

fish ham. Japanese product made from a red fish such as tuna or marlin, pickled with salt and nitrite, mixed with whale meat and pork fat and stuffed into a large sausage-type casing.

fish meal. The surplus fish, waste from filleting (fish-house waste) and fish unfit for human consumption are dried in vacuum, by steam, or hot air, and powdered. Whole fish is ground and cooked below 100°C to avoid loss of protein, and the oil is extracted. About 2% oil is retained in the meal, but for the manufacture of fish flour this residue oil is removed by alcohol extraction. Prior to the extraction of the oil, which may be up to 16%, fish meal contains upto about 23% protein, and up to about 30% minerals, including calcium, phosphorus, iron, and copper. The proteins have all the essential amino acids to supplement cereal foods for poultry raised by commercial methods where the birds lack access to normal feeding. The fish meal made from white fish is termed white fish meal as distinct from the oily type. The latter is sometimes of very poor quality and is then used as fertilizer.

fish oil. The oil obtained by boiling the fish and skimming off the oil, or by solvent extraction from the fish meal. The crude oil has a brownish colour and an offensive odour, but it is usually decolorized and deodorized. Oil content of fish varies between 0.5-16%, depending on the type of fish, the season, and the location of catchment. Fish in cold waters tend to have more oil than those in warm waters. There is only a small difference in the composition of oils from different species. They usually contain 20-30% of saturated acids and 70-80% unsaturated acids. The average specific gravity is about 0.92. Much of the commercial oil is obtained from the cod, herring, menhaden, sardine, and salmon. Japan fish oil consists of a mixture of sardine and herring oils. Fish oil is of the nondrying class, and is used for lubricants, leather dressings, soaps, and heat-treating oils, but is also used for blown oils or for fractionating for use in paints and in plastics.

fish paste. A paste which legally must contain not less than 70% fish.

fish protein concentration. Deodorised, decolourized, defatted fish meal also known as fish flour. Cheap source of protein for enrichment of foods.

fish sausage. Japanese product made from chopped fish fillet, spiced, flavoured and with preservatives plus fat and starch and the whole packed into sausage casing.

fish, fatty. All fatty fish, such as herring, salmon, trout, mackerel, tuna, having similar composition. Average composition per 100 g fillet is: 20% protein; 10% fat; 40 mg calcium; 3.7 mg zinc; 1.2 mg iron; 30 µg vitamin A; 0.08 mg vitamin B_1; 0.21 mg vitamin B_2; and 2.7 mg nicotinic acid.

fishmeal. The fish protein in the form of meal contains relatively high concentration of lysine and methionine and other essential amino acids, and consequently is especially valuable in supplementing cereal grain and oilseed proteins used in feeding poultry and swine. Most of the vegetable proteins fail to supply completely the dietary amino acid requirements of these animals. In addition, fish meal is rich in a number of minerals and vitamins. The oil fraction of fishmeal is composed of unsaturated triglycerides and phospholipids with high iodine value. In the presence of atmospheric oxygen, these two components autoxidize during storage of fishmeal. The autoxidation reaction is exothermic and results in the formation of primary and secondary oxidation products, that is, hydroperoxides, nonvolatile carbonyls, etc. As the autoxidation reaction progresses, the high molecular mass polymerized compounds are also formed. One of the results of the autooxidation reaction is the decrease in the degree of unsaturation of the meal-oil fraction. The oxidative deterioration of fishmeal during storage is well recognized as conductive to decline in nutritive value. Antioxidants, such as butylated hydroxytoluene and 6-ethoxy-2,2,4-trimethyl-1,2-dihydroquinoline, are generally added to fishmeal after the drying operation so as to regard the progress of the auto-oxidation reaction during storage. Autooxidation commences during the drying operations. More powerful antioxidants are required to improve storage capabilities. A more effective antioxidant is tertiary butyhydroquinone, approved as a direct food and feed additive.

fixation. 1. In general, the act or process of making secure or permanent. The examples are found in microscopy, where the term is applied to the preparation of slides from specimens or sections cut from them; in photography, the term is applied to the removal from photographic film or other media, after exposure, of the unchanged light-sensitive substances, to prevent further change and hence marring the picture.

2. In immunology, the term is applied to the method of preventing hemolysis by the complement; in perfume and flavor formulation, to the use of high boiling components to make the evaporation of the mixture uniform; and in chemistry, it refers to reactions and processes by which free nitrogen enters into chemical combination.

flamber. To light spirit poured over a dish, e.g. brandy on the Christmas pudding.

flash 18. A method of canning foods under pressure 18 pounds per square inch above atmospheric pressure. The food is sterilised at 121°C and then canned at that temperature, not requiring further heat. The advantages claimed are improved taste and texture compared with the conventional canning, and the possibility of using large containers without overheating the food.

flash evaporation. Very rapid evaporation, especially as applied in industrial processes, in which liquids are heated under pressure is subsequently suddenly reduced causing the liquid, which is then superheated, to evaporate rapidly. Also known as flash drying.

flash pasteurization. A pasteurization technique in which a heat-labile liquid such as milk, is briefly subjected to temperature around 375-383 K.

flash photolysis. Photolysis generated by very short but high-intensity flash of light. Flash photolysis is a method of investigating the mechanism of extremely rapid photochemical reactions involving formation of free radicals.

flash point. With reference to frying oils, the temperature at which the decomposition products can be ignited, but will not supported combustion. When they will support combustion, this is known as fire point. Cottonseed oil: smoke point 232°C, flash point 330°C. These points are lowered by the presence of free fatty acids. Flash point varies with different fats and ranges between 290-330°C.

flash pasteurization. A process in which the material is held at a higher temperature than in normal pasteurization, but for a shorter period. There is less development of the cooked flavour in the shorter period. For milk, ordinary pasteurization involves heating to 60°C for 30 seconds; in the flash process, it is heated to 74°C for a few seconds only.

flats. The whole milk American Cheddar cheese in the shape of cylinders 25-30 cm in diameter and 13-15 cm in height, and weighing 12-15 kg. When two blocks of this cheese are packed in a box, one on top of the other, they are called "twins." When packed separately, they are called "singles."

flat sours. Bacteria that render canned food sour, without gas production, i.e. the ends of the can are not swelled out but remain flat. They are thermophilic, facultative anaerobes, that attack carbohydrates with the production of acids, lactic, formic, acetic, but without gas formation. Economically they are the most important of the thermophilic spoilage agents; some species can grow slowly at 25°C and thus spoil products after long storage periods. Type species is *Bacillus stearothermophilus.*

flatworms. Two main groups of parasitic worms making up the flatworms are the tapeworms (*cestodes*) and the flukes (*trematodes*). Many varieties or species of both classes comprise the flatworm group, and all may be found at one time or another in animals and man. As a rule, only one species of flatworm at a time will be found in the body, but there are exceptions. Depending upon which species of tapeworm infects the host, the symptoms, the only evidence is the presence of

proglotids (series of segments containing male and female reproductive systems, but no alimentary canal) in the feces, in the other cases, loss or increase of appetite may indicate parasites. The other infestations may cause abdominal pain, nausea, vomiting, diarrhea, dizziness, anemia and general weakness. The flukes produce a number of infections which occur in man and animals. Chief among these are liver and blood infections, caused by the liver fluke and blood fluke etc. The blood flukes are also known as schistosomes.

flavedo. The coloured outer peel layer of citrus fruits, also called the epicarp or zest. It contains the oil sacs and numerous yellow plastids (green in the unripe fruit, containing chlorophyll; yellow in the ripe fruit, containing carotene and xanthophyll).

flavin. The colour obtained from the quercitron (bark (species of oak, *quercus tinctoria*); largely permitted in food in most countries. Insoluble in water but soluble in alkalies to give yellow colour, changed to brown in air. Also known as quercitron.

flavin adenine dinucleotide. FAD. The flavin nucleotide, riboflavin adenosine diphosphate, which is a coenzyme form of the vitamin riboflavin and which functions in dehydrogenation reactions catalyzed by flavoproteins; it is abbreviated as FAD in its oxidized form and as $FADH_2$ in its reduced form. The reactive part of FAD is its isoalloxazine ring. FAD, like NAD^+, is two electron acceptor. However, unlike NAD^+, FAD accepts both the hydrogen atoms lost by the substrate. Flavin adenine dinucleotide is synthesized from riboflavin and two molecules of ATP. Riboflavin is phosphorylated by ATP to give riboflavin 5'-phosphate (also called flavin mononucleotide). FAD is then formed by the transfer of an AMP moiety from a second molecule of ATP to riboflavin 5'-phosphate. It comprises phosphorylated vitamin (B_2) molecule linked to the nucleotide adenine monophosphate (AMP) It is usually tightly bound to the enzyme forming a flavoprotein. It functions as hydrogen acceptor in hydrogenation reactions and is reduced to $FADH_2$, which in turn is oxidized to FAD by the electron transport chain, thereby generating ATP. A key part of the structure of FAD is its isoalloxazin ring which is able to gain two hydrogen atoms, thus producing the reduced form $FADH_2$. FAD is the prosthetic group of some membrane-bound flavoprotein dehydrogenases such as succinate dehydrogenase. It is also the prosthetic group of some oxidases that react directly with oxygen, the two hydrogen atoms of $FADH_2$ reacting to give hydrogen peroxide.

flavin mononucleotide. FMN. A derivative of riboflavin (vitamin B_{12}) that is the immediate precursor of FAD and functions as a coenzyme in various oxidation-reduction reactions. It is the prosthetic group of the membrane-bound NADHdehydrogenase. A complex flavoprotein which is the first complex involved in electron transport chains for oxidation of NADH by oxygen. Hydrogen atoms of $FMNH_2$ are released as protons, the electrons being transferred to the iron-sulphur centre of the enzyme complex.

Flavobacterium meningosepticum. Facultatively anaerobic, oxidase-positive, nonmotile, long, thin, Gram-negative rods that produce yellow colonies. They utilize glucose and other carbohydrates fermentatively; found in soil and water. They cause nosocomial infections, particularly epidemics of meningitis in premature infants.

flavonoid. 1. Compounds widely distributed in nature as pigments in flowers, fruit, vegetables and tree barks. Structurally the flavone nucleus consists of a benzoid ring fused to gamma-pyrone carrying a second benzenoid ring and bearing a number of hydroxyl groups. Flavonoids are flavone glycosides with rhamnose or rhmnoglucose attached at position 3 to 7.

Flavonoids are divided into flavonols: hydroxyl group replaces H in flavone nucleus; Flavanones, one double bond reduced in the 2,3 position; Flavanals, hydroxyl group in place of the O and reduction of double bond at 4 and reduction of 2,3 double bond; Isoflavones, benzenoid ring at attached to C_3 instead of 2. The term "bioflavonoid" is sometimes used instead of vitamin P. Three most important classes are antocynins, the flavons, and the flavon-3-ols, or flavonols. Other classes are chalcones, isoflavons, an leuco-anthocynidins. The various flavonoid classes are biogenetically related, all being derived from a common precursor. In contrast to the alkaloids, flavonoids are rather inactive pharmacologically. An economically significant property of flavonoids is their contribution to taste and flavour in foods.

flavoproteins. The yellow conjugated proteins in which prosthetic group is either flavin mononucleotide of flavin adenine dinucleotide. Flavoproteins are enzyme of the dehydrogenase type in the electron-transport chain. The prosthetic groups of flavoproteins are flavin coenzymes FAD and FMN. These cofactors, in contrast to the nicotinamide nucleotide coenzymes, are much more firmly associated to the protein moiety, and in some cases (such as succinic dehydrogenase) are covalently bonded to that protein. In their simplest form, flavin cofactors accept 2 electrons and a proton from NADH or 2 electrons and 2 protons from an organic substrate such as succinic acid. The flavoproteins of mitochondrial respiratory chain are more complex in that they contain or are closely associated with nonhaem iron (NHI) proteins. Thus, NADH dehydrogenase of beef heart mitochondria contains 1 FMN and 8 iron atoms per particle weight of 200,000. The iron is present as nonhaem iron and is associated with acid-labile sulphur atoms. Because the flavin cofactors can accept one electron at a time forming a semiquinone, the flavoproteins represent a point in the respiratory chain where electrons can be transferred one at a time rather than in pairs.

flavor. *See* flavour.

flavour. 1. A term almost synonymous with taste. Though much research has been expended on analyzing this sense, no correlation between flavour and chemical type or structure has been determined. The basic tastes are bitter, sweet, salty, and sour; beyond this, the problem is physiological and psychological, rather than chemical. Taste, like odour is a property widely used by chemist for identification purposes.
2. A substance having a strong characteristic taste, often obtained by extraction from the leaves, twigs, or flowers of plants; many are now made artificially. Among the more common natural flavoring materials are vanillin and chocolate, oil of wintergreen, peppermint, clove, and cinnamon (from plant leaves or blossom), oil of bitter almond (from nuts), and citrus flavors (from seeds of oranges, lemons, etc.).

More than 2,000 natural and many more synthetic flavouring agents are known. Also spelled as flavor.

flavoured milk drinks. The most popular of the dairy-made flavoured milk drinks is chocolate milk, which enjoys a sales volume ranging from 5-10% of total homogenized milk sales, depending upon region and season of the year. Product is generally available in two types: Chocolate milk (3.5% fat); and chocolate milk drink (2.0% fat). Generally, these drinks contain about 6% sugar, 1.25% cocoa, (2% chocolate liquor), 0.1% stabilizer, along with traces of vanilla and salts. Cocoa is more frequently used than chocolate liquors. Pasteurization ranges vary with individual dairies. Typical time-temperature conditions include 73.9°C for 15 seconds; 62.8°C for 26 minutes for inactivating bacteria. Creaming can be minimized by employing somewhat higher temperatures for longer times, such as at 73.9°C for 20-30 minutes; or at 80°C for 16 seconds. In Europe, chocolate milk is commonly sterilized at 118.3°C for 10-20 minutes.

flavour potentiator. Substance that enhances the flavours of other substances without itself imparting any characteristic flavour of its own, *e.g.*, mono sodium glutamate, ribotide, as well as small quantities of sugar, salt and vinegar.

flavour profile. Method of judging flavour of foods by examination of a list of the separate factors into which the flavour can be analysed - the so-called character notes.

flavours, synthetic. these are generally mixtures of esters, such as banana oil, that is, ethyl butyrate and amyl acetate; apple oil, that is, ethyl butyrate, ethyl valerianate, ethyl salicylate, amyl butyrate, glycerol, chloroform and alcohol; pineapple oil, that is, ethyl and amyl butyrates, acetaldehyde, chloroform, glycerol, alcohol.

flaxseed. *Linus usitatissimum.* The cultivation of flaxseed reaches back to the remotest periods of history. Both the seeds as well as the cloth woven from this plant fabric have been found in ancient Egyptian tombs. In fact, the first linen mentioned in the Bible has been proven by historians and archaeologists to have been spun from flax. The flax is a little plant with turquoise blue blossoms, a tall, erect annual 40-60 cm in height. The stems are usually solitary, quite smooth, with alternate, linear, sessile leaves nearly in inch long. The seed vessels with their five-celled capsules are referred to in the Bible as bolls, with the expression in Exodus 9:31. In order to help in the separation of the fibre from the stalks, the bundles are placed in water for several weeks, and then spread out to dry. From the crushed or milled seeds comes linseed oil and meal. The oil is applied to wood surfaces in thin layers to form a hard, transparent varnish. Internally the oil is used by some veterinarians as a purgative for sheep and horses or a jelly from the boiled seeds is fed to young calves.

flaxseed drying. Flaxseed should have about 8% moisture content or below for safe storage because of a high fat conetne. Flaxseed can be dried with unheated as well as heated air. Flaxseed with 18% moisture can be dried with 79.4°C air without detrimental effect on germination. If the moisture content is 9-11%, it is more economical to use air at 65.5°C for drying.

flint corn. *Zea indurata.* A variety of corn which shrinks uniformly as it matures, and does not have a dent formation. Flint corn has long cylindrical ears with hard smooth grains of various colours. Traditionally, flint types have been preferred by Argentine growers. The term flint derives from the hard surface layer of starch over the kernel, with the soft starch being deposited in the centre.

Florence oil. Name given to high purity grade olive oil.

Floridean starch. A glucosan resembling glycogen, obtained from red algae (*Florideae*).

flotost cheese. A boiled-whey cheese made in Norway; it is similar to Myost but is little richer.

flour. Generally refers to the ground wheat berry although also used for other cereals and applied to powder dried materials such as fish flour (deodorised dried fish) potato flour, etc. The ground wheat yields wholemeal flour (100% extraction), whiter flours are obtained by separation of the bran and the germ from the starchy endosperm. The white flour is used in the ordinary white loaf is 70-72% extraction fortified to contain not less than 0.24 mg vitamin B_1 1.6 mg nicotinic acid, and 1.65 mg iron per 100 g plus some amount of *creta praeparata* (chalk).

flour enrichment. The addition of certain vitamins and minerals to flour.

flour strength. A property of the flour proteins enabling the dough to retain gas during fermentation to give a bold loaf. Strong flour is higher in protein content, and greater ability to absorb water. A weak flour gives a loaf that lacks volume.

flour, high ratio. Flour of very fine and more uniform particle size, treated with chlorine to reduced the gluten strength. It is used for making cakes since it is possible to add up to 140 parts of sugar to 100 parts of this flour, whereas only half this quantity of sugar can be incorporated into cakes with ordinary flour.

flour, self-raising. Flour to which have been added chemicals that produce carbon dioxide in the presence of water and heat; the dough is thus aerated without prolonged fermentation. Usually weaker flours are used. chemical agents used include sodium carbonate, calcium acid phosphate or sodium pyrophosphate, or a mixture of these two. Legally self-raising flour must contain not less than 0.4% available carbon dioxide.

flow quenching. A rapid flow technique in which the enzyme and the substrate are mixed in the usual manner, but the mixture then flows into a second mixing chamber rather than into an observation cell. The enzymatic reaction is stopped rapidly in the second chamber by mixing a chemical quenching reagent with the enzyme and the substrate. A reactant or a product of the reaction is then determined by any convenient method.

flue curing. A high heat is provided through a central heating system or flues on the floor of the barn for the drying of tobacco. Hot air, usually heated by gas, oil, or coal, is evenly distributed throughout the barn with a blower or fan. Flue-cured tobacco is kept in the barn for about a week until a honey yellow colour develops.

fluid bed dryer. A bed of solid particles is supported on a cushion of hot air jets (fluidized) and the material may be conveyed in this way, while being dried. The method achieves intimate mixing without mechanical damage: it is applicable to particles of a size sufficiently small to become impervious when packed closely and sufficiently large to float on an air cushion (as distinct from fine powders), *e.g.*, cereals, tabletting granules, salt, coffee and dried vegetables.

flummery. Another name for frumenty.

fluorescence. The ability to absorb light at one wavelength and radiate part of it at another wavelength. Is used analytically for quantitative measurement by fluorimetry; the intensity of fluorescence being proportional to the amount of material present. For example, vitamin B_2 and thiochrome, prepared from vitamin B_1 fluoresce.

fluoridation. Process of adding traces of fluoride to drinking water to arrest or prevent dental decay.

fluorine. An element of the same family as chlorine, bromine and iodine (the halogens). Although it ordinarily occurs in small amounts in plants and animals it is not thought to be essential to either and no deficiency symptoms have ever been produced. Drinking water ranges in fluoride content between 0.05 and 14 mg/L, and water containing concentrations around 1 mg/L helps to protect teeth from decay, although the mechanism of this effect is unknown. Quantities of this order are added to drinking water in enlightened areas to confer this protection. In larger amounts, it causes chalky white patches to appear on the surface of the teeth, known as mottled enamel. Excessive doses of fluorine are toxic and give rise to fluorosis.

foam spray dryer. Products which can entrain air or a gas, such as certain food and biological material including skim milk, cream, and juices, are foamed then forced through an atomizing nozzle in a conventional spray dryer. Air or nitrogen are the gases which are commonly used. Foam spray-dried products have less heat-induced changes, such as flavour and discoloration, as compared with conventional spray-dried products. A product with density less than conventional is obtained which is about equal to the density of instantized or agglomerated powder.

foam-mat drying. A method of drying food. Liquid concentrate is whipped to a foam with the aid of a foaming agent, spread on a tray and dried in a stream of warm air. It reconstitutes very rapidly with water because of the fine structure of the foam. It has the further advantage that the foam-dried materials hold less water at a given relative humidity than do spray-dried foods and are less liable to cake.

fodrin. A spectrin-like protein that lines the cortical cytoplasm of neurons and which appears to link actin filaments to the membrane. Fodrin is thought to down-regulate the number of receptor bindings sites on neuronal membranes. Its breakdown by the Ca^{2+} dependent protease, calpain 1, leads to the exposure of more receptors. Studies to date have been concerned with glutamate receptors, but there may well be a similar fodrin-mediated mechanism underlying the down and up-regulation of other types of neuronal receptors. It has been suggested that the increase in receptor number arising from fodrin breakdown plays a part in memory storage.

α-foetoprotein. Albumin-like proteins that is the main proteins component of fetal plasma. It is a glycoprotein (molecular mass ~70000), and is synthesized chiefly in the liver. It is not entirely fetal-specific, since its synthesis in the adult liver occurs during pregnancy and in cases of liver injury or disease. Its presence in the adult plasma may be used in the detection of liver carcinoma, although the effects of poisonous substances such as carbon tetrachloride also include α-foetorproteins production.

foggiano cheese. A ewe's milk cheese prepared in Italy; it is similar to Cotronese and Moliterno cheese.

folic acid. $C_{19}H_{19}N_7O_6$. petrolyglutamic acid. A water soluble vitamin. Milk contains about 1 mg/L of folic acid. Folic acid has been of therapeutic value in the treatment of macrocytic anemia, leucopenia, and thrombopenia. Green leafy vegetables are excellent sources of this vitamin. Folic acid is a vitamin of the B-complex that, with vitamin B_{12} is required as a cofactor in the enzymatic transfer of one-carbon groups in the metabolism of proteins and nucleic acids. Rapidly growing tissues (*e.g.,* intestinal mucosae, haemopoietic system, embryos) have the greatest requirements of folic acid. Folic acid is synthesized by some plants and by microorganisms in the reticulorumen and large intestines, although the later require adequate supplies of *p*-aminobenzoic acid (PABA). It is moderately stable to air and heat but is degraded by light, alkalies, and acids. It has three major components; glutamic acid, *p*-aminobenzoic acid, and a pteridine derivative. The deficiency of folic acid causes a type of anemia in which the red blood cells do not mature properly. Folic acid is important in metabolism in various coenzyme forms, all of which are specifically concerned with the transfer and utilization of single carbon (C_1) group. Before functioning in this manner folic acid must be reduced to either dihydrofolic acid (FH_2) or tetrahydrofolic acid (FH_4). It is important in the growth and reproduction of cells, participating in the synthesis of purines and thymine.

Synthesis of folic acid occurs in the rumen, but some researchers believe that newborn lambs require a dietary supply. In species affected by a deficiency of folic acid, a characteristic macrocytic, hyperchromic anemia (known as megaloblastic anemia) occurs. There are bone marrow changes and red cells are large and immature. Leucopenia (reduction of white cell numbers) also may occur. In poultry, a deficiency retards growth, with poor feathering and a depigmentation of colored feathers. Most natural animal feeds contain more than adequate supplies of folic acid. Supplementation is usually confined to poultry. Supplementation ranges from 0.2-0.5 g per ton of feed.

Folic acid occurs in foods as a variety of derivatives of petroyl glutamic acid; the active form appears to be formyltetrapteroylglutamic acid (previously called folinic acid and citrovorum factor). The various forms isolated have given rise to a number of names including Wills factor, *Lactobacillus casei* factor, *Streptococcus lactis* R factor or rhizopterin, leucovorin, vitamin M, vitamin B_{c9} factors U, R and S. The nomenclature adopted by the International Union of Pure and Applied Chemistry does not agree with that of the International Union of Nutritional Sciences. Generic description folic acid (folacin). The specific compounds, petroylglutamic acid (folic acid); pteroyldiglutamic acid (folic acid glutamate); pteroyltriglutamic acid (folic acid diglutamate); tetrapteroylglutamic acid (tetrahydrofolic acid). It is found in fresh dark green vegetables, kidney and liver. The assay is certain and amounts are expressed as folate equivalent being the amount of folic acid activity measured by *L. casei* assay without pre-treatment to liberate combined forms. Its recommended intake according to the US National Research Council is 0.4 mg per day.

Folle Blanche grape. A variety mainly grown in France for production of white wines. The variety is also cultivated in California and is some times used in the production of California "Chablais" and California Champagnes.

follicle-stimulating hormone. FSH. The gonadotrophic protein hormone secreted by the anterior lobe of the pituitary gland, that stimulates the growth of ovarian follicles in the female and spermatogenesis in the male. In the absence of FSH, the testes are atrophic and sperm production is absent. FSH also stimulates estradial production in isolated Sertoli cells. Plasma FSH concentrations increase through puberty from the low levels of infancy.

fondant. Minute sugar crystals in a saturated sugar syrup; used as the creamy filling in chocolates and biscuits and for decorating cakes. Prepared by boiling sugar solution with addition of confectioners' glucose or an inverting agent and cooling rapidly while stirring.

food. Substances taken in by mouth which maintain life and grown, *i.e.*, supply energy, and build and replace tissue. Food is used to maintain certain essential biological processes in living organisms, notably to furnish cell and tissue-building materials, and to provide heat and energy, as well as to supply auxiliary substances needed for the functioning of these processes. The basic food requirements of animals and man are fats, carbohydrate, proteins vitamins, and minerals, all of which are obtained by the ingestion of plants or their assimilated forms (meat, milk). The energy stored in the food is made available by oxidation, hydrolysis, and similar chemical reactions.

food chain. The flow of energy and matter in living organisms through a producer-consumer sequence.

food from microorganisms. Many microorganisms are high in protein and can be used as sources of protein food for humans and animals. In many cases, microbial cells contain greater than 50% protein, and in at least some species, this is complete protein. The only organism presently used as a source of single-cell protein is yeast, but algae, bacteria, and fungi have also been considered. The desirable properties that an organism should possess, to be useful as a source of single-cell protein include: rapid growth; simple and inexpensive medium; efficient utilization of energy source; simple culture system; simple processing and separation of cells; non-pathogenic; harmless when eaten; good flavor; high digestibility; and high nutrition content.

food infection. The gastrointestinal illness caused by ingestion of microorganisms, followed by growth and disease occurrence in the consuming organism.

food intoxication. Food poisoning caused by microbial toxins produced in the food prior to consumption.

food phosphate factor. A term applied to the resistance of bacteria to thermal destruction; defined as the ratio of resistance to heat when present in a food, to the resistance when in phosphate buffer (at pH 6.98). The protective action of the ingredient of food renders the bacteria more resistant than in buffer. Factor 360 is the thermal death time at 100°C of the most resistant strain of *Clostrium botulinum* that has been isolated.

food poisoning. A general term usually referring to a gastrointestinal disease caused by the ingestion of food contaminated by pathogens or their toxins. It may be due to :
(a) contamination with harmful bacteria;
(b) toxic chemicals;
(c) allergic reaction to certain proteins;
(d) chemical contamination.

Staphylococci multiply enormously, producing toxins that cannot be destroyed by reheating. People with staphylococci food poisoning are miserably sick with cramps, diarrhea, and vomiting. This kind of illness can be most dangerous for young children and people with poor health. The other common kind of food poisoning is botulism, which is due to a toxin produced by a bacterium called *Clostridium botulinum*. The outbreaks of this type of food poisoning are generally due to improperly processed canned food. The third type of food poisoning can be due to *salmonella* infection. Many animals harbor various types of salmonellae, and outbreaks are usually traced to animal products. The organism is usually destroyed by cooking but not by freezing or drying. The symptoms of *salmonella* food poisoning are much like those of staphylococcus poisoning but are not due to toxin but to intestinal infection. The shigella organisms are related to the salmonellae and have been found to be the cause of bacillary dysentery. It has been found that the bacterium called *Clostridium perfringens*, a normal inhabitant of the human intestine, can cause trouble if it gets into food. It can cause the very dangerous wound infection known as gas gangrene. Food can also be contaminated by a number of other bacterium.

food preservation. The prevention of chemical decomposition and the development of harmful bacteria in foods. It is generally affected by the sterilization of food (*i.e.*, by destruction of bacteria in it) by heating in sealed vessels, *i.e.*, canning; or by making the conditions unfavorable for development of bacteria, by pickling, drying, freezing, smoking, etc. See *also* freezing.

food scientist. One who studies the basic chemical, physical, biochemical, and biophysical properties of foods and their constituents.

food technologist. One who applies food science to the processing of foods to preserve them, improve flavour, texture, appearance and other desirable properties, and manufactures foods from basic materials.

food vacuole. A storage reservoir for food in protists and some animals.

food web. A network of many interlinked food chains, encompassing primary pro-ducers, consumers, decomposers, and detritivores.

forcemeat. Savoury seasoned stuffing for fish, meat and poultry made of sage, parsley, onion and thyme.

formaggi di pasta filata. A group of Italian cheeses which when plastic and hot are kneaded, pulled, and shaped. Some of the common types are Provolone, Caciocavallo, Mozzarella, Provatura and Scamorze.

formula 21. A slimming preparation composed of methyl cellulose and glucose, with flavour and colour. The average composition per 100 g is: vitamin B_1 1.1 mg; vitamin B_2 2.7 mg; nicotinic acid 10.9 mg; reduced iron 10.9 mg, and calcium 675 mg.

forskolin. A diterpene obtained from the roots of the plant *Coleus forskohlii*. An alternative name for forskolin is coleonol. Forskolin is a valuable experimental tool because it has a powerful and specific action to stimulate the adenylate cyclase of eukaryotic cells, and so elevate the concentration of cyclic AMP. In stimulating the enzyme it bypasses all known membrane receptors and it does not act via the guanine nucleotide subunits. It therefore probably acts directly on the catalytic subunit of the enzyme.

Fortifex. A protein-rich baby food containing about 30% protein. It is made from maize, defatted soya flour with added vitamins A, B_1, B_2, calcium carbonate and methionine.

fortification. A term used in the food industry to describe the addition of essential nutritional factors such as vitamins, minerals, proteins, etc., to certain food products to replace losses incurred in the processing of raw materials, and to meet standard nutritional requirements. It is practiced especially with milled wheat flours, prepared mixes, meat and fish by-products, margarine, and infant foods. In cases where food is baked after fortification, a large percentage of the vitamins so added may be inactivated by heat.

fortified wines. The wines which have been strengthened during or after fermentation, by the addition of spirits, so that their alcohol content is about 20%, almost double that of the beverage wines. In France, fortified wines are known as '*Vine Liqueur*' and wines with naturally enhanced alcohol content are called '*Vins Liquoreux*'. The fortified wines are Sherry, Port, Vermouth, Maderia, Marsala, Malaga, Angelica, Californian Tokay and a number of wines of more or less local interest, such as the French V.D.N., the wines of the Greek islands and so on. Wines with more than 18% alcohol are not subject to many of the ills which may attack the lighter beverage wines, for although the bactericidal properties of alcohol are often exaggerated, the organisms which attack wine either die or are very poorly themselves in liquids containing as much alcohol as the fortified wines.

foxtail millet. *Setaria italica.* A variety of millet widely grown in India, China, Japan, and Manchuria. In China, this millet is next to rice and wheat as a cereal for human consumption. In some regions, such as Armenia and Turkey, this millet is used as substitute for proso millet in regions of very poor soils and during extended hot, dry periods. Foxtail millet is frequently mixed with proso millet in such areas. Foxtail millet is an annual grass and is slender and erect, reaching a height of from 0.3-1.8 m. The panicle is roughly cylindrical, dense, and bristly, and from 5-30 cm in length. The seed hulls have a wide colour range from white through red and orange, as well as green and dark purple, depending upon variety. Seeds are from 2-3 mm long and from 1-2 mm in width. Varieties planted in the United States include Common, Goldmine, Hungarian, Kursk, Siberian, and White Wonder. Foxtail millet, particularly the German variety, is widely sold as seed for caged and wild birds. Also known as German millet; Italian millet; and Hungarian grass.

fractional test meal. Method of examining secretion of gastric juices of patients. The stomach contents are sampled at intervals via a stomach tube after a test meal of gruel. It is usual to test for total and free acidity, and in addition peptic activity may be measured.

frangipane. Originally a jasmine perfume, which gave its name to an almond cream flavoured with the perfume. The term is used for cake-filling made from eggs, milk and flour with flavouring; and also, for the pastry filled with an almond-flavoured mixture.

frappe. 1. An ice consisting of water, sugar, and flavouring material frozen to slushy consistency and served in that condition. It can be prepared as follows: Juice of 3 dozen lemons and one dozen oranges, 0.5 litre grape juice, 1 kg sugar, and water enough to make 15 litres. This is made in the same manner as an ice except that it is not hardened. Since frappes are served in a soft condition they ought preferably to be frozen just prior to serving. Many other fruit mixtures pleasing to taste can easily be developed.

2. Egg-white and sugar syrup whipped until so aerated that the density reaches 5 pounds per gallon.

freeze concentration. Concentration of a liquid by freezing out pure ice leaving a more concentrated solution; of interest in the concentration of fruit juices, vinegar and beer.

freeze dryer. A unit for removing moisture in which vacuum is usually maintained around a product. The vacuum is maintained such that the water is frozen in the substance, and moisture is removed by sublimation of the solid ice to water vapour. The freeze dryer is used for drying products which otherwise would be damaged if higher temperatures were used.

freeze drying. A method of drying in which the material is frozen and subjected to high vacuum. The ice sublimes off as water vapour without melting. Materials dried in this way are damaged little if at all. Freeze-dried food is very porous since it occupies the same volume as the original and so rehydrates rapidly. There is less loss of flavour and texture than with most other methods of drying. Controlled heat may be applied to the process without melting the frozen material 'that is accelerated freeze drying.

Free-Zee. A registered trade-mark for a chocolate coated frozen confection on a stick consisting of either:
(a) ice cream,
(b) ice milk,
(c) vegetable fat frozen dessert, or
(d) sherbet.

freezer burn. A change in the texture of frozen meat, fish and poultry during storage due to sublimation of the ice.

freezing. A technique used to check the microbial growth in the foodstuffs. Freezing does not kill all bacteria. The Gram-positive bacteria, yeasts, molds, and microbial spores are relatively resistant to killing by freezing; whereas Gram-negative bacteria are more susceptible to freezing, but a proportion of the cells survive. For instance, 30-70% of *E.coli* and 50-80% of *pseudomonas* population are killed by freezing. Some of the effects of freezing on microorganisms are:
(a) loss of cytoplasmic gases, such as oxygen and carbon dioxide;
(b) change of pH in the cell;
(c) loss of cellular electrolytes;
(d) denaturation of some of the proteins; and
(e) metabolic injury.

Microorganisms can grow during freezing of food. Consequently, many procedures and mechanical innovations have been devised to enhance rapid freezing.

Freisa. An Italian red wine usually of high quality and made from grape of the same name. Vineyards are located in the hills of piedmont between Turin and Castle Monferato.

French dressing. Temporary emulsion of oil and acid in distinction to mayonnaise which is a stable emulsion. Heavy French dressing is a similar product stabilized with pectin or vegetable gum.

frenching. Break up the fibres of meat by cutting, usually diagonally or in a criss-cross pattern.

fribourg chese. A hard cheese made similar to Swiss cheese in Switzerland and the Po valley.

friesian clove. A spiced cheese of partially skimmed cow's milk made extensively in the Netherlands.

frigi-canning. A process of pre-serving food by controlled heating, sufficient to destroy the vegetative form of micro-organism (and possibly to damage spores sufficiently to prevent germination) followed by sealing aseptically and storing at a low temperature but not a freezing point.

fromage fort cheese. A variety of cheese prepared in France by melting well-drained skim milk curd, subjecting it to a pressure and burying in dry ashes to remove excess whey. The curd is then grated and allowed to ripen for 8-10 days after which milk, butter, salt, pepper and wine are added and the mixture is further ripened.

Froment. Trade name for a wheat germ preparation. The average composition per 100 g is: protein 28.5%; fat 7.7%; carbohydrate 44.4%; vitamin B_1 0.45 mg; vitamin B_2 0.2 mg; vitamin E 8 mg; iron 2.7 mg; and food energy 1.5 MJ.

Frost's cellular test. A test devised by W. D. Frost for determining whether or not milk has been pasteurized. The sample of milk is mixed with an equal quantity of methylene blue stain. The mixture is allowed to stand for a least

10 minutes and then is centrifuged. It is then spread on a slide, dried and examined under a microscope. Slides from raw milk show a blue background with unstained leucocytes as clear areas, whereas slides of milk which has been heated to 55° C and held for 20 minutes of longer show well stained nuclei of leucocytes against a clear background.

frozen cream. Sweet cream which has been frozen and held at low temperatures for later use in dairy manufacturing. Because ice cream is largely consumed during hot weather, many ice cream manufacturers follow the practice of buying at low price during surplus months of good quality cream and storing it as frozen cream until needed. Good quality fresh cream, which tests at least 40% fat and has been pasteurized, should be used. It is usually stored in straight sided tins or in fibre containers and kept at a low temperature. These containers should not have exposed iron or copper.

fructofuranose. Fructose formulated as the five membered furan ring.

fructopyranose. Fructose formulated as the six-membered pyranose ring.

fructosan. A complex built of units of fructose. e.g., inulin.

fructose. $C_6H_{12}O_6$. A six-carbon sugar, differing from glucose in containing a ketonic group (on carbon 2) instead of an aldehydic group (which glucose has on carbon one). Found as the free sugar in some fruits and in honey and combined with glucose as sucrose. It is prepared by the hydrolysis of inulin from the Jerusalem artichoke. Alternative names fruit sugar and laevulose; 173% as sweet as sucrose. Fructose rotates polarized light to the left hence the name leavulose, in distinction from glucose which rotates polarized light to the right.

fructose-1,6-diphosphate. FDP. A metabolite that is cleaved in glycolysis to two triose phosphates, glyceraldehyde-3-phosphate and dihydroxyacetone phosphate.

fructose-1,6-diphosphate phosphatase. A regulatory enzyme which, together with phosphofructokinase plays a key role in regulating the flow of carbon up and down the glycolytic sequence. Regardless of the source, however, the phosphatase is strongly inhibited by AMP.

Fruhstuck. A Limburger type of cheese made in a round mold about 8 cm in diameter. During curing, yeasts and moulds grow on the surface, followed by the so-called red cheese bacteria and smear development. It is wrapped in foil or parchment and cured.

fruit. As common used in the food industry, the word fruit signifies tree fruits, such as apple, apricot, cherry, peach, pear, plum, of deciduous trees; or the important family of citrus fruits; or the bushberries, blackberry, raspberry, and strawberry, among others. The term generally refers to fleshy seed-bearing part of plants (including tomato, usually called a vegetable). Fruits generally contain negligible protein and fat; carbohydrate content varies from 3% in melon to 25% in banana. Carbohydrate occurs as glucose, fructose, sucrose, starch, pectin and cellulose. Cellulose adds bulk to the diet; During ripening of fruit starch changes to sugars. Fruits are a good source of potassium and vitamin C, and some are a useful source of carotene and iron.

Botanically a fruit is the ripened ovary of the flower, with or without other associated parts and, thus, this definition greatly broadens the number of food commodities that fall under the umbrella of fruits. There are many kinds of fruits. Usually, they are separated into two classes dry fruits and fleshy fruits. The fruit begins its existence as the ovary of the flower. After pollination and fertilization have occurred, embryos begin to develop in one or many ovules inside the ovary. As this growth continues, the ovule gradually becomes a seed, and the ovary wall or pericarp may grow larger or thicker, may store relatively large amounts of food, or may undergo other changes. Eventually the seeds reach maturity, and about the same time, the fruit ripens. The final form of the fruit is characteristic of the particular species of plant.

Three layers of cell tissue are sometimes recognizable as the ovary matures. The outermost layer is the exocarp, which is usually a thin layer, often an epidermis only one cell thick. The innermost layer is the endocarp. Between these two is the mesocarp, in which the vascular tissues ordinarily occur. The relative thickness and appearance of these layers vary greatly in different fruits. During the growth of the ovary into a fruit, other flower parts or adjacent stem tissue may also change and become an integral part of the fruit. In a strawberry, for example, the red pulp is not the ovary, but a very much enlarged and modified stem tip, the receptacle of the flower. A large part of the pineapple is stem, not ovary.

Fruits are generally classified as simple, multiple, or aggregate according to the arrangement of the carpels from which the fruit developed.

Simple fruits develop from one carpel or several united carpels.

Aggregate fruits, such as magnolia, raspberry, and strawberry, consist of a number of separate carpels of one gynoecium.

Multiple fruits consist of the gynoceia of more than one flower. The pineapple, for example, is a multiple fruit consisting of an inflorescence with many previously separate ovaries fused on the axis on which pineapple flowers were borne (the other flower parts are squeezed between the expanding ovaries.)

Simple fruits are by far the most diverse of the three groups. When ripe, they may be soft and fleshy, dry and woody, or papery. There are three main types of fleshy fruit; the *berry,* the *drupe,* and the *pome.* In the berry, examples of which are tomatoes, dates, and grapes, there are one to several carpels, each of which is usually many-seeded. The inner layer of the fruit coat is fleshy. In the drupe, there are also one to several carpels, but each usually contains only a single seed. The inner coat of the fruit is stony and usually tightly adherent to the seed. The coconut is a drupe whose outer covering is fibrous rather than fleshy, but in temperate regions we usually see only the seed with the adherent stony inner coat of the fruit. Other familiar drupes are the peach, cherry, olive, and plum. A highly specialized sort of fleshy fruit is the pome, which is characteristic of one subfamily of the rose family. The pome is derived from a compound inferior ovary in which the fleshy portion comes largely from the enlarged base of the perianth. Apples and pears are pomes.

Dry simple fruits are classified as dehiscent or indehiscent. In dehiscent fruits, the tissues of the mature ovary wall (the pericarp) break open freeing the seeds. In indehiscent fruits, the seeds remain in the fruit after the fruit is shed from the parent plant. There are several sorts of dehiscent simple dry fruits. The follicle is derived from a single carpel that splits down one side a maturity, as in columbines and milkweeds.

In the pea family, the characteristic fruit is a legume. Legumes resemble follicles but split along both sides.

In the mustard family (Brassicaceae), the fruit is called a silique and is formed of two fused carpels. At maturity, two halves split off, leaving the seeds attached to a persistent central portion. The most common sort of dehiscent simple dry fruit is the capsule, which is formed from a compound ovary in plants with either a superior or an inferior ovary. Capsules shed their seeds in a variety of ways.

In the poppy family, Papaveraceae, the seeds are often shed when the capsule splits longitudinally, but in some members of this family they are shed through holes near the top of the capsule. Indehiscent simple dry fruits are found in a great variety of plant families. Most common is the achene, a small single-seeded fruit in which the seed lies free in the cavity except for its attachment by the funiculus. Achenes are characteristic of buttercups and buckwheat. Winged achenes, such as those found in the elm and ash, are termed samaras.

In the grass family (Poaceae), the achenelike fruit (*caryopsis*) is derived from a compound ovary and the seed coat is firmly united to the fruit wall.

In the Asteraceae, the achenelike fruit is derived from a compound, inferior ovary and is called a cypsela. Acorns and hazelnuts are examples of nuts, which resemble achenes but have a stony coat and are derived from a compound ovary.

Finally, in parsley family (Apiceae) and the maples, as well as a number of other unrelated groups, the fruit is a schizocarp. The schizocarp is derived from a compound ovary but splits at maturity into a number of one-seeded portions.

fruit juice drying. The principal non-citrus fruit juices which are usually dried include apple, grape, and strawberry. Drying is preceded by concentration in an evaporator. Excessive heat treatment in the evaporator must be avoided to prevent off-flavours. Generally, for fruit juices (including berry), a falling-film evaporator operating below 55.6°C, usually less than 2 hours, does not produce excessive off-flavour. Of these products, strawberry is the most heat sensitive. Heat damage in the evaporator is carried to the dryer. Spray drying is most commonly used. Puff drying, foam-mat drying, and foam spray drying offer other methods. Products leaving the spray dryer are normally at 2-4% moisture. To dry further, a dehumidified air for final drying, or in-package drying, is used. Sweetened (50% of juice solids in sugar) fruit drinks (apple, grape, and tart cherry) of an instantizing quality can be made in a turbulent film evaporator in a vacuum, which produces small flakes upon cooling, the sugar being a drying agent.

fruit wines. In Northern Europe, especially in those parts which fall just outside the wine-belt, such as Poland, Northern Germany and much of Russia, fruit wines are made in very large quantities. The fruit-drink industry specifies that fruit wines shall have a certain minimum amount of alcohol and maximum acid. Commercial fruit wines are made from red, white and black-currants, gooseberries, strawberries, blackberries, raspberries, whortleberries, elderberries, sloes and several kinds of cherries. The alcohol content of these varies between 7 and 14%. The fruit wines of Poland have been described as being high in alcohol content and of good quality and Rumania has a high reputation for her fruit wines, especially those from red and white currants made in Dobruja. Russia makes a wide range of fruit wines, including that from mountain ash berries and rose-hips which is described to have a peculiar but pleasant taste. Imitation of grape wines such as Port are also described as being made from whortleberries. Generally, the vinification methods employed for the fruit wines are very similar to those normally used for grape-wine. Juice is usually diluted, and this, as well as the addition of sugar, which is universal, renders it liable to bacterial attack. Sulphuring is practised and it is necessary to be wary of the attentions of the air-borne organisms if open vats are used. A mouse-like odour and corresponding taste easily result from carelessness. The wines made from tropical fruits are innumerable, but their preparation is local and scantily recorded. Banana wine of 10-12% alcohol content is widely made in Central Africa.

fruit, canned. The fruit is usually canned in a sugar solution and hence the energy content is greater than that of the fresh fruit. Vitamin loss is about 50%, for example, peaches lose half of the carotene, B_1, B_2, nicotinic acid and vitamin C in canning.

fruits with starch reserve. Typical of fruits with a starch reserve are apple, banana, and pear. It has been shown, for example, that invert sugar and sucrose increase throughout the growing period of the apple fruit, but starch reaches its maximum when ripening processes begin. During the course of ripening, therefore, the starch is hydrolyzed to sugar. During early stages of ripening, the soluble pectin substances also develops. The sugars in a ripe apple consist mainly of glucose, fructose, and sucrose. Fruits like apple, pear, and banana, with their carbohydrate reserve, can be harvested in the mature green and permitted to finish their ripening process during storage. Other fruits, like citrus, raspberries, cherries, among others, do not develop a carbohydrate reserve and must, therefore, be ripened on the tree.

fruits without starch reserve. Fruits which do not accumulate a large carbohydrate reserve are typified by citrus fruits, blackberries, and raspberries, cherries, peaches, plums, strawberries, and others. During ripening on the tree or bush, these fruits show an increase in sugars and a decrease in acids. Following harvest, fruits without a starch reserve may develop a characteristic color, soften (in some types), and lose a slight amount of acid through respiration, but they will not show any increase in sugar. A good variety of orange has been shown to contain 10.6% soluble solids (mainly sugars) and 0.85% acids when acceptable to consumers. Several exceptions or variations from the general rule can be found in this second group. Lemons, for example, do not undergo the same changes during ripening as those in oranges and grapefruit. The lemon fruit, during growth and maturation, does not increase in sugar. Free acids in the juice increase during ripening and predominate over sugars in the ripe fruit. In the avocado, total sugar content decreases during maturation. With the loss of sugar, there is a concomitant increase in oil. Dates are unique not only because of the high sugar content in ripe fruits, but also because different varieties accumulate different kinds of sugar.

frumentry. Whole wheat stewed in water for 24 hours until the grains have burst and set in a thick jelly, then boiled with milk.

frying. A cooking process which involves rapid evaporation of water. In case of meat nearly all the extractives are left in the meat and the losses are smaller than in roasting. About 10-20% loss of vitamin B_1, 10-15% loss of B_2 and nicotinic acid. Fish loses about 20% vitamin B_1 on frying.

fudge. Carmel in which crystallization of the sugar (graining) is deliberately induced by the addition of fondant saturated syrup containing sugar crystals).

fumarase. The enzyme catalyzing the reaction between fumaric acid and water to form L-malic acid in the citric acid cycle. The enzyme has been crystallized from pig heart. It is a tetramer of four identical polypeptide chains.

fumeol. Refined smoke with the bitter principles removed: used for preparing liquid smokes for dipping foods such as fish to give them a smoked flavour.

fumigant. A chemical substance, applied in gaseous or vapor state and within a confined space, for eradicating all but the most resistant forms of animal life. Thus, fumigants and the procedures of fumigation represent a severe hazard to the lives of humans and domestic and farm animals if they are not treated in the most professional and expert manner. In food production, storage, and distribution, fumigation is frequently done:

(a) On citrus trees and other plantings around which portable tents or boxes can be constructed, for reaching pests, such as scale insects, which cannot be controlled by the normal use of spray or dust insecticides;

(b) in greenhouses in which, after a while, pest populations build up to a point where normal control methods no longer suffice;

(c) on nursery stock to eradicate scale insects, and to destroy any pests which may be present on stock brought in from other countries or regions and, in particular, of subterranean pests which are not readily visible;

(d) in food-packing and processing plants, warehouses, and consumer outlets, again where pest populations have a tendency to built up and where total eradication is periodically required to minimize pest damage;

(e) in all manner of food-storage facilities, notably those concerned with various grains and dried fruits, in which extremely resistant species of beetles, weevils, and other insects tend to habituate and increase their populations unless destroyed with fumigation power periodically;

(f) in a variety of transportation facilities, such as trucks, railway containers, shipments, where the problem is similar to that of the warehouse, and very important to avoid shipping (or receiving) damaging pests species from one region to the next;

(g) of seeds prior to planting;

(h) of soil that may be infested with ants, grubs, nematodes, wireworms and other soil-inhabiting pests; and

(h) occasionally in food-serving facilities, where long neglect and lack of cleanliness and normal pest controls have been lacking. Open field fumigation to control cinch bugs and grasshoppers no longer is common. **fungal diseases.** The disease caused in animals and humans as a result of fungal invasion. Most fungi are harmless, but a few are pathogenic causing skin and systemic infections. Those which are pathogenic to the skin, hair and nails produce superficial fungal diseases. Those which invade the body produce deep fungal diseases. The most common among the superficial fungal diseases is the ringworm or tinea; tinea of the body (*Tinea corporis*); tinea of the groin (*Tinea cruris*); infection of the feet (*Tinea pedis*); tinea of the nails (onychonychosis); tinea of hair and scalp (*Tinea capitis*). Among various fungal diseases the most common are: coccidiomycosis (bones and skin); blastomycosis; sporotrichosis etc. **fungi.** A major group of eukaryotic organisms constituting the taxon Mycota (Fungi). Some authorities do not regard fungi as plants and include them with other organisms of uncertain affinities in the kingdom. Fungi are classified in the taxonomic division Mycota or Fungi. They can either exist as single cells or make up a multicellular body called a mycelium, which consists of filaments known as hyphae.

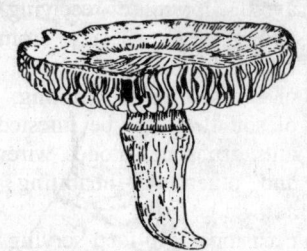

Most fungal cells walls composed chiefly of chitin. Fungi exist primarily in damp conditions on land and, because of absence of chlorophyll, are either parasites or saprophytes on other organisms. The Mycota can be subdivided into four main classes, *Phycomycetes, Ascomycetes, Basidiomycetes, and Fungi Imperfecti*. The principal criteria used in classification are the nature of the spores produced and the presence or absence of cross walls within the hyphae.

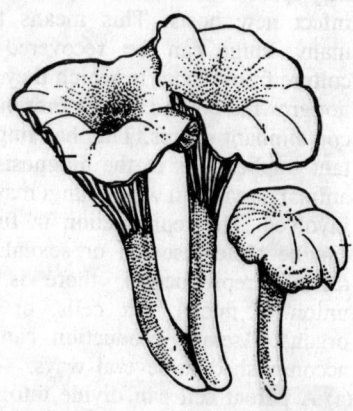

Most fungal cells are multinucleate and have rigid cell walls composed chiefly of chitin. Originally (and sometimes still) classified with green plants, fungi are now placed by many authorities in a separate taxonomic kingdom. A few groups of fungi that produce motile water-borne spores are transferred by some to the kingdom Protista, which contains the protozoa and most algae.

Most fungi live as saprophytes, of which a number are also able to infect animals. Fungi are also a major cause of plant disease, and many plant pathogens can survive only as parasites. Several fungal diseases are of considerable veterinary importance, such as ringworm, phycomycosis, blastomycosis, and my-cotic abortion. Moreover, fungi of different groups produce various toxic substances, some of which are released into the material on which fungus is growing. These substances include antibiotics, which are exploited therapeutically, and mycotoxins, which cause diseases known as mycotoxicosis. Mycelial fungi characteristically produce large numbers of microscopic, often air-borne, spores by which means they spread and colonize new sites or infect new hosts. This means that many fungi can be recovered in culture from places in which they are not growing but are merely present as contaminant spores. This has important implications in the diagnosis of animal diseases in which fungi may be involved. The reproduction in fungi can be either asexual or sexual. In asexual reproduction, there is no union of nuclei, sex cells, or sex organs. Asexual production can be accomplished in several ways:

(a) A parent cell can divide into two daughter cells by central constriction and formation of a new cell wall.

(b) A hypha can fragment to form cells that can behave as spores, called arthrospores. If the cells are surrounded by thick a thick wall before separation, they are called chlamydospores.

(c) Somatic vegetative cells or spores may bud to produce new organisms.

(d) In many cases, fungi can directly produce spores. This is most common method of asexual production. Sexual reproduction in fungi involves union of compatible nuclei.

Many fungal species are self-fertilizing and produce sexually compatible gametes on the same mycelium. Other species require outcrossing between different but sexually compatible mycelia. Depending on the species, the sexual fusion may occur between haploid gametes, gametangia, or hyphae. Sometimes, both the cytoplasm and haploid nuclei fuse to produce the haploid zygote.

In Pilobolus, a Zygomycete that grows on dung, the sporangia are shot toward the light. The sporangium is oriented toward the light so that all light rays entering the subsporangial swelling converge on a basal photorecptive area. Light focused elsewhere promotes maximum growth of the sporangiophore on the side away from the light. The high turgor pressure of the sap in the vacuole of the subsporangial swelling splits it and blasts the sporangium off to a distance of 2 m or more. When it has been fired off, sporangiophore collapses. The sporangium adheres where it lands, and if this happens to be a blade of grass, it may be eaten by a herbivore. It then passes through the digestive tract of the herbivore unharmed and is deposited in the dung to begin the new   cycle.

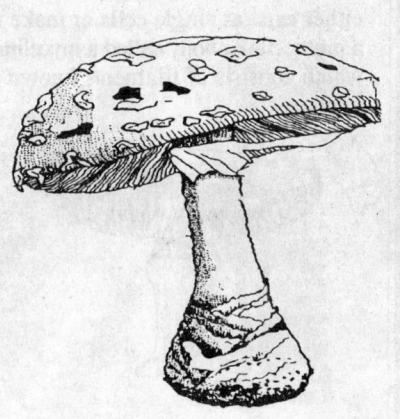

Varieties of penicillium, aspergillus etc. are the cause of deterioration in foods in the presence of oxygen and relative humidity of at least 70%. On the other hand varieties of penicillin such as *P. cambertii* and *P. rocquefortii* are desirable in certain cheeses. Among the edible fungi are mushrooms, *Agaricus compestris*. Experimentally, varieties such as Graphium, Fusarium and Rhizopus are grown on waste carbohydrates as a potential food; their fibrillar structure offers textural advantages in foods manufactured from them.

funicular. A condition in drying a porous body where moisture in the pores forms a continuous connection. The funicular condition precedes the pendular condition.

furanose. A sugar having a five-membered ring containing four carbon atoms and one oxygen atom.

fusel oil. Alcohol fermentation produces about 95% alcohol and 5% fusel oil, a mixture of organic acids, higher alcohols (propyl, butyl and amyl), aldehydes and esters. It is present in low concentration in wines and beer, and higher concentration in pot-still spirit. On maturation of the liquor the fusel oil change and imparts the special flavour to the spirit.

fusidic acid. A steroid antibiotic that inhibits protein synthesis by blocking the GTP-dependent reactions that are catalyzed by the enzyme translocase.

fusion protein. Protein molecule produced by recombinant DNA technology, usually when a novel gene is inserted into recipient plasmid vector in such a way that a terminal stop codon in a plasmid gene is deleted. Thus translational read-through occurs with the new fusion protein beginning with a plasmid sequence and continuing with the protein sequence of the inserted novel gene.

Fusobacterium nucleatum. Anaerobic, nonmotile, Gram-negative rods with long slender shape and pointed ends; normal inhabitants of mouth and upper respiratory tract. They are susceptible to penicillin, and are occasional cause of abscesses and blood stream infections.

fustic. Colouring matter obtained from the tree *Chlorophora tinctoria* or *Maclura tinctoria*. Two colour agents present, morin, sparingly soluble in water but soluble in alcohol, and maclurin, more soluble. Both are yellow but the colour changes in the presence of alkalies and metals.

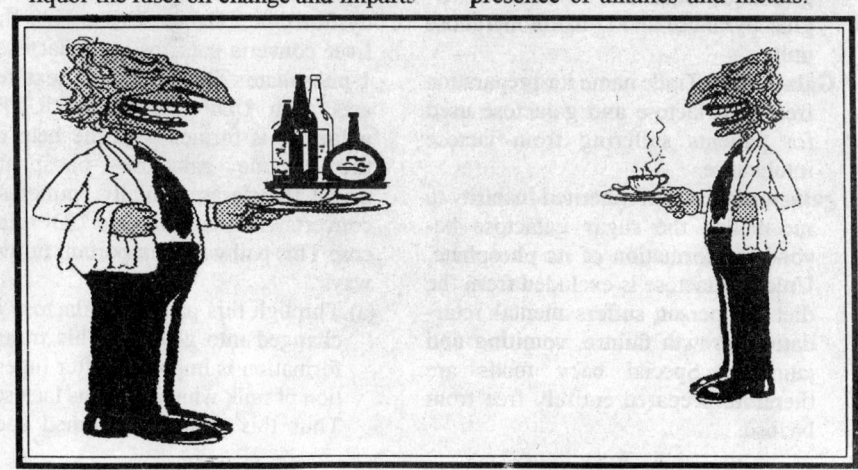

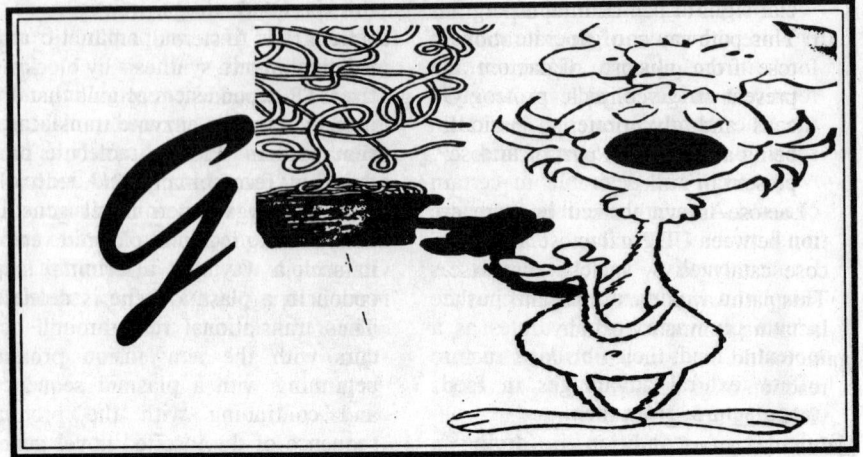

gaffelbitar. A semi-preserved herring preparation in which microbial growth is checked by the addition of salt at a concentration of 10-12%, and sometimes by the addition of benzoic acid as preservative. Anchovy is a similar product.

gaiskasli cheese. A soft goat's milk cheese prepared in Germany and Switzerland which ripens in 3 weeks.

galactoglucomannan. Any of a group of polysaccharides which are prominent components of the coniferous woods; galactoglucomannan consist of D-glucopyranose and D-mannopyranose units.

Galactomin. Trade name for preparation free from lactose and galactose used for patients suffering from lactose intolerance.

galactosaemia. An inherited inability to metabolize the sugar galactose beyond the formation of its phosphate. Unless galactose is excluded from the diet the person suffers mental retardation, growth failure, vomiting and jaundice. Special baby foods are therefore prepared entirely free from lactose.

galactose. $C_6H_{12}O_6$. A six-carbon sugar differing from glucose only in the position of the hydroxyl group on carbon four. It occurs mainly linked with glucose to form lactose (milk sugar), and is also present in the galactolipids of nerve tissue. It is about 32% as sweet as sucrose.

galactose metabolism. Liver is the only organ where galactose is metabolized. So much so that after an oral load of galactose, if galactose does not disappear quickly from the blood, it can be taken as an indication of liver dysfunction. Galactokinase in the liver converts galactose to galactose-1-phosphate. This molecule next reacts with UDP-glucose and UDP-galactose is formed with the help of the enzyme galactose-1-phosphate uridyl transferase. Finally epimerase converts UDP-galactose to UDP-glucose This pathway is important in two ways:

(a) Through this pathway galactose is changed into glucose. This transformation is important after ingestion of milk which contains lactose. Thus this pathway assumed special significance in infants.

(b) This pathway can generate galactose from glucose. Galactose is present in glycolipids, proteoglycans and glycoproteins, besides, being a constituent part of lactose, present in milk.

Lactose is synthesized by a reaction between UDP-galactose and glucose catalyzed by lactose synthatse. This pathway is thus important in the lactating mammary glands.

galactoside. A glycoside formed by the reaction of galactose with an alcohol; yields galactose on hydrolysis.

galactosyltransferase. Any one of a group of enzymes that help to make mature complex oligosaccharides from more simple sugars. Many of these complex sugars are finally attached to proteins, and much of this assembly occurs in vesicles of the Golgi apparatus. Indeed these enzymes are used as specific markers for the Golgi vesicles.

galactotoxin. A poisonous substance of ptomaine (a crystallizable, nitrogenous basic substance, produced by bacteria in dead animals or in vegetable matter) generated in milk by the growth of certain microorganisms.

galactozymase. The enzyme system responsible for the inducible fermentation of galactose in *Escherichia coli*; consists of galactokinase, galactose-1-phosphate uridyl transferase and UDP-glucose epimerase.

galanin. A 29 amino acid neuropeptide isolated from porcine upper small intestine. It is present in nerve fibres in the mucosa, smooth muscle, intramural ganglia and around blood vessels of the gastrointestinal tract.

galantine. A dish of white meat or poultry, boned, rolled cooked with herbs glazed with aspic jelly; it is usually served cold.

galenicals. Crude drugs, infusions, decoctions, and tinctures prepared from medicinal plants.

gallates. Salts and esters of gallic acid, found in many plants; used in making dyes and inks and medicinally as an astringent. Propyl, acetyl and dodecyl gallates are legally permitted antioxidants; 100 mg/L permitted in fats and vitamin oils, 80 mg/L in butterfat for manufacturing, 1,000 mg/L in essential oils for flavouring.

gallbladder. Organ situated in the liver the stores the bile manufactured by the liver.

gallstones. Stones formed in the gall bladder or in the bile duct. In the latter they obstruct the flow of bile and the result is jaundice. The stones consist of cholesterol and calcium salts of bilirubin, carbonate or phosphate; also called biliary calculi. Treatment includes a low-fat diet.

gallup number. A index of the hardness of butter fat. It is the number of grams (of mercury) required to forced a plunger of 5 mm diameter and weighing 50 g through a disc of butter fat of 6 mm thickness at 20°C.

Gambian bologi. *Basella alba*. A strongly growing, climbing plant with very thick, succulent leaves and fruits that turn black when ripe. Propagation is by means of seeds. Native growers usually plant in double rows about 60 cm apart, with the plants 30-38 cm apart in the rows. A fertile soil, with subsequent application of fertilizer, is required. When the plants reach a height of about 30 cm, they are supported by sticks. Also known as native spinach or broad-leaved bologi.

gamma radiation. The electromagnetic radiation emitted by excited atomic nuclei during passage to a lower excitation state. Gamma radiation ranges in energy from about 10^{15}-10^{11}

joule (10 keV-100 MeV) corresponding to a wavelength range of about 10^{10} to 10^{14} m. Gamma radiation are an example of ionizing radiation, which causes biological damage by producing hyperreactive ions and other molecular forms when the rays transfer their energy to microorganism. Gamma radiation, for example, are used for killing pathogens such as *Salmonella* in food products. Such applications are analogous to the use of heat in the pasteurization process. Complete sterilization is impractical because higher doses of radiation would produce undesirable changes in color, flavor, or consistency of the food. A large number of biological materials (such as penicillin) and numerous disposable plastic items (such as hypodermic syringes) can be sterilized effectively with gamma radiation without altering the material. Sterilizing plastic with gamma radiation is an alternative method to sterilizing with ethylene oxide, and it has the advantage that the sterilized objects can be used immediately without extended wait required after ethylene oxide sterilization.

gammelost cheese. A Norwegian, semi-soft, blue-mold ripened cheese with a sharp aromatic flavour. Lactic starter is added to skim milk and after souring for a day or two the milk is warmed to 50° C After maintaining for about 30 minutes at this temperature, the curd is dipped into cloth bags and pressed. The curd is removed, packed in cloth lined forms and placed in boiling whey for 3-4 hours. The next day the cheese is pierced and inoculated with a *Penicillum roquerforti* or related mold. The main ripening molds are: *Mucor, Rhizopus and Penicillium*. The cheese is cured for 4 weeks at 15-18° C.

gammon. Hind legs of bacon pig, cured while still part of carcass.

garden bean. Any of numerous varieties of beans grown for human consumption, the pods of which are picked in an immature state. Prompt picking of the pods prolongs the bearing period of the plant. The plants are grown mainly for their pods, not their seeds. String (stringless) beans with green, yellow, or purple pods fall into the category. Not a precisely used term.

garden mint. *Mentha spicata.* There are many species and types of this most popular of culinary herbs. Spearmint, or garden mint, is the most commonly grown domestic mint, which according to variety, may have dark green or grey-green leaves with smooth, decorative, or frilled edges.

Eau-de-cologne mint (*M. citrata*) has the scent of orange flowers and numbers orange, lavender, and bergamot mints among its varieties.

Water mint (*M. aquatica*) and horse mint (*M. longifolia*) grow in the wild and have an overpoweringly strong aroma.

Round-leafed mint (*M. rotundifolia*) has a distinctive appearance and numbers apple mint, Bowles, and pineapple mints in its list of varieties.

Most species are native to the Mediterranean region and western Asia, and now grow wild throughout northern Europe and in parts of North America. They grow wild in the garden, too, if their roots are not contained (in a bottomless container sunk into the ground, say) and their colonization process curtailed by vigilant thinning and cutting back. Mint sauce, in which the chopped herb is mixed with vinegar as a accompanied to roast lamb, is the traditional herald of a British spring. A spring of mint can be added when cooking new potatoes, peas, marrow, and many other vegetables.

Mint is chopped into softened butter for serving with lamb; and into apple jelly as a preserve to serve with a variety of poultry, meats and grilled fish. Sprigs of mint are also used as a garnish, and to flavour fruit salads and summer drinks, particularly mint julep. Mint tea, served hot or cold with a slice of lemon, is a refreshing and reviving tisane. The dried leaves may be used in pot pourri.

garden thyme. *Thymus vulgaris.* A sun-loving herb, at its aromatic best when growing wild on the sun-baked hills around the Mediterranean. It is grown in gardens in less favourable climates, it will be aromatic, but less powerfully so. It is a decorative herb, covered for two or three of the summer months with delicate pale mauve flowers, themselves highly fragrant, attractive to bees, and with many culinary uses. Different species offer a range of flavours: try *T. citriodorus,* lemon thyme, for a distinctly citrus aroma, and *T. herba-barona,* caraway thyme, for a spicy flavour. The English wild thyme referred to by Shakespeare is *T. drucei.*

Thyme is traditionally used with parsley in stuffing for chicken and pork, and, with the addition of a bay leaf, in bouquets garnis for use in soups and casseroles. It is especially goods with oil and wine or vinegar in marinades for meat and fish, and with vegetables such as courgettes, aubergines, sweet peppers, and tomatoes. It both dries and freezes well, so no kitchen need ever be without it.

Lemon thyme may be used in custards, fruit salads, and syrups. The essential oil - thymol - is a strong antiseptic. Thus an infusion may be used as a mouthwash, a gargle, and a wash for cuts and abrasions. The dried leaves especially those of lemon thyme, are used to scent linen, and are an important ingredient in pot pourri, herb, and sleep pillows.

garlic. Family: *Liliaceae.* Genus: *Allium.* Species: *Allium sativum.* A member of the onion family, the garlic bulb is an indispensable flavouring in cooking and is widely used throughout the world. It is a native of Asia, it is easily grown and widely cultivated in warm climates throughout the world. It can be grown successfully but in cooler conditions the bulb never reaches its maximum flavour potential. Garlic is a close kin to onion and was widely used throughout antiquity as an aphrodisiac of sorts, a plague repellent, an antidote to ward off demons and vampires with and an embalming agent, not to mention being a popular culinary spice as well. The leaves are long, narrow and flat like lawn grass. The bulb is of compound nature, consisting of numerous bulblets or cloves, grouped together between the membranous scales and enclose within a whitish skin, which holds them as in a sac.

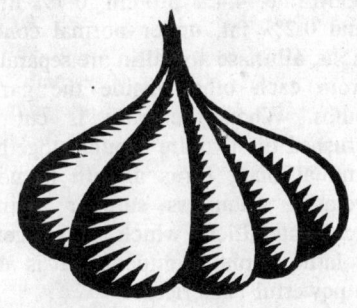

The bulb has expectorant and antiseptic properties and contains an antibiotic, allicin. Garlic salt is dried powdered garlic mixed with salt with the addition of starch to prevent caking. The garlic cloves may be finely chopped or crushed with a garlic press and used to complement the flavour of meat, fish, vegetables, salad dressings, sauces, and egg dishes. In southern Europe, sauces such as *aioli* (garlic mayonnaise) and *skordalia* are made from raw garlic, and in one French dish, chicken is cooked surrounded by whole cloves of garlic and salt. The aftertaste of garlic is offensive on breath; chewing fennel seeds can alleviate this problem. Whole cloves, peeled, may be preserved in jars filled with olive oil; the flavoured oil may then be used as a salad dressing. Garlic has positive health-giving properties. It may be used as an antiseptic; to tone up the digestive system; to reduce blood pressure; and to clear catarrh and bronchitis. It has also been used as a diuretic and as a combatant to diseases such as typhoid.

Fresh garlic contains about 0.2% volatile oil, allin, alliinase (an enzyme that breaks down allanin), calcium, phosphorous, iron, potassium, thiamin, riboflavin, niacin and vitamin C. Garlic contains 70% water, 23% carbohydrate, 4.4% protein, 0.7% fibre and 0.2% fat, under normal conditions, alliinase and allin are separated from each other inside the garlic bulbs. When the bulb is cut or crushed the two are brought together and alliinase turns allanin (a non-volatile, odourless sulphur amino-acid) into allicin, which is a pungent, volatile sulphur compound. It is also a powerful bactericide.

Garlic has a wide variety of biological effects, although not all active chemical constituents of garlic are known. It seems that the volatile sulphur-containing compounds are considered to be responsible for most of garlic's beneficial effects. Allicin, at a concentration of only 1 in 100,000 inhibits the growth of various bacteria, fungi and amoebas. Garlic oil, juice or extract has anti-fungal and anti-bacterial qualities which inhibit some microbes and are deadly to others. Garlic kills amoebas that cause amoebic dysentery, and trichomonades. It inhibits the growth, or prevents the formation, of experimentally induced tumours in mice and rats. It lowers the blood sugar level in rabbits and the blood cholesterol in rabbits and humans. It reduces the blood pressure and prevents the formation of arteriosclerosis. The Japanese scientists have shown how garlic can increase the assimilation of B vitamins. One of the Russian scientists reported that he could stopped the movement of bacteria in four minutes, by the introduction of garlic oil and the Russians use garlic vapour in most of their hospitals. To treat snake and insect bites, simply rub a crushed clove a garlic gently over the bitten area. Garlic is useful in an oil for ear pains and congested-middle-ear problems. It also acts as a digestive aid. If treating serious infections chew at least 4-6 cloves daily until such time as the infection is under control. Despite its many beneficial qualities, garlic may induce blisters, irritation and edermatitis, especially eczema in some individuals, so keep this in mind when handling or using garlic.

garlic drying. The garlic bulb is sliced and dried on trays in a cabinet or tunnel, similar to onions. Garlic is dried to about 6.5% moisture and is made into powder or granules.

garlic flavours, encapsulated. The spray-dried product containing garlic oil and/or garlic oleoresin or extract encapsulated either in gum acacia or a modified starch. The flavouring strength of these products depends on the manufacturer and range from equal to 10 times stronger than that of garlic powder.

garlic oil. The oily mass obtained by the distillation of crushed fresh garlic cloves. Garlic oil contains allyl compounds that are absent from onion oil. It has been reported that diallyl thiosulfinate is the major component in solvent extracted garlic, which is the source of the following constituents: allyl alcohol (5.4%), methyl allyl disulphide (1.2%), diallyl disulphide (5.7%), dimethyl trisulphide (2.4%), methylallyl trisulphide (1.5%), diallyl trisulphide (1.0%), and, in addition, two fractions (representing about 78.9%) of the extract were investigated and thought to be diallyl disulphide (66%), diallyl sulphide (14%) and diallyl trisulphide (9%).

garlic powder. A cream to creamy/white coloured powder prepared by the dehydration of selected cloves of garlic, and has a strongly persistent and characteristic odour and flavour when rehydra-ted. The flavour character is retained well on storage but, as garlic powder is very hygroscopic, containers should be kept well closed or product becomes hard and lumpy and loses its flavouring strength. The comparison of flavour level between fresh and dehydrated garlic is approximately 1:5. Garlic powder is widely used in dry sausages, salami, etc., and if used with discretion, it produces a distinct, pleasing and not overpowering flavour. The dehydrated product is not necessarily ideal as a flavouring, since many of the finer aromatic components are lost during dehydration, overall profile changes due to partial caramelization of the sugars present and the enzymatic potential for producing further aromatic constituents is reduced. Garlic powder tends to have a "boiled" note that is not present in the fresh material.

garlic salt. A mixture of garlic powder and salt; an anticaking agent such as starch or tricalcium phosphate may be present to maintain free-flowing properties. Standardized dispersion of garlic oil (usually at 0.1-0.25%) on salt or other suitable edible carriers are also available for use in blended seasonings and are generally preferred.

garlic, oleoresin. A dark brown soft extract prepared by the vacuum concentration of the expressed juice and the aqueous extraction of the press-cake. It contains about 5% garlic oil. The flavouring strength is about two to three times that of fresh garlic and eight times that of garlic powder, although the determination of these equivalents is very difficult other than directly in an end product.

garner bin. A holding container placed ahead of a dryer which receives wet grain. The garner bin discharges grain to the wet grain chamber of the dryer, either by gravity or augers.

gas storage. Method of storing fruit and vegetables in fresh condition, applied mostly to apples and pears. Storage in gas at 4.5°C doubles the life of the fruit compared to 4.5°C without gas. Gas mixture varies with the type of fruit. Bramley seedlings produce their own gas by respiration, while Cox's Orange Pippin requires 2.5% oxygen, 5% carbon dioxide and 92% nitrogen. Some varieties require good ventilation and can not be gas-stored. Eggs can be stored for even 9 months in 60% carbon dioxide atmosphere. Control of the growth of microorganisms also achieved by gas, e.g., obligate aerobes, like moulds, inhibited by storage in nitrogen or vacuum; addition of carbon dioxide limits growth of bacteria in cold store and delays germination of mould spores. Chilled beef in 10% carbon dioxide can be stored 60-70 days. Ozone has been found to be useful in storage of eggs and soft fruits at level of few parts per million.

gastric secretion. Gastric juice consists of the enzymes pepsin, rennin and lipase, together with mucin and hydrochloric acid. The acid is secreted by the parietal cells. The pepsin is secreted by the chief cells, and the mucin by the mucous cells. Pepsin requires an acid medium to function and breaks down proteins to proteoses. Sole function of rennin is to coagulate milk. The small amount of lipase present splits only a very small proportion of the fat.

gastrin. A polypeptide hormone secreted by the duodenum in response to gastric dilatation or the ingestion of peptides and amino acids. Gastrin promotes gastric acid and pepsinogen secretion, motility of the pyloric antrum, and gastric mucosal growth.

gastritis. Inflammation of the stomach; may be the result of eating undesirable foods, drinking too much alcohol, and infections with bacteria or viruses, allergies, or as a complication of other diseases. The general symptoms of gastritis include haematemesis, uneasiness, anorexia (lack of desire for food), fever chills, nausea, vomiting, diarrhea, cramps, and tenderness in the abdomen, headache and muscular pain. Poisoning by contaminated foods or by chemicals may also be the cause of gastritis. The cases of gastritis are more frequent in damp and hot climatic conditions.

Gavi. A dry, white, Italian wine made from the Cortese grape in vineyards located near the town of Gavi in Piedmond. The wine is fresh, light of pale colour and best when consumed young.

gavot. A cheese made from the milk of goat, sheep, or cow, in Hautes-Alpes, France.

gefillte fish. German stuffed fish. The dish is of Russian or Polish origin, where it is commonly refereed to as Jewish fish. The whole fish is served and the filleted portion chopped and stuffed back between the skin and the backbone. More frequently today, the fish is simply chopped into a pulp and made into balls. In the UK, it has been legally referred to as "fish cutlets in fish sauce" instead of a fish cake. Also spelled gefilte and gefultee.

gefilte. See gefillte.

gefultee. See gefillte.

gelatin. A colourless to pale-yellow, water-soluble protein obtained by boiling collagen with water and evaporating the solution. Gelatin is a heterogenous mixture of water-soluble proteins of high average molecular weight obtained by treating specific animal tissues like skin, tendons, ligaments and bones with hot water. Gelatin is not found in nature but derived from collagen by hydrolytic action. For preparation of Gelatin, the insoluble collagens are converted into soluble gelatin which is then purified and concentrated to a solid form. Commercially, gelatin is obtained from by-products of slaughtered cattle, sheep, and hogs. The starting materials, e.g., bones, are defatted with an organic solvent. Sometimes these are decalcified with hydrochloric acid. The material is then heated with water at 85°C to convert collagens to Gelatin. The solution is decolorized, filtered by electroosmosis, concentrated under reduced pressure, allowed to set into gel in shallow trays and dried rapidly in drying-rooms at 30, 40, 50 and 60°C for some weeks. Gelatin consists of the protein glutin which on hydrolysis gives a mixture of amino acids. Approximate amino acid contents are: glycine (25.5%), alanine (8.7%), valine (2.5%), leucine (3.2%), isoleucine (1.4%), cystine and cysteine (0.1%), methionine (1.0%), tyrosine (0.5%), aspartic acid (6.6%), glutamic acid (11.4%), arginine (8.1%), lysine (4.1%) and histidine (0.8%).

Nutritionally, gelatin is an incomplete protein lacking tryptophan. The gelatinizing compound is known as chondrin and the adhesive nature of gelatin is due to the presence of glutin. There are several grades used for different purposes, e.g., 40 mesh for confectionery; crumble gelatin for table jellies; 10 mesh for pharmaceutical capsules. As a protein it is of poor nutritive value, since it lacks tryptophan. Also spelled as gelatine.

gelatin cubes. A novel way of attracting trade by introducing a very appealing and attractive speciality, such as fruit flavoured gelatin cubes, which impart a new, distinct, and delicious flavour and colour to ice cream. The fruit-flavoured gelatin is made a little firmer than the usual jelly pudding and then cut into cubes. These true fruit cubes of gelatin have been used in bricks, week-end species, ice cream bars, and bulk ice cream. They are good for decorating and do not discolour the cream.

gelatin in dairy products. An acid solution of mercuric nitrate is prepared in twice its weight of nitric acid of 1.42 sp. gr., and this solution is diluted to 25 times its bulk in water. To 10 ml of the milk (or cream) to be examined, is added an equal volume of the acid mercuric nitrate solution, the mixture is shaken, 20 ml of water is added and the mixture is shaken again and allowed to stand for about 5 minutes, then centrifuged. If much gelatin is present, the centrifugate will be opalescent and cannot be obtained quite clear. To a portion of centrifugate, an equal volume of saturated aqueous solution of picric acid is added. A yellow precipitate will be produced in presence of any considerable amount of gelatin, while smaller amount will be indicated by cloudiness. In the absence of gelatin, the centrifugate remain perfectly clear.

gelatin sugar. A popular name for glycine.

gelatine. See gelatin.

gentobiose. A disaccharide of the D-glucose, in which the glucose molecules are linked by means of a β-1,6 glycosidic bond.

Geranium family: *Geraniaceae.* Mostly herbs and some small shrubs are represented in this family. Scented leaves in some species, a flower and a beaked or lobed fruit are some of the characteristics. The leaves usually have palmate venation and stipules. They are alternate or opposite, and compound or simple with lobes or divisions. The bisexual flower has 5-15 stamens in whorl of 5 and 1 pistil with 3-5 carpels in a superior ovary. Adhering to the ovary axis, the 3-5 styles aid in an unusual seed dispersal mechanism. The fruit is a septicidal or loculicidal capsule.

The family include: *Pelargonium zonale* (geranium, of commerce), *P. crispus* (lemon-scented geranium), *P. graveolens* (rose-scented geranium), *P. fulgidum* (spice-scented geranium), *P. tomentosum* (peppermint-scented geranium); *Geranium* (crane's-bill, wild geranium), *Erodium* (stork's-bill).

Gerardmer cheese. *See* Gerome cheese.

Gerber test for fat. A test for butterfat in milk and milk products using sulphuric acid and amyl alcohol as reagents. The sulphuric acid dissolves the solids other than fat, liberates the fat, and creates heat to keep the fat in a liquid conditions. The amyl alcohol prevents the charring of the fat, after chemical liberation from the otter milk solids, is separated by centrifugal force as in Babcock test.

germ. In reference to cereals that part of the grain which gives rise to the new plant; comprises 2.5 - 3.5% of the berry (except maize - 8%). It consists of the embryo proper (plumule and radicle) and the scutellum, a membrane separating the germ from the endosperm. The average composition is: 6-11% fat; 17-27% protein; 4-5% ash; and 2-4% fibre. It is rich in vitamins of the B group and E. The scutellum contains the greater part of the thiamine of the grain (about 50%) but only small amounts of the riboflavin and nicotinic acid. In low-extraction flour much of the germ is removed with consequent reduction in the nutritive value.

Gerome cheese. A soft cheese made in France and Switzerland; prepared from a mixture of cow's milk and goat's milk. The mixture, when cured may have a greenish tint. Also known as Gerardmer cheese.

Gervais cheese. A French cream cheese of the Neufchatel group, made from a mixture of whole milk and cream. The cheese is usually consumed while fresh but may be kept for several days.

gex cheese. A hard rennet cheese made from cows' milk and belonging to the class of blue-mold cheese, known in France as Fromage Persille. It has been made in the town of Gex for about 85 years. The ripened cheese weigh about 5-6 kg. The Penicillium type mold is not introduced into the interior of the cheese as is done in the case of Roquefort. The 3-4 months ripening takes place in caves or cellars.

ghee. The name given in India and other neighbouring countries to butter from which the water has been driven off by heat, the salt and curd being allowed to settle and the fat filtered off. Butter production, of course, is not limited to cow milk. It can be made from fat from the milk of buffalo, goat, or sheep. Ghee has somewhat the similar chemical composition as butter fat but with a lower Richert-Meisel value.

gherkin. *Cucumis anguria.* Young green cucumber of small variety, used for pickling.

Giardia lamblia. An intestinal parasitic protozoan having eight flagella and two prominent nuclei, thus having a distinctive appearance. It is found in nearly all untreated water supplies. Ingesting a few cysts of *Giardia lamblia* may cause giardiasis. *Giardia* goes through its life cycle within the intestines of humans and other animals. The cysts are shed along with feces into the water supply, where they await the next warm-blooded animal that takes a drink.

gibberellins. Derivatives of gibberellic acid, originally found in the fungus *Gibberella fujikuroi* growing on rice. They were first isolated and identified chemically in Japan in the 1930s. In 1956, the first successful isolation of gibberellin from a plant rather than a fungus (seeds of the bean *Phaseolus vulgaris*) was made. Since that time, gibberellins have been isolated from many species of plants, and it is now generally believed that they probably occur in all plants. They are present in varying amount sin all parts of the plant, but the highest concentrations are found in immature seeds. More than 40 gibberellins now have been isolated from plant tissues and identified chemically. They vary slightly in structure and also in activity. The best studied of the group is GA_3, which is also produced by Kurosawa's fungus. The gibberellins have dramatic effects on stem elongation in intact plants. A marked increase in the growth of the shoot is the most general response seen in higher plants; often the stems become long and thin and the leaves pale in color. The gibberellins stimulate both cell division and cell elongation and affect leaves as well as stems. Some plants, such as mustard (*Brassica juncea*) or the biennial henbane (*Hyoscyamus niger*), from rosettes before flowering. (In a rosette, leaves develop but the internodes between them do not elongate.) In these plants, flowering can be induced by exposure to long days, to cold (as in the biennials), or to both. Following appropriate exposures, the stems elongate, a phenomenon known as bolting, and plants flower. Application of gibberellin to some of these rosette plants causes bolting and flowering without appropriate cold or long-day exposures. The juvenile stages of some plants are different from their adult stages. Ivy offers a very familiar example. If sufficiently adult plants of ivy are growing on a building or a wall near you, compare the growing on a building or a wall near you, compare the upper branches, with the lower ones. The form of the leaf is different. Also, the behaviour is different. The juvenile branch roots readily; the

adult one does not. The adult branch flowers; the juvenile one does not. If you take an adult branch and nip off the apical meristem, the axilliary buds will develop and form new adult branches. If you apply gibberellin to such a bud, however, it will grow into a typical juvenile branch. Gibberellins have been shown to stimulate pollen germination and the growth of pollen tubes in a number of genera, including lilies, petunias, and peas. Like auxin, gibberellins can cause the development of parthenocarpic fruits, including apples, currants, cucumbers, and eggplant. In some fruits, such as the mandarin orange, the almond, and the peach, the gibberellins have been effective where auxin was not. Auxins and gibberellins together, in some instances, produce fruit more than twice as large as those obtainable by the application of either one alone. The seeds of most plants require a period of dormancy before they will germinate. In certain plants, dormancy usually cannot be broken except by an exposure to cold or to light. In many species, including lettuce, tobacco, and wild oats, gibberellins will substitute for the dormancy-breaking cold or light requirement and promote the growth of the embryo and the emergence of the seedling. In barley and other grass seeds, there is a specialized layer of cells, the aleurone layer, just inside the seed coat. These cells are rich in protein. Which the seeds begin to germinate, triggered by the inhibition of water, the embryo releases gibberellins. In response to the gibberellins, the aleurone cells synthesize hydrolytic enzymes, the principal one of which is α-amylase, the enzyme that breaks down starch into sugar. The enzymes digest the stored food reserves of the starchy endosperm, which are released in the form of sugars and amino acids, absorbed by the scutellum, and then transported to the growing regions of the embryo. In this way, the embryo calls forth the substances needed for its growth at the moment it requires them. The investigators believe that gibberellins activate certain genes, causing the synthesis of specific messenger RNA molecules, which, in turn, direct the synthesis of the enzymes. It has not been proved, however, that gibberellins act directly on the gene, although it has been shown that both RNA and protein synthesis take place and are necessary for the appearance of the enzymes. Whatever the details of the mechanism of gibberellin action in aleurone cells, it is clear that the aleurone layer cells constitute a highly differentiated tissue poised to respond to the demands, mediated by the gibberellins, of the growing embryo. This is one of the best-described examples of how hormones integrate the biochemistry and physiology of the different tissues of a whole plant. It is not known whether the way in which gibberellin works in these seeds is related to its effects on other plant organs.

Gilcrease phosphatse method. A method for determining phosphatase in milk in which phenol liberated from disodium phenyl phosphate is detected by Folin-Ciocalteu's reagent. The colour is evaluated by means of permanent colour standards.

gin. One of the most popular of the distilled liquors, which may be sweetened or unsweetened grain spirit, that is flavoured with the essential oil of juniper berries, from which it derives its name. Francis De La Boe, the originator of this botanical flavoured beverage, gave it the French name, *Jenievre* which means juniper berries. This was later known as "Geneva" and is finally abbreviated to the English, "Gin". Even so, it is sometimes referred to Geneva by the illiterate though it has no connection with the Swiss city. However, in South America it is sometimes known as Ginebra which is Spanish name for Geneva city. Although the juniper berry has traditionally been the most popular flavoring agent for gin, other substances have been used to a limited extent. These include coriander, angelica root, anise, caraway seeds, lime, lemon, and orange peel, and licorice, among others. It is quite popular for many fruits (small blue-black, plumlike fruits from the blackthorn) which impart a reddish colour to the gin.

Possibly of all alcoholic beverages, gin enjoys the most stained reputation. Part of this stems from the fact that the world gin has been and is still sometimes used incorrectly to designate any inferior liquor. Despite the apparent relative simplicity of gin as a product, it is interesting to observe that quality gin, like any other alcoholic beverage of quality, is not easy to manufacture.

There are notable differences between gin of various distilleries. This is due to the fact that this spirit is not always sold to the public at the same strength. Some are sweetened with sugar, some flavoured. The use and proportion of the botanical in the gin formula is left to the producer and the character and quality of the gin will depend to a great extent on the skill of the craftsman in formulating the recipe. To assure a greater degree of product uniformity, some producers formulate their aromatic ingredients on the basis of the essential oil content in the raw materials. Gin derives its main flavour from juniper berries. In addition to this, other botanicals may be used, including angelica roots, anise, coriander, caraway seeds, lime, lemon and orange peel licorice, calamur, cardamom, cassia bark, orris root, and bitter almonds. Malt produced from barley is added to a mixture of grains in a large vessel in which fermentation takes place. The liquid is distilled atleast 3 times in a pot still to produce a distillate known as Malt Wine. The final Geneva is prepared by rectifying the malt wine to which juniper and other ingredients are added. The entire process is proprietary. Gin can also be made by introducing the flavouring ingredients directly into the mash prior to distillation. More commonly, the flavouring agents are either added directly to the base of the still, allowing for liquid extraction, the vapors thus carrying flavorants with them as they rise in the still. Or, the flavouring ingredients can be suspended in a basket near the head of the still or placed on trays near the top of the still where the extraction proceeds by the vapours of alcohol. To produce a smoother product, some distillers add a few plates near the top of the still to effect a degree of rectification. Still other distillers, to prevent any thermal degradation of flavouring agents, will operate the still under a vacuum, where the temperature is maintained in the region of 54°-60°C. So-called compounded gin involves simple procedure of adding essential oils directly to grain spirits. In order to ensure that no undesirable flavours are imparted to the gin, the grain spirit must be as neutral as possible. High grade 'silent' (i.e.,

extra neutral) molasses spirit (not below 168-169° proof) obtained by still distillation and subsequent pasteurization to remove fusel oils and aldehydes, is redistilled after dilution to prove strength with juniper berries, coriander and other flavouring agents in pot-stills fitted with gin-heads. Some gin-stills possess a refinement section above the pot for flavour stability and enrichment. The essential oils are distilled over the entire distillation cycle by the application of indirect steam-heat. The first and the last portion is discarded and only the heart of the run which represents approximately an 85% recovery of the original alcohol concentration, is used. The mixture of fore shots and tailings is re-rectified for sale as industrial alcohol. To avoid thermal decomposition of the delicate flavours and to acquire a degree of softness, some distillers conduct distillation under reduced pressure at a temperature of about 8-10° C. Details relating to the flavouring materials employed in gin production are kept as trade secrets.

Gin contains about 40-50% alcohol and hence higher in alcohol content than whisky or brandy. The ingredients are reduced to a granular form and immersed into a pot which is filled with grain-neutral spirits at approximately 100° proof.

ginger. Rhizome of *Zingiber officinale*; it is an erect perennial herb with an aromatic, knotty rootstock which is thick, fibrous and whitish or buff-coloured in appearance. The plant reaches a height of more than 1 metre, the leaves growing about 15-30 cm long. It is extensively cultivated in the tropics such as India, China, Haiti, Nigeria and Jamaica, and is used as a flavouring; pungency due to non-volatile compounds including gingerol, zingerone and shogool. Preserved ginger made from young fleshy rhizomes boiled with sugar and packed in syrup. The average composition per 100 g is: 2.5 g protein; 0.8 g fat; 1 g carbohydrate; 2.2 g fibre; 2.5 mg iron; 0.8 mg nicotinic acid; 4 mg vitamin C; and 0.25 MJ food energy.

ginkgo. The maidenhair tree, *Ginkgo biloba*, is easily recognized by its fan-shaped leaves with their openly branched, forking (dichotomous) pattern of veins. The leaves on the numerous spur shoots are more or less entire, whereas on the long shoots and in seedlings they are deeply lobed. Unlike most gymnosperms, *Ginkgo* is deciduous, its leaves turning a beautiful golden color before falling an autumn. *Ginkgo* is the sole living survivor of an evolutionary line that probably extends back to the late Palaeozoic era and was common during much of the Mesozoic era. The class Ginkgoinae was once widespread but seems to have been represented by relatively few species. It is especially resistant to air pollution and so is commonly cultivated in cities. Like the cycads, the *Ginkgo* bears the ovules and microsporangia on different individuals. The ovules of *Ginkgo* are borne in pairs on the end of short stalks and ripen to produce seeds in autumn. In *Ginkgo*, fertilization within the ovules may not occur until after the ovules have been shed from the tree. Embryos are formed during the later stages of maturation of the seeds, which occur on the ground. The seeds have a rancid odour as a result of the butyric acid in their fleshy coats, and for this reason only male trees are usually cultivated on streets or in parks or gardens. The microscoporophylls are clustered in conelike structures, each microsporophyll bearing two microsporangia.

ginseng. Family: *Aradiaceae.* Genus: *Panax.* Species: *ginseng*; *Panax quinque folius* (American ginseng). Ginseng can refer to any of 22 different plants. Some of these are members of the same family (Araliaceae) or even genus (*Panax*), Still others are completely unrelated to ginseng either botanically or chemically and are often passed off as frauds trading on the good reputation and high price of the original root. Ginseng has been defined as an adaptogen, that is a substance that increases the body's resistance to outside stresses of various kinds without causing it to deviate from its normal functions. It achieves this balancing effect by normalizing the physiological functions of the individual as a whole and not by acting on one specific part or function of the body. To the untrained eye, ginseng looks pretty much like any other root: brown, gnarled and about as large as a little finger. But the root sometimes resembles part of a human body, hence its other common name of manroot. It has been found that it contains numerous saponins, which are thought to be its active constituents. Oriental ginseng also contains variable amounts of starch, steroids, pectin, sugars, vitamins, including B_1 to B_{12}, nicotinic acid, pantothenic acid and biotin, minerals, including zinc, manganese, calcium, iron and copper; choline, fats; and trace amounts of volatile oil. American ginseng differs from Oriental ginseng chemically because it contains ginsenosides not panaxoside.

Chinese consider ginseng as the king of all tonic and use it to stimulate the entire body energy to overcome stress and fatigue and to recover from weakness and deficiency. It has a very beneficial effect on the heart and circulation and is used to normalize blood pressure, reduce blood cholesterol and prevent atherosclerosis. It nourishes the blood and so is used to treat anemia. It reduces blood sugar levels and thus is useful in managing diabetes and controlling hypoglycemia. American ginseng, which was introduced in China during the eighteenth century, acts as a fever breaker and is considered to benefit the lungs, dissipate heat, quench thirst and promote body secretions. It too is a tonic but it is used for different conditions, including coughs resulting from lung deficiencies which are make by short difficult breathing and a dry throat, loss of blood, thirst, fever, irritability, tiredness, toothache and hangover.

A tea made from the root is used to stop thirst and assist in cases of sunstroke. Put a teaspoon of ginseng powder in a cup of boiling water, leave for 5-10 minutes, and then drink the tea and eat the sludge.

Both ginsengs are available in tablet or in extract or powder form. For long-term use, decoct 400-800 mg of the dried root daily. Up to 2000 mg of the root may be taken daily for three weeks in any moth for short-term use. Ginseng should never be mixed with caffeine.

gladiola drying. The curing of gladiolas is very similar to curing of onions. By curing at 32.2 to 34.9°C with relative humidity above 80% a disease-resistant surface layer is developed and some rot fungi are killed. Good results have been obtained by curing at 26.7-32.2°C for 48-72 hours with a relative humidity between 50-80%, using air velocities up to 1 m/s. It is a common practice to store the corms at 4.4-10°C after curing and cleaning.

glazing. The decoration performed on food products such as cakes and pastries. Glazes are mainly of two types, the concentrated sugar mixtures that dry to a thin, translucent to nearly opaque layer, and are typically applied to doughnuts, and the high moisture, nearly transparent, almost gel-like materials used on fruit cakes. There are also types called finishes that are poured over fruit cakes,, rum cakes, and other bakery products, that require a flavouring and moistening sauce to attain their maximum palatability. All these types are used on products that have already been baked and they are usually applied by pouring or dipping. Particulate materials may be included in, or sprinkled on, the glaze. There is no clear dividing line between glazes and thin water icings. The main purpose of using glazes to increase the visual appeal of products, but they may also and positive flavor notes and textural contrast. Flavours that would be at least partially dissipated in the oven, such as vanilla, can exert their full impact when included in glazes. The high sugar content give an initial effect of sweetness that is widely appreciated. An additional function of the high moisture type of glaze is to retard the drying of fruits on flans and tarts and of fruit cakes, etc.

gliadin. One of the proteins of wheat, differentiated by its solubility in 70% alcohol; a prolamin.

gliding bacteria. A variety of bacteria that exhibit gliding motility. These organisms have no flagella, but are able in some manner to move when in contact with surfaces. Some gliding bacteria are very similar to cyanobacteria and have been considered to be their non-phototrophic counter-parts. All gliding bacteria are Gram-negative.

gliding motility. A type of motility in which a microbial cell glides along when in contact with a solid surface. The mechanism of gliding by gliding bacteria appears complex, and it is likely that more than one mechanism is responsible. Gliding motility is generally much slower than flagellar motility, but absolute rates of gliding are somewhat dependent on cell length.

globe artichoke. Family: *Compositae.* Genus: *Cynara.* Species: *Cynara scolymus.* A large proportion of the carbohydrate in artichoke is insulin which is converted to sugars during storage, so the calorie content ranges between 10-53 for every 100 grams after storage. Artichokes are an excellent cholagogue, stimulating liver-cell regeneration, and are diuretic, and are used for gall-bladder and biliary disease, and for chronic liver condition and have long been used for diabetes mellitus and atherosclerosis. Since they have cholesterol-reducing properties they are also useful for high blood pressure and some types of heart complaint. A decoction made of the leaves is used as medicine.

globins. Basic proteins that differ from histones since they are rich in histidine, deficient in isoleucine and contain average amounts of arginine and tryptophan. Globins are simple proteins themselves but are often found as the protein portion of conjugated proteins, *e.g.*, globin from haemoglobin.

globoside. A ceramide oligoglycoside that contains simple sugars, amino sugars, and N-acetyl amino sugars.

globular proteins. A major group of proteins which perform a multitude of functions. A typical globular protein may be described as an extensively folded and compact polypeptide chain with little if any space for molecules of water in its interior. The polypeptide chain may have extensive α-helicity as in myoglobin, or it may have little as in cytochrome c and possess β-extended form of β-keratin.

Gloucester cheese. A firm, smooth, waxy, close textured, hard cheese made in Gloucester, England. It is similar to Derby cheese in character and in making procedure. When the cheese is about one month old, it is coloured red or brown. Well developed blue molds are often found on the sides.

glucagon. A hormone, secreted by the islets of Langerhans in the pancreas, that increases the concentration of glucose in the blood by stimulating the metabolic breakdown of glycogen. It thus antagonizes the effects of insulin.

glucaric acid. Alternative name for saccharic acid, the dicarboxylic acid derived from glucose.

glucide. Name occasionally used for saccharine.

glucitol. Obsolete names for sorbitol. Also known as glycitol.

glucoascorbic acid. Homologue of ascorbic acid containing an extra -CHOH group. Acts as an antagonist to the vitamin; its administration can cause scurvy in animals that do not normally require to vitamin in the diet.

glucocorticoids. The 21-carbon steroid hormones that are secreted by adrenal cortex and that acts primarily on carbohydrate, lipid, and protein metabolism. Glucocorticoids include corticosterone, cortisone, and cortisol, and lead to protein catabolism, gluconeogenesis from amino acids thus formed, lipid mobilization, and an increase in ketone bodies. In addition, glucocorticoids also have antiallergic and anti-inflammatory effects. Some of them are used in replacement therapy, and they are also used as anti-inflammatory drug and immunosuppressants.

glucofuranose. Glucose formulated as the five-membered furan ring.

glucogenic amino acids. The amino acids whose carbon chain can be metabolically converted into glucose or glycogen.

gluconeogenesis. The biosynthesis of new carbohydrate precursors from nonsugar precursors; the most important being pyruvate, lactate, citric acid cycle intermediates, and a number of amino acids. As is true for all biosynthetic pathways, gluconeogenesis proceeds by an enzymatic pathway, that differs from the corresponding catabolic pathway, that is independently regulated, and that requires input of chemical energy in the form of ATP. The biosynthetic pathway from pyruvate to glucose, which in vertebrates takes place largely in the liver and secondarily in the kidney, employs eight of the glycolytic enzymes, which function reversibly and are present in large excess. There are, however, three irreversible steps in the downhill glycolytic pathway that cannot be used in gluconeogenesis and are bypassed by alternative reactions catalyzed by quite different enzymes. The first bypass consists of the conversion of pyruvate into phosphoenolpyruvate via the formation of oxaloacetate; the second is the dephosphorylation of the fructose 1,6-diphosphate by fructose diphosphatase; and the third is the dephosphorylation of glucose 6-phosphate by glucose 6-phosphatase. For each molecule of D-glucose made from pyruvate the terminal phosphate groups of four molecules of ATP and two of GTP must be used. Gluconeogenesis is regulated at two major sites:

(a) thecarboxylation of pyruvate by pyruvate carboxylase, which is stimulated by the allosteric effector acetyl-CoA, and

(b) the dephosphorylation of fructose 1,6-diphosphate by fructose diphosphatase, which is inhibited by AMP but stimulated by citrate.

gluconeogensesis. Formation of glucose and glycogen from non-carbohydrate sources via glucose.

gluconic acid. The acid derived from glucose from glucose by oxidizing the hydroxyl group on carbon atom number one. The acid produced when carbon six is oxidized is glucuronic acid; the oxidation of both carbon one and six yields saccharic acid.

glucono-delta-lactone. Lactone of gluconic acid; slowly liberates acid at a controlled rate; used in chemically leavened bread, i.e., to liberate carbon dioxide from bicarbonate instead of using yeast. Also used in bland-flavoured sherbets and to reduce fat-absorption in products sucn as dough-nuts.

glucophore. A radical or atomic grouping which is supposed to impart a sweet taste to many compounds in which it appears.

glucosamine. Amino derivative of glucose. It is a constituent of many complex polysaccharides.

glucosan. A complex of glucose molecules, e.g., starch, cellulose and glycogen. Insulin is a complex of fructose molecules and is a fructosan. The general name for the polysaccharide complexes made up from simple hexose units is hexosans.

glucose. A hexose sugar, which, with its

phosphate esters (glucose-1-phosphate and glucose-6-phosphate), plays a central role in the metabolism of all living organisms, particularly as a source of energy. The concentration of glucose in the blood is under close hormonal control and brain is very sensitive to changes in its level. Excess glucose is stored as glycogen, principally in the liver and skeletal muscle. Liver glycogen acts as a hormonally regulated reservoir of blood glucose, being mobilized by phosphorylase to replace depleted glucose or being synthesized when blood glucose is in excess. Defects in this mechanism lead to diabetes melitus. Abnormally low blood glucose (hypoglycaemia) or excessively high blood glucose (hyperglycaemia) can both cause pathological effects.

glucose metabolism. The process through which glucose is broken down in living tissues to provide energy. The overall reaction follows the equation:

$$C_6H_{12}O_6 + 6O_2 = 6\ CO_2 + 6\ H_2O +$$

3.9 kcal/g of glucose, but in detail the process involves about 20 stages. The first series of stages does not require oxygen and is referred to as glycolysis or glucose fermentation. The glucose is converted through a number of sugar phosphates to 3-carbon sugars (trioses) and then to pyruvic acid. The latter is oxidized in a series of reactions known as the Kerbs or tricarboxylic acid cycle ultimately to carbon dioxide and water. The energy is liberated from the glucose at certain of these stages. Surplus blood glucose is stored in the muscles as glycogen, and when energy is required the latter is converted first to glucose and then follows the metabolic pathway.

glucose syrup. A clear, viscous, colourless syrup produced by the partial hydrolysis of starch, usually maize or potato. The product is of variable composition depending upon the degree of hydrolysis and includes glucose, maltose, dextrins and trisaccharides. It is widely used as sweetening agent in confectionery, and particularly useful in sugar confectionery since it prevents crystallization of the sugar on cooling. Also known as corn syrup (especially in US), starch syrup, confectioner's glucose and liquid glucose.

glucose tolerance. The ability of the body to deal with a large dose of glucose; used as a test for diabetes mellitus. The fasting subject ingests 50 g of glucose and the blood sugar is measured at intervals. In the normal individual the fasting sugar level is approximately. 80-100 mg per 100 ml, rises to about 150 mg, and returns to the starting level within 1-1.5 hours. In diabetic individuals, the glucose concentration rises to a higher value and does not drop back as rapidly as is the case for normal individuals. The plotted results form a glucose tolerance curve.

glucose-T_m. A term used in measuring the efficiency of the kidneys; it is the maximum rate of reabsorption of glucose by the kidney tubules. T_m is the maximum reabsorption capacity.

glucosides. Complexes of substances with glucose. General name for such complexes with other sugars is glycosides.

glucostatic mechanism. Theory that appetite depends on the difference between arterial and venous levels of glucose; when the difference falls to 8 mg, the hypothalamus is stimulated and hunger results.

glucuronate pathway. A metabolic pathway for the conversion of glucose to xylulose-5-phosphate that is operative in higher plants, mammals, crustaceans, and yeast; it is apparently not a major pathway for the oxidation of glucose. The pathway serves to provide vitamin C in plants and in those animals capable of synthesizing this vitamin. Also known as the glucuronate-gluconate pathway; the glucuronate-xylulose cycle.

glucuronic acid. A derivative of glucose which, in the liver, can be added (from UDP-glucuronic acid) to other molecules to detoxify them and make them more water soluble, for example bilirubin diglucuronide. Many toxic substances are excreted from the body combined with glucuronic acid as glucuronides. It is also present in various complex polysaccharides.

glutamate receptors. Receptors specifically sensitive to and operated by glutamic acid. Glutamate receptors are coupled to Na^+ channels. Influx are sensitive to both D- and L- isomers.

glutamate, sodium. Sodium salt of the amino acid, glutamic acid. First introduced as a flavouring agent under the Japanese name of Aginomoto. It enhances the flavour of some foods, especially meat and vegetables, apparently by stimulating the taste buds. Frequently added to soup mixes and meat products. Commercially, it is manufactured from sugar beet pulp and wheat gluten. Glutamic acid has two acidic groups and it is the mono sodium salt, known as MSG, that has this flavour property.

glutamic acid. $HOOC\text{-}CH_2\text{-}CH_2\text{-}CH\text{-}(COOH)\text{-}NH_2$. A dicarboxylic amino acid which probably function as an exciting neurotransmitter in certain regions of the spinal cord (dorsal horns), cerebellum (granule cells) and possibly other regions. Additionally, it plays a role in intermediary metabolism. It is involved in transmination reactions in the body; its amide is glutamine. The sodium salt, monosodium glutamate or MSG, originally known as Aginomoto, is used to enhance the flavour of savoury dishes and is frequently added to canned meat and soups.

glutamic dehydrogenase. An enzyme which catalyzes the reversible oxidative deamination by NAD^+ of L-glutamate to form α-ketoglutaric acid, ammonia, and NADH.

glutamine synthetase. An enzyme that is ubiquitous in nature and catalyzes a major reaction in the assimilation of ammonia. The first step in the reaction is believed to be the formation of a γ-glutamylphosphate-enzyme complex. In the second reaction, ammonia, a good nucleophile, attacks the complex and displaces the phosphate group to form glutamine and inorganic phosphate. The enzyme is highly specific, since aspartic acid cannot replace glutamic acid as a substrate.

glutamine. Amide of the amino acid, glutamic acid; formed by the addition of ammonia to glutamic acid. It occurs in plants, where it appears to function as a storage depot for ammonia, and as part of the urea cycle in animals.

glutathione. A widely distributed tripeptide, γ-glutamyl-cysteinyl-glycine, that serves as a coenzyme for some enzymes and is thought to function as an antioxidant in protecting sulphydryl groups of enzymes and other proteins. Reduced glutathione is synonymous with glutathione and is abbreviated as GSH; oxidized glutathione is a dimer of two glutathione molecules, linked by means of a disulphide bond. It serves as a hydrogen acceptor in reactions such as the formation of disulphide linkages and thiol groups in proteins. The sulphydryl (-SH) group of cysteinyl residue is important in maintaining the correct reducing condition within the cell by oxidizing disulphide bonds. More than 90% of the cellular glutathione is in the reduced form. It is particularly important in the protection of red blood cells against the harmful action of peroxides, as the selenium-containing enzyme glutathione peroxidase.

glutelin. 1. A major protein of wheat gluten. It is insoluble in water and neutral salt solutions but soluble in dilute acids and alkalies. Maize glutelin is one of the two main proteins of the maize (corn) kernel, along with zein. 2. A general name for a class of proteins which are insoluble in water, alcohol or neutral salt solutions, but readily dissolve in dilute acids and alkali. Glutelins are mixture of various similar proteins.

gluten. A mixture of two proteins, gliadin and glutenin, occurring in the endosperm of wheat grain. Their amino acid and composition varies but glutamic acid (33%) and proline (12%) predominate. The composition of wheat glutens determines the 'strength' of the flour and whether or not it is suitable for biscuit or bread making. Certain people are sensitive to gluten (coeliac disease) and must have gluten-free diet. Too much gluten gives too strong a dough and it is "weakened" by the addition of an enzyme, or malt flour rich in the enzyme, to break down a limited amount of the gluten. Prepared from flour by washing out the starch. Gluten in the undamaged state with its extensible properties is called vital gluten. Overheating destroys these properties and the result is devitalized gluten.

gluten-free foods. Food formulated without any wheat or rye protein (although the starch may be used) for subjects suffering from coeliac disease.

glutose. A hexose sugar carrying a keto group on carbon-3; not metabolized and non-fermentable.

glycamines. Derivatives of sugar alcohols in which the -CH$_2$OH group is replaced by -CH$_2$NH$_2$, e.g., ethanolamine, and ribamine (part of vitamin B$_2$).

glycan. A polysaccharide made up of a single type of sugar unit. As a class the glycans serve both as structural units (e.g., cellulose in plants and chitin in invertebrates) and energy stores (e.g., starch in plants and glycogen in animals). The most common homoglycans are made up of D-glucose units and called glucans.

glycerides. Esters of glycerol with fatty acids. As glycerol possesses three hydroxyl groups it can combine with three molecules of fatty acid to form a triglyceride or simple fat. If all three molecules of fatty acids are the same, a simple triglyceride is formed, e.g. tristearin, triolein; mixed glycerides may be formed such as distearo-olein and stearo-oleo-palmitin.

glycerin. See glycerol.

glycerol. 1,2,3-propanetriol. An alcohol with three -OH groups. Glycerol is biologically important as the alcohol involved in lipid formation (these particular lipids being called glycerides). These glycerides are the fat stores of the body and enter into metabolic pathways, particularly when carbohydrate levels are low. Digestion of lipids occurs in the small intestine after being emulsified under the influence of bile salts. They are then converted back to the fatty acids by pancreatic lipase, (i.e., the reverse of the reaction above) and enter metabolic pathways via reaction with coenzyme A. Also known as glycerin.

glyceryl lacto-sterate. A compound formed by glycerolysis of hydrogenated soya bean oil followed by esterification with lactic acid, which results in a mixture of mono and diglycerides and their lactic mono esters. It is used as an emulsifier in shortenings. Also known as lactostearin.

glycine. One of the 20 common amino acids found in proteins. It is found in the free form in all tissues of the body. It is an important constituent of the diet, but is also available from the breakdown of peptides and proteins of nucleotides and nucleic acids. Glycine can be formed from carbohydrates by way of 3-phosphoserine and serine, and is readily interconvertible with serine in the central nervous system by the enzyme serine hydroxymethyl transferase, which utilizes tetrahydrofolic acid as cofactor. It probably functions as an inhibitory neurotransmitter in the lower brain stem and spinal cord of vertebrates, especially at the endings of interneurons in the spinal cord. Strychnine blocks the inhibitory action of glycine. Tetanus toxin inhibits its release. Glycine also plays a role in intermediary metabolism.

glycine receptors. The receptors specifically sensitive to glycine. Glycine receptors present on spinal cord neurons are coupled to Cl⁻ channels. Influx of Cl⁻ through these channels causes hyperpolarization of the postsynaptic cell. Glycine receptors are blocked by the strychnine.

glycinin. Globulin protein in soya bean.

glycitol. Obsolete name for sorbitol.

glycocoll. Obsolete name for the amino acid glycine.

glycogen phosphorylase. The enzyme that catalyzes the successive hydrolytic removal of glucose residues, in the form of glucose-1-phosphate, from the non-reducing end of glycogen; this reaction is the first step for the utilization of glycogen in glycolysis.

glycogen synthetase. An enzyme which catalyzes only the synthesis of α-1,4 linkages. For example, new glucosyl units are added to the non-reducing terminal residues of the glycogen. The activated glucosyl unit of UDP-glucose is transferred to the hydroxyl group at C-4 terminus of glycogen to form an α-1,4-glycosidic linkage. In this elongation reaction, UDP is displaced by this terminal hydroxyl group of the growing glycogen molecule. This reaction is catalyzed by glycogen synthetase. Glycogen synthetase is inactivated by phosphorylation of a specific serine residue.

glycogen. A starch polymer which is classed as a polysaccharide and is found chiefly in the liver of animal organisms where it acts as a reserve of energy, It can be broken down to simpler forms by the action of enzymes, a reaction called glycolysis. It is composed of many glucose units linked in a similar way to starch. Glycogen is readily hydrolyzed in a step-wise manner to glucose itself. It is stored largely in the liver and in muscle but is found widely distributed. After a meal, most of the glucose contained in food is absorbed via the intestine and blood and converted to glycogen in the liver (glycogenesis). The concentration of glucose in the blood is then normally regulated by the conversion of glycogen back to glucose (glycogenolysis). The liver can store about 100 g of glycogen. Since glycogen is rapidly broken down to glucose immediately an animal is killed, meat and animal liver do not contain glycogen, the only dietary sources are oysters, cockles, muscles, scallops, clams, whelks and winkles that are eaten virtually alive and contain about 5% glycogen.

glycogenesis. Synthesis of glycogen from glucose, as, for example, occurs in the muscle where glucose is stored as glycogen; facilitated by insulin.

glycogenic amino acid. An amino acid that can serve as a precursor of pyruvic acid, glucose, and glycogen in metabolism.

glycogenolysis. Breakdown of glycogen into its glucose subunits. The hormones adrenaline (epinephrine) and glucagon induce glycogenolysis in the liver via a cascade of intracellular secondary messengers. Binding of the hormones to their receptors stimulates adenyl cyclase which increases the concentration of cyclic AMP. This activates protein kinase which phosphorylates the phosphorylase β-kinase which, in turn, activates glycogen phosphorylase α-kinase. It is this enzyme that breaks down glycogen into its glucose subunits.

glycoleucine. An obsolete name for norleucine.

glycolipids. Complex lipids that consist of compounds of fatty acid with carbohydrates and contain nitrogen but no phosphoric acid; found in brain tissues. These formed by the combination of carbohydrate and lipid molecules. Glycolipids are important constituents of the cell membrane. The carbohydrate region of the molecule protrudes away form the cell; this region contributes to the negative surface charge of most cell types.

glycolysis. The series of biochemical reactions by which a molecule of glucose is converted into two molecules of pyruvate (or lactate) with the production of usable energy in the form of two molecules of ATP. It is central to the generation of energy in the cell and can operate under either anaerobic conditions (*e.g.*, leading to the excretion of lactate by strenuously exercising muscle) or aerobically in conjunction with the Krebs cycle to produce carbon dioxide along with 38 molecules of ATP. Lactic acid is one of the products formed. It involves the conversion of glucose into pyruvate, with the release of some energy in the form of ATP. Glycolysis occurs in cell cytoplasm. In anaerobic respiration, breakdown proceeds no further and pyruvate is converted into ethanol or lactic acid for storage or elimination. In anaerobic respiration, glycolysis is followed by the Krebs cycle. Glycolysis alone yields only two molecules of ATP per molecule of glucose in anaerobic respiration. In aerobic respiration there is a net yield of six (the conversion of NADH back to NAD yields further four ATP molecules, and can occurs only when oxygen is present). In aerobic condition pyruvate and NADH are further oxidized in the mitochondria. In anaerobic conditions (*e.g.*, in anaerobic muscle or fermentative bacteria) the NADH reduces the pyruvate to lactate in a reaction catalyzed by lactate dehydrogenase. In some fermentation reactions the pyruvate may be further metabolized before its products are used to oxidize the NADH, and in some cases the NADH may be oxidized to NAD^+ with convomitant formation of hydrogen gas. Also known as Embden-Meyerhof pathway.

glycoproteins. The proteins that consist of a protein covalently linked to a carbohydrate polymer *via* an N or O-acyl-glycosyl amine linkage. These are differentiated on the basis of their carbohydrate composition and the linkage of the carbohydrate to the protein. Glycoproteins fall in to three basic groups:

(a) plasma glycoproteins over 40% of which are found in the blood sera;

(b) mucin glycoproteins that are associated with various secretions such as saliva and make up in the highly characteristic blood group substances associated with surface layers of cells; and

(c) mucopolysaccharides, which consist of a short peptide chain to which long unbranched polysaccharides are attached and which are found widely distributed in cartilage, eyes, tendons, skin, etc. A most unusual function of glycoproteins is found in the freezing resistance of some Antarctic fish which survive in an environmental temperature of 271 K, because of the presence in their blood at a concentration of about 2.5%, of a group of freezing point depressing glycoproteins ranging in molecular mass from 10,000-20,000.

glycosaminoglycans. Molecules consisting of chains of complex carbohydrates characterized by their content of amino sugars and uronic acids. When these chains are attached to a protein molecule, the compound is known as a proteoglycan. They are associated with the structural elements of the tissues such as bone, elastin, and collagen, Their property of holding large amount of water and occupying space, thus cushioning or lubricating other structures, is assisted by the large number of -OH groups, and the negative charge on the molecules, which, by repulsion, keep the carbohydrate chains apart. Some of the examples of this type are: hyaluronic acid, chondroitin sulphate, and heparin.

glycosidase. Enzyme able to break glycosidic bonds in carbohydrates, and commonly found in lysosomes.

glycoside. Any of a member of a large class of carbohydrate derivatives characterized by the replacement of the hydrogen atom of the hemiacetal hydroxyl group by an alkyl or aryl moiety, the aglycon. The glycosides are stable compounds and, do not undergo many of the reactions of sugars, *e.g.*, they show no reducing properties, they do not mutarotate etc. The non-sugar part of a glycoside is known as the aglycon, Natural glycoside constitute a large and biologically important class of sugar derivatives. Many natural pigments and dyestuffs, poisons and drugs, are glycosides. Glycosides are classified according to the sugar formed during their hydrolysis such as: glucosides, fructosides, rhymnosides, galactosides, mannosides, arabinosides, xylosides, sorbosides, glucoheptosides, etc., or as aldosides, or ketosides if formed from aldoses or ketoses. Other classifications are based upon the nature of the non-sugar or aglycone group formed when glycosides are hydrolyzed.

glycyrrhizin. A triterpenoid glycoside (a saponin of the corresponding glycyrrhetinic acid with an attached disaccharide) from liquorice root. It is about 50-100 times as sweet as sucrose but with undesirable aftertaste. It has been described as a noncaloric extract of liquorice root. Ammoniated glycerrhizin is the most common form of the sweetener. It is said to be 100 times sweeter than sugar, but its strong liquorice flavour appears to be inseparable from the sweetening effect, so its use in bakery products is attended with difficulty. It has been applied mostly in tobacco and pharmaceutical manufacture, but a few confectionery products have also been made with it. has foam-enhancing properties that can be useful in beverage formulation.

glyoxylate cycle. A modification of the Krebs cycle, occurring in some micro-organisms, algae, and higher plants, in regions where fats are being rapidly metabolized, *e.g.,* in germinating fat-rich seeds. Acetyl groups, formed from the fatty acids are passed into the glyoxylate cycle, with the eventual formation of mainly carbohydrates. With the help of this cycle plants and some bacteria are able to use acetyl-CoA not only for energy production but also for anabolic reactions (forming metabolites for synthesis of amino acids and carbohydrates). Remember that Krebs cycle reactions cannot use acetyl-CoA for formation of carbohydrates or amino acids (fatty acids cannot be changed into the carbohydrates or proteins). Acetyl-CoA is only used of oxidation in the Krebs cycle.

The reactions start with condensation of acetyl-CoA and oxaloacetate to form citrate which then isomerizes to isocitrate.

Isocitrate is cleaved by isocitrate lyase into glyoxylate and succinate.

Glyoxylate condenses with second molecule of acetyl-CoA to form malate.

Finally, malate is oxidized to oxalo-acetate. In whole cycle two molecules of acetyl-CoA are used and succinate appears as a bye-product. The reaction malate to oxaloacetate generates NADH for providing ATP. Succinate provides skeleton for anabolic purposes. This pathway is especially important in seeds which can form carbohydrates from metabolism of fatty acids. Also known as glyoxylate bypass.

GMS. Abbreviation for glyceryl monostearate.

goat. One of the valuable animals which provides milk and flesh for food and skins and hair for clothing. There is a prejudice against goat's milk in many countries, but it is sweet and nourishing, and justifies the term, "the poor man's cow," which is applied to the animal. However, there is increasing realisation of the value of the milk of goats for invalids and undernourished children.

gold thioglucose. A compound used to cause obesity in experimental animals by stimulation of the appetite through damage to the hypothalamus.

golden-brown algae. *Class: Chryso-phyceae.* The other generally recognized class of Chrysophyta consists of about 1100 species. Until recently, they were thought to be primarily freshwater group, but within the past decade they have proved to be of extraordinary importance in the marine plankton, particularly the *nannoplank-ton.* This nannoplankton comprises components of the plankton so small that they pass through an ordinary plankton net, which has mesh openings of 0.040-0.076 mm Some of the nannoplankton consist of minute di-noflagellates and diatoms, but representatives of the Chrysophyceae are often abundant. In fact, it is now thought that the Chrysophyceae may be the major food-producing organisms in the ocean. Some of the golden-brown algae lack cell walls, whereas others have a well-defined wall rich in pectic substances. Many species have superficial or internal siliceous or organic scales or skeletal structures, which may be exceedingly elaborate. Many golden-brown algae are motile, having two flagella, whereas others are amoeboid and lack flagella. Except for the presence of chloroplasts, the amoeboid cells are indistinguishable from amoeboid protozoa (phylum Sarcodin), and the two groups may be closely related. Reproduction in the golden-brown algae is largely asexual and involves zoospore formation.

goldenseal. *Hydrastis canadensis.* A small, perennial plant, usually cultivated for the mass herb product, but also occurring wild in rich, shady woods and damp meadows. A thick, knotty, yellow rootstock sends up a hairy stem, about 30 cm high, with a pair of five-lobed, serrated leaves near the top terminated by a single greenish white flower.

goose. A large web-footed bird, related to the duck and the swan. The domestic goose, of which there are many varieties, all nearly alike. It lives chiefly on land. It is valued for the table, for its quills and for its fine, soft feathers, which are used in making pillows and matresses. A rich delicacy called gras is obtained from the livers of fattened geese. In the spring these geese are seen flying northward in V-shaped flocks, and as cold weather approaches, they return to the South. Other species are gray goose, or graylag, of Europe and Northern Asia, and pigeon goose, of Australia.

gooseberry. Berry of shrub, *Ribes grossularia.* The average composition per 100 g is: protein 1%; fat 0.5%; calcium 20 mg; iron 0.5 mg; vitamin B_2 0.02 mg; nicotinic acid 1 mg; vitamin C 35 mg; and food energy 0.18MJ.

gooseberry, cape. Fruit of *Physalis peruviana,* also called golden berries.

Goosefoot family: *Chenopodiaceae.*

Plants in this family are mainly salt-tolerant annual or perennial herbs with vesicular hairs on the leaves that store salt as sodium or potassium chloride. Betalain pigments are also present. Tiny, wind-pollinated flowers form in dense clusters.

The family include: *Beta vulgaris* (beet, sugar beet), *Beta vulgaris* var. *Cicla* (Swiss chard, rhubarb chard), *Spinacia oleracea* (spinach), *Tetragonia expansa* (New Zealand spinach); *Chenopodium album* (lamb's quarters); *Kochia* (cypress spurge).

Gorgonzola cheese. A semi-hard, rennet curd, mold-ripened cheese made chiefly in Italy. It is ripened in cool valleys in the Alps for atleast one year. It is cylindrical in shape, crumbly in texture, streaked with mold, and at its best the flavour resembles that Roquefort. The interior of the cheese is mottled with blue-green veins like those in Roquefort. In Italy the mold is called *Penicillium glaucum* rather than *P. roqueforti,* the name used in the US, but is the same mold, at least in some instances. The surface of the cheese formerly was protected by covering it with a reddish coat resembling clay, which is prepared from barite or brick dust, lard or tallow, and coloring matter. Now, however, tinfoil and stout containers are used. The cheeses, which are cylindrical and flat, are from 21.6-38 cm in diameter and from 16.5-20.3 cm thick, and weigh between 6.4-7.7 kg. Milk is warmed to about 30°C, and enough rennet added to coagulate it in 15-20 minutes. The curd is cut slowly, allowed to settle, collected in a cloth, and hung up to drain overnight in a room in which the temperature is between 15.6-20° C. Curd is prepared similarly from morning milk and is drained but not cooled.

Expandable wooden hoops, 20.3-30.5 cm in diameter and 26.7-30.5 cm deep, are lined with cloth and placed on rye straw or drain mats on a drain table. The two lots of curd are cut into rather large slices or portions, and mold powder is sprinkled in as the portions are placed alternately in the hoops. The warm (morning) curd is placed mainly in the bottom and at the periphery and piled up on top, with cool (evening) curd between. This distribution of the curd is considered a critical part of the making process. It aids in developing mechanical openings in the interior of the cheese and in binding the surface and making it smooth. The piled-up curd is covered with the edges of the cloth lining, and the cheese is turned. It is repressed and turned every 2 hours at first and less frequently thereafter for a day. The cloth is removed and the cheese is replaced in the hoops, left on the straw or drain mat, and turned twice daily for several days. It is salted heavily at first and lightly later, a total of 8-12 times in 1-3 weeks. The temperature of the room is held at about 10°C. The cheese is dried and initial curing takes place in a room in which the temperature is between 11.1°-15.6°C, and the relative humidity is 75-80%. During this period of about 20-30 days, the cheese is turned and rubbed by hand every other day and kept clean. It is scraped with a knife occasionally. Cheese then is moved to a room in which the temperature is from 8.9-10°C, and the relative humidity 85-90%, where the second stage of curing takes place. This period lasts 2 months. If the cheese was not punched earlier, it is punched at this stage. Final curing takes place in a room in which the temperature is from 4.5°-6.5°C, and the relative humidity is even higher than in the other curing rooms. The entire curing period is at least 90 days, frequently is 6 months, and may be a year.

gossypol. The toxic substance found in cottonseed, which must be removed before the seed-cake can be used as foodstuff. It is a bright yellow pigment of undetermined composition found in pigment gland in the seed. If present in chick diet it causes the eggs to discolour on storage.

gotu kola. *Centella asiatica, Hydrocotyle asiatica.* A slender perennial is found throughout tropical regions of the world. Its nearly smooth surface kind kidney-shaped or heat-shaped leaves accompanied by dark-purple flower petals make for a somewhat exquisite plant. But efforts to domesticate it have often failed, because its apparent obstinance requires human persecution in order to spread. Thus, when gotu kola is sprayed with herbicides, only the leaves die, while the root actually seems to thrive on these harmful chemicals. After one good spraying, the plant usually proliferates like crazy.

gouda cheese. A variant of Edam cheese, made in southern Holland. The diameter of the top and bottom surfaces is about 16 cm and the cheese slopes outward to the middle where the diameter is usually about 35 cm, and 10 cm deep. It is made in much the same way as Edam. Milk is set at 35°C, cut, cooked at 38-40°C and drained. The curd is brine or dry salted and is aged at least two to three months. Baby Goudas of about one pound are quite popular in the United States. Federal Standards recommends that themMoisture should not be more than 45% and fat content not less than 46% in the solids.

gourds. The vegetables of the family

Cucurbitaceae, including cucumber, marrow, pumpkin, squash, gourd and melon. Calabash or bottle gourd (*Lagenaria vulgaris*), ash gourd (*Benicasa hispida*), snake gourd (*Trichosanthes anguina*), cucumber (*Cucumis sativus*), vegetable marrow (*Cucurbita pepo*), pumpkin, (*Cucurbita moschata*), squash (*Cucurbita maxima*), coocha or chayote (*Sechium edule*), cantaloupe melon (*Cucumis melo*), water melon (*Citrullus vulgaris*). All contain more than 90% water and about 1% protein and have little food value apart from vitamin C at 10 mg per 100 g. In addition yellow pumpkin contains 900 mg vitamin A per 100 g. Melons are sometimes grown for their seeds which contain 20% oil and about 20% protein. The fruit is berry with soft fleshy pericarp or with a hardened pericarp and classified as pepo. Before Linnaeus, pepo was the name for pumpkin. Pepos that are dried or ornamental use or hollow vessels are commonly called gourds. Separate male and female unisexual flowers are most common. Male flowers have unusual stamens. While there may be 1-5, there are usually 3 stamens with one stamen having a 1-chambered anther of 2 pollen sacs and 2 stamens with 2-chambered anthers of 4 pollen sacs each. The female flower's pistil has an inferior ovary of 3-5 carpels, usually united into 1 chamber (locule) of ovules in parietal placentation.

gournay. A soft, rennet Neufchatel-type cheese deriving its name from Gournay, France, the village in which it is made.

Graham bread. Whole-wheat bread in which the bran is very finely ground. Graham cakes are made from whole meal flour and milk.

grain dryer. A device which reduces the moisture content of grain, with or without heated air, but including an air moving device, appropriate ducts for air distribution, a chamber for drying, often with conveying or materials handling devices to move grain to and from the dryer.

grain whisky. All whiskies are made from grains but the term 'grain whisky' is reserved for the spirit made with a little help from malt. Unlike malt whisky it is distilled in a patent-still of the coffee-type. It has very much less flavour than a malt whisky and the two types are blended to give ordinary Scotch. The method of producing grain whisky is more or less similar to the making of malt whisky. Whisky as it comes from the still, whether not or patent, is an unattractive beverage. It has no colour and is harsh in taste. The colour of whisky is scarcely at all due to extraction from the casks it is matured in; caramel is added to produce a fairly standard and a popular shade. The blending of malt and grain whiskies is more than a mere mixing. There is some interaction between the constituents which tempers the crudeness of the taste. However, the amelioration takes place chiefly during ageing period, when the whisky is stored in oak barrels in unheated warehouses for several years; Scotch whisky must be matured for at least three years before selling. The casks are usually old sherry casks. The legal minimum of three years is always exceeded in practice and eight or ten years would be nearer to truth. After twenty years in wood, whisky tends to deteriorate, but once bottled, whisky does not changes significantly.

grain. The fruit, dry, indehiscent, and containing one seed, of which the testa is united closely to the fruit wall. Cereal protein generally lacks the amino acid lysine which makes it imperfect unless married up to another source of protein rich in this particular essential amino acid, such as soyabean products. 22 amino acids are needed to build protein and of these eight cannot be made by the body but have to be ingested. Vegetable proteins do not supply all eight essential amino acids but happily the amino acid in short supply in one food is often available in excess in another. So pulses like dried beans, peas and lentils which are high in lysine and low in tryptophan make the ideal partner for grains high in tryptophan and low in lysine. Hence the evolution and importance of dishes like beans on toast, humus with pitta bread, rice or chapatis with dhal, beans and tortillas, rice and bean curd all of them perfect protein combinations. To ensure a good protein balance on vegetarian diet choose 60% grains, 35% pulses or nuts and seeds, and 5% green leafy vegetables, as well as plenty of raw fruit and vegetables to make up the balance of other nutrients. Some of the grains used as food include:

Barley. *Hordeum vulgare.* Originated in western Asia, where it was one of the first grains to be cultivated. As human food, the larger, white-seeded variety of barley is pearled, or ground in a revolving drum until the hull and germ are removed. This reduces the grains to small, starchy balls which are then used to thicken soups. Pot, or hulled, barley is ground enough to remove only the husk.

Buckwheat. *Fagopyrum vulgare.* Native to central Asia, Thought of as a cereal grain, but is really in a family of its own. Mainly used for making flour for pancakes. Groats, or kaska, are kernels with the hulls removed. They are eaten as breakfast food or as thickeners for soup, gravy and dressing.

Corn. *Zea mays.* Native to America; commercial varieties are either yellow or white in colour. Popcorn is distinguished by its small, hard kernels with tough outer covers, while flour corns have soft, starchy kernels. The other recognized types include dent, flint, sweed, pod and waxy corn. The basic products of refined or processed corn are starch, oil, syrup, hominy grits, cornmeal and flour. Indian corn is popular for its unusual variety of colours. For instance, the Hopi of northern Arizona have a least 20 varieties, with multiple legends and religious beliefs being attached to each particular colour.

Millet. *Panicum milliaceum.* Native grain of the East Indies. It is the common name applied to a variety of cultivated grasses with small white or golden kernels. Among the most popular are foxtail and pearl millet. Since it lacks gluten, it's good for people who must avoid this protein.

Oats. *Avena sativa.* It developed from the wild grasses of eastern Europe and Asia. Today there are 3 general classes and nearly 100 varieties grown. They are equal to corn as a tissue builder. Steel cut oats are simply cracked oat kernels, while rolled oats have been flattened or rolled into thin flakes.

Rice. *Oryza sativa.* An ancient grain cultivated for over 4,000 years. Originated in Southeast Asia. Each whole grain has an outside hull, a brownish-coloured covering called bran and a finer, lighter-coloured layer called polish which surrounds the kernel. Commercial varieties are classified on the basis of size and shape of the kernel, short, medium and long-grain. All have the same food value, but long-grain costs more since more kernels break during milling. Brown rice is simply rice that has not had the bran and polish removed.

Rye. *Secale cereale.* It developed from a wild variety still growing in the mountains of eastern Mediterranean countries. It is deficient in the glutinous protein that give wheat dough the elasticity necessary for good leavening, so pure rye bread is heavy and compact by comparison.

Triticale. *Triticum secale.* A hybrid grain produced by cross-breeding wheat and rye. First bred in the 1930s by Swedish agronomists and has since become very popular in the US and Canada.

Wheat. *Triticum aestivum.* One of history's first cultivated grains in western Asia. Now covers more of the earth's surface than any other grain crop. For marketing purposes, five classes of wheat based on usage and habit of growth were established, hard red spring, soft red winter, hard red winter, durum and white. Generally, the harder translucent varieties are valued for the production of flours while durum is prized for the manufacture of macaroni, spaghetti and noodles.

Wild rice. *Zizania aquatica.* Native to the Great Lakes region of the US and Canada. Although used in the same way ordinary rice is, this really isn't a true "rice" as such. Wild rice has a gustier, chewier, and somewhat smokier taste to it than conventional rice does.

Gram stain. A set of two stains that are used to stain bacteria; the staining depends on the composition and the structure of the bacterial cell wall.

This differential staining procedures divides bacteria into Gram-positive and Gram-negative groups based on their ability to retain crystal violet when decolorized with organic solvents.

gram, Indian. Name given to small dried peas, e.g. green gram (*Phaseolus aureus*), black gram (*Phaseolus mungo*), red gram (*Cajanus indicus*).

Gram-negative bacteria. Designating a bacterium that does not retain the initial Gram stain but retains the counterstain. Gram-negative bacteria possess a relatively thin cell wall that is not readily digested by the enzyme lysozyme, and in which peptidoglycan layer is converted with lipopolysaccharide.

Gram-positive bacteria. Designating a bacterium that retains the initial Gram stain and is not stained by the counterstain. Gram-positive bacteria generally possess a relatively thick and rigid cell wall that is readily digested by the enzyme lysozyme, and that consists of a layer of peptidoglycan.

grana cheese. A class of Italian cheese with granular body, sharp flavour, and grating characteristics. This class of cheese has excellent keeping quality even under adverse conditions. Grana-type cheeses are said to have been made in the Po Valley as long ago as 1200 AD, at which time that was the most important cheese-making center in Europe. According to Italian authorities, there are two main types of Grana cheeses:

(a) Grana Lombardo, which is made largely in the Province of Lombardy (north of the Po); and

(b) Grana Reggiano, which is made largely in Reggio, in the Province of Emilia (south of the Po).

There are numerous subvarieties of

each type, named usually according to the place of manufacture. Lodigiano (named for Lodi) is similar to Lombardo; Emiliano (for Emilia) and Parmigiano (for Parma) are similar to Reggiano, and there are others. The subvarieties differ principally in method of manufacture (acidity of the milk, cutting the curd, cooking temperature, curing period, etc.), and in shape and size. Considerably quantities of both types of grana cheeses are exported from Italy, usually under the name Parmesan (common name outside of Italy, and sometimes in Italy, for these cheeses).

granite mosses. The genus *Andreaea* consists of about 50 species of small, blackish-green or olive-brown tufted rock mosses, which in their own way are as peculiar as *Sphagnum*. Although the gametophyte closely resembles that of the true moss, it arises from a protonema that is platelike instead of filamentous. Just as in *Sphagnum* the sporophyte lacks a true stalk, and it is elevated above the leaves on a stalk of gametophytic tissue. The minute capsules of *Andreaea* are marked by four lines of weaker cells along which the capsule splits. The capsule remains intact above and below the dehiscence lines. The resulting four valves are very sensitive to the humidity of the surrounding air, opening widely when dry and closing when moist.

granula curd. A cheese made in a manner resembling the regular cheddar process, except that it not matted or milled. The curd is cooked firm whey is drained, curd is stirred until proper acidity develops and the curd is salted and pressed. Some salt may be added immediately after dipping to prevent the curd from matting. The moisture should not exceed 39%, and

the fat, should not be less than 50% in the solids.

Grape family: *Vitaceae*. Vines with tendrils that develop opposite the leaves are characteristics in this family. The tendrils may be twining, as a grape *(Vitis)*, or end in attaching discs, as in the Virginia creeper *(Parthenocissus)*. Flower clustres also develop at the node opposite a leaf. The flowers are bisexual or unisexual on the same plant (monoecious). Usually there are 4-7 sepals, 4-7 petals, 4-7 stamens, and 1 pistil, which develops into a berry fruit. The family includes: *Vitis* spp. (grapes- wine, jellies; dried grapes- raisins, currants); *Cissus* spp. (grape ivy), *Parthenocissus quinquefolia* (Virginia creeper), *P. tricuspidata* (Boston ivy).

grape sugar. Alternative name for glucose.

grapefruit. Fruit of *Citrus maxima*. The pith contains a bitter glucoside naringin. The average composition per 100 g of the grapefruit is: protein 0.4%; fat 0.1%; iron 0.3 mg; vitamin A 3 mg; vitamin B_1 0.03; vitamin B_3 0.01 mg; nicotinic acid 0.2 mg; vitamin C 28 mg.; and food energy 0.1 MJ.

Grapenuts. Trade name for a breakfast cereal made from wheat. The average composition per 100 g is: protein 12%; fat 3%; carbohydrate 75%; calcium 49 mg; iron 5.5 mg; and food energy 1.5 MJ.

grapes and raisins. *Vitis species.* Grapes are readily identifiable as a fruit, with their trailing, climbing, tendril-clasping, wide-leafed vines and pale green to reddish purple fruit. Nearly half of this plant's innumerable grapes are native to North America. Many of our present species evolved from their cousins in the wild, such as the fox grape which kept the Lewis and Clark Expedition from near starvation. The average composition per 100 g of the grapes is: protein 0.7%; fat 0.45%; iron 0.5 mg; vitamin A 20 mg; vitamin B_1 0.05 mg; vitamin B_2 0.05 mg, nicotinic acid 0.2 mg; vitamin C 4 mg; and traces of cobalt and zinc; and food energy 0.25 kJ.

Grass family: *Poaceae (Graminae).* The grass flower is unlike any other plant family's flowers. Within a spike (a), the flower unit is called a spikelet. An exaggerated separation of the structures is shown in the spikelet diagram. The primary axis of the spikelet is called the rachilla. At the base of the spikelet are 2 bracts called first glume and second glume. The next bracts are called lemmas and may have a bristle-like appendage. A soft inner bract is called the palea. The remaining parts comprise a floret. Each spikelet may have one or more florets, which are unisexual or bisexual. There are no sepals or petals, instead there are 2-3 lodicles. Lodicles enlarge with turgor pressure and cause the lemmas and palea to expand, exposing the stamens and/or stigmas at pollination time. Grasses are wind-pollinated. There are usually 3 stamens with freely moving (versatile) anthers and 1 pistil with 2, usually feathery, stigmas. The pistil's ovary is superior and contains 1 ovule. The fruit is usually a grain or a berry in some bamboos. Grasses are annual or perennial herbs except for bamboo, which is woody. Roots and fibrous and adventitious roots arise from stem nodes. The stems, called culms, are usually hollow and round with 1 leaf to a node. Leaves are alternate in 2 rows up the culm. The leaf consists of a blade and a sheath, which encircles the culm, and has parallel venation. Where the leaf blade diverges from the culm is often a membranous appendage, the ligule. The family include: *Avena sativa* (oats), *Hordeum* (barley), *Oryza sativa* (rice), *Saccharum* (sugarcane), *Secale cereale* (rye), *Setaria italica* (millet), *Sorghum bicolor* (sorghum), *Triticum* (wheat), *Zea mays* (corn); *Bambusa* (bamboo); *Agrostis* (bentgrass), *Dactylis* (orchard grass), *Phleum* (timothy), *Setaria* (foxtail grass), *Sorghum, Zea; Agrostis, Cynodon* (Bermuda grass), *Festuca* (fescue grass), *Poa* (bluegrass), *Stenotaphrum* (St. Augustine grass), *Zoisia* (zoysia grass); various grasses (insulation materials, newsprint, ethyl alcohol).

grass tetany. Name given to the magnesium deficiency in cattle.

grated cheese. *See* grating cheese.

grating cheese. A hard, dry, low moisture cheese which is grated into foods as a condiment. A grating cheese of the Grana type is usually well aged. This type of product is usually prepared by grinding hard, dry, low-fat well-aged natural cheese to a powder. Italian varities of cheese, the Parmesan type are usually used. The cheese should be cured for at least six months before it is grated. After it is grated, it may be dried further on trays in a current of hot, dry air; then it is packed in moisture-and-air-proof containers. Some manufactures prepared a so-called "grated" cheese by adding nonfat dry milk solids and cheese colour to dry (usually low-fat) American-type cheese, grinding the mixture, and then drying it. This product, however, usually lacks full flavor. Federal Standards recommends that the moisture should not be more than 39%; and the fat content not less than 50% in the solids. Also known as grated cheese.

grayling. A family of fishes related to

the salmon. Graylings are more slender, however, have larger scales and are more graceful and active, resembling the trout in their habits. They are fine game fish, and their flesh is considered a great delicacy. The common European species is found in Scandinavia, Russia, the Orkney Islands and as far south as Switzerland. The largest specimens weigh four or five pounds. There are three American species, found only in Arctic streams and in Michigan and Montana. They never exceed a length of eighteen inches. The graylings of Michigan are being exterminated by the brown trout, their mnatural enemy.

grayanotoxins. The toxins contained in the leaves of plants of the family *Ericaceae*, such as the rhododendron. There are several active components including grayanotoxins I and III, and α-dihydrograyanotoxin II. Other components are almost inactive. They produce a reversible increase in sodium permeability in excitable membranes rather like that produced by batrachotoxin.

grease butter. A farmer classification of butter which includes butter below cooking grade.

Green. A popular term for the cheese which is newly made and which has not been ripened or cured. Also called Fresh Cheese. It lacks the characteristic cheese or pasteurized process cheese flavour.

green algae. *Division: chlorophyta.* The most diverse of all the algae, both in form and in life history. The group comprises at least 7000 species. Although most green algae are aquatic, they are found in a wide variety of habitats, including the surface of snow, in green patches on tree trunks, and as symbionts in lichens, protozoa, and hydra. Of the aquatic species, a few groups are entirely marine, but the great majority are found in fresh water. Many green algae are microscopic, but some of the marine forms are large; *Codium magnum* of Mexico, for example, sometimes attains a breadth of 25 cm and a length of more than 8 m. This group has a long fossil record, with some simple forms reported from rocks nearly a billion years old. The Chlorophyta are similar to the bryophytes and vascular plants in several important characteristics. They contain chlorophylls a and b, store their food as true starch, and have firm cell walls composed, in most genera, of cellulose, with hemicelluloses and pectic substances incorporated into the wall structure. For these reasons, they are believed to be directly related to the evolutionary line from which the bryophytes and vascular plants evolved. Within the Chlorophyta, three fairly distinct lines of progressive evolutionary specialization have been recognized: the volvocine line, the tetrasporine line, and the siphonous line.

This life history of *Cladophora* differs significantly from those of the other green algae. In them, meiosis is zygotic and the only diploid cell in the life cycle is the zygote. In *Cladophora,* meiosis is sporic. Two types of individuals exist, one haploid, the other diploid. The diploid individual arises from the zygote by mitosis and produces sporangia with *spore mother cells.* Meiosis occurs within the sporangium, each spore mother cell giving rise to four spores (zoospores in *Cladophora*). The haploid zoospores develop into unisexual (either + or -), haploid filaments. These filaments produce gemetangia and gametes (a zygote is produced and the cycle is completed. As mentioned previously, this type of life cycle, in which diploid, spore-producing individuals (*sporophytes*) alternate with haploid, gamete-producing individuals (*gametophytes*), is called an alternation of generations. In *Cladophora*, the two generations are similar in size and morphology. *Cladophora* thus has an isomorphic alternation of generations. Among the marine green algae is *Ulva*, commonly called sea lettuce. Cell division occurs in three planes, but only once in one plane, giving rise to a glistening, flat *thallus* (a simple, relatively little differentiated vegetative body) two cells thick and up to a meter or more long. The thallus is anchored to the substrate by a holdfast produced by protuberances of the basal cells. Each cell of the thallus contains a single nucleus and chloroplast. *Ulva* is anisogamous and has an isomorphic alternation of generations similar to that of *Cladophora*. An example of a green alga with a heteromorphic alternation of generations is siphonous marine Derbesia (*Halicystis*). The gametophyte is a bladder up to 3 cm in diameter, the sporophyte a freely branched filament. The two generations are so different in appearance that they were long placed in separate genera. *Derbesia* is an excellent organism for classroom use, being easy to culture and handle. Such green algae as *Chlamydomonas* and *Spirogyra* may be considered to have an alternation of generations in which the sporophyte generation is represented only by the zygote. At the other extreme, *Codium* is diploid, with its gametes being the only haploid cells in the life cycle, as in animals, and so clearly has no alternation of generations.

green beans. *Phaseolus vulgaris.* Green beans (snap or string) belong to the same *Phaseolus* species kidney, navy and lima beans do, except that they are picked while still green in their pods. These green beans were first introduced by Native Americans to early colonists and became an instant hit with them. Green beans are one of the safest vegetables to serve guests with finicky tastes and picky eating habits.

green bean drying. Snap beans or green beans are used for edible pods or seeds in the pods which can be dried. Split green beans are dried a tray or on a belt a temperature of 62.7-65.5°C for 6 hours, followed by bin drying at 46.1°C for about 2 days to produce a product at 2-5% moisture content. Higher temperatures can be used if the time is reduced. An improved quality of product can be obtained by freezing the beans prior to drying.

green BS, brilliant. *See* Green S.

green crop dryer. A device used to remove moisture from forage crops, which is identified as a low temperature green crop dryer if the hottest air in contact with the crop does not exceed 176.6°C. The device is known as a high temperature green crop dryer for hotter temperatures of air in contact with the crop, which usually exceed 315.5°C.

green pea drying. Green peas are edible peas which are difficult to dry and rehydrate by conventional methods. Peas are slit prior to blanching, sulfiting, and dehydrating. Tunnel, cabinet, and continuous belt dryers are used for green peas. Temperatures of 82.2°C and 71.1° are used in the first and second stage of the tunnel dryer, with peas on trays. An initial temperature of 87.7-93.3°C is used for a continuous belt dryer. Peas are removed from the dryer at 8% moisture and finished to 4% in a bin dryer using air at 48.9°C.

green revolution. Until recently, the major food plants of the world, like the wild ancestors from which they arose, were genetically very diverse. In fact, since the beginning of agriculture, more than 10,000 years ago, huge reserves of variability have accumulated in the important crop plants by the processes of mutation, hybridization, artificial and unconscious selection, and adaptation to a wide range of conditions. Thus for crops such as wheat, potatoes, and corn, there are literally thousands of known strains. This genetic variability provides an important safety factor. If one strain were to prove unusually susceptible to a particular pathogen, for example, others could be found that were genetically resistant from which new varieties could be bred. As a result of the Green Revolution, however, crop plants have become more and more uniform and hence more vulnerable to destruction. In 1970, for example, the southern corn leaf blight fungus, *Helminthosporium maydis*, destroyed huge quantities of corn. These losses were apparently related to the appearance of a new race of the fungus that is highly virulent for corn of a type that is used extensively in hybrid seed production. Such dangers increase as the improved strains being developed continue to replace the many distinct types that existed before. Indeed, it is already becoming difficult to locate seeds of many of these previous strains. It is now generally agreed, by both critics and supporters of the Green Revolution, that aggressive research programs are needed in connection with our crop plants, first to monitor the appearance of new strains of plant pathogens and second to maintain the genetic diversity of these crops. Varieties threatened with extinction must be sought out throughout the world and preserved in suitable gene banks.

green S. Food colour; sodium salt of di-(*p*-dimethylaminophehyl)-2-hydroxy-3,6-disulphonaphthyl-methanol anhydride. Also known as Wool green S; Brilliant acid green BS.

Grenache grape. A red grape cultivated in California, France, Germany, Israel, and Spain. It is used in the preparation of sweet and heavy dessert wines, in some vin roses, and California Ports. A white variety is much less widely grown. Also known as Alicante.

Grignolino grape. A native Italian red wine grape of highly regarded quality. The color of the wine is somewhat different from the usual reds, having a crimson coloration. Some Grignolino grapes have been planted in southern California where they are used for producing vin roses.

grilling/broiling. Rapid roasting on a grid-iron. With meat the expressed juices mostly evaporate before they have time to drip away, and so leave most of the extractives on the surface. Grilling causes minimum losses of vitamins. The losses: for meat- B_1 30%, B_2 15%, nicotinic acid 20%; for fish- 50% B_1.

grinder cheese. A Swiss cheese which does not meet the requirements for higher grades but is used in the manufacture of pasteurized process cheese or pasteurized process cheese foods.

Grissini. Italian "finger rolls" or stick bread 15-35 cm long.

grist. Cereal for grinding.

groats. Oats from which the husk has been entirely removed; when crushed, Embden groats result.

groundcherry. A plant that is closely related to the tomato and can be grown wherever tomatoes do well. The kind ordinarily grown in gardens produces a yellow fruit about the size of cherry. The seeds may be started indoors or sown in rows in the garden. Also known as husk tomato.

groundnut. *See* peanut.

groundnut oil. Three principal methods are used for recovering the oil content of the groundnut. The earliest method used, but now largely replaced in most of the countries with advanced processing technology, was hydraulic press. For this operation, the raw groundnuts (peanuts) are shelled and crushed, usually without any presorting or grading. The nuts are heated with open steam and placed on press cloths, which are approximately 0.6 m squares. The optimum moisture content of the groundnuts (peanuts) prior to pressing is about 5%. The nuts on each cloth are about 5 cm deep. These loaded cloths are placed in tiers of perhaps about 1 m in height and then subjected to a hydraulically generated pressure of about 9.8×10^6 kg/m^2. The hydraulic pressure process leaves about 7% oil in the residual cake.

In expeller pressing, the machine used is somewhat similar to a meat grinder on a very large scale. The process is continuous. The mass of material is forced forward by a large screw. Expelled oil passes through perforations in the sides of cylindrically shaped chambers. Provided the raw peanuts are of an edible quality and the expelling operation is conducted under sanitary conditions, the residue may be ground into so-called peanut flour. If these conditions are not met, the resulting meal may be used for livestock feed. The expeller process leaves about 5% oil in the residue. In the solvent oil extraction process, particularly suited to large-scale operations, hexane is used as the oil solvent. In principle and concept, this process is quite similar to that used in obtaining soy oil from soybeans. Oil in the residue from this process is about 1%. In the hydraulic and expeller processes, fine particles of peanut may be incorporated in the extracted oil. These are removed from filtration. The recovered oil also contains some free fatty acids. These are neutralized by treatment with sodium hydroxide, after which the oil is deodorized by passing superheated steam through it. A precipitate known as "foots" is produced and this is removed by centrifugation and filtration. The use of this oil for cooking in the home and in restaurants is so familiar that no explanation is required. Groundnut oil is used in the manufacture of mayonnaise and for this purpose should be refined so as to retain its nature color. When used for shortening, the oil is hydrogenated and frequently blended with other vegetable fats. The oil also is used in a number of nonfood products, such as face creams, shaving creams, hair lotions and other cosmetics. Groundnut oil is sometimes used to adulterate olive oil. Physical properties of refined groundnut oil are: melting point 0.56°-2.22°C; smoking point 227°C; iodine number, 90-94; free fatty acid content, 0.0137-0.0422% (weight); peroxide number, 3.5-8.0 mm per kg and saponification number, 188-191.

gruyere cheese. 1. A kind of Swiss Cheese made in the Gruyere district of southern France. Also called Emmental and Schweitzer cheese. It is similar to Swiss cheese except that it has smaller eyes and a sharper flavour, and a second fermentation takes place which produces a smear growth on the surface.

2. Trade name of Swiss cheese processed and packaged in tinfoil. It differs from ordinary Swiss cheese in having no gas holes. The Federal Standards recommends that the moisture should not be more than 39%, and the fat content not less than 45% in the solids.

guaiac. *See* guaiac gum.

guaiac gum. A gum resin of the true *lignum vitae* trees; used in the preparation of varnishes; as a chemical indicator; and to prevent rancidity and loss of flavour in preserved and dehydrated foods. It is an effective antioxidant, although its chief use is in medicine as a stimulant and laxative. The resin comes in greenish-brown tears, and a good quality product is 90% soluble in alcohol. Also known as guaiacum.

guaiacum oil. An essential oil distilled from the wood of the guayacan tree of Paraguay, used in medicine, soaps, and perfumes. It is light grey in colour, and is solid at temperatures below 45°C. The odour is that of a combination of tea leaves and roses. It is also called guaiacwood oil. The wood yields 5-6% of the oil. Azulene, a blue dye, is extracted from guaiacum oil, from eucalyptus oil, and from some balsams. The azulenes derive names from the source, as guaiazulene, but they all have the empirical formula $C_{15}H_{18}$, the molecule having two rings and five double bonds. The synthetic material is known as vetivazulene.

guaiacwood oil. *See* guaiacum oil.

guanine. One of the purine bases found in DNA and RNA. Guanine has a purine ring structure.

guanylate cyclase. An enzyme containing a haem moiety that catalyzes the production of cyclic guanosine-3',5'-monophosphate (cyclic GMP) from GTP. Guanylate cyclase occurs in at least two forms: one is in the cytosol and another is associated with the particulate fraction of broken cells. Endogenous activators of guanylate cyclase include EDRF, unstable intermediates in prostaglandin synthesis, and the inhibitory transmitter mechanism of NANC innervation of the bovine retractor penis and related smooth muscles. Cyclic GMP, like cyclic AMP, mediates smooth muscle relaxation. However, it is often produced during smooth muscle contraction elicited by a smooth muscle stimulant. In these instances it acts as negative modulator that limits the site of the contraction. The activating stimulus to the enzyme may be EDRF released by the contraction from the endothelium of vascular tissues, or arachidonic acid peroxide or prostaglandin endoperoxide released during the PI response.

guar gum. *Cyamopsis tetragonoloba or C. psoralioides.* A polysaccharide of galactose and mannose, used as a stabilizer in ice-cream preparations, salad dressings, processed cheese, etc., and as a "cloud" stabilizer in fruit drinks. The part used in the endosperm of the seed. The endosperm constitutes 35-42% of the seed; it is separated from the other components of the seed (seed coat or hull and embryo or germ) during processing. The endosperm left is then ground to a fine powder, which is commercial guar gum. The major producers of guar gum are India and Pakistan.

guarana. Dried paste prepared from the seeds of the climbing shrub, *Paullinia cupana* (S. America); rich in caffeine; used in S. America as a beverage similar to cocoa.

guava. Fruit of *Psidium guajava,* tropical shrub.

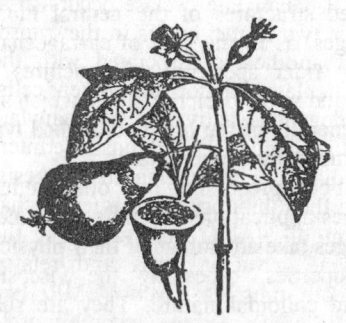

It is usually eaten raw or preserved as guava jelly. The average composition per 100 g is: water 80%; protein 1%; fat 0.5%; carbohydrate 12%; iron 1 mg; vitamin A 65 mg; vitamin B$_1$ 0.04 mg; vitamin B$_2$ 0.05 mg; nicotinic acid 1 mg; vitamin C 215 mg; and food energy 0.25 MJ.

gudgeon. A fresh-water fish, belonging to the carp family. Neither of its jaws is furnished with teeth, but there are two triangular bones at the entrance of the throat, which act as grinders. These fish are marketed as food fish.

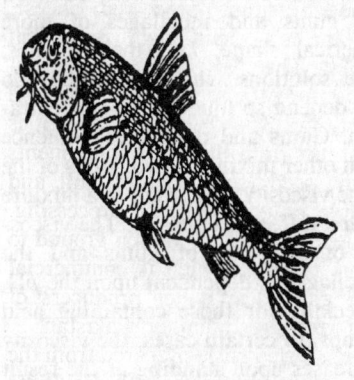

Guinea green. FD&C green no. 1. A triarylmethane type dye which has a structure similar to that of Fast Green.

It is a dull green powder, which is very soluble in water, glycerol and the glycols and slightly soluble in ethanol (95%). The colour is light-fast, had good stability in a wide range of pH, and is stable in solutions of sodium benzoate, but fades badly in the presence of sulphur dioxide Guinea green is no longer permitted for use in food in the US.

Gukuhara orange. A variety of sweet orange, it is sometimes seedy. Fruit is of medium size, and of deep orange colour, with a high juice and soluble solids content. It is believed to be a bud mutation of the Joppa orange. Juice of the Fukuhara is frequently blended with satsuma mandarin concentrate. The Gukuhara orange has a juice yield of 53.9%.

gum, Arabic. Exudate from the stems of several species of Acacia, also known as gum acacia (best product comes from *Acacia senegal*); it is used as thickening agent, as stabilizer often in combination with other gums, in gums drops and soft jelly gums and to prevent crystallization in sugar confectionery.

gum, British. Dextrin, partly hydrolysed starch.

gum, chewing. Based on chicle, the partially evaporated milky juice of latex of the Sapodilla tree, plus sugar, balsam of Tolu and flavour.

gum, tragacanth. Obtained from the trees of *Astralagus* species; used as stabilizer.

gums. The substances capable of disperse in water to form a viscous, muciganous mass. Gums find numerous application in food processing as stabilizing emulsions (for salad dressings, processed cheese) as a thickener and in sugar confectionery. Gums may be extracted from seeds (guar gum, locust, quin;e, psyllium), sap or exudates (gum Arabic, karaya (sterculia), tragacanth, ghatti, bassora or hog gum, shiraz, mesquite, anguo) and seaweeds (agar, kelp, alginate, Irish moss) or they may be made from starch or cellulose (dextrins and methyl, carboxymethyl, etc. cellulose) or they may be synthetic, such as vinyl polymers. Most of these (apart from dextrins) are not digested by the human body and have no food value.

The extracellular plant gums and mucilages (gum Arabic, karaya gum, and tragacanth) generally have a more complex structure than the intracellular types. They are made up of a number of different sugar-building units linked together by a variety of glycosidic bonds. They possess central core or nucleus composed usually of D-galactose and D-glucoronoic acid units joined by glycosidic bonds which are relatively stable to hydrolysis by acids. To this central nucleus, there are attached as side chains those sugar units which are removed by milk acid hydrolysis. Thus, in the case of gum Arabic, the acid-resistant portion of the molecule is composed of D-glucuronic acid and D-galactose and to this nucleus are attached units of L-arabinose, L-rhamnose, and D-galactopyranosyl (1-3) L-arabinose. The neutral mucilages and gums, such as mannans, galactomannans, and glucommannas extracted from seed and roots, have relatively simple structure. The kinds of building units are fewer and the molecules are much less branched. The galactomannans are usually composed of a backbone of linear chains of D-mannose units joined together by the 1,6-glycosidic bonds, to which are attached at regular intervals side chains of D-galactose residues. The glucomannans are essentially linear polymers

united by 1,4 linkages. The algal polysaccharides are relatively simplified structures of the neutral mucilages, as in the case of carrageenan. A wider spectrum of structures is found in the bacterial gums, which are generally of the highly branched type exuded by higher plants.

Food processing and other industries applications of gums and mucilages take advantage of their physical properties, especially the viscosity and colloidal nature. They are substances of high molecular mass. For example, gum Arabic has a molecular mass in the range of 250,000-300,000. The gums and mucilages which possess relatively linear molecules, such as gum tragacanth, form more viscous solutions than the more spherically shaped gums, such is gum Arabic, when at the same concentration. Consequently for some applications, the gums with linear molecules are more economic to use. Due also to the elongated molecular shape of the seed gums and mucilages, the viscosity of their aqueous solutions varies widely with concentration. They exhibit structure viscosity. In contrast, the gums and mucilages of more spherical shape, i.e., the exudates, give solutions whose viscosities do not depend so much upon concentration. Gums and mucilages influence each other mixing of two. gums of the same viscosity may result in a mixture with a different viscosity. The viscosity of solutions of gums and the mucilages is dependent upon the pH, especially for those containing acid groups. in certain cases, the viscosity decreases upon standing as the result of enzymatic breakdown of the molecules. The molecules can undergo large changes in shape and size under the osmotic influence of opposing ions. Some of them, such as carrageenan from Irish Moss, can be fractionated by dilute salt solutions (potassium chloride) and the poly-β-glucosan from barley grain may be precipitated with ammonium sulphate.

Gums and mucilages may be found either in the intracellular parts of plants or as extracellular exudates. Those found within plant cells represent storage material in seeds and roots. They also serve as a water reservoir and as protection for germinating seed. The polysaccharides found as extracellular exudates of higher plants appear to be produced as a result of injury caused by the mechanical means or by the insects. It has not been well established whether the exudates are formed at the site of the injury, or whether they are generated elsewhere and then transported to the injured area. The true exudates, such as gum Arabic and the East African and Indian gums are picked by hand. Seldom are commercial samples pure.

The gums are classified according to the grade, which, in turn, depends upon colour and contamination with foreign substances, such as wood and bark. The exudates are processed simply by grinding, their only prior treatment being sorting and sometimes bleaching in the sun. In some cases, they are purified by extraction with water and precipitated by alcohol. Gums and mucilages present in roots, tubers and seaweeds are usually extracted with hot water, dried, and marketed as powder. Those gums found on the inner side of the seed coat as a vitreous layer (such as locust bean, guar bean, etc.) are obtained by suitable process.

gurjun balsam. An oleoresin obtained from various species of the *Diptero-carpus* tree, about 50 varieties of which grow in India, Burma, Sri Lanka, and the Malay Peninsula. It is a clear liquid with a greenish fluorescence. The specific gravity is 0.955-0.965. Gurjun balsam is used in lacquers and varnishes that are capable of resisting elevated temperatures. Also known as wood oil. Sometimes, it is called East Indian copaiba.

Burmese trees form two groups yielding products known as kanyin and in oil. Kanyin oils are brown in color, while the In oils are whitish and heavier. Gurjun balsam may consist of either or both of these products. Commercial gurjun oil is obtained by steam distillation of the balsam, and has a specific gravity of 0.900-0.930. It is soluble in alcohol.

Capaiba balsam is a resin obtained from the copaifera tree, a species of Dipterocarpus, of South America. Maracaibo copaiba and Paracopaiba are the principal varieties. They are dark yellow or brown in colour, and are soluble in alcohol. The resin is used as a plasticizer, in varnishes, tracing paper, and in pharmacy. The specific gravity is 0.940-0.990.

gussing cheese. An Austrian skim milk cheese resembling the Brick cheese of the US; its process of manufacture is also similar to the Brick cheese, except that skim milk is used.

Gutadel grape. A kind of grape vine which requires sites that are well sheltered against wines and with a rich, deep humus soil, found most readily in the Baden region of Germany. Its ripening period falls between that of the Muller-Thurgau and Silvaner varities. The wine prepared from this variety of grapes is light, pleasing, and agreeable. The soft, sweet Gutadel grape is also appreciated as a dessert grape.

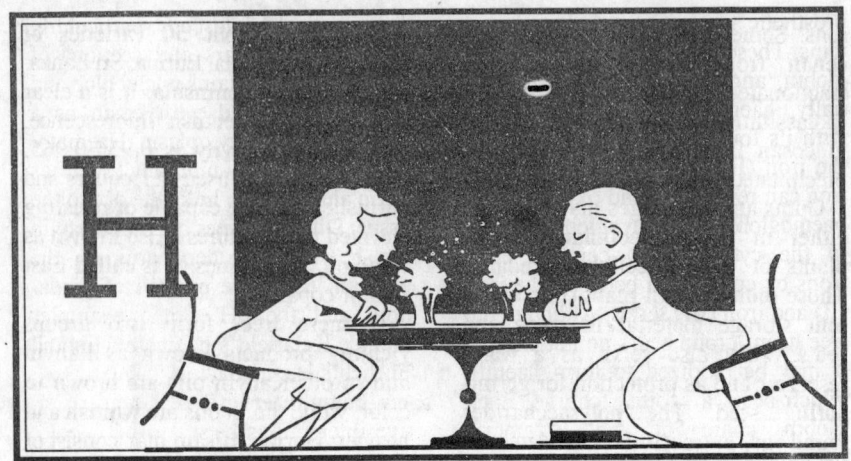

H.T.S.T. Abbreviation for High Temperature Short Time Pasteurization.

hackberry. The name of a number of trees of rapid growth which belong to the same family as the nettles. The best known species is a large tree sometimes 40 m high. It has a rough bark and nearly horizontal branches, and it may be used in much the same way as the elm. There are two species, of which the smaller, more generally known as the sugar berry.

haddock. *Melanogrammus aeglefinus.* An important food fish, of the cod family, though less valuable than the cod. It is smaller than the cod, which it much resembles, and it has a dark line along much resembles, and it has a dark line along its side and a dark spot just behind the head. It commonly weighs from 1-2.5 kg, though sometimes as much as 4.5 kg. It ranges in length up to nearly 1 m. Its distribution in the northern Atlantic is similar to that of the Atlantic cod. Haddock differs from all other codfishes by a black spot above the pectoral fin. The lower jaw is very short and the barb is small. Its chief diet consists of invertebrate, bottom-dwelling organisms and herring spawn. As a pure shelf inhabitant, haddock is rarely found below 200 m. The age of this medium-size fish is about 14 years. Like Atlantic cod, haddock undertake periodic migration between the feeding grounds and the spawning sites. In the northeastern Atlantic, the chief spawning sites are in the northern North Sea and off the Norwegian coast. Haddock reach sexual maturity after 3-4 years, spawning in the spring, somewhat later than Atlantic cod. The haddock has lower fertility, but the development period of the eggs is shorter than in the Atlantic cod. The initially pelagic young are often found under the umbrellas of large medusas before changing to bottom dwelling in the fall of their first year of life. Their length at that time is about 10 cm. Unlike other codfishes, which migrate toward the shallow coastal waters, haddock spend their first years in the open sea.

haem. An iron-containing molecule that binds with proteins as a cofactor or prosthetic group to form haemoproteins. These are haemoglobulin, myoglobin, and the cytochromes. Essentially, haem comprises a porphyrin with its four nitrogen atoms holding the iron (II) atom as a chelate. This iron can reversibly bind oxygen (as in haemogloblin and myoglobin) or (as in the cytochromes) conduct electrons by conversion between the iron (II) and iron (III) series. Although the free haem group bears no net charge, it may be oxidized to form haemin which bears a positive charge. Each globin chain of the tetrameric haemoglobin molecule carries a separate haem group, an iron atom being carried centrally by each haem. If oxygen binds to one haem group, an allosteric shape change is initiated in the haem, its attendant globin, and finally in the whole haemoglobin complex. Also spelled as heme.

haemagglutination inhibition. The inhibition of haemagglutination; used for assaying haemagglutinating viruses by adding antiviral antibodies to a mixture of virus particles and red blood cells.

haemagglutinin. A protein substance present in certain viruses, such as the influenza virus, which has the property of producing agglutination of red cells owing to its specific action on mucopolysaccharides of the membrane of those cells. The phenomenon of haem-agglutination is one of the means most used to show that certain viruses are present, in particular those of influenza and mumps.

haematin. A derivative of haemoglobin formed by removal of the protein part of the molecule and oxidation of the iron from the ferrous (II) to the ferric form (III).

haematoxylin. A compound used in its oxidized form (haematein) as a blue dye in optical microscopy, particularly for staining smears and sections of animal tissue. It stains nuclei blue and is frequently used with eosin as a counter-stain for cytoplasm. Haematoxylin requires a mordant, such as ferric alum, which links the dye to the tissue. Different types of haematoxylin can be made up depending on the mordant used, the method of oxidation, and the pH. Some examples include Kelafield's haematoxylin and Ehrlich's haemotoxylin.

haem-haem interactions. The cooperative interactions between the haemes of the subunits of hemoglobin with respect to the binding of oxygen.

haemin. Oxidized form of haem in which trivalent iron replaces the divalent iron atom at the centre of the porphyrin ring. Haemin is the crystalline form in which haem can be isolated and studied in the laboratory. The iron present is the trivalent state (iron (III)). Haemin can be made to crystallize by heating haemoglobin gently with acetic acid and sodium chloride.

haemocyanin. A blue copper-containing blood pigment found in many molluscs and arthropod. Haemocyanin is the second most abundant blood pigment after haemoglobin and functions similarly in acting as an oxygen-carrier in the blood.

haemoerythrin. A red oxygen-carrying blood pigment similar to haemoglobin in containing iron. However, whereas haemoglobin is the blood pigment in all vertebrates and a wide range of invertebrates, haemoerythrin is confined to several closely related minor groups of invertebrates, e.g., brachiopods.

haemoglobin C. Type of haemoglobin with an abnormal β-globin chain, in which lysine has replaced glutamic acid at position 6.

haemoglobin H disease. If three of the four genes that code for α-globin on chromosome 16 in all human cells, are deleted, result is severe anemia that must be treated by transfusion. This state is called haemoglobin H disease.

haemoglobin S. Type of haemoglobin with an abnormal β-globin chain, in which valine replaces glutamic acid at position 6 from the NH_2-terminus of the β-peptide chain. Such β-globin, renders the molecule less soluble and the red blood cells containing the pigment tend to adopt a sickle shape. Haemoglobin S is the pigment present in the cells of individuals suffering from sickle cell anemia.

haemoglobin. The pigment of the red blood cells (erythrocytes) that performs two major biological functions:

(a) transport of oxygen from the respiratory organ to peripheral tissues; and

(b) transport of carbon dioxide from peripheral tissues to the respiratory organ for subsequent excretion. It consists of a basic protein, globin, linked with haem. Its approximate molecular mass is 64,500 and it contains four haem groups, and hence four iron atoms, per molecule.

The most important property of haemoglobin is its ability to combine reversibly with one molecule of oxygen per iron atom to form oxyhaemoglobin, which has a bright red color. The iron is present in the divalent state (iron (II)) and this remains unchanged with the binding of oxygen. Oxygen molecules diffusing across the red cell membrane, are readily attached to haemoglobin in the lungs and equally readily detached in the tissues. This is the mechanism by which blood transports oxygen through the body. There are variations in the polypeptide chains, giving rise to different types of haemoglobins in different species. The binding of oxygen is governed by partial pressure; high pressure favours formation of oxyhaemoglobin and low pressure favors release of oxygen. It also depends on pH. The affinity of oxygen decreases as the pH is lowered (more acid, as a result of dissolved carbon dioxide). This dependence is known as the Bohr effect.

In addition to transporting oxygen from the lungs to peripheral tissues, it facilitates the transport of carbon dioxide from tissues to the lungs for exhalation. Haemoglobin can bind carbon dioxide directly when oxygen is released, and about 15% of the carbon dioxide entering the blood is carried directly on the haemoglobin molecule. However, as carbon dioxide is absorbed in blood, carbonic acid is formed which dissociates into bicarbonate and a proton. To avoid the extreme danger of increasing the acidity of blood, a buffering system must exist, to absorb the excess liberated protons. Haemoglobin binds 2 protons for every 4 oxygen molecules lost. In the lungs, as oxygen binds to deoxygenated haemoglobin, protons are released.

haemolysin. One of a group of the metabolic products of bacteria, some plants as well as animals, such as snakes, toads, bees, spiders, etc., which have the power of producing hemolysin. Certain of these exist normally in blood serum or are produced during immunization. Some of the haemolysins have been shown to be enzymes that attack the phospholipid of the host cell membrane.

Because the phospholipid lecithin is often used as substrate, these enzymes are called lecithinases or phospholipases. Since the cell membranes of all organisms, both prokaryotes and eucaryotes, contain phospholipids, haemolysins that are phospholipases sometimes destroy bacterial as well as animal cell membranes. Some haemolysins are not phospholipases, however. Streptolysin O, a haemolysin produced by *streptococci*, affects sterols of host cell membrane, and its action is neutralized by addition of cholesterol or other sterols.

haemolysis. 1. The separation of hemoglobin from the stroma of the blood and its appearance in the serum, This is effected by hypotonic solutions, a number of chemical compounds (ether, chloroform, alkalies, and especially saponins) and by hemolysins. 2. The actual destruction of red blood corpuscles.

haemophilus influenzae. A Gram-negative organism that morphologically ranges from coccobacillus to a filamentous rod. It is a part of the normal microbial flora of the respiratory tract of humans and many animals. Two strains may be present in the respiratory tract; the encapsulated and non-encapsulated. The encapsulated strain, called *H.influenzae type b*, is the more virulent and also the more predominant type in children under four years of age. Older children and adults rarely carry the type b strain, which is one of the major causes of meningitis in children under four years of age but disease in adults is rare.

haemosiderin. Brown granular pigment composed of iron-protein complex, present in various tissues. It is a storage form of iron that can be mobilized for haemoglobin synthesis but is only present when there are ample store of ferritin. It accumulates in the spleen, liver and bone marrow in diseases where there is excessive destruction of blood. Siderosis also occurs on poor diets rich in iron.

Haff disease. A paralysis due to the excessive consumption of various freshwater fish (probably inadequately cooked) which contain the antivitamin antithiamin. Occurs in Sweden and is the human equivalent of Chastek's paralysis which effects foxes.

Hagberg test. Measure of α-amylase activity of flour derived from the change in viscosity of flour paste.

hagfish. An eel-like fish, allied to the lampreys, that lives as a parasite upon other fishes. The mouth is large and adapted to sucking; there are no jaws; the eyes are rudimentary. A single fang upon the palate enables the hafgish to rend its prey, which are small cod, halibut, flounder and such. The skeleton is composed entirely of cartilage. The body is covered with a leathery skin that secretes slime.

haggis. Traditional Scottish dish; made from liver, heart and lungs of sheep, cooked with suet, oatmeal and seasoning, then filled into a bag made from sheep's stomach and boiled for several hours. Said to have been originated by the Romans when originated by Romans when campaigning in Scotland; when breaking camp in an emergency the food was wrapped in the sheep stomach.

hake. Family: *Merluccidae.* A marine fish related to the cod family. The North American silver hake abound off the northeastern banks, where they are caught with cod. They are usually eaten fresh, though some are smoked and dried. The average weight is 2 kg. A species of hake is found on the Pacific coast. The fish which is closely related to the codfish, but has a special systematic position due to their unusual distribution. The family has just one genus, *Merluccius*. Its slender body, skull structure, and the large-toothed mouth give this carnivorous fish a garlike appearance. There are two dorsal fins and one long anal fin, which is almost the mirror image of the second dorsal fin in shape, size, and position. The hake (*Merluccius merluccius*) is found in the north eastern Atlantic off the western and southwestern coasts of Europe, along the continental shelf. Living in deep water has enabled the hakes to penetrate the tropical Atlantic and inhabit oceanic regions in the southern hemisphere with temperate to subtropical conditions. This accounts for the large South Atlantic populations of stockfish (*Merluccius capensis*) off southwestern Africa and Merluccius hubbsi from the coasts of southern Brazil and Argentina. There are also Pacific species, *Merluccius gayi* and *M. productus*, off the western coasts of North and South America. Their presence has been explained by a presumed migration around Cape Horn. The New Zealand species, *Merluccius australis*, may also have come by this route. Hakes can be over 1 m in length, but there are small- and medium-sized species as well. They are predators, feeding chiefly on herring and other schooling fishes. The European hake seeks its prey at night in the upper water levels; during the day it is less active and is near the floor, at which time it can be caught easily, even with a dragnet. This species spawns in spring, apparently without preferred spawning sites. The floating eggs then drift within the hake distribution region.

halawa. *See* halva.

half-value dose. The dose of radiation or toxic compound that produces deaths in 50% of the cells, or loss of infectivity of 50% of the virus particles, in a test group within a specified time; analogous to the median lethal dose for animals.

halibut *Hippoglossus*. The largest of the flatfishes and an important article of food. Some specimens reach a very large 2-3 metres in length, and weigh over 100 kg. In rare cases, halibut grow to be giants. The largest halibut ever recorded 4.7 m long and weighed 330 kg. The average length and weight of those which are presently brought to fish markets are much smaller. Those which weigh about 30 kg are most desired for food, as the flesh is then tenderized. The halibut lies on its left side, with its right side, in which are both eyes, uppermost. It is white beneath and dark brown above. Halibut prey upon smaller fish and crustaceans, and are themselves devoured by seals, whales and sharks. Not a true arctic species, halibut exists so far north only because it stays warm in the Gulf streams. This powerful fish is rather elongated, with a tapered head and curved caudal fin edges. The eye-side of the body has a uniform gray-brown to dark olive-brown hue. The underside is white, and the powerful jaws have sharp teeth. While young halibut occur in shallow water, between 35-70 m, the adults are found in depths of nearly 700-1000 m. They usually live there above sandy or gravel bottom, very rarely above mud or rocky floors During summer, halibut prefer the banks of moderately deep to shallow water along the coasts. In winter they

retreat to deeper water.
halibut-liver oil. One of the richest
natural sources of vitamins A and D;
contains about 5 g vitamin A and 8
mg vitamin D per 100 g.
hallucinogen. Any of a group of
cyclic organic compounds which cause
various aberrations of perception and
feeling, as will as a undesirable
physical reactions. Many of these
compounds are from natural sources
and encompass six distinct types. The
best-known of these are derivatives
of lysergic acid, chiefly the diethyl-
amide (LSD-25), which is one of the
most powerful; mescaline, a phenyl-
ethylamine: and tetrahydrocannobinol
group occurring in marijuana and its
concentrated form, hashish.
halophilic bacteria. The bacteria *Halo-
bacterium halobium*; which conserve
energy derived from absorbed sunlight by an entirely different principle
from that employed by true photosynthetic organisms. These unusual bacteria live only in brine ponds and salt
lakes, where high salt concentration
results from water loss by evaporation. They can live in NaCl concentrations lower than 3M. These bacteria are aerobes and normally use
oxygen to oxidize organic fuel molecules. However the solubility of
oxygen is so low in salt ponds, in
which the concentration of NaCl may
exceed 4M, that halobacteria must
sometimes call on another source of
energy, namely sunlight. The plasma
membranes surrounding the cells of
H. halobium contain patches of light
absorbing pigments, called purple
patches. These patches are made of
closely packed molecules of bacteriorhodopsin (molecular mass ~26,000),
which contain a molecule of bound
retinal or vitamin A aldehyde as
prosthetic group. When the cells are
illuminated, the excited bacteriorhodopsin molecules undergo transient bleaching. As the light excited
bacteriorhodopsin in the membrane
revert to their initial ground state, the
energy released is harnessed to
translocate H^+ ions from the inside to
the outside of the cells, to form an
acid outside the pH gradient across
the cell membrane. Because its concentration is higher on the outside, H^+
ions tend to diffuse back into the cell
through an ATP-forming enzyme in
the membrane, similar to ATP synthetase of mitochondria and of chloroplasts. As the H^+ ions pass through
bacterial ATPase, they supply energy
required to make ATP from ADP and
phosphate. Thus bacteria can conserve light energy in the form of ATP,
to supplement their ability to carry
out oxidative phosphorylation when
oxygen is available. However halobacteria do not evolve oxygen, nor do
they carry out phosphoreduction of
$NADP^+$. Bacteriorhodopsin, relatively
a small protein molecule, is the
simplest light driven H^+ pump known.
Halphen reagent for cottonseed oil. A
solution of 1 g sulphur in 100 ml
carbon disulphide, used in detecting
cottonseed oil. 1 ml of this reagent is
heated with 1 ml of the oil to be tested
and 1 ml amyl alcohol for 15 minutes,
in a concentrated aqueous solutiion
of sodium chloride. A red colour is
given by cottonseed oil.
Halphen ·reagent for linseed oil. A
solution of sufficient bromine in 10 ml
carbon tetrachloride to bring the
volume to 15 ml, used in detecting
linseed oil. 1 ml of the reagent is
added to about 0.5 ml of the oil tested
and 30 ml ether at 300K. A turbidity
which appears in 2 minutes is given
by linseed oil.
halva. 1. A sweetmeat composed of an

aerated mixture of glucose, sugar and crushed sesame seeds; because of the seeds, the sweet contains 25% fat. Also spelled halwa, halawa and chalva.
2. An Indian sweet-dish made from sugar, ghee, and wheat flour. It may have different bases such as carrots, potatos, etc.

halwa. *See* halva.

ham. The whole hind leg of the pig removed from the carcass and cured individually, sometimes the process is secret. Hams cured or smoked in different ways have different flavours, York, Bradenham, Suffolk and Westphalian hams. The average composition per 100 g after cooking is: protein 15%; fat 40%; iron 2.4 mg; vitamin B_1 0.6 mg; vitamin B_2 0.2 mg; nicotinic acid 3.6 mg; and food energy 1.8 MJ.

Hamlin orange. A variety of sweet orange, nonblood type. Shape of the fruit is oblate to globose; the size is medium, with a diameter ranging from 6.4-7.3 cm. The rind is smooth and glossy, usually thin. The fruit ranges from seedless to a few seeds. Its colour is light orange, and the juice content is about 53%; soluble solids, 10%. Tree is a heavy bearer, with consequent tendency for fruit to be small and times. When properly cultured, and in good seasons, the quality of the Hamlin is considered excellent. The fruit provides a fine blend of sweetness and acidity. Hamlin juice concentrate packed in November-December tends to be of poor color. This is compensated by blending the juice with concentrate from Pineapple or Valenica varieties. The Hamlin enjoys plantings in Algeria, Argentina, Brazil, Iran, and Mexico.

Hammarsten's casein. Casein prepared by the method of hammarsten. Fat-free milk is diluted with water and precipitated with acetic acid. It is washed three times with water by decantation; dissolved in ammonium hydroxide and reprecipitated, this repeated twice. The final precipitate washed with alcohol and ether and finally extracted with ether in a Soxhlet.

hand cheese. A small, sour-milk, surface-ripened cheese, which is so named because originally it was molded in final shape by hand, and still is in some parts of Europe. It is very popular among Germanic peoples and is made in several, countries. There are many local names for hand cheese. For example, in Austria, it is known as Olmutzer, Quargeln and Olmutzer Bierkase. In Russia it is called Livlander. Mainzer Handkase or Harzkase, Alte Kuhkase, or Berliner Kuhkase, Ihlefeld, Satz, and Thuringia Caraway cheese, are some of the names in German markets.

The curd is prepared much as cottage cheese curd with or without rennet, heated to 50°C for 3 hours and then drained after which the curd is mixed thoroughly or ground in a curd mill and salted. It is sometimes flavoured with caraway seed. Then the cheese is hand molded or pressed into small forms of desired shape and dried in a warm room. It is cured for 6-8 weeks in a moist room at about 15°C. Well ripened Hand cheese has a sharp, pungent flavour and aroma. The cheese is kept clean while curing. When surface ripening has begun, it is wrapped and packed in boxes. It is cured for 6-8 weeks at a temperature of 10°C. At higher temperatures, they cure too rapidly. Well-ripened Hand cheese has a very sharp, pungent flavour and aroma; the consumer sometimes must become accustomed to it before it is found agreeable.

haptoglobin. A serum protein, in the alpha globulin class, that binds free haemoglobin in the plasma and prevents its loss via the kidneys. Instead, the bound haemoglobin is transported to the liver, bone marrow, and spleen for degradation. In the event of haemolysis, circulating haptoglobin is depleted; estimates of plasma haptoglobin concentrations are therefore used to detect recent haemolytic events.

Hardy pear. *Beurre Hardy.* A variety of pear mainly used for canning. Very few of this variety are sold fresh. the fruit is medium to large in size, having shape that is obtuse-pyriform, symmetrical. Its skin is usually granular, tender, dull greenish-yellow, often with some russeting, dots numerous and sometimes conspicuous; the flesh is somewhat granular, buttery, juicy. it is rich in aromatic flavour when properly grown and handled, but inclined to be bitter in taste if picked too early and susceptible to core breakdown if left on tree too long. Fruit is somewhat too soft to withstand commercial handling. Tree is of good growth habits, vigorous and productive, often used as an intermediate trunk stock on quince; semi-dwarf on quince; fairly susceptible to blight.

Harris rennet test. A test to determine the strength of rennet solutions. A sample is taken from the cheese vat at 30° C and placed in a conical glass graduate. The time is noted and a small amount of rennet mixed with traces of water is added. The mixture is stirred with a thermometer for 5-10 seconds and the time noted when the milk first thickens. This test is now more or less obsolete.

haslet. Pigs' offal, minced with herbs and spices and baked.

hawkweed. A large family of plants injurious to crops. The flowers, usually yellow, are clustered on the end of a stalk about twice the length of the leaves, which grow from the ground. The weed may be exterminated from fields with salt, and also by ploughing under the planting the land to hoed crops.

hawthorn. Family: *Rosaceae.* Genus: *Crataegus.* Species: *Crataegus oxyacantha.* A thorny shrub or small tree of the rose family, found wild in many parts of Europe, in North Africa and Western Asia, where it is native. The real hawthorn has been introduced in North America. It is in general use in many places as a hedge and is cultivated for the white and rose-colored blossoms, which make the country landscape very beautiful. The tree bears a small red fruit, called a haw, which affords a winter food for birds. The American thorn apple belongs to the same genus. Hawthorn is rich in vitamin C, and flavone glycosides. It appears to act as an adaptogenic agent. It is of specific use in hypertension associated with myocardial weakness, arteriosclerosis, paroxysmal tachycardia and angina pectoris. It has a toning effect on the muscles of the vasculature. The twin, almost paradoxical, effects on the heart-first dilating the coronary blood supply, and then slowing down and stabilizing the contraction of heart muscle, meat that it has wide applications for all sorts of heart disturbances. A decoction of the berries is used for treating sore throats, and in India it has been used to relieve kidney complaints, and for nervous conditions, insomnia, giddiness and stress, as well as to treat rheumatism. It is also used to avoid cholesterol build-up.

hay. A skim milk cheese made in the department of Seine-Inferieure, France, and known there as Fromage de Foin. The name comes from the fact that it is characteristic aroma. It remains buried in hay for 6-12 weeks after which it is ready for sale.

hay diet. A system of eating based on the fallacy that carbohydrates and proteins should not be eaten at the same meal. Since protein, in the absence of adequate carbohydrate, is oxidized to provide energy and therefore not available for tissue building, this diet is not only faddish but foolish.

hay drying. The removal of moisture from long, chopped, ground, or baled hay, using forced unheated air or forced heated air. The product is dried from green cut at 60-80% moisture, wet basis, using heated air, up to 150-815°C, often in a rotary dryer with chopped or ground forage, reducing the moisture content to 5-10%. This process is often referred to as dehydration. In a belt or conveyor dryer the temperature of the air is usually limited to 176.6°C. Partial drying of cut long forage in the field, often crushed or lacerated, reducing the moisture to 25-50% in 1-4 days, followed by forced unheated air drying of chopped, long, or baled hay in storage is often practiced. Drying must occur rapidly enough to avoid mold formation, depending on the moisture content. An air flow of 0.15-0.26 m³/tonnes static pressure is needed. Supplemental heat can be used for these systems. A major problem in drying is maintaining uniform air flow through the stored hay.

haybox cooking. The food is cooked for only a short time, then placed in a well-lagged container, the haybox, where it remains hot for many hours and so cooking continues without further usage of fuel. Also known as the fireless cooker.

haze. Term in general use in brewing to indicate cloudiness of the beer. Chill haze appears at 0°C and disappears at 20°C but there is no fundamental difference. Due to gums derived from the barley, leucoanthocyanins from the malt and hops, and glucose, pentoses and amino acids.

hazelnut. Family: *Corylaceae*. Genus: *Corylus*. Species: *Corylus avellana* (common European); *Corylus americana* (American).

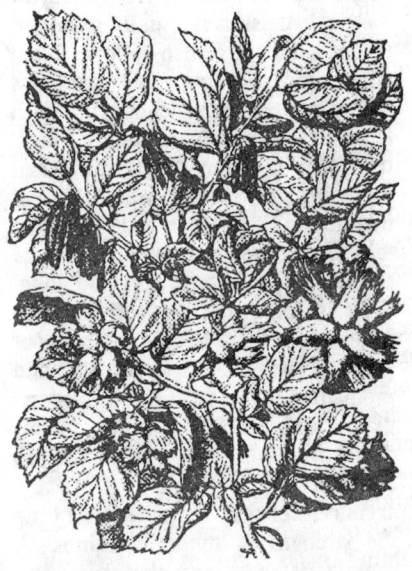

Most nuts have an alkaline reaction on the digestive system but peanuts, walnuts, hazelnuts, cobnuts, filberts and Barcelona are all acid-forming and so need to be eaten in moderation. They are god for the teeth and gums and for body-building. Hazelnuts, like hawthorn, are known to improve the heart and proven hardening of the arteries, but their alleged aphrodisiac virtues may mean that those with shaky hearts had better stay off them.

headcheese. Chopped, cooked edible parts of meat or meat products. Also known as Mock brawn.

health foods. Substances whose consumption is advocated by various reform movements including vegetable foods, whole grain cereals, food processed without chemical additives, foods grown on organic compost, "magic" food (honey, molasses, yoghurt, etc.) and pills and potions.

heart sugar. A classical name for inositol.

heat damage. A general term which might apply to any of several undesirable changes in a food or biological material during drying. The most common example is browning of food products by overheating. Other examples are checking, splitting, cracking, charring, and burning. Browning occurs as a result of a reaction between the free amino groups and lactose in milk, which can be delayed or reduced by storing at low moisture content. For dehydrated potatoes the rate of browning is greatest at 15-20% moisture. Browning increases with an increase in temperature. The deterioration of quality of a product is a result of excessive heat exposure. The heating may occur as a result of excess moisture, in the field or in storage, or during drying. Heat damage is manifested by discoloration, darkening, checks, etc., and may result in lowering the grade for cereal grains.

heat dryer. A heat pump is a refrigeration system which can be used for heating or cooling designed an a manner which enables a surface to deliver usable heat to a space during heating and drying or to cool the same space. When operating as a heating system, the evaporator (cooling coils) absorbs heat from an outside space and delivers it with the heat from compressing the refrigerant, to the condenser which releases heat to the space being heated. When operating as a cooling system, the evaporator absorbs heat from the conditioned space and rejects it to the outside media, basically. It is similar to a conventional refrigeration system. A system making use of rejected heat cannot properly be called a refrigeration system because cooling is not the primary objective of the cycles. For drying, heat is added at the condenser and moisture is removed at the evaporator. The heat pump dryer is used for temperature sensitive products.

heat exchanger. Equipment for heating or cooling liquids rapidly by providing a large surface area and turbulence for the rapid and efficient transfer of heat. It is used for continuous pasteurization and also for the subsequent cooling.

heat pipe dryer. A dryer using a heat pipe as a means of recovering heat from the exhaust air. A heat exchanger pipe transports heat by evaporation and condensation of a liquid in an enclosed pipe. Using a heat pipe in a concurrent (heating), counterflow (cooling) dryer, a 20% saving in energy is reported; for a fixed bed dryer, a 10% saving in energy is reported.

heat wheel. A device for recovery of heat. The device consists of a wheel or rotor which turns slowly (1-3 rpm) in a housing made of two compartments. One compartment is for the cold air being heated; the other is for the hot air being cooled. In one revolution the rotating wheel is heated by the hot air or gas and gives up heat to the incoming cold air or gas. The wheel may rotate in a vertical or horizontal plane. The wheel has a large heating surface formed by plates, tubes, or cells. Also known as Ljungstrom regenerator.

Heath family. *Ericaceae.* Shrubs are the most common form in this family, but some plants are perennial herbs, trees, or vines. Most prefer acidic substrate and many have fungus-root (mycorrhizal) associations. Leaves are simple, alternate, sometimes opposite or whorled, and often leathery and evergreen. Flowers are bisexual, borne singly or in clusters. The 4-5 sepals are distinct or joined at the base. There are usually 4-5 petals joined in a funnel or urn-shape, but in some genera the petals are separate. Stamens are the same or twice the number of petals. The single pistil has a superior ovary of 4-10 carpels with ovules usually in axile placentation, and 1 style and 1 stigma. Fruit types are capsules, berries, or drupes. The family include: *Gaultheria* (wintergreen), *Gaylussacia* (huckleberry), *Vaccinium* spp. (cranberry, blueberry); *Arbutus, Erica* (heath), *Kalmia* (mountain laurel), *Leucothoe* (leatherleaf), *Pieris* (andromeda), *Rhododendron* spp. (rhododendron, azalea); *Arctostaphylos* (bearberry), *Monotropa* (Indian pipe), *Pyrola* (shinleaf); *Andromeda glaucophylla* (bog rosemary), *Kalmia angustifolia* (lamb-kill), *K. latifolia* (mountain laurel), *K. polifolia* (swamp laurel), *Leucothoe* spp., *Lyonia mariana* (stagger-bush), Menziesia ferruginea (fool's huckleberry), *Rhododendron* spp.

heavy chain. One of two polypeptide chains that are linked to two light chains to form the immunoglobulin molecule. The molecular mass of a light chain is about 25,000 and that of heavy chain is about 50,000. The heavy chains of the IgG, IgA, IgM, and IgD immunoglobulins are denoted, respectively, as γ, α, μ, and δ-chains.

Hedonic scale. Term used in tasting panels where the judge indicates the extent of his like or dislike or the food.

heifer. Young cow the has never had a calf.

held butter. Butter that has become cold storage butter by virtue of the laws of the state in which such butter is sold.

hemiacetal. A molecule formed by the addition of nucleophilic alcohol to aldehyde group; chemically it behaves as alcohol as well as ether. The formation of pyranose ring in D-glucose is the result of an intramolecular reaction between aldehydic carbon atom 1 and free hydroxyl group at carbon atom 5, rendering the former asymmetric. D-glucopyranose therefore, can exist as two different stereoisomers, designated α and β, known as anomers.

hemicellulose. A fraction of cellulose containing relatively few monomer units, compared with normal cellulose; as the name suggests, it is a sort of 'half-cellulose'. It is a minor component of wood; and is sometimes also known as β- or γ-cellulose. High percentages occur in corn cobs and in other agricultural wastes. It comprises a group of alkali-soluble polysaccharides that are important constituents of plant cell walls and also act as food reserves in some plants. They include mannans, glucans, xylans and galactans.

hemidesmosome. Cellular structure morphologically resembling half a desmosome, occurring on the basal aspect of epithelial cells and assumed to serve a comparable adhesive function, in this case, anchoring the cells to the basal lamina. Recent evidence indicates certain compositional differences form a true desmosome but these may turn out to be minor.

hemiketal. A molecule formed by the reaction of ketone group with hydroxyl group. D-fructofuranose, 5-membered furanose ring contains a hemiketal linkage formed by an intramolecular reaction of hydroxyl group on carbon atom 5 of D-fructose with the ketone group at carbon atom 2.

hemiterpene. One of a class of substances related to terpenes of the formula C_5H_8, e.g., isoprene.

hepatoflavin. Name given to substance isolated from liver, shown later to be riboflavin.

hepatotoxicity. The toxicity manifested in the liver. The hepatotoxic effects of drugs and other chemicals may take the form of cholestatic jaundice (e.g., with tolbutamide), of hepatocellular damage (e.g., with chloroform), or of carcinogenesis (e.g., nitrosamines).

herb. A very widely used and extremely general term to describe thousands of plants. Usually, for a plant to qualify as an herb, it possesses a root, stem, and leaf structure, usually flowering; which dries up at the end of the growing season-with the exception of the root crown and root system. However, herb may or may not have a life cycle that extends over one growing season. Some writers use the term herb to distinguish a plant from heavier and more woody shrubs, small trees, etc. Other writers may confine the term to a select group of plants, usually grown on a small scale, for flavouring and seasoning prepared foods. The adjective used is herbaceous. The word herb is also commonly used in the sense of a small plant, parts of which, often the leaves or roots, are used as flavoring ingredients of soups, sauces, stews, casseroles, etc. In this connection, the term potherb is more descriptive. Such potherbs include basil, rosemary, sage, tarragon, and thyme.

herbalism. The practice that deals with herbs, parts of which are used for the benefit of man as medicines or food, or for their scent of flavor.

herbicides. Chemicals used in agriculture and gardening to destroy weeds, and sometimes in war a defoliants to expose areas of dense bush. Their relevance to microbiology lies in their toxicity to man and animals. The include chlorophenoxy compounds such as 2,4-D and 2,4,5-T, substituted dinitrophenols such as dinitro-o-cresol (DNOC), bipyridyl compounds such as paraquat, certain carbamates (e.g., propham), substituted ureas (e.g., monuran), triazines (e.g., atrazine), aniline derivatives (e.g., alachlor) and benzoic acid derivatives (e.g., ambiben). Paraquat and 2,4,5-T are dealt with in separate entries because of their special toxicity problems.

Hermitage. One of the famous wines, made from both red and white grapes, in the Rhone Valley of France. Approximately one-third of the wine is white and yielded by *Roussanne* and *Marsanne* grapes, while the remaining two-thirds is red, made from the Syrah grape. About 80% of Hermitage wines are red, the colour being described as ruby with a tint of purple. The flavour and bouquet is reminiscent of the raspberry, the Remaining 20% are white wines noted for their longevity. The latter are usually served after gentle cooling. The production of Hermitage wines is on a very small scale.

Herrgardsost. A popular, medium firm, mild, nutty cheese of Sweden which has a pliable body and a pleasing aroma. The cured cheese contains eyes similar to those of Gruyere, or smaller than the Swiss cheese. The curd is settled under the whey in rectangular portions and is pressed in the vat similar. Cheese in this country is called Herrgard or Irowa Swiss.

herring family. Herring is *Clupea harengus.* Sprat is *Clupea sprattus;* young are brislings. Pilchard is *Clupea pilchardus;* young are sardines. Kippers, bloaters and red-herrings are salted and smoked herrings; bucklings are hot-smoked herrings. Gaffelbitar are preserved herring. The sardine is the smaller fish of this family. The Norwegian herring, *Clupea harengus,* or sea herring, is sardine of Maine, eastern Canada, and the North Sea. The herring is an abundant fish, but it is objectionable as food because of the quantity of sharp bones. In the very small sardines the bones are soft and edible when cooked. *See also* herring oil.

herring oil. A fish oil obtained by extraction from several species of fish of the herring family, *Clupeidae.* In Norway the oil is produced by boiling the whole fish, pressing, and separating the oil from the water centrifugally. A process used in the US is to grind the whole fish into liquid form, remove the oil, and condense the remaining solution until it is 50% solids, which is marketed as homogenized condensed fish for use as poultry feed. In California and western Canada, the sardine is a much larger fish, the pilchard, *Sardinia coerulea,* usually about 20 cm long. The pilchard, or California sardine, once constituted about 25% of the entire fish catch of the United States by weight, but since 1948 the number of sardines in California waters has decreased greatly. The oil yield is about 125 L/metric ton of fish, but much of sardine oil is a by-product of the canning industry. The oil content of herring is 10-15% of the total weight of the fish, being low in the 1-year-old fish and reaching a peak in the third year. The fish builds up its oil in the summer. In winter the herring tends to stay close to the bottom, or at great depths, and uses up much of its oil. Much of the fish oil of South Africa is from the pilchard, *C. sagax.* In France, Spain, and Portugal the European pilchard, *C. pilchardus,* and the *C. sardinus* are used. The oil from the latter has a high iodine value. The Japanese herring is the *C. pallasi.* Herring oil, or sardine oil, is employed as a quenching oil in heat-treating, either alone or mixed with other oils; in soaps; printing inks; lubricants; and for finishing leather. It is also fractionated to use in blends for paint oils. The herring oil contains about 25% of clupanodonic acid, $C_{21}H_{35}COOH$; 20% arachidonic acid, $C_{19}H_{31}COOH$; 18% palmitoleic acid, $C_{21}H_{35}COOH$; 20% arachidonic acid, $C_{19}H_{31}COOH$; 18% palmitoleic acid, $C_{15}H_{29}COOH$; 13 linoleic, 9 oleic, 8 palmitic, and 7 myristic acids. The specific gravity is 0.920-0.933; iodine value 123-142; and saponification value 179-194. It can be made clear and odourless by hydrogenation. Sardine oil is richer in hydrocarbons than most marine oils; it also contains some stearic acid, higher percentages of palmitic and linoleic acids. Pilchard oil is quite similar, but has less oleic acid. Both of these oils contain about 15% of tetracosapoly-enoic acid, a 24-carbon acid, also occurring in herring oil.

hesperidin. A substance, at one time called vitamin P, since it affects the fragility of the capillary walls. It is found in the pith of the unripe orange and other citrus fruits; chemically a complex of glucose and rhamnose with the flavanone, hesperitin.

Hess test. A test for capillary fragility in scurvy. A slight pressure is applied to the arm for five minutes and a shower of petechiae appear on the skin below the area of application.

heterobasidiomycetes. The subclass of basidiomycetes consists of the rusts, smuts, and jelly fungi. The jelly fungi are mostly saprobes and like Homobasidiomycetes, produce basidiocarps. The rusts and smuts are parasitic on vascular plants. They do not form basidiocarps, but produce their sproes in clusters, or *sori*. As a group, the Heterobasidiomycetes are characterized by their septate (multicellular) basidia. The rusts and smuts are of tremendous economic importance, causing damage to crops throughout the world each year. The life cycles of the rusts may be very complex, and these pathogens are a continual challenge to the plant pathologist whose task it is to keep them under control. Until recently, the rusts were thought to be obligate parasites on vascular plants, but now several species have been maintained in artificial culture. Some smuts are also capable of completing their development under these conditions. *Puccinia graminis*, the cause of black stem rust of wheat, will serve to illustrate one of the life cycles of the parasitic Heterobasidiomycetes. It is one of some 7000 species of rusts. Numerous strains or races of *P. graminis* exist and, in addition to wheat, they parasitize other cereal grains such as barley, oats, and rye, and various species of wild grasses. *P. graminis* is a continual source of economic loss for the wheat grower.

heterocyclic compound. An unsaturated cyclic compound containing one or more atoms other than carbon as part of the ring structure. The rings may be hexagonal or pentagonal, the latter appearing in the furan, purine, and pyrrole families of heterocyclics. Substance of cyclic structure, as acid anhydrides, lactides, lactams, lactons, cyclic ethers, and cyclic derivatives of dicarboxylic acids which are formed by the elimination of water from aliphatic compounds, are not considered among the heterocyclic substances. The derivatives of pyridine, quinoline, thiophene, thiazole, pyrone, etc., which contain heterocyclic ring that persist in the compound through chemical reactions, are considered the true members of this class.

heterofermentative lactic acid bacteria. Lactic acid bacteria that produce in fermentation less than 1.8 moles of lactic acid per mole of glucose; in addition to lactic acid, these organisms produce ethanol, acetate, glycerol, mannitol, and carbon dioxide.

heteropolysaccharides. The polysaccharides containing two or more different monosaccharides. Some of the monosaccharides that are bound together by glycosidic bonds to form heteropolysaccharides include arabinose, glucose, and xylose. These are usually tasteless and insoluble compounds of high molecular mass.

hexamic acid. Trade name for cyclohexyl sulphamic acid (free acid of cyclamate); a synthetic sweetening agent; 27 times as sweet as sugar; it is used in effervescent drinks.

hexauronic acid. The acid derived from a hexose sugar by the o idation of the group on carbon atom number six.

The hexauronic acid derived from glucose is glucuronic acid.

hexokinase. An enzyme that catalyzes the conversion of glucose to glucose-6-phosphate. This is the first stage of glycolysis. The enzyme has been crystallized from yeast and has a molecular mass of 1,11,000. The yeast enzyme can be dissociated in to subunits, two polypeptide chains of 55,000 molecular mass each containing an active site. This enzyme exhibits rather broad specificity in that it will catalyze the transfer of phosphate from ATP not only to glucose, but also to fructose, mannose, glucosamine, and 2-oxyglucose. The relative rates of reaction depend on the concentration of the sugars in the reaction mixture; fructose is phosphorylated most rapidly at high concentrations. The multisubstrate hexokinase is also found in brain, muscle, and liver.

hexon bases. The amino acids lysine, arginine, and histidine which contain six carbon atoms.

hexosans. The general name for complex polysaccharides built up from simple units of hexose sugars.

hexose monophosphate shunt. An alternative pathway in the metabolism of glucose to the Embden-Meyerhof-Parnas pathway. The glucose-6-phosphate formed in the main route can be converted to phosphogluconic acid, then to pentose phosphate and to sedoheptulose-7-phosphate. The latter then joins the main pathway. Since pentoses are formed it is also referred to as the pentose cycle and the direct oxidative pathway.

hexose monophosphate shunt. The metabolic pathway that requires the input of six molecules of glucose-6-phosphate and leads to the complete oxidation of one molecule of glucose-6-phosphate to carbon dioxide, water, and phosphate. The pathway functions to generate reducing power in the form of NADPH, allows for the inter-conversion of monosaccharides, and is linked to the fixation of carbon dioxide in photosynthesis.

hexose. A six-carbon sugar such as glucose and fructose.

hexoses. Sugars with six carbon atoms.

hickory. The name given to several species of timber trees, belonging to North America, but to some extent introduced into Europe. They are remarkable for stateliness and general beauty, and they grow to heights of seventy to eighty feet. The wood is heavy, strong and tenacious, and is used for making such things as carriage shafts, handles of golf clubs, whip handles and cogged wheels. The wood is liable to decay more quickly then some other woods, owing to exposure and the onslaught of worms. It makes a valuable fuel, for it develops great heat. The shagbark species yields the hickory nut of commerce. This fruit, a hard-shelled nut, divided into four parts, has a delicate flavour.

high dried. A term once applied to fish which have been dried throughout so as to store long periods as distinguished from those dried on the surface for keeping a short time. The term may also be used for the dry fruits.

high frequency heating. Heat results from the passage of a high frequency current, i.e., radio frequency at 5 million cycles per second. If a foodstuff (non-conductor) is placed between the electrodes heat is generated inside the material due to the very high electrostatic stresses and molecular movement. The process, in effect, heats from the inside outwards in contrast to normal oven heating and is applied to bakery products, for example, to biscuits after baking to reduce the final moisture content. Also called radio frequency heating and electronic heating.

high-density lipoprotein. Any of the various lipoproteins which contain about 30% protein, 30% neutral lipids, and 40% phospholipids; these lipoproteins have molecular mass in the range of 100,000-400,000, and a density of about 1.062-1.21 g/L.

high-energy phosphate donor. A high-energy compound that can function as a phosphoryl group donor to a low-energy phosphate acceptor by way of the ADP-ATP phosphoryl group carrier system.

hiochic acid. A growth factor isolated 1956 in Japanese rice wine (sake) and later shown to be identical with mevalonic acid.

hirudin. Blood anticoagulant found in buccal glands of the leech. It functions by interfering with thrombin.

Hi-soy. Trade name for full-fat soya flour; it has high protein content; popular in many countries.

histamine. Compound formed from the amino acid histidine by decarboxylation and also found in ergot. It has powerful pharmacological effects on the body; constricts the smooth muscle of the bronchioles as in asthma (hence the use of antihistamines in this condition), lowers blood pressure by dilating the vessels, and powerfully stimulates secretion of acid in the stomach (used as a test for achlorhydria).

histidine. One of the common 20 amino acids in protein structure. Histidine has a basic side-chain and is a precursor of the amine histamine. Histidine compounds present in the body include ergothioneine, in red blood cells and liver; carnosine; and anserine.

histohaematin. Or myohaematin, earlier name for cytochrome.

histone acetylase. Enzyme responsible for histone acetylation.

histone. A basic, globular, and simple protein that is characterized by its high content of arginine and lysine. Histones are found in association with nucleic acids in the nucleic of many eucaryotic cells; they are classified into four major groups, denoted I-IV, on the basis of their arginine and lysine content. They are believed to be involved in the condensation and coiling of chromosomes during cell division and have also been implicated in nonspecific suppression of gene activity. Histones do not occur in vertebrate sperm cells or in bacteria and blue-green algae. In prokaryotic cells, histones are entirely absent. However, the anionic charges of each nucleotide phosphate in DNA may be neutralized by the binding of cations such as Mg^{2+} or polyamines such as cadverine, putrescine, and spermine.

HMT. Hexamethylene tetramine. Preservative permitted in some countries.

hogget. The popular name for one-year-old sheep.

hohenheim cheese. A kind of soft cheese which is cylindrical in shape, 10-15 cm in diameter, and weighing about 200 g. It is made in Hohenheim, Germany from partly skimmed milk.

holocellulose. A mixture of cellulose and hemicellulose in wood, the fibrous residue that remains after the extractives, the lignin, and the ash-forming elements, having been removed.

holoenzyme. A catalytically active complex made up of an apoenzyme and a coenzyme. The former is responsible for the specificity of holoenzyme while the latter determines the nature of the reaction.

holoside. A name given to complexes of sugars (or osides) that yield only sugars on hydrolysis. As distinct from heterosides that yield other substances as well as sugars on hydrolysis, e.g., tannins, anthocyanins, nucleosides.

hominy. Prepared maize kernels. Lye hominy, pericarp and germ removed by soaking in caustic soda. Pearled hominy, degermed hulled maize. Corn grits are called ground hominy.

homoacetogenic bacteria. The obligate anaerobes that utilize carbon dioxide as a terminal electron acceptor, producing acetate as the sole product of anaerobic respiration. All homoacetogenic bacteria that produce and excrete acetate in energy metabolism are Gram-positive and many are classified in the genus *Clostridium*. A few other Gram-positive bacteria and many different Gram-negative bacteria utilize the acetyl-CoA pathway for autotrophic purposes, reducing carbon dioxide to acetate, which then serves as a source of cell carbon.

homobasidiomycetes. The subclass basidiomycetes to which the mushrooms, shelf fungi, stinkhorns, earthstars, bird's nest fungi and puffballs belong. All members of Homobasidiomycetes produce basidiocarps, which are comparable to the ascocarps of the Ascomycetes. In addition to the presence of basidiocarps, the Homobasidiomycetes are characterized by their club-shaped, aseptate basidia, each of which usually bears four basidiospores on minute, projections, or *sterigmata*.

homocyclic. A ring or nucleus composed of atoms of the same element which is usually carbon. This is true of cycloparaffins, cycloolefins, benzene and its derivatives, and cyclic terpenes. The term carbocyclic is also used for rings composed only of carbon.

homocysteine. An intermediate in the synthesis of cysteine, in addition to being precursor of methionine in the activated methyl cycle. Serine and homocysteine condense to form cystathionine. This reaction is catalyzed by cystathionine synthetase, a PLP enzyme. Cystathionine is then deaminated and cleaved to cysteine and α-ketobutyrate by cystathioninase, another PLP enzyme. It may be noted that the sulphur atom of cysteine is derived from homocysteine, whereas the carbon skeleton comes from serine.

homogenizing. A process for reducing the size of particles in a liquid and useful in the preparation of numerous food substances, including milk, ice cream, salad dressings, various fruit juices, flavor concentrates, infant foods, among others. A reduction of particle globule size in a mixture of two immiscible liquid makes an emulsion possible. If an emulsifying agent is present, a more stable emulsion can be produced and coalescence of the dispersed phase is prevented. The homogenizer is also used to produce dispersions by reducing the particle size with solid-in-liquid mixtures. As in the preparation of an emulsion, a dispersing agent in a needed to maintain a homogenous mixture. Typically, a homogenizer consists of a high-pressure, positive-displacement pump and an adjustable orifice. The pump is a piston or plunger type, usually consisting of three plungers, although some homogenizers are made with five or even seven plungers. The cylinder for each plunger has an inlet and discharge valve. The plunger pump must push the product through the homogenizing valve (adjustable orifice). For 2-stage homogenization, two valves are arranged in series. A number of mechanisms have been proposed as the what actually breaks up the particles in the homogenizer:

(a) As the product enters the area between the lapped surfaces, it is suddenly accelerated to velocities as high as 9144 m/minute at a pressure 340 atmospheres. When acceleration is sudden, the particle (especially the liquid particles) is stretched or elongated to the point of breaking.

(b) At this high velocity, there are shear forces between layers of liquid under flow that break up particles.

(c) Cavitation may be the major causes of homogenization. When the pressure energy is converted into velocity energy, the vapor pressure of the product exceeds product pressure, resulting in the formation of vapor cavities which collapse upon leaving the valve at higher pressures. This collapsing, or implosion, of cavitation exerts tremendous force, breaking up the particles. Most homogenizers are designed to incorporate one or more of the foregoing principles.

homoitherms. Animals that maintain constant body temperature irrespective of the surrounding temperature; also known as warm-blooded animals.

honey. Syrupy liquid manufactured by bees from the nectar of flowers (essentially sucrose). The flavour and colour depend on the flower from which the nectar was obtained and the composition also varies with the source. It is composed principally of two sugars, fructose and dextrose. If the ratio of fructose to glucose is high

there is a tendency for the honey to crystallize. The colour is from greyish white (rarely) to darkish yellow, largely depending on the food on which the bees feed.

Honey is used to some extent in ice cream making as a substitute for other sugars. However, on account of certain strong flavours it does not combine well with certain fruit flavours. Honey is non-irritating to the digestive tract, is easily and rapidly assimilated, has a gentle laxative effect, and a slight sedative value, is easier for the kidneys to process than any other sugar and because it is predigested, it can enter straight into the bloodstream and therefore give a powerful boost of energy. The hygroscopic nature of honey make it a natural healer, since germs need water to breed.

It is also an excellent antiseptic and antibiotic. The research has shown that the bees manufacture several kinds of antibiotics and inject them into the honeycomb and beeswax. According to some naturopaths, honey can be used for dressing burns as it draws moisture away from the burn and encourages healing which is further accelerated by the antiseptic and antibiotic values. Just because honey is a natural food, it does not means we should use it without restraint. Bears who come to the hives of wild honey-bees are the only animals in nature with decayed teeth. There have been claims for thousands of years that honey helps rheumatism, arthritis, sleeplessness and bed-wetting, and encourages potency.

The composition of honey depends upon the source and other factors, but a typical analysis would be: water 17.1%, 38.5% fructose, 31% glucose, other carbohydrates 12.8%, protein

0.3%, ash 0.2%, and no fat. There is a very small amount of sucrose present in honey. In honey more than 90 organic compounds have been identified, including carboxylic acids, aldehydes, alcohols, and phenols. It can be said that honey contributes about the same sweetness as an equal amount of invert syrup, but any other generalizations about its flavor There is a considerable history of adulteration of honey with invert sugar and corn syrup, but this practice seems to have been pretty well suppressed by government action in recent years. Truthfully labeled commercial mixtures of honey mixed with sucrose, glucose, invert syrup, etc., are available to those who find this form of the flavoring material convenient. The minerals in honey are important and include iron, copper, sodium, potassium, manganese, calcium, magnesium and phosphorus, as well as the vitamins B_1, B_3, B_6 and B_{12}, pantothenic acid, biotin and folic acid. There are also large amounts of vitamin C, varying according to the types of nectar. The sugars include dextrose, levulose, sucrose and maltose, and the acids include citric, malic, succinic, formic, butyric, lactic, pyroglutamic and amino. Honey also contains several enzymes.

An excellent cough mixture can be easily made at home by macerating a large chopped onion (weighing about 50 g) in 250 g honey for 24 hours, straining through muslin and bottling.

Cider vinegar and honey diluted in hot water make a good gargle for ulcerated throats and taken on an empty stomach first thinning in the morning will gradually relieve chronic constipation.

Chinese and Japanese reports on the successful treatment of stomach and duodenal ulcers using honey are very impressive.

An unidentified ingredient of raw honey causes a reaction known as honey botulism in babies. This is really a misnomer since botulism is caused by spoiled food, but the severe gastric stress is real enough and raw honey should not be feed to babies until they are at least a year old and then only in tiny amounts.

Although honey appears to be a simple and commonly available substance, it is relatively complex and requires some rather exacting conditions where it is processed. In the processing of honey, care must be taken of:

(a) moisture content which, if in excess, causes the honey to ferment over a period of time;

(b) the tendency of the glucose to crystallize out of the liquid phase, a process known in the trade as granulation; and

(c) the presence of nitrogenous substances, even if in very small amounts, to cause the honey to darken with age.

Raw honey as taken from the comb, prior to heating or any processing, contains a number of enzymes, including diastate, inulase, catalase, and invertase, the latter catalyzing the inversion of sucrose. There are also suspended solids pollen grains, small particles of beeswax, traces of minerals. The glucose present is in the form of a supersaturated solution and thus the glucose is capable of crystallizing out whenever seed crystals are present. Raw honey is naturally seeded with fine glucose crystals and thus, after a few days is not processed, will granulate. The degree of granulation at equilibrium is determined by the extent of glucose supersaturation, expressed by the glucose: water ratio (commonly called dextrose: water ratio). When this value is about 1.7 or less, the honey is essentially considered as nongraining honey. When the value is greater than 2.1, this indicates a rapidly graining honey. There are incidentally naturally nongranulating honeys, such as gallberry, the sages, and tupelo. For an average granulating type honey, heating will delay granulation by 6-18 months, but after this time span, large crystals will form in conformance with the phenomena of crystal growth. Thus, if a liquid honey of reasonable stability is required, early heating of the raw honey is needed. It is possible to redissolve large crystals later, but much more heat is required.

In processing raw honey, premature regranulation of a final product can occur should the processed honey pick up seed crystals from processing equipment. For this reason, most processors will examine examples of final product with polarized light, an excellent method for detecting traces of introduced crystals. Depending upon end-product objective, granulation is not always negative because some markets prefer a crystalized honey. Both temperature and water affect the possible fermentation of honey. There are naturally sugar-tolerant yeast present in raw honey as contaminants. When water content is less than 17.1%, fermentation will not occur for a year or more even if the yeast count is very high. At a water content of about 18%, a yeast concentration of about 1000 cells per gram will cause fermentation; as will the presence of only 10 cells per gram cause fermentation if the water content is 19% or greater. However, this is also linked with temperature. The ideal range for fermentation to occur is 10-37.8°C. Because of deterioration of other qualities of the honey, storage above 38°C in the interest of delaying or preventing fermentation is not common. Advantage is taken however, of storing honey below 10°C as a means to inhibit fermentation. The ability of honey to ferment was taken advantage of many centuries ago in the preparation of honey wine, often called mead. In processing, amber or golden types of honey that usually possess a powerful, distinctive flavour are much more sensitive to heat than lighter-coloured types. The former honeys contain higher concentrations of various nitrogenous materials that are subject to Maillard or browning reaction.

FDA regulations prohibit additions of any sort. The lip-smacking honeys, though, come from fig blossoms and wild flowers found in and around the hills of Athens, Greece. They are undeniably the sweetest in the world. Bee pollen is the male sexual grains of seed-bearing plants, which bees carry with them back to the hive. Pollen is comparable to spermatic cells in humans and animals. When bees enter the hive and brush it off, the substance falls to the bottom where it is later swept up by the beekeeper and sold to the health food industry for human consumption. Propolis is a resinous substance, gathered by the bees, from the leaf buds or bark of trees (especially poplars). Bees use this stuff to seal any holes or cracks in the hive, to fix the comb of the roof and to protect the hive from outside contaminants. When the honeycomb is constructed inside the hive, some of the cells are made to slightly larger dimensions. These are known as the royal cells.

The eggs which are laid in these cells by the queen bee are designed to produced potential queens from the female grubs, which will be fed on royal jelly. This food is a sticky substance secreted by the glands near the mouth of the honeybee. It's a pearly-white, gluey kind of mass containing a high supply of protein and invert sugars like glucose and levulose. Beeswax is the wax obtained from the honeycomb of the bee. After the honey is removed from the honeycombs the combs are washed rapidly and thoroughly with water. They are then melted with hot water or steam, strained and run into mold to cool and harden.

As a basis for purchasing pure liquid honey meeting US Grade A standards, the certain specifications have been recommended by the National Honey Board Food Technology Program, which include:

Color. Most application call for an extra-light, amber, or light amber honey. Amber and dark amber honeys are suitable for use in dark breads, fruit cakes, brownish, etc.

Moisture. The maximum moisture content is 18.6% for both Grade A and Grade B. A range of 17.07% to 18.6% is often specified. The moisture content of honey influences its viscosity and should be monitored for accurate pumping and metering.

Refractive index. This test provides a rapid, accurate, and simple measurement of the water content of honey. A range of 1.400-1.494 at 20°C is often specified.

Flavour and odour. Honey to be used in bakery products should possess a typical honey flavour and aroma with no objectionable taste and odor notes.

Packaging. Honey is shipped in various containers, such as metal drums, tote bins, pails, and tankers. When shipped in bulk tankers, the temperature of the honey should not exceed 40°C and the tankers should be equipped with in-line strainers. Honey can be pumped, stored, and metered with the same kind of equipment used for corn syrup.

The viscosity of honey decreases as its temperature increases, and holding honey at 25˙45°C facilitates transfer by fluid handling systems. Temperatures over 45°C should be avoided, since they can affect the flavor and odor of the product. The glucose to fructose ratio of honey influences the tendency of honey to crystalline and granulate. Heating redissolves the glucose crystals and reverses granulation. The colour of honey can be affected by several factors, including the kind of flowers from which the bees collect nectar. Among the floral sources, sweet clover, alfalfa, white clover, tupelo, tulip-polar, and buckwheat honeys, in that order, will result in very light to dark gold loaves.

honeycombing. The formation of splits and voids in a wet material due to uneven shrinkage during drying.

honeydew honey. During periods of prolonged drought bees may supplement their nectar supplies with honeydew, the sweet fluid excreted on leaves by leaf-sucking insects. The resultant honey is dark with an unpleasant taste.

Honeysuckle family: *Caprifoliaceae.* Distinguishing features of this family include opposite leaves without stipules and the pistil's inferior ovary of 3-5 carpels, which develop into a berry or drupe fruit. Plants in this family are mostly woody shrubs and vines.

The family include: *Kolkwitzia* (beauty-brush), *Linnaea borealis* (twinflower), *Lonicera* spp. (honeysuckles), *Symphoricarpos* (snowberry), *Viburnum lantana* (wayfaring tree), *V. lentago* (nannyberry, sheepberry), *V. dentatum* (arrow-wood), *Weigela; Sambucus* (elderberry).

honey wine. *See* Mead.

hop cheese. 1. A kind of German cheese, also called Hopfen. After the cheeses are made they are placed in a well ventilated room and allowed to dry. They are then packed and cured in hops.

2. A perennial climbing plant, *Humulus lupulus.* The female flowers contain bitter resins and essential oils used in brewing beer. The vine has many angular, rough stems growing up to 7 metres in length from a branched rootstock. The leaves are rough, opposite, serrate and 3-5 lobed. Attractive yellowish-green flowers adorn the vine, with the male flowers arranged in hanging panicles and the female ones in catkins. The name hops generally pertains to the scaly, cone-like fruit that develops from the female flowers.

hop drying. Hop or hops, the ripe cone-like flowers of a plant Humulus lupulus, containing an aromatic oil used in beer manufacture, are often dried, particularly for commercial use. After picking and sorting, hops are placed into a bulk holder and into pokes. The pokes are carried or moved by trolley to the green stage room and placed adjacent to the kinds for loading. Each poke is then carried into the kiln and placed on lifter cloths on the floor. After the kiln is loaded sulphur is burned in pans in the plenum chamber. The hops are dried in a batch unit and then tipped into piles from the lifter cloths. After

conditioning for several hours the hops are made into bales. The hops may be dried in bulk boxes about 0.6-1 m deep, through which heated air is moved.

hordein. A protein in barley; one of the prolamines.

horehound. *Marrubium vulgare.* A plant of the mint family, with whitish, downy leaves and stem. A perennial found in waste places, in meadows and pastures and along, railroad tracks and roadsides in coastal areas of the US and Europe. A tough, fibery rootstock sends up many bushy, square, downy stems. The leaves are somewhat distinctive, being wrinkled, rough on top and woolly-like underneath. The flowers are small and nearly white, possessing an aromatic smell and bitter flavour. The leaves also are fragrant and in various forms are used as a popular remedy for roughs and colds.

horizontal agitated batch vacuum dryer. A horizontal cylinder which has radial paddles, which is heated, in which the material to be dried is stirred or agitated in contact with the heated metal wall. Units can be operated under vacuum or at atmospheric pressure. A ribbon or scroll agitator blade may also be used.

horizontal belt dryer. An apparatus which carries the materials to be dried on a moving horizontal belt through drying air. A cooling section may follow the drying section. The air may be forced through the product on a perforated, slotted, or screened belt or over a shallow layer of product of the belt.

horizontal chamber. The part of a spray dryer into which atomized products are forced in a horizontal direction, through which air is moved for moisture removal, and from which the dried products are removed. Horizontal chambers may be in the shape of a box, horizontal cylinder, or other shape in which the major axis of the chamber is in a horizontal direction.

horizontal tube evaporator. An evaporator for removing water from a liquid, usually under vacuum, in which heat is transferred to the product in the evaporator through horizontal tubes.

Horlicks. Trade name for preparation of malted milk, for consumption as a beverage when added to milk. The average composition per 100 g is: protein 14.4%; fat 8.0%; carbohydrate 70.8%; calcium 272 mg; iron 1 mg; and food energy 1.7 MJ.

hormonal control of metabolism. Insulin and the somatomedins enhance the active transport of amino acids across cell membranes. Insulin inhibits gluconeogenesis from amino acids and it promotes protein synthesis. Thyroid hormones also promote a positive nitrogen balance by stimulating protein synthesis. Thyroid hormones also promote a positive nitrogen balance by stimulating protein synthesis. Glucocorticoids, like methylprednisolone, enhances gluconeogenesis from amino acids. Therefore, the high-dose glucocorticoid therapy leads to thinning of skin and osteoporosis. During fasting, glucocorticoids predominate and insulin virtually disappears. Protein in skeletal muscle and in viscera is lost daily by gluconeogenesis process to provide glucose.

hormones, sex. Male hormones, or androgens, include testosterone and androsterone; female hormones, or oestrogens, include oestradiol, oestrone and progesterone. Chemically all are steroid in structure. The synthetic female hormones, stilboestrol and hexoestrol, are similar in biological activity but quite different chemically.

Apart from clinical use the oestrogens have been widely used in chemical caponization of cockerels and to enhance the growth rate of cattle.

hormones. The chemical messengers that coordinate the activities of different cells in multicellular organisms. The hormones are molecules synthesized by specific tissues; and are secreted directly in to the blood, which carries them to their sites of action. They specifically alter the activities of certain responsive tissues. Hormones are chemically diverse and can exert their specific effects in different ways:
(a) by influencing the rate of synthesis of enzymes and other proteins;
(b) by affecting the rate of enzymatic catalysis; and
(c) by altering the permeability of cell membranes.

Hormones are regulators of physiological processes within the body, exerting control over such processes as metabolism, growth, reproduction, pigmentation, electrolytic and osmotic balance among other processes. Hormones display not only great variations in function but also in their chemical nature. They vary widely in chemical nature. Some are steroids such as estrogen, progesterone, cortisone, etc., while others are amino acids (thyroxine), polypeptides (vasopressin), low-molecular mass proteins, and conjugated proteins. Amino acid and steroid hormones have been isolated and many, including insulin have been synthesized. The other types are prepared directly from the endocrine organs of animals.

Hormones occur in very low resting concentrations in the blood, $i.e.$, from $10^{-6}M$-$10^{-9}M$. When the secretion of the hormone is stimulated, its concentration in the blood rises. On cessation of secretion, the hormone concentration quickly returns to the resting level. Hormones have a short life-time in the blood. Once their presence is no longer required, hormones are quickly inactivated by enzyme action. The various types of hormones are:

(a) thyroid hormone,
(b) parathyroid hormones,
(c) adrenal cortical hormones,
(d) pituitary hormones,
(e) thyrotrophic hormones,
(f) growth hormones,
(g) gonadotrophic hormones, and
(h) sex hormones.

The first step in the action of a hormone is its binding to a specific molecule or set of molecules, called hormone receptor, which is located on the cell surface or in the cytosol of the target cell. The receptors for the water-soluble peptide and amine hormones, which do not penetrate cell membranes readily, are located on the outer surface of the target cells. The receptors for the lipid-soluble steroid hormones, which readily pass through the plasma membrane of their target cells, are specific proteins located in the cell cytosol. Cyclic AMP plays a critical role in the action of many hormones by serving as a second messenger inside the target cell. Such hormones bind to specific receptors on the plasma membrane of the target cell and stimulate adenylate cyclase. This membrane-bound-enzyme catalyzes the synthesis of cyclic AMP from ATP. A guanyl-nucleotide-binding protein (G protein) couples hormone receptors to adenylate cyclase. The activation of adenylate cyclase leads to an increased amount of cyclic AMP inside the cell. Cyclic AMP then activates a protein kinase which phosphorylates one or more proteins.

For example, the phosphorylation of glycogen synthetase and phosphorylase kinase in muscle and the liver results in decreased synthesis and enhanced degradation of glycogen. This reaction cascade amplifies the initial hormonal stimulus.

hornbeam. A small, bushy tree often used in hedges, as it survives cutting and in age becomes very stiff. The wood is white, tough and hard and is used by carpenters and wheelwrights in making various articles, but it does not withstand the action of water or the weather well and should not be used in exterior construction. The inner bark yields a yellow dye. The American hornbeam is a small tree sparingly diffused over the whole US, where it is called leverwood; ironwood and blue beach.

horse-chestnut. A large family of handsome trees and shrubs, with snowy white, yellow or red flowers and fanshaped leaves which grow on opposite sides of long stems. It was first known in Tibet. Some of the trees grow to be 30-40 m high. The seeds are large, brown and highly polished, and the bitter meats have been used as horse feed, hence the name. The trees of the North America species are not as large as the true horse-chestnut, and their wood is of little value. The horse-destnut is in no way related to the chestnut which produces the table nuts.

horse radish. Root of *Armoracia lapathifolia*. The plant belongs to the mustard family, whose whitish root possess a pungent taste and odour and when grated is used with vinegar as a relish. It is also employed medicinally as a stimulant. Horse-radish is now cultivated in many parts of the world, but was first known in Southern Europe.The pungency is due to volatile oil (allyl isothiocyanate and butyl sulphocyanide) liberated by the enzyme myrosinase from the glucoside sinigrin.

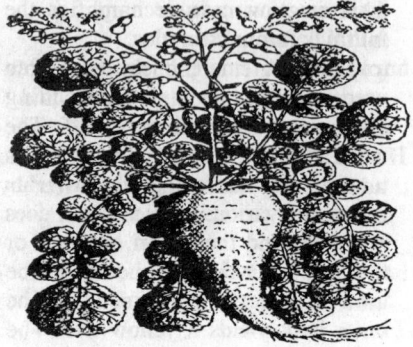

Country people frequently eat horseradish with bread for it is one of nature's natural accompaniments to bread. Wild horseradish is tougher and has a more pungent flavour than the garden variety which, freshly picked, is preferable. It is used as a condiment.

horse meat. The average composition per 100 g of the horse meat is: protein 15%; fat 3%; calcium 7 mg; iron 2 mg; vitamin A B$_1$ 0.07 mg; vitamin B$_2$ 0.06 mg; nicotinic acid 3.2 mg; and food energy 0.5 MJ.

horseradish. Family: *Cruciferae.* Genus: *Armoracia or Cochlearia. Species: Armoracia rusticana* or *Cochlearia armoracia.* A perennial plant native to south-eastern Europe and western Asia, and occasionally is found wild but usually is cultivated in other parts of the world. The long, white, cylindrical or tapering root produces 1 m high stem in the second year. The dried, powdered root found in many herb formulas today is practically worthless. The real benefits lay in the freshly dug root. When grated, however, the strong volatile oils are released, so it is necessary to cover the grated root with apple cider vinegar and refrigerate it in a glass jar with a tight-fitting lid. It will keep for at least 3 months this way or the entire root can be packed in damp sand and kept in a cool corner. The large fleshy roots are strongly aromatic, so much so that they can, like raw onions, make your eyes water as you prepare them. Unusually, for a herb, the large coarse leaves have no aroma and no known uses. A food processor is ideal for grating the peeled root. It can be stored in vinegar or oil in a screw-topped jar, mix it with cream, soured cream, yoghurt, mayonnaise, or cream cheese and dressings for sauces to serve with meat, fish, and potatoes. It is especially good with beef and smoked trout. Fresh horseradish contains a glycoside named sinigrin, which is decomposed in the presence of water by the enzyme myrosin, producing mustard oil. It is also extremely rich in vitamin C, and has antiseptic and antibiotic substances, as well as calcium, magnesium, phosphorus, potassium and traces of iron and zinc. It is a strong circulatory stimulant and has an excellent antiseptic action, notably on the lungs and urinary system, acting as a diuretic. It promotes healing, stimulates stomach secretions and is a powerful solvent of excess mucus, especially in the nasal and sinus cavities, and therefore wonderful for colds, coughs, persistent bronchial catarrh and bronchitis. Applied externally in a muslin poultice, it will stimulate the circulation over inflamed joints or tissues and, like cayenne pepper, is a vital ingredients in formulate which are designed to help poor circulation. It can also be applied as a poultice for pulmonary and urinary infections, urinary stones, and any condition where there is excessive fluid in the body. Horseradish may cause blisters on some skins (so test on a little patch first), and large internal doses may produce inflammation of the gastrointestinal mucosa. Like all members of the cabbage and mustard family, it tends to depress thyroid function, so it should to depress thyroid where the thyroid levels are sluggish.

horseradish drying. The roots of horseradish may be dried and used as a flavoring, seasoning, or condiment. After slicing the roots may be dried in a two-stage tunnel dryer, with inlet temperatures of 68°C and 57.2°C for the first and second stages, respectively, to about 8% moisture content. The product may then be dried in a bin dryer to 5%. Powder or granules are usually made from the dried slices.

horsetail grass. *Equisteum arvense.* A perennial plant which is common to moist loamy or sandy soil all over North America and Eurasia. It is a strange-looking sort of plant with creeping, string-like rootstock and roots at the nodes that produce numerous hollow stems, which are of two types. A fertile, flesh-coloured stem grows first, reaching a height of 15-20 cm and bearing on top a cone-like spike which contains spores; this stem quickly dies. A green, sterile stem grows up to 50 cm high and features whorls of small branches. In the dinosaur era, horsetails reached incredible heights of up to 12 metres or more and resembled skinny lodgepole pines, but lacking the green boughs. During the Middle Ages clumps of the plant were often used as scouring pads to clean iron cookware and pewter dishes due to a high silicon content. Also known as shave grass.

horticulture. The cultivation of vegetables, fruits and ornamental plants. It is divided into four classes: (a) fruit growing in orchards; (b) truck farming; (c) floriculture, or the raising of flowers and ornamental plants; and (d) landscape gardening.

Hortvet freezing test. Test for the adulteration of milk with water by measuring the depression of freezing point; normal range - 0.53 to 0.55°C.

hotbed. A small section of soil, usually enriched by fertilizer, and covered with a glass-topped frame to exclude cold air. It is generally employed to force the growth of plants in early spring, with the expectation of transplanting them in open ground after frosts have disappeared. The heat in a hotbed results from the rays of the sun through the glass and from fermentation. The usual fertilizer is manure, but other fertilizing agents may be employed. Sometimes hotbeds are used during the entire growth of vegetables or flowers,to force them to early maturity, to take advantage of high prices for such products marketed out of season.

hot sauce. A tomato sauce with hot flavour due to cayenne.

Hotis test. A test used for detecting mastitis in infected milk. The method consists in adding 0.5 ml of sterile 0.5% aqueous solution of bromocresol-purple to 9.5 ml of milk carefully collected directly from the animal. After the sample is mixed, it is incubated for 24 hours at 37.5° C and the results observed. The characteristic change in the colour of the sample after incubation, together with the occurrence of flakes or balls of growth, indicates the presence of *S.*

agalactiae.

Hovis. Trade name of a wheat germ-enriched loaf. The average composition per 100 g is: protein 9%, fat 2.2%, carbohydrate 48%; calcium 105 mg; iron 2.8 mg; vitamin B_1 0.3 mg; nicotinic acid 2.0 mg; and food energy about 1 MJ. Phytic acid phosphorus 38% of total P (which is 200 mg per 100 g of the bread) compared with white bread, in which phytic acid P is 15% of total P (which is 80 mg per 100 g bread.

Hubl-Wijs value. The amount of iodine or bromine, in grams, absorbed by 100 grams of unsaturated fatty acids. The value for butterfat is 26.0-38.0. It is also known as the bromine or iodine value.

hull. *See* husk.

humectants. Substances that have affinity for water, with stabilizing action on the water content of a material, are termed humectants or moisture-retaining agents. Ideally, a humectant maintains within a rather narrow range the moisture content caused by humidity fluctuations. These materials are widely used in certain food products and have taken on increasing importance in the case of relatively recent concepts in intermediate-moisture foods (IMF). Traditionally, humectants have been used in various food and notably in tobacco products for many years. Humectants are used to retain moisture in foods like coconut and marshmallows which otherwise would quickly become dry and tasteless. For example, flaked coconut is kept moist in the container by adding glycerine and glycerol monosterate. Among commonly used humectants are: glycerin, sodium chloride, molasses, sorbitol, potassium polymetaphosphate, sucrose, triacetin, propylene glycol. Phosphates are added to the pickling solutions used to treat cured meats, such as ham, bacon, and corned beef, by soaking or injection. Their principal purpose is for moisture binding to reduce the loss of fluids during curing and cooking. In addition, they also convey several other benefits in clouding color and flavor retention, tenderness, juiciness, and prevention of rancidity. Sodium tripolyphosphate (STPP) is widely used for this application, occasionally mixed with relatively small amounts of sodium hexametaphosphate (SHMP). Fresh meat which is to be frozen can be treated with phosphate by dipping or soaking to retain moisture, preserve flavor, and prevent freezer burn and after-thaw drip. Many products are made by chopping or dicing meat and reforming it into loaves, rolls or other fabricated shapes. Adding phosphate, in addition to providing moisture retention, solubilizers a portion of the protein, which then comes to the surface of the meat and thickens during cooking to bind the individual portions of meat together. Poultry and seafoods can be treated similarly to the red meats. Seafood readily loses large amounts of its fluid content. Molasses is an excellent humectant for a number of food products, particularly if the molasses flavour is compatible with the product.

humulone. One of the two resins found in hops, the other being lupulone. Humulone is a mixture of humulone, cohumulone and adhumulone. The resins are responsible for the bitter flavour of the hops used in brewing.

husk. In reference to cereal grain this is the outer woody cellulose covering. In wheat it loosely attached and removed during threshing; in rice it is firmly attached. High in fibre content and of limited use as animal feed. Also known as hull.

hyaluronic acid. The mucopolysaccharide, which, in animal tissues, binds water in the interstitial spaces, and holds the cells together and acts as a shock-absorber in the joints; also present in the vitreous humour of the eye. Its viscosity is reduced by the enzyme hyaluronidase by which it is depolymerized.

hyaluronidase. Group of carbohydrase enzymes that depolymerize mucopolysaccharides such as hyaluronic acid. They are found in bee-sting, bacteria, testes, leeches. Also known as spreading factor because the enzyme breaks down the hyaluronic acid under the skin and permits the spread of substance there. For this reason it is used clinically to aid the absorption of drugs administered subcutaneously or intramuscularly, and to permit the subcutaneous injections of relatively large volumes of solution as, for example, in glucose feeding by this route.

hybrid corn. A variety of corn. Since the early 1900s, when the development of hybrid corn (maize) was first seriously undertaken on a commercial scale, a long list of achievements of plant geneticists and plant breeders has been recorded. The hybrid varieties are planted throughout the world; today have replaced the older traditional varieties. These were open-pollinated varieties. Many of the hybrids used today are derived from these earlier varieties that were considered reasonably satisfactory in their own time. Inbred lines, developed by self-pollinating maize (corn and selecting desirable plants for further inbreeding, are the parents of hybrids. An official definition of hybrid corn is that it must be a first-generation cross of inbreeds or crosses of the inbreeds, or, in another definition; the first generation of a cross that involves 2 or more inbred lines. An inbred variety of corn (maize) is a variety developed from inbreeding, generally from inbreeding a minimum of seven generations. Inbreeding is done by putting a plastic bag over the shoots before the emergence of any silks and a sack over the tassel of the same plant for the collection of the pollen. This is followed by placing the pollen from the tassel on the silks of the ear produced by the same stalk so that the original kernel planted becomes both the male and female parent of the kernels produced on that ear. If the next year's kernels from this ear are planted and the same process repeated-and if this is done each year for 7 years-an inbred variety is then produced which will retain its purity, even though the pollen from one plant may have fertilized another plant of the same inbred variety.

hydrocolloid. A hydrophilic colloidal material used largely in food products as emulsifying, thickening and gelling agents. They readily absorb water, thus increasing viscosity and imparting smoothness and improved body texture to the product, even in concentrations of less than 1%.

hydrocooling. Vegetables are washed in cold water then, while still wet, subjected to vacuum. The evaporation of the water chills the vegetables for transport. The term is also applied to vegetables washed in ice water without the vacuum treatment.

hydrogen peroxide. H_2O_2. Anti-microbial agent; can be used at 0.1% concentration to preserve milk (Buddeized milk), but destroys vitamin C, methionine and tryptophan. Its use is not permitted in many developed countries. It readily loses active oxygen, the effective sterilising agent, and so forms water.

hydrogenated oils. Liquid oils can hardened by hydrogenation. Treatment with hydrogen in the presence of a nickel catalyst cause saturation of the double bonds of the fatty acid chain and a rise in melting point. Cottonseed, maize, sunflower, and whale oils are commonly hardened and used in margarine and cooking fats.

hydrolases. A class of enzymes that control hydrolysis; *e.g.*, esterases, phosphatases, glycosidases, and peptidases. Hydrolases play an important part in rendering insoluble food material into a soluble form, which can then be transported in solution. Also, these enzymes catalyze the transfer of water molecules between receptor and donor molecules. Proteolytic enzymes (proteases) are a class of hydrolases. The plant cell walls has associated with a significant number of hydrolases including invertase, phosphatases, nucleases, and peroxidases.

hydrophilic. 1. With the literal meaning of 'water-loving', this term refers to substances that tend to absorb and retain water; this results in swelling. Often accompanied by formation of gels. Hydrophilic agents are widely used as stabilizers and thickeners in food products, pharmaceuticals, and coatings for textiles, paper, etc. The term should not be confused with hydroscopic.

2. The term is also used for surfaces of solids which are readily wetted by water or on which water is adsorbed easily.

hydrophobic. Literally meaning 'water-hating,' this term describes substances which repel water and thus are difficult to 'wet' or emulsify. Most notable of these are fats, waxes, and oils, but this property is also found in many solids in finely divided form. In liquids, this property is often due to differences in surface tension.

hydrostatic sterilizer. A continuous sterilizer used for the large-scale (8,000/minute) production of canned foods. The principle is that the pressure is developed beneath an adequate depth of water.

hygroscopic. Readily absorbing water, as when table salt becomes damp. Materials like calcium chloride and silica gel absorb water so readily that they are used as drying agents.

hypercalcaemia. An abnormally high concentration of calcium in the blood. This rarely occurs because blood calcium is normally strictly regulated by two hormones (parathyroid hormone and calcitonin) and any tendency to hypercalcaemia is soon corrected.

hypercalcinuria. An excessively high calcium concentration in the urine, usually occurring as a result of hypercalcaemia.

hyperchloraemia. An abnormally high concentration of cholesterol in the blood. In humans it is associated with atherosclerosis and cardiovascular disease, whereas in animals its significance is an an indicator of liver and thyroid disorders.

hypoglycin. A derivative of propionic acid, that is metabolically converted into a substance which, in the form of its CoA ester, is a powerful and specific inhibitor of the oxidation of short-chain acyl-CoAs, particularly of butyroyl-CoA. As a consequence butyroyl-CoA undergoes hydrolysis to yield free butyrate, which accumulates in the blood in abnormal amounts and indirectly causes lowering of blood sugar level.

hypothermia. Literally low temperature; used in connection with reduction of the body temperature (down to 28°C) to permit surgery of the heart or brain.

hypotonic. Designating a solution with an osmotic pressure less than that of a specified other solution, the latter being hypertonic. Water will move across a semipermeable membrane by osmosis into another solution of higher solute concentration. Cells expand in a hypotonic solution.

hypoxanthine. One of the rarer bases found in nucleic acids. It is deamination product of adenine and is normally recognized as such by DNA repair enzymes and removed from the DNA sequence. Also known as 6-hydroxypurine.

hyssop. Family: *Labiatae*. Genus: *Hyssopus*. Species: *Hyssopus officinalis*. A plant of the mint family, the common species being a perennial, shrubby plant, rising to the height of about 60-70 cm. It is a native of Siberia and the mountainous parts of Austria, but it is common in other parts of the world. It flowers from June to September, having tiny blue blossoms which cluster on spikes. The leaves have an agreeable aromatic odour, and are slightly bitter. Hyssop was once valued for its reputed medicinal qualities. The hyssop of Scripture, the symbol of spiritual purification from sin, is believed by most authorities to be the caper. It has a slightly bitter flavour with overtones of mint, and was so widely known in ancient times. The fresh or dried leaves and flowers may be added to soups, ragouts, casseroles, and sausages. Fresh leaves may be used sparingly in salads. The herb is an ingredient of Chartreuse liqueur. Hyssop contains about 0.2-1% volatile oil (a flavonoid glycoside, diosmin) and 8% tannin. The leaves account for the aromatic fragrance of the plant because they contain most of the volatile oils. Medicinally, the use of hyssop is recommended for coughs, colds, bronchitis, and as a gargle for sore throats. Fresh and dried leaves were used as a strewing herb, and may be used in pot pourri, in insect-repellent sachets. Hyssop acts as a peripheral vasodilator and diaphoretic. It is also relaxing, an expectorant and a carminative. It is a tonic, stomachic astringent and mild spasmolytic. It is specifically employed in bronchitis and the common cold to improve appetite and stimulate gastric secretions, and as a gargle to soothe sore throats. It actively reduces perspiration and may be applied externally to cuts or bruises round the eye in poultice form. It is particularly effective for coughs, colds and respiratory infections in children, especially those of a nervous or tense disposition. It has a bitter, rather minty flavour with a musky odour. It has been used for treating the common cold, and is most effective when mixed with elderflower, peppermint and yarrow.

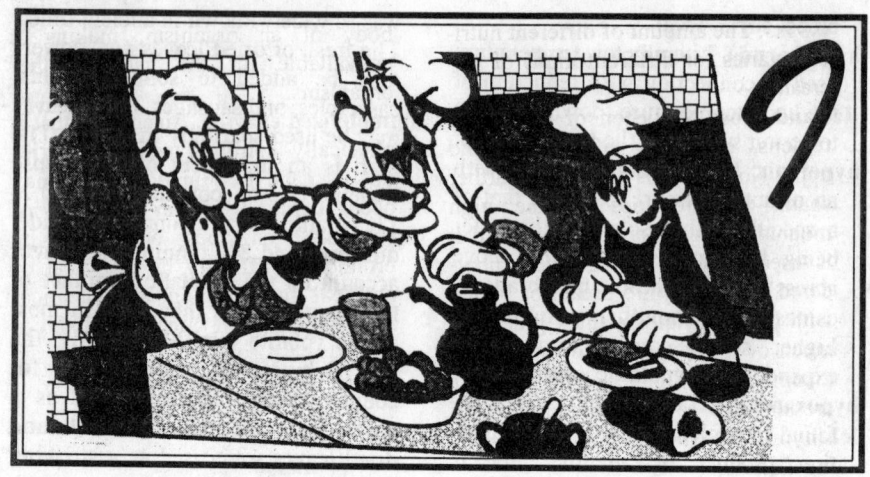

ibotenic acid. A substance obtained from the mushrooms *Amanita pantherina* and *A. muscaria*. It has insecticidal action, and it potentiates barbiturates in mammals. In rats it produces lesions of the nucleus basalis magnocellularis which is thought to be the rodent equivalent of the nucleus of Meynert in man. The nucleus of Meynert is one of the main sources of cholinergic input to the cerebral cortex, and it is severely degenerated in the Alzheimer's disease. Ibotenic acid has therefore been used in attempts to produce an animal model of Alzheimer's disease.

ice cream mix, dry. Ice cream mix consists of the ingredients which make up the ice cream before it is frozen and before air is incorporated. The mix consists of milk fat, milk solids not fat, egg yolk, sugar, stabilizer, flavors, fruits, nuts, and water. Ice cream and ice cream mix contain from 35-40% total solids, with the remaining 60-65% water. The water can be removed from ice cream mix by drying to less than 3% in a spray dryer. The dry mix is reconsti-tuted by adding 1.65 parts of water to 1 part of mix, following which it can be frozen.

ice-cream. A frozen confection of fat, milk and sugar. In the UK, ice-cream legally must contain not less than 5% fat and 7% milk solids-not-fat. "Non-drip" ice-cream contains 0.06-0.75% added mixed triglycerides (mono and di-) which holds together the looser globules of water and gives a "drier" non drip product.

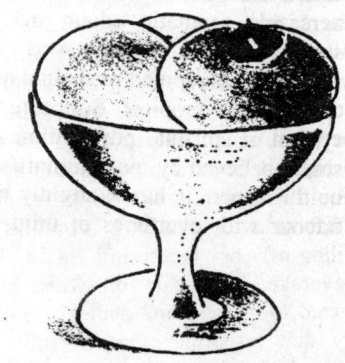

The typical composition is: water 62%; protein 4%; fat 11%; sugar 20%; calcium 137 mg; and food energy

0.85kJ. The amount of different nutrients varies for different kinds of ice-creams.

Iceland moss. A lichen of the Arctic regions, especially of Iceland and upper Norway. It is also found farther south, on the tops of the high mountains. In Iceland and Lapland it is used as food, being dried, powdered and made into bread, or boiled with milk. It yields a thick glue, and much of it is exported for use in the manufacture of paper-sizing and for dressing the wrap in weaving.

ichthyosarcotoxin. Poisoning from eating fish.

ichthyotocin. A peptide hormone of nine amino acids that is secreted by the posterior lobe of the pituitary gland and that is related to oxytocin in its structure and in its function.

ileum. Last portion of the small intestine, after the jejunum and before the small intestine joins the large intestine or colon.

ilha cheese. A cows' milk cheese made in the Azores Islands and imported to a great extent into Portugal. It is moderately firm, 25-30 cm in diameter, and about 10 cm thick.

imitation half-and-half. The coffee whiteners prepared from vegetable oils blended with a sweetener and a protein substance, such as casein or soy protein. Proteins are held to between 1 and 6% to avoid flavour problems. Important to the quality of liquid whiteners are: stability (remain uniform after standing; absence of oiling-off or feathering in a hot beverage; nonseparation when subjected to freeze-thaw cycles); viscosity that resembles that of milk or cream; a uniform whitening ability; and a bland, odor-free flavour.

immobilization. The incorporation of a simple, soluble substance into the body of an organism, making it unavailable for the use of other organisms.

immobilized enzyme. An enzyme that is physically confined while it carries out its catalytic function. This may occur naturally, as in the case of particulate enzymes, or it may be produced artificially by chemical or physical methods. In the chemical methods, the enzyme is linked covalently to a support. These methods include attachment of the enzyme to a water-insoluble support, incorporation of the enzyme into a growing polymer chain, or cross-linking of the enzyme with a multifunctional low-molecular mass reagent. In the physical methods, the enzyme is not linked covalently to a support. These methods include adsorption of the enzyme to a water-insoluble matrix, entrapment of the enzyme within either a water-insoluble gel or a microcapsule, or containment of the enzyme within special devices equipped with the semipermeable membranes.

immune response. The response of the body to contact with an antigen that leads to the formation of antibodies and sensitized lymphocytes. The response is designed to render harmless the antigen and the pathogen producing it. The various features of the immune response are:

(a) Many but not all foreign macromolecules elicit the immunological response; those that do not, are called immunogens.

(b) In virtually every case, an immune response directed against a foreign macromolecule occurs only if the animal is challenged with the foreign substance.

(c) There is a high specificity in the immune response; antibodies or activated T cells made against one antigen generally do not react against other antigens.

(d) Not all immune reactions are beneficial, some such as those involved in hypersensitivities and autoimmune reactions, are harmful.

(e) Antibodies are formed against a variety of foreign macromolecules, but ordinarily not against macromolecules of the animal's own tissues; thus the animal is able to distinguish between its own and foreign macromolecules.

(f) Microorganisms and viruses that invade the host contain large number of different macromolecules that can act as antigens. Thus immunological response can be made the basis of specific immunization procedures for the prevention and control of specific diseases.

immunity. The state of relative insusceptibility of an animal to infection by disease-producing organisms or to the harmful effects of their poisons (toxins). Immunity depends on the presence in the blood of antibodies and white blood cells (lymphocytes), which produce an immune response. Inherited (natural) immunity is that with which an individual is born. The acquired immunity is of two types: active immunity, which arises when the body produces antibodies against an invading foreign substance (antigen), either through infection or immunization of serum taken from an individual already immune to a particular antigen. Active immunity tends to be long-lasting, while passive immunity is considered to be short-lived. Immunity based on antibodies is called humoral immunity and immunity based on activated T cells is called cellular immunity.

immunogens. The substances that, when administered to an animal in appropriate manner, induce an immune response. The immune response may involve either antibody production, the activation of specific immunologically competent cells, or both. An enormous variety of macromolecules can act as immunogens under appropriate conditions. These include virtually all proteins and lipoproteins, many polysaccharides, some nucleic acids, and certain teichoic acids. Although the specificity of the immune response is comparable to the specificity of the enzyme and substrate, antibodies or activated T cells can sometimes react with the heterologous antigens.

immunostimulants. Substances that increase the intensity of the immune response. So-called adjuvants, which are administered together with the antigen, come into this category. Adjuvants include pertussis vaccine (often used to enhance the antigenic activity of diphtheria vaccine), nucleic acids and Freund's complete adjuvant.

immunosuppressants. Agents that suppress the immune response. These include cytotoxic drug (such as cyclophosphamide, metotrexate, azothioprine, cytaribine and actinomycin D) which inhibit proliferation of lymphocytes, anti-inflammatory steroids which act at recognition phase of immune response as well as on the proliferative stage, and cyclosporin A.

immunotoxins. Hybrid molecules containing an antibody component of defined fine speciality coupled to a cytotoxic moiety. The cytotoxic moiety is usually an anti-cancer agent (such as α-amanitin, methotrexate, the A chains of ricin or abrin $^{125}I^{-}$ or ^{131}I). The antibody component might be a monoclonal antibody.

IMP. Integrating major pneumotachograph. Apparatus for measuring energy expenditure indirectly from oxygen consumption. It meters the expired air and removes a proportion for analysis.

in vitro. An experiment (usually of a biochemical nature) that is carried out in laboratory equipment rather than on living organisms. The opposite meaning is given by the expression *in vivo.*

in vivo. An event or process occurring naturally or spontaneously within a living organism.

inanition. The process of exhaustion and wasting due to complete lack of or non-assimilation of food; a state of starvation.

incanestrato, (basketed) cheese. A pasta filata cheese made in Sicily, to which various spices are added. A kind known as "Majocchino" is made in the region of Messina of cows', goats', or sheep's milk, and contains olive oil. It is first pressed by hand and allowed to ferment for 2-3 days, when it is cooked in whey, then pressed, salted and spiced. The curd is pressed in wicker baskets, the imprint of which remains on the cheese.

Incaparina. A protein-rich dietary supplement. One of the versions consists of about 38% cottonseed flour, 29% ground corn, 39% sorghum, 3% Torula yeast, 1 % calcium carbonate and 1350 µg vitamin A per 100 g. Incaparina 9A includes about 58% maize and 38% cottonseed flour; in formula 14 the cottonseed is replaced by soya. All versions contain 27.5% protein.

Indian hemp. *Cannabis indica;* active principle unknown, stimulates and deranges the mental processes. Also known as hashish.

Indian mandarin. A variety of mandarin that is closely related to the Ponkan. It is orange in colour and is of fair quality; it ripens in early mid-season, and tends to puff excessively.

Indian pipe. *Monotropa uniflora.* Family: *Monotropaceae.* A flowering plant which grow up to 15 cm. The flowers are 1-2 cm long. The stamens are brownish-yellow. At first the flower nods on its stem. After fertilization a capsule, containing hundreds of tiny seeds, forms and becomes erect. The Indian once used these plants for a medicinal tea. They are widespread in Canada and the US, but quite rare, growing only where conditions are suitable.

Indian rice grass. Perennial, growing wild in USA, *Oryzopsis hymenoides;* tolerant to drought. Seeds resemble millet, small, round, dark in colour, covered with white hairs; used for flour; now used almost exclusively for forage.

Indican. Indoxyl potassium sulphate.

indicator. Usually refers to a pH indicator. Various dyes such as litmus, methyl orange, phenolphthalein, change colour at a specific degree of acidity or alkalinity and this colour change is used as an indicator of pH.

indigo carmine. Blue food colour, disodium salt of indigotin-5:5'-disulphonic acid. Indigotine is the colouring principle of natural indigo obtained from the Indigo fern. Permitted food colour in most countries but its use is limited by its low stability and solubility.

indigotine. FD&C blue no. 2. Indigotine or indigo carmine is a bright blue powder which is only moderately soluble in water (1.6 % at 25°C), a little less so in glycerol; (1 % 1 at 25°C) and very poorly soluble in either the glycols or ethanol (95 %). It has poor stability and fades in acidic medium. It is fully acceptable for use in foods.

indirect heater. A heat exchanger used for heating a fluid, which for drying is usually air, in which the products of combustion and air heat a wall through which heat is transferred to heat air on the opposite side, without mixing with the air being heated. Steam heated and hot water heat exchanges for dryers are indirect heaters.

indirect-fired dryer. A type of dryer in which the products of combustion do not come in contact with the product being dried. Sometimes called an indirect dryer. Heat exchangers are often used in which a wall separates the products of combustion and drying air.

indoxyl. A substance found in the urine which is a metabolic derivative of the amino acid tryptophan. It is excreted as indoxyl potassium sulphate, known as indican, and is thus one of the means whereby sulphur is excreted from the body.

induction heating. A method of heating in which a material which conducts electricity is heated by electric current induced in the material by an alternating magnetic field. Electric heating is accomplished with an electric alternating current of high value and voltage of low magnitude. The frequency of the induction coil varies over a large range depending on the method of obtaining the effect. Uniform heating is obtained in the normal frequency range: standard, 480, 960, 3000, and 9600 cycles/s; with a spark gap, 20,000-40,000 cycles/s; and electronic, 450,000 cycles/s. High frequency induction gives surface heating at about 100,000-500,000 cycles/s. Induction occurs as a result of current flow induced.

induction period. A term frequently used in connection with fats. It is the lag period during which the fat shows stability to oxidation because of its content of antioxidants, natural or added, which are preferentially oxidized. After this induction period there is a sudden and large consumption of oxygen and the fat becomes rancid.

infection. The invasion of a host by a microorganism with subsequent establishment and multiplication of the agent. An infection may or may not lead to overt disease.

infection thread. A tubular structure formed during the infection of a root by nitrogen-fixing bacteria. The bacteria enter the root by way of the infection thread and stimulate the formation of root nodule.

infectious disease. Any change from a state of health in which part or all of the host's body cannot carry on its normal functions because of the presence of an infectious agent or its products.

infectious disease cycle. The chain or cycle of events that describes how an infectious agent grows, reproduces, and is disseminated. The development of an infectious disease is associated with a cycle of events concerned with the:
(a) characteristics of the microbial agent;
(b) source or the reservoir of the microbial agent;
(c) transmission of microbial agent;
(d) susceptibility of host; and
(e) mechanisms of exit of the infectious agent from the body and its dissemination to a new host.

infrared dryer. A device for removing moisture from products in which the energy for moisture removal is supplied primarily from an infrared energy source. The design must carefully consider the surface area to be radiated, method of exposing the surface area, and removal of moist air. The infrared energy does not penetrate the solid product, can rapidly heat and possibly scorch the product, and can be more rapidly absorbed by the air between the product and heat source if the air is nearly saturated with water.

inherent moisture. The chemically combined and absorbed moisture of a product, such as in coal, as separate from the surface or free moisture. In bituminous coal the inherent moisture is 10-30% and lignites, 30-45%.

inhibition, competitive. With reference to enzymes means inhibition by a substance chemically similar to the substrate, which competes with the true substrate for the active surface of the enzyme. Thus malonic acid competitively inhibits succinic dehydrogenase, of which the true substrate is the chemically similar succinic acid. The inhibition is reversed with a sufficiently high concentration of the true substrate. Sulphanilamides act as bacteriostats because they compete for a vitamin essential to the bacteria, namely, p-aminobenzoic acid.

inosite. Obsolete name for inositol.

inositol triphosphate. A hydrolysis product of the phosphatidylinositol-4,5-diphosphate that is released into the cytosol in response to the action of certain agonists. In the cytosol if function as a second messenger for mobilizing intracellular Ca^{2+} ions.

inositol. Essential nutrient for microorganisms and many animals and so classed as a vitamin, although there is no evidence of its essentially for man. Its deficiency causes alopecia in mice and "spectacle eye" (denudation around the eye) in rats. Chemically hexahydrocyclohexane $(CHOH)_6$; there are nine stereoisomers of this compound but only one, meso-or myo-inositol, is of major interest. It occurs widely in plant and animal tissues as an essential part of the structure and in combination in phosphatides. Its hexaphosphoric acid ester is phytic acid. The insecticide gammexane is hexachlorocyclohexane, and appears to function by competing with inositol. The obsolete names are inosite and meat sugar.

in-package desiccation. Nearly dry products with less than 5% moisture can be dried further with drying agents (desiccants) placed in the package or container with the product. Desiccants are used which have a substantial moisture absorption ability at low relative humidities (below the relative humidity in equilibrium with a moisture content below 5%). Desiccants with absorption ability at low relative humidities (below the relative humidity in equilibrium with a moisture content below 5%). Desiccants with absorption/adsorption characteristics similar to calcium oxide are used. The desiccants is placed in a container (usually a small package) which will prevent the desiccant from contaminating the product and which will permit water vapor to pass into the desiccant. The rate of desiccation is related to:

(a) adsorption property of desiccant,
(b) size of package of adsorbant,
(c) size of particle and porosity of product,
(d) size and shape of product container, and
(e) location of desiccant in product package.

An inert gas, such as nitrogen, may also be a part of the in-package environment.

instant. A term used with reference to dried foods that reconstitute rapidly when added to water, *e.g.*, instant milk, tea, coffee, soups. Instant tea and coffee are simply the dried forms of the liquid preparations. Instant milk is the dried form that has been further treated, "instantized", so that it reconstitutes more rapidly than ordinary dried milk. The treatment consists of moistening the dried product and redrying. Instant coffee was first prepared in 1906 by Mr. G. Washington, an Englishman living in Guatemala.

insulin. A hormone which controls the carbohydrate metabolism; secreted by the pancreas gland. Diabetes mellitus is due to under-production or over destruction of insulin. The hormone is a protein and is digested if given by mouth so must be administered by injection. It cannot be synthesized and is prepared from animal pancreas. There are four types used clinically; standard (quick-acting), protamin-zinc-insulin (12-14 hours), globin insulin 8-10 hours), and modified protamin insulin (28-30 hours). Insulin was the first protein whose amino-acid sequence was fully determined. It is a polypeptide produced by the β-cells of the islets of Langerhans of the pancreas. Its secretion is stimulated by high blood levels of glucose and amino acids after a meal. Glucose uptake is then stimulated by the action of insulin on various tissues (*e.g.*; muscles, liver, and fat). It also stimulates glycogen and fat synthesis. Insulin is used therapeutically in the treatment of diabetes mellitus. Underproduction of insulin results in the accumulation of large amounts of glucose in the blood and its subsequent excretion in the urine. This condition, known as diabetes mellitus, can be treated successfully by insulin injections. Insulin decreased blood glucose level by increasing glucose utilization and decreasing glucose formation. Glucose utilization is increased in the following ways:

(a) In the presence of insulin, tissues start getting energy from glucose instead of fatty acids and ketone bodies. Even the formation of these fuel molecules (fatty acids and ketone bodies) is reduced. This is , partly, because lipolysis in the adipose tissue is, inversely, related to glucose utilization in this tissue. There are plasma membrane receptors for insulin in tissues. Insulin binds to these receptors to produce its effects. It increases glucose transport into the insulin sensitive cells except in the liver cells which are permeable to glucose without insulin. Activities of glycolytic enzymes, glucokinase, phosphofructokinase and pyruvic kinase are increased by insulin. Pyruvate dehydrogenase appears to be activated.

(b) Insulin promotes glycogenesis both in the liver and muscle. It activates synthase by activating phosphatase which dephosphorylates synthase.

integral proteins. A class of proteins which are tightly bound to a lipid bilayer and may include a large number of functional proteins that participate as transport carriers, drug and hormone receptor sites, antigens and a large number of membrane-bound enzymes. For example, cytochrome b_5 is classified as integral protein of the endoplasmic reticulum of eucaryotic cells as in the NAD-cytochrome b_5-reductase, which is tightly coupled to the hemeprotein, and cytochrome oxidase which is embedded in the inner membrane of the mitochondrion.

intercropping. The growing of two kinds of crops on the same plot of land at the same time. This is often desirable in an area where available land for cultivation is limited. In order to achieve success in this practice, the soil must be in a very fertile condition because the resulting planting density imposes a severe drain upon the food reserves of the soil. Often, above-average quantities of fertilizers and organic materials are required to maintain a satisfactory rate of growth of both crops. The most suitable combinations of plants for intercrop planting are those which have a definite difference in their rates of growth. Thus, crop that takes several months to mature may be interplanted with advantage with a crop that matures in half of that time. The harvesting of this rapidly growing crop will allow the more slowly maturing plants to develop fully, taking advantage of both the increased area available and the food reserve residues in the soil.

Interdonato lemon. A variety of lemon having fairly large fruit somewhat similar to the *Femminello Ovale*, but less susceptible to *mal secco* disease. The variety is reasonably juicy and early maturing.

interesterification. Fats are mixtures of triglycerides with various fatty acids esterified to the glycerol. By dry heat at 45-95°C there is an exchange of the fatty acids between the glycerol molecules - interesterification - with a consequent change in physical properties of the fat; *e.g.*, lard is not a good creaming fat until it has been so treated.

intermediate hydrogen carrier. The oxidation of many substances in the living cell involves their loss of hydrogen. Hydrogen is passed on to an intermediate hydrogen acceptor, under the influence of an enzyme, and thence along a chain of acceptors to the ultimate hydrogen acceptor, which is oxygen (thus forming water). For example, lactic acid is dehydrogenated (oxidized) to pyruvic acid, under the influence of a specific enzyme, and the hydrogen is passed on to Coenzyme I (an intermediate hydrogen carrier) thence to cytochrome (another intermediate hydrogen carrier) and finally to oxygen.

intermittent drying. Moisture removal by periodic operation of the fan and/ or application of heat, so that the greater concentration of moisture in the center of the product may diffuse toward the surface during "resting" periods. If the total time for drying is not critical from the standpoint of product quality, the energy for drying by fan and heater operation can be reduced by intermittent operation.

international units. Used as a measure of the comparative potency of natural substances, such as vitamins, before they are obtained in sufficiently pure form to measure by weight. An international unit is arbitrarily defined in terms of a reproducible standard, *e.g.*, 1 I.U. of vitamin A was originally 1 microgram of the purest then known preparation of carotene, later 0.6 microgram of β-carotene.

intestinal juice. The digestive juice produced by intestinal glands lining the small intestine. It contains the enzymes "erepsin" (aminopeptidase and dipeptidase), amylase, maltase, lactase, sucrase, lipase, esterase, nucleases, nucleotidase, and the activator enterokinase (activates trypsinogen and chymotrypsinogen of the pancreatic juice to trypsin and chymotrypsin). Also known as succus entericus.

intestine, small. That part lying between the stomach and the large intestine, comprising duodenum, jejunum and ileum. The site of the greater part of digestion of food and absorption of the products. Only water is absorbed in the large intestine.

intrinsic factor. Vitamin B_{12} from the diet (formerly known as the extrinsic factor) appears to require an unidentified substance from the gastric mucosa (known as intrinsic factor) either to aid its absorption or to form a complex called the haemopoietic factor. This complex or the B_{12}, is stored in the liver and is essential for the synthesis of the nucleoproteins of the red blood cells. In pernicious anaemia there appears to be a deficiency of the intrinsic factor and the vitamin B_{12} is not absorbed. Treatment is by administering B_{12} intravenously, or orally in conjunction with dried hot mucosa (which contains intrinsic factor) or by injecting the complete haemopoietic factor as liver extract.

inulin. A plant polysaccharide, composed of fructose. It serves as a food reserve of many higher plants; especially in the *compositae*. This starch, unlike potato, is easily soluble in warm water and has been used in physiologic investigations such as a test of renal function.

invariant amino acid site. Amino acid residue, within the primary structure of proteins belonging to a family with similar or identical biological function, which is preserved in the proteins from different organisms.

inversion. Applied to sucrose, means its hydrolysis to glucose and fructose.

invertase. Enzyme that splits sucrose into the invert sugars, glucose and fructose. Also known as sucrase or saccharase. Saccharases are widely distributed in plant tissues and the digestive juice of animals and are of two types, glucosaccharases (in animals and the mould, Aspergillus) and fructosaccharases (in yeast). They respectively attack the glucose and the fructose and of complex sugars. As sucrose is glucose-fructoside, it is attacked by any of the saccharases.

invisible shrinkage. That loss or reduction in weight which occurs in excess of the water removed, which varies from 0.1-1.0% of the weight. Most of the commercial concerns use values from 0.1-0.8% loss to represent invisible shrinkage. Also called invisible loss. These losses occur as a result of respiration, handling, product particles, dust, etc.

iodine. A trace element required at the level of 150 micrograms per day. It is part of the hormone thyroxine produced by the thyroid gland, and a prolonged shortage of iodide in the diet leads to goiter. It is plentifully supplied by sea foods and by vegetables grown in soil containing iodide. In certain areas where the soil water is deficient in iodide, goiter occurs in defined geographical regions. Iodine is not essential to plant growth but is present in plants in amounts varying with the level in the soil.

iodine number. *See* iodine value.

iodine value. A measure of the degree of unsaturation of a fat by the extent of the uptake of iodine (grams iodine per 100 g of fat) by the unsaturated double bonds in the fatty acid chain. Some of thee examples of iodine values are: butter 22-38, lard 54-70, coconut oil 8-10, cottonseed 104-114, linseed 170-202. Drying oils are highly unsaturated and have high iodine numbers, as linseed oil. Also known as iodine number.

iodized salt. The common salt containing added potassium (or sodium) iodide. It also contains a small amount of magnesium carbonate to improve the free-running qualities; i.e., 15-30 parts of iodide per million of salt.

ion-exchange resins. Various resins, such as Permutit, Zeocarb, Amberlite, Dowex, will adsorb ions under one set of conditions and release them under other conditions. The best-known example is in water-softening, where the calcium ions are removed from the hard water by the resin, and liberated from the resin by the addition of salt (regeneration). The ion-exchange resins are used for purification of chemicals, metal recovery and analysis.

ipecac. A medicinal substance of a nauseous odour and a repulsive, bitterish taste. it is the dried root of several kinds of plants growing in South America, which bear the name ipecacuanha. The active principle of ipecac is called emetine. The medicinal preparation is a white odourless powder, which in small doses causes violent vomiting. It has been found useful in treating bronchitis and other diseases where an expectorant is needed, and an in treating disorders in which it is desired to stimulate the activity of the skin, as in small and repeated doses ipecac stimulates the secreting organs of the skin.

Iris family: *Iridaceae.* The 3 sepals of flowers in this family are coloured and petal-like and may differ in size, shape, and color from the 3 petals. The bisexual flower has 3 stamens and a single pistil with an inferior ovary of 3 fused carpels. The leaves sheath at the base, overlapping each other transverse, in an equitant manner, unique to this family. Plants are perennial herbs with underground storage organs or rhizomes, bulbs, or corms. The fruit type is a loculicidal capsule.

The family include: *Belamcanda* (blackberry lily), *Crocus, Freesia, Gladiolus, Iris, Ixia, Sisyrinchium; Crocus sativus* (saffron: style-stigma).

Irish moss. Name given to several species of seaweed which grow off the rocky coasts of most parts of Europe and in some North American waters. The weeds are used medicinally and as food. The principal commercial species is from two to twelve inches long, is flexible, reddish brown in color and has numerous forked brances. Preparing it for market consists in washing, bleaching in the sun and drying. Nutritious soups and jellies are made friom it. Carrageen is one of its local names.

iron. An essential nutrient for animal and plant growth. It is contained in the protein haemoglobin, which gives the colour to red blood cells and is responsible for oxygen transport from the lungs. Iron deficiency leads to anemia. Iron is also fou.id in other porphyrins and in cytochromes, which are important components of the electron-transport chain. It is also required as a cofactor for certain enzymes, e.g., catalase and peroxidase. Certain iron-containing proteins are essential for the fixation of nitrogen by bacteria. The average adult has 4-5 grams of iron of which 60-70% is present as haem in the circulating haemoglobin, and the remainder present in various enzymes (e.g., catalase, cytochrome oxidase), in muscle myoglobin or stored. About 15% of the iron is stored in the liver as ferritin, in other tissue as haemosiderin, and as the blood transport complex called transferrin (average blood level 50-180 micrograms of iron per 100 ml plasma). The losses of iron: in faeces 0.3-0.5 mg per day, in sweat as skin cells 0.5, traces in hair and urine, total loss 0.5-1.5 mg per day; diet contains 10-15 mg of which 0.5-1.5 mg is absorbed.

The recommended intake of iron is 12 mg for adults, 15 mg during pregnancy and lactation and for adolescents, 7.5-10.5 mg for children rising to 13.5 mg in 11-14 year old group. Absorption of iron is aided by vitamin C and reduced by phosphate and phytic acid.

The average content of some foodstuffs is: liver, 6-15 mg per 100 g, cereal, up to 10 mg, nuts 1-6 mg, eggs 2-3 mg, meat 2-3. Iron is added to flour so that it contains not less than 1.65 mg per 100 g of iron. Fortified cereals provide 35% of the iron the diets of many European countries. The prolonged deficiency of iron gives rise to nutritional anaemia.

iron caseinate. Preparation of iron and casein; also known as iron nucleoalbuminate.

iron chink. Machine used to behead and eviscerate salmon before canning (in the early days the work was done by Chinese labour).

iron oxides. Iron oxides occur naturally, but are mostly manufactured by either treatment of a solution of ferrous sulphate or chloride with an alkali followed by oxidation of the precipitated hydroxide in a current of air at 30°C for 12-16 hours, or by wet oxidation of ferrous sulphate liquor in the presence of iron and soda ash followed by calcination. The FAO/WHO (1963) defines six grades, namely:

(a) CI Pigment Yellow 42 and 43 - Ferrite yellow, Goethite or Mars yellow;

(b) CI Pigment Brown 6 and 7 - brown iron oxides and brown magnetic oxide;

(c) CI Pigment Black 11 - iron oxide black, magnetic iron oxide;

(d) Iron oxide, Brown native Red hematite;

(e) Red iron oxide - Rubigo, Indian red or iron sequioxide; and

(f) iron oxide, brown precipitated. Of the above, CI Pigment 11 (CI 77499) is the most widely used for colouring chocolate, cake mixes, meat paste, etc.

iron vitellinate. Preparation of egg yolk and iron.

iron, reduced. Metallic iron in finely divided from produced by reduction of iron oxide. The form in which iron is sometimes added to foods, such as bread. Latin name *ferrum redactum.*

iron-sulphur proteins. Proteins that contain iron-sulphur clusters and participate in single-electron transfer reactions; best known are the ferredoxins. They are involved in the functioning of such diverse enzymes as NADH dehydrogenase, succinate dehydrogenase, pyruvate dehydrogenase in anaerobes and nitrogenase. Three known types of iron-sulphur proteins are those in which:

(a) a single iron atom is linked to four cysteine sulphur atoms as in rubredoxin;

(b) two iron atoms are linked to four cysteine sulphur atoms and to two bridging, acid-labile sulphur atoms as in plant-type ferredoxin; and

(c) four iron atoms are linked to four cysteine sulphur atoms and to four bridging, acid-labile sulphur atoms as in bacterial-type ferredoxin and in high-potential iron-sulphur proteins.

irradiation. In respect of food, apart from ultra-violet irradiation, refers to ionizing radiation which kills off various microorganisms- so-called cold sterilization. Complete sterilization requires high dosage that causes changes in flavour, colour and texture. Smaller doses useful to inactivate Salmonella in egg, parasites in meat, for disinfection of grain. Also useful to prolong storage life by suppression of sprouting in potatoes and root vegetables.

isano oil. An oil obtained from the kernel of the nut of the *Ongokea klaineana* of tropical Africa. It is a pale-yellow viscous oil that has little drying power, but when heat-treated sets up an exothermic action to produce a varnish oil. Anda-assu oil, also used in Brazil for paints, is from the seeds of the plant *Joannesia princeps*. The seeds yield 22% of a clear yellow oil with an iodine value of 142 which is bodied by heating.

isigny cheese. A variety of American cheese which originated 45 years ago during an attempt to make Camembert cheese here. It is slightly larger than Camembert, though of similar shape. When ripe, it resembles mild Limburger.

isinglass. Protein membrane from the swim bladder of certain species of sturgeon; practically pure collagen. When specially prepared is used to clarify beer, as it slowly precipitates and carries with it any suspended particles.

islets of langerhans. Areas of the pancreas from which the insulin is secreted.

isoascorbic acid. Also known as erythorbic acid, a geometric isomer of ascorbic acid with only slight vitamin C activity.

isocitrate dehydrogenase. An enzyme which catalyzes the reversible oxidation of isocitrate to oxoglutarate. In the presence of Mn(II) ions; the oxalosuccinate first formed is decarboxylated.

Two forms of the enzyme are known, one in mitochondria requiring NAD as coenzyme, the other, a soluble form, requiring NADP. It is the latter, present in serum and most richly in liver, heart and skeletal muscle, with which we are concerned.

isoelectric point. Proteins and amino acids carry both negative and positive charges on the molecule, and are therefore called amphoteric. At a certain degree of acidity, depending on the particular protein or amino acids, the substance becomes electrically neutral, *i.e.*, the isoelectric points, Proteins are usually least soluble and therefore precipitated from solution at the I.E.P.

isoenzymes. Different forms of an enzyme, usually occurring in different tissues. The isoenzymes of a particular enzyme catalyze the same reaction, but they behave in different manners on electrophoresis. The formation of isoenzymes usually involves different arrangements of subunits arising from two different genetic loci to form the active polymeric enzyme. The isomeric forms all have the same molecular mass but differing structural configurations and properties. Large numbers of different enzymes are known to have isomeric forms; for example, lactate dehydrogenase has five forms. The isomeric forms are usually associated together giving a blend of their properties. Isoenzymes are demonstrated by separation by electrophoresis. They are usually made up of at least two types of genetically distinct polypeptide chains. These may occur in various proportions thus giving rise to enzymes differing in affinity for substrates, inhibitors, etc. Also spelled as isozyme.

isoionic protein. A protein that has an equal number of protonated basic groups and deprotonated acidic groups; operationally defined as a protein from which all bound ions have been removed by electrolysis or by mixed-bed ion-exchange chromatography. Such a protein contains no ions other than those arising from dissociation of solvent.

isopentenyl pyrophosphate. A compound derived from acetyl-CoA, is the activated building block precursor of many important biomolecules that contain isoprene units. They include vitamin A, E, and K; the carotenoids; gutta-percha; the phytol side chain of chlorophyll, many essential oils, such as fragment principles of lemon oil, eucalyptus, and musk, as well as the hydrocarbons found in turpentine. This compound is the precursor of many isoprenoid compounds in which isoprene units are joined in different ways to form long chains or rings.

isoprene. The unit that forms part of the structure of the terpenes and the carotenoids.

isoriboflavin. An analogue of riboflavin containing the two methyl groups in the 5,6 instead of the 6,7 positions. It competes with the vitamins and of inhibits growth.

isotonic. A term referring to the solution(s) having equal osmotic pressure; an isotonic salt solution is one containing the same concentration of sodium chloride as occurs naturally in body fluids (about 1%). For this reason, such a solution can be used effectively to restore osmotic balance in tissues when too much water has been lost from the body as a result of injury. It is also called physiological salt solution.

Italase. The trade name for a lipolytic enzyme solution which is extracted from the gland found in the mouth of milk-fed calves. This solution is used in the making of Italian types of cheese instead of rennet paste. This enzyme has to coagulating power, so rennet extract must also be used.

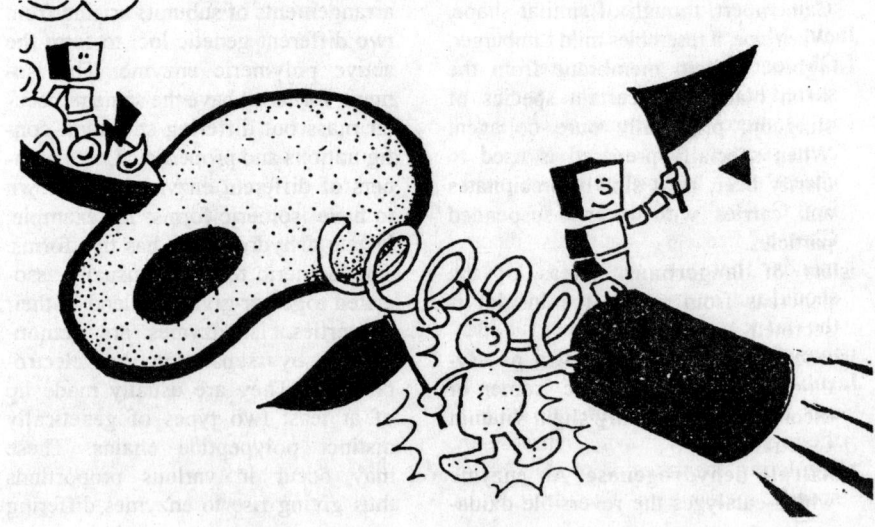

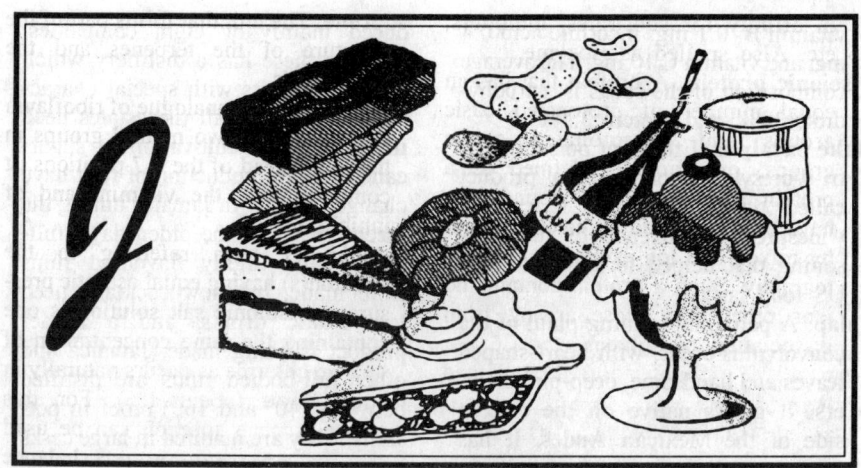

jack bean. *Canavalia gladiata var. ensiformis.* A bean-like plant of Leguminosae, but not of the genus Phaseolus. It is raised for edible seeds as well as for ornamental use. The plant is cultivated in tropical regions, where it is used for stock feed. If picked before the pods exceed about 10 cm, the jack bean can serve as a reasonably palatable snap bean. The jack bean has received consideration as a possible coffee substitute.

Jack, Monterey cheese. A variety of Cheddar cheese manufactured by the stirred curd method. It was made first in Monterey, California. After sufficient stirring, the curd is wrapped in cheese cloth and rolled before pressing. Generally, it is called Monterey Cheese. Federal Standards recommends that the moisture content should not be more than 44%; while the fat content should not be less than 50% in the solids.

Jacob-Monod hypothesis. An hypothesis that offers a scheme to explain the regulation of enzyme synthesis by regulating the rates of production of specific messengers. The idea centres around a control mechanism, a portion of the DNA molecule, called operon. At one end of the operon is a sequence of nucleotides, the operator, which interacts with a repressor, which is genetically determined by a regulatory gene. This interaction represses copying of the structural genes, whose expression gives rise to specific messenger RNAs. Regulation enzyme synthesis in this way, by an interaction of two circuits allows the cell to select the genetic information required for expression at a particular time.

jaggery. Coarse dark sugar made from the sap of the coconut palm; or raw sugar cane juice; used in India and Pakistan as sweetening agent; it is also used to prevent oxidative rancidity of fats since it contains a natural antioxidant. Also known as gur.

Jak fruit. Tropical fruit that grows from the trunk and large boughs of *Artocarpus integrifolia, heterophyllus* and *integra.* Both pulp and seeds are eaten. The average composition per 100 g pulp is: carbohydrate 10%; protein 2.5%; vitamin A 130 µg;

vitamin B_1 0.1 mg; nicotinic acid 0.4 mg; and vitamin C 10 mg. The average composition of the seeds is: carbohydrate 30%; and protein 3.5%.

Jake paralysis. Effects of poisoning by tri-*o*-cresyl phosphate in a product called "Jamaica ginger". It was the widespread occurrence of this poisoning that helped to stimulate new US food laws.

jalap. A perennial twining plant of the convolvulus order, with heart-shaped leaves and handsome, deep-pink flowers. It grows native on the eastern side of the Mexican Andes. It has irregular, dark-brown roots, ranging in size from half an inch to three inches in diameter, which yield a resinous substance containing convolvulin. From this a purgative medicine is made. The roots are the part used medicinally. They are brown and wrinkled when placed on the market, but white and juicy when fresh.

jam. Fruit preserved and set to a gel by reaction between acid, pectin and added sugar. The solution of pectin in the fruit is caused to conglomerate by the sugar and forms a network of fibres enclosing liquid, *i.e.*, jelly. This only occurs under acid conditions, pH 2.5-3.5, optimum sugar concentration 67.5%. Normally 0.5-1% pectin used in jam manufacture. Legally jam must contain not less than 68% soluble solids (or 65% if hermetically sealed). Minimum fruit content: blackberry, strawberry and greengage 38%; blackcurrant 25%; damson, redcurrant, strawberry and gooseberry 35%; gooseberry, raspberry, loganberry, 30%; and marmalade 20%.

Jamaica rum. Jamaica was the first commercial producer of rum and is still one of the most important. More than a sixth of the cultivated land is under sugarcane and sugar is produced mainly by eight companies. Each of these has a distillery which produces spirits with special characteristics. Almost all the estates need irrigation. The cultivation of sugarcane and the production of rum have changed greatly in Jamaica during the recent years. In the olden days, full-bodied and highly flavoured rums were made, but now cocktails need less exotic drinks, and a milder product is being made. Jamaica and other full-bodied rums are distilled between 140° and 160° proof in potskills. They are matured in large casks known as "Puncheons". Unlike the light-bodied rums which are cultured yeast for inoculation, Jamaica rums depends on natural fermentation, sometimes refereed to as "wild" fermentation. In this method, the mask is inoculated by the yeast that is present in the air and in the raw material. The flavour of rum depends on the amount of esters added. A lower Ester rum called "Common Clear Rum" was made here since the olden days. In the latter part of the 19th century, a high Ester rum was made by the exported to the Continent, especially to Germany. Higher Esters rums were made by keeping the mash more acidic than usual and also by allowing a longer fermentation. This was not consumed in the continent, but was shipped to the darkest part of Africa as 'Jamaica Rum'. Jamaica Rum is still the most highly flavoured rum, with the exception of Martinique product. It has three or four times as much esters as the US, rum. Jamaica rum is highly-prized by many. In Jamaica, rum may not be distilled above 88% alcohol and only pure water and caramel from burnt sugar are allowed to be added. Rum is diluted with water before bottling it to various places. The rum for the English market has only 35% alcohol. Legally, it has to be kept in casks for ageing for at least three years.

Japanese heartnut, (walnut). *juglans sieboldiana cordiformis.* A nut, either heart-shaped or the shape of a guinea egg and having a flavour like that of the American butternut. It is used in ice cream, often in the place of the pecan. These nuts have a hard thin shell which is easily removed without breaking the nut.

Japanese medlar. *See* loquat.

Japanese millet. *Enchinochloa crusgalli* var. *frumentacea.* A variety of millet often present (as a weed) where other millets are cultivated. It is purposely planted as a catch crop in parts of Australia for hay and pasture. Some limited planting have been made in the US. Japanese millet is a minor crop in some regions of Egypt, Japan and India, where it is used for human consumption. Closely related to Japanese millet is the Shama millet (*E. colonum*) or jungle grass, which is grown in India. Japanese millet tolerates a wide variety of soils and prefers temperate and humid climates. The appearance of Japanese millet is much like barnyard grass or water grass. The stem of the plant is thick, coarse, and leafy. A flat, branched head is produced at the end of each stem. The plant reaches a height of from 0.6-1.2 m. Also known as billion dollar grass (US); Japanese barynard millet; and Sawan millet (India).

Japan plum. *See* loquat.

jasmine. *Jasminum officinale.* A vinelike plant that is indigenous to the warmer regions of the eastern hemisphere and is currently grown in some gardens India and the southern US. Some species of jasmine also appear as evergreen or deciduous shrubs. The vine leaves are usually opposite, dark green and pinnate. Both the vines and the shrubs produce extremely fragrant flowers which are of considerable value in the perfume industry. The unique aroma has been described as being a "delicate, sweet odour so peculiar that it's without comparison one of the most distinct of all natural odours." The common jasmine has become naturalized in sub-tropical latitudes throughout the world. In cool climates it is cultivated as a garden shrub. It grows from 2-3 m, has fragrant white blossoms and resembles of evergreens. The flowers are used in making oil of jasmine, a delicate perfume. Cape jasmine is the name commonly applied to the gardenia, not a true jasmine, but a subtropical plant belonging to the madder family. The flowers are large, white and fragrant, and the leaves are very beautiful.

J-chain. Polypeptide chain (molecular mass ~35,000) linking, by means of disulphide bonds, the μ-chains of the pentameric IgM molecule of α-chains of the dimeric secretory IgA molecule.

jejunum. Second portion of the small intestine, between the duodenum and the ileum.

jelly. A colloidal suspension that has set; may be made from gelatine, pectin, agar, usually flavoured with fruit juice or synthetic flavour.

Jensen-Kirschner value. A measure of the butyric acid in fats. It is represented by the number of millilitres of N/10 alkali required to neutralize a distilled Ag_2SO_4 filtrate from 100 ml of Reichert-Meissl distillate. The presence of butyric acid is especially characteristic of milk fat, and this determination is helpful in detecting the adulteration of milk products. A low value indicates the probable adulteration of milk fat with some other fat. Normal butter fat has a Jensen-Kirschner number of 20-26.

jerked beef. Dried meat of S. America, similar to biltong.

jerked venison. Meat prepared by cutting lean meat into strips of 5-7.5 cm in thickness and then dipping into boiling brine. The meat is thoroughly smoked, followed by searing over a hardwood fire. After this, the meat is dried in the sun. When properly prepared, the meat is not attacked by insects.

Jerusalem artichoke. Family: *Compositae*. Genus: *Helianthus*. Species: *Helianthus tuberosus*. Jerusalem artichoke is extremely nourishing, and high in carbohydrates, producing levulose sugars which diabetics can eat. It is a good catarrhal cleanser.

Jesuit's bark. Alternate name for cinchona bark; source of quinine.

jet dryer. An apparatus for moisture removal in which high velocity air is impinged on the product. For drying veneer, microwave heating to 93.3-148.9°C using air at 15.3-22.6 m/s, with 0.12-0.25 veneer, the drying occurs approximately twice as rapidly in a jet dryer as in the conventional dryer. A yellow popular 0.25 cm thick material veneer dries in 15-20 minutes in a conventional dryer and 7 minutes in a jet dryer.

Jew-fish. The name given to two species of large fishes well known in American waters. The one, known also as the guasa, or black grouper, sometimes reaches the weight of seven hundred pounds. It has a large, flat head and huge mouth and is olive-green in colour. This fish is common around Mexico, Florida and the West Indies. It often weighs 200 kg, is from 2-3 metres long and has flesh of excellent quality for the table.

Jochberg cheese. A cheese made in the Tyrol from a mixture of cows' and goats' milk. It is 50 cm in diameter, 10 cm in height.

Johnston-Ogston effect. The changes in the values of the sedimentation coefficients and of the apparent concentrations that are obtained for two or more components when they are present in a mixture as compared to the values obtained when each component is present alone. The effect is due to the dependence of the sedimentation coefficient on concentration, and it leads to a decrease in the observed sedimentation coefficients for both the slow and the fast components in a mixture. The apparent concentration, which is proportional to the area under the ultracentrifuge peak, will be increased for the slow component and will be decreased for the fast component.

Jonathan. Calcined, ground oat chaff used as adulterant for maize and other cereals.

jowar. Indian name for millet. Also spelled as jower.

Jubilee watermelon. A variety of watermelon of oblong shape with bright-red, firm, and sweet flesh. The rind is light green with dark-green stripes and is thick and tough. Jubilee is a Garrison type originally, with moderate resistance to Fusarium wilt, but some seed stocks are now susceptible. There is good resistance to anthracnose (Race 1). The fruit weighs from 13.5-15.8 kg. Its seeds are black. From planting to maturity of this variety takes about 90 days.

jujube. The fruit of the tree of the same name. Of the genus (*Zizyphus*), there are about 40 species of this genus of trees and shrubs, all of which bear edible fruit. *Z. Jujuba* is the only species that is known to be consumed and to be seriously cultivated for its yield of fruit. Some South American species, such as Z. *Joazeiro* which grows in Brazil, is reported to be relished by sheep and cattle. The tree is considered tropical and semitropical, but it is quite hardy. The tree is found today in southern Mediterranean Europe and northern Africa, North and South America, but is probably most extensively cultivated in China. The delicate, light-green foliage of the tree has made it popular as ornament as well as source of fruit. The fruit of the common jujube is of a reddish-brown colour and is small (shape and size of an olive). When fully ripe, the fruit is somewhat dry and partially wrinkled, having a pleasing acid flavour. The tree tolerates a variety of soils with exception of heavy clays. Relatively little irrigation is required except in semiarid areas. In orchards, the trees are planted at a distance of 4.5-6 m apart. The trees do not blossom out until June and thus are essentially frost immune. Propagation is by seed. The trees bear after

about 4 years. The fruit is easily dried by brief exposure is sunlight, which turn is a dark colour and increase the wrinkling of the skin. Consumers of the fruit in southern Europe prefer it as a dessert fruit when ripe, and eat it later in the season in the dry form as a sweetmeat. Traditionally, the fruit has been considered by many persons as a pectoral and thus it has been incorporated in cough tablets and syrups. The average composition of per 100 g of the raw jujube is: water 80.2%; protein 1.2 g; fat 0.2 g; carbohydrates total 27.6 g; fibre 1.4 g; ash 0.8 g; calcium 29 mg; phosphorus 37 mg; iron 0.7 mg; sodium 3 mg; potassium 269 mg; vitamin A 40 IU; thiamine 0.02 mg; riboflavin 0.04 mg; niacin 0.9 mg; and vitamin C 69 mg.

julienne. The vegetables cut into thin, match-like strips. Also a clear, vegetable soup.

junket. Precipitated protein of milk (casein only) carrying the fat with it and leaving behind the clear whey. The precipitation is carried out with the enzyme rennin.

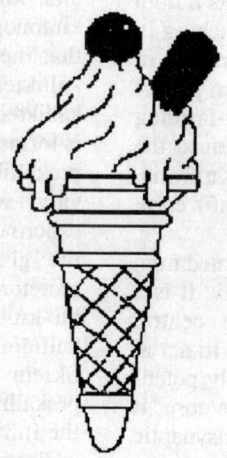

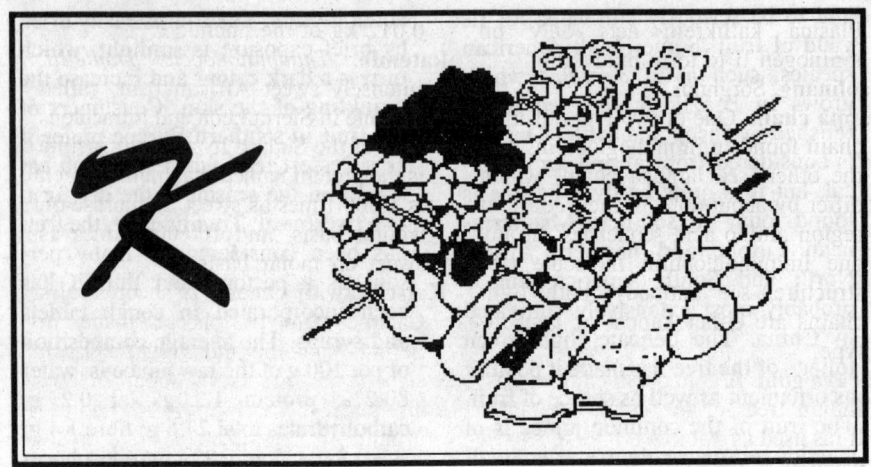

Kadarka grape. A native variety of Hungarian red wine grape. Its plantings are extensive. The Zinfandel is no longer regarded as identical with the Kadarka. The Kadarka is used in production of a number of red wines in Hungary.

kaffir beer. A beer brewed from Kaffir corn grain (sorgbhum), kaffircorn malt, and various maize products.

kaffir corn. A cereal grain belonging to the sorghum group, used chiefly as a food for live stock. It contains a high percentage of starch, but is lacking in saccharine. Kaffir corn is raised in large quantities in the western part of the US, especially in the dry-farming sections. It is so called because the seed was first brought from Kaffraria, in Africa. Also spelled as kafir corn.

kafir corn. *See* kaffir corn.

kainic acid. An amino acid isolated from the seaweed *Digenea simplex*. It is a powerful stimulant of the central nervous system and appears to act at glutamate synapses. It greatly potentiates glutamate, and in large doses it causes destruction of postsynaptic cells that possess glutamate receptors. It is used as a pharmacological tool by neurobiologists to inactivate particular nerve centres in the brain.

kajmak. The Turkish word "Kajmak" means cream and is used to designate a product made in Serbia and sometimes known as Serbian butter. It is similar to a cram cheese. The flavour varies between that of goats' milk cheese and Roquefort.

kallikreins. The enzymes which act on kininogens to produce kallidin and/or bradykinin. They are also called kinionogenases. It has been shown that the pancreas is a rich source of kallikrein. There are two type of kallikrein enzyme. Glandular kallikrein is formed from a precursor (glandular prekallikrein) in certain glands (salivary, sweat, lachrymal glands and exocrine pancreas) and released from the glands into the blood during secretory activity. The enzyme acts on kininogens I and II to produce kallidin and bradyinin. Plasma kallikrein is formed from plasma prekallikrein (Fletcher factor) under the influence of the enzyme plasmin or Factors XII of the clotting cascade.

Plasma kallikrein acts only on kininogen II to form bradykinin.

kaolinang. Sorghum.

kappa chain. One of two types of light chain found in immunoglobulins (for the other, see lambda chain) which differ by about 60% in their constant region amino acid sequences. In any one immunoglobulin molecule (for structure, see antibody) both light chains are either kappa- or lambda-type.

karaya gum. A gum obtained from East Indian trees of the genus *Sterculia.* It ius used as stabilizer, *e.g.*, in frozen water ices; also used in combination with other stabilizers. Sometimes it is employed as a mild laxative. Also known as sterculia gum.

Karell diet. For patients with severe cardiac failure. It is a low-calorie fluid diet consisting of 800 ml milk given in four feeds; it provides 2.3 MJ food energy; 28 g protein; and 0.45 g of sodium and is given only for 2-3 days.

Karo syrup. Trade name for a dextri-maltose preparation made from maize starch; used as a carbohydrate modifier in milk preparations for infant feeding. It consists of a mixture of dextrin, maltose, glucose and sucrose.

karut. A very hard, dry, skim, milk cheese made in Afghanistan and northwestern India.

kaskaval. A loaf-shaped rennet cheese weighing 2-3 kg made in Bulgaria, Romania and Transylvania from partially skimmed sheep's milk.

katal. The amount of enzymatic activity that converts 1 mole of substrate per second; the katal (kat) is related to an enzyme unit (U) by the relationship: $1 \text{ kat} = 6 \times 10^7 \text{U}$.

In some cases conversion of 1 mole of substrate is equivalent to the number of reaction cycles which equals the number of carbon atoms in 0.012 kg of the nuclide C^{12}.

katemfe. *Thaumatococcus Daniellii.* Intensely sweet African fruit, called katemfe in Sierra Leon and miraculous fruit of the Sudan. Its active principle is the protein named thaumatin, which is 1,600 times as sweet as sucrose on weight basis, and 100,000 times as sweet on molar basis.

Katschkawalj cheese. A sheep's milk Cacio-cavallotype cheese made in Serbia, Rumania and Bulgaria. Each slab of cheese weighs about 2.5 kg.

kauri gum. A fossil gum dug from the ground in New Zealand and New caledonia, used in varnishes and enamels to increase the body and increase the elasticity and hardness. It is also used in adhesives, and the lower grades of chips are used in linoleum. It was first known as New Zealand gum, and first spelled cowrie, although cowrie is the name of a genus of mollusk shells found in the Indian Ocean and formerly used as money in China.

Kauri is a product of kauri tree exudations buried for long periods, but it also comes from the conifer tree *Agathis australis.* There is little extraction of the gum from the present kauri forests, whose wood is employed for lumber, but some bush gum is obtained by collecting the deposits in the forks of branches. Range gum is found in clay deposits, and some is transparent. Swamp gum is brown in colour and varies from hard to friable. The fossil gum has a specific gravity of 1.05, a melting point of 1823-232°C, and is soluble in turpentine, benzol, and alcohol. The kauri tree grows to a height of 30 m and great diameters, and yields a yellowish-brown, straight grained wood free from knots and much prized as a useful softwood. It weighs about

577 kg/m³.

kava kava. *Piper methysticum.* A tall, leafy shrub of the South Pacific has been used for many centuries among the islands of Oceania as a social beverage for many different occasions. The infusion prepared from the rhizome or stem of the plant is still used in many social ceremonies, to welcome visitors, commemorate marriages, births and deaths and to remove the curses.

kebab. General name for the Muslim preparations of meat, usually two or three kinds, grilled on charcoal; the pipes of meat are interspersed with vegetables.

kebobs. Indian dish; of rice, split pulse, onions, eggs, etc.; European dish of fish, rice, eggs, etc. In northern parts of India, it is called khichri.

Kefalotyi cheese. A hard, grating-type goat's or ewe's milk cheese of Greece and Syria. A goat's milk cheese of this type is also made in the Ozarks, Missouri and Arkansas.

kefir. The name giveeen to a kind of fermented or cultured milk characterized by acid and alcohol production. It is usually made from the milk of sheep or goats, although cow's milk may also be used. The fermentation is brought about by adding Kefir grains to the milk. The golden yellow trains, resembling miniature cauliflowers, consists of casein, yeasts, and bacteria. They increase in size in the fermenting milk and after fermentation is well under way they may be strained out, dried, and kept for long periods of time for inoculating fresh batches of milk. Fermentation is usually carried on in closed bottles so that the gas is retained and the milk becomes effervescent. Kefir is a well known drink in Southeastern and Central Europe, and has gained some popularity in America. Also known as Khapon, Kaphir, and Hippe, Kepi, etc.

Kellogg's special K. Trade name for an enriched breakfast cereal based on maize. The average composition per 100 g is: 18 g protein; 0.8 g fat; 73 g soluble carbohydrate; 0.4 g fibre; 7 mg iron; 1.4 mg vitamin B_1; 1.8 mg vitamin B_2, 19 mg nicotinic acid; and 1.5 MJ food energy.

kelp. Family: *Fucaceae*. Genus: *Fucus.* Species: *Fucus vesiculosis* and others. The common name of kelp applies to a broad range of seaweed of many different species. But for those using herbs a lot, kelp probably refers to seaweed of the brown algal order Laminariales which posses large, flat, leaf-like fronds. A class of brown algae called bladderwrack is generally used the most often for producing kelp products. All sea vegetables absorb nutrients through their entire surface from the sea-water they float in, and since they average 39% salt, other forms of salt should be eliminated or curtailed whenever sea vegetables are used. They are usually extremely high in protein, and as sea-water is a solution of all the minerals vital to human health, they are an excellent source of minerals. Kelp is a rich source of organic iodine, helps to correct minerals deficiencies and is a good protector in food, valuable in overcoming poor digestion and goitre, and in rebuilding and maintaining the function of all the glands. It is useful as an adaptogen in thyroid disease of any description. Arame supplies vitamins A, B_1 and B_2. Hiziki is especially high in calcium and also supplies vitamins A, B_1 and B_{12}, and iron. Wakeme is high in iron, calcium and magnesium and rich in vitamins A. B_1 and B_{12}, and iron. Nori is extremely high in protein, containing 35%, and is high in vitamin A. Dulse is high in Protein and vitamin A and supplies vitamins B_6, B_{12}, C and E.

Kempner diet. A diet low in salt comprising rice, fruit, fruit juices, sugar and vitamins, containing about 8.4 MJ as food energy, 15-30 g protein and 100-150 mg sodium per day for patients suffering from congestive heart failure, cirrhosis of the liver, hypertensive disease, toxemia of pregnancy and certain kidney disorders.

kephalins. Or cephalins; phosphatides similar to lecithins but composed of glycerol, fatty acids, phosphoric acid and ethanol amine (instead of choline). Found in brain and nerve tissue, part of cell structure.

keratins. A group of fibrous proteins occurring in hair, feathers, hooves, and horns. Keratins have the coiled polypeptide chains that combine to form supercoils of several polypeptides linked by disulphide bonds between adjacent cysteine amino acids. Aggregates of these supercoils from microfibrils, which are embedded in a protein matrix. This produces a strong but elastic structure. They are characterized by their high content of several amino acids, especially cystine, arginine, and serine. They are generally harder than the fibrous collagen group of proteins; the softer keratins are components of the external layers of skin, wood, hair, and feathers, while the harder types predominate in such structures as largely due to the extent of cross-linking by the cystine molecules, which makes them difficult to dissolve.

The keratins are sulphur-containing proteins; there are two types: α-keratins and β-keratins. The former have a coiled structure with many cysteine links. α-keratin is the major protein of skin, hair, and nails. Its secondary structure is predominantly in the form of an a-helix held together by hydrogen bonds. Several of these helices are then twisted together to form long fibres. β-keratin is found in silk and the beaks of birds. It is arranged almost completely in a pleated-sheet structure. Because of this, it does not stretch when wet, when heated, or after treatment with disulphide reducing agents. When a-keratin is exposed to moist heat and stretched, it is converted to β-keratin. The hydrogen bonds stabilizing the a-helical structure are broken under these conditions and an extended parallel β-pleated sheet conformation is formed.

keratitis. Inflammation of cornea of the eye.

keratolysis. See keratolytic agents.

keratolytic agents. Agent that promotes keratolysis, i.e., softening or peeling of the horny (keratin) layer of the epidermis. Keratolytic agents are applied topically and include resorcinol, salicylic acid and sulphur.

keratoplastic agents. Agents that promote the growth of the superficial layers, the keratin, of the epidermis. Such agents include coal tar, ichthamol, and tretinoin.

kermes. A brilliant red natural dyestuff similar in colour to cochineal, having a beautiful tone and being very fast. It is one of the most ancient dyes, but is now largely replaced by synthetic dyestuffs. Kermes is an insect found on the kermes oak tree, *Quercus coccifera*, of southern Europe and North Africa. The body of the animal is full of a red juice, and the colouring matter, kermesic acid, $C_{18}H_{12}O_9$, is separated out in brick-red crystals. The yield is about 100 g from 100 kg of kermes. It has only about one-tenth the colouring power of cochineal.

Garouille is the root bark of the kermes oak. It contains 18-32% tannin, and is used for making sole leather. The colour is darker than oak tannin.

Kerner grape. A relatively recent development, out of the Trollinger and the Riesling vine. The grape grows in all soil conditions. Favored regions in Germany include the Wurttemberg, Rhenish Palatinate, and Francoia areas. The wine is lively, pleasing, Rieslinglike, with a light muscat bouquet. Of the total vineyard areas in the whole Germany, this grape represents about 2% of total.

Kesp. Trade name for textured vegetable protein made from spun fibres from field bean (*Vicia faba*). It is marketed frozen in the wet form.

keto acids. Several α-keto acids are important metabolic intermediates; these include pyruvic acid and α-ketoglutaric acid. Keto acids are usually produced from the corresponding amino acids in transamination reactions. β-Keto acids in bound form are intermediates in fatty acid oxidation metabolism.

ketogenic diet. A diet poor in carbohydrate (20-30 g) and rich in fat; causes accumulation of the ketone bodies in the tissues; used to be used in the treatment of epilepsy.

ketonaemia. Accumulation in the blood of ketone bodies.

ketone bodies. Name given to the penultimate products of the fatty acid metabolism. The three substances-acetoacetate, β-hydroxybutyrate, and acetone; that are produced by the liver under certain conditions, particularly when blood glucose levels are low. They can be oxidized at only a limited rate, and when their production rate is excessive, as in diabetes and starvation, they accumulate in the blood (ketonaemia), and are excreted in the urine (ketonuria). There develops an excess of acetyl groups (produced, *e.g.*, from the breakdown of fatty acids) over oxaloacetate, an intermediate in the Krebs cycle. Two molecules of acetyl CoA condense to form acetoacetyl CoA, the precursor of acetoacetate, β-hydroxybutyrate, and acetone. Enzymes responsible for ketone body formation are associated mainly with the mitochondria. The ketone bodies (other than acetone) can be metabolized by other tissues and are a normal source of energy within the animal body. These are formed by the condensation of acetyl CoA which result from fatty acid oxidation. They include such substances as β-hydroxybutyrate and acetone. Two reactions take place in extrahepatic tissues by which ketone bodies are utilized. These activate acetoacetate-CoA. The aceto-acetyl-CoA formed by these reactions is split to acetyl-CoA by thiolase and oxidized in the citric acid cycle. Overproduction, known as ketosis, occurs in diabetes and starvation and leads to acidosis and eventual coma. If the body has little or no carbohydrate as a respiratory substrate, ketosis occurs, in which more ketone bodies are produced than the body can use.

ketonic rancidity. Certain moulds of *Penicillium* and *Aspergillus* species attack fats containing short carbon chains and produce ketones with a characteristic odour and taste, so-called ketonic rancidity. Fats such as butter, coconut and palm kernel are most susceptible.

Ketonil. Trade name for protein-rich food low in phenylalanine for feeding patients with phenylketonuria.

ketose. Monosaccharide that contains a

ketone group. The simplest example is dihydroxyacetone (a triose having three carbon atoms) and one of the most abundant in nature is fructose (a hexulose having six carbon atoms). The C-2 ketone in hexuloses can react rapidly and reversibly with the C-5 hydroxyl group to form an intramolecular ring structure consisting of four carbon atoms and an oxygen atom (furanose); it is the predominant form of hexuloses in solutions.

ketosis. An excessive accumulation of ketone bodies in the tissues, blood, and urine. Ketone bodies are formed by the oxidation of fatty acids by the liver. The simplest form of ketosis occurs in starvation and involves depletion of available carbohydrate coupled with mobilization of free fatty acids. Thus, ketosis arises as a result of a deficiency in available carbohydrates.

ketosteroid. One of a group of steroids that are known as either 17-ketosteroids or neutral-17-oxosteroids and that represent degradation products of steroids; they are excreted in the urine and provide an index of androgen production in the body. These compounds react with m-dinitrobenzene to form a chromogen with a characteristic absorption spectrum. These compounds are 17-ketosteroids; they have a keto oxygen in the 17-position of the chemical formula. Essentially none of the other steroid hormones besides androgens are 17-ketosteroids. The primary androgenic hormones which are precursors of ketosteroids are testosterone, which is secreted by the Leydig cells of the testes, and dehydroisoandrosterone, which is derived from the adrenal cortex. Because testosterone and dehydriosoandrossterone are metabolized by the tissues and appear in urine as ketosteroids, the rate of secretion of ketosteroids in urine is a very reliable index of the rate of androgen production in the body.

key enzyme. An enzyme that is unique to a metabolic pathway which has several enzymes in common with other pathways.

khaskhas. A wild plant the extract of whose seeds is mainly used for flavouring sharbat and similar drinks. It has also been tried as a mosquito repellant.

khichri. See kebobs.

khushkhash. Israeli term for the bitter orange.

kidney beans. Family: *Leguminosae*. Genus: *Phaseolus*. Species: *Phaseolus vulgaris*. Kidney beans are rich in protein and are particularly high in iron and vitamin A. They produce a gummy substance which helps to slow the passage of sugar through the gut and reduce the cholesterol in the bloodstream. For a warning about the toxic factor in kidney beans.

kidney clearance test. Test of kidney function by measuring the ability to excrete inulin, area, or a dye, in the urine. The quantity excreted per minute divided by the amount present in 1 ml of plasma is the urinary clearance.

killed vaccine. A vaccine that consists of originally infectious bacteria or viruses that have been rendered noninfectious; a vaccine of either killed bacteria or of the inactivated viruses.

kiln. An oven which is heated for curing, baking, dehydrating, and/or drying products such as sand, tile, wood, brick, and some food products. The products may be treated in a batch or moved continuously through a stationary kiln or a rotating cylinder through which heated air is forced and the product is moved.

kiln-dried lumber. Lumber dried to a specified moisture content, usually between 6 to 19% moisture content, using heated air under controlled conditions.

kininogens. The polypeptide precursors of plasma kinins (kallidin and bradykinin). Kininogens are derived from the plasma α_2-globulin fraction. There are two kininogens, kininogen I (molecular mass 57000) and kininogen II (molecular mass 19700).

kinins. 1. Chemical substances which stimulate differentiation of plant cells that otherwise may have lost permanently the power of differentiation. The kinins contain adenine, which seems to give these substance their biological activity. 2. Group of blood-borne polypeptides that cause smooth muscle contraction and blood vessel dilation, the best known is bradykinin.

kinnow. A fruit classified as a tangor, that is, a cross between a mandarin and a sweet orange (King X Willowleaf). The fruit is of medium-size and is oblate. The rind is thin and quite adherent, but peelable. The surface is smooth, glossy, and yellow-orange. The flavor is rich and distinctive. The Kinnow is also grown in Arizona and in Pakistan and India.

Kirigscherkase cheese. *See* Krutt cheese.

kitol. An inactive form of vitamin A found in whale which is converted into retinol by heating at 200°C.

kiwifruit. An egg-shaped fruit with a fuzzy brown outer skin and sweet, green flesh, the odd but appealing kiwi is a native of New Zealand, which leads the world in its production. Long regarded by horticulturists essentially as an ornamental plant, the Chinese gooseberry or yang-tao plant (*Actinidis chinensis*). Over the years, the fruit has been variously called Ichang gooseberry, monkey peach, kiwi and kiwi berry, in addition to the names already mentioned. The name now commonly accepted in many world markets for the fruit is kiwifruit.

The exotic interior of the kiwifruit represents a sunburst of neat white streaks radiating from a cream-coloured core, past tiny black seeds and into the shimmering green flesh. Sweet-tart in taste, kiwifriut appears to be a succulent blend of strawberry, banana, melon and pineapple flavours.

The growing seasons for the kiwifruit in New Zealand and California are complementary and thus extend the market availability over much of the year. Many people proclaim it as a dessert and snack fruit, as well as a source of juice, as an ingredient of shortcakes, pies, and cakes, as a beverage additive, and as a cooked fruit for adding to ice creams, cream pies, and milkshakes. The fruit also contains enzymes, similar to papain in papaya, that are useful in tendering meats.

Klim. Trade name for a variety of dried milk.

klipfish. Salted and dried cod mainly produced in Norway. The fish is boned, stored in salt for a month, washed and dried slowly. It is known is bacalao in S. America.

Klondike watermelon. A popular market and shipping melon, particularly in California. The striped Klondike is medium large, oblong, thick, 40-46 cm long and from 20-25 cm in diameter. The average weight is 12kg). The rind is light-green with irregular dark-green stripes and is medium-thin and tough. The flesh is scarlet, very sweet, with excellent flavor. Seeds are small, black-very sweet, with excellent flavour.

kloster. A soft-ripened Romadur-type cheese made in Germany from whole cow's milk. It has a somewhat unusual shape.

knot grass. A plant of the buckwheat family, one of the most widely-distributed plants in the world. Its many branched, trailing stems with knotty joints form a thick mat, even on hard or trampled ground. Tiny flowers, two or three in number, grow from the axils of the leaves. Several species of knotgrass yield a valuable blue dye.

kohlrabi. Family: *Cruciferae*. Genus: *Brassica*. Species: *Brassica caulorapa*. A variety of cabbage, cultivated for the stem, which swells into a peculiar bulblike growth just above the ground. This part is cooked in about the same way as the turnip, and it tastes much like the rutabage, or Swedish turnip. Kohlrabi is rich in potassium, fibre and vitamin C and contains a reasonable amount of carbohydrate. It has a good reputation as a blood cleanser and is recommended for toxemia and accompanying poor complexions. It is also useful for dental health, and healthy bone and nail development, as well as for kidney and bowel irritation, especially if eaten raw.

Koji process. A process by which molds are cultured on surface of moist bran.

koji. A fungal proteolytic enzyme preparation from the mould *Aspergillus oryzae* traditionally grown on steamed rice. It is used to prepare products such as miso by the proteolysis of soya and soya sauces. It was introduced from China to Japan about 1700 years ago.

kola nut. *Cola acuminata*. The dried seed or kola nut comes from evergreen trees with long, leathery leaves and growing up to 20 m in height. They are native to western Africa, Indonesia and other tropical climates. The fruit consists of 4-5 leathery or woody pods each containing 1-4 seeds. The seeds are dried and their outer coats removed. Although not actually a nut as such, yet it's called that due to its hard consistency when dried, thus resembling a nut in appearance.

Kolosarver cheese. A kind of cheese made from buffaloes' milk, resembling Trappist cheese when ripened.

Kommenost cheese. *See* Kuminost cheese.

Kopanisti chese. A Greek, blue-mold, sharp peppery variety of cheese which is kneaded by hand into orange-sized balls. These balls develop mold and are kneaded with salt and mold until thoroughly mixed. The cheese are cured for 1-2 months.

Koppen cheese. A sour-milk cheese made by herders between Bohemia and Silesia varities. The cheese block weighs about 1 kg, and is conical or cylindrical in shape, and possesses a sharp pungent flavour.

Kosher gouda cheese. A variety of gouda cheese bearing a stamp whereby the Jewish trade for whom it is made can identify it.

Kosher cheese. A kind of cheese typically made without animal rennet for the Jewish trade. Sometimes a starter is used, or the milk is allowed to sour naturally. The soft varieties such as Kosher Cream, Cottage, and Gouda are popular. All cheese for this market bear an identifying Kosher stamp. The selection and preparation of kosher is done in accordance with traditional Jewish ritual and dietary laws. The only kosher flesh foods are from animals that chew the cud and have cloven hoofs, such as cattle, sheep, goats and deer, and the hindquarters must not be eaten. The only fish permitted are those with fins and scales; birds of prey and scavengers are not kosher. Moreover, the animals must be slaughtered according to ritual before the meat can be considered kosher. From Hebrew 'Kosher' meaning 'right'.

Krebs cycle. A cyclic series of biochemical reactions that is fundamental to the metabolism of aerobic organisms, *i.e.*, animals, plants, and many microorganisms. The enzymes of the Krebs cycle are located in the mitochondria and are in close association with the components of the electron transport chain. In this cycle of reactions, the pyruvate, produced by glycolysis, is oxidized to carbon dioxide and water, with the production of large amounts of energy. Since the oxidative enzymes of the Krebs cycle are located in the mitochondria, the first step is the transport of pyruvate from the cytoplasm into the mitochondrial matrix. Then the pyruvate is dehydrogenated and decarboxylated by a four enzyme complex to form acetyl-CoA. This reaction requires thiaminepyrophosphate, lipoamide, FAD, NAD, and coenzyme A. It is inhibited by arsenite and mercury. This conversion is irreversible under cellular conditions. Krebs cycle consists of nine reactions that oxidize two carbon atoms to carbon dioxide. First, acetyl-CoA condenses with oxaloacetate, forming citrate, which isomerizes to isocitrate with cis-aconite as the intermediate. This reaction can be inhibited by fluoroacetate after the inhibitor is converted to fluorocitrate. This inhibitor is called 'suicide inhibitor' as it leads to irreversible inhibition of an essential enzyme. In the next reaction, isocitrate is dehydrogenated and decarboxylated, producing NADH and α-ketoglutarate. Then α-ketoglutarate is also dehydrogenated and decarboxylated to form succinyl-CoA and another NADH. In the next reaction succinate is formed from succinyl-CoA and at the same time, GDP is phosphorylated to GTP in the presence of enzyme succinyl-CoA synthetase. Further, succinate is converted to fumarate, producing $FADH_2$. This reaction is inhibited by malonate. Finally, fumarate is converted to malate, which is then converted to oxaloacetate, completing the cycle. In the Krebs cycle each pyruvate molecule yields 15 ATP molecules. Since two pyruvate molecules enter the cycle from glycolysis, 30 are produced in all. Also known as citric acid cycle; tricarboxylic acid cycle.

Krebs solution. A physiological salt solution for bathing isolated mammalian tissues.

Its composition is: (mmol/L): NaCl, 94; KCl, 4.7; $MgSO_4.7H_2O$, 0.45; $CaCl_2$ 2.5; KH_2PO_4, 1.2; $NaHCO_3$, 22; glucose, 13; pyruvic acid, 3.1; fumaric acid, 5.3; glutamic acid, 3.1; (the acids are converted to the sodium salts by the $NaHCO_3$). The solution is bubbled with 5% carbon dioxide in oxygen.

Krebs-Henseleit solution. A physiological salt solution used for maintaining mammalian tissues, especially when nerve evoked responses are to be recorded.

Its composition is (mmol/L): NaCl, 118; KCl, 4.7; $CaCl_2$, 2.5; $MgSO_4.7H_2O$, 1.2; NaH_2PO_4, 1.2; (but sometimes replaced by KH_2PO_4), $NaHCO_3$, 25; glucose, 11.1. It is bubbled with 5% carbon dioxide in oxygen.

Kreis test. A chemical test for the oxidative rancidity of fats. Fat is treated with a solution of phloroglucinol in ether and hydrochloric acid; a pink colour develops in rancid fat, due to the presence of epihydrin aldehyde.

Krutt cheese. A sour skim milk cheese made in the Asiatic Steppes, from the milk of cows, goats, ewes or camels. The curd is drained, made into small balls and sun dried. Also known as Kirigscherkase cheese.

Kryavac. The trade name for a heat shrinking plastic film used in wrapping cheese for curing. The process involves placing the cheese in an appropriate sized Kryavac bag, removal of air by vacuum, sealing the bag, and finally shrinking the film by immersion in hot water. A viscous whey that was quite generally used in Holland for making Edam cheese. The whye contains a lactic acid bacterium *Streptococcus hollandicus,* which causes the viscous condition and produces acid at the same time.

kryptoxanthin. Alternative spelling of cryptoxanthin.

Kuhbacher-Kumbach cheese. A kind of soft, ripened cheese made in upper Bavaria, Germany from whole or partly skimmed cow's milk. It is cylindrical in shape and weighs 1-3 kg.

kulthi. *M. uniflorum.* A palnt whose seeds are used as food in some parts of India and and other regions of southeast Asia; also used as fodder and for green manuring.

Kuminost cheese. A variety of special Scandinavian cheese made from whole or partially skimmed milk. This Colby-like curd is formed into 2 kg loaves and flavoured with cumin or caraway seed. Also known as Kommenost cheese.

kummel. A liqueur prepared from caraway seeds, fennel and orris root. Alcoholic strength varies from 60-75% of proof spirit.

kumquat. A citrus fruit of the genus *Fortunella;* widely distributed in S. China; resemble citrus fruits, but very small, acid pulp, and sweet, edible skin.

kurrat. Plant closely related to leek.

kynurenine. A di-amino acid formed as an intermediate in tryptophan metabolism both in mammals and in lower forms. In mammalian livers there is an enzyme system which catalyzes the oxidative opening of the pyrrole portion of the indole ring, with the production of kynurenine and formic acid. By the complex transformations, kynurenine may be converted into eye pigments in insects; it is also intermediate in the conversion of tryptophan to nicotinic acid in mammals. Kynurenine is obtained from N-formylkynurenine, the reaction is catalyzed by kynurenine formylase. Further metabolism of kynurenine involves conversion to 3-hydroxy-kynurenine, which is converted to 3-hydroxyanthranilate; the reaction is catalyzed by kynureninase, a pyridoxal phosphate enzyme.

kynurenines. The major metabolites of tryptophan on the pathway other then those which result in serotonin and tryptamine. The kynurenines include kynurenine itself, 3-hydroxyky-nurenine, 3-hydroxyanthranilic acid, anthranilic acid, quinolinic acid, picolinic acid, xanthurenic acid, nicotinic acid and nicotinamide.

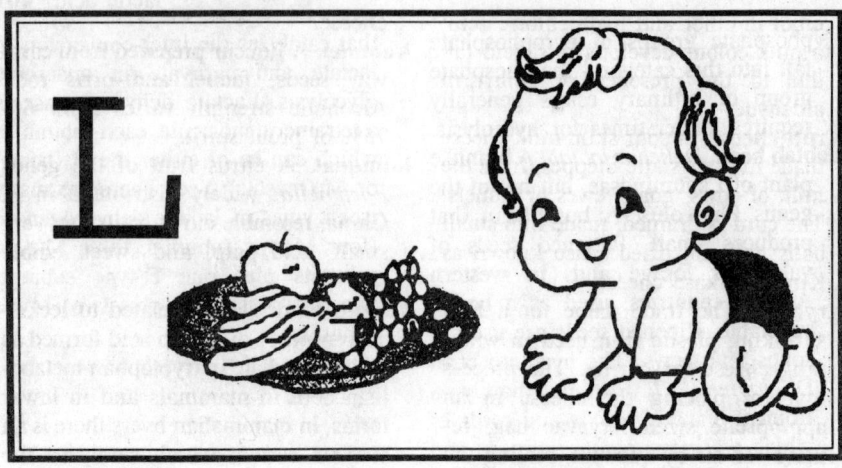

labelled substances. In order to follow the progress of a substance, food stuff or drug, through the body, it is sometimes marked or labelled so that it can readily be distinguished. Such labels may be chemical radicals that are abnormal and can therefore be distinguished, e.g., the introduction of phenyl groups into fatty acids, or, more recently, the use of radioactive substances.

labiatae. The botanical name of the mint family, a very important and extensive group of plants, so named because most of the flowers present prominent upper and lower lips. The name is derived from the Latin labium, meaning lip. The labiate have a four-lobed ovary, which changes into four seed-like fruits. There are about 3,000 species, mostly herbs or small shrubs, with opposite or whorled leaves and usually square stems. They are found throughout the world in temperate latitudes. Many, such as lavender and thyme, are valued for their fragrance; others, such as mint and peppermint, for their stimulating qualities, and still others, such as savory, basil and

marjoram, as aromatics. Many of them posses bitter tonic qualities, and not a new bear beautiful flowers, that make them favorite garden plants.

labile. Susceptible to change by one or more of numerous factors. For example a food ingredient, such as an additive, may undergo alteration when subjected to excessive temperature or heat; or to an excessively acidic or alkaline environment; or to an oxidizing or reducing environment; or by exposure to light or other forms of radiation. Thus, a substance may be referred to as heat labile, light labile, etc. Frequently, a substance that is labile with respect to acids may be stable under alkaline conditions; or a substance that is labile with respect to oxidants may be quite stable in a reducing atmosphere. In a very general way, the term stable is the antonym of labile.

labile phosphate group. A phosphate group that is readily liberated from a compound by hydrolysis at 100°C in 1N hydrochloric acid for 5-10 minutes. The terminal phosphate group of nucleoside triphosphates and the phosphate groups of pyrophosphate fall into this category; the phosphate group of ordinary esters generally requires longer times for hydrolysis.

lablab bean. *Dolichos lablab.* A beanlike plant of Leguminosae, but not of the genus Phaseolus. A bush bean that produces small, flattened seeds of value for forage and, in western African countries, used as a boiled vegetable. Ripened seeds are used in soups and stews. The hyacinth bean *D. lablab cultratus*, is mainly a tropical plant, the pods and seeds of which are consumed by humans and animals. Many varieties of *Dolichos* are planted for ornamental purposes.

laccase. Enzyme in bacteria, potato, and mushrooms that converts polyphenols to quinones.

lacerator. A machine for breaking or shredding forage plants at or slightly after the time of harvest in the field to hasten drying. Flails are commonly used.

lacquer. In reference to tinned food, a layer of gum and gum resin coated on to the tin-plate and hardened with heat. The layer of lacquer protects the tin lining from attack by acid fruit juices.

lactalbumin. One of the proteins of milk; it contains about casein 3%, lactalbumin 0.5% lactoglobulin 0.25%. It is not precipitated from acid solution as casein, hence during cheese-making the whey contains the lactalbumin and lactoglobulin. They are precipitated by heat, and a whey cheese can be made in this manner.

lactase. An enzyme found in mammals, honeybee larvae, and some plants. It is β-galactosidase which hydrolyzes lactose to galactose and glucose. This enzyme is very active in suckling infants.

lactate dehydrogenase. LDH. Enzyme that catalyzes the inter-conversion of lactate and pyruvate in anaerobic glycolysis. Lactate dehydrogenase is a tetrameric molecule, each subunit of which can be of either the H (heart) or M (muscle) type. There are many isoenzymes of lactate dehydrogenase (four M-type subunits, three M-type subunits plus one H-type subunit, two M-type subunit plus two H-type subunits).

lactein bread. An alternate name for milk loaf, *i.e.*, loaf to which skim milk powder has been added.

lactic acid bacteria. A group of Gram-positive, usually nonmotile, nonsporulating bacteria that ferment carbohydrates in the presence or absence of oxygen, with lactic acid always a major end product. The members of this group lack porphyrins and cytochromes, do not carry out electron-transport phosphorylation, and hence obtain energy only by substrate-level phosphorylation. They are highly tolerant to acidic conditions and grow anaerobically. Most lactic acid bacteria can obtain energy only from the metabolism of sugars and related fermentable compounds, and hence are usually restricted to habitats in which sugars are present. They usually have limited biosynthetic ability, and their complex nutritional requirements include needs for amino acids, vitamins, purines, and pyrimidines. Lactic acid bacteria are involved in the formation of yogurt, cheese, and silage. They can occur as spoilage organisms and some are pathogenic, causing infections of the nasopharynx. They include members of the genera *Lactobacillus, Streptococcus* and *Leuconostoc*.

lactic acid. An α-hydroxy carboxylic acid, $CH_3CH(OH)COOH$, with a sour taste. Lactic acid is produced from pyruvic acid in active muscle tissue when oxygen is limited and subsequently removed for conversion to glucose by the liver. During strenuous exercise it may build up in the muscles, causing cramp-like pains. It is also produced by fermentation in certain bacteria and is characteristic of sour milk. It is also produced by fermentation in silage, pickles, sauerkraut, cocoa, tobacco; its value here is in suppressing the growth of unwanted organisms. In mammalian muscle metabolism the first stages of breakdown of glucose and at pyruvic acid. In severe exercise this is reduced to lactic acid which can accumulate in the muscles. Similarly formed in meat muscles from glycogen immediately after death. It is used as an acidulant (as well as citric and tartaric acids) in sugar confectionery, soft drinks, pickles and sauces.

It exists in two optically active forms. The dextro form, which has been called sarcolactic acid, is produced from glycogen in muscle, contributes the lactic acid found in blood, and can be converted into glycogen in the liver (Cori cycle). It has a configuration corresponding to that of L-alanine (which is also dextrorotatory) and is designated L-lactic acid, is produced by fermentation by some bacteria. It is also the end-product of glycolysis in anaerobic skeletal muscle during exercise. It is released into the blood stream, hence by way of the heart, where it becomes a substrate for gluconeogenesis. Release of the glucose so produced into the bloodstream and thence to muscle completes the Cori cycle. Lactic acid is also the major product of fermentation by lactic acid bacteria. The acid produced by the fermentation of milk sugar and re-

sponsible for the flavour of sour milk and precipitation of the casein curd in cottage cheese. Also known as 2-hydroxypropionic acid.

lactic dehydrogenase. An enzyme which occurs in heart (H_4) and skeletal muscle (M_4). The heart enzyme is active at low levels of pyruvate (and lactic acid) and is inhibited by concentrations of pyruvate exceeding $10^{-3}M$. The muscle enzyme does not achieve its maximum velocity until pyruvate concentration is $3 \times 10^{-3}M$ but maintains its activity in much higher concentrations of pyruvate. Tissues such as the heart which are continually contracting are found to have H_4-lactic dehydrogenase, while flight muscles of chicken and pheasants which make sporadic short flights have predominantly M_4-lactic dehydrogenase.

lactide. Any of the various compounds formed by reaction between two molecules of the α-hydroxy acid, with the loss of two molecules of water and the formation of a ring compound containing two oxygen atoms in the ring.

Lactobacilli. The typical rod-shaped, varying from long and slender to short bent rods. *Lactobacilli* are often found in dairy products, and some strains are used in the preparation of fermented food products. For example, *L. delbrueckii* is used in the preparation of yogurt, and *L. acidophilus* in the production of acidophilus milk. The *lactobacilli* are usually more resistant to acidic conditions than are the other lactic acid bacteria, being able to grow well at pH values around 4-5. Because of this, they can be selectively isolated from natural materials by the use of carbohydrate-containing media of acid pH, such as tomato juice-peptone sugar. The *lac-*

tobacilli are rarely if ever pathogenic.
lactochrome. Pigment in milk. Lacto-
flavin. Obsolete name for vitamin B$_2$;
it is so named because it was first
isolated from milk.
lactollin. Protein found in small traces
in bovine milk; of unusual composition, lacking methionine and with little
alanine.
lactone. Compound formed by loss of
water from a molecule of a hydroxy
acid to form a ring compound or inner
ester, for example, gluconic acid forms
gluconolactone.
Lac-tone. Trademark for a protein-rich
baby food (26% protein) made in
India from peanut flour, skim milk
powder, wheat flour and barley flour
with added vitamins and calcium.
lacto-ovo-vegetarian. One whose diet is
composed of vegetables, fruit, milk
and eggs but no flesh foods.
lactose. Milk sugar, 4.8% of milk. A
disaccharide that is hydrolyzed by
acid or the enzyme lactase, to glucose
and galactose. Fermented by microorganisms to lactic acid hence the
souring of milk by lactobacilli. It is
used pharmaceutically as tablet filler
and as medium for growth of microorganisms. Ordinary lactose is alpha
lactose (16%) of the sweetness of
sucrose); if crystallized above 93°C is
changed to the beta form, which is
more soluble and sweeter than the
alpha form. Since it has a potentially
free carbonyl group on the glucose
residue, lactose is a reducing disaccharide. Lactose is manufactured by
the mammary gland and occurs only
in milk. For example, cow's milk
contains about 4.7% lactose. It is less
sweet than sucrose (cane sugar). The
first step in its metabolism is by way
of hydrolysis to the component
monosaccharides. Lactose is an excellent example of an inducer compound.

The inducible enzyme is β-galcto-
sidase and it catalyzes the conversion
of lactose into galactose and glucose.
Indirectly, *E. coli* utilizes lactose.
First, a galactoside permease which
permits entry of lactose into the cell
must be induced; and second, the β-
galactosidase which hydrolyzes the
disaccharide to galactose and glucose
must be induced. A third enzyme,
thiogalactoside transacetylase, is also
induced, but its function is not fully
understood. Thus, when *E.coli* is
grown in the presence of lactose as
the sole carbon source, these three
enzymes are induced in large quantities in a coordinated manner.
lacto-serum. Grandiloquent word for
whey.
lactulose. Disaccharide ketose, galacto-
sidofructose, found in human milk;
stimulates growth of *Lactobacillus
bifidus* in intestine of babies fed on
breast milk and so termed bifidus
factor.
ladled butter. Butter which has been
collected in lumps, rolls or wholesale
packages and reworked.
laevulose. Alternative name for fructose.
Lagos bologi. *Talinum triangulare.* A
small, pink-flowered annual plant with
club-shaped succulent leaves. Propagation may be by seeds or cuttings
and the culture is similar to that of the
Sierra Leone species, except the
plants are spaced at from 15-23 cm
apart. The soil must be well dug or
hoed before planting, with application
of manure or compost and subsequent dressings of fertilizer.
lag period. The delay in cell-free protein
synthesis that occurs when synthetic
polyribonucleotides are used as messenger RNA and that is thought to be
caused by the absence of an initiating
codon in the polyribonucleotide.
lamb. Meat from sheep younger than

12-14 months. Genuine spring lamb, 3-6 months; spring lamb up to 1 year. The average composition per 100 g of lamb meat is: protein 12.8%; fat 7.1%; calcium 7 mg; iron 1.5 mg; vitamin B_1 0.12 mg; vitamin B_2 0.15 mg; nicotinic acid 3.8 mg; and food energy 0.5 MJ.

Langres cheese. A kind of soft rennet cheese deriving its name from the village of Langres, France. It is mainly consumed locally. Each block of Langres cheese weighs about 1 kg, is about 20 cm high, and 12 cm in diameter.

lanoline. The fat from wool. It mainly consists of a mixture of cholesterol oleate, cholesterol palmitate and cholesterol stearate and therefore not useful as food; it is used in various cosmetics.

Lapland cheese. A variety of cheese made by the Laplanders from the milk of reindeer. It is round, flat, and dump-bell shaped in cross-section, and resembles the very hard variety of Swiss cheese.

lard. The material prepared from pig fat by various rendering operations. It has a distinctive natural flavour that is thought to be desirable in some foods. In its unmodified forms, it has a tendency for early development of rancidity. Lard is classified on the basis of the rendering method as either hard. Lard sold commercially to bakers and other food processors is generally the type called refined pure lard, and it can be made by any of the preceding methods. The characteristics of lard are governed by the composition of the hog fat from which it is made, by the method of rendering, and by the refining and modification methods application to the extracted fat. Variations in hardness of the lard depend upon the body location of the fat that has been rendered. For example, internal fats such as leaf fats, are always higher in melting point than fat taken from locations nearer the surface of the animal. The refiner controls and standardizes his product by selecting and blending different fats. Special grades are produced by segregating certain fats and by using special rendering methods. Pure leaf lard, which has the highest melting point of the unmodified lards, is made only from fat taken from the body cavity. If a still firmer fat is required, hydrogenated lard flakes can be added to the natural fats. By varying the amount of hydrogenated material, a wide range of melting points can be obtained.

lard compounds. Blends of animal fats, such as olesterin with vegetable oils to produce products similar to lard in consistency and texture. Vegetable shortenings made from mixtures of partially hardened vegetable fats with the consistency of lard are referred to as lard substitutes.

lard, neutral. Highest quality pig fat, prepared by agitating the minced fat with water at a temperature below 50°C. Kidney fat provides No. 1 quality; while back fat provides No. 2 quality.

larding. Method of adding fat to lean meat to that it does not dry during long slow cooking. Narrow strips of bacon fat, 4 cm long and 2 cm wide, are threaded into the surface of the meat with a special larding needle. The strips are called lardoons.

lateral ducts. Tubes, channels, or pipes extending, usually horizontally, from a main duct located at one side or center of a drying chamber, which distribute air through the product being dried under a pressure system, or collect air from the product for a suction system. The spacing and size of the lateral ducts depends on quantity of air flow, product, and depth of product. The cross-section of the 'duct is selected to provide velocity not exceeding 5.8-7.6 m/s. Openings are provided so that the air velocity from duct is about 0.25 m/s.

lathyrism. Disease caused by excessive intake (50% of the diet) of the chick pea, *Lathyrus sativus;* characterized by degeneration of the spinal cord and thrombosis of the spinal artery; common in India. The cause and mechanism of the disease is unknown, no toxic substance has been found in the chick pea, unlike the toxin found in the sweet pea that causes odoratism in the rat.

Latin lettuce. A variety of lettuce which has coslike or romainelike leaves which are shorter than typical cos leaves, and they form a loose, open head. The leaves are leathery and tougher than true cos. Also known as Gallega, this cultivar is used mainly in breeding as a source of lettuce mosaic resistance.

laucine. An essential amino acid; rarely limiting in foods. Chemically amino isocaproic acid.

laudanum. The name originally given to preparations of, or containing opium. The name laudanum, which is now obsolete, and is restricted to the simple alcoholic tincture of opium.

Laurel family. *Lauraceae.* Aromatic bark and leaves, and small flowers with parts in whorls of 3 are characteristics of this family, as are stamens with flap openings. Plants are mostly evergreen, except in the temperate zone, and are in the form of trees, shrubs, or vines. Usually, the leaves are alternate and have entire margins. The flowers are usually bisexual and develop as clusters in the leaf axils.

A single flower has 6 sepal-petal parts and 12 stamens in 3 whorls. But one or two stamen whorls may be sterile "honey leaves" called staminodes. The single pistil usually has an ovary above over flower parts (a superior position, containing 1 ovule in parietal placentation, 1 style and 1 stigma. For fruit types, there are drupes or berries, which are enclosed at the base by the persistent sepal tube.

The family includes: *Cinnamomum camphora* (camphor), *C. zeylanicum* (cinnamon bark spice), *Lindera benzoin* (spicebush), *Laurus nobilus* (bay laurel, bay tree and sweet bay), *Persea spp.* (avocado), *Sassafras* (Sassafras); *Laurus, Lindera, Umbellularia california* (California laurel); *Persea americana* (avocado); *Beilschmiedia, Endiandra* (walnut bean, orient salnut), *Litsea* (pond spice), *Ocotea rodioei* (greenheart, was used to make the original gates of the Panama Canal locks), *O. bullata* (South African stinkwood).

lauric acid. $CH_3(CH_2)_{10}COOH$. One of the long chain fatty acids; it occurs as the triglyceride in seeds of the spice-bush and to lesser extent in butter, coconut oil and palm oil.

lauter tub. In the brewing process, a tank where insoluble spent brewers grains are removed after mashing is completed.

lavender. *Lavandula angustifolia.* A traditional cottage-garden plant, its grey-green spiky foliage and the mauve-blue flowers providing colour throughout the year. It is native to the Mediterranean region and grows in profusion in the sun-baked *maquis* region of France. The fresh lavender flowers may be used to flavour syrup for jellies and fruit salad, and milk and cream for desserts. They may also be candied to decorate cakes and puddings. Fresh or dried flowers are used in rinsing water for clothes and hair. Bunches of lavender are said to ward off insects, and an infusion of the flowers may help relieve insect bites. Because of their sweet, pungent smell, the dried flowers and seeds are a frequent ingredient of pot pourri, herbal sleep pillows, and sachets. Dried lavender stems are used to weave decorative baskets and bowls.

laver. Name given to edible seaweed. Laver-bread is made from the seaweed *porphyra* by boiling in salted water and mincing to a gelatinous mass. It is made into a cake with oatmeal or fried. In S. Wales, it is known as Bara lawr.

lax. Scandinavian term for salmon; this term is used for smoked salmon in US. Also known as lox.

laxative. Any substance that accelerates the passage of food through the intestine. If it alters peristaltic activity it is termed a purgative, other types stimulate or depress the muscular activity of the gut. Cellulose act as a purgative by retaining water and increasing the volume of intestinal contents, Epsom salts function similarly through osmotic pressure. Castor oil is hydrolyzed by lipase to liberate ricinoleic acid which irritates the intestinal mucosa.

LD_{50}. Lethal dose 50, or median lethal dose; the amount of a pharmacological or toxic substance (such as ionizing radiation) that causes death in 50% of a group of experimental animals. For each LD_{50} the species and weight of the animal and the route of administration of the substance is specified. The usual method of determining the LD_{50} is to administer a range of doses (on a body weight basis), each to a group of 30 animals. The percentage mortality in each group may be plotted against the dose; a sigmoid curve is obtained. The dose corresponding to 50% mortality (the LD_{50}) can be obtained from the graph. The percentage kill plotted against logarithm of the dose is also a sigmoid curve, but if the percentages are converted to probits, the sigmoid curve is stretched into a straight line. Logarithm of the LD_{50} then corresponds to a probit of 5.

lead. Lead, one of the seven metals of antiquity, has accompanied all civilizations since their beginnings. It was in use before the time of the Hebrew exodus from Egypt. Discovery of metallic lead may have resulted from the accidental dropping of galena into a campfire. There are numerous references to the metal in the scripture. The book of Jeremiah contains an allusion to the process of cupellation, the procedure whereby silver is separated from argentiferous galena: 'The bellows are burned, the lead is consumed of the fire; the founder melteth in vain, for, the wicked are nock plucked away. Reprobate silver shall men call them . . .' Judging by his many metaphors in metallurgical terms, Jeremiah probably had considerable metallurgical experience.

Probably the greatest portion of the lead is used to make battery oxides and lead alkyls. Exposure to lead may account in part, for his rather saturine comments. Lead is mentioned in the tribute lists of the Pharoh Thomes III. Ancient peoples used lead for making rings and other ornaments, dishes and trays; and as a core for bronze statuettes and figures; sinkers for fishing nets, etc. probably the first use of galena was an eyepaint.

Lead poisoning was recognized in antiquity. Hippocrates (370 BC) was said to have recognized lead colic in a lead worker. Nicander in his book on poisons (first century BC) mentions litharge (lead oxide) and the symptoms of intoxication following its use. The Greeks and Romans are said to have used lead extensively in cooking. Bronze pots gave food a bitter taste, but lead sweetened it. Olive oil was often stored in lead-lined vessels. Wine was prepared in lead-line pots. The systems of Roman aqueducts were lead lined. Horace, about 25 BC, questioned the purity of water in relation to lead pipes and rather wisely prefers that from a murmuring book! Following the fall of Rome in the fourth century AD, lead used declined and remained at a comparatively low level for about 600 years. Around the tenth century, lead ores began being mined in eastern Germany. Lead exposure escalated.

Lead is of no dietary interest except that it is toxic and its effects are cumulative. May be present in food from traces naturally present in the soil, from shell fish that have absorbed it from seawater, as lead arsenate used as insecticide and from lead glazes on vessels. Traces are excreted in the urine. Symptoms of chronic poisoning can start with muscular weakness, constipation, pale skin and colic. The formation of a blue line marking the gums is characteristic of lead poisoning along with anaemia, anorexia and damage to the nervous system causing muscle tremors and paralysis. Lead also causes damage to the kidney, blindness (temporary or permanent) because of nerve damage, convulsions and death if treatment cannot halt the damage and exposure continues. Acute poisoning is similar, causing abdominal pains, diarrhoea, vomiting and possibly developing into convulsions and paralysis.

Sweetening of wine with lead salts, a common practice in continental Europe despite the imperial edicts, made lead colic an endemic 'disease' over the centuries. 'Devonshire colic', discussed by Sir George Baker in 1767, was thought to be due to the lead introduced during the manufacture and storage of cider. Lead colic, very common in colonial America, was also associated with the distilling of rum in lead heads and pipes.

Lead is a general protoplasmic poison that is cumulative, slow acting and subtle, and produces a variety of symptoms. Like other heavy metals, it has an affinity for sulphur. Though it exerts much of its activity through sulfhydryl inhibition, lad interacts with carboxyl and phosphoryl group also. The elements interferes with heme synthesis. Lead may be absorbed into the body by ingestion, inhalation and through the skin. Absorption is governed by chemical structure. Inorganic lead salts do not penetrate the intact skin but an be absorbed through cuts and abrasions. Significant quantities can also be absorbed from a bullet or shot wound. Lead shot (buckshot) is considered particularly dangerous, because of its larger surface area permitting greater absorption. Organic lead compounds for example tetraethyl lead, rapidly penetrate the intact skin. Absorption into bodily tissues is more rapid than with inorganic compounds. Because of greater lipid solubility large amounts of organic lead gain access to nerve tissue. Major routes of lead absorption are the respiratory and gastrointestinal tracts. Most industrial exposures in foundries, smelters, or areas where lead salts are processed follow inhalation of lead dusts of fumes. Absorption is dependent upon particle size and solubility. It had demonstrated that lead can be absorbed from all portions of the respiratory tract, including the nasal passages.

The classic studies indicate that under normal circumstances, 300 m*g are ingested daily by an adult. Ingestion of 600 µg of lead daily can result in lead intoxication. The World Health Organization suggests that the daily lead intake should not exceed 5 µg. kg (body weight). Following absorption into the blood stream, 95% of the lead circulates loosely bound to the erythrochtes. Only 5% is in the plasma. Previously, it was thought erythrocyte lead was bound primarily to the cell membrane. Recently, however, it has been observed that the lead is bound primarily to the haemoglobin in the cell. While examining the lead-binding properties of erythrocytes obtained from both normal and lead-exposed adults. it has been discovered the existence of a low molecular mass protein in the latter. This protein was not found in the erythrocytes of unexposed individuals. It was found, further, that white lead binds primarily to the haemoglobin in normal cells, appreciable binding of lead to the low molecular weight protein present in the erythrocytes of lead-exposed individuals occurs. The elucidation of the characteristics of the protein may assist in explaining the vagaries of different methods of blood lead analysis. Lead disappears from blood into tissues at a rate which follows first-order kinetics. Lead diffuses from red cell to plasma, then to the extracellular space, and then into the intracellular spaces or tissue cells. The liver and kidney, among the soft tissue, contain the highest concentrations. Lead diffuses from the soft tissue; part is stored in the bone, part is excreted. During the early period of lead deposition, especially in growing bone, concentration is greatest in the epiphyseal portion. Skeletal lead is fairly inert. It leaves the skeleton very slowly. Under certain conditions, however, such as a disturbance in acid-base fluid balance or a respiratory infection, lead may suddenly be mobilized from the bones, and symptoms of an acute lead intoxication may be precipitated. In the stable state more than 90% of the total body lead is stored in the skeleton. The form in which it is stored is becoming more clearly defined. X-ray diffraction studies indicate that lead assumes a position within bone crystal either by displacing other cations or by occupying lattice interstics. However, the possibility that lead may also be bound to organic components or be deposited as a discrete crystal of an insoluble compound are not excluded. At very low concentration led is an effective nucleating agent for inducing the formation of calcium phosphate crystals. The mechanism may be important in trapping lead at the surface of bone crystal.

Lead also follows the metabolic pathways of calcium. Deposits in bone and tissue comprise the body burden of lead and represent the cumulative difference between the quantities absorbed and excreted. The total body burden rises with age.

During the early years of the industrial revolution, lead smelters, for example, contributed much lead to the atmosphere because of inefficient smelting processes and poor design of furnaces. Prior to 1880 the loss was 2% compared to 0.5% before 1920 and about 0.06%, currently.

The lead content in foods varies with the site of production and processing; the degree of industrialization. For example, the wine manufactured from the grapes grown near the highways, are found to have higher lead contents, compared to the the wine manufactured in regions which are less polluted. Foods with pH below 6 leach lead, antimony and other metals from this alloy. The increased use of pewter during the bicentennial prompted examination of representative products available locally. 4% acetic acid was left in contact with the metal cups for two hours, and were determined.

Human beings, plants and animals absorb lead from the most diverse sources. From sewage water it gets into ground and river water; from waste gases it gets into the atmosphere, and from there into foodstuffs and beverages. By far the greatest volume is inhaled with the air we breathe, however. While 5-15% of the lead contained in the food we consume is absorbed by the intestines, the absorption by the lungs of lead from exhaust fumes in the air we inhale amount to almost 100%. Damage done by elements to lead released into the atmosphere is extremely difficult to eliminate. Particularly worrying, therefore, is the long-term buildup of lead in the environment. The ground on both sides of busy streets and highways is seriously contaminated with lead to a distance of 0.5-1 km. The oceans of the world today have a lead content more than 50 times above the natural level. Soluble lead salts, and insoluble lead compounds which can be rendered soluble by metabolic processes, are toxic. At the outset the symptoms of lead poisoning are: general upset,

loss of appetite, loss of energy, etc. Later on, the persons affected lose weight and suffer from anemia. In woman the menstrual cycle is disturbed. Characteristic changes in the blood count set in; and the red blood cells appear granulated. In every case a blue line appears around the gums, and there is a slategray discoloration produced by a build up of the metal in the oral cavity. The blue line, which is frequently the first specific sign of lead poisoning, may last a long time, well after the cause of the poisoning has been removed. At a later stage, more serious symptoms of lead poisoning, sometimes verging on the fatal, will manifest themselves in such forms as lead colic, feeble pulse and high blood pressure, cirrhosis of the kidney (nephritis), acute or nagging pains in the muscles, and finally bring fever (encphalopathy) accompanied y severe headaches, epileptic-type fits and psychosis. Also established are nervous ailments displaying symptoms of paralysis, arthritis, allergies and other skin reactions, anemia and various metabolic disorders. In cases of chronic lead poisoning severe damage can also be done to the chromosomes, which transmit hereditary factors. Typical lead poisoning with clearly diagnosable symptoms mainly affects persons working in the lead industry, who in the course of their activity have absorbed large quantities of the heavy metal. Less prominent but probably more problematic is gradual poisoning of the environment by smaller quantities of lead and the chronic lead poisoning of people, who from childhood onward, are exposed to higher accretions of lead throughout their lifetime. It must also be noted that the lead concentrations well below the levels that may give rise to physical symptoms can still touch off marked behavior disturbances.

The hazards of leaded paints to young children has been a point of discussion for years. The plaster beneath paint and the putty on the window frames have been ignored. Putty, with its lead content of approximately 30%, is quite palatable to children. Glazed earthenware is a notorious as a source of lead poisoning. Many incidents, including fatalities, have been reported in the following the use of glazed earthenware in preparing and storing foods, especially acidic foods. Ceramic dishes and cups, irrespective of their country of origin, are suspect until they are shown by analysis to be safe. Strong spirits in decanters made from leaded glass may enhance the flavour but could present somewhat of a hazard. Pewter were, even modern pewter, is more wisely used for display purposes or for serving dry foods.

The occupational exposure to lead should be controlled in such a manner so that no employee is exposed to lead at a concentration greater than 50.0 $\mu g/m^3$ of air, determined as a time-weighted average (TWA) concentration limit for up to a 8-hour workshift in a 40-hour workweek. The ambient water quality criterion for lead is recommended to be identical to the existing drinking water standard which is 50 $\mu g/L$. Analysis of the toxic effects data resulted in a calculated level that is protective to human health against the ingestion of contaminated water and contaminated aquatic organisms. The available data for lead indicate that acute and chronic toxicity to saltwater aquatic life occur at concentrations as low as 668 and 25$\mu g/L$, respectively; and

would occur at even lower concentrations among the species that are more sensitive than those tested. The exposure to inorganic lead is defined as exposure to the compounds of lead such as its oxides, and salts (inorganic salts such as lead soaps but excluding lead arsenate).

Occupational exposure to inorganic lead should be controlled in such a manner so that no person is exposed to lead at a concentration greater than 0.1 mg/m^3 of air, determined as a time-weighted average (TWA) concentration limit for up to a 10-hour workshift in a 40-hour workweek. All persons subjected to exposure to inorganic lead should be offered biological monitoring at least every 6 months. If blood level of 0.06 mg Pb/100 g or greater is found, and confirmed by a second sample taken within 2 weeks, steps to reduce absorption of lead should be taken as soon as high levels are confirmed.

leaf area index. LAI. The ratio of the leaf surface area of a plant to 1 m^2 of the ground surface beneath it. For example, if the LAI is equal to 3, the plants have developed a leaf surface three times larger than the soil surface beneath, that is, the leaf surface covers an area of 3m^2. Ratios greater than 1:1 occur because plants can produce many layers of leaves, or grow in dense bunches. High LAI values are usually found in undisturbed plant communities while low LAI values are typical of agricultural crops and pioneer communities.

leafy liverworts. The leafy liverworts are a diverse group that include more than two thirds of all known liverworts. The plants are usually well branched and form small mats. Their leaves are often two-lobed, and each grows by means of two distinct apical growing points. The leaves are often arranged in two rows, with a third row of reduced leaves along the lower surface. The leaves of liverworts, like those of mosses, are generally only a single layer of nondiffentiated cells thick. The antheridia and archegonia of the leafy liverworts are characteristically enclosed in a cuplike structure formed by the fusion of two or three leaves. The leafy liverworts are especially abundant in the tropics and subtropics, in regions of heavy rainfall or high humidity, but they are also present in large numbers in temperate latitudes. See also liverworts.

lean body mass. Measure of body composition excluding adipose tissue, i.e., cells, extracellular fluid and skeleton.

leaven. Sour dough, soured by wild yeast. Old method of fermenting bread before commercially prepared yeast was available. It is still used in rye bread.

lectins. Sugar-binding proteins of glycoproteins of non-immune origin which are devoid of enzymatic activity towards the sugars to which they bind and which do not require free glycosidic hydroxyl groups in these sugars for their binding. Lectins have the properties of agglutinating certain cells, stimulating mitotic division in lymphocytes and/or precipitating complex carbohydrates. They are isolated from a wide variety of natural sources including seeds, roots, bark, fungi, bacteria, sea-weeds, sponges, molluscs, fish eggs, body fluids of invertebrates and lower vertebrates, and mammalian cell membranes. Their precise physiological roles are unknown but they are valuable tools in biological studies, such as blood-grouping, mitogenic stimulation of lymphocytes, fractionation of cells, isolation and purification of carbohydrate containing molecules, and certain histochemical studies. Concanavalin A (obtained from jack beans) is a well-known example of a lectin. It has an affinity for the terminal α-D-mannosyl and α-D-glucosyl residues. There is some evidence to indicate that lectins may serve to protect plants against certain pathogenic fungi and insect predators. Lectins are highly specific carbohydrate-binding proteins or glycoproteins that will agglutinate cells and/or precipitate complex carbohydrates. Also known as phytohemagglutinins; phytolectins.

leek. Allium porrum L. is popularly regarded more as a very flavourful vegetable than as a source of flavour. It is widely eaten throughout Europe and Canada, but is less popular in the US, and other parts of the world. The plant is a biennial having a thick bulbous base and tightly packed leaves, which form the fleshy "stem" of the vegetable. The inner leaves and the lower parts of the outer leaves are etiolated by exclusion of light during growth. The flavour is much more delicate the onion and has a pleasant green character. The American wild leek is Allium tricoccum L. The average composition per 100 g is: 1.9 g protein; 6 g carbohydrate; 1 mg iron, 0.4 mg zinc, 6 µg vitamin A (bulb only, leaves 300 µg); 0.1 mg vitamin B_1; 0.6 mg nicotinic acid; 18 mg vitamin C; and food energy 0.13 MJ.

leek drying. Leek, a plant of sturdy stem and large drooping leaves, is used primarily for making soups. The leek plant is diced and dried in a continuous dryer on a belt, at about 4.9 kg/m² or less and sulphited. Temperatures of air from 82-54°C are used as the leek moves through the dryer.

leek oil. The oil obtained by the distillation of freshly crushed whole leek in a yield that may vary widely between 0.005 and 0.02%, depending on the wetness and maturity of the vegetables at the time of distillation. 67 components have been identified in steam-distilled leep oil and concluded that propanethiol, allyl methyl sulphide, methyl propyl sulphide, dipropyl disulphide and methyl propyl trisulphide had distinctive leek-like odour.

Legionella pneumophilia. Gram-negative, short to filamentous rod, motile by a single flagellum; the microorganisms found in aquatic ecosystems; the reservoir is usually contaminated air-conditioning cooling water or a contaminated potable water system. More than 22 species of *Legionella* that cause febrile illness, are known. *Legionella pneumophilia* can be isolated directly from natural sources on several media, including charcoal yeast agar and modified Mueller-Hinton agar enriched with iron and the amino acid cysteine. *Legionella pneumophilia* requires cysteine for growth and utilizes other amino acids as its major source of carbon and energy.

legumin. Globulin protein in pea, bean and lentil.

Leicester cheese. A kind of rennet cheese made in Leicester, UK. It resembles Cheshire cheese and Cheddar cheese, which are usually cured for about one year.

lemon. Family: *Rutaceae*. Genus: *Citrus*. species: *Citrus limonum*. Lemon was used by ships' crews to prevent scurvy and other diseases after the passing of the 1867 Merchant Shipping Act which determined that every vessel visiting a country where lemons could not easily be obtained had to carry enough lemons on broad to

give 25 g of the juice daily to every crew member. Heated lemon slices can be applied to boils, and the fresh juice will help acne, eczema, sinus congestion, pyorrhoea and erysipelas if dabbed on externally. It is helpful for dandruff if applied directly to the scalp and included in the rinse-water. Lemon juice is a wonderful natural antiseptic and destroys bacteria very quickly. It is rich in vitamin C, B-complex vitamins and vitamin P, with calcium, copper, iron, phosphorus, potassium, sulphur and traces of sodium. Lemon juice also contains significant amounts of fructose and citric acid. The average composition per 100 g is: protein 0.5%; fat 0.25%; calcium 26 mg; iron 0.5 mg; vitamin B_1 0.02 mg; nicotinic acid 0.1 mg; vitamin C 30 mg; and food energy 0.06 MJ.

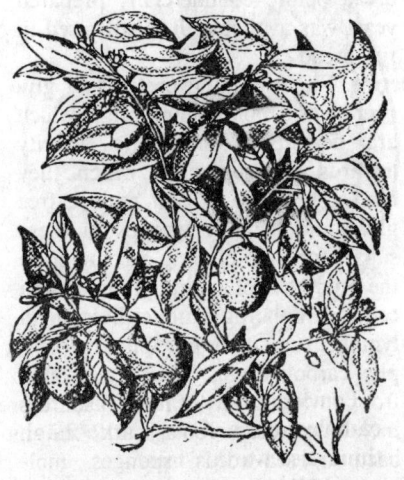

It may be noted that the calcium content falls significantly when the peel is removed. Most interesting of all it is an excellent anti-acid as it actually becomes alkaline when it reaches the stomach. It produces potassium carbonate which neutralizes excess acidity in the bodily fluids. It is far more effective than the readily available commercial anti-acid tablets and should be diluted with a little water and sipped before each meal. Lemon juice is also helpful for liver ailments, asthma, colds, fever, headaches, pneumonia, rheumatism, arthritis and neutritis. It also helps to prevent the accumulation of fatty deposits, so is useful if you are trying to lose weight. Canned or frozen unsweetened lemon juice is similar in nutrients to the fresh lemon, except that it has much less vitamin C, but is light years away in taste. Concentrated lemon juice has five times the strength of fresh.

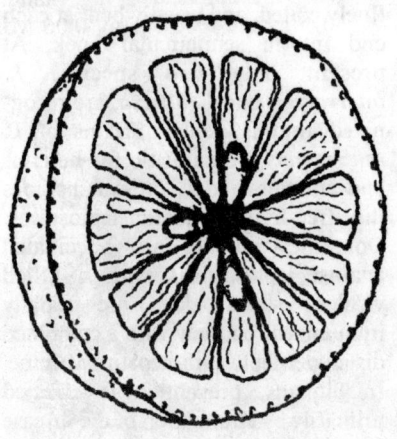

Lemonade concentrate has more carbohydrate and very little of anything else worth while.

lemon balm. Family: *Labiatae.* Genus: *Melissa.* Species: *Melissa officinalis.* It is an attractive herb with yellow or variegated leaves smelling strongly of lemons. It is a great addition to any garden since it maintains a strong attraction for bees. Indeed, it used to be said that a swarm of bees would never desert a hive if a lemon balm plant was close by. A tisane made from the leaves, known as melissa tea, is said to relieve tiredness, soothe hcadaches, and have a calming effect on the nerves. In this capacity, it was a popular drink with Victorian ladies. The fresh leaves may be used in salads, candied for cake decoration, and used to garnish fish and other dishes.

Add them at the last minute to summer drinks and fruit salads, after long infusion they turn unpleasantly brown, and, in recipes, as a lemon peel substitute. An infusion of the leaves make a refreshing skin toner and can be used in water to rinse clothes. The dry leaves lend a refreshing lemony scent to pot pouri blends. The fresh plant contains 0.1% essential oil, 5% tannin, a bitter principle, resin and a succinic acid.

The Arabs introduced it as a medicinal plant especially of benefit in anxiety and depression, and it has been used as a sedative and tonic tea over since. It is a particular favourite of mine for treating all sorts of children's illness. One reason for this is the helpful fact that it tastes quite acceptable and goes down easily. Lemon balm is used in conjunction with other remedies to treat nervous tachycardia and restlessness. It has some hypotensive action and is useful for the sort of people who find themselves in place and life situations they are not ready to accept, and who consequently become dispirited. The fresh leaf rubbed on to a bite will soothe it.

lemon curd. Cooked mixture of sugar, butter, eggs and lemons. Legally, it contains 4% fat, 0.33% citric acid, 1% dried egg or equivalent, 0.125% oil of lemon or 0.25% oil of orange, and not less than 65% soluble solids.

lemon oil. The peel oil, 0.15-0.3% of the weight of the fruit; it contains 90% limonene, along with phellandrene, terpinene, camphene, bisabolene, cadinene, citral, etc.

lemon verbena. *Aloysia triphylla.* One of the most delightful of scented plants, lemon verbena has a strong citrus aroma that is at its most powerful in the early evening. A native of South America, it thrives best in hot climates, where it will grow up to 1.5 m tall and almost as wide. It is, therefore, a good choice as a back-of-the-bed plant in sunny borders. The strong citrus aroma is used to flavour stuffing for meat, poultry, and fish, in fish dishes and sauces, fruit salads, poached fruit, soft drinks, and cream sweets. The herb may be substituted for lemon grass in Southeast Asian dishes. Fresh or dried leaves may be used medicinally, as a mild sedative and as a help for indigestion and flatulence, or may be infused to make a mild skin toner and skim freshener. The dried leaves are an invaluable ingredient in pot pourri, particularly when used to scent bed linen or in a herbal sleep pillow.

Lenhartz diet. For peptic ulcer patients; mainly fluid diet including raw eggs, milk, boiled rice and vegetable purees fed at frequent intervals.

lentils. Family: *Leguminosae.* Genus: *Lens.* Species: *Lens esculenta.* They fall into the same group as peas and beans. They are a valuable source of protein in Third World countries. They are generally made into a complete protein by being served with rice or chapatis. They are about 25% protein and 54% carbohydrate, and contain some vitamin A and B together with good traces of iron and calcium. Because lentils are so high in calories they are extremely good nourishment and are helpful for low blood pressure and anemia. In parts of the Middle East lentil soup is used for ulcerated stomachs and any ulceration in the digestive tract. There is a green variety and an orange-red variety that is commonly imported into Europe from Egypt and India. They are frequently used as a soup thickener in the powdered form. Lentils lose much of their essential amino-acid content during cooking.

Leptospira. The genus containing strictly aerobic spirochetes that use long-chain fatty acids (such as oleic acid) as electron donor and carbon sources. With few exceptions these are the only substrates utilized by leptospiras for growth. The leptospira cell is thin, finely coiled, and usually bent at each end into a semicircular hook. At present only two species, *L. interrogans* and *L. biflexa*, are recognized in this genus. Strains of *L. interrogans* are parasitic for humans and animals, and *L. biflexa* includes the free-living aquatic leptospiras. Domestic animals are vaccinated against leptospirosis with a killed virulent strain; dogs are usually immunized routinely with a combined distemper-leptospira-hepatitis vaccine. In humans, prevention is effected primarily by elimination of the disease from animals.

lethal synthesis. The process whereby an enzyme catalyzes a reaction with a compound, other than its normal substrate, and leads to the formation of a product which then acts as an inhibitor of a different enzyme.

lettuce. Family: *Compositae.* Genus: *Lectuca.* Species: *Lactuca sativa.* The plant is very leafy and contains a milk-white latex. In young plants the leaves are crowded on a short stem, forming a close rosette. In older plants, the stem elongates greatly and bears a panicle of heads of yellowish flowers. The achenes are flat, ribbed, and contracted into a slender beak bearing numerous soft white or brownish pappus hairs which radiate outward like a parasol.

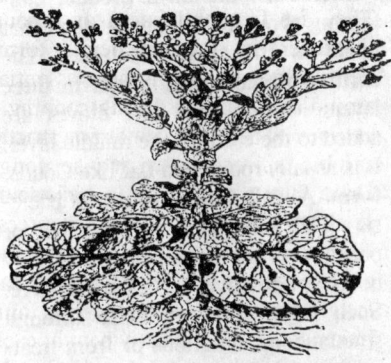

Many varieties have been developed in cultivation. Although there are minor culinary uses of lettuce, as in soups, the vegetable is predominantly raised for its value as a salad vegetable. Lettuce is popular because of its fresh, pleasant taste in combination with its low caloric value. Based upon nutrient values, lettuce is comparable with the artichoke, asparagus, celery, and cauliflower. Lettuce is mostly self-fertilized. The anthers dehisce from the inside as the style elongates and the floret opens. Thus, the pollen from a particular floret has a great advantage over foreign pollen. The pollen in heavy and sticky, and crossing, when it occurs, is accomplished by insects, but probably not by wind.

The physiology of lettuce seed germination has been studied extensively. It has been shown that seeds of some lettuce cultivars, which are subject to dormancy, react to red and far-red light. Red light converts a substance called phytochrome to a state which activates the germination process. Far-red light or darkness converts phytochrome to another state which inhibits germination. The process is reversible. Lettuce seed has a relatively short life and are stored at room temperature, it may lose viability in 2 or 3 years; sometimes in as little as one year. At 10°C and 50% relative humidity, lettuce seed will survive about 10 years. Cultivated lettuce is usually divided into six types:

(a) Crisphead,
(b) butterhead,
(c) cos or romaine,
(d) looseleaf or cutting,
(e) stalk or stem, and
(f) Latin.

Cultivars of these types were developed long before plant breeding became more scientific, and it is unlikely that any sophisticated genetic techniques were involved in their development. Lettuce is not a very valuable food: the vitamin C is only one-seventh of that of cabbage. The average composition per 100 g is: protein 0.9%; fat 0.1%; calcium 18 mg; iron 0.29 mg; vitamin A 42 µg; vitamin B_1 0.04 mg; vitamin B_2 0.05 mg; nicotinic acid 0.1 mg; vitamin C 5 mg; and food energy 0.05 MJ.

Cos lettuce has slightly more calories, protein, carbohydrates and fibre than Iceberg as well as more calcium, phosphorus, iron, potassium and vitamins A and C. Butterhead lettuce has half the vitamin A of, and less vitamin C than, Cos (or Romaine). The latter contains a substantial amount of vitamin E. Because all lettuce is high in iron it is recommended for anemia as well as urinary infections, constipation, obesity, rheumatism and arthritis and, if taken in heroic doses, for insomnia.

Iceberg lettuce is so common that is really does not require any kind of a physical description to speak of. To the ancient Egyptians, however, at least one kind of romaine-type lettuce that grew on the island of Kos off the Turkish coast, held sexual symbolism. The long, stiff leaves were thought to resemble a man's sexual organ and the milky juice from them the semen emitted during ejaculation.

leucocytes. White blood cells, normally 5,000-9,000 per cubic mm; includes polymorphonuclear neutrophils, lymphocytes, monocytes, polymorphonuclear eosinophils, and polymorphonuclear basophils. A white cell count determines the total; a differential cell count estimates the numbers of each type. Fever, hemorrhage, violent exercise, cause an increase - leucocytosis; starvation and debilitating conditions cause a decrease - leucopoenia.

leucocytosis. Increase in the white cells in the blood.

leucopoenia. Decrease in the white cells in the blood.

leucosin. One of the water-soluble proteins of wheat flour.

leucovorin. Growth factor for *Leuconostoc citrovorum,* related to folic acid.

levitin. One of the proteins of egg yolk, about one-fifth of the total, the remainder being vitellin. Rich in sulphur and accounts for half of the sulphur in the yolk.

levulose. Levulose is a name applied in earlier years to D-fructose. This name had the advantage of calling attention to the levorotatory property of one of the two simple sugars derived from sucrose by hydrolysis, in contrast to the dextrorotatory property of the other hydrolysis product which was called dextrose (now D-glucose). These names dextrose and levulose are not acceptable chemical names partly because both sugars have optical antipodes for which the names levo-dextrose or dextro-levulose would seem unfortunate.

leyden, (Komijne kaas) cheese. A hard spiced variety of cheese made in the Netherlands; the farm product containing about 10% more fat than that made in the cheese factories. The curd is placed in the hoops in three layers. Cumin seed and cloves are added to the curd for the middle layer. It is usually round and flat like Gouda.

L-form. A wall-deficient form of bacteria. The loss may be complete or partial and the parent organism may be Gram-positive or Gram-negative. Such organisms can arise through spontaneous mutations or from treatments such as growth in isotonic or hypertonic media containing penicillin. If all the traces of peptidoglycan disappear, bacteria cannot resynthesize it because preexisting wall is necessary to construct new peptidoglycan. In such case, the L-form may be stable; that is, it may continue to grow and may reproduce after the penicillin treatment has ceased. Other L-forms sometimes synthesize a wall once again. L-forms are not closely related to mycoplasmas.

Lichenes. A group consisting of organisms that are symbiotic associations between a fungus (usually one of the *Ascomycetes*) and an alga (from the *Chlorophyta* or *Cyanophyta*). The fungus usually makes up most of the plant body and the cells of the alga are distributed within it. The alga photosynthesizes and passes most of its food to the fungus and the fungus protects the algal cells. The lichen reproduces by means of fungal spores, which must find a suitable alga on germination. Lichens are generally slow growing but are capable of living in very cold regions. They are also capable of living in dry environments where, other kinds of plants cannot grow. They may form a flattened crust or be erect and branching. Lichens consist of a tight association of many fungal cells, within which the algal cells are embedded. The shape of the lichen is determined primarily by the fungal partner, and a wide variety of fungi are able to form lichen associations. The diversity of algal types is much smaller, and many different kinds of lichens may have the same algal component. Some lichens contain cyanobacteria instead of algae as the phototrophic component. Many lichens grow as epiphytes, especially on tree trunks. Some of the species of lichens are very sensitive to air pollution and quickly disappear in areas experiencing heavy air pollution and have been used as indicator species. One reason for great sensitivity of lichens to air pollution is that they absorb and concentrate materials from rainwater and air and have no means for excreting them, so that the lethal concentrations are easily reached.

licorice root. *Glycyrrhiza glabra.*

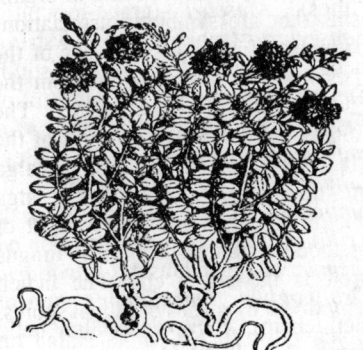

Licorice is a perennial plant found wild in southern and central Europe and parts of Asia, and cultivated in the US and Canada to some extent. The woody rootstock is wrinkled and brown on the outside, yellow on the inside and tastes sweet. Fresh licorice is considered to be best, with roots neither too large nor too thin, tender and of uniform consistency. It has been found to be useful in treating hoarseness of voice and throat.

Liederkranz cheese. The trade name of a soft, surface-ripened variety of cheese that is made in Ohio from cow's whole milk. It is rectangular in shape. The cheese is somewhat similar to Limburger in body, flavour, aroma and degree of ripening. The milk is pasteurized, starter is added, and the milk is set with rennet at a temperature of about 30°C. The curd is cut with 1.3 cm curd thrives, and when it has firmed sufficiently it is dipped into perforated metal forms. After the whey has drained off, the cheeses are removed from the forms, salted with dry salt, and then cured at a temperature of about 7°C for 3-4 weeks. The surface-growing microorganisms produce progressive ripening from the surface inward. The cheeses, which are rather perishable, are wrapped in tinfoil for marketing. They may be wrapped and shipped after curing for 12-15 days. They are about 6.4 cm long 3.8 cm. wide, and an inch thick, and they weight 142 to 170 gm. The average composition is: moisture 54%; fat 24.2% (fat in the solids, more than 50%); protein 16.8%; and ash 3.9%.

ligases. A class of enzymes which catalyze the formation of covalent bonds using the energy released by the cleavage of ATP. Ligases are important in the synthesis and repair

of many biological molecules, including DNA. Degree of bond formation by ligases is proportional to the amount of ATP available in the cell at a particular instant. Their representative subclasses include:
(a) enzymes catalyzing formation of C-N bonds, *e.g.*, glutamine synthetase; and
(b) enzymes catalyzing formation of C-C bonds, for example, acetyl-CoA carboxylase.

light chain. One of the two polypeptide chains that are linked to two heavy chains to form the immunoglobulin molecule. The molecular mass of a light chain is about 25,000 and that of a heavy chain is about 50,000. The light chains of type K and type L immunoglobulins are known, respectively, as κ(kappa) and λ(lambda) chains.

light strand. 1. A polynucleotide chain that is either not labeled with a heavy isotope or that is labeled with a light isotope.
2. The naturally occurring polynucleotide chain of a duplex that has a lower density than the complementary chain.

lignin. The noncellulosic portion of wood, of which it constitutes from 25 to 35%. It is an amorphous organic polymer whose function is to hold the cellulose fibers together. It is a complex polymer of somewhat variable composition, made up from alcohols, sugars, aromatic amino acids and phenolic substances. It is one of the main constituents of wood. Lignified tissues include sclerenchyma and xylem. Lignin is deposited during secondary thickening of cells walls. The degree of lignification varies from slight in protoxylem to heavy in sclerenchyma and some xylem vessel, but values of 25-35% lignin and 50% cellulose are average. Lignin is characteristically stained yellow by aniline sulphate or chloride, and red by phloroglucinol with hydrochloric acid.

lignoceilulose. Alternative name for lignin.

lignoceric acid. Long-chain fatty acid containing total of 24 carbon atoms (tetracosanoic acid); present in the cerebrosides and sphingomyelins.

Lily family: *Liliaceae.* Lily flowers have 3 sepals and 3 petals that look alike (tepals), 6 stamens, and a single pistil with a superior ovary of 3 fused carpels. Fruit types are septicidal or loculicidal capsules or berries. This large family of about 3,500 species consists mostly of perennial herbs with narrow, parallel-veined leaves and underground storage organs such as rhizomes, bulbs, corms, or tubers. Some plants are evergreen succulents, as in Aloe and Haworthia or vines as in Smilax.

The family include: *Allium* spp. (onion, shallot, leek, garlic, chives), *Asparagus officinalis: Alloe: Colchicum* (colchicine), *Urginea* (red squill); *Convallaria majalis* (lily-of-the-valley), *Frittillaria, Gloriosa, Haworthia, Hemerocallis* (day lily), *Hosta, Hyacinthus* (hyacinth), *Kniphofia* (torch lily, red-hot-poker), *Lilium* spp. (lilies), *Muscari* (grape-hyacinth), *Sansevieria* (snake plant, bowstring-hemp, leopard lily), *Scilla* (squill, *Smilax* (greenbriar), *Tulipa* (tulip); *Erythronium* (dogtooth violet), *Maianthemum* (false lily-of-the-valley), *Lilium, Polygonatum* (Solomon's seal), *Smilacina* (false Solomon's seal), *Trillium, Uvularia* (bell-wort); *Amianthemum* (stagger-grass), *Convallaria, Ornithoglum umbellatum* (star-of-Bethlehem), *Veratrum* (false hellebore), *Zygadenus* (death camas).

lima bean. Family: *Leguminosae.* Genus:

Phaseolus. Species: *Phaseolus lunatus.* A variety of beans which occurs as both a bush and pole bean and of high economic value. Three principal types are:
(a) large lima bean (large and flat);
(b) Dreer lima bean, seeds of which are smaller than the large lima, rounded, and rather closely crowded in the pod. Along with the sieva bean, the Dreer lima bean is sometimes referred to as a dwarf lima bean or dwarf butter bean; and
(c) small lima or sieve bean (*Phaseolus lunatus*).

The plant is quite widely used as forage for livestock. Lima beans are particularly rich in iron and so excellent for treating anemia. Being high in protein they are good for body-building and in South America are given to people suffering from hemorrhoids.

Limburger cheese. A soft, rennet curd, surface ripened, variety of cheese made form fresh, whole or partly skimmed milk. It is made similar to Brick cheese in the US, except that the curd is much softer. After cutting, draining and salting, the cheese is ripened from one to two months. The ripening room should have a relatively high humidity and a temperature of about 16°C. When ripe the cheese possesses a very strong odour and flavour. Limburger was first made near Limburg, Belgium, and is now made in large quantities in many parts of Europe and United States. Surface-ripening organisms are responsible for the characteristic flavour and aroma. Film yeasts predominate at first followed by *B. linens* and the reddish yellow smear. Federal standards recommends that moisture should not be more than 50%; and fat not less than 50% in the solids.

lime (fruit). *Citrus aurantifolia.* One of the two principal sour fruits produced by citrus trees, the other being the lemon. Of all citrus crops, lemons and limes rank third in total world production accounting for about 9% of total tonnage. It is a much poorer source of vitamin C than the lemon. The lime is a hesperidium, that is, a berry with a tough, leathery rind. The lime has distinctive flavedo and albedo, that is, the green outer layer and the whitish inner portion of the rind characteristic of all citrus fruits. The lime also has oil glands in the fruit segments and juice vesicles. The fruit develops parthenocarpically (without requiring fertilization) and visible pollen is lacking. Like lemon trees, lime trees may blossom much of the year, with the heaviest opening or blooms following a cool winter, or a rather long dry period. Lime trees are of medium size, much branched, thick-headed, with small thorns, and require very little pruning. Pruning is often limited to that required to avoid overlapping of branches of one tree of the next.

Limes fall into two main categories; acid types of sweet type. The acid type is better known and is the only type grown commercially in the US. The acid type is further divided into:
(a) Mexican group; and
(b) Tahiti group. The lime (*Citrus aurantifolia* Christm.) is of the family *Rutaceae* (rue family) and of the subfamily Aurantiodeae. *C aurantifolia* is one of 16 recognized species of the genus Citrus.

The classification and naming of citrus fruits has posed difficulties for many years and new research findings are tending to upset prior systematics. Some authorities place the Tahiti lime in a separate category

(*C. latifolia*); others consider it to be a hybrid rather than a true lime. The average composition per 100 g of the lime juice is: protein 0.32%; fat 0.1%; calcium 15 mg; iron 0.18 mg; vitamin B_1 0.01 mg; vitamin C 10 mg; and food energy 0.07 MJ.

limit dextrin. When a branched polysaccharide such as glycogen is hydrolyzed enzymatically (*e.g.*, by phosphorylase) glucose is split off step by step until the branch point is reached. The hydrolysis then stops leaving what is termed a limit dextrin. Further hydrolysis requires different enzymes.

Limmisax. Trade name for saccharine.

Limmits. Trade name for a slimming preparation which is composed of whole-meal biscuits with a vitamin-methylcellulose mixture as filler; contains vitamin A, B_1, B_2, nicotinamide, C and D with iron, calcium, iodide and phosphorus. It is intended to replace a meal or meal with a reduced calorie diet. Six biscuits contain about 4.2 MJ of food energy.

limonin. Bitter principle in the albedo of Valencia orange. Similarly, isolimonin is the bitter principle of the Navel orange. Both are present in a non-bitter, water-soluble state, and are liberated into the juice during extraction. On standing they slowly hydrolyze and the juice becomes bitter. Limonin is not present in the ripe fruit.

linoleic acid. $C_{17}H_{31}COOH$. A straight-chain fatty acid with 18 carbon atoms and two double bonds (a diene), with double bonds at 9-10 and 12-13 carbons. Also known as octadeca-dienoic acid.

linolenic acid. $C_{17}H_{29}COOH$. A straight-chain fatty acid containing 18 carbon atoms with three double bonds at 9-10, 12-13 and 15-16 carbons. It is a major component of linseed oil and its high degree of unsaturation is responsible for the drying properties of the oil. At one time included with the essential fatty acids. Also known as octadecartrienoic acid.

linseed. Family: *Linaceae*. Genus: *Linum*. Species: *Linum usitatissimum* (fibre and seed flax). Linseed oil was used in food preparation by the Greeks and Romans and continues to be used in this way in Central Europe. Its flavour deteriorates on exposure to the air but if it is refined and deodorized it is palatable and a good source of protein (33%) as well as being high in minerals, such as phosphorus and calcium. It is also an extremely useful poultice and a good chest rub. It can be applied to boils and furuncles and to ease chest pains of a bronchitic or pulmonary origin.

The seeds themselves, which are rich in mucilage, act as a gentle bulk laxative and are useful as a tonic for spastic constipation if taken with plenty of liquid. Take up to 6 g of crushed seed, three times a day. They contain a cyanogenic glycoside called linamarase but there is no fear of poisoning because it breaks up in the stomach only partially. Linseed has the dual ability to expand in the gut so exciting peristalsis, while at the same time reducing irritation and blocking reabsorption. Linseed also deodorizes the bowel by slow release of tiny amounts of hydrocyanide.

Lintner value. A measure of the diastatic activity using soluble starch as a substrate and measuring the effect by Fehling's solution; applied to flour, malt extract, etc.

liothyronine. An alternative name for the L-triiodothyronine, the most potent of the hormones of the thyroid gland. It is used as an aid to weight reduction by stimulating the metabolism of the body.

lipase. Enzyme that hydrolyzes fat to glycerol and fatty acid. It has a low specificity and may attack any triglyceride or long-chain ester. It is present in the intestinal juice and in many seeds and grains. Sometimes responsible for development of rancidity in stored foods. Lipases from different sources, *e.g.*, digestive juices or seeds, appear to be similar but attack the substrates at different rates.

lipid digestion. In the small intestine fat is hydrolyzed by pancreatic lipase. As such pancreatic lipase is inactive and is activated by calcium salt and bile salts. Bile salts are essential for emulsification of fat. Soluble proteins also help in the emulsification land absorption of fatty acid. Intestinal juice also contains lipase which can act upon any fat unaffected by pancreatic lipase. Partially hydrolyzed lipid is readily absorbed in the last portion of duodenum and proximal part of jejunum. Lipids are also absorbed by pinocytosis process, lipids pass through the membrane by diffusion. Lipids, whether absorbed as such or resynthesized in the epithelial cell enter the lymphatic vessels as a milky emulsion called chyle. The minute droplets of fat are chylomicron. Chylomicron consists of triglycerides, phospholipid. Free fatty acid and they are surrounded by a thin layer of protein. These particles passes through lymphatic duct of abdominal cavity and then enters into the blood.

lipids. General term embracing fats and oils and waxes, as well as the complex compounds, the phosphatides and cerebrosides, *i.e.*, all naturally occurring compounds of fatty acids which are insoluble in water and soluble in nonpolar organic solvents, such as chloroform, ether, benzene, etc. Lipids are broadly classified into two categories:

(a) complex lipids, which are esters of long-chain fatty acids and include the glycerides (which constitute the fats and oils of animals and plants), glycolipids, phospholipids, and waxes; and

(b) simple lipids, which do not contain fatty acids and include the steroids and terpenes.

Lipids have a variety of functions in living organisms. Fats and oils are convenient and concentrated means of storing energy. Phospholipids and sterols, such as cholesterol, are major components of cell membranes. Waxes provide vital waterproofing for body surfaces. Terpenes include vitamins A, E, and K, while steroids include the adrenal hormones, sex hormones, and bile acids. Lipids can combine with proteins to form lipoproteins, *e.g.*, in cell membranes. In bacterial cell walls, lipids may associate with polysaccharides to form lipopolysaccharides. Lipids are generally classified into various groups such as:

Simple lipids: 1. Triglycerides or fats and oils and fatty acid esters of glycerol, *e.g.*, corn oil, cottonseed oil, lard, butter.

2. Waxes are fatty acid esters of long-chain alcohols.

3. Steroids are lipids derived from partially or completely hydrogenated phenanthrene, *e.g.,* cholesterol and ergosterol.

Complex lipids: 1. Phosphatides or phospholipids are lipids which contain phosphorus and, in many instances nitrogen; *e.g.*, lecithin, cephalin.

2. Glycolipids are lipids which contain carbohydrate residues; such as sterol glycosides, cerebrosides, and plant phytoglycolipids.

3. The sphingolipids are lipids containing the long-chain amino alcohol sphingosine and its derivatives, e.g., ceramides, sphingomyelins. Lipids are transported in the blood in the form of lipoproteins, which are synthesized in the liver.

Lipids encompass the following broad bands of biological roles:

(a) basic structural units of cellular membranes and cytologically distinct sub-cellular bodies such as chloroplasts and mitochondria;

(b) compartmentalizing units for metabolically active proteins localized in membranes;

(c) a store of chemical energy and carbon skeletons; and

(d) primary transport systems of non-polar material through biological fluids.

There are also the more physiologically specific lipid-hormones and lipid-vitamins. On a molecular level, lipids are also classified into simple lipids and compound lipids. The simple lipids include neutral lipids or glycerides, which are esters of glycerol and fatty acids, and the waxes which are esters of long chain monohydric alcohols and fatty acids. Compound lipid have one of the fatty acid parts replaced, such that complete hydrolysis gives only two fatty acids; the phospholipids or phosphatides are particularly important examples. In these a fatty acid group is replaced by a phosphate in which P-O-H hydrogen can be further replaced by a wide range of derivatives.

lipoamide. The dipeptide-like structure, formed by linking a molecule of lipoic acid through its carboxyl group to the ε-amino group of a lysine residue, that is part of the enzyme for which lipoic acid serves as a coenzyme.

lipocaic. Unidentified factor in the pancreas that prevents the deposition of fat in the liver.

lipochromes. Plant pigments soluble in fats and organic solvents, e.g., chlorophyll, carotenoids.

lipofuscin. An insoluble pigment that accumulates in some ageing tissues. It is formed from malondialdehyde which polymerizes with itself and some other tissue breakdown products. Malondialdehyde is formed during the auto-oxidation of membrane polyunsaturated lipids in a chain reaction started by free radical formation.

lipoic acid. A sulphur-containing fatty acid consisting of fatty acid chain bridged by a disulphide linkage found in a wide variety of natural materials. It is an essential component in metabolism, although it is active in extremely minute amounts. Lipoic acid is classified with the water-soluble B vitamins. It is one of the coenzymes involved in the decarboxylation of pyruvate by the enzyme pyruvate dehydrogenase. This reaction has to take place before carbohydrates can enter the Krebs cycle during aerobic respiration. Good sources of lipoic acid include liver and yeast.

lipoids. A term applied to a group of substances, including fats and esters possessing analogous properties, e.g., lecithins, phosphatins, sterols. Also known as lipins.

lipolysis. The breakdown of storage lipids in living organisms. Most long-term energy reserves are in the form of triglycerides in fats and oils. When these are needed, e.g., during starvation, lipase enzymes convert the triglycerides into glycerol and the component fatty acids. These are then transported to tissues and oxidized to provide energy. Lipolysis is under hormonal control, and is effected in the body, largely in the gut, by the lipase enzymes. Hormones (e.g., ACTH and adrenaline) increase lipolysis from adipose tissue thus making more fatty acid available in the blood plasma.

lipolytic. A term denoting fat-splitting. Lipases are called lipolytic enzymes.

lipolytic enzyme. An enzyme that catalyzes the hydrolysis of fats and other esters to yield alcohols and acids. Also known as lipase; stearolytic enzyme.

lipolytic rancidity. Some microorganisms produce lipases,which are also present in tissues. In stored foods they hydrolyze the fats to free fatty acids, so-called lipolytic rancidity. As the enzyme is destroyed by heat this type of rancidity occurs only in uncooked foods.

lipomodulin. An antiphospholipase protein closely related to, and possibly a precursor of, macrocortin.

Lipomul. Trade name for a mixture of 10% glucose and 40% vegetable oil.

lipopolysaccharides. The conjugate polysaccharides in which the non-carbohydrate part is a lipid. Lipopolysaccharides are a constituent of the cell walls of certain bacteria. The lipopolysaccharides are important for several reasons other than the avoidance of host defenses. Since the core polysaccharide usually contains charged sugar and phosphate, it contributes to the negative charge on the bacterial surface.

lipoproteins. A large group of conjugated proteins characterized by their high content of lipid. The lipid components consist of triacyl glycerol, phospholipid, and cholesterol (or its esters) in remarkably consistent proportions within each class of lipoproteins. The protein components in turn, have a relatively high propor-tion of nonpolar amino acid residues which can participate in the binding of lipids. They occur in the organism as either soluble complexes, e.g., in serum, or in insoluble complexes such as are present in nervous tissue or in subcellular components of cells. Lipids are ubiquitous in the animal organism and are probably always associated with protein; it is doubtful that any lipid exists in the completely free state. The soluble lipoproteins in serum constitute the most widely studied group of this class of conjugated proteins. Normal human serum contains 0.5-0.7% lipid. These lipids-cholesterol, cholesterol esters, phosphatides and triglycerides, are either insoluble or only slightly soluble in aqueous solutions, although in serum they are present in solution in relatively high concentrations. It is the association of the lipids with protein that enables these water-soluble materials to exist in a soluble form. The lipoproteins of plasma are soluble in isotonic solution but are insoluble in water, and thus behave like euglobulins. Some lipoproteins are used to transport fats to metabolic sites while others are used to form the structures of cell membranes. They are found in membranes of mitochondria, nuclei, endoplasmic reticuli, and microsomes. The electron transport system in mitochondria appears to contain large amounts of lipoproteins. Lamellar lipoprotein systems occur in myelin sheath of nerves, photoreceptive structures, chloroplasts, and membranes of bacteria. They function in lipid transport between sites of fat deposition and liver, and between liver and small intestine.

lipovitellenin. A lipoprotein complex of egg comprising about one-sixth of the solids of the yolk.

Liptauer cheese. A sharp-tasting variety of cheese made in Hungary. It is similar to Brinsen cheese; condiments are often added to it.

liqueurs. Prepared from distilled alcohol by the addition of fruit flavours and sugar.

liquified herring. Herring reduced to liquid state by enzyme action at slightly acid pH; used as protein concentrate for animal feed.

liquorice. Liquorice root and extract are obtained from the plant. *Glycyrrhiza glabra;* stick liquorice is the crude evaporated extract of the root. The plant has been grown in the Pontefract district of Yorkshire since sixteenth century, hence the name of Pontefract cakes for the sugar confection of liquorice.

Lisbon lemon. A variety of lemon having elliptical-oblong shaped fruit, tapering to an inconspicuous neck. From the apex, it tapers to a prominent, symmetrical, often pointed nipple. The texture is generally smoother and less markedly ribbed than the Eureka. The rind is of medium thickness and the surface is finely pitted. The color is yellow at maturity. The juice is of good flavour, very acidic and easily extracted. The seed content is variable, ranging from a few to none.

The tree is densely foliated, thorny, more vigorous, more upright growing, and more productive than the Eureka. Lisbon is also more resistant than Eureka to frost, heat and wind. Lisbon has been accepted as the most desirable variety in the desert or very warm locations. The variety produces more of one-bloom crop than Eureka, and with a shorter harvesting period.

litchi. *Litchi chinensis.* Of the family Sapindaceae (soapberry family), the litchi tree is probably native of China, and is the best known for its fruit (usually spelled lychee) and which, when dried, is called the litchi nut. The flavour of the fresh litchi may be described as slightly acidic and strongly suggestive of the Royal Ann cherry, particularly when cooked. One authority has described the fruit as delicious, perhaps, as that of any fruit in existence. In its dried form, there is little resemblance to the fresh fruit, the dried form often being likened to that of a raisin. The litchi tree has pinnately compound leaves, the leaflets of which are lanceolate and leathery. The small flowers are borne in panicles, and have no petals. The fruit is roughly spherical, 2.5-4 cm in diameter, with a hard, brittle rind. Within this rind is a fleshy, translucent pulp, the aril, which is the part that is eaten. The fruit contains a single seed. The average composition per 100 g is: 0.9 g protein; 0.5 g fat; 16 g carbohydrate; 0.04 mg vitamin B_1; 0.04 mg vitamin B_2; 0.3 mg nicotinic acid; 50 mg vitamin C; 0.5 mg iron; and food energy 0.28 MJ. Also spelled as lychee.

lithium. Lithium, the lightest of all metallic elements, was discovered in 1817 by Johann Auguste Arfvedson, a Swedish investigator working with Berzelius. Emil Rosenberg, a Philadelphia physician, circa 1876, demonstrated the element's presence, along with that of sodium, potassium, and calcium, in tissue and other biological materials. Its occurrence is rather widespread. Lithium is found is most rocks of igneous origin. The concentration of lithium in sea water is about 0.1 mg/kg. However, high concentrations are found in certain brines such as Searle's Lake in California or Great Salt lake in Utah. The latter is estimated to contain four million tons of lithium chloride.

Lithium is found in plants and in all animal tissues and fluids. The mean lithium concentration in normal tissue is: lymph nodes, 0.13-0.27 µg/g wet weight; lung, 0.05-0.07 µg/g; brain, 3-5 ng/g; testis, 2-4 ng/g; and human blood, 4-8 ng/g. It has been estimated the total dietary intake of lithium by an adult to be about 2 mg per day. Some researchers consider an intake of 54-160 µg per day to be more likely. The function of lithium is unknown. No biochemical or physiological system has been found to be lithium dependent. However, the element is tolerated in considerable quantity when compared with the limits for other non-essential metals, for example, beryllium, is neighbour in the periodic table. Lithium enters into various biochemical activities. Enzymes activated by potassium are inhibited by lithium, and the action of calcium and of magnesium are also antagonized. Lithium affects carbohydrate metabolism at several points, namely, hexokinase activity, activation of liver adenyl cylase and protein kinase, glycogen synthesis, and pyruvate kinase activity. A lithium ion can replace both sodium and potassium in some active transport mechanisms. *In vivo*, as well as *in vitro*, studies indicate that the passive diffusion of lithium resembles that of sodium. While therapeutic doses do not appear to alter sodium or potassium concentrations very much, the ion does induce changes in calcium metabolism. Serum calcium concentrations are elevated above normal, and urinary calcium is decreased in the presence of lithium ions. Lithium became an important agent in the therapeutics of psychiatry. Lithium seemed to have a specific effect upon mania. Lithium chloride had been utilized as a salt substitute in the 1940s, but by 1950 the practice was discontinued following reported of serious side effects and fatality resulting from the salt's use.

Ionic lithium is almost completely absorbed from the gastrointestinal tract. Peak concentrations in the plasma are attained within two to four hours following an oral dose; absorption is complete in approximately eight hours. Lithium does not seems to bind to plasma proteins. It passes through the blood-brain barrier slowly and achieves a concentration in the cerebrospinal fluid equivalent to 40% of that in plasma. Lithium levels in saliva are several times greater than those in plasma. The ion is also excreted in the milk of lactating women receiving lithium therapy. Lithium is primarily eliminated from the body via the kidneys. Approximately 95% of a single dose is excreted in urine 4%, in sweat, and only 1% via faeces. Nausea, vomiting, profuse diarrhoea, and lethargy are among the characteristic symptoms of lithium intoxication. Some patients may experience confusion, and exhibit hyperreflexia, tremors and dysarthrias. In acute incidents, seizures may ensue and progress to coma and death. Other side effects arising from lithium therapy include hypotension, cardiac arrythmias, proteinuria, edema, polyuria and polydipsia. The latter two symptoms may be quite marked in certain patients and renal failure can develop. The occurrence of changes in the size and function of the thyroid has been noted and well documented. Plasma or blood lithium levels must be monitored rather closely, for the salts have a low therapeutic index. A dose that may be adequate for one patient may be potentially lethal for another. Furthermore, dose requirements for an individual patient are also dependent upon changes in body physiology.

litmus. A colorant used primarily as pH indicator. The colouring principle is azolitmin $(C_7H_7HO_4)$ which is pH sensitive, giving the well-known colour change from red in acid to blue in alkaline media.

Livarot cheese. A soft rennet cheese made in France and deriving its name from the village in which it is made. It is much like Camembert cheese. When ripe, the cheese is wrapped with liache leaves (*Typha latiofolia*). In about four months, it is coloured with annatto and marketed.

liver. The edible organ of many animals used as food. It is extremely valuable source of nutrients. Fish liver oils are the major source of vitamins A and D. Composition of animal liver (after cooking); protein 30%; fat 16%; carbohydrate 4%; iron 20 mg; zinc 12 mg; vitamin A 13 mg; vitamin B_1 0.3 mg; vitamin B_2 3.5 mg; nicotinic acid 15 mg; vitamin C 20 mg; vitamin D 0.5 µg; and food energy 1.2 MJ.

liver factor 2. Obsolete name for pantothenic acid.

liver filtrate factor. Obsolete name for pantothenic acid.

liver, fatty infiltration of. Under the influence of liver poisons, and in the absence from the diet of substances containing methyl groups, there is a flow of fats to the liver, the so-called fatty liver. This is prevented by lipotropic substances, which include choline, methionine, and a pancreatic extract called lipocaic. The affliction is aggravated on a high-fat diet and is found clinically on chronic low-protein diets.

liverworts. *Class: Hepaticae.* Liverworts are small plants that are generally less conspicuous than mosses. Their name dates from the ninth century, when it was thought, because of the liver shaped outline of the gametophyte in some genera, that these plants might be useful in treating diseases of the liver, the medieval "Doctrine of Signatures," the theory that the outward appearance of a body signals its special properties. Wort simply means herb and so appears as part of many plant names. The gametophytes of some liverworts are flattened, dorsiventral (having distinct upper and lower surfaces) thalli, which grow from an apical meristem. The gametophytes of most species, however, are leafy and grow from a single apical cell, which resembles an inverted pyramid with a base and three sides. Daughter cells are cut off from this single cell. The rhizoids of liverworts are single-celled, unlike those of mosses, which contain several cells each. The gametophytes generally develop directly from spores.

The sporophytes of liverworts are, in general, less complex than those of mosses, and their capsules have very different mechanisms for the release of spores.

Thallose liverworts. They are nonleafy liverworts which display a wide variety of forms, including members of the order *Marchantiales*, a familiar and widespread group comprising some 450 species. They can be found on moist, shaped banks and in other suitable habitats such as flowerpots in a cool greenhouse. The thallus is many cells thick, about 30 at the midrib and approximately 10 in the thinner portions, and is sharply differentiated into a thin, chlorophyll-rich upper (dorsal) portion and a thicker, colourless lower (ventral) region. The lower surface bears two kinds of rhizoids, as well as rows of scales. The upper surface is divided into raised regions, each of which marks the limits of an underlying air chamber and has a large pore that leads to this chamber. Each chamber and has a large pore that leads to this chamber. Each chamber has a number of strands of tissue that are rich in chloroplasts, but the walls and floor of the chamber are colourless. There is also some differentiation among the layers of colourless cells below the chamber, particular cells being specialized for storage of starch. On the basis of sporophyte structure, *Riccia* and *Ricciocarpus* are among the simplest of liverworts. *Ricciocarpus,* which is amphibious, is bisexual, that is both sex organs arise on the same plant. Although some species of *Riccia* are amphibious, most are terrestrial. *Riccia* gametophytes may be unisexual or bisexual. The sporophytes are deeply embedded within the dichotomously branched gametophytes of *Riccia* and *Ricciocarpus* and consist of little more than a sporangium. No special mechanism for spore dispersal occurs in these sporophytes. When the portion of the gametophyte containing mature sporophytes dies and decays, the spores are liberated.

One of the most familiar of liverworts is *Marchantia,* a fairly widespread terrestrial genus, which grows on moist soil and rocks. Its dichotomously branched gametophytes are larger than those of *Riccia* and *Ricciocarpus.* Unlike the latter two genera, in which the sex organs are distributed along the upper, or dorsal surface of the thallus, *Marchantia* has its gametangia restricted to specialized erect structures called game-

tophores. The gametophytes of *Marchantia* are strictly unisexual, and the male and female gametophytes can readily be identified by their gametophores, which are quite distinct from one another. The antheridia are borne in disk-headed stalks *(antheridiophores)* and the archegonia on an umbrella, headed stalks *(archegoniophores).* The sporophytes of *Marchanita* are more highly differentiated than those of *Riccia* and *Ricciocarpus,* consisting of a foot, a short stalk or seta, and a capsule or sporangium. In addition to spores, the mature sporangium contains elongate cells, called *elaters,* with spirally arranged hygroscopic (moisture-absorbing wall thickenings. The walls of these cells are sensitive to very slight changes in humidity, and by twisting action they aid in spore dispersal after the capsule dehisces into a number of petal-like segments. Fragmentation constitutes the principal means of asexual reproduction in the liverworts. Another fairly widespread means of asexual reproduction in the liverworts and mosses is the production of *gemmae,* minute, lens-shaped bodies that can give rise to new plants. The gemmae are produced in special cuplike structures called gemma cups located on the dorsal surface of the gametophyte. Gemma cups are produced by *Marchantia,* but not by *Riccia* and *Ricciocarpus.*

livestock. Mammals, such as beef, goats, sheep, and swine that are raised as sources of human food. Some authors, speaking in very broad terms, may infrequently include poultry within the meaning of livestock. Generally, livestock connotes meat animals on the hoof. Dairy animals (cows and goats) usually are also included because in the long term, retired dairy animals are slaughtered for meat.

livetin. A water-soluble protein fraction of egg yolk.

lobelia. *Lobelia inflata.* A hairy annual or biennial herb with light-blue flowers, which grows about 15 cm high. The plant is native to North America and ranges from Labrador to Georgia and west to Arkansas.

lobster. Shellfish of various tribes of the suborder *Macrura.* True Lobster (with claws), species of *Homarus.* Norway lobster, Scampi or Dublin Bay Prawn-*Nephrops norvegicus.* Squat Lobster-family *Galatheidae.* Crayfish, fresh-water-families *Astacidae, Parastacidae* and *Austroastacidae.* Crawfish, spiny lobster, rock lobster or sea crayfish (without claws)-species of family *the Palinuridae.* Langouste-*P. vulgaris.*

Locasol. Trade name for a low-calcium milk substitute. The average composition per 100 g is: protein 22.6%; fat 20%; carbohydrate 52%; calcium 44 mg (dried milk calcium 960 mg); iron 1.5 mg; and food energy 2.0 MJ.

Locke solution. A physiological salt solution originally devised for perfusing the isolated mammalian heart.

It has the following composition (mmol/L): $NaCl$, 154; KCl, 5.4-5.6; $CaCl_2$, 1.1-2.2; $NaHCO_3$, 1.8-6.0; glucose, 5.5-11.1. The solution is saturated with air/oxygen.

Locksoy. Name given to fine drawn rice Chinese macaroni.

locust bean. 1. Carbob seed, 2. African locust bean, *Pakia* spp; the average composition per 100 g is: 26 g protein; 10 g fat; 47 g carbohydrate; food energy 1.6 MJ; 300 mg calcium, 4 mg iron, 0.06 mg vitamin B_1; 0.2 mg vitamin B_2; and 3 mg nicotinic acid.

locust bean gum. A gum obtained from the ground endosperms of *Ceratonia siliqua* (family *Leguminosae*). The gum is also known as carob flour and is obtained by milling bean kernels of locust trees which are found principally in tropical America, Africa, and the Mediterranean region. The gum contains galactose and mannose in a complex polymer and may be regarded as a polysaccharide or complex sugar. The ratio of mannose to galactose is 3:1 and the gum contains about 6% protein and is somewhat similar in many respects to guar. Locust bean gum has many technical and industrial uses, and, in the food industry, finds application as a stabilizer, thickener, and emulsifier. The gum finds wide use in pet foods and jellies. The gum is a white-to-yellowish white, nearly odorless, powder and is dispersible in either hot or cold water, forming a sol with a pH between 5.4-7.0. This can be converted to a gel through the addition of small quantities of sodium borate.

Lodigiano cheese. A kind of Grana or Parmesan grating cheese made in Italy. The cylindrical cheese has a dark oiled surface and a yellow interior. The cheese which has eyes, is sharp, fragrant and sometimes slightly bitter. It may be cured as long as three or four years.

Lodmann reaction. The transfer of phosphate from adenosine triphosphate to creatine, to form adenosine diphosphate and creatine phosphate. The first source of energy on muscle stimulation is adenosine triphosphate, leaving the diphosphate. This is resynthesized to the triphosphate by creatine phosphate which thus serves as the reserve of energy.

Lofealac. Trade name for food low in phenylalanine; employed for the treatment of phenylketonuria.

loganberry. A kind of berry that is cross between the European raspberry and the Californian blackberry; the vitamin C content is 400 mg/kg..

logarithmic phase. In reference to bacteria means the most rapid period of growth when the numbers increase in geometric progression. Under ideal conditions bacteria can double in numbers every 20 minutes.

Lombardo. An Italian Grana or Parmesan cheese similar to Lodigiano. This sharp aromatic cheese with a granular texture is used for grating.

Lonalac. Trade name or a milk preparation free from sodium.

long tube vertical evaporator. LTV. A device for removing water in the form of a vapor from a liquid solution, in which the heat from the steam is transferred through vertical tubes of considerable length to the product being evaporated. The long tube vertical (LTV) evaporator may have either a falling film or rising film.

longhorn cheese. A kind of cylindrical-shaped Cheddar cheese approximately 12 cm in diameter and weighing about 5 kg. It is characterized by a more open texture, high moisture and faster ripening than larger types of Cheddar.

lonzein. Rice from which the husk has been removed; also known as brown rice, hulled rice and cargo rice.

loop dryer. An apparatus for drying fabric without tension in which the cloth passes over a roller in a chamber with warm circulating air.

loose-leaf lettuce. A variety of lettuce in which cultivars form clustres of the leaves rather than heads. The loose-leaf type is grown in home gardens because these cultivars have less exacting growth requirements than other types of lettuce. They are used mainly for the culture in commercial greenhouse during winter. The loose leaf-type cultivars are poorly adapted to shipping. The principal cultivars

are Prize Head; Grand Rapids; Salad Bowl; Black Seeded Simpson; and Oakleaf. Also known as bunching-type lettuce.

loquat. *Eriobotrya japonica.* The fruit of the tree of the same name. The loquat tree is of the family *Malaceae* (apple family) and of the order *Rosaceae* (rose). In its natural state, the tree may achieve height of 6-9 m, but in cultivation, it seldom exceeds 3.5 m. The tree is quite densely clothed with deep-green, oblong-obovate or elliptical-shaped leaves that are toothed and wrinkled and usually from 15-25 cm long. The flowers (fragrant, white, woolly) are borne on woolly panicles. The trees do not bloom until late summer or early fall, after which fruit is set, but the fruit does not ripen until the following spring. The fruit, which can be eaten raw or in preserved form (jams, jellies, pie fillings, etc.) is a downy, pale-yellow to deep-orange, oval or pyriform pome that may be up to 7.5 cm. long. The smooth, thin skin tends to be tough. The subacid edible flesh of the fruit is from a creamy to deep-orange color and contains several (from two to nine) rather large 19m in length brown-colored seeds. The seeds are sometimes used as condiments in cookery because of their pleasing flavor. The flavour of the flesh of the fruit is variously described as suggestive of cherry or plum. Although the loquat tree tolerates several kinds of soils and microclimates, some authorities believe that it grows best when planted near the seacoast. In orchards, the trees are planted about 6.6 m. apart. Propagation can be from seed, but budding and grafting are generally practiced. The average composition of loquat (raw) per 100 g is: water

86.5%; food energy 50 calories; protein 0.4 g; fat 0.2 g; carbohydrates 12.4 g; calcium 20 mg; phosphorus 36 mg; iron 0.4 mg; sodium traces, potassium 348 mg; and vitamin A (IU) 670 mg. The loquat is sometimes called the Japan plum; Japanese medlar.

lord, leaf. A preparation made from the residue of kidney and back fat after the preparation of neutral lard (at 50°C) by treating with water above 100°C in an autoclave.

Lorraine cheese. A kind of small hard cheese made in Lorriane, Germany. It is seasoned with salt, pepper, and pistachio nuts, and is a local delicacy. It weighs about 100 g and is quite expensive.

lotus. *Nelumbium nuciferum.* A sacred lotus of India and China; water plant whose rhizomes and seed are used for food. Other water plants of the same family whose seeds and rhizomes are eaten are water-lilies, *Nymphaea.* The average composition per 100 g is: 1.7g protein; 11 g carbohydrate; 1.5 mg iron; 0.05 mg vitamin B₁; 20 mg vitamin C; and food energy 0.21 MJ.

lovage. Family: *Umbelliferae.* Genus: *Ligusticum.* Species: *Ligusticum scoticum.* Lovage is rich in an essential oil (umbelliferone), as well as starch, a variety of resins, and vitamin C. An infusion, which is quite tasty when included in soup, will act as a tonic and diuretic and is mildly stimulating. It was once used as an emmenagogue to induce menstruation. Lovage is strongly antiseptic and acts as a good natural deodorant if added as an infusion to bath water. Lovage was much used as a herb in Britain during the Middle Ages, and then, like so many others, went out of fashion for several centuries.

It is the tallest of the unbellifers,

reaching over 1.8 m, and makes an attractive back-of-the-border addition. All parts of the plant, that is, leaves, steams, and seeds, can be used in the kitchen, and so it well repays its keep. The leaves may be used to flavour soups, casseroles, sauces, and marinades, or lightly cooked as a green vegetable. The stems are candied as angelica, and the seeds are often used to flavour bread, savoury scones, and biscuits.

low temperature grain drying. The drying of grains at moisture contents not exceeding 25% such as shelled corn and soybeans with a limited amount of heat ($\Delta T < 6°C$), the temperature increase of heated air less than 28°C supplied by electricity or fossils fuel, in a storage not exceeding 4.6-6.1 m depth, circulating air through a perforated floor and grain with a fan with a flow of 0.005-0.015 m^3/m^2s. Typically, a 10 hp motor-fan would be used. With electric heat, a 10-15 kW heater would be used to heat the air providing a temperature rise of at least or approximately 27.8°C. From 0.3-0.5 kWh was used to remove each 1% (point) of moisture per bushel. The fan should normally be operated continuously. A humidistat may be used to control the fan, turning it off during periods of high humidity.

low-density lipoprotein. A lipoprotein that contains approximately 60% neutral lipid, 20% phospholipid, and 20% protein; such lipoproteins have molecular mass of the order of 2×10^6, a density of about 1.02-1.06 g/L, and a flotation coefficient of about 0-20S.

lox. *See* lax.

LSM. Trade name for a low sodium milk-contains 50 mg per litre, ordinary milk contains 500 mg sodium per litre.

lucerne. *Medicago sativa* L. Essentially a forage crop but eaten by man to a small extent.

Lucozade. Trade name for a glucose beverage; it contains about 17.9% carbohydrate.

Lue gim gong orange. A variety of sweet orange. A subvariety of the Valenica. The variety was introduced by a Chinese horticulturist (Lue Gim Gong) in about 1886. At one time, it was regarded as a hybrid of Valencia and the Mediterranean Sweet orange. Later, botanists decided that it is a nuclear seedling of Valencia. The qualities are similar to those of the Valencia and most consumers have difficulty in distinguishing between the 2 fruits. It is marketed during same period as the Valencia.

Lugol'ssolution. A solution containing 5% iodine in 10% potassium iodide.

Luneberg cheese. A varirty of cheese made in the Voralberg Mountains of western Austria. Saffron is used in colouring. When ripe, the cheese resembles a cross between the Emmentaler and Limburger types of cheese.

lupine. Of the family Leguminoseae (pea family), three are about 100 varities of lupines of which are the most important are: *Lupinus hirsutus*, the blue lupne; *L. albus*, the white lupine; *and L. luteus*, the yellow lupine. These plants are of old world origin, but are found widely distributed over the continents. The lupines serve several functions in food production as pasturage for livestock, as feed in the form of silage and hay, as a soil-enrichment crop (all leguminous plants fix nitrogen from the air land thus enrich the soil with this element), and as a table vegetable in a number of European countries. The lupine bean contains a protein substance of rather bitter taste, most of which can be removed through long soaking in water. However, the very limited acceptance of the lupine in countries a protein substance of rather bitter taste, most of which can be removed through long soaking in water. However, the very limited acceptance of the lupine in countries such as the US, where it has not been traditionally served as a human food, probably stems from the characteristic flavor of the lupine bean. Some lupines are used ornamentally. As with most forage-type crops. worldwide reporting is quite inadequate. The Food and Agriculture Organization of the United Nations ceased reporting lupine production in its annual production review as of 1975. The US Department of Agricultural annual statistics do not report lupines. Lupines make excellent winter growth. The grazing value of the sweet blue and sweet yellow varieties has been recognized by cattlemen in Florida and southern Georgia. Hungry livestock may be poisoned by grazing the bitter, hinge-alkaloid varieties if good forage is not available. The situation is similar to that on western ranges, where livestock, mainly sheep, have been poisoned by grazing certain other lupine species that are native to the western states. Although lupines are generally free from insect attack, several pests occasionally attack the plant, including root weevil *(Sitonia explicita)*, the lupine maggot *(Hylemya lupini)*, and the larva of white-fringed beetles *(Graphognathus* spp.).

Lur brand. A brand of butter distributed by the Danish butter Mark Society which adopted the Lur as a collective mark for all butter exported by its members. The Lur mark represents two pairs of "Lurs" or trumpets, such as were used by Scandinavian Vikings during the bronze age.

lutein. Alternative name for xanthophyll.

luteol. Alternative name for xanthophyll.

Luxus Konsumption. A theory that normal people manage to keep their weight within reasonable limits by burning off any excess of food, while obese people suffer a failure of this mechanism.

lyases. A group of enzymes that remove groups from their substrates (not by hydrolysis), leaving double bonds, or which conversely, add groups to double bonds. The class also includes the decarboxylases, aldolases, dehydratases, fumarase, etc.

lychee. See litchi.

lycopene. Red pigment found in tomato, pink grapefruit and palm oil; It is a carotenoid with long chain hydrocarbon having 13 double bonds, 11 of which are in conjugation, with no vitamin A activity. The synthetic material is sometimes used as a food colour.

lycophytina. The five living genera and approximately 1000 living species of Lycophytina are the representatives of an evolutionary line that extends back to the Devonian period. It seems likely hat the progenitors of the Lycophytina were Zosterophyllum-type plants. The lycopods early split into two major groups. One group remained herbaceous and is still represented in today's flora. The second (the lepidodendrids) became woody and treelike and was among the dominant plants of the coal-forming forests of the Carboniferous period. The lepidodendrids became extinct in the Permian period, about 280 million years ago. Some of them bore seedlike structures analogous to those of modern seed plants.

lycopodium. One the most familiar living representatives of the Lycophytina are the club mosses, Lycopodium. The approximately 200 species of this genus extend from arctic regions into the tropics but rarely form conspicuous elements in any plant community. Most tropical species are epiphytes and are thus rarely seen, but several of the temperate species form mats which may be evident on forest floors. Because they are evergreen, they are most noticeable in winter. The sporophyte of Lycopodium consists of a branching rhizome from which aerial branches and adventitious roots arise. The leaves of Lycopodium, which are usually arranged in spirals, are microphylls, and the stem and root are protostelic. Lycopodium is homosporous. The sporangia occur singly upon the upper surface of fertile microphylls called sporophylls, modified leaf or leaflike organs that bear sporangia. In some species, the sporophylls are similar to ordinary microphylls and are interspersed among the sterile microphylls. In others, nonphotosynthetic sporophylls are grouped into cones (strobili) at the ends of the aerial branches. Upon germination, the spores of Lycopodium give rise to bisexual gametophytes, which, depending on the species, are either green, irregularly lobed masses or branching, subterranean, and nonphotosynthetic variable structures. Like the gametophytes of Psilotum and Tmesipteris, those of the species of Lycopodium with subterranean gametophytes contain a symbiotic fungus. The development and maturation of archegonia and antheridia in a Lycopodium gametophyte requires 6-15 years. Some subterranean forms reportedly live for as long as 25 years, and they may even produce a series of sporophytes in successive archegonia as they continue to grow. Water is require for fertilization, the biflagellated sperms swimming through water to the archegonium and then down its neck. Following fertilization, the zygote develops into an embryo, which grows within the venter of the archegonium. The young sporophyte may remain attached to the gametophyte for a long time, but eventually it becomes an independent plant.

lymph. The fluid found in the lymphatic vessels; it is similar in composition to tissue fluids but that draining the intestine and liver contains more proteins. Lymph contains clotting factors but clot formed is much looser than that of blood.

lymphatics. Vessels through which the lymph flows.

lymphocytes. Spherical cells of 7-12 mm in diameter, with a large, round nucleus and very scanty cytoplasm, and do not contain a well developed endoplasmic reticulum. Most lymphocytes are found in normal blood, and the collections of lymphocytes are also abundant beneath the mucous membranes in respiratory and gastrointestinal tracts. The lymphocytes are primarily responsible for the specific immune response.

lyophilization. A method of freeze-drying used to preserve microbial cultures as well as some foods such as coffee, milk, meats, and vegetables. Their light weight and stability without refrigeration make freeze-dried foods popular with hikers. Although drying stops the microbial growth, but it does not kill bacteria and fungi in the foodstuffs. Numerous cases of salmonellosis have been traced to dried eggs.

lysate. Product of cell lysis; often used to refer to a suspension of phage particles released by the lysis of host

bacteria, or to a cell-free homogenate following the action of detergent or mechanical means to break the cells.

lysine. One of the common amino acids. It possesses a basic side-chain, and is found in many common proteins, but is conspicuously low (or lacking) in certain cereal proteins such as gliadin from wheat and zein from corn. Lysine is one of the amino acids which is nutritionally essential for rats, chicks and human beings. Its supplementary use for improving the adequacy of proteins of bread has been advocated and has some justification in the light of the fact that bread is often too prominent a constituent of the diet, especially of those who are not able to afford more expensive foods.

lysis. The rupture or physical disintegration of a cell.

lysosomes. Subcellular organelles which are believed to contain digestive enzymes capable of breaking down many of cellular constituents. Disruption of the lysosomes and liberation of these enzymes may occur under certain conditions, and can lead to lysis of cell. The lysosome membrane protects the rest of the cell from these enzymes. Lysosomes play a part in many cellular reactions to disease, and some drugs have the property of stabilizing the lysosomal membrane, thereby preventing the damage that ensues from the release of its enzymes. Collectively, the lysosomal enzymes act on a number of biopolymers. Thus, the proteases have a wide capacity for the hydrolysis of proteins, the acid nucleases for RNA and DNA, and the acid glycosidases for polysaccharides. A family of acid phosphatases are also present. The median value for the *p*H optimum for these enzymes is around pH 5. Thus, the lysosomal matrix must be acidic for the enzymes to be reactive. The lysosomal membrane has high specific activity for NADH dehydrogenase and serve as a hydrogen ion pump. All the enzymes other than the esterases and the NADH dehydrogenase, are present in soluble proteins in the matrix of lysosome. In autophagic processes, cellular organelles such as mitochondria and the endoplasmic reticulum undergo digestion within the lysosome. The enzymes are active at postmortem autolysis. The biogenesis of a primary lysosome occurs at the periphery of the Golgi body with the lysosome enzymes, presumably synthesized at the ribosomal sites, being collected in Golgi vesicles and then organized as primary lysosomes. Biopolymers may move in to the cell by endocytosis. Primary lysosomes are believed to merge with the phagosomes to form a second type of lysosome, the digestive vacuole, in which under pH conditions the biopolymers are broken down to basic units which diffuse out of the vacuole in to the cytoplasm to be incorporated again in to cellular components. The residual, undigested fragments in the vacuole are then expelled by the cell in to the surrounding fluid *via* the third type, namely the residual body. At times, the primary lysosome engulfs cellular organelles such as mitochondria to form autophagic vacuoles, the fourth general type. On the death of a cell, lysosomal bodies disintegrate, releasing hydrolytic enzymes in to the cytoplasm with the result that cell undergoes autolysis.

lysostaphin. A bacteriolytic enzyme which is specific for members of the genus *Staphylococcus*. It lyses viable and killed staphylococcal cells and isolated cell walls. The unit of lysotaphin has been designated as the amount required to reduce the optical density of a standard suspension of *S. aureus* FDA 209P 50% in 10 minutes at 37°C. Lysostaphin has proved to be active *in vitro* against all of the more than 500 coagulase-positive isolates of *S.aureus* tested. It has proved inactive against all of 72 viable isolates of 53 species of 21 genera of bacteria other than staphylococci. Coagulase-negative staphylococci are attacked at a more variable rate than coagulase-positive isolates. Efforts are being made to correlate this variable lysotaphin susceptibility of coagulase-negative staphylococci with their relative virulence.

lysozyme. An enzyme that catalyzes the hydrolysis of β-1,4-glycoside links of N-acetylneuraminic acid residues in sialic acids of the cell walls of many bacteria. It is effective against Gram-positive organisms whose peptidoglycan is exposed and accessible to the enzymes. It is present in lachrymal secretion, saliva, nasal mucus, gastric secretion and milk, and serves to protect against bacterial infection. It was the first enzyme to have its three-dimensional structure determined.

lyxoflavin. Substance isolated from human heart muscle, similar to riboflavin but containing the sugar lyxose; its function is not yet fully understood.

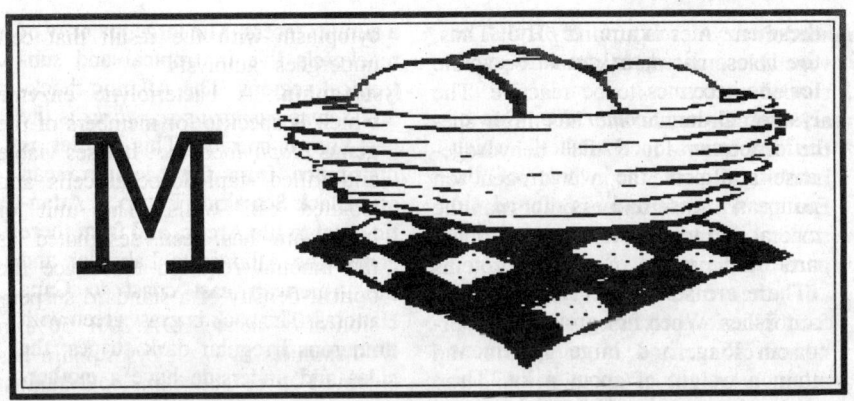

Macadamia nuts. Family: *Proteaceae*. The edible nuts of the macadamia tree (Macadonia spp.) are believed to be native to Australia (New South Wales). Out of a total of over 80 known species and varieties, only a few are cultivated. These include *M. integrifolia* (smooth-shell type) and *M. tetraphylla* (rough-shell type). The smooth-shell type is produced in the large quantities by a wide margin. The macadamia nut, when hulled, averages about 2.5 cm in diameter.

The nuts occur in long grape-like open clusters and, when mature, they fall to the ground. It appears to have excellent acceptability from the standpoints of flavor and texture. A relatively high cost has prevented its widespread application to commercial bakery products, but it does have a prestige image that may be a considerable advantage in marketing upscale goods. The nuts in their husks fall from the trees when mature and are gathered by hand. The husks are removed by mechanical devices leaving the nuts in a very hard and thick shell. Because the nuts deteriorate rapidly, they must be gathered within a short period and dried to a moisture content not exceeding 3.5%. Drying can be performed in forced air dryers at ambient temperatures or at temperatures below 40°C for a few days and then at 50-55°C.

Removing the nutmeats from the hard shells is difficult and can lead to a considerable number of damaged kernels. Cracking machines force open the shells, and automatic separators shake out the loose kernels.

The kernels are graded according to their density by immersing them in solutions of known specific gravity and separating those that float and those that sink.

Grade 1 kernels will float in tap water at room temperature.

Grade 2 kernels have a specific gravity higher than 1.0 but no higher than 1.25.

Grade 3 nuts are those that have a still higher density.

Macadamia nuts are cooked either by immersion in oil or by dry roasting. The colour, texture, and flavour of Grade 1 dry roasted and oil roasted nuts are about equal, because of their high content of oil, but Grade 2 nuts dry out and become cull when dry roasted.

macedoine. A mixture of fruits or vegetables, sliced, or cut into even-shaped pieces.

mackerel. Order: *Scombridae*. One of the important food fishes, which inhabits almost the whole of the European seas and is found in tropical and temperate zones in other parts of the world.

There are several species, but the food fishes. When full-grown it is 25-40 cm long, and large specimens attain a weight of about a kg. The mackerel is variegated blue and green. The term mackerel sky has reference to the wavy stripes on the back of the fish, a mackerel sky being one in which the clouds suggest wavy parallel lines.

Mackerel has an elongated fusiform (spindle-like) body which is only slightly compressed. The tail typically has one to three longitudinal keels; it is long and rather thin. Scales are absent or tiny, sometimes forming a corselet on the front of the body. A wavy lateral line is present. The large head is tapered. The wide mouth opening extends at least to beneath the eyes; the jaws have large or small sharp teeth. The wide gill opening has four gill arches. There are 31-61 vertebrae, and the vertebral column is well ossified. There are 33 genera with a large number of species. All mackerels are epipelagic (high-sea) fishes. Many of them undertake extensive feeding migrations; a few species swim to coastal waters to spawn, while others are never in shallow water.

The anatomy of these extremely fast swimmers reflects their great swimming ability; the pectoral and pelvic fins are recessed into shallow grooves. They click into place with a jerk of the fin base. The dorsal fin has a similar recess. The large majority of mackerels live in tropical and subtropical regions. The Atlantic mackerel *Scomberomorius scombrus* is the best-known species. This species is distributed from the Mediterranean and Black Sea along Europe's Atlantic coast to the Arctic, and from there across the Atlantic to Labrador and the American east coast to Cape Hatteras. The back is grass green with numerous irregular dark stripes; the sides and underside have a mother-of-pearl hue with a reddish shimmer; the first and second dorsal fins are widely separated. The tail shaft lacks a median keel. The bony eye rings are well developed. There is no swim bladder. Like many other mackerels, the Atlantic mackerel occurs in dense schools just beneath the water surface, and sometimes there are so many of them together that they churn up the water at the surface. Since they lack a swim bladder, they can dive very quickly, as when evading predators, such as sharks, tuna, and dolphins.

They feed chiefly on small crustaceans, juvenile herring, sardines, and anchovies, as well as sand lances. After the winter rest in deep waters, sexually mature mackerel seek coastal waters in April and May, where they spawn during the early summer months (March to April in the Mediterranean). One female can lay up to 500,000 eggs, each of which has an oil bubble and floats on the water surface. They young hatch after about 6 days, and grow very rapidly. After 2 years, they are already over 20 cm long and at the end of the third year, they are about 30 cm long and reach sexual maturity.

Since they are highly valued because of their very tasting meat,

Atlantic mackerels are commercially fished just about wherever they occur. Of all the numerous saltwater food fishes, the Atlantic mackerel has presented marine researchers with one of the most fascinating and elusive puzzles.

macon. Bacon made from mutton.

Maconnais cheese. A variety of cheese made in France from goat's milk.

Macqueline cheese. A kind of soft rennet cheese of the Camembert type, made around Snelis, France.

macrocortin. An endogenous glycoprotein which is inhibitor of the enzyme phospholipase-A which catalyzes the release of arachidonic acid from membrane phospholipids. The synthesis and release of macrocortin is stimulated by the glucocorticoids which inhibit eicosanoid synthesis by this mechanism. Macrocortin is so named because it is a large molecule originally obtained from rat macrophages, and because it mimics the effects of glucorticoids; (alternative names are renocortin and lipomodulin although lipomodulin may not be identical with macrocortin).

macrocytes. Large red cells found in the blood in pernicious anemia, due to disturbed development of the red blood cells. Hence macrocytic anemia.

madder. A genus of plants native in almost all tropical regions. From the roots of a species, is obtained a beautiful red coloring matter, which in one shade is known as 'Turkey red'. The chief colouring matter in the different madder dyes is called alizarin. Common madder is a native of Southern Europe and Asia, though cultivated in most European countries. It has black fruit and small, greenish-yellow flowers. Cinchona trees and coffee trees are members of this family. The madder family has

about 6,000 species.

Madeira. A variety of wine made from the grapes of the vineyards in Madeira owes its characteristic flavour to the system of ageing.

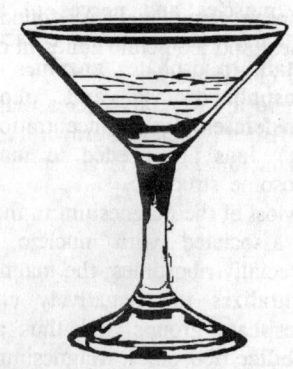

The wine is casked in pipes and stored in hot rooms for several months. The better-quality wines are kept for long periods (six months or more) in a relatively cooler atmosphere, whereas the common wines are kept for a shorter time at higher temperatures, even as high as 45°C. This darkens the wine a little and imparts the flavour of slightly-decomposed sugar. It is generally said that no wine lasts longer than a Madeira and a good Madeira never reaches senility. By far the largest consumers of Madeira are the Scandinavian countries.

madurose. The sugar derivative of 3-O-methyl-D-galactose, which is characteristic of several actinomycete genera that are collectively known as *maduromycetes.*

magma. In food technology, the name given to a mixture of sugar syrup and sugar crystals produced during sugar refining.

magnesium. An element which is essential for plant and animal growth. It is contained in the chlorophyll molecule and is thus essential for photosynthesis. In animals it is found in bones and teeth; magnesium carbonate is found in large quantities in the skeletons of certain marine organisms, and is found in smaller quantities in the muscles and nerves of higher animals. It is an essential cofactor for certain phosphate enzymes, *e.g.*, phosphohydrolase and phosphotransferase. High concentrations of Mg^{2+} ions are needed to maintain ribosome structure.

Most of the magnesium in the cells is associated with nucleic acids, especially ribosomes; the magnesium neutralizes the negatively charged phosphate groups and thus act to stabilize ribosomes. Magnesium deficiency can lead to filament formation in ordinary unicellular forms, to ribosome degradation, and to a decrease in nucleic acid synthesis. Magnesium also binds to the negatively charged teichoic acids.

The rate of absorption from the intestine exerts an important role in magnesium metabolism. Whereas *in vitro* studies show that magnesium absorption is positively correlated with the concentration of magnesium, it does not appear to be a purely passive process. The magnesium absorbed in excess of body needs is excreted primarily by the kidney. Urinary excretion is controlled primarily by a filtration-reabsorption mechanism so that magnesium appears in the urine only when glomerular filtration exceeds tubular reabsorption. Acute renal failure is accompanied by hypermagnesemia.

In some species, considerable endogenous magnesium is lost by way of the feces, the amount depending upon the magnesium status of the animal and upon other dietary factors, such as the digestibility of the diet. The endogenous fecal magnesium in calves has been estimated at about 3.5 mg/kg of body weight. In contrast with the metabolism of calcium, no one endocrine gland exerts a primary regulatory function on magnesium.

Thyroparathyroidectomy in dogs causes only a temporary lowering of plasma magnesium. Adrenalectomy causes a rise, whereas hyperaldosterinism produces a fall in the plasma level. Administration of deoxycorticosterone or aldosterone to sheep lowers the magnesium concentration in plasma. Magnesium-deficient animals exhibit a higher metabolic rate than normal, and the toxic effect of excess thyroxine is partially overcome by increasing the dietary level of magnesium.

Although magnesium activates isolated enzymes, in most cases an absolute requirement is difficult to establish because the enzymes are partially active without added magnesium. The stimulating effect is not always specific for magnesium. In some cases, manganese or calcium also will activate the system. Magnesium is particularly concerned with enzyme-catalyzed reactions involving the cleavage of phosphate esters and transfer of phosphate groups. Magnesium ions activated phosphatases and phosphorylation reactions involving adenosine triphosphate (ATP). Among the latter group glucokinase, phosphoglucokinase, phosphofructokinase, myokinase, creatine transphosphorylase, arginine transphosphorylase, and flavokinease, may be mentioned. It has been suggested that an ATP-Mg complex is the active substrate inasmuch as ATP forms a 1:1 complex with magnesium and maximum activation occurs when the ATP:

Magnesium ratio is 1. Alkaline phosphatases, pyrophosphatases and ATPase are activated by magnesium, as are enolase, certain peptidases, and pyruvic oxidase. Since magnesium is tied to ATP utilization, it follows that magnesium plays a role in important metabolic processes, including the synthesis of protein, fat and nucleic acids, and in the trapping and utilization of energy derived from catabolism of carbohydrate and fat. There is little change in the magnesium concentration of soft tissues from deficient animals even at the point of expiration. This does not preclude the possibility that a small component of the cell, such as the nucleus or a cell particulate, is deprived of its critical level, but the dramatic drop in extracellular magnesium suggests that a function outside the cell is of greatest significance. It appears that tetany and convulsions in deficient animals result from a derangement of neuromuscular transmission.

Magnesium ion possesses strong pharmacological properties depressing both the central and peripheral nervous systems. These effects are counteracted by calcium. In the presence of normal calcium levels, a reduction of extracellular magnesium is believed to increase the release of acetylcholine and to decrease the rate of its hydrolysis. Such effects would increase the irritability of neuromuscular system.

Magnolia family: *Magnoliaceae*. The family of plants which is considered to be among the most primitive of the flowering plants because it consists of woody shrubs and trees that may be deciduous or evergreen, and the flower parts (sepals, petals, stamens, pistils) are spirally arranged and usually without a definite number. The alternate leaves are simple and usually have smooth (entire) margins. Stipules enclose young buds and are shed as the leaves expand. Bracts enclose flower buds. Flowers are often large and showy and usually bisexual. Sepals and petals look alike or there may be three sepals and six to many petals. Many stamens are spirally arranged around a raised axis with many pistils. Each pistil has an ovary of one carpel containing one to many ovules in parietal placentation and 1 style and stigma. Fruit types in this family include follicles, samaras and berries.

The family includes *Liriodendron tulipifera* (tulip tree, yellow poplar), *Magnolia* spp. (magnolias); *Liriodendron, Magnolia acuminata* (cucumber tree), *M. denudata* (Yulan magnolia), *M. grandiflora* (bull-bay), *M. stellata* (star magnolia), *M. tripetala* (tripetala (umbrella tree), *M. virginiana* (sweet-bay), *M. x soulangeana* (saucer magnolia, a hybrid between *M. denudata* and *M. liliflora*, has large, deep pink, sterile flowers *Michelia fuscata* (banana shrub), *Talauma, Illicium vernum* (Chinese anise, star anise), and *Kadsura*.

Maile cheese. A kind of sheep's milk cheese of Crimea, which may be kept in a salt brine for as long as a year.

Maillard reaction. Two processes in food can produce a brown colour.

One is the enzymatic oxidation of phenolic substances, such as occurs at the cut surface of an apple. The other is a reaction between proteins or amino acids and sugars, and is variously known as the Maillard reaction, the browning reaction and non-enzymatic browning. It takes place on heating or on prolonged storage and is one of the deteriorative processes that take place in stored foods. It is accompanied by a loss in nutritive value since the part of the protein that reacts with the sugar is the free amino part the sugar is the free amino part of the lysine. This complex is not digested and there is thus a reduction in the biologically available lysine.

Mainauer cheese. A kind of cheese named for an island in Lake Constance between Germany and Switzerland. The cheese is similar to Raddolzeller cream cheese and to Munster. The cheese is cured in the similar manner as the Munster cheese.

Mainzer hand cheese. A kind of German cheese made by the usual hand process, which is ripened in a cellar for about 6-8 weeks.

maize flour. Highly refined and very finely ground maize meal from which all bran and germ has been removed.

maize rice. Finely cut maize with bran and germ partly removed: also called mealie rice.

maize, flaked. Partly gelatinized maize used for animal feed. The grain is cracked to small pieces, moistened, cooked and flaked between rollers.

maize. Family: *Gramineae*. Genus: *Gea.* Species: *Zea mays* var. *indenta* (dent corn); *Zea mays* var. *rugosa* (sweet-con). Grain of *Zea mays,* also called Indian corn. Maize is a staple article of the diet in many areas but its protein is of poor quality (lacking both lysine and tryptophan), and this, together with its low content of available nicotinic acid and the possible presence of a toxic factor can give rise to pellagra. The average composition per 100 g of maize is: protein 9.4%; fat 4.4%; iron 2.4 mg; food enbergy 1.56 MJ; vitamin A 145 μg; vitamin B_1 0.42 mg; vitamin B_2 0.1 mg; and nicotinic acid 2 mg.

Of all the varieties of maize two are of commercial importance, *Zea indurata* (Flint corn) and *Zea dentata* (dent corn). Sweet corn, pod corn, popcorn and waxy corn are other varieties. Sweet-corn is best eaten as fresh as possible as the older it gets the more the vitamins C, A and B are depleted (in that order). It needs to be particularly well chewed to be properly digested and is believed to help anemia and constipation. It depresses the action of the thyroid gland and so is best suited for those who live in hot climates.

maize processing. The majority of starch produced is manufactured from corn. The processing is done by what is commonly referred to as the corn wet milling industry. Shelled corn is delivered to the wet-milling plant by truck or railroad box-car (2000 bushels; 51 metric tons) and unloaded into a pit for short-term storage, after which it is sampled and weighed. The corn passes through mechanical cleaners, designed to separate unwanted substances, such as pieces of cob, sticks, husks, as well as pieces of metal and stones. The cleaners agitate the kernels over a series of perforated metal sheets; the smaller foreign materials drop through the perforations, while a blast of air blows away chaff and dust, and electromagnets draw out nails and bits of metal. Combing out of in-line storage bins; the corn is given a second cleaning; before going into very large "steep" tanks. At this point, the use of water becomes an essential part of the corn-refining processes.

The cleaned corn is typically moved into large wooden or metal tanks holding 50-150 metric tons. At this stage, the grain is soaked for 36-48 hours in circulating warm water at

49°C containing a small amount of sulphur dioxide to control fermentation and to facilitate softening. The steeping process removes some of the soluble and toughens the germ as well as softening the protein matrix surrounding the starch granules. Steepwater, modified or unmodified, is an excellent nutrient for the production of antibiotic drugs, vitamins, amino acids, and fermentation chemicals. Steepwater is also an effective growth supplement for animals feeds. The steepwater is concentrated by evaporation. From steeping process, the softening kernels go through degerminating mills, which are designed not for fine grinding, but rather for tearing the soft kernels art into coarse particles, freeing the rubbery oil-bearing germ without crushing it, and loosening the bran.

The wet, macerated kernels are then sluiced into the flotation tanks known as germ separators, or centrifugal hydrocyclones. The germs, lighter than the other components of kernel, float to the surface and are skimmed off. This germ, which contains most of the oil in the kernel, is processed subsequently to recover he corn oil by expellers and solvent extraction. By oil expellers or extractors (heat and pressure) and by means of solvents, almost all oil is removed as another byproduct to be settled, filtered, refined, and otherwise processed into clear, edible oil for salad dressing and frying; and also as soap stock for soap manufacture. The residue of the germ, after oil extraction is ground and marketed as corn germ meal, or may become a part of corn gluten feed or metal. The remaining mixture of gluten and starch is pumped from shakers to high-speed centrifugal machines which, because of the

difference in specific gravity, separate the relatively heavier starch from the lighter gluten.

Having been separated from the kernels, the starch is now readily for washing, a part of the starch produced is routed to starch dryers, after which it is packed for marketing. At any given time, the remainder of the starch (often the majority of it) is passed on for conversion into other products.

In one process, the starch is mixed with water and heated in the presence of weak hydrochloric acid, which breaks the starch down chemically by hydrolysis. If the hydrolysis is interrupted before final conversion, a noncrystalline corn syrup is obtained. Many varieties can be made by supplemental use of enzymes to meet specific functional requirements. The solids content is varied to suit the requirements of users. Corn syrup is used in a wide variety of food products, including baby foods, breakfast foods, cheese spreads, chewing gum, chocolate products, confectionery, cordials, frostings and icings, peanut (groundnut) butter, sausage; as well as for numerous industrial products.

maze starch. *See* maize processing.

Malaga wines. The wines made from the vineyards in Malaga, on the south coast of Spain. Fermentation of the must lasts for six weeks and then 5% of spirit and 'Vino Tierno' (a wine made from grapes which have been dried off in the sun to half their weight) are added to improve the alcohol, and about 8% of 'Arrope' (an unfermented grape must, evaporated over an open fire until it has the consistency of syrup and a clear brown colour and has a sweet, bitterfish acid taste) is added to enhance the body of the wine, and then enough 'Pantomima' (similar to Arrope but is evaporated almost to a paste so that it is very dark) to enrich the colour. Malaga wine is of almost of the colour of a strong infusion of coffee and has all the properties of body, alcohol, colour and bouquet which have been donated to it.

maleic hydrazide. 1,2,-dihydro-3,6-pyridazinedione. A compound used on several food items. In the case of onion and potato, the compound slows or stops sprouting while the commodities are in storage. The compound also 'is used to promote dormancy in connection with citrus trees as well as increasing protection from frost.

Some of the popular commercial names of maleic hydrazide are: De-Cut, De-Sprout, Maintain-3, Regulox, Retart, Royal MH, Slo-Gro, Sprout-Off, Sprout-Stop, Stunt-Man, Sucker-Stuff, Supper-Desprout, Super Sucker-Stuff, Vondalhyde, Vondrax.

malic acid. $HOOC-CH_2-CHOH-COOH$. An acid which got its name because of its occurrence in unripe apples (Latin *malum*, apple). The L-form is an intermediate in carbohydrate metabolism and, in the citric acid cycle, is convertible into oxaloacetic acid in one direction, and fumaric acid in the other. The rotatory power of malic acid changes from slightly positive to negative when a concentrated solution is diluted. Also known as hydroxysuccinic acid.

malic dehydrogenase. An enzyme which catalyzes the oxidation of L-malic acid to oxalacetic acid, the fourth oxidation-reduction reaction in the tricarboxylic cycle. The malic dehydrogenase of the mitochondrial matrix is distinct from the isoenzyme counterpart in the cytosol. The cytosolic malic dehydrogenase plays an important role in the production of NADPH from NADH in the cytosol.

malic enzyme. The enzyme that catalyzes the anaplerotic reaction whereby pyruvic acid is carboxylated to malic acid.

Mallow family: *Malvaceae*. The flower's column of fused stamenal filaments is a common feature in this family. The leaves are usually palmately veined and alternate. There are about 1,500 species of herbs, shrubs and trees, belonging to this family. The flower is bisexual with 5 valvate sepals, 5 separate petals, numerous stamens, and 1 pistal with 2 to many carpels. Fruit types include a loculicidal capsule, often with hairy (comose) seeds, a schizocarp, and a berry.

The family include: *Gossypium hirsutum* (cotton, cottonseed oil), *Hibiscus esculentus* (okra); *Abutilon* (flowering maple), *Althea rosea* (hollyhock), *Callirhoe* (poppy mallow), *Hibiscus* spp. (queen-of-the-border, swamp mallow, rose-of-China, roselle, rose-of-Sharon), *Lavatera* (tree-mallow), *Malope, Malva* spp. (hollyhock mallow, curled mallow, musk mallow), *Sidalcea* (false mallow, miniature hollyhock); *Malva neglecta* (common mallow, cheeses), *Abutilon theophrasti* (velvet-leaf).

malt extract. A mixture of breakdown products of starch, containing mainly maltose (malt sugar). It is prepared from barley or wheat. The grain is allowed to sprout, when the enzyme diastase (or amylase) develops and hydrolyses the starch to maltose. The mixture is then extracted with hot water and this malt extract contains a solution of starch breakdown products together with diastase. Malt extract may be the concentrated solution or evaporated to dryness.

For brewing, barley low in protein and rich in diastase is used an mixed with extra unmalted barley to provide more starch for the yeast fermentation.

malt flour. Germinated barley or wheat, dried and milled. It is quite rich in diastase and added to flour of low diastatic content for bread-making, and also used to make a malt loaf.

malt whisky. Scotland, the chief centre for the production of malt whisky produces three varieties of it. The whisky is produced with the raw material got from the neighboring regions.

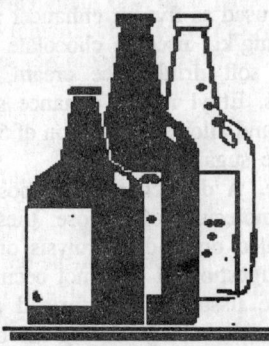

By the action of photosynthesis from the carbon dioxide of the air, starch is produced in the vine. This starch is then turned to sugar by the agency of enzymes in the plant. The resulting sugary pulp adheres to the grape-stones and is the food on which the seeds depend until they can get nourishment from the soil. The grains of cereals secrete certain enzymes which make the starch of the grains available to the germinating seed by turning it to sugar. These enzymes are called diastase. As the grain ripens, the amount of diastase also increase until much more than necessary is available. At this point, the tiny plume which will become the stem of the new barley plant is about as long as the grain. This takes about nine to fourteen days depending on the type of barley. The distiller now takes the enzymes to saccharify his grain by the process of 'malting'.

Malt is almost all made from barley. The grain is first cleaned from dust and chaff and then it is spread out on the malting floors and allowed to sprout. Its temperature is strictly kept at 22°C and it is turned back and forth to prevent overheating. After this, the sprouted grain is taken to the next kiln and gradually heated. This is done, so that the growth will stop but the enzymes will not be destroyed. The malt is now spread on perforated floors and heated with a peat fire to a temperature of 45°C gradually. The malted barley now dry, resembles ordinary barley but has the reek of peat fire. It has swollen a little and it contains a large amount of enzymes. Next it is matured for some weeks in bins, then ground up finely. Then the grist which is produced is mixed with hot water in tanks called "mash tuns". At this stage, the starch must be converted into sugars by the diastase and extracted by the water and so the temperature is very important. It is stirred constantly and kept warm. This process is called mashing. The mash tun has a perforated false bottom and when all the sugar has been extracted, the sweet liquor and the worts is drawn off, leaving the grain husks in the tun.

The next stage, the fermentation, carried out in fermenting backs is similar to the fermentation of a grape-must. The worts are cooled to about 22°C and yeast is added.

Cooling coils are fitted in the backs to control the temperature. Fermentation takes about two to three days, the alcoholic liquid, known as wash, contains about 10% alcohol and is something like very strong beer.

malt. *See* diastase.

Malta blood orange. A variety of sweet, blood-type, orange produced mainly in India and Pakistan. This variety is seedy and matures at midseason, and possesses good colour and flavour. Juice content is about 40%; soluble solids content, about 10%. The Malta orange is similar, but is a nonblood type. Considerable experimentation with the Malta blood has been carried out in Florida. In the Florida climate, the fruits do not develop the same, desirable red colouration. However, some authorities believe that this variety may be suitable for frozen-concentrated orange juice and possibly superior to Hamlin and Parson Brown.

maltase. Enzyme that splits maltose (malt sugar) into two molecules of glucose; present in the pancreatic juice and intestinal juice.

malting. The germination of the grain until the starchy food-store (endosperm), available for the development of the germ of the grain, has suffered some degradation by enzymes. Malting is carried out in three steps :

(a) *Steeping.* It consists of immersing the carefully selected barley in water until a moisture content of 42%-46% (wet weight basis) is achieved.

(b) *Germination.* The steeped barley is set to germination in darkness at relatively low temperatures (12-15°C).

(c) *Kilning.* It involves the drying and partly cooling of green malt in a stream of warm air.

A good malting barley must have the following biochemical properties:

(a) It must contain very little of the harsh and bitter-tasting substance present in the husk.

(b) During germination, it must produce sufficient quantity of hydrolytic enzymes, especially hemicelluloses and proteases.

(c) It must yield a high percentage of its dry substance, 'extract' after malting and mashing.

maltol. 3-hydroxy-2-methyl-4H-pyran-4-one. A compound with a fragrant, caramel-like odour and bitter-sweet taste used as flvaour enhancer at 50-350 mg/kg; used in chocolate products, soft drinks, ice cream, table jellies. Ethyl maltol enhance sweetness and allows a reduction of 5-15% of the sugar present.

maltose. A disaccharide composed of two molecules of glucose; these are liberated on acid hydrolysis or during digestion. It does not occur free in the tissues but is formed as an intermediate stage during the breakdown of starch to glucose. Its sweetness is about 33% that of sucrose. Maltose occurs in barley seeds following germination and drying, which is the basis of the malting process used in the manufacture of beer and malt whisky. The enzyme maltase converts maltose into glucose in small intestine; the optimal conditions for the activity of this enzyme is at pH 5.8-6.2. Also known as malt sugar.

Malvasia grape. A variety of grape which is native of Greece and considered of ancient origin. The white vaiety of Malvasia grape is now found in several parts of the world, including California, France,

Mammee apple. *Mammea americana.* A minor fruit of the large tree, which is a member of a small group of tropical trees native to the American tropics. The tree, which rises to a height of from 12-18 m bears a fruit that is from 10-15 cm in diameter. The shape is oblate to spheroidal. The colour is russet and the skin is quite thick, pliable, and leathery. The flesh is of a bright-yellow colour, with a firm texture, but it furnishes generous quantities of juice. Some authorities state that the flavour is reminiscent of the apricot. The fruit can be served fresh or, as preferred by Europeans, it can be made in jams and preserves.

manatee. An animal found on the coasts of South America, Africa and Australia. It frequents the mouths of rivers and feeds on algae and such land vegetation as it can reach at high tide. The animal is assisted in feeding by a peculiar upper lip, which is cleft in two and furnished with strong bristles. It has no hind limbs, and the fore limbs, or swimming paws, have nails, by means of which the animal drags itself along the shore. Manatees are large, awkward animals, attaining a length of from 2 to 6 metres. The skin is grayish-black, and is sparsely covered with hairs. The flesh and oil are valuable. Also known as sea cow.

manganese. An element required by microbial cells in trace amounts. It can serve as alternate cofactor for magnesium during magnesium deficiency, particularly in magnesium-requiring enzymes. Microbial oxidation of manganese occurs among many soil and marine species. Soil bacteria and fungi reduce insoluble salts of manganese (Mn^{4+}) to soluble manganese (Mn^{2+}) compounds. This type of reduction is characteristic of some bacteria that inhabit the roots of some plants, and makes manganese available in a soluble form. The sheathed bacteria, such as *Leptothrix* and *Sphaerotilus*, oxidize manganese and accumulate it within the sheath as deposits of manganese oxides.

Manganese is required for the synthesis of secondary metabolites such as antibiotics. Peptide antibiotics produced industrially by species of *Bacillus*, for example, cannot be synthesized in the absence of manganese. Peptide antibiotics, which are produced during sporulation, are believed to act as carriers of calcium and thus may help the cell to accumulate the divalent cation. Manganese is an element that activate certain enzymes such as arginase and alkaline phosphatase, although no deficiency has ever been observed in man. It is essential for animals and deficiency causes perosis (slipped tendon) in chicks, sterility in rats and bone malformations in rabbits. Also essential for plants. Green foodstuffs and tea are rich sources of manganese.

mangelwurzel. *Beta vulgaris rapa.* Cross between red and white beetroot, used as cattle food. Its average composition is: water 75.4-94.3%; nitrogenous substances 0.47-3.65%; fat 0.02-0.45%; N-free extract 5.75-10.0%; fibre 0.39-2.14%; ash 0.59-2.77%; sucrose 3.5-8.7%. Also spelled as mangoldwurzel.

mango. *Mangifera indica.* The name of a genus of evergreen trees, which are natives of India and Malay Peninsula, though they have been introduced into numerous tropical countries. In India there are nearly 150 varieties. In its native state the common mango tree grows to a height of about 10-15 metres and has a spreading top with dense foliage, the leaves being 15-20 cm long. The flowers are small, reddish-white or yellow and are borne in dense clusters. The fruit is kidney-shaped and varies considerably in size and color with different species. The best varieties of fruit are highly prized for eating. Some are sweet, and others are slightly acid. The unripe fruit is frequently used for sauces and pickles. By cultivation the mango has been extended to most of the West India Islands and to Florida and California. Mango are usually orange-coloured with edible flesh surrounding central stone, the depth of colour is an index of vitamin A activity which can be up to 7.5 g/kg. The average composition per 100 g is: 0.5 g protein; 15-20 g carbohydrate; 0.5 mg iron; 250 µg vitamin A; 0.03 mg vitamin B_1; 0.05 mg B_2; 0.25 mg nicotinic acid; and vitamin C 35 mg; and food energy 0.3 MJ.

mangoldwurzel. *See* mangelwurzel.

mangosteen. *Garcinia mangostana.* A tropical fruit of Indian origin, the size of an orange with thick purple rind and sweet white pulp in segments. The fruit has an outer rind enclosing a number of delicate, white locules like those of an orange. The sweet and juicy locules are the edible parts of the fruit. In the location where it is grown, it is sometimes referred to as the queen of tropical fruit. The juicy flesh has a flavour suggesting both the peach and pineapple to some eater of the fruit; to others, the flavour suggests strawberry and grape. In contrast to the white flesh, the rind of the mangosteen is dense, thick, darkly coloured. This rind is sometimes used medicinally for its astringent properties. Limited interest has been expressed in the US, both as a fruit in its own right, as well as a potential colorant source. The rind contains a substantial amount of red pigment. The major pigment is cyanidin-3-sophoroside, and a minor pigment, cyanidin-3-glucoside.

mangrove. A genus of trees or shrubs which grow in tropical regions along the muddy beaches of low coasts, where they form impenetrable barriers for long distances. They throw out numerous roots from lower part of the stem and also send down long, slender roots from the branches, like the Indian banyan tree. The seeds germinate in the seed vessel, the root growing downward till it fixes itself in the mud. Mangrove trees thus are responsible for shore lines being extended into the water, for their roots catch flying particles and hold mud washed up by the waves. The fruit of some species is said to be sweet and edible, and the fermented juice is made into a kind of light wine.

Maniacal. Trade name for sodium alginate.

Manitoba maple. *Acer negundo* L. Family:Aceraceae. A tree of the Maple Family. The Manitoba maple is a fairly small tree, usually reaching heights of 9-18 m with a diameter of 0.8 m. Each compound leaf is about 15-40 cm long, with individual leaflets 5-15 cm in length. The leaves are light green above and paler beneath. They change to yellow or red in the fall. The bark is light gray-brown and you can color the twigs green, brown, or purplish. Shade the twigs with white, to represent the white blooms that often cover them. Male and female flowers occurs on separate trees and appear before or with the leaves. The male flowers grow in clusters while groups of female flowers are attached to a central stock. Winged seeds develop by fall and remain attached well into winter. Manitoba maple grows well in moist soils along river banks, but it also does well in drier locations.

Manitoba maple is a fast-growing tree. This has made it a popular choice for prairie shelter-belts and as an ornamental. The wood is soft and weak and is not of great commercial value, although it is used to make rough boxes and crates, woodenware, and inexpensive furniture. It is also used for pulpwood.

Like other maples, syrup and sugar can be made from its sap and the Plains Indians are thought to have used it for this. Songbirds eat its seeds, as do squirrels. Because its wood is weak, the branches of Manitoba maples are susceptible in high winds. If a snapped branch leaves a hole in the trunk, cavity-nesting songbirds will readily use it as a nest site. Also known as box elder; ash-leafed maple.

Manketti oil. An oil with about two-thirds the drying power of linseed oil. It is light-yellow viscous oil from the seed nuts of the tree *Ricinodendron rautanenii,* of southwest Africa. Chia-seed oil is a clear amber-coloured oil extracted from the seeds of the plant *Salvia hispanica* of Mexico. It has a higher drying value than linseed oil. The seeds yield about 30% oil, which contains 39% linolenic acid, 45% linoleic, 5% palmitic, 2.7% stearic, with some arachidic, oleic, and myristic acids. The specific gravity is 0.936, iodine value 192, and acid value 1.4. The seeds scatter easily from the pods and are difficult to collect.

Mann's acid test. A method for measuring the acidity of milk. The apparatus necessary for the test is a 50 ml burette graduated to 0.1 ml. It has a rubber tube and pinch cock at the lower end. Also needed are a 17.6 ml pipette, a glass stirring rod, a white cup, phenolphthalein indicator, and 0.1N sodium hydroxide. To operate the test: With the pipette 17.6 ml of the milk sample are placed in the white cup, 3-5 drops of indicator are added and stirred thoroughly. The burette is filled with the NaOH and the height at which the alkali stands in the tube is observed. Slowly and with constant stirring the alkali is run into the sample. When a faint pink colour appears, all the acid has been neutralized and the burette is again read.

manna. Dried exudate from the manna-ash Tamarisk tree (*fraxinus ornus*). Abundant in Sicily and used as a mild laxative for children. The average composition is: 40-60% mannitol, 10-16% mannotetrose, 6-16% mannotriose, plus glucose, mucilage and ⁊ fraxin. This is thought to be the food eaten by the children of Israel in the wilderness.

mannitol. $CH_2OH(CHOH)_4CH_2OH.$ The polyhydric alcohol containing six carbon atoms; derived from mannose or fructose. It is the main soluble sugar in fungi and lichens and an important carbohydrate reserve in brown algae. Mannitol is used as a sweetener in certain foodstuffs.

mannose. $C_6H_{12}O_6.$ A monosaccharide, stereoisomeric with glucose, that occurs naturally only in polymerized forms called mannans; found in plants, fungi, and bacteria, serving as food energy stores.

manteca. A whey butter of Italy produced as a by-product of Caciocavallo and Provolone, is enclosed in a bag of plastic curd. Heated plastic-curd (made like Scamorze) is formed into a bag of butter is put in the curd bag and the edges are sealed. The cheese is shaped like small Cacicavallo which is usually smoked. Also known as manteche.

Manur cheese. A variety of cheese made in Servia from either sheep's or cows' milk. The milk is first heated to the boiling temperature and then cooled until the fingers can be held in it. A mixture of buttermilk and fresh whey with rennet is added. The curd is lifted from the whey in a cloth and allowed to drain, then it is kneaded like bread, lightly salted, and dried.

maple. *Aceraceae.* A family of trees peculiar to the northern and temperate parts of the world. There are about 100 species are known, distributed through Europe, North America and different parts of Asia. The 2 genera (*Diperonia* from China and *Acer*) in this family are small to large deciduous trees found mainly in the north temperate zone. The flower in some species is bisexual, but usually is unisexual with both male and female flowers on the same tree (monoecious) or separated on different trees (dioecious). Unisexual flowers may have vestigial organs of the opposite sex. There are usually five sepals, 5 petals or none, 4 to 12 stamens, and 1 pistil with a superior ovary. The two fused carpels of the ovary develop into a double samara fruit. The sugar, or rock, maple is the most important species; this yield maple sugar, an important product of Vermout, New York and other states, and some parts of Canada. Its leaf is the emblem of Canada. The knotted parts of the sugar-maple furnish the pretty birds eye and curled maple of cabinet-makers. Some other American species are the white maple; the red, or swamp, maple; the striped maple, or moosewood; the mountain maple, the vine maple and the large-leaved maple. Two species are common in UK, the great maple, often wrongfully called sycamore, and the common maple. Bird's-eye maple, a peculiar formation of sugar maple caused by a defect in the growth of the wood. The defect is the result of injury to the bark. A piece of bird's eye maple shows a number of small, round spots not unlike bird's eyes, and when polished it is very attractive. Curled maple, another variation from the ordinary wood, has wavy ripples instead of a straight grain. Both forms are used in making high-grade furniture.

The maple family include: *Acer saccharum* (sugar maple), *A. macrophyllum* (big leaf maple); *A. saccharum* (sugar maple), all maple species yield sap with a high sugar content; *A. saccharum* (sugar maple), *A. platanoides* (Norway maple), *A. pseudoplatanus* (syacamore maple), *A ginnala* (amur maple), *A. japonicum* (fullmoon maple), *A. palmatum* (Japanese maple, with red leaves throughout growing season).

maple syrup. Sap of certain varieties of the maple tree, *Acer saccharum* (USA and Canada). Evaporated either to syrup or finally to sugar. Maple syrup, 62.6% sucrose, 1.5% invert sugar.

maple syrup urine disease. An inborn error of metabolism in which unusually large amounts of the three amino acids, leucine, isoleucine and valine, are excreted in the urine; the urine smells like maple syrup. There is progressive cerebro-degeneration leading to early death.

maracle berry. *Richardella dulcifica* (also known as *Synepalum dulcifum*); tropical fruit from west Africa containing a taste-modifying substance that causes sour food to taste sweet. Hence the name miracle berry, and miraculin for the active principle, a glycoprotein.

margarine, kosher. Made only from vegetable fats since ordinary margarine can include animal fats that may not be kosher also the margarine is fortified with carotene (which is derived from vegetable (which is derived from vegetable sources) instead of retinol (which can be obtained from non-kosher sources).

margarine. Emulsion of fat and water flavoured with the butter aroma-diacetyl and acetyl methyl carbinol (or containing milk soured with selected organisms to develop the butter aroma). Fats commonly used are a blend of several of the following; groundnut, cottonseed, whale, sunflower and soya (all hardened to some degree) and coconut palm and palm kernel. Generally is composed largely of vegetable oils and some animal fats emulsified with skim milk, ordinary milk or cream. It may also contain a special emulsifier and some starter distilled with other desired flavour ingredients. Butterfat is also used in margarine. However, most manufacturers rely upon emulsifying the oils they use with nonfat milk solids. This may be used in the form of fluid skim milk or in the dried form. The skim milk should, of course be pasteurized and lactic acid starter used to develop from 6/10 to 7/10% acidity. The general composition of this product is about 80% vegetable oil, 18% skim milk and approximately 2% of salt, coloured with carotene, annatto or coal-tar dyes; not more than 10% butter fat may be added. In many countries margarine is fortified with vitamins A and D. Also called oleomargarine (US), butterine and lardine.

Ever since margarine came on the market there has been noticeable rivalry between butter and margarine manufacturers and not surprisingly the average person is confused as a to what he or she should eat Vegetables oil used to make margarine have first to be solidified by a process called hydrogenation. They are then mixed with skimmed milk and reworked to add salt and remove excess water. The solidification process used frequently turns the unsaturated fats into saturated fats, so raising the cholesterol content of the product. Many margarine producers have claimed to have solved this problem and now produce a low-cholesterol margarine made with polyunsaturated fats. However, before we get too excited about this perhaps we ought to take a look at how margarine is made.

Hydrogenation is the next step after refining, hydrogen gas is introduced to liquid oil in the presence of a metallic catalyst, usually nickel or cadmium. This succeeds in bonding hydrogen ions on to the oil molecules, saturating them and transforming them form a liquid to a solid. The resulting hydrogenated oil actually has the same molecular structure as plastic when examined under a microscope. Any label that states 'high in polyunsaturates' plays down the fact that hydrogenation is in itself a saturation process. What this really means is that the oil was high in polyunsaturates before it was hydrogenated so that margarine could be made from it. Butter is saturated and has cholesterol but it is at least a real food. Margarine has approximately the same amount of calories as butter and normally it has added vitamin A and D. US government regulations specify the minimum amount of vitamin A (1500 IU) which must be added to a pound of margarine. Margarine in tubs is likely to have more polyunsaturated fats than margarine in stick forms because it may not be solidified. Low-calorie margarines contain more water and half the amount of fats than their polyunsaturated sister. These margarines though usable for spreads cannot be used for cooking.

marigold. *Calendula officinalis.* The sunshine-gold marigold flowers are a familiar sight in cottage and country gardens and in colourful window boxes. The plant is a native of southern Europe but flourishes in cool, temperate climates. It was once treated for its many culinary uses; the petals have a pungent, spicy flavour, and the leaves have a rather bitter aftertaste. A hardy annual, the marigold has a long flowering period, though not usually as long as its French popular name, *tous les mois,* would suggest. The petals, with their slight aromatic bitterness, are used in fish and meat soups, rice dishes, cakes desserts, and salads and, commercially, as a colouring for cheese and butter. In medieval times, the whole flowers were popular as a garnish. Medicinally, the petals were used to heal wounds and to treat conjunctivitis, while the leaves were felt to relieve the effects of bee and wasp stings. An infusion of the petals may be used as a hair rinse to lighten fair hair, and the petal made into a nourishing cream for the skin. When used together with alum, the petals give a yellow dye.

marinade. Preparation of olive oil, lemon juice, vinegar and mixed herbs in which fish or meat is steeped before cooking.

marinate. To pickle in salt, *e.g.,* anchovy and Bismarck herrings.

marjoram. Family: *Labiatae.* Genus: *Origanum.* Species: *Origanum Majorana* (sweet or knotted marjoram); *Origanum onites* (pot marjoram); *Origanum vulgare* (wild marjoram or oregano). Dried leaves of a number of aromatic plants of different species.

The most widely accepted marjoram herb is *Origanum majorana* (perennial bush) and a sweet marjoram *majorana hortensis* (annual).

Spanish wild marjoram is *Thymus matichina.* The volatile oils contain terpenes and terpene alcohols; used as seasoning for poultry and meats.

Sweet marjoram is a tender, bushy perennial herb with woolly hairy leaves, which gets up to 50 cm in height. The herb is native to the Mediterranean countries but is cultivated as an annual in colder climates. The dried flowering herb yields a faint sage-like odour and leaves a slightly minty aftertaste in the mouth.

Oregano, as such, is not just one or two well-defined species but rather any one of over 20 known species that yield leaves or flowering tops having the flavour recognized as being oregano. European oregano is a hardy perennial herb with erect, more or less hairy, branching stems and hairy leaves. The herb can grow to over 60 cm tall, and is acrid and pungent with a strong sage-like aroma somewhat reminiscent of thyme. Sweet marjoram contains 2% essential oil, as well as mucilage, bitter substances and tannic acid. The chemical constituents of pot marjoram are much the same but oregano contains only 0.5% essential oil, of which 15% is thymol.

Marjoram is a weak expectorant and anti-spasmodic, carminative, aromatic, a weak hypertensive, antiseptic and diaphoretic. It accelerates the healing process by increasing the white blood cells so that there are more of them to fight infection. It is very useful in most simple gastrointestinal disorders, and a weak tea is an excellent digestive aid. It is particularly useful for children's colic.

marker enzyme. An enzyme, the intracellular location of which is known, so that an assay of the enzyme can be used an aid in following the isolation and purification of subcellular fractions.

marmalade. Originally, name given to a jam made from the Portuguese marmelo or quince. Now, the name given to jam made from citrus fruits such as orange, lime, lemon, grapefruit.

Marolles cheese. A kind of soft, cow's milk cheese of the Point Peveque type made in France. Several types and shapes are made and are known by different names. The Boulette type is pear-shaped, while the Dauphin is half moon shaped and flavoured with certain herbs.

Marsala (wines). The wines made from the grapes of the Marsala vineyards in Italy, where wine has been made for more than twenty centuries.

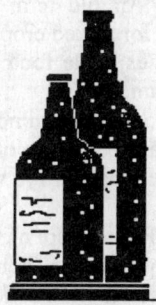

After the wine has been manufactured, it is mixed with *Vino Cotto*, which is the evaporated must, a dark coloured thick, sweet liquid. Then it is fortified, usually by adding a must to which alcohol has been added. Vino Cotto is made by mixing 'must, evaporated over an open fire, and fresh must with alcohol added. Good

Marsala wine is matured in casks for 2-5 years. It is a dark, almost treacle-sweet wine, and is not to everyone's taste. It contains about 20% of alcohol and 5-6% of sugar. The taste of burnt sugar is derived from Vino Cotto.

Marshall rennet test. A test used for determining the ripeness of milk for cheese making, made first after adding starter and again after an elapse of time. A special cup is filled with milk to a point marked zero. Dilute rennet extract is then added and mixed with the milk. In the bottom of the cup is a hole, out of which the milk will run until coagulation takes place. The time required to coagulate the milk is shown by the scale on the wall of the cup. This test is more sensitive to slight changes in acidity than the acidity test. The cheese maker use this test to indicate the increase in acidity after the addition of starter. After a change in the units or portion of a unit, the cheese-maker has an indication of the increase of acidity and he will then set the milk.

marshmallow. *Althaea officinalis.* A member of the hollyhock family, marshmallow has small but attractive flowers carried without steams. It is grown throughout Europe, in Australia, Asia and eastern north America.

The mucilage, which comprises about 30% of the roots, steams, and leaves, was used to make the confection known as marshmallow, but now substitutes are used commercially. The young leaves and shoots may be shredded and added to salads and soups; the roots may be parboiled, then fried in butter. In earlier days, the plant was used in self-help medicine for sprains, brushes, and muscular pain. An infusion of the dried roots was used to treat sore throats and ulcers, while an infusion of flowers was used as a mouthwash. A soft is sweetmeat prepared from an aerated mixture of gelatin or egg albumin with sugar or starch syrup. It differs from nougat in containing less glucose and more water. Originally, it was made from the root of the marshmallow plant (*Althaea*) which provides a mucilaginous substance as well as starch and sugar.

Marshmallow is a perennial plant growing a height of nearly 1.2 metres in some cases. It is both cultivated as well as found growing wild in damp and wet places everywhere. The rootstock is white and sweetish like unto a parsnip, but with considerable mucilage to it. The plant sends up several unbranched, woolly stems with serrate, pubescent leaves. The axillary flowers are about 2 inches in width and can be either light red to white or royal purple in colour.

marsh marigold. *Caltha palustris.* Family: *Ranunculaceae.* A flowering plant. The flowers are 3-4 cm across. The plant grows to 50 cm high, with heart-shaped leaves. The sepals, stamens, and pistils are bright yellow. The leaves are shiny green. When seeds are produced they are able to stay afloat for a long time and are widely distributed in the wet growing areas. The petal-like parts are sepals which surround the many stamens and pistils. They grow in loose clusters above the leaves. The plants have a bitter taste and contain a poisonous substance. They are usually avoided by animals. Since the poison is destroyed by cooking people do prepare a delicious vegetable from the leaves and stems. However, marsh marigolds cannot be used in salads.

marsmus, nutritional. Severe wasting of the body of infants because of gross dietary deficiency. Symptoms include atrophy of muscles and subcutaneous fat. Together with kwashiorkor, marsmus is one of the major problems of infant nutrition in the developing countries. Also known as total under nutrition

marzipan. Name given to a sweetmeat or cake decoration composed of 25% ground almond paste and 75% sugar; also called almond paste.

mash. The soluble materials released from germinated grains and prepared as a microbial growth medium.

mash tun. Vessel used in brewing in which the malt is extracted from the sprouted barley with hot water.

mashing. 1. A process in which cereals are mixed with water and incubated in order to degrade their complex carbohydrates to more readily utilizable forms such as simple sugars.

2. In the brewing of beer, the malted barley is heated with water both to extract the soluble sugars and to continue enzyme reactions started during malting.

maslim. 1. An old term still used in Scotland, for mixed crop of beans and oats used as cattle food. Also known as mashlum.

2. In Yorkshire and north of UK, it refers to a mixed crop of 2-3 parts of wheat and 1 part of rye which is used for bread.

masscuite. The mixture of sugar crystals and syrup mother liquor obtained during the crystallization stage of sugar refining.

mastication. The process of dividing the food by the combined action of the jaws and teeth, the tongue, the palate and the muscles of the checks. By it the food, besides being finely divided, is mixed with the saliva. Imperfect mastication is a source of indigestion.

masticatory substances. Chewiness is one of several components experienced by the consumers, though it may be highly undesirable in a piece of roast beef, this property is the predominant rewarding factor of some food products, notably certain kinds of novelties, such as chewing gum. Biting and deformation resistance can be created or improved by the use of a number of essentially rubber-like substances. They are termed as masticatory substances. Chewiness is the main advantage contributed by such substances and thus other ingredients, such as sweeteners, flavors, colorants, etc., and admixed with them to result in an overall attractive product for particular consumers.

During the last several decades, naturally derived masticatory substances have been displaced to a considerable degree by synthetic materials-for reasons of availability, economics, and frequently, better controls over purity. These developments essentially paralleled the development of the synthetic rubbers for industrial uses.

mate. A preparation made from the dried leaves of *Ilex paraguayensis*. It contains caffeine and tannin. Also known as yerba mate; Paraguay tea; Brazilian tea.

matoke. Name given to the cooked (steamed) green banana.

maturation factor. Substance in the liver which aids maturation of red blood cells. It may be vitamin B_{12} or combination of B_{12} with the intrinsic factor produced by the stomach.

Matzka process. The process of sterilization by the combined use of silver ions (oligodynamic process) and limited supply of heat. It may be noted that the Katadyn process employs silver ions alone. In the presence of the silver the pasteurization temperature is reduced to only $15\text{-}20°$ C. This process is suitable for fruit juices.

matzos. Although matzos or matzoth, the Jewish specialty which is traditionally consumed during Passover, is an unleavened bread in the sense that no fermentation is permitted, it does undergo a moderate amount of volume increase during cooking, as a result of the expansion of entrapped air bubbles and evolution of water vapor within the dough piece. If it were not for this leavening effect, the product would be much less palatable. The matzos is essentially prepared from a mixture of flour, salt, and water, although some commercial varieties are flavoured with onion and garlic. The product is baked in very thin sheets at moderately high temperatures until a moisture level of 2% to 5% is reached. Docking is essential to prevent permanent separation of the top and bottom surfaces during baking. It is desirable have a substantial contribution of radiant (top) heat in the oven to brown the tops of the wafers so as to produce some flavour in this otherwise quite insipid product. Shelf-life is good (about the same as soda crackers) if the matzos are protected from moisture absorption.

maw. Fourth stomach of the ruminant.

may apple. A common plant of North America, sometimes called mandrake. It belongs to the barberry family. Two large leaves are borne on a stem a foot or more high. From the fork between them grows a large, handsome flower, with waxy petals, which produces a yellowish, slightly acid, pulpy fruit, about the size of a pigeon's egg. From the root a powerful drug is prepared.

maysin. Coagulable globulin protein of maize.

McEwen solution. A physiological salt solution. The essential difference from Krebs-Henseleit solution is the inclusion of sucrose to reduce edema formation in the tissues. It is used to bathe isolated mammalian tissues, especially when nerve-evoked responses are to be recorded.

It has the following composition (mmol/L): NaCl, 130; KCl, 5.6; $CaCl_2$, 2.2; $MgCl_2$, 0.5; NaH_2PO_4, 1.0; $NaHCO_3$, 25.0; glucose, 11.1; sucrose, 13.0. It is bubbled with 5% carbon dioxide in oxygen.

Mead. Name of one of the most ancient fermented products and wines. Although regarded by some people as a curiosity in modern times, there is some demand for mead in various parts of the world and it is still made, largely on a regional basis. Present makers of the wine have found that the addition of a nitrogenous yeast food to the diluted honey is desirable for successful fermentation; and that phosphates also can be helpful. The honey of pleasing, mild flavour is diluted with water to 22° Balling. Citric acid (5 g), diammonium monohydrogen phosphate (1.5 g), potassium bitartrate (1.0 g), and magnesium chloride and calcium chloride (0.25 g each) are added to each litre of the diluted honey. These constituents dissolve in the honey with mild heating. It is also suggested that about 100 parts per million of sulfur dioxide (or 200 ppm of potassium metabisulphite or sodium bisulphite) be added per 378.5 litres be added to the diluted honey. Then, 2-3% of pure wine yeast starter (Burgundy, Champagne, etc.) be added. Some makers grow this yeast in pasteurized diluted honey or in pasteurized grape or sugar juice. During fermentation, cask or tank should be provided with a fermentation bung to avoid acetification. After settling for several weeks, the new wine is racked.

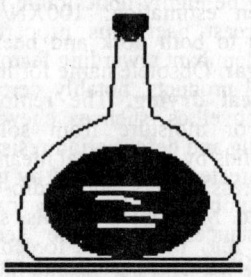

The wine is then filtered, using a filter aid and aged a few months in a fully filled, tightly sealed cask, after which it is racked, polish filtered, and bottled. It is then ready for the table. The wine may be sweetened to 5° or 10° Balling by adding honey or sugar, then filtered and flash pasteurized at to 63°C, after which it should be bottled hot and cooled with a water spray. Fortification to 18-20% can be accomplished by adding high-proof brandy. Also known as honey wine.

mealie(s). Maize.

meat bar. Dehydrated cooked meat and fat; a modern form of pemmican; the average composition per 100 g is: 7.5% water; 50% protein; with 2.5 MJ as food energy.

meat extract. The water-soluble part of meat that is mainly responsible for flavour. Commercially is made during the manufacture of corned beef; minced meat is immersed in boiling water, when the water-soluble extractives are partially leached out. This soup is concentrated and produces the meat extract (called No. 1 extract) of commerce. (Exhaustive extraction of the meat produces Direct Extract, containing more gelatin.) Rich in the B vitamins (particularly B_2, nicotinic acid and B_{12}), meat bases, and potassium.

meat factor. Factor used to determine the fat-free meat content of sausages and similar meat products from a nitrogen estimation: 100XN/3.4; it applies to both pork and beef.

meat sugar. Obsolete name for inositol.

mechanical drying. The removal of water or moisture from solids or semisolids by mechanical means, e.g., filter press, rollers, and hydro-extractors, etc. Mechanical means, such as rollers, may be used to forced moisture to the surface of the product, such as with forages and paper, which facilitates subsequent moisture removal.

medicinal paraffin. A mineral oil of no nutritive value as it is not affected by digestive enzymes and passes through the intestine unchanged; used as a mild laxative because of its lubricant properties; if taken at the same time as the fat-soluble vitamins, these go into solution in the oil and pass through the digestive tract unabsorbed.

Mediterranean mandarin. A fruit of unknown origin; one of the older varieties of mandarin which is grown throughout the Mediterranean and near Eastern region. Production of this variety is also important in Argentina and Brazil. In Italy, it is grown in Palermo, Catania, and Taranto regions. There is substantial production in the Argos-Nauplion region of Greece. The fruit is of medium-size, moderately oblate. Commonly, it will have a small naval-like structure. The fruit is yellowish-orange when mature. The thin rind is not leathery and is quite loosely adherent. An essential oil in the leaves and rind presents a distinctive aroma. A noticeable feature of the tree is the small, narrow, lanceolate leaf.

Mediterranean orange. A variety of sweet orange, nonblood type. One of the early sweet oranges produced in the Mediterranean region. The Mediterranean Sweet orange has participated in a number of cross-breeding experiments, notably in producing crosses with the Shamouti. There is considerable production of the Mediterranean Sweet orange in Italy.

melangeur. Mixing vessel consisting of rollers riding on a rotating horizontal bed; used to mix substances of pasty consistency (hence melangeuring).

melangolo. An Italian term for the bitter orange.

melanin. Any of a group of polymers, derived from the amino acid tyrosine, that cause pigmentation of eyes, skin, and hair in vertebrates. Melanins are produced by specialized epidermal cells called melanocytes, and protect the skin from the harmful effects of ultraviolet radiation. The hereditary albinism is caused by the absence of the enzyme tyrosinase, which is necessary for melanin production. The colours range from black through brown to yellow, orange, or red. In animals melanin occurs in melanophores (pigment cells) in the skin, usually below the epidermis. In melanin synthesis, tyrosine is converted to DOPA by the action of copper containing enzyme tyrosinase.

melezitose. 3-α-D-glucosido-D-fructose. Trisaccharide composed of two glucose and one fructose; hydrolyzed to glucose plus the disaccharide turanose.

melibiose. 6-(α-D-galactose)-D-glucose; a disaccharide.

mellorine. US term for ice-cream made from non-butter fat.

melons. A fruit generally grown in hot and dry conditions. Some of thee common varieties are:

Cantaloupe. A variety of muskmelon having a warty rind and reddish-orange flesh.

Casaba. A variety of muskmelon or winter melon with a yellow rind. First introduced to Smryna in Asia Minor.

Honeydew. A sweet, smooth-skinned, white variety of muskmelon.

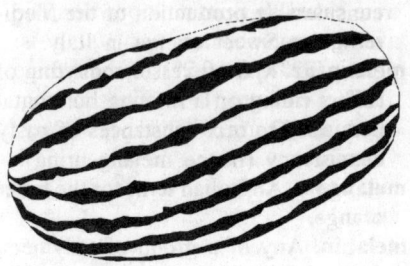

Watermelon. Large oblong or round-ish fruit of a vine of the cucumber family. It has a hard green or white rind, and a pink or red pulp with a copious sweet juice. Some scientists who specialize in the evolution, migration and use of plants by indigenous cultures believe that these melons were brought to the western hemisphere around 2,000 BC by emigrants from central Iraq.

membrane, semi-permeable. One that allows the passage of small but not large molecules, *e.g.*, pig's bladder is permeable to water but not salt, collodion is permeable to salt but not protein molecules. The exchanges of water and salts between tissues of the body and red blood cells is possible because of the semi-permeable nature of the walls.

menaquinone. 2-methyl-1,4-naphtho-quinone. A generic descriptor of substances with vitamin K activity; formerly called menadione.

menhaden. Genus: *Brevoortia,* the men-haden is one of the most important commercial fishes in North America. Of the four species of menhaden occurring along the coasts of the US,

two contribute nearly all of the commercial catch. The Atlantic coast catch consists principally of the Atlantic menhaden (*B. tyrannus*), which ranges from Nova Scotia to northern Florida. The Gulf menhaden (*B. patronus*), which range from the west coast of Florida to Mexico, contributes most of the catch from the area. Two other species, the yellowfin menhaden (*B. smithi*), which occurs mainly along the east and west coasts of Florida, and the fine scale menha-den (*B. gunteri*) from the western Gulf of Mexico, are of relatively minor importance. Other species are known. Menhaden are small, oily herring-like fishes closely related to shad, alewife, herring, and sardine. The largest authenticated specimen was about 48 cm long, but most of those caught are less than 30.5 cm in length and weigh somewhat less that 0.45 kg. The average size of Gulf menhaden at any particular age is considerably less than that of the Atlantic species.

menhaden oil. An oil obtained by steaming for boiling the fish *Brevoortia tyrannus,* caught along the Atlantic Coast of the United States. It was first called porgy oil, the Maine name for the fish. Other names for fish are whitefish, fatback, and mossbunker. The fish, when fully grown, are 30-38 cm long, weighing about 0.5 kg. They yield up to 15% oil, although fish from warm southern waters yield less oil. An annual catch of 1.5 billion fish yields 10.2 million gal (38.6 million litres) of oil and 103,000 tons of meal. Menhaden is not a desirable food fish because of its oily nature. The oil contains about 27% oleic acid, 20% arachidonic acid, 16% clupanodonic acid, 17% palmi-toleic acid, 7% myristic acid, and 1% stearic acid. It has an iodine number of 140-180, and a specific gravity of 0.927-0.933. The inedible oil is used for dressing leather, mixing in cutting oils, and for making paint oils. It is also hydroxylated with acetic acid and used for making paint oils. It is also hydroxylated with acetic acid and used for making polyisocyanate and alkyd resins.

Menhaden oil polymerizes easily, and the drying power is good, but it does not give an elastic film as do the vegetable oils. Its strong odour is due to the clupanodonic acid esters. The residue fish meal, is sold for poultry feed and fertilizer. The meal is not as rich in vitamins A and D as that from some other fish, but as much as 15% can be used in poultry feed without producing a fishy taste in the eggs. Most edible oil is hydrogenated and blended in margarines and shortenings.

mentha arvensis. The essential oil prepared from the herbaceous plant (*Mentha arvensis* L.) of the Labiatae family. The name *mentha arvensis* is applied to both the plant and the oils derived from it. The oil is the source of menthol. Other names for *mentha arvensis* include corn mint and wild pennyroyal. The use of menthol in foodstuffs is not permitted in some countries. In years past, *M. arvensis* oil has been a common adulterant of true peppermint oil. The essential oil can be dementholated by crystallization at low temperature, followed by centrifugation, and redistillation (rectification). the use of the rectified oil is permitted in some countries for use as a flavoring agent in products, such as candies and bitter chocolate. menthol-like, minty, cooling, but not quite as smooth as true peppermint oil.

mercapturic acid. Complex of cysteine with naphthalene or various haloge-nated aromatic hydrocarbons (such as bromobenzene) whereby the latter compounds are detoxicated and excreted in the urine.

meringues. Confections made by beating together a mixture of sugar and white of eggs.

Meritene. Trade name for food concentrate based on skim milk powder. The average composition per 100 g is: protein 32%; fat 0.2%; carbohydrate 58.7%; calcium 1 g; iron 15 mg; vitamin A 2 mg; vitamin B_1 2.3 mg; vitamin B_2 4.3 mg; nicotinic acid 22 mg; vitamin C 80 mg; vitamin D 15 µg; and food energy 1.5 MJ.

Merlot wine. A well-regarded red grape wine, somewhat comparable in quality with the Cabernets in Bordeaux region. Merlot wines tend to be somewhat more mellow than the Cabernets. The Merlot is also cultivated in California, Chile, Italy, and Switzerland.

mesomorph. Description given to a well-covered individual with well-developed muscles.

mesophiles. Microorganisms that grow best at temperatures between 25 and 40°C; usually will not grow at temperatures below 5°C.

mesquite. A small tree or shrub allied to the accacia. It is common in Mexico, Texas and other parts of the southwest of North America, where in dry regions is often appears as about the only conspicuous form of vegetation. It yields a gum resembling gum arabic, but much inferior. Its seeds are sometimes eaten, and from the mucilage of its pods a drink is made.

metabolic inhibitors. A term usually referring to the agents that inhibit ATP production in the mitochondria. Additional metabolic inhibitors include compounds that act to disorganize mitochondrial structure (*e.g.*, high doses of thyroxine), the antibiotic antimycin A (not used therapeutically) which inhibits the reaction between cytochromes B and C arsenates which interact with ADP and so prevent ATP production, and the plant alkaloid which inhibits the release of ATP from the mitochondria.

metabolic rate. Rate of utilization of energy.

metabolic water. The water produced in the body by the oxidation of foods; for example, 100 g of fat produce about 107.1 g of water; 100 g of starch produce 55.1 g of water; while 100 g of protein produce 41.3 g of water.

metabolism. Highly integrated network of enzyme-catalyzed reactions that occurs in all living organisms. Although it includes all such reactions, the term in sometimes used more specifically to refer to those reactions involved in the degradation of a particular compound. Metabolic reactions involve the breaking down of molecules to provide energy (catabolism) and the building up of more complex molecules and structures from simpler molecules (anabolism). Cells extract energy from their environments and convert foodstuff in to cell components by the highly integrated network of chemical reactions.

The most valuable thermodynamic concept for understanding the energetics of metabolism is free energy, which is a measure of the capacity of a system to do useful work at constant temperature and pressure. A reaction can occur spontaneously if the change in free energy is negative. The change in free energy for a reaction is independent of path and depends only on the nature of the reactants and their activities. ATP, the universal measure of energy in biological systems, is an energy-rich molecule because it contains two anhydride bonds. The electrostatic repulsion between these negatively charged groups is reduced when ATP is hydrolyzed. Also, ADP and Pi are stabilized by resonance more than is ATP. The hydrolysis of ATP shifts the equilibrium of a coupled reaction by a factor of about 10^8. The basic strategy of metabolism is to form ATP, NADPH, and macromolecular precursors. ATP is consumed in muscle contraction and other motions of cells, active transport, and biosyntheses. NADPH, which carries two electrons at a high potential, provides reducing power in the biosynthesis of cell components from more oxidized precursors. ATP and NADPH are continuously generated and consumed.

Hormones play an important role in integrating metabolism. In particular, insulin, glucagon, apinephrine and norepinephrine have large effects on the storage and metabolization of fuels and on related facets of metabolism. Metabolism is regulated in a variety of ways. The amounts of some critical enzymes are controlled by regulation of the rate of protein synthesis and degradation. In addition, the catalytic activities of some enzymes are regulated by allosteric interactions and by covalent modification. Compartmentalizing and distinct pathways for biosynthesis and degradation also contribute to metabolic regulation. The energy charge, which depends on the relative amounts of ATP, ADP and AMP, plays a role in metabolic regulation. A high energy charge inhibits ATP-generating (catabolic) pathways, whereas it stimulates ATP-utilizing (anabolic) pathways. The metabolic patterns of the brain, muscle, adipose tissue, and the liver are very different. Glucose is essentially the sole fuel for the brain in a well-fed person. During starvation, ketone bodies (acetoacetate and 3-hydroxybutyrate) become the predominant fuel of the brain. Muscle uses glucose, fatty acids and ketone bodies as fuel and it synthesizes glycogen as a fuel reserve for its own needs. Adipose tissue is specialized for the synthesis, storage, and mobilization of triacylglycerols. The diverse metabolic activities of the liver support the other organs. The liver can rapidly mobilize glycogen and carry out gluconeogenesis to meet the glucose needs of other organs. The liver plays a central role in the regulation of lipid metabolism. When fuels are abundant, fatty acids are synthesized, esterified, and sent from the liver to adipose tissue in the form of very low density lipoprotein.

In the fasting state, however, fatty acids are converted in to ketone bodies by the liver. The activities of these organs are integrated by hormones. Insulin signals the fed state; it stimulates the formation of glycogen and triacylglycerols and the synthesis of proteins. In contrast, glucagon signals a low blood glucose level; it stimulates glycogen breakdown and gluconeogenesis by the liver and triacylglycerol hydrolysis by adipose tissue.

metabolite. A substance that takes part in a metabolic reaction, either as reactant or product. Metabolites are thus intermediates in metabolic pathways. Some are synthesized within the organism itself, whereas others have to be taken in as food.

metalloenzyme. Enzyme consisting of a protein molecule complexed with one or more metal atoms. Carboxypepti-dase A, for example, contains an atom of zinc.

metalloproteins. Proteins especially in solution, readily participate in a greater variety of chemical reactions than any other class of compounds of biological interest. This reactivity is a function primarily of the many polar side chains containing -OH, -COOH, $-NH_2$, -SH and other groups, all of which can, to varying extents, interact with metal ions. It is not surprising then that in general all proteins can bind metals, some of them very tightly indeed. A negatively charged protein molecule exerting a nonspecific electrostatic attraction on metal ions would not quality as metalloprotein. Nor will we consider such insoluble artificial compounds as those obtained by treatment of collagen with trivalent chromium during the tanning process or by precipitation of proteins with $Zn(OH)_2$, even though the action of chromium on zinc may here be fairly specific. Further, metal ions such as those of magnesium or manganese, are often found as important coenzymes.

metallothionein. One of a group of proteins that bind heavy metals, especially copper, cadmium and zinc. They have two important functions: homeostasis, ensuring that metal-requiring enzymes are provided with these atoms; protection, binding excess heavy metal and thus, by the excretion of the complex, reducing the heavy metal content of the cell or tissue. These proteins are probably ubiquitous and are remarkable in that they are specifically inducible by heavy metals which they bind. They are characterized by their low molecular mass and high glycine content.

Metcalf bean. *Phaseolus restusus.* A low-spreading or trailing annual with a large, deep-running root. The pods are oblong, short, and flat. The plant grows best at high altitudes of about 1200 metres and has been suggested as a forage plant for dry, high-altitude regions.

Metercal. Trade name for a "slimming" preparation comprising all the dietary essentials limited to 900 kcal (3.8 MJ), per day intake, in powder, liquid and biscuit form. Its major constituent is skimmed milk with added protein and full range of vitamins.

methaemoglobin. The oxidized form of haemoglobin (unlike oxyhaemoglobin which is a loose and reversible combination with oxygen) which cannot transport oxygen to the tissues. Present in small quantities in normal blood, increased after certain drugs and after smoking; found rarely as a congenital abnormality. It can be formed in blood of babies after consumption of the small amounts of nitrate found naturally in vegetables grown in certain areas and in some drinking water since the lack of acidity in the stomach does not prevent reduction of nitrate to nitrite.

methanol dehydrogenase. The enzyme responsible for the oxidation of methanol to formaldehyde in methylotrophic bacteria. It has an unusual prosthetic group, pyrroloquinoline quinone. It is also unusual in being a dehydrogenase that interacts with the electron transport chain at level of cytochrome c, thus by passing the quinones and b-type cytochromes which are usually involved in the oxidation of organic molecules. The result of this arrangement is that only one molecule of ATP is synthesized for every molecule of methanol oxidized to formaldehyde.

methionine sulphoximine. Substance formed by reaction between nitrogen

trichloride (Agene) and the amino acid methionine when flour is treated with agene as a bleaching agent. It causes running fits in dogs; although it has never been shown to be toxic to man, the use of Agene as a bread improver was abandoned in UK in 1955.

methionine. One of the 20 common amino acids, and possessed by a nonpolar side-chain. It is an essential amino acid for humans. In the form of S-adenosylmethionine, it is the principal source of methyl groups in the body. In addition to direct utilization, the methyl group is also oxidized. S-adenosylmethionine, an active methionine, is formed by the condensation of L-methionine with ATP. This activated S-methyl group may transfer to various acceptors.

Methocel. Trade name for methyl cellulose.

Methofas. Trade name for methyl hydroxypropyl cellulose.

methyl alcohol. The first member of the alcohol series. It is a highly toxic substances and leads to mental disturbance, blindness and death when consumed over a period. It is present in methylated spirits, to which it is added to denature the ethyl alcohol and render it undrinkable. Since methylated spirits is duty-free alcoholic addicts often drink this despite the presence of the toxic methyl alcohol.

methylated spirits. Ethyl alcohol containing methyl alcohol, coloured with a dye and given a repulsive smell by the addition of pyridine. Its toxicity is due to the presence of the methyl alcohol.

methylene blue. Blue dye that becomes colourless when reduced, the so-called leuco- form; it is used in cell respiration experiments to indicate when oxygen is being consumed. When methylene blue or resazurin is added to milk the bacteria present take up oxygen and change the colour of the dye. Methylene blue becomes colourless; while the resazurin changes to blue-purple pink-white. The speed of the change indicates the bacterial content. Pasteurized milk must not reduce dye in half an hour.

Meulengracht diet. A special diet for the peptic ulcer patients; sieved foods such as meat, chicken, vegetables, at 2-hour intervals. It differs from Sippy and Lenhartz diets in having much higher protein content. The intention is to neutralize and acid in the stomach by the buffering effect of the protein.

Meunier grape. A variety of grape related to the Pinot Noir grape, the Meunier grape, is highly regarded, but not quite on same level as the Pinot Noir grape. It is planted in the Burgundy and Champagne districts of France as well as in California. The Meunier grape is sometimes confused with the Pinot Noir grape in California.

mevalonic acid. β-δ-dihydroxy-β-methyl-valeric acid; growth promoting factor for *Lactobacillus acidophilus* distinct from lipoic acid, can replace acetate which is an essential factor for this organism. It is an intermediate stage in the biosynthesis of sterols and terpenes (including carotene).

Meyer lemon. A variety of lemon which is favorite for gardens in many parts of the world. It was introduced from China where it has been grown for centuries as an ornamental pot plant in the region around Bejing. The variety is quite cold-hardy and bears heavily. It has the acid content and other characteristics of the true lemon, although the rind is lacking in lemon aroma. The fruit is very juicy and may

have a nipple at each end.

Michaelis constant. A measure of the kinetics of enzyme reaction. Defined as the substrate concentration at which half the limiting velocity of the reaction is reached. It is a characteristic of the enzyme and is useful as a means of following the stages of purification of an enzyme.

microaerophile. A microorganism that requires low levels of oxygen for growth, around 2-10%, but is damaged by normal atmospheric oxygen levels.

micro-aerophiles. Microorganisms that can grow in extremely low concentrations of oxygen. It can thus spoil the foodstuffs intended to be stored in the absence of air, if traces are left.

microbial culture. A sensitive means for detecting the presence of a potential pathogen, involving specific methods for each organism and for each part of the body to be examined. Anaerobes are cultivated in media from which all oxygen is excluded. Depending on the case, blood, urine, feces, or tissue may be sampled and cultured. In case of the important sexually transmitted disease gonorrhea, bacterial culture provides the most assured means of diagnosis.

microbial enzyme production. The use of microorganisms to produce large amounts of certain enzymes on commercial basis. Microorganisms produce a large variety of enzymes, most of which are produced only in small amounts and are involved in cellular processes. However, certain enzymes are produced in much larger amounts by some organisms, and instead of being held within the cell, they are excreted into the medium. Extracellular enzymes are usually capable of digesting insoluble nutrients such as cellulose, protein, and starch, the products of digestion then being transported into the cell, where they are used as nutrients for growth. Some of these extracellular enzymes are used in the food, dairy, pharmaceutical, and textile industries, are produced in large amounts by microbial synthesis. They are useful because of their specificity and efficiency when catalyzing reactions of interest at moderate temperature and pH. Similar reactions achieved by chemical means would generally require extreme conditions of temperature, pressure, and pH. Enzymes are produced commercially from fungi and bacteria. The production process is usually aerobic, and culture media similar to those used in antibiotic fermentation are employed. The enzyme itself is generally formed in only small amounts during the active growth phase but accumulates in large amounts during the stationary phase of growth. The microbial enzymes produced in the largest amounts on industrial basis are the bacterial proteases, used as additives in laundry detergents, Other important enzymes manufactured commercially are amylases, and glucoamylases, which are used in the production of glucose from starch; and rennin, which is used in cheese production.

microbial insecticides. Several microbes are either insect pathogens or they produce toxins that affect insects and consequently are being considered or are used as insecticides. Microbial insecticides offer several potential advantages. In general, they are specific, affecting only a limited group of insects, and relatively short-lived in the environment. But the main disadvantage is that their insecticidal action is short-lived. The most widely used microbial insecticide is the bacterium *Bacillus thuringiensis*, although viruses, fungi, and other bacteria have potential for widespread use. *B. thuringiensis* is marketed with the commercial name 'Thuricide'. It appears that the insecticidal agent is not the bacterium itself but a protein toxin that it produces. In the susceptible insects the toxin disrupts the gut cells and induces paralysis. It is effective against several caterpillar insects. *B. popilliae* is effective in the control of the Japanese beetle and has been produced commercially. *Bacillus sphaericus* has been shown to be toxic to several species of mosquitoes. As research continues and expands, it is likely that many new microbial insecticides will be developed.

microbial lipids. The principal lipids found in the microbial membrane are glycerophospholipids. The fatty acid components of microbial lipids are most frequently chains containing 15-19 carbon atoms. The chains are usually straight, but occasionally they are cyclic. Any unsaturation of the molecule is usually at carbon atom 2 of the fatty acid.

microbial polysaccharides. The polysaccharides produced by a wide variety of microorganisms. Those of primary industrial interest are found on the outside of the microbial cell wall and membrane, are called exopolysaccharides. They occur in two distinct forms: attached to the microbial cells that synthesize them as discrete physical structures termed as capsules; or secreted from the cell into the surrounding environment in the form of soluble slime. An important use of microbial polysaccharides is in the recovery of tertiary oil by the petroleum industry. Pumping an aqueous polysaccharide solution into an oil well that has had most of the readily accessible oil removed significantly enhances the production of the well.

The chemical structures of microbial polysaccharides fall into two classes: those composed of a single repeating structural unit, known as homopolysaccharides; and those constructed of two or more monomers, known as the heteropolysaccharides. Homopolysaccharides of microbial origin are less abundant than heteropolysaccharides.

Dextrans, that are polymers of glucose are essentially the only group of microbial homopolysaccharides to have significant industrial applications. The heteropolysaccharides, which are composed of neutral sugars and, commonly, uronic acids, have many industrial applications. Dextrans are α-linked polymers of glucose produced by several bacterial species including *Klebsiella* spp., *Acetobacter* spp., streptococci, and *Leuconostoc mesenteroides*. Xanthan is produced by the *Xanthomonas campestris*.

The alginates are currently produced commercially from the brown algae. Curdlan is homopolysaccharide compound of β1,3-linked glucose units produced by *Alcaligenes faecalis*.

Pullulan is a homopolysaccharide produced by fungus *Aureobasidium pullulans*. Although the present production of microbial polysaccharides is relatively small, the potential market is large, and new polysaccharides are continuously being developed. *See also* curdlan; pullulan.

microbiological assay. Biological assay using microorganisms; used for vitamins and amino acids in particular. The principle is that the organism is inoculated into a medium containing all the needed growth factors except the one under examination, the rate of growth is then proportional to the amount of this particular factor added in the test substance. Rate of growth determined by turbidity or by titrating the acid produced after incubation for 2-3 days.

microbiostasis. The inhibition of microbial growth and reproduction.

microbodies. Unlike plastids and mitochondria, which are bounded by two membranes, *microbodies* are spherical organelles bounded by a single membrane. They range in diameter from 0.5-1.5 µm. Microbodies have a granular interior, sometimes with a crystalline, proteinaceous inclusion. The Microbodies are generally associated with one or two cisternae of rough endoplasmic reticulum, which usually are smooth on the surfaces facing the microbodies. Some microbodies, called *peroxisomes,* play an important role in glycolic acid metabolism associated with photosynthesis. Others, known as *glyoxysomes,* contain enzymes necessary for the conversion of fast into carbohydrates during germination in many seeds.

microcapillary. Capillaries in a solid with a radius less than 10^{-7} m in which the saturated vapor pressure of moisture depends on the curvature of the meniscus. The rules governing transfer are molecular in nature and molecules move under thermal motion. Neither laminar nor turbulent flow develops. Micropores in grain, such as corn, have a surface area of 26.3 km^2 for about 0.1 kg dry grain.

micrococci. The obligate microbes that are found in the soil and water. Samples of water or soil incubated on agar plates will often reveal them as pigmented types. They are morphologically similar to the staphylococci and appears in clusters. They differ from streptococci in that acid is produced by aerobic oxidation and not by fermentation.

microcyclus. Ring-shaped and non-motile organotrophic bacteria; they resemble very tightly curved vibrios and are widely distributed in aquatic environments. A phototrophic counterpart to *microcyclus* has been discovered and placed in the genus *Rhodocyclus*.

microencapsulated enzyme. An enzyme that is immobilized in a microcapsule, equipped with a semipermeable membrane, such that substrates and products, but not the enzyme, can diffuse across the membrane.

microgram. μg. One-thousandth part of a milligram; *i.e.*,

$$1\mu g = 10^{-3} \text{ mg} = 10^{-6} \text{ g}$$

micron. μm. One-thousandth part of a millimetre; unit of measurement of bacterial size.

$$1\mu m = 10^{-3} \text{ mm} = 10^{-6} \text{ m}$$

micronutrient. A nutrient required by organisms in relatively small quantities. Micronutrients are typically found in cofactors and coenzymes. They include vitamins and trace elements such as copper, nickel, cobalt, vanadium, and zinc.

microorganism. An organism that is too small to be seen with the naked eye. An extraordinary variety of organisms such as viruses, bacteria, many algae, and fungi, and protozoa, are the conventional microorganisms.

Microorganisms are indispensable components of our ecosystem and make possible the carbon, nitrogen, oxygen, and sulphur cycles that take place in the terrestrial and aquatic systems; they are at the base of all ecological food chains. Also, microorganisms have harmed humans and disrupted society since the beginning of recorded history. Term including bacteria, moulds and yeasts classified as Fungi or Mycetes, a subdivision of *Thallophyta* or flowerless plants.

microwave drying. The process of removing moisture from a product in which the product is heated with microwave energy. Microwave heating is with energy at a frequency in the range of 900-18,000 megacycles/s. As compared to drying with electric resistance heating, a vacuum microwave dryer is about 50% more efficient. Microwave drying can be used for a wide range of products, from fine to large particles, and can be carried out at low temperatures.

Mignot cheese. A kind of soft rennet cheese similar to Point Pveque cheese, that has been made for a century in the Department of Calvados, France. Two types are made, white and passé, the former being a fresh cheese and the latter, a ripened cheese.

milk biosynthesis. The synthesis of milk takes place in specialized secretory cells of the mammary gland under the control of many hormones including estrogen and progesterone concerned with mammary development, prolactin with the initiation of lactation, and oxytocin with the release or letdown of milk into the collecting passages. Milk as normally removed from the mammary gland contains white blood cells (leukocytes), some bacteria, and portions of sluffed-off secretory and other cells lining the inter-mammary passages.

The mechanisms concerned with the selective assimilation of certain blood components into milk are not known. The secretory cells require all of the usual essential amino acid and a proportion of some of the nonessential acids to synthesize the milk proteins. Genetic polymorphs of several of milk proteins exist in the same species, differing from one another by only a few amino acid residues. The secreting cells is characterized by a high ratio of metabolized glucose proceeding *via* the pentose phosphate or oxidative shunt pathway instead of by glycolysis. One effect is for the NADPH$_2$ generated to enhance reductive synthesis such as takes place in the cells in the formation of the even chained fatty acids from acetate by the step wise condensation of acetyl-CoA units, with malonyl-CoA also involved. The synthesis of lactose involves the formation of uridine diphosphate glucose-1-P, its conversion to UDP-galactose and the condensation with glucose to form lactose. In many regards, the constituent ingredients are probably more readily appreciated if milk is conserved to have been a part of the actual tissue itself rather than only as a specific product of it.

milk drying. Milk and milk products are dried to provide a product of less volume for handling and storage and a product which will keep longer. The most common dairy products dried are nonfat dry milk (NDM), whole milk, whey, cream, and buttermilk, plus several manufactured products such as cheese, ice cream mix, malted milk, and other beverages. Drying is usually preceded by evaporation of 2:1 to 3:1. Drying is done in a spray dryer or on a drum dryer. The spay dryer is most commonly used for food products because flavour of product is superior for reconstitution as compared to the drum-dried product. With the spray dryer there is generally less heat effect, better stability, and dispersibility of product. Foam spray drying produces a product of low density and improved dispersibility

during reconstitution. Instantiating of dried milk products is the particular value for beverage products. The product is dried to 3 to 5%. Inlet air is heated to 121-260°C which leaves the dryer at 79.4-98.9°C. The dry product should be cooled quickly to 32.2-43.3°C.

milk fat. The fat found in milk is a mixture of mixed triglycerides. It contains significant amounts of at least sixteen different fatty acids ranging from four to twenty carbon atoms. It also contains the fat-soluble vitamins A and D and some cholesterol. The well known saturated fatty acids in milk include: arachidic, butyric, capric, caproic, caprylic, lauric, myristic, palmitic and stearic. Of the polyunsaturated fatty acids in milk, arachidonic and linoleic have been proved essential for growth of animals as has linolenic acid found in vegetable oils. Among polyunsaturated fatty acids are, oleic, decenoic, palmitoleic, and vaccinic.

milk ice. A milk sherbet. A semi-frozen product made of the same ingredients as water ice, with the addition of milk or milk products. It contains milk, sugar, fruit, juice, and may or may not contain added colour, flavour, fruit, acid, and stabilizer.

milk scum. A pellicle forming on the surface of hot milk in the open air. The cause of the formation of scum is due chiefly to the drying of the upper layer of liquid.

milk starter cultures. The purposeful addition of bacteria to milk, to effect unique organoleptic characteristics in the product as well as to aid its preservation. Not only do the starter culture acidify the milk, but also they produce specific flavoring compounds during fermentation, and the enzymes liberated by the lysed cells during subsequent ripening period also contribute to the flavour. Starter cultures are used in the production of milk products such as buttermilk, yogurt, some types of butter, and a variety of cheese. The starter cultures employed in fermented milk and cheese production fall into two categories based on the temperature of fermentation.

Some common starter cultures employed include *streptococcus lactis, streptococcus cremoris, streptococcus thermophilus, lactobacillus acidophilus, lactobacillus bulgaricus* and *propionibacterium freundenreichii*. t may be recalled that the cheese and fermented milk manufacture is prone to bacteriophage development in the starter cultures during scale up or in the fermentation vat.

milk stone. An accumulated precipitate of milk proteins, fats, and minerals on metal dairy equipment or a combination of these substances with hard water salts and alkaline detergents. Also, the deposit of calcium and magnesium phosphates, protein, etc., produced when milk is heated to temperatures above 60°C. Milk stone may be prevented by using soft water, by rising all equipment with cold water immediately after use, and by avoiding excessively high temperatures. Milk stone is best removed by the use of organic acids, citric and acetic acid having been used with success.

milk thistle. *Silybum marianum.* A robust annual or biennial, reaching a height of 0.3-1.2 metres. The glabrous leaves have undulate margins and sharp spines, are brilliant dark green above and markedly streaked with white along the veins. The flower heads are a reddish-purple with bracts ending in sharp spines. Milk thistle yields seeds that contain an important compound called silymarin, which holds enormous medical potential in the treatment of liver diseases.

milk, accredited. The milk untreated by heat, from cows examined at specified intervals for freedom from disease.

milk, acidophilus. A preparation similar to cultured buttermilk but soured by *L. acidophilus* instead of acid-producing streptococci.

milk, adulterated. Milk, the composition of which has been altered by the subtraction of some ingredients or by the addition of various substances; usually with fraudulent intent or as a means of escaping legislative regulations of standard milk quality. The most common forms of adulteration detected are:

(a) addition of water;

(b) skimming of milk (skim milk);

(c) addition of water and skim milk;

(d) addition of colouring matter to restore colour lost by skimming or watering;

(e) addition of thickening agent in order to restore body and viscosity;

(f) addition of preservative in order to keep milk saleable for longer periods of time; and

(g) reconstituted milk.

milk, buddeized. Milk preserved by the addition of hydrogen peroxide. It is not permitted in many countries.

milk, citrated. Milk to which sodium citrate has been added to combine with the calcium and inhibit and curdling of caseinogen which would normally occur in the stomach. It is claimed, with little evidence, to be of value in feeding infants and invalids.

milk, designated. Legally, milk may be designated pasteurized or sterilized and also Tuberculin Tested. The special designation "accredited" has been abolished.

milk, dried. Milk that has been evaporated to dryness, usually by spray or roller-drying. May be whole or full-cream milk (26% fat), three-quarter cream (not less than 20% fat), half-cream (not less than 14% fat), quarter cream (not less than 8% fat), or skim milk (1% fat).

milk, evaporated. Concentrated to about 45% of its original volume by evaporation. Legally must contain not less than 7.8% fat and 25.5% total solids. Also known as unsweetened, condensed milk.

milk, filled. Milk from which the natural fat has been removed and replaced with at from another source. The reason may be economic, if the butterfat can be replaced by a cheaper one, or, more recently, to replace a fat poor in the essential food acids with a vegetable fat rich in these factors.

milk, freezing-point test. The sample of milk is cooled below its freezing point and seeded with a crystal of ice. The temperature rises to the freezing point of milk as the whole freezes, normally between -0.53 to 0.56° C. When milk has been adulterated the freezing point rises nearer to that of water. The freezing point's above -0.53° C are indicative of adulteration.

milk, frozen or fresh frozen. Milk is pasteurized, treated with an ultrasonic vibrator at 5 million cycles per second for 5 minutes and frozen. It will keep for a year, and when thawed is indistinguishable from the original milk.

milk, half-cream. Usually refers to the dried product sometimes recommended for small and premature babies who are said by some pediatricians to be unable to digest the fat of whole milk. The fat is reduced by two methods:
(a) simple skimming of half the fat, when the protein content is proportionately increased from 26% to 29%; and
(b) by dilution with lactose when the protein is simultaneously diluted to 19%. Both types of half-cream milk are on the market for infant feeding.

milk, homogenized. After pasteurization, the milk is treated mechanically to break the fat globules into minute droplets which are evenly distributed throughout the milk. Homogenized milk therefore does not have a cream line.

milk, humanized. Cow's milk that has had its composition modified to resemble human milk. The main change is a reduction in protein content often achieved by dilution with carbohydrate and restoration of the fat content.

milk, irradiated. Milk that has been subjected to ultraviolet radiation for a short duration, when 7-dehydrocholesterol present naturally, is partially converted into vitamin D.

milk, long. A Scandinavian soured milk which is viscous because of "ropiness" caused by bacteria.

milk, long-life. Trade name for milk sterilized for a very short time 2 seconds) at ultra-high temperature (137°C). Also known as UHT milk.

milk, malted. A preparation of milk and the liquid separated from a mash of barley malt and wheat flour evaporated to dryness.

milk, non-fat. U.S. term for skimmed milk.

milk, sterilized. Legally, milk that has been filtered, homogenized and maintained at a temperature not less than 100°C until it complies with the turbidity test.

milk, sweetened, condensed. Milk that has been evaporated to less than one-third volume, and sugar added as preservative; it may be full cream or skimmed.

milk, toned. Dried, skim milk added to a high fat milk such as buffalo milk, to reduce the fat content but maintain the total solids. If the fat were diluted simply by adding water the milk would not be "toned up".

milk, turbidity test. This test is employed to distinguish sterilized milk from pasteurized milk. During sterilization, the milk is held at 104-116°C for 20-40 minutes, when all the albumin is precipitated. In the test the filtrate from an ammonium sulphate precipitation should remain clear on heating, indicating that no albumin was present in solution and the milk had therefore been sterilized.

milk. The secretion of the mammary gland of a number of animals is used as food in different parts of the world, e.g., cow, buffalo, goat, ass, mare, ewe. Milk contains a reasonable variety of vitamins except for E. It also contains minerals, particularly phosphorus and calcium, and it is a good emergency food for people whose diets are obviously deficient but not in specific ways that can be easily identified or corrected (provided they are not milk-intolerant). But for most of us on a reasonably rich and balanced diet milk should be used modestly particularly as it encourages heavy catarrhal secretion. Milk left in glass bottles for more than 2 hours can lose up to 80% of its vitamin A and 9% of its riboflavin, but the greatest loss of nutrients occurs in plastic containers. Milk packed in these and left under fluorescent lights of the shops can lose up to 14% of its riboflavin within 24 hours. Waxed cartons, on the other hand, block out most of the destructive light. Milk heated in an open saucepan loses 7%

of its riboflavin and boiling reduces the vitamin C content by 22%.

The vitamin content of milk varies according to the seasons. Vitamin A can vary from 235 IU in winter to 350 IU in summer and likewise the B vitamins fall in winter and rise in summer.

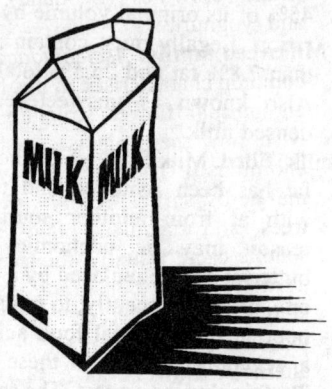

The milks differ considerably in composition. The average composition of cow's milk per 100 g is: protein 3%3; fat 3.5-4%; carbohydrate 4.6-5%; calcium 114 mg; phosphorus 100 mg; iron 0.04 mg; vitamin A 40 mg; vitamin B_1 0.045 mg; vitamin B_2 0.15 mg; nicotinic acid 0.08 mg, vitamin C 2 mg; vitamin D 0.05 mg; and food energy 0.28 MJ. Legally milk is not considered genuine if the fat is less than 3% and the other solids less than 8.5%.

milk-alkali syndrome. Weakness and lethargy caused by prolonged adherence to a diet rich in milk per day and alkalis.

Milk-Nickel. A registered trademark for a chocolate coated frozen confection on a stick consisting of either milk or vegetable fat frozen dessert.

milks, fermented. In various countries milk, from the ass, mare, cow, goat and buffalo, is fermented with a mixture of bacteria and yeasts when the lactose is converted to lactic acid and, in some drinks, to alcohol. Such type of fermented milks include busa (Turkestan), cieddu (Italy), dadhi (India), kefir (Balkans), kumiss (Steppes), leben (Egypt), mazun (Armenia), taette (N. Europe), skyr (Iceland), mast (Iran), crowdies (Scotland), kuban, and yoghurt.

Milkweed family: *Asclepiadaceae.* The common characteristic in this family is an unusual flower structure. Otherwise, how these plants appear varies enormously. There are sturdy perennial herbs, shrubs, dainty vines, small trees, and succulent plants that resemble cacti. Usually, the stems have a milky, latex-containing sap, and simple leaves in an opposite or whorled arrangement, but sometimes alternate. Flowers occur singly or in various types of clusters. The fruit is a follicle that splits along one seam.

The family includes: *Asclepias tuberosa* (butterfly-weed), *A. curassavica* (blood-flower), *Ceropegia woodii* (string-of-hearts), *Hoya carnosa* (wax-plant), *Huernia, Oxypetalum caeruleum* (blue milkweed), *Stapelia* (carrion-flower), *Stephanotis floribunda* (Madagascar-jasmine); *Asclepias syriaca* (common milkweed).

mill drying. The process of adding heat to the air circuit of the grinding mill to reduce the moisture content of the product. The procedure is also known as attritor drying and grinder drying. Products may be dried before, during, or after milling.

millerator. Wheat-cleaning machine consisting of two sieves, the upper one retaining particles larger than wheat, the lower one rejecting particles smaller than wheat.

millet. Family: *Gramineae.* Genus: *Pennisetum* (bulrush millet); *Panicum* (common millet); *Setaria* (foxtail millet). Species: *Pennisetum typhoideum* (bulrush millet); *Panicum* (common millet); *Setaria Italica* (foxtail millet).

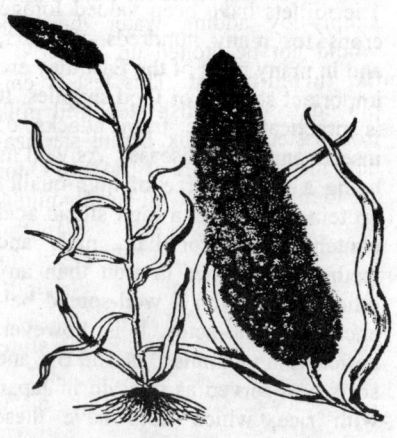

Millet is a common name for various species of grasses that produce roundish grains smaller than wheat and rice and high in fibre content. It is one of the most ancient of food grains, and is an important grain in Asia, being used as a food by a third of the population of the world. Nearly 161,876 million square metres are cultivated to this grain in India alone. Common millet (*Panicum* and *Setaria* species) also known as China, Italian, Indian, French, hog, proso, panicled and broom corn millet; grows very rapidly, 2-2.5 months from sowing to harvest. The average composition is: protein 10%; fat 2.5%; carbohydrate 73%; Red, finger, South India millet or ragi is *Eleusine coracana.* It contains about 6% protein, 1.5% fat, 75%carbohydrate. Bulrush millet, pearl millet, bajra or Kaffir manna corn is *Pennisetum typhoideum* or *americanium;* the staple food in poor parts of India. The approximate composition of this variety is: protein 11%, fat 5% carbohydrate 69%.

Other species are Kodo or haraka millet *Paspalum scrobiculatum*) and jajeo millet (*Acroceras amplectens*). The millets have been valued forage crops for many hundreds of years, and in many parts of the East they are important sources of food supplies. It is practically free from attacks of insects and plant diseases. As well as being a good source of high-quality protein, millet has a high silicic acid content (good for hair, nails and teeth). It is richer in iron than any other cereal, with a well-spread balance of amino-acids. It is, however, deficient in vitamins C, A and B$_{12}$, and so is best served as they do in Japan with rice, which does have these vitamins.

German millet, also known as foxtail millet and Hungarian grass, is from the grass *Setaria italica*. The seed contains phosphates and many minerals and vitamins A and E. It is an important food in Europe and Asia, but in North America it is a forage corp.

White millet, or proso millet, from the grass *Pancium miliaceum,* is one of the richest grains in food value, but is employed in the United States only as a birdseed. It is much used in Russia as a food. The millet from the plant *Sorghum vulgare* is a staple food in India.

Sanwa millet, from the *Echinochloa frumentacea,* is an important food in Japan. The plant will produce as many as eight forage crops per year.

Million's test. (For proteins). A test for the hydroxyphenyl group and therefore for tyrosine, but since every protein contains some tyrosine it is used as a general protein test. The reagent consists of mercury in nitric acid and gives a white precipitate with proteins which turns red on heating.

milt. The soft roe of the male fish. Also the name given to the spleen of animals.

mincemeat. Legally 30% dried fruit and peel, 30% sugar, 2.5 % fat, 0.5% acetic acid, not less than 65% soluble solids. In US, a heavily spiced mixture of chopped meat, apples and raisins.

mineral salts. The inorganic salts, including sodium, potassium, calcium, chloride, phosphate, sulphate, etc.

mineral waters, natural. Spring waters impregnated with carbon dioxide; some slightly alkaline; various minerals present in dilute solution. Legally, the amount of dissolved substances and the undissolved solids must be mentioned on the bottle containing mineral water.

mineralocorticoids. An obsolescent term for the steroid hormone of the adrenal cortex which controls the excretion of salt and water by the kidney.

miners' cramp. Cramp due to the loss of salt from the body caused by excessive sweating; occurs in tropical climates and with severe exercise-mining often combines the two. It may be prevented by consuming proper amount of salt, *e.g.,* salt tablets in the tropics and for athletes.

mint. Family: *Labiatae.* Genus: *Mentha.* Species: *Mentha viridis* (garden mint or spearmint); *Mentha piperita* (peppermint). The mints all contain similar chemical constituents though there are considerable variations in the relative proportions of these compounds among them. They all contain a volatile oil, ranging from about 0.3-0.4% in peppermint, through 0.7% in spearmint, to 1-2% in corn mint. Among a number of aroma chemicals present in the volatile oil, are menthol and carvone. In addition to volatile oils, mints also contain numerous biologically active constituents as well as flavonoids like rutin, resins, tannin and azulene. It has been noticed that menthol causes allergic reactions in many sensitive persons and these reactions may include flushing, contact dermatitis and headache. Newly borns may be sensitive towards menthol ointments applied to their nostrils to treat cold symptoms. Since peppermint and corn mint both contain sizeable amounts of menthol, be cautious when using these mints on children and be particularly cautious when using their oils. Menthol applied locally in its oil form to adults, however, has been reported to stop headache, neuralgia and itching. Pennyroyal oil is an abortificant and should not be used.

Many varieties of the species are used to flavour meat, fish, tobacco, etc. Oil of peppermint is distilled from stem and leaves of *Mentha piperita* and used both pharmaceutically and as a flavour. Peppermint. *Mentha piperita.* Spearmint. *Mentha spicata.* Both kinds of mints are closely related perennial aromatic herbs with runners by which they are propagated. The leaves of spearmint are sessile (no petioles), while those of peppermint are petioled. Both grow to about 1 m height and are cultivated worldwide. Each species has numerous varieties that produce essentials oils, which yield a menthol aroma and taste to varying degrees.

Mint family: *Lamiaceae (Labiatae).* Mint plants have square stems, mostly opposite leaves, and usually present are aromatic oils that account for the distinct and characteristic odours. Flowers have 5 fused petals that diverge into 2 lips (bilabiate). The single pistil has a superior, 4-lobed ovary, and a style that arises between the ovary lobes from the base of the flower (gynobasic style). The fruits produced are 4 nutlets. Usually, plants in this family are annual or perennial herbs, although shrubs, trees, and vines are also represented. The family include: *Majorana* (marjoram), Mentha spp. (mints), Nepeta (catnip), *Ocimum* (basil), *Origanum* (oregano), *Rosmarinus* (rosemary), *Salvia officinalis* (sage), *Satureja* (savory), *Thymus* (thyme); *Ajuga* (bugloss), *Coleus, Lavandula* (lavender), *Leonotis* (lion's-ear), *Molucella* (bells-of-Ireland), *Monarda* spp. (bergamot, Oswego tea, beebalm), *Physostegia* (false dragonhead). *Salvia splendens* (scarlet sage).

Mintzitra cheese. A kind of soft cheese made from ewe's milk in Macedonia.

miotin. Unidentified urinary excretion product of biotin, together with triotin and rhiotin.

miracle fruit. *Synsepalum dulcificum* Schum. A tropical red berry considered as a possible source of anthocyanins for food colorings, and as a source of a non-nutritive sweetener. The intensely red colour of the skin is due mainly to the presence of cyanidin-3-monoglycosides. The latter use is currently under a thorough investigation, including toxicological testing. Should the fruit be approved as a sweetener, further processing of the skins for their content of anthocyanins may be economical.

mirepoix. Bed of vegetables used to give flavour to braised meats and also soups and sauces.

Mish cheese. A kind of soft, ripened Egyptian cheese usually made from skim milk cheese to which whole milk and other flavouring and nutritive substances are added. The mixture is stored under microaerophilic conditions in an earthenware pot, called "Ballas" for a period of about one year before it becomes "Mish." When it is well ripened it has a sharp, pungent taste with a somewhat butyric odour resembling Romano and Roquefort cheese.

Miso. Name of an old Japanese food prepared by the fermentation of cooked soybeans or koji, with soybean and salt by *Aspergillus oryzae*. It differs from matto and tempeh in that it is prepared from a mixture of soybeans and rice in varying ratios with added salt. The rice is first mixed with *A. oryzae* and, after mixing with soybeans, the fermentation is allowed to proceed for periods of up to 1 year. Final protein content ranges between 10-17%. It is used mainly in soups.

Mitzithra, pot. The whey from Feta cheese is mixed with fresh milk, usually ewe's milk and curdled. It is made near Athens, Greece, and is eaten fresh.

mixed acid fermentation. The fermentation of glucose that is characteristic of *E. coli* and related bacteria and that yields formic, acetic, lactic, and succinic acids, as well as a number of other products.

mixed-function oxidases. A term used to describe liver microsome enzymes that catalyze oxidation reactions. They utilize molecular oxygen for the direct oxidation of the substrate, and they act on a wide range of substrates to cause cleavage of O-C or N-C bond.

moisture determination. The moisture content is usually expressed on a dry weight basis. Oven drying, distillation, titration, electrical properties, and hygroscopic methods are used to determine the moisture content. The most exact method for much research is the oven drying method, using a temperature of 100-103°C with small samples of 15-20 g until a constant weight is obtained.

moisture gradient. The variation of moisture content in a solid material or drying bed at a given time in the drying process. The moisture gradient may be expressed in percent moisture per unit distance.

moisture migration. The movement of moisture in stored products as a result of moisture and temperature changes. Moisture migration may occur with a product generally considered safe for storage. Moisture may accumulate on cold surface, usually at the top of stored products. The moisture content of the top layer may increase from 12-30% due to moisture migration. Greater moisture accumulation, and therefore greater losses, occur as a result of:
(a) high moisture content at the beginning of storage of materials,
(b) tall structure, and
(c) large difference in atmospheric and grain temperatures, when produce is placed in storage during warm weather followed by cold weather.

molasses. Syrup produced by washing raw sugar. It is boiled till as much sugar as possible crystallizes out. Molasses is a general term that has different meanings to the raw sugar manufacturer, the sugar refiner, and the baker. The various grades and types of molasses that are offered to the food manufacturer can be loosely defined as concentrated cane juice with:
(a) some of the sucrose removed;
(b) some of the sucrose inverted;
(c) various processing aids added; and
(d) various reaction products accumulated.

All types of molasses tend to be dark brown in colour, acidic in reaction, and bitter in flavour. The syrupy residue, so rich in non-sugars that no more sucrose can be crystallized out, is called molasses. Edible molasses is a heavily-bodied liquid derived from sugar cane. It is available in various types and grades depending upon milling and refining processes. The characteristic flavour of molasses is derived directly from the cane. The quality of molasses is determined by a number of factors, including the maturity of the sugarcane, the amount of sugar extracted, and the particular processes used. For most applications, the finest type of molasses is unsulfured molasses from the West Indies that has a lighter, clear color and delicate flavor. This type of molasses is sweeter than other grades.

Whole cane juice molasses is, ostensibly, all the juice as pressed from the cane, concentrated by boiling. Since sucrose will dissolve to give a concentration of only about 67% in water and at this concentration is not sufficiently stable microbiologically to allow safe storage and distribution, manufacturers of molasses invert part of the sucrose to give a total solids concentration of about 78-80% in the finished product. At this Brix level, molasses will resist fermentation by most microorganisms and can be distributed through normal channels without spoiling. This type of syrup is relatively light in color. Though mild in flavour, it is sweeter than a saturated solution of sucrose, Some of these kind of syrups are treated with sulphur dioxide. Other grades of molasses are collected in the sugar manufacturing process as liquids removed from the mass of crystallized sucrose that forms at various stages in the procedure.

First strike molasses is the syrup removed from the first crystallization. It can be sold as syrup or subjected to a further crystallization of sucrose after various treatments have been applied.

Molasses removed from the second crystallization step is called second strike molasses.

Third strike molasses is removed from the third crystallization vessel, etc. The molasses becomes progressively darker, more bitter, and lower in sucrose content as the number of "strikes" proceeds. Furthermore, nonfermentable carbohydrates, minerals, and other unwanted materials accumulate in the syrup, and some can have unwanted physiological effects.

Blackstrap molasses is the end point in the sequence and it is generally considered unfit for human consumption. Three principal advantages for the use of molasses by food processors are:

(a) It is a natural source of sugar which contributed to sweetness and, because of the invert sugar present, has a higher sweetness level on a total sugar basis than an equivalent amount of sucrose.

(b) It is a natural flavouring and can be used as the major flavouring in a formulation. Molasses is an excellent mask for certain undesirable flavours. At low levels, molasses can enhance the flavour of mocha, vanilla, and butterscotch, offering potential uses in puddings, cakes, and similar products. Similarly, molasses enhances the flavour of ham glazes and saucers for fish dishes, and frozen foods.

(c) Molasses offers natural nutrients, mainly the substantial quantities of readily available simple sugars.

(d) Molasses has significant humectant and water activity properties. Molasses has a high sugar content, consisting of noncrystallizing combination of invert and sucrose solids, both of which have substantial moisture control properties.

In addition, molasses has a nonsugar fraction (colloids, dextrans, pectic substances, salts, which amplifies the humectancy and water activity beyond that associated with the sucrose and invert present.

mold. Any of a large group of fungi that cause mold or moldiness and that exist as multicellular filamentous colonies; also the deposit or growth caused by such fungi; molds do not produce macroscopic fruiting bodies.

molecular sieve drying. A method of moisture removal, usually from gases but also from organic liquids, using a class of adsorbents known as aluminosilicates or zeolite. Previously molecular sieves were made with naturally occurring zeolites. There is now an increasing use of synthetic crystalline zeolites. The adsorbent has a high porosity of uniform size of pores, thus providing a large surface area. The adsorbents have high adsorptivity at low water vapor pressure. The zeolite pellets used for drying are dried in a rotary dryer or tunnel dryer.

Molisch reaction. Test for carbohydrates. The reagent is a 5% solution of α-naphthol in alcohol; two drops added to the test solution and concentrated sulphuric acid poured down the side of the tube to form a lower layer. Violet zone appears at the junction.

molybdenum. An element that is part of the enzyme xanthine oxidase and so may possible be a dietary essential in small traces although there is no evidence for this. It is toxic in small doses and "teart" in cattle is associated with feeding on pastures containing molybdenum. It is essential to plants. On an average, most soils contain about 2 mg/L molybdenum. However, a few soil are sufficiently rich in the element to yield a herbage containing a molybdenum concentration that is toxic to grazing animals. Other soils are so molybdenum deficient that the crop yield as poor. The latter soils are acidic. Striking responses in crop yield, especially with pasture legumes, have been reported following the addition of small quantities of molybdenum ores or salts. Trace amounts of the metal are found in fresh and sea waters, 0.35 ppb and 0.01 mg/L, respectively.

Molybdenum is present in all marine animals and plants as well as land animals and plants. It is essential to all organisms except perhaps some algae. The first evidence of a biological role for molybdenum was reported in 1930, when it was indicated that the element was an essential nutrient for azobacter. Subsequently, irregular, occurrence in low concentrations in all plant and animal tissues examined. It has been found that molybdenum is necessary for all nitrogen-fixing organisms. Later it was demonstrated that it was required by higher plants independent of its role in symbiotic nitrogen fixation. Scientists discovered the essential role of this trace metal in animals nutrition when they demonstrated that the flavoprotein enzyme xanthine oxidase contains molybdenum, as well as iron. Aldehyde dehydrogenase contains both metals, while, nitrite reductase contains molybdenum only. Iron and molybdenum are functional in the nitrogenases. Later it was demonstrated the essentiality of molybdenum in diets of lambs and fowl. Deficient molybdenum intake apparently reduced the growth rate in experimental animals and depleted the liver of xanthine oxidase. It is thought that a deficient molybdenum intake may produce xanthine renal calculi in sheep.

Under naturally occurring conditions uncomplicated molybdenum deficiencies have never been reported in either farm animals or man. There seems to be little evidence as yet that this trace metal plays a significant role in any aspect of human health or disease. In truth the metal has been studied very little in clinical situations. The mechanism of molybdenum action in caries formation is not yet known. It may modify the tooth morphology. According to a study conducted in high and low molybdenum-containing soil regions in California, a reduced prevalence of caries in children in the molybdenosis region was not observed. However, there was definitely higher level of molybdenum in the outer enamel of premolars obtained from the high molybdenum region. Furthermore, tooth enamel showed increasing molybdenum content with increasing age of tooth donors. Human dental enamel has been found to be relatively rich in molybdenum, ranging between 0.7 and 39 µg molybdenum g⁻¹. Molybdenum concentrations in the tissue of all species of animals is of a low order of magnitude, comparable to manganese. Concentrations in the liver are highest, followed in descending order by the kidney, spleen, lung, brain and muscle. Levels were not found to change significantly with age. Human blood molybdenum levels, among apparent controls reported from various regions, do show variations. Studies indicate that levels range between 0.5 µg/ml and 1.59 µg/ml, for the most part. Approximately 3% of the population had blood molybdenum concentrations of more than 10 µg/ml. The molybdenum levels in serum and packed blood cells have been found to be ten-fold less, about 1.1 ppb and 0.6 ppb, respectively. Judging from studies on sheep and cattle blood levels are dependent upon the molybdenum content in the diet. Levels could be raised by adding molybdenum supplements. Changes were reflected also in molybdenum concentrations in tissues and wool.

Foods vary greatly in their molybdenum contents. Legumes, cereal grains, leafy vegetables, liver and kidney are good sources of molybdenum. Fruits, root and stem vegetables, muscle meats, and dairy products are poor. Since molybdenum in grain is mainly concentrated in the outer layers, refined grain products are a poor source. Copper is also lost in the milling process. Daily molybdenum intakes of 10-15 mg had been reported to occur in certain regions of Armenia. It would be of interest to study those and other areas again utilizing currently available instrumentation. At this point minimum molybdenum requirements cannot be estimated. Molybdenum, copper and sulphate interact. It was first noted that the metabolism of one is dependent upon concentrations of the other more than thirty years ago, when scientists found increasing the molybdenum intake an effective treatment for copper poisoning among sheep in Australia. Later it was discovered that the inhibiting effect of molybdenum on copper retention to be dependent up to the inorganic sulphate content in the diet. Within certain limits blood molybdenum levels in sheep were found markedly and inversely dependent upon inorganic sulphate intakes. Studies with sheep indicate that sulphate limits molybdenum retention by reducing intestinal absorption, as well as by increasing urinary excretion.

Molybdenum is excreted in urine primarily as molybdate ion. Sulphate, it was postulated, if present in sufficiently high concentration interfered with and prevented the transport of molybdenum across membranes. The mechanism of interference is still known. Apparently, the sulphate effect is quite specific. Citrate, permanganate, selenate, silicate, and tungstate did not show similar activity. Diuretics were found to increase urine volume but not molybdenum excretion. The formation of a stable copper-molybdenum-protein compound in plasma that may explain the lower tissue uptake of copper in the presence of a high copper level in plasma has been described. The role of organic sulphur in the copper-molybdenum-sulphur interrelationship in ruminant nutrition is quite important. It was observed and plasma molybdenum levels were increased by molybdenum supplements; unaffected by molybdenum and sulphur given together; and slightly decreased by sulphur supplements alone. The latter also reduced replenishment of plasma copper pools. Molybdenum and sulphur supplements given together totally inhibited replenishment of plasma copper pools, but molybdenum alone was without apparent effect.

Manifestations of molybdenum toxicity (molybdenosis) vary among different species. High molybdenum uptakes from diet result in growth retardation and weight loss in different animals observed. However, diarrhoea is observed only among cattle. Molybdenosis in cattle occurs in many parts of the world where the soil molybdenum content is excessive. Though all cattle are susceptible, young cattle and milking cows are affected kore severely, while sheep in those areas, are only slightly affected, and horses not at all. The condition, which can lead to death, has been treated successfully with copper sulphate and potassium sulphate. Disturbances in phosphorus metabolism resulting in joint abnormalities, osteoporosis, lameness, and spontaneous bone fractures in farm animals, have been reported in areas of high molybdenum soils. Decreased reproduction of cattle in such areas has been observed when supplemental copper was not added to their diets. Similar effects of excess molybdenum intake have been observed experimentally in rats. Molybdenum in the latter has also been shown to induce thyroid hypofunction. Toxic manifestations of molybdenum in humans are unknown or unrecognized. The available data suggest that this trace element and its compounds are of low order of toxicity. Reports that very high molybdenum intakes alter uric acid metabolism in man are yet to be substantiated. Some compounds of molybdenum combined with ferrous sulphate, have been utilized to a limited degree as a hematinic in treating iron deficiency anemias.

Monachello lemon. A variety of lemon of relatively minor importance; mainly produced in Italy. The fruit is small, not very juicy, and generally of poor quality. The variety does not have good resistance to *mal secco* disease.

Moncenisio cheese. A variety of Italian blue-mold, Gorgon-zola-type cheese.

Moncenisio cheese. A kind of pasta filata cheese originally made in Calabria, is now made in many parts of Italy. The cheese is made by the same process as Caciocavallo cheese and is similar to Cotronese cheese.

Mondseer-Schachtelkase cheese. A variety of popular, Munster-type cheese of Austria which is made from whole or partly skimmed milk. The smear-ripened cheese is sharp and acidic in flavour, quite similar to a mild Limburger. The whole milk cheese is called Mondseer Schlosskase.

monellin. Active sweet principle from Serendipity Berry.

Monk's head. *See* Bellelay cheese.

monoamine oxidase. MAO. A mitochondrial enzyme located between the outer and inner mitochondrial membranes. The outer membrane is freely permeable to the substrates for the enzyme. Monoamine oxidase activity is present in nearly all tissues, and is particularly high in intestinal mucosa and liver. MAO catalyzes the oxidative deamination of catchlamines and a wide range of other amines to form corresponding aldehyde derivatives. FAD is a prosthetic group. There are two forms of the enzyme, known as MAO-A and MAO-B, with different substrate specificities and inhibitor sensitivities. Both forms of the enzyme have been found to be active against tyramine. MAO-A, but not MAO-B, is active against benzylamine and 2-phenylethylamine (and possibly dopamine, although this is controversial). In fact these specificities are relative rather than absolute, and the two enzyme forms are better distinguished by their sensitivity to inhibitors. MAO-A is relatively selectively inhibited by clorgyline, whereas MAO-B is relatively selectively inhibited by servilence.

monophagia. Desire for one type of food.

monosaccharide. A carbohydrate that cannot be split into smaller units by the action of dilute acids. Monosaccharides are classified according to the number of carbon atoms they possess: trioses have three carbon atoms; tetroses, four; pentoses, five; hexoses, six; etc. Each of these is further divided into aldoses and ketoses, depending on whether the molecule contains an aldehyde group or a ketone group. For example glucose, having six carbon atoms and an aldehyde group, is an aldodexose whereas fructose is a ketohexose. These aldehyde and ketone groups confer reducing properties on monosaccharides: they can be oxidized to yield sugar acids. They also react with phosphoric acid to produce phosphate esters (*e.g.,* in ATP), which are important in cell metabolism. Monosaccharides can exist as either straight-chain or ring-shaped molecules. They also exhibit optical activity, giving rise to both dextrorotatory and levorotatory forms.

monosodium glutamate. A chemical used as a flavour enhancer in various manufactured foods. The excessive amounts of this compound may cause intoxication; the clinical symptoms include burning sensation in the chest, neck, abdomen, and extremities plus a sensation of lightness and pressure over the face. Recently, the presence of this compound in the manufactured foods has been questioned by many health authorities.

Monostorer cheese. A ewe's milk cheese made in Transylvania, Rumania. The cheese are brine-salted for two days and cured for 8-10 weeks.

Mont cenis cheese. Large cheese blocks resembling imitation Roquefort varieties such as Gex. It is 45 cm in diameter and weighs about 10-12 kg. It was originally made in south-eastern France, but is quite popular in north-eastern Europe. A penicillium mold is sometimes incorporated in the curd.

Montasio cheese. A kind of strong rennet cheese made in certain parts of Austria and Italy. After the cheese is pressed, it is salted for a month (about 3% of the weight of the cheese is the weight of salt applied). Fresh cheese is nearly white; old ones are yellow, granular, and have a characteristic odour.

Montavoner cheese. A kind of Austrian sour milk cheese; dried herbs are added during the process of making.

Monterey, Jack. A variety of high-moisture, fast-curing cheese developed in Monterey. The cheese is made similar to Colby. Water at 28°C is added to the granular curd. The curd is placed in bags for draining and is pressed in these bags. The finished cheese is about 25 cm in diameter. Federal Standards recommends that the moisture should not be more than 44%, while the fat content should not be less than 50% in the solids.

Monthery cheese. A kind of soft cheese made in France from cows' milk to which rennet has been added in curdling. During the process of ripening, white mold, and later peculiar blue mold with red spots, appear on the outside surface of the cheeses.

Moore's diamond grape. A variety of native North American grape planted in the eastern US and Canada, and used for producing a tart, pale wine.

Morio-Muscat grape. A variety of grape which is a hybrid of Silvaner and Weisser Burgunder (Pinot Blanc). It ripens fairly early and gives a very good yield. The vine grows particularly well in the Rhenish Palatinate and the Rheinhessen wine-producing regions of Germany. Its wine has a strong muscat bouquet, which can become very potent in very ripe wine.

Moro orange. A variety of sweet, blood-type orange produced mainly in Italy. The fruit is distinctive in that pigmentation develops early and strongly in the flesh, although rind pigmentation may be inferior. The flesh is more intensely colored than any fruit in Italy and can become almost blue-black. The aroma of the fruit is distinctive, reminiscent of raspberry or violet at maturity. The variety is produced mainly for the fresh market.

morphactins. A group of plant growth regulators (morphologically active substances) that affect plant morphogenesis and growth. They consist of modified carboxylic acids and inhibit shoot elongation and cell division in apical meristems. These and other effects are believed to result form antagonic or synergistic interactions with other endogenous plant growth substances. Morphactins usually inhibit shoot elongation, but may stimulate lateral bud growth. In roots however they stimulate primary and inhibit lateral root growth. They have other effects, generally inhibiting development and abolishing phototropic and geotropic responses.

morphine. The main alkaloid of the opium poppy *Papaver somniferum*, and the prototype narcotic analgesic drug. Drugs producing the type of analgesia produced by morphine are known as morphine-like drugs. They are more commonly called narcotic analgesic drugs. Also known as opioids or opiates.

Mosambi orange. A variety of sweet orange that is produced mainly in India on Decan Plateau near Bombay. The fruit has a light-yellow rind at maturity. The surface is ridged. Because of the comparatively low acidity of the fruit, it is regarded by some persons as insipid. The fruit is very popular in India and Pakistan. This early-ripening fruit is believed to have been introduced into India From Mozambique.

motza. A kind of unleavened bread on Passover bread made as thin, flat, round or square water biscuits, and, according to the injunction in Exodus, eaten by Jews during the eight days of Passover in place of leavened bread. Also spelled as motzo.

motzo. *See* motza.

mould bran. A fungal amylase preparation produced by growing mould on moist wheat bran; used as source of starch-splitting enzymes.

moulds. Fungi that produce branched filaments, mycelia; reproduce by spores. They grow rapidly under appropriate conditions and the reproductive cycle from spore to spore can be completed in 24 hours. Include white *Mucor*, grey-green *Penicillium*, black *Aspergillus*, and also mushrooms and toadstools. Their growth is inhibited by propionates and sorbic acid. Many varieties of moulds are of technological importance, such as *Aspergillus niger* for citric acid manufacture, various *Penicillia* for cheese ripening, and antibiotic production.

Mouse. A frozen dessert consisting of whipped cream to which sugar and natural flavouring have been added.

mozzarella cheese. A kind of soft, plastic curd cheese earlier made in Campania in Southern Italy; now available throughout Europe and many other countries including India. This variety of cheese was originally made from buffalo's milk but is now made from cow's milk. The making procedure is similar to Caciocavallo and Scamorze. The cheese is eaten fresh. The curd may be wrapped in flexible wrappers and sold to the consumer or it may be sold fresh, to the dealer who completes the heating and kneading. Much of the Mozzarella is used in cooking, particularly in Pizza, pasta and macaroni.

M-protein. 1. A galactoside carrier protein in the permease system of *E. coli*. 2. A structural protein present in the M line of the myofibrils of striated muscle.

mucilage. A gum-like substance frequently present in the cell walls of aquatic plants and in the seed coats of certain other species. Mucilages are hard when dry and slimy when wet. Like gums they probably have a general protective function or serve to anchor the plant. Some organisms (*e.g.*, certain bacteria) are completely covered with mucilage and in such cases it probably prevents water loss.

mucin. Naturally occurring complexes of protein and carbohydrates; highly viscous.

mucopolysaccharides. The complexes of sugars, sugar acids and aminohexoses, *e.g.*, hyaluronic acid, heparin. Compound with protein they form mucoproteins. Mucoproteins. Complexes of protein with mucopolysaccharides; they function as lubricants in the eye, respiratory tract and intestines. Animal connective tissues contain a group of closely related acidic carbohydrate polymers which are located in the extracellular matrix and are collectively known as mucopolysaccharides. They are heteropolysaccharides formed by the chain condensation of a pair of monomeric sugar units in an alternating sequence, and as a result, these large polymers are invariably built up from disaccharide repeating units. Castilage has the highest content of chondroitin. Several polysaccharides of this type have been isolated and designated as chondroitin sulphate A, B, and C.

mucoproteins. Conjugated proteins in which the proteins portion is combined with a relatively large amount of carbohydrate (conventionally more than 4% measured as hexosamine); the carbohydrate portions are complex polysaccharides such as mucopolysaccharides. Glycoproteins are very similar in structure, but have less carbohydrate (less than 4%).

mucosa. Name given to the moist tissue lining, for example, the mouth (buccal mucosa) intestines and respiratory tract. The intestinal wall has two sides, the inner or mucosal side, and the outer, so serosal side.

Muesli. A dish, which is complete food, perfectly balanced, rich in calcium, phosphorus and other trace minerals and abundant in all the vitamins.

mulberry. *Morus nigra* (also white mulberry, *Morus alba*). A genus of trees and shrubs distinguished by large leaves and fruit which in form and structure resembles the blackberry. These trees originated in Persia. Of the several species, the common black mulberry is the best known and has been cultivated for centuries because of its fruit, which is used as dessert and also preserved in the form of a syrup or light jelly.

The white mulberry is the most interesting, because it furnishes food for silkworms. The red mulberry bears a fruit of a rich, deep-red colour.

The paper mulberry, now much cultivated, belonged originally to Japan, where its bark is used in the manufacture of paper.

The Russian mulberry is a small, hardy shrub that grows very rapidly and has been introduced into the Western US as a hedge plant. The average composition per 100 g is: 15 g carbohydrate; 1.4 g protein; 10 mg vitamin C; and 0.24 MJ food energy.

mullein. *Verbascum thapsus.* Mullein is aligned with snap dragon in the same family of *Scrophulriaceae.* With its tall, stately spires of primrose-yellow flowers, mullein is likely to be one of the tallest and most attractive plants in the border. It is a native of Europe and Asia. It was a familiar plant in cottage gardens which it had a number of folk names, including torches, hag taper, Adam's flannel, and Aaron's rod. The plant is not fragrant and has no culinary uses. In folk medicine the leaves were used to treat coughs, catarrh and asthma, and were a mild sedative. The dried flowers are infused in water to make a lightening hair rinse. If the leaves are used in an infusion, it must first be strained through a fine cloth to remove the minute hairs. Mullein flowers are stalkless with their sulphur-yellow corollas forming irregular cups an inch across, having five rounded petals enclosed in woolly calyxes. All manner of insects are attracted to this plant due to the easy accessibility of the nectar. By this means the plant is able to propagate itself elsewhere. The unique leaves are large and numerous, 15-20 cm long and upto 4 cm wide, becoming smaller as they ascend towards the stem. Mullein can reach heights greater than 2 metres and prefers clearings, fields, pastures and waste places from the Atlantic to the Pacific. This herb is common sight along many highways and railroad tracks, but should not be picked in these places due to frequent spraying with noxious chemical herbicides.

multienzyme system. The structural and functional entity that is formed by the association of several different enzymes which catalyze a sequence of closely related reactions; the aggregate may contain one or more molecules of a given enzyme.

multipurpose food. Indian multipurpose Food is prepared from peanut flour and chick-pea flour alongwith calcium carbonate, and vitamins A, B_1 and B_2 and contains as high as 40% protein; while the American multipurpose Food is based on soya products.

multi-stage drying. The procedure for removing moisture from products in more than one step. It is accomplished by either moving the product from one drying chamber to another, perhaps with different drying conditions, or by changing the drying conditions of product being dried in a particular chamber. The purpose of multistage drying is to avoid damage to the product (such as cracking of rice) to maintain desirable product conditions during moisture transfer, and to provide more economical drying.

multivitamin milk. A term used for milk which has been fortified with essential vitamins and minerals. As advertised by some companies each quart supplies minimum daily requirements of vitamin A, vitamin B_1, B_2 and niacin, vitamin D, calcium and phosphorus, iron and iodine.

Munchener beer. A sweet, dark-brown coloured larger beer which has peculiar aroma caused by the melanoidins formed during the drying of malt. The water used for brewing this beer has more calcium carbonate and less calcium sulphate. Munchener beer requires a low dosage of hops.

mung bean. Family: *Leguminosae*. Genus: *Phaseolus mungo*. Mung beans are rich in vitamins A, C and E and contain calcium, phosphorus and iron.

Munster cheese. A kind of semi-hard, rennet-curd, cheese which originated in Munster, Germany. The cheese is cylindrical in form, and in flavour a cross between Brick and Limburger. Its ripening takes about 2-3 months, and the process of manufacture is somewhat similar to that of brick cheese, but has less surface smear and undergoes less surface ripening during curing. Federal Standards recommends that the moisture content should not be less than 46%; not more than 50% in the solids.

Murcott mandarin. A variety of mandarin sometimes called the Murcott Honey or Smith, this variety is a medium-size, oblate, orange-colored fruit with a thin, smooth rind that is tightly adherent. However, it is fairly easy to peel. The flesh is an orange color and juicy. Flavor is rich and sprightly. There are few seeds. The fruit is very attractive with a good shipping quality. For processing, the concentrate prepared from the Mucrott has a bitter aftertaste and thus not over 10% of the juice can be blended with other citrus juices. The colouring power of the juice is high, well exceeding that of the Valencia orange. The origin of the variety is obscure.

Muscadelle grape. A white wine grape cultivated principally in the Bordeaux district of France. It is sometimes planted in with the vines of the Semillon and Sauvignon Blanc. The grape provides a Muscat flavour to finished wine. The variety also has been planted in South Africa.

Muscat grape.

of this grape exist, ranging in colour from yellow to blue-black. Thus a number of wines and other uses are made of it, include sweet red dessert wines and use as a blend with some Sauternes. The muscat is also popular as a table and raisin grape. Its plantings are widespread, including Alsace, Austria, California, Cyprus, France, Greece, Hungary, Israel, Italy, Portugal, Spain, Tunisia, and many other Mediterranean countries.

Muscatles. A sweet wine made from the same grape. Made by drying the large seed-containing grapes grown almost exclusively in amalaga (Spain). They are partially dried in the sun and drying completed indoors; they are left on the stalk and pressed flat for sale.

muscle. The contractile cellular unit of skeletal muscle is the fibre. This is a long cylinder in shape and composed of many myofibrils. Chemically the muscle fibre is composed of three proteins, myosin, actin and tropomyosin. The muscle fibre is surrounded by a thin membrane, the sarcolemma. Within the muscle fibre surrounding the myofibrils is the sarcoplasm or cytoplasm. Individual fibres are separated by a thin network of connective tissue, the endomysium and bound together in bundles by larger sheets of connective tissue, the perimysium. Muscle tissue also contains the structural elements, such as collagen reticulin and elastin.

muscovado. The impure sugar left after evaporating the juice from the sugar cane and draining off the molasses. It is moist and dark brown in colour, and is often used in making cakes.

mushroom drying. The mushroom, a fungi devoid of chlorophyll, whole or cut into pieces, is blanched then dried. When mushrooms are air dried, air temperature not in exceeding 65.6°C is used to dry to the level of 5% moisture content. Freeze drying is often used in which mushrooms are dried to the level of 3%.

mushroom sugar. α-α'-trehalose; found in most species of fungi, yeasts, many bacteria and the blood of insects.

mushroom. Family: *Agaricaceae*. Genus: *Agaricus*. Species: *Agaricus campestris*.

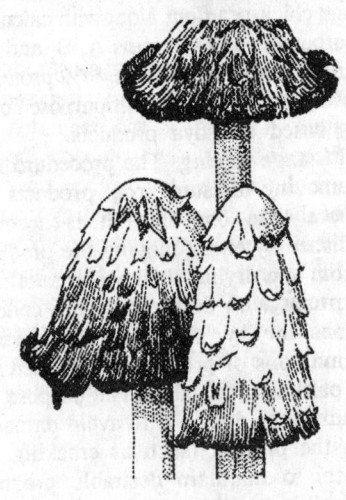

The common name for numerous species of fungi many of which are edible. Mushrooms are fungi that live in darkness, feeding off other organic matter. Lacking chlorophyll, they are unable to photosynthesize nourishment from sunlight. They have no roots, leaves, flowers or seeds. These mysterious characteristics have fascinated and tempted man since prehistoric times. Mushrooms are found in all parts of the world, and most species are of a very rapid growth. Certain classes are commonly known as toadstools and puffballs. While many varieties are edible, some are deadly poisonous.

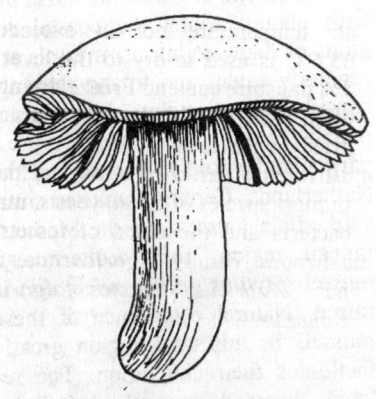

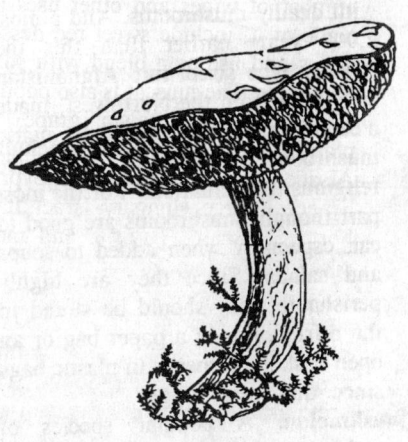

The parts of a typical mushroom are the cap, the gills, the ring and the stem. The cap is the expanded top, frequently umbrella-shaped. The gills are the thin plates on the under side of the cap, usually extending from the stem to its circumference; they bear the spores by which the mushroom is propagated. The ring is a growth around the stem, just below the gills, and is formed by part of the covering of the cap, left when the mushroom expands into its perfect form. The stem may be wanting altogether, as in the case of puffballs, or it may be short and thick or long and slender. The cap also takes a great variety of forms, some of them fantastic in the extreme. In young plants of some species, the cap, before breaking away from the mushrooms are often said to be in the "button stage." Mushrooms take a great variety most brilliant or rainbow tints, and in some species several colours blend, making beautiful specimens when growing, but they soon wither when picked. Certain species are unpleasant or even disgusting in appearance, and all are clammy and cold to the touch. Some species growing on the trunks of trees become hardened with age,

and one of these forms, the well-known touchwood, or punk, has the property of shedding light in the dark.

Edible mushrooms are cultivated for market in India, US and in many parts of the Europe. They thrive best in a moist atmosphere, from which bright sunlight is excluded. Gardeners usually grow them in beds of soil mixed with decaying horse manure. The beds are long and narrow and are usually covered, to protect them from the sun.

As an article of food, mushroom contain but little nutrition and are regarded as a delicacy rather than a staple. Of the species commonly found, the golden pezia, clavaria formosa and polyporus are edible; the russulus acts as an emetic, and the fly mushroom is poisonous. Since it is difficult for those not thoroughly familiar with the species to distinguish between poisonous and edible mushrooms, these plants should never be eaten unless selected by some one whose knowledge can be relied upon. Any mushrooms whose stalks have a swollen base, surrounded by a saclike or scaly envelope, should be avoided, especially if the gills are white, as should those with a milk-white juice. The ancient Roman emperor, Nero, poisoned his captain of the guards with deadly mushrooms. And almost 2,000 years earlier than this the Aryans, who swept into Afghanistan and India from the Northwest, made a ceremonial drink from the fly agaric mushroom in order to experience religious hallucinations. For the most part though, mushrooms are good to eat, especially when added to soups and salads. Since they are highly perishable, they should be stored in the refrigerator in a paper bag or an open basket, but never in plastic bags since they turn soggy.

muskmelon. A popular species of melon, so called because it has a delightful flavor suggestive of musk. The term muskmelon, sometimes used for the fruit, is simply a misnomer. Of the several varieties, two are in great demand, cantaloupes and nutmeg melons. The former have a hard, scaly rind, sometimes containing deep furrows. They ripen later than the nutmeg melons. The latter have softer rinds, more or less netted. The distinction between these forms is not known to most people, and the name cantaloupe is applied for the most part to both kinds. Muskmelons, like other members of the gourd family, grow on vines. They require a warm soil of moderate fertility. As a table fruit they are about as nutritious as peaches, pears or oranges.

mussels. *Mytilida.* They enjoy a worldwide distribution and are extremely adaptable. Their meat is tasty and contains a high percentage of vitamins, protein, minerals, and other important nutritive substances. Boiled mussels can be made into a variety of simple dishes, curried with rice, mixed with spaghetti, or made into a fish pie with potato. Along the coastal regions of many countries, mussels are regularly eaten, and inland they are considered tasty tidbits. Mussels are popular throughout Europe, and are a particular favorite in France and the Netherlands. Certain countries cultivate edible mussels. In the Mediterranean region, the Mediterranean mussel *(Mytilus galloprovincialis)* is raised. Natural occurrence of these mussels in this tidal region greatly facilitates their cultivation. The related bearded mussel (*Modiolus barbatus*) is also a valued food time in the Mediterranean countries. A principal predator of the mussel is the starfish.

must. A general term for the juices of fruits, including grapes, that can be fermented for the production of alcohol.

mustard. Family: *Cruciferae.* Genus: *Brassica.* Species: *Brassica hirta* or *alba* white mustard); *Brassica nigra* (black mustard); *Brassica juncea* (mustard greens). An extensive order of plants, embracing about 1,800 species. The plants are easily distinguished. The seeds of some species are ground into powder and are used medicinally and in cookery, while almost the entire plant of others (cabbage, cress, turnips, radish, horseradish) are used for the table. *Brassica nigra,* black mustard, which can reach a height of 3 m and was the main type grown commercially until some 40 years ago.

The pungency of the herb is due to an essential oil which forms only when the dry mustard powder is mixed with water. It is not present in the dry seed, which is why the seed does not have the 'bite' of made mustard, nor in the dry powder.

Mustard powder should be mixed with cold water. Boiling water kills the enzymes and produces a bitter flavour. Pungent taste and tear-producing properties of mustard seeds are due to the presence of nitrogen and sulphur-containing compounds called isothiocyanates. These are formed from two glucosides, called sinigrin (present in brown mustard) and sinalbin (present in white mustard). These are normally found in ground mustard seeds when the seeds are dried and it is only when they are wet that special enzymes like myrosin break down these glucosides to form isothiocyanates. Legally (UK) mustard condiment must yield not less than 0.35% allyl isothiocyanate after maceration with water for 2 hours at 37°C. English mustard contains not more than 10% wheat flour and water. Apart from the varying amounts of sinigrin and sinalbin, all the mustards have similar chemical constituents. They contain 25-37% fat, with protein and mucilage and numerous other biologically active compounds. Brown mustard yields a volatile oil (about 1%) composed almost exclusively of allyl isothiocyanate which is formed from the breakdown of sinigrin. Both brown and white mustard seeds are used in treating rheumatism, arthritis, sciatica, lumbago and neuralgia, and they are also used in emetics, diuretics, stimulants, appetizers and rubefacients. In China, 10-20% solution made from white mustard seeds has been successfully injected into various acupoints of people suffering from chronic bronchitis. Plasters made of white mustard can be applied to painful joints. The application is continually renewed until just before blisters are raised. Black mustard can be added to hot water as a footbath to ease chilblains. It should be taken sparingly internally because it can cause inflammation.

Dry mustard powder is added to salad dressings to give them pungency, added to egg and cheese dishes, and can be rubbed over the skim meat before roasting. White mustard seed is a preservative used in pickling, either alone or as an ingredients in mixed pickling spice. Ready-made mustards vary according to regional traditions. Dijon mustard is made from black mustard seed mixed with wine and spices; Bordeaux mustard, which is dark brown, contains the seed husks; English ready-made mustard is usually a mixture of the black and white seeds, without the husk, blended with wheat flour. Whole-grain mustards, with their coarse granular texture, are becoming more popular. A mustard bath, where the powder is mixed with hot water, is comforting for sore and aching feet and relaxing and reviving for the entire body.

Mustard greens are recommended as a tonic for anemia, constipation, rheumatism, arthritis, acidity, kidney and bladder ailments, and bronchial inflammation and are recommended particularly for pregnant women and nursing mothers, to rid the system of accumulated poisons. Mustard greens are rich in vitamins A, B and C and contain bulk fibre which produces a mildly laxative effect. A wonderful all-round reviver is a hot mustard footbath taken simultaneously with iced compresses applied to the head. A tea made from the seeds and used as a gargle loosens mucus congestion.

Dijon mustard is made exclusively from B. nigra or juncea with vinegar, grape juice or wine and not coloured.

Violet mustard is obtained by colouring with grape juice. Mustard leaves eaten raw in salads (mustard and stress) are seed leaves of Synapsis alba; much of the commercial product is a strain of rape (*Brassica napus*), a different strain from that used for edible oil.

Mustard family. *Brassicaeae (Cruciferae).* Cruciferae, the old family name, refers to the cross form (cruciform) of the 4 diagonally opposed petals. The flowers also have 4 sepals. Stamen number and lengths and the single pistil's ovary with a false partition are notable characteristics found in this family. The specialized type of fruit produced from the ovary is a narrow silique or a round silicle, in which seeds are separated into 2 chambers by a partition and covered on each side by a valve. The family consists of annual, biennial, or perennial herbs with pungent oils in the sap. The leaves are alternated and simple and usually have forked or star-like, 1-celled hairs.

The family include; *Armoracia* (horse-radish); *Brassica oleracea* (wild cabbage) selected varieties as food are *capitate* (head of leaves, cabbage), *acephala* (without a head, kale), *botrytis* (cluster of white flower buds, cauliflower), *gemmifera* (axillary buds-Brussels sprouts), *italica* (green flower buds, broccoli), *caulorapa* (swollen stem, kohlrabi); *B napobrassica* (rutabaga); *Nastrutium* (water cress); *Raphanus* (radish); Brassica spp. (wild mustards), *Capsella bursapastoris* (shepherd's purse), Lepidium pepper-grass), *Draba* (hoary cress), *Thlaspi* (penny cress); *Arabis* (rock cress), *Aubrieta, Aurinia saxatillis* (basket-of-gold), *Hesperis* (rocket), *Iberis* (candy-tuft), *Lobularia* (sweet alyssum), *Lunaria annua* (honesty, money plant, *Matthiola* (stock); *Isatis tinctoria* (dyer's woad).

mustard oil. An edible oil employed as cooking medium in many parts of India, Bangladesh, and Pakistan. The seeds are often contaminated with seeds of epidemic dropsy since the sanmexicana) which contains an alkaloid, sanguinarine. The contaminated mustard oil is the cause of epidemic dropsy as the sanguinarine inhibits the oxidation of pyruvic acid which accumulates in the blood.

mutagen. An agent that causes an increase in the number of mutants in a population. Mutagens operate either by causing changes in the DNA of genes, so interfering with the coding system, or by causing chromosome damage. Various chemicals such as nitrous acid, have been identified as mutagens. Chemical mutagens often act by altering the hydrogen-bonding properties of the bases. The chemical mutagens include alkylating agents, base analogs, and intercalating agents. The base pairs are incorporated into DNA in place of the natural base, while intercalating agents result in the addition of nucleotides. Certain base analogs are also useful in treating diseases. For example, azidothymidine (AZT), an analog of thymidine, inhibits the replication of human immunodeficiency virus (HIV) and is employed in the treatment of AIDS. Certain types of radiation, such as ultraviolet radiation and X-rays, are powerful mutagens. Irradiation of cells with UV light causes covalent bond formation between adjacent thymine molecules on the same strand of DNA, resulting in formation of thymine dimers. The covalent bonds distorts the DNA strand so much that the dimer cannot fit properly into the double helix and the DNA is damaged. DNA cannot be replicated beyond this site of damage nor can genes be transcribed.

mutton. A general term for the meat of sheep older than one year. The average composition per 100 g of mutton is: protein 12%; fat 21%; calcium 7 mg; iron 1.5 mg, zinc 1.8 mg; vitamin B_1 0.12 mg; vitamin B_2 0.13 mg; nicotinic acid 3.5 mg; and food energy 1 MJ.

mycobacteriaceae. Members of the family *Mycobacteriaceae*, in which the principal genus is *Mycobacterium*; are non-spore forming and do not usually form mycelia. Filaments may form that are extremely fragile. One of their unusual property is their slow growth rate. Many mycobacteria are found in soil and water, but some are obligate parasites in warm and cold-blooded animals. The most important human pathogens are *Mycobacterium tuberculosis* and *M. leprae*, the causative agents of tuberculosis and leprosy, respectively.

mycoplasmas. A trivial name for all bacteria of the class *Mollicutes* and the order *Mycoplasmatales*; Bergey's manual lists two families- *Mycoplasmataceae* and *Acholeplasmataceae*, but a third family- *Spiroplasmataceae* has also been added. All mycoplasmas lack cell walls and cannot synthesize peptidoglycan precursors; most require sterols for growth; they are the smallest organisms that are capable of independent reproduction. They are found in plants, animals, and insects, and one species, *Thermoplasma acidophilum*. The mycoplasmas have complex nutritional requirements and are the only prokaryotes that cannot synthesize fatty acids. Morphologically, the mycoplasmas are pleomorphic. Motility among the mycoplasmas except for spiroplasma, appears to be of a gliding nature and is believed to be associated with the specialized polar structure such as stalks, blebs, or tapered tips. These structures apparently help the organism to attach to surfaces and to push forward in a gliding movement. Very few species of mycoplasma are agents of disease in humans. They are important research tools because of their limited genetic information, minimal biochemical activity, and reduced size. They possess a minimum set of structures that are necessary for self-replication, a cell membrane, DNA, and ribosomes.

mycotoxins. The poisonous substances produced by the fungus which cause disease (mycotoxicosis) when eaten by an animal. Mycotoxins are among the many fungal products known as secondary metabolites- they have no obvious vital metabolic function for the organism. The production of any particular mycotoxin is often restricted to one or a few closely related species of mould, and occur only in a limited range of conditions.

myelin. A complex material formed of protein and phospholipid that is laid down as sheath around the axons of certain neurons, known as myelinated (or medullated) nerve fibres. The material is produced and laid down in concentric layers by neurilemmal cells at regular intervals along the nerve fibre. Myelinated nerve fibre conduct impulses more rapidly than nonmyelinated fibres.

Myoacets. Trade name for a range of distilled monoglycerides.

myogen. Protein of muscle, about 20% of the total; an albumin, not present in the muscle fibrils but only in the sarcoplasm in which the fibrils are embedded.

myoglobin. A complex protein in muscle, similar to the haemoglobin of the blood (but one fourth of its molecular weight), composed of iron-containing pigment, haem and the protein, globin. It serves as a storage mechanism for oxygen for the cells as it can reversibly add oxygen to form oxymyoglobin. The globin is denatured by heat to a brown pigment, hence the change from the red colour of raw meat to brown on cooking. When meat is cured with nitrite the myoglobin is converted into bright red nitric oxide-myoglobin or nitrosomyoglobin.

myosin. Major fraction, about two-fifths, of muscle protein. A globulin, insoluble in water but soluble in salt solution. Combines with the protein actin, to form actomyosin; the complex dissociates in the presence of ATP.

myristic acid. $CH_3(CH_2)_{12}COOH$. A long chain saturated fatty acid, which occurs as triglyceride in nutmeg butter, coconut, butter, lard, spermaceti and wool wax.

myrobalan extract. A liquid or solid extract from the dried, unripe fruit of several species of *Terminalia*, especially *T. chebala* of India and China. The *Phyllanthus emblica* of India also yields the fruit. The dried fruit resembles a plum, and contains about 30-40% tannin in the pulp. The fruit is graded and marketed as myrobalans chiefly on the basis of color, the lighter the color the higher the grade. The best grades of fruit are oval, pointed, and solid in structure. Inferior grades are round and spongy. The bimlies from Madras are rated best. Liquid myrobalan extract contains 25-30% tannin, and solid extract contains about 53%. It is used in tanning light leathers, and gives a quick tan. The natural acidity of myrobalan plums the leather, but when used alone on heavy hides it makes a porous leather. It is used with other tannins.

myrosinase. Glycosidase enzyme in mustard seed that hydrolyses myrosin or sinigrin to glucose and allyl isothiocyanate (mustard oil).

myrrh. *Commiphora myrrha.* A gum resin which exudes from a small balsam tree growing in Arabia and Eastern Africa. The gum exudes from the bark in oily yellowish tear which harden and turn dark. It has used by the ancients as a fumigant. Nowadays, it is used in medicine as a tonic, a stimulant, a mouth wash and a gargle. The best myrrh is exported from Turkey. Shrubs yielding myrrh gum grow upwards to 10 m in height and are native to north-eastern Africa and south-western Asia. The part used is the exudation from natural cracks in the bark or from man-made incisions. The exudation is a pale yellow liquid while soon hardens to form yellowish-red or reddish-brown tears or masses which are then collected.

Mysore flour. A blend of 75% tapioca flour and 25% peanut flour; it is used as a partial substitute for cereals in large-scale feeding trials in Tamil Nadu and Karnataka states of India.

Mysost. A by-product obtained from the cheese industry of Norway, Sweden, Denmark, and US. There is considerable variation in the composition of the whey used in different factories and in different localities, and in the manufacturing procedure and the composition of the cheese; and it is known by different local names. It has a butter-like consistency, and a milk sweet taste, but somewhat lacks flavour. In some instance a small proportion, usually not more than

10%, of buttermilk or whole milk, or even cream is added to the whey. It is strained, put into a kettle, brought to a boil, and the albumin which rises to the top is skimmed off. As soon as the whey evaporates to one-fourth the original volume, the albumin is returned to the whey and stirred well. When the mixture is of the consistency of heavy cream, it is quickly poured into a container and stirred with a paddle until cooled, to prevent sugar crystals from forming. It is then molded. Mysost is prepared from cow's milk whey. Gjetost is prepared from goat's milk whey; while Primost is prepared from goat's milk and contain more fat (buttermilk or cream).

myxobacteria. A group of Gram-negative, aerobic soil bacteria characterized by gliding motility, a complex life cycle with the production of fruiting bodies, and the formation of myxospores. Myxobacteria are found in the soil, in decaying vegetation, on the bark of trees, and in animal dung. Under appropriate conditions a swarm of vegetative cells aggregate and form fruiting bodies, within which some of the cells become converted into resting structures called myxospores. It is the ability to form complex fruiting bodies that distinguishes the myxobacteria from all other prokaryotes. Since the vegetative cells of fruiting myxobacteria look like those of non-fruiting gliding bacteria, it is only through observation of the fruiting bodies that these organisms can be identified. The fruiting bodies of the myxobacteria vary from simple globular masses of myxospores in loose slime to complex forms with a fruiting-body wall and a stalk. The fruiting bodies are strikingly coloured. In the genus Stigmatella, light greatly stimulates fruiting body formation, and it is thought that light catalyzes the production of a pheromone that initiates the aggregation step. The fruiting myxobacteria are classified primarily on morphological grounds using characteristics of the vegetative cells, the myxospores, and fruiting body structure. Phylogenetically, the gliding myxobacteria belong to the purple bacterial group.

myxospores. The special dormant spores formed by the myxobacteria. Under proper environmental and nutritional conditions either the myxospores are released to germinate or encysted vegetative cells are released to reproduce immediately. The spores possess unique structures called polar capsules, which contain filaments that are either coiled within the capsule or extruding from the cell. After the host ingests these spores, the polar filaments are extruded and used to attach to the host tissue, such as epithelium of intestinal tract. During the period of attachment the ameboid unit within the spore, called a spiroplasm, is released, and it migrates to specific organs where it develops into a multinucleated unit.

myxoxanthin. A carotenoid pigment found in algae possessing vitamin A activity.

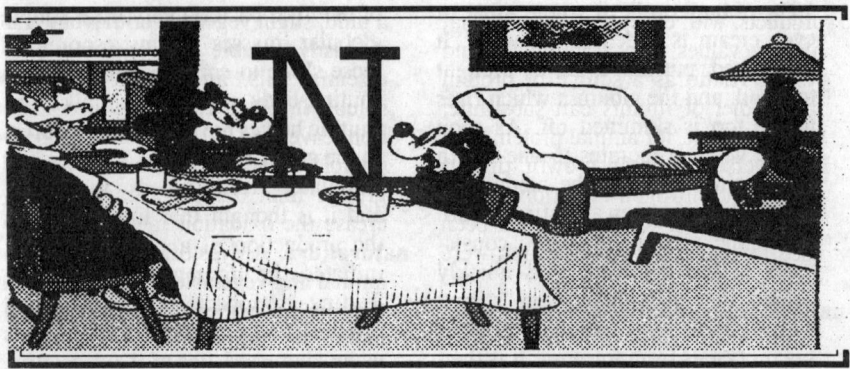

Naii tofu cheese. A kind of Mongolian Cheese made by the natural lactic fermentation of milk. After the whey is separated, the coagulated casein is taken out to be boiled and stirred up in a kettle until its serum evaporates and its viscosity increases. It is then put in a swollen box and cooled for a short time to be again coagulated; and, then, when it is taken out and dried in the sun, it is ready to be preserved in a receptacle.

nano-. A prefix meaning one-billionth part; for example, a nanosecond is one-billionth second; a nanometre is one-billionth metre, *i.e.*, 1 millimicron or 10 angstrom units.

α-naphthol test for carbohydrates. A standard test for carbyhydrates in solution. Molisch's reagent, α-naphthol in alchohol, is mixed with the test solution. Concentrated sulphuric acid is added and a violet ring at the junction of the two liquids indicates the presence of carbyhydrates. Also known as Molisch's test.

naphthoquinone. The basic part of the molecule of vitamin K; various forms of this vitamin are referred to as substituted naphthoquinones.

narcotic drug. Literally, a drug that produces narcosis; *i.e.*, reversible insensibility or stupor. In practice the term is often used to mean a dependence-producing drug. No contradiction arises when dependence-producing dugs of morphine type, for example, are referred to, because these drugs to produce depression of the cetral nervous system. However, the term is sometimes less appropriately applied to dependence-producing drugs such as cocaine or amphetamine which stimulate the central nervous system.

naringin. The complex of glucose, rhamnose and naringenin; the glucoside found in the pith of the grapefruit, especially when unripe, but no other citrus fruit. It often crystallizes in tiny beads from canned grapefruit segments and concentrated juice, particularly if the fruit was not fully ripe. It is very bitter, and is much stronger than quinine and can be detected at dilution of 1:50,000. Iit is hydrolyzed by the enzyme naringinase to the glucoside, prunin, which is less bitter, and to naringenin, which is not bitter. Thus, the bitter grapefruit and juice can be debittered.

natto. A product obtained from the fermentation of cooked soybeans by *Bacillus subtilis.* The essential amino acid composition docs not differ much from that of most other soybean products, with exception of somewhat higher values for tryptophan and lysine. Alatto as a source of protein in the diet of infants can substitute, at least in part, for animal protein with no adverse effects on growth, digestibility, and nitrogen retention. Natto, in the form of a powder, also has been used for making biscuits which were well accepted by children.

natural antioxidants. Many substances naturally occurring in foods and food ingredients act as fat antioxidants to some extent. They are usually of limited practical value for one or more of the following reasons:

(a) they are of low potency;

(b) they are accompanied by flavours, odours, or colours that are undesirable in most foods;

(c) they would be inordinately expensive to produce in commercial quantities; and

(d) their legal status as ingredients is questionable; for example, the tea extract evidently owes its antioxidant properties to galic acid.

A widely promoted natural antioxidant is mixed tocopherols, a material derived from vegetable oil distillates. The term 'mixed' indicates that alpha-beta-, gamma-, and delta-tocopherols may be present. It is said these additives, or some of them, as an additional advantage increase the vitamin E content of the finished product. It is said by the manufacturer that the ingredient may be described on the label as natural mixed tocopherols, a natural source of vitamin E, used to protect freshness. A commercial preparation of mixed tocopherols containing 70% of these compounds is described as a reddish brown, slightly viscous liquid having a refractive index of 1.559 at 20°C and a specific gravity of 0.92 at 25°C. It has

a mild, slight vegetable oil flavour and is easily soluble in vegetable oils, essential oils, and ethanol but insoluble in water. Recommended addition leaves are 0.015-0.045% of tocopherols, based on fat as 100%. Leaves greater than 0.1% may actually increase the oxidation rate.

natural dye. A dyestuff extracted from animal and vegetable tissues in which they are performed or exist in combination, as indigo, alizarin, logwood, carmine.

natural immunity. The ability of a living system to resist a disease without having had the disease and without being vaccinated against the disease. It is the nonspecific immunity resulting from the genetic constitution of the host. A natural immunity is based on the body's own defense and immunity system. The term is generally used to indicate an immunity to a disease that most people will contract when they are exposed to it. *See also* non-specific immunity.

natural starters. Portions of naturally soured clean-flavoured milk, or skim milk, cream, or buttermilk from a previous churning of good butter, added to the cream for butter-making in an effort to control the development of flavour in the cream and in the butter made from it. Their bacterial content is varied and therefore results are uncertain.

natural ventilation. The use of wind or change in temperature and humidity of the air to obtain air moyement to ventilate buildings or to remove moisture from grain. Natural ventilation can be accomplished by:

(a) air movement through the storage, as with eat corncribs;

(b) down-draft or pressure ventilator;

(c) an up-drift or suction ventilator;

(d) an A-type frame or vertical duct

which provides an air movement through the center of the bin or crib; and

(e) tubes made of steel spring or screened channels placed horizontally in the bin.

Neapolitan ice cream. A class of ice creams which is noted for its generous content of egg yolks. To each gallon of regular mix 10-20 egg yolks are added. These fresh egg yolks should be thoroughly beaten to break up all structure before they are added. To maintain proper sweetness in the mix, add 50 g of sugar for every 10 egg yolks used. A custard can be made by cooking the egg yolks in the regular mix in a jacketed kettle to 65° C and holding that temperature, with constant stirring, until custard is formed.

neat's foot. Ox or calf's foot used for making soups and jellies. Now called cow's heels.

neat's-foot oil. Oil obtained from the knuckle bones of cattle; it is used in leather working and for canning sardines.

negative control. The prevention of a biological activity by the presence of a specific molecule; the prevention by a repressor of either inducible enzyme synthesis or initiation of messenger RNA synthesis are two examples.

Neisseria. The Gram-negative, nonmotile, aerobic diplococci that inhibit the mucous membranes of animals. Some species are part of the normal flora of the human throat, others can cause sexually transmitted diseases, eye infections, and meningitis. *Neisseria gonorrhoeae* is the causative agent for the sexually transmitted human disease, gonorrhea. This bacterium was first observed in the pus cells from the genital exudate of the infected patients. It grows in the mucous membrane of the human urogenital tract where it can cause sufficient tissue damage to result in sterility of the patient. It is often referred to as the gonococcus. *Neisseria meningitidis* is the inhabitant of the nasopharynx of human carriers. A small percentage of these carriers develop cerebrospinal meningitis after the bacteria are transmitted by the blood to the central nervous system.

nematicides. The chemicals used to control nematodes; they are toxic to plants and must therefore be applied from one week to several months before planting. The rate of application is usually 200-450 kg/ha. The compounds most widely used as nematicides are methyl bromide, ethylene dibromide, 1,3-dichloropropene, methyl isothiocyanate, formaldehyde, carbon disulphide and chloropicrin. The first four are generally used when nematodes are the primary target and the last three when control of soil fungi is also required, but they are all effective general sterilants in sufficiently high dosage. 1, 2-dibromo-3-chloropropane has sufficiently low phytotoxicity to permit its use under favourable and controlled conditions for control of nematodes in citrus orchards. The toxicant is introduced into the soil along one side of each row of trees in one year and along the other side in the next in order to reduce direct chemical damage. All these compounds disperse through the soil in the vapour phase and, if good nematode control is to be achieved, distribution within the soil must be very good. If a non-volatile nematicide is to be used this distribution must be achieved mechanically or by the use of heavy irrigation following treatment with a water-soluble compound.

The first method involves introduction of a dust formulation into the soil and stirring to the necessary depth with a powerful rotary hoe. This method is effective only on easily-worked, friable soils, and is expensive. It has been applied to potato land using an inorganic mercury salt as the nematicide.

The second method can be applied only to good-structured, free-draining soils in which the compound can be washed down quickly and uniformly. If slow downward leaching under natural rain is to be relied on, the compound must not be significantly adsorbed on soil colloids. This imposes an almost impossible condition for complex non-ionized substances. Metham sodium is commonly used as a drench and acts by breaking down into methyl isothiocyanate. A number of organophosphorus compounds are also very useful for this type of application, for example, One of the most effective compounds for incorporation into topsoil by rotary cultivation is dazomet. However, applying a nematicide to soil in the autumn creates difficulties and non-phytotoxic granular material are being sought which can be applied to seedbeds in the spring. Some organophosphorus compounds are promising but the most effective substances are oxime carbamates such as aldicarb. At 7-14 kg/ha this compound prevents nematode injury to crops and stops them multiplying. The leaf and stem-dwelling nematodes may be controlled by several organophosphorus pesticides. Parathion is effective on chrysanthemums. Thionazin is used on bulbs and corns. Diclofenthion is less poisonous to men and animals. *See also* nematodes.

nematodes. The *Nemathelminthes*, including the class nematodes, are one of the two phyla of worms (the other is the *platyhelminths*) that include these that are obligate parasites of man. Examples of parasitic roundworms include Trichuris (whipworm), enterobius (threadworm), Ascaris (giant intestinal worm), Necatur (hookworm), and Onchoceca (blinding filaria). They are small worm-like organisms, generally about 1 mm long, which either live on plant roots as ectoparasites or enter the plant tissues via the roots and become endoparasites in leaves and stems. There are many species which are ubiquitous and do vast damage to crops, not only by feeding on the plants and causing them to become stunted, unyielding and less resistant to diseases, but also by actively transmitting virus diseases and allowing entry of fungi and bacteria through the damaged roots. Many produce galls. Their eggs remain dormant in the soil for long periods and often hatch out only under the influence of chemical substances secreted from the roots of the growing plants. The full nematode fauna of soil and the precise damage they do are imperfectly known as yet. Because the eggs are often protected by cysts they are very invulnerable to attack of any kind and so chemical control is a difficult problem. The principal method of control is still crop rotation but this has its limitations, and the modern tendency towards monoculture has exacerbated the problem. An attractive method of control would be chemicals which would cause the eggs to hatch in the absence of host plants, but this has not yet been achieved. The natural hatching factors are complex oxidized sugars, quite unsuitable for commercial production. The most widely used methods for controlling nematodes involve rather drastic and expensive treatment of the soil before sowing or planting.

Most soil nematodes are not deep-dwelling and are usually eliminated, so the results in practice are better than might be expected. Some nematodes have seasonal migratory habits and it is important in these cases that treatment is carried out when they are not in the deep layers of the soil. The damage done by nematodes to crops is much more serious if they are present during the early life of the transplant or seedling of elimination from the initial rooting zone may give the most satisfactory results.

nematode-trapping fungi. Some species of *Fungi Imperfecti* that reside in the soil are predaceous. These fungi have evolved a number of mechanisms for capturing small animals, such as nematodes, that they use for food, primarily as a source of nitrogen. For example, some species (*Dactylella bembicoides*) secrete a sticky substance on the surface of their hyphae. When a passing soil nematode comes in contact of the sticky hyphae, it becomes attached. Another species, namely, *Arthrobotrys dactyloides*, snares nematodes using specialized rings, each of which consists of three cells. When a nematode enters a loop, it triggers the release of osmotically active material in the cells, and water rushes in by osmosis. Turgor pressure increases and the cells swell rapidly, blocking the opening rapidly like a noose. Once triggered, the ring can garrote the nematode in less than a tenth of a second. When the nematode has been trapped, fungal hyphae grows into its body and digest it.

neohesperidin. A sweetener made by processing a substance found in rinds of grapefruit and some other citrus fruits. L-sugars are stereoiosomers of common natural D-sugars such as D-glucose, although these compounds stimulate human taste buds, the body cannot metabolize them and so they contribute sweetness without calories. Sucralose, a chlorinated derivative of sugar, is said to be about 600 times sweeter than sucrose, Neosugar is a derivative of sucrose produced by a fungal enzyme and it, too, is non-metabolizable.

neohesperidin dihydrochalcone. A synthetic compound, 1,000 times as sweet as sucrose; it is formed by the hydrogenation of naturally occurring flavonoid, neohesperidin.

neomycin. Antibiotic isolated from *Streptomyces fradii,* used to some extent in controlling infections in food processing.

neroli oil. An oil prepared from blossoms of the bitter orange by steam distillation. Yellowish oil with intense odour of orange blossom.

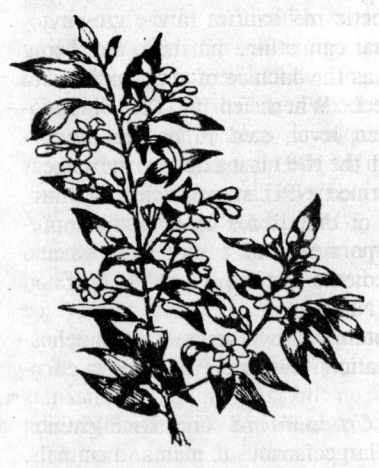

Nescafe. Trade name for a dried and

blended, instant coffee; it contains more potassium than any other commonly available food.

Nessler reagent. An alkaline, aqueous solution of potassium mercuric iodide, used in the detection and determination of ammonia, various amines, and other substances. Yellow or brown colours or precipitates are obtained. A number of methods are available for the preparation of this reagent.

net dietary protein energy ratio. The protein content of a diet or food expressed as protein energy multiplied by net protein utilization divided by total energy. Before the change from calories to joules this was termed net dietary protein calories per cent.

net protein utilization. Measure of quality of protein in terms of the amount of dietary protein retained in the body under specified experimental conditions. Previously expressed as a percentage, *i.e.*, egg protein and human milk and NPU 100; wheat protein 50; now expressed as ratio, 1.0 and 0.5 respectively. By convention measured at 10% dietary protein level, NPU_{10}, at which level the protein synthetic mechanism in the growing animal can utilize all the protein so long as the balance of amino acids is correct. When fed at 4% dietary protein level, said to be that level which the NPU is maximum, the value is termed NPU standardized. If the food or diet is fed as it is, i.e. not incorporated into a diet with other ingredients, the value is NPU operative (NPU_{op}).

net protein value. Product of net protein utilization and protein content per cent.

nettle. *Urtica diocia.* The name given to a large family of plants, most of them covered originated in Europe and now found all over the world. The square, bristly stem grows from 1-2 m high and bears pointed leaves which are downy underneath, and small, greenish flowers that grow in clustres from July to September. The main excuse of many a cook who leaves an unsightly clustre of nettles is that he likes them in soup. The young leaves are good lightly cooked like spinach, and in soup garnished with croutons and cream. They are also used to make beer. In self-help medicine the leaves were used to treat rheumatism, as a diuretic, and as a soothing aid to skin problems. The root fibre was at one time used to make twine, and bunches of fresh leaves were hung in the home to deter flies. One variety of nettle is used in China to make Chinese grass-cloth, and various other species are used for textile purposes. A yellow dye is made from neetle roots; green dye is produced from the leaves and stalks.

Neuberg ester. Name given to fructose-6-phosphate, one of the intermediates in glucose metabolism.

Neufchatel cheese. A kind of soft cheese, made originally in France, from either whole or skim milk, or a mixture of milk or cream. It may be eaten fresh or cured. When eaten fresh it is used like cream cheese. To cure this type of cheese, it is placed in curing rooms and cellars where it is kept clean and turned frequently. Microorganisms, such as *Mycoderma casei*, *Penicillium candidum* and *P. camemberti* and the so-called red cheese bacteria, grow on the surface during this period. In 3-4 weeks the cheese is wrapped in parchment or tinfoil and is ready to be marketed. In the US, Neufchatel is made from pasteurized milk or pasteurized milk and cream mixture in the same way as cream cheese, but with less moisture and fat. Federal Standards recommends that the moisture content should not be more than 65%; while fat not less than 20 and not more than 33% of the finished products.

neuraminic acid. A compound, derived from mannosamine and pyruvic acid, the acetylated form of which is a major building block of animal cell coats. It is an important constituent of many phospholipid membranes. It is a glycolipid and is particularly abundant in the plasma membranes of neurons.

neuraminidase. The enzyme that catalyzes the cleavage of N-acetylneuraminic acid from mucopolysaccharides; the enzyme is present on the surface of certain viruses and destroys the receptor activity of many cells for these viruses.

neuropeptide Y. A polypeptide containing 36-amino acids, first isolated from porcine brain. It coexists with noradrenaline in certain sympathetic nerve endings. It has been suggested that neuropeptide Y may function as a cotransmitter with norarenaline. It is a powerful vasoconstrictor and it as been proposed that it produce those vasoconstrictor responses to sympathetic nerve stimulation that are resistant to α-adrenoceptor blockade (note that this role has also been attributed to ATP). Neuropeptide Y inhibits cyclic AMP accumulation in cerebral blood vessels.

neurotensin. A tridecapeptide originally isolated from the bovine hypothalamus, but later found to have a characteristic distribution in the gastrointestinal tract, mainly within mucosal N-cells in the terminal ileum. Its pharmacological action include vasodilation, reduced gastric acid secretion, delayed gastric emptying, inhibition of gut motility, and stimulation of exocrine pancreatic secretion.

neurotoxin. The toxic substances with selective toxic actions on nervous tissue. Thy may be naturally occurring or synthetic. Tetrodotoxin B-bungarotoxin and dendrotoxin are examples of naturally occurring neurotoxins. Semicarbazide (which selectively depletes GABA systems), 6-hydroxydopamine (which selectively destroys noradrenergic nerve fibres) and 5,7-dihydroxytryptamine (which destroys serotoninergic nerve fibres) are some of the examples of synthetic neurotoxins.

neutral. A general term usualiy referring to an aqueous solution in which the concentration of hydronium ions and hydroxyl ions is exactly equal; such a solution has a pH value of 7.0 at room temperature; which is the pH of pure water.

neutral lipids. The lipids which do not possess a hydrophilic end and do not form micelles or bilayers with water; e.g., cholesterol esters and triglycerides.

neutrophil. A white blood cell (leukocyte) containing granules that do not stain with either acid or basic dyes. Neutrophils have many lobed nucleus and are therefore called polymorphonuclear leukocytes or polymorphs. Comprising about 70% of all leukocytes, they engulf and digest foreign particles, such as bacteria, using enzymes from their granules. This is the body's first line of defence against disease. They can pass out of capillaries by an amoeboid process (diapedesis) and wander in the tissues, gathering in large numbers at the site of an infection, where they may die, forming pus.

New zealand spinach. *Tetragoniaceae expansa.* Family: *Azoaceae* (carpetweed). A large plant with thick, succulent leaves and stems, that grows with a branching, spreading habit to a height of 0.6 m or more. This spinach is not related to common spinach, but is frequently grown as a substitute for spinach in areas where the weather is hot. The plant thrives in hot weather in seasons when ordinary spinach cannot withstand the heat. The soil requirements are the same as those for spinach. However, because of their larger size, these plants require more space to grow. Usually plantings are made in rows at least 0.9 m apart, with the plants about 0.5 m apart in the rows. As prompt germination may be difficult the seeds usually are soaked for 1-2 hours in water at 49°C before planting. They may be sown 2-4 cm deep as soon as danger of frost has passed. Successive harvests of the tips made by made from a single planting, as new leaves and branches are readily produced. Care must be taken not to remove too large a portion of the plant at one time.

N'gart oil. An oil obtained from the seeds of a climbing plant of Africa, and is equal in drying power to linseed oil. Lallemantia oil is obtained from the seeds of *Lallemantia iberica*, of south-eastern Europe and Asia; it resembles linseed oil in physical properties.

niacin. The vitamin nicotinic acid occurs in some foods partly in a bound form as niacytin, which is not available is the body (nor to bacteria) until it has been hydrolyzed. It is a complex of nicotinic acid with glucose, xylose, arabinose, and cinnamic acid derivatives.

nickel. An element present in most foodstuffs, but at levels below (and often well below) 1 mg/kg. Little is known about the chemical form of nickel in food, although it is probably partly complexed with phytic acid. Dietary contributions have been reported ranging from less than 200 to 900mg/day. A typical diet might contribute about 400 mg/day. Nickel concentrations of 100 mg/L and 50mg/L have been reported in wines and beers respectively.

It has been reported that about 10-20% of the nickel content of cigarettes (typically around 3 mg per cigarette) can be inhaled. This appears to be mainly as a volatile nickel compound, nickel carbonyl. A typical weekly intake for someone who smokes 20 cigarettes a day might be 40-80 mg of nickel.

Nickel is almost certainly essential for animal nutrition, and consequentially it is probably essential to man. Absorption of nickel through the gastrointestinal tract seems to be very low, *i.e.*, 1% or even less, although higher absorption values have been reported. There is little evidence of accumulation of nickel by various tissues. No significant accumulation of nickel was observed in rats fed nickel in drinking-water at a concentration of 5 mg/L. It is clear that at least in the animal body a mechanism controls excessive intake of nickel. Certain disease states in man do give rise to elevated nickel in tissue; the reasons, however are not understood. Nickel is readily excreted, mainly in the faeces, with smaller quantities in the urine and sweat.

The levels of nickel found in food and water are not considered a serious health hazard however, high doses (1600 mg/kg in the diet) were shown in early animal studies to cause minimal toxic effects. Certain nickel compounds have been shown to be carcinogenic in animal experiments. However, soluble nickel compounds are not currently regarded as either human or animal carcinogens. As in the case of other divalent cations, nickel can react with DNA and at high concentrations can result in DNA damage as shown in vitro mutagenicity tests. Dermatitis is most commonly associated with industrial exposure. However, the same effects have been observed from dermal contact with coinage or jewellery. High-level occupational exposures have been associated with renal problems, and effects such as vertigo and dyspnoea have been observed.

Occupational exposure to nickel should be controlled so that no employee is exposed to nickel at a concentration greater than 15 mg/m³ of air, determined as a time-weighted average (TWA) concentration limit for up to a 10-hour workshift in a 40-hour workweek, over a working lifetime.

Many compounds of nickel are water-soluble, therefore contamination of water can arise; significant problems are associated with industrial discharge to rivers of effluents containing nickel compounds. Level as high as 1 mg/L have been reported in surface-waters although the levels are generally much lower, e.g., 5-20 mg/L. For the protection of human health from the toxic effects of nickel ingested through water and contaminated aquatic organisms, the ambient water criterion has been set to be 7.1 mg/L; while for the protection of human health from the toxic properties of nickel ingested through the contaminated aquatic organisms alone, ambient water criterion has been determined to be 140 mg/L.

nicotinamide adenine dinucleotide. NAD.
A coenzyme, derived from the B vitamin nicotinic acid, that participates in many biological dehydrogenation reactions. NAD is characteristically loosely bound to the enzymes concerned. It normally carries a positive charge and can accept one hydrogen atom and two electrons to become the reduced form, NADH, which is generated during the oxidation of food, especially by the reactions of the Krebs cycle. It then gives up its two electrons (and single proton) to the electron transport chain, thereby reverting to NAD⁺ and generating three molecules of ATP per molecule of NADH. NADP (nicotinamide adenine dinucleotide phosphate) differs from NAD only in possessing an additional phosphate group. It functions in the same manner as NAD although anabolic reactions generally use NADPH (reduced NADP) as a hydrogen donor rather than NADH. The enzymes tend to be specific for either NAD or NADP as coenzyme. Living organisms carry out a variety of chemical reactions which are catalyzed by enzymes, e.g., hydrolytic, isomerization, transfer, synthetic, an oxidation-reduction reactions, there are about 200 that are known, and in many cases, electron carriers known as coenzymes are involved. Examples of such coenzymes are nicotinamide adenine dinucleotide (NAD) and a closely related compound nicotinamide adenine dinucleotide phosphate (NADP). Both coenzymes are reduced by the transfer of two hydrogen atoms from substrates to the coenzymes, such transfer being catalyzed by substrate-specific enzymes known as dehydrogenases. The reduced products formed are designated NADH and NADPH, respectively. In the case of NADP, there is an additional

phosphate group on the ribose next to the adenine, which is of importance in determining the specificity of combination with different dehydrogenases. However, both of these compounds are functionally similar as far as oxidation and reduction are concerned.

nicotinate, sodium. Sodium salt of nicotinic acid; used, among other purposes, to preserve the red colour in fresh and processed meats.

nicotine. 3-(1-Methyl-2-pyrrolidinyl) pyridine. The main alkaloid present in tobacco leaves *Nicotiana tabacum* and *N. rustica*. The naturally occurring form in tobacco is the (-)-S-isomer which is pharmacologically more active than the (+)-R-isomer.

nicotinic acid. One of the water-soluble B-group of vitamins with no numerical designation; sometimes called vitamin PP (pellagra-preventative). It is found in meat, liver and yeast; that present in cereals often largely unavailable; added to flour in many countries. Its deficiency in man causes pellagra.

Nicotinic acid is unique among the B vitamins in that it can be synthesized in animal tissues from the amino acid tryptophan. Other routes of synthesis exist in plants and certain microorganisms. The major pathway of tryptophan metabolism in the animal involves its oxidation to kynurenine and subsequent hydroxylation of the benzene ring and cleavage of the 3-carbon side chain to form alanine and 3-hydroxyanthranilic acid. This compound can be further oxidized to carbon dioxide and water or it can be converted to quinolinic acid, which then condenses with the 5-phosphoribosyl-1-pyrophosphate with the simultaneous evolution of carbon dioxide to yield nicotinic acid ribotide. The ribotide can be hydrolyzed to

yield free nicotinic acid, or it can be converted to NAD or NADP, the coenzyme forms of niacin. Niacin functions in metabolism as an integral part of the pyridine nucleotides NAD and NADP. These coenzymes act as hydrogen donors and acceptors for the biological oxidation-reduction reactions in the metabolism of carbohydrates, amino acids and lipids. Animals tissues do not retain large amounts of nicotinic acid. The excessive amounts are excreted in the urine, in man chiefly as the methylated compounds N^1-methylnicotinamide (N^1-Me) and the 6-pyridone of N^1-Me. Small amounts of free nicotinic acid and nicotinamide are found in human urine, and ingestion of large doses of nicotinic acid results in excretion of nicotinuric acid, which is the glycine conjugate of nicotinic acid.

Dogs, rats, cats and pigs, like man, excrete niacin as N^1-Me; however, the herbivora, rabbits, guinea pigs, sheep and goats excrete other forms. Chickens excrete ornithine derivatives of nicotinic acid. Radioactive carbon dioxide results from the administration of ^{14}C-nicotinic acid to mice, rats and dogs. Very little radioactivity is found in the feces of these animals. Also known as niacin. The recommended daily intake of nicotinic acid is 10 mg.

Nieheimer cheese. A kind of sour milk cheese, named after the city of Nieheim in Westphalia, where it is made. Salt, caraway seed, and sometimes beer are added to it during the initial ripening period. Following this, the cheese is covered with straw and ripened.

Niftee. The registered trademark for a chocolate coated frozen confection on a stick consisting of either ice milk or vegetable fat frozen dessert; it is popular in many countries.

nightshade. A plant belonging to the genus known to botanists as Solanum, and found in all continents. The plants have slightly narcotic properties, and some are poisonous. One species is the beautiful bittersweet, a woody vine with flowers resembling potato blossoms and having clusters of tomato-red berries; another is the black night shade, having white, bell-shaped flowers and black berries; still another is the deadly nightshade, or belladonna, which has black berries the size of cherries, and is poisonous. It yields a valuable drug, for which it is widely cultivated in parts of Europe. *See also* nightshade family.

Nightshade family: *Solanaceae.* There is no single characteristic common only to this family. The number of features are present. Flower petal lobes tend to overlap or have creases in a petal tube, which in bud is folded to the petals. Numerous ovules develop into numerous seeds in the berry or capsule fruit. The leaves are mostly alternate and simple, but size and shape vary greatly throughout the family. Usually the leaves are hairy and have a characteristic odour. Plant form ranges from herb to shrub to tree to vine.

This family include the following: *Capsium* spp. (bell pepper, chillies, cayenne pepper, paprika), *Lycopersicon esculentum* (tomato), *Solanum tuberosum* (potato); *Browallia, Datura arborea* (angel's trumpet), *Nicotiana Nierembergia, Petunia, Physalis alkekengi* (Chinese lantern), *Schizanthus, Solandra* (cup-of-gold); *Atropa belladonna* (deadly nightshade, belladonna, atropine), *Datura stramonium* (jimson weed), *Nicotiana* (tobacco, nicotine insecticide), *Physalis heterophylla* (ground-cherry), *Solanum dulcamara* (bitter night-shade), *S. nigrum* (black nightshade), *S. pseudocapsicum* (Jerusalem-cherry).

Nikl-Stikl. The registered trademark for a chocolate coated frozen confection on a stick consisting of either (a) the iced milk; or (b) the vegetable fat frozen dessert.

ninhydrin. A reagent used for the detection of amino acids. A blue colour is produced with proteins and all amino acids except for proline, which gives a yellow color. Ninhydrin also reacts with imino acids to give yellow color.

nioigome. A kind of perfumed rice.

NIOSH. Abbreviation for the U.S. *N*ational *I*nstitute for *O*ccupational *S*afety and *H*ealth. It evaluates all available research data and criteria and recommends standards for occupational exposure.

nisin. An antibiotic isolated from lactic streptococci group N. The non-toxic, polypeptide, inhibits some but not all clostridia; not used medically. The only antibiotic permitted in UK in food preservation (in certain foods). It is naturally present in cheese, being produced by a number of strains of cheese starter organisms. It has been found to be useful to prolong storage life of cheese, milk, cream, soups, canned fruits and vegetables, canned fish and milk puddings. It is used at 2-4 µg/g of processed cheese and 1-5 µg/g of canned peas. It also lowers the resistance of many thermophilic bacteria to heat and so permits a reduction in the time and/or temperature of heating in the processing of canned vegetables.

nitrates. The oxyanionic species containing nitrogen; occurs naturally in many foods; used sometimes in combination with nitrites to cure meat such as bacon, ham and luncheon meat. During pickling processes nitrate is partly reduced to nitrite which combines with meat pigment, myoglobin, to form red nitrosomyoglobin. Nitrite and its breakdown products inhibit growth of pathogens. Nitrites can react with amines in foods to form nitrosamines, many of which are carcinogenic. Permitted content in cured meats in UK is restricted to 500 mg/L sodium or potassium nitrate and 200 mg/L nitrite.

nitrifying bacteria. Bacteria able to grow lithotrophically at the expense of reduced inorganic nitrogen compounds. Several genera have been recognized on the basis of morphology and the particular steps in the oxidation sequences that they carry out. No lithotrophic organism is known that can carry out the complete oxidation of ammonia to nitrate; thus nitrification of ammonia in nature results from the sequential action of two separate groups of organisms, the ammonia-oxidizing bacteria, the nitrosifyers, and the nitrite-oxidizing bacteria, the true nitrifying bacteria.

nitrogen. An essential element found in all amino acids and therefore in all proteins, and in various other important organic compounds, *e.g.,* nucleic acids. Gaseous nitrogen forms about 80% of the atmosphere but is unavailable in this form except to a few nitrogen-fixing bacteria. Nitrogen is therefore usually incorporated into plants as the nitrate ion, NO_3^-, absorbed in solution from the soil by roots. In animals, the nitrogen compounds, such as urea and uric acid, form the main excretory products.

In nutrition, the term nitrogen is used to refer to ammonium salts and nitrates as plant fertilizers, to proteins and amino acids as animal nutrients, and to urea and ammonium salts as excretory products. In other words all nitrogen-containing substances are loosely referred to as nitrogen.

nitrogen assimilation. Once the nitrate is within the cell, it is reduced back to ammonium. This reduction process requires energy, in contrast to the nitrification process which involves oxidation (of NH_4^+) and which releases energy. The ammonium ions formed by the reduction process are transferred to carbon-containing compounds to produce amino acids and other nitrogen-containing organic compounds. This process is known as amination. The incorporation of nitrogen into organic compounds takes place largely in the young, growing root cells. The initial stages in the metabolism of nitrogen appear to occur right in the root; almost all the nitrogen ascending the stem in the xylem is already in the form of organic molecules, largely amino acids.

nitrogen balance. Condition in which intake equals output, as in the normal adult. In negative balance the excretion exceeds the intake; positive balance is the reverse. Growing children and convalescents are in positive nitrogen balance; patients with wasting diseases are in negative balance. Alternatively known as nitrogen equilibrium.

nitrogen fixation. Nitrogen can be obtained by microorganisms either from inorganic or organic compounds. The most common inorganic nitrogen sources are nitrate and ammonia, but other inorganic sources used by certain microbes include cyanide, cyanate, thiocyanate, cyanamide, nitrite, and hydroxylamine.

Nitrogen fixation involves the activity of the enzyme nitrogenase, a large two-component protein containing iron and molybdenum. Nitrogenase in the root nodules has characteristics similar to enzyme of free-living N_2-fixing bacteria, including O_2 sensitivity and ability to reduce acetylene as well as the molecular nitrogen. Nitrogenase is localized within the bacteroids themselves and is not released into the plant cytosol. Bacteroids are totally dependent on the plant for supplying them with energy sources for molecular nitrogen fixation. The major organic compounds transported across the peribacteroid membrane and into the bacteroid proper are citric acid cycle intermediates, in particular the C-4 acids succinate, malate, and fumarate. These serve as electron donors for ATP production and as the ultimate source of electrons for the reduction of molecular nitrogen (N_2). Although the precise reductant for molecular nitrogen fixation in the bacteroid is not known, the biochemical steps in the conversion of molecular nitrogen to NH_3 are probably similar to those in free-living nitrogen-fixing systems, suggesting that pyruvate is the direct electron donor to bacteroid nitrogenase. The first stable product of nitrogen fixation is ammonia, and several evidences suggest that assimilation of ammonia into organic nitrogen compounds in the root nodule is primarily carried out by the plant. Although bacteroids can assimilate some ammonia into organic form, the levels of ammonia assimilatory enzymes in bacteroids are quite low. By contrast, the ammonia assimilating enzyme *glutamine synthetase* is present in high levels in the plant cell cytoplasm. Hence, ammonia transported from the bacteroid to the plant cell can be assimilated by the plant as the amino acid glutamine. Besides, glutamine, other nitrogenous compounds, in particular other amino acid

amides, such as asparagine and 4-methyleneglutamine, and urea derivatives such as allantoin and allantoic acid, are synthesized by the plant and subsequently transported to plant tissues.

nitrogen mustards. A group of alkylating agents that alkylate various nucleophilic cell constituents, *e.g.*, the 7N of guanine which is the main purine base of DNA that is alkylated.

nitrogen, metabolic. Nitrogen of the faeces derived from internal or endogenous sources, as distinct from nitrogen residues from dietary sources (exogenous nitrogen). This nitrogen consists of unabsorbed digestive juices, the shed lining of the gastrointestinal tract and bacteria from the intestine, and continues to be excreted on a protein-free diet.

nitrogenous base. Heterocyclic compound, containing both carbon and nitrogen in a ring structure; found as a component of nucleosides, nucleotides and nucleic acids. The term is usually applied to purine and pyrimidine bases, but in a broader sense it can refer to other nitrogen-containing heterocyclic groups such as flavin and nicotinamide occurring in nucleotide coenzymes.

nitrosomyoglobin. The red colour of cured meat. It is formed by the reaction of nitric oxide from the pickling salts (saltpeter) with the muscle pigment, myoglobin. Fades in light to yellow-brown metmyoglobin.

nitrous oxide. A gas used as propellant in pressurized containers, for example, to eject cream or salad dressing from containers.

Noekkelost cheese. A Norwegian spiced cheese similar to Kuminost and Dutch Leyden. The cheese is usually made from partly skimmed milk. Paraffin-covered loaf. Also known as Nogelost.

Nogelost. *See* Noekkelost cheese.

non-esterified fatty acids. NEFA. Free fatty acids in the blood, about 10% of the total blood fatty acids, usually 0.5-1.0 µmole/L. They have a rapid turnover rate and may be the primary fuel of working muscles. The fuel for sudden bursts of hard exercise is glycogen, but for long-continued work the free fatty acids are said to be the source of energy. Also known as unesterified fatty acids.

non-pareils. The silver beads used to decorate confectionery, made from sugar coated with silver foil or aluminium-copper alloy.

non-specific immunity. The mechanism for destroying the foreign and potentially harmful macromolecules, microorganisms or metazoa which do not involve the recognition of antigen and the mounting of specific immune response. Such mechanisms include the action of lysozyme or interferon, phagocytosis and chemical and physical barriers to infection.

nor-. Chemical prefix to the name of a compound indicating one methyl group less, *e.g.*, noradrenalin contains a methyl less than adrenalin, similarly norleucine, norvaline.

noradrenaline. A catecholamine, which is secreted as hormone by the adrenal medulla, that regulates heart muscle, smooth muscle, and glands. It is also secreted by nerve endings of the sympathetic nervous system in which it acts as a transmitter of impulses. In the brain, levels of noradrenaline are related to mental function; lowered levels lead to mental depression. Also known as norepinephrine.

nordihydroguaiaretic acid. NDGA. A substance of plant origin (creosote bush) used as an antioxidant for fats.

Norite. A variety of activated carbon used to decolorize solutions.

normal enzyme. An enzyme, substrates of which are metabolites normally occurring within the organism, as distinct from a drug-metabolizing enzyme, the substrates of which are compounds foreign to the organism.

notatin. Enzyme glucose oxidase isolated from the mould *penicillium notalum*. It oxidizes glucose to gluconic acid and at the same time forms hydrogen peroxide; specific for glucose and used for quantitative estimation of this sugar and for removing traces of glucose from foodstuffs. Its property of using free oxygen is made use of by adding the enzyme as a stabilizer, *e.g.*, 0.5 g added to a barrel of beer after fermentation.

notexin. A polypeptide neurotoxin from the Australian tiger snake. It acts to prevent the release of acetylcholine from cholinergic nerve fibre endings. It may be noted that the toxin notechis II-5 is chemically related and comes from the same source, and has a similar action to notexin.

Nougat. Sweetmeat made from a mixture of gelatin or egg albumin with sugar and starch syrup, and the whole thoroughly aerated.

Novadelox. Trade name for benzoyl peroxide used for treating flour.

novain. Old name for carnitine.

n-propoxy. The registered trade name for 1-n-priopoxy-2-amino-4-nitrobenzene, a benzene derivative, and not a sugar. Its sweetening properties were reported as 4000 times that of sucrose. It is easily obtained in the pure state as crystals which are orange in colour and very slightly soluble in water. Its use in ice cream should be subject to the same supervision and restriction as that placed on saccharin.

NPU. Abbreviation for Net Protein Utilization.

NPV. Abbreviation for Net Protein Value.

nubbing. A term used in the canning industry for topping and tailing of the gooseberries.

nucleases. The enzymes which breakdown nucleic acids: DNase degrades DNA and RNase degrades RNA. Nucleases have been classified into two categories depending on their mode of attack:

(a) endonucleases, which attack polynucleotides at many points within the chain generally producing only a small proportion of mononucleotides;

(b) exonucleases, which catalyze a step-wise attack producing exclusively mononucleotides.

An exonuclease may initiate its attack at either the 3'- or 5'-hydroxyl end of a polynucleotide (or oligonucleotide). Such enzymes generally require that a free hydroxyl group be available at the site at which attack begins. Substitution of the hydroxyl group with, for example, a phosphoryl or acyl group renders a normally susceptible substrate resistant to enzymatic attack. Nucleases may show specificity for the pentose moiety of the polynucleotide chain.

One category is specific for polynucleotides containing ribose. Among these enzymes (the ribonucleases) are pancreatic ribonuclease (and the analogous enzymes from liver and spleen), ribonucleases from the plant sources including pea leaf, tobacco leaf, and rye grass, and from bacterial sources, including *B. subtilis*, *E. coli* and *Aspergillus oryzae* (Takadiastase). The high degree of specificity of these enzymes for polynucleotides containing ribose is readily accounted for, that cleavage of internucleotide bonds by pancreatic ribonuclease proceeds first by a very rapid intramolecular *trans*-phosphorylation to form the cyclic 2',3'-phosphate ester followed by slower hydrolysis of the cyclic ester to form the 3'-phosphomonoester. In one instance (the leaf enzyme), pyrimidine cyclic 2',3'-phosphates are actually resistant to further hydrolysis. A mechanism involving the obligatory participation of a 2',3'-cyclic phosphate intermediate ensures the specificity of these nucleases for polyribonucleotides. The ribonucleases cited above are all endonucleases.

nucleic acids. Extremely complex compound of high molecular mass which occurs in the nuclei of biological cells; when associated with a protein, the combined molecule is called a nucleotide. They can be partially hydrolyzed to sugar derivatives (ribosides) of purines and pyrimidines (nucleosides), or to nucleotides (phosphate esters of these compounds).

There are two main types of nucleic acid: ribonucleic acid (RNA) consisting of phosphoric acid, two purines (adenine and guanine), two pyrimidines (cytosine and uracil), and the sugar ribose; and deoxyribonucleic acid (DNA) which differs in containing desoxyribose as the sugar, and thymine in place of uracil. RNA and DNA are believed to play a key role in the synthesis of proteins in the body and in the transmission of hereditary characteristics. Nucleoproteins are present in some foods such as fish and are useful as a source of protein, but they are not essential to the diet and the nucleic acids are readily synthesized in the body.

nucleo-albuminate, iron. A preparation of iron and casein, also called iron caseinate.

nucleoprotein. A generic term applied to

various association products between proteins, polynucleotides and nucleic acids. Such aggregates form many of the fundamental structures of eukaryotic cells, including ribosomes and chromosomes. Since nucleic acid such as DNA carries a net negative charge, largely resulting form its phosphoric acid residues, it is associated mainly with basic proteins such as histones and protamine which neutralize the charge. Examples of nucleoproteins are the chromosomes, made up of DNA, some RNA, and histones (proteins), and the ribosomes (ribonucleoproteins), consisting of ribosomal RNA and proteins.

nucleosidase. Enzyme that hydrolyzes a nucleoside to a free nitrogenous base (a purine or a pyrimidine) and a pentose (ribose or deoxyribose).

nucleoside. An organic compound consisting of a nitrogen-containing purine or pyrimidine base linked to a sugar (ribose or deoxyribose). A covalent bond joins C-1 of the sugar either N-1 of a pyrimidine or to N-9 of a purine in a β-glycosidic bond. Common nucleosides derived from RNA are cytosine, uridine, adenosine and guanosine (containing ribose); those from DNA are deoxycytidine, thymidine, deoxyadenosine and deoxyguanosine (containing deoxyribose). Other nucleosides (naturally occurring or synthetic) act as cytotoxic drugs (e.g., cytosine arabinoside), or have antibiotic (e.g., puromycin, cordycepin) or antiviral properties.

nucleosome. A complex of histones and DNA found in eucaryotic chromatin; the DNA is wrapped around the surface of bead-like histone complex.

nucleotide. An organic compound consisting of a nitrogen-containing purine or pyrimidine base linked to a sugar (ribose or deoxyribose) and a phosphate group. Phosphorylation at the 5'-carbon of the pentose is usually implied, although 2'- and 3'- phosphates, and 3',5'-cyclic phosphates occur. Nucleotides are the monomeric units of DNA and RNA, those in DNA being deoxycytidylic acid (deoxycytidine monophosphate, dCMP), thymidylic acid (thymidine monophosphate, TMP), deoxyadenylic acid (deoxyadenosine monophosphate, dAMP) and deoxyguanylic acid (deoxyguanosine monophosphate, dGMP). Nucleotides commonly found in RNA are cytidylic acid (cytidine monophosphate, CMP), uridylic acid (uridine monophosphate, UMP), adenylic acid (adenosine monophosphate, AMP), and guanylic acid (adenosine monophosphate, GMP).

nuoc mam. Name of a kind of fermented fish sauce prepared in Vietnam and Cambodia. The fish is digested by autolytic enzymes in the presence of added salt to inhibit bacteria.

nut drying. Drying of nuts is necessary to prevent molding, discoloration, and undesirable chemical changes of the nut meat, and to provide a product which will shell easily. Some nuts may crack if dried too rapidly. Dryers may be used to dry nuts which have been re-wet. Usually the nuts dry 30-40% on the tree to 5% for normal storage, in appropriate weather conditions. Otherwise, the nuts may be dried in a bin with forced air. Forced natural or slightly heated air can be used for drying re-wet nuts. To avoid the undesirable effect of heated air, the air may be dehumidified over an evaporator plate before forcing over wet nut products. The nut meats may be 6-10% moisture upon shelling. The moisture content must be reduced to 3-5% to provide product with safe-keeping quality. Forced heated air is used for drying, but the temperature must be kept below that which would otherwise cause migration of the oil to the surface, cause off-flavors, or undesirable taste and appearance, usually below 48.9°C. Nut meats may be dried with an internal rotating drum dryer, continuous belt dryer, or tray dryer.

nutmeg. *Myristica fragrant.* The kernel of the seed of an evergreen tree growing principally in the islands of the East Indies, used commercially as a spice.

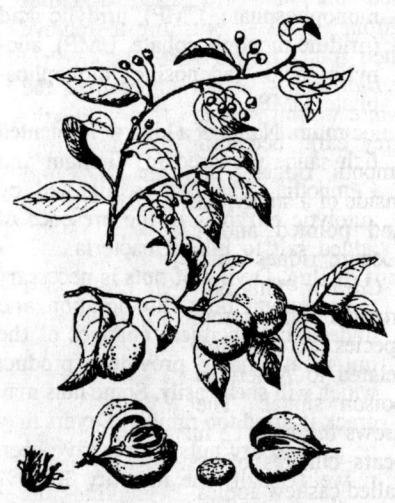

The fruit is pear-shaped and about 5 cm in diameter. When thoroughly ripe, it splits open to two nearly equal longitudinal sections, presenting to view the nut or seed, surrounded by a crimson jacket, the mace of commerce. When the thin hard shell of the nut is taken off, the wrinkled, oval kernel is exposed; this is the nutmeg of commercial value. The nutmeg tree has been introduced into Sumatra, India, Brazil and the West Indies. It reaches a height of about 7-10 metres, and produces numerous branches.

The colour of the bark is a reddish-brown; that of the young branches, a bright green. The nutmeg is aromatic, is pleasing to the taste and smell and is much used in cookery. It yields, by distillation with water, a transparent oil, called oil of mace or oil of nutmeg. The fruit of the nutmeg tree is fleshy like an apricot. The net-like aril is mace, which on drying turns from red to yellowish or orange brown. The dried brown seed, after the shell is broken and discarded, is nutmeg.

nuts. Nuts are a concentrated storehouse of food - low in water and high in unsaturated fat, as well as protein which sees the developing plant through the first few days of its life. They need to be combined with other vegetable proteins in the same way as grains and beans in order to make a complete protein containing all eight amino-acids including isoleucine and lysine which nuts lack. Nuts are thought to be very fattening and are avoided by slimmers. However, if chewed thoroughly, they are very filling and an excellent source of energy, so a quantity containing not too many calories can be very satisfying. Nuts are a good source of B vitamins, unsaturated fatty acids, lectin and minerals. The B vitamins include folic acid, which is destroyed in the body by some drugs and by processing or heat-treating food. This vitamin is essential for proper growth. Nuts also contain niacin, for healthy nerves, and thiamin needed for the conversion of glucose to energy. A good source of thiamin is the red skins around peanuts. (However, strictly speaking, the peanut is not a nut, it is a bean, a member of the legume family.) The only nut to contain any vitamin C is the coconut, which contains traces in its flesh and milk. Fat-soluble vitamin E is also present in nuts which have not been heat-treated. It may be noted that the vitamin E acts as a natural antioxidant and prevents the essential fatty acids in the nut and other foods from being destroyed by oxygen. The vitamin E is carried in the essential fatty acids in the nut. Nuts also contain lecithin, a natural emulsifier which allows fat to be broken down in particles small enough to pass through arterial walls, rather than being deposited and so promoting arteriosclerosis.

Nuts contain many valuable minerals, including magnesium for healthy nerves, potassium for regulation of fats, and zinc for reproductive health. They also contain some dietary fibre, but not as much as grains and beans. Coconuts and almonds have more fibre than other nuts. Technically Brazil nuts are seeds and almonds are fruit. Although it is not, strictly speaking, a nut, the peanut is commercially treated as such.

The most common varieties of nuts are the hazelnut, the chestnut, the English walnut, the hickory nut, the pecan and the Brazil nut. The Brazil cut and the coconut are products of tropical climates. Nuts are valuable for food, since they contain suitable proportions of fat and other nutritive matter. When eaten in connection with other food, they are found to be digestible and healthful, and they are now extensively used in the manufacture of "prepared foods." Some of the edible nuts include:

Almond. Botanically classified as and related to fruits like peach and plum. The outer shell is leathery, but the seed inside the fruit, which can be either sweet or bitter, is the nut itself. Bitter almonds contain amygdalin or

laetrile, and the oil contains mostly benzaldehyde, the same anti-cancer factor found of figs and mushrooms.

Brazil nut. This is one of the very few commercially available nuts which are never cultivated. It grows wild in the dense South American Amazon rain forest, the trees often towering up to 45 metres or higher. The nut is contained in a pod similar in shape to a coconut which holds 12-30 of stem. When ripe these pods fall with such force they can bury themselves under the ground. Once removed from the pod the nuts are dried and put through a heavy brushing to remove their rough brown skin.

Butternut. The nut comes from the white walnut, a small tree with ash-grey bark, becoming separated into smooth ridges. The nut is found inside of a sticky, hairy husk, is thick and pointed and has very rough, obscure ridges on it.

Cashew. This nut is the fruit of a tropical and subtropical evergreen, a species, interestingly enough, that's related to American poison ivy and poison sumac. The evergreen tree grows to about 12 metres height and bears clusters of pear-shaped fruits called cashew apples. Below this fruit hangs the crescent-shaped cashew nut. The kernel ha two shells, an outer one that's thin, flexible and somewhat leathery and an inner which is hard like most nuts and must be cracked open. Between both of these shells is a brown oil that's so toxic it has a extreme blistering effect on the skin. For this reason, the oil must be burned off before it can even be touched.

Chestnut. A magnificent tree growing almost to 30 metres with a very broad spread. The nuts grow 2-3 together in a spiny burr about the size of a baseball. When ripe the burr opens and the nuts are removed. This is the only nut usually served as a vegetable.

Coconut. The fruit of coconut palm, a very important economic product fount throughout the tropics. Unopened coconuts keep at room temperature for 2 months. The white meat inside the shell can be eaten raw or fried. Also, it can be grated and squeezed into a very rich, fatty milk.

Filbert and Hazelnut. These brownshelled nuts are actually fruits of the same bush that differ only in their shape. To tell the difference between them, hazelnuts are shorter and rounder than filberts. They have the sweetest meats of all the nuts and are mainly used in desserts and candies as a rule.

Hickory. A tall, slender, straight tree belonging to the walnut clan. Also known as shagbark hickory. The outer husk of the nut is thick and woody, splitting to the bottom when the nut is ripe. The nut has prominent ridges, is quite sweet and edible.

Macadamia. The nut has a honeybrown shell that is extremely hard to crack open. The crisp, creamy-white nutmeg has a slightly sweet flavour to it. Also called Queensland nut since it's native to Australia.

Peanut. Botanically classified as an underground pea of the legume (bean) family, peanut is also called ground nut or goober in the South. It is native to Brazil, the peanut comes in two varieties, the small, round Spanish kind used for candy, butter and oil, and the larger, oval-shaped Virginia type which is generally used whole. In US, about half of the entire peanut crop is used for making peanut butter.

Pinenut. Comes from various pines (mostly the pinion). A very sweet-flavoured, high-protein kind of a nut that varies in size, shape (cylindrical to round) and colour (white to pale yellow).

Pistachio. The tree is part of the poison sumac family and contains green nuts with ivory-beige shells that split open upon ripening. Those with red shells have been coloured with vegetable dye, and those with white shells have been coated with salt.

Walnut. There are two types, black and English. The former have a strong flavour, and their dark-brown shells are somewhat difficult to open. The latter or more popular kind are white on the inside an golden tan to amber on the outside. Their light-brown shells are easy to open. Black walnut is chiefly used for medicinal purposes by the American herb industry, white the English kind are consumed raw or cooked.

It may be noted that the Brazil nut (*Bertholletsia excelsa*), cashew nuts (*Anacardium occidentale*), walnut (*Juglans regia*) - all have high fat content, 45-60%, high protein content 15-20%, 15-20% carbohydrate, much of which is in the form of pentosans and other indigestible forms. The chestnut (*Castanea sativa*) is something of an exception with 3% fat and 3% protein, being largely carbohydrate 37%. A number of nuts are grown specially for their fat content, such as groundnuts, coconut, and palm.

Nutrela. Trade name for a food product made from soybeans; available as chunks and as granules. It contains more than 50% proteins along with minerals and vitamins.

nutrients. Essential dietary factors such as vitamins, minerals, amino acids and fats. Sources of energy are not termed nutrients so that a commonly used phrase is "energy and nutrients" (calories and nutrients).

nutrition. The study of foods in relation to the needs of living organisms.

nutritionist. According to the US Department of Labour, one who applies the science of nutrition to the promotion of health and control of disease instructs auxiliary medical personnel; participates in surveys.

nutritive ratio. Measure of the value of a feeding ration for growth (or milk production) compared with its fattening value. It is the sum of the digestible carbohydrate, protein and 2.3 X fat, divided by digestible protein. (Calorie value of fat is 2.3 times carbohydrate and protein.) Ratio 4-5 for growth, 7-8 for fattening.

nutritive value index. Term used in animal feeding; intake of digestible energy expressed as energy digestibility multiplied by voluntary intake of dry matter of a particular feed divided by metabolic weight (weight to power of 0.75), compared with standard feed.

nutro-biscuit. A biscuit baked from a mixture of 60% wheat flour and 40% peanut flour; contains about 16-17% protein; developed in India.

nutro-macaroni. A mixture of 8-10 parts wheat flour, 20 parts defatted peanut meal (total 19% protein); developed in India.

Nuworld. The commercial name for a cheese ripened by a white mutant of *Penicillium roquefortii*. The flavour is similar to Blue-veined cheese. It is characterized by the presence of creamy-white mold throughout the cheese. It contains not more than 46% of moisture and its solids content not less than 50% of milk fat. Federal Standards recommends that the moisture content should not be more than 46%; while fat not less than 50%.

nux vomica. The fruit of a species of strychnos, which is found in various parts of the East Indies. It is about the size and shape of a small orange and has a very bitter, acrid taste. It is a virulent poison, and an extremely poisonous drug is prepared from it.

Ny'lander reagent. A solution of Rochelle salt, bismuth subnitrate, and sodium hydroxide, in water. This reagent is used for testing glucose in urine. A black colour on boiling indicates the presence of glucose.

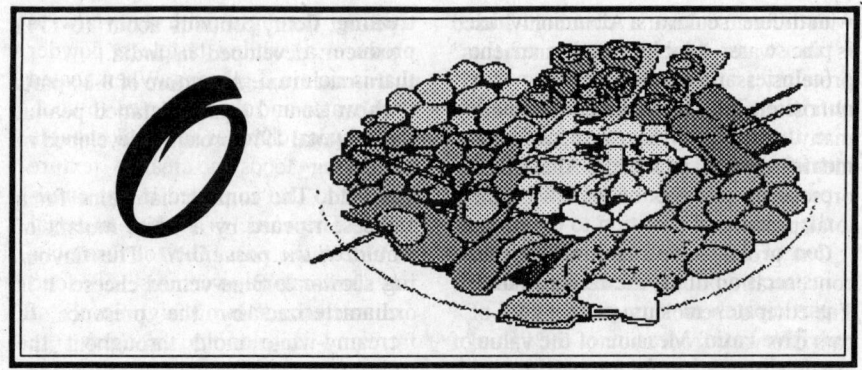

oats. Famiiy: *Gramineae*. Genus: *Avena*. Species: *Avena sativa*. One of the most important fodder crops cultivated, especially valuable as a grain for horses. Oats is also used extensively in making cereal foods for the table, notably oatmeal and rolled oats. Such preparations are excellent breakfast food for cold weather, because the grain of which they are made is a good heat producer. Oatmeal and similar preparations are especially recommended for children. The grain belongs, with wheat, rye, barley and other cereals, to the grass family. The cultivated species are divided into numerous varieties, distinguished from one another by colour, size, form of seeds, quality of straw, period of ripening, adaptation to particular soils and climate and other characteristics. The grain thrives especially well in a cool, moist climate, and while it is widely distributed and hardy, it cannot be successfully cultivated in hot, arid regions.

Whole oats, including hulls, yields about 65% nitrogen-free extract, on a dry basis. Starch and other carbohydrate polymers make up about 90% of this material. Reducing sugars in the extract are quite low, usually less that 0.1%, while total sugars are often near 1.4%. Whole oats contain about 14% pentosans, mainly araban and xylan. The highest concentration of pentosans is in the hulls although the groats will have around 4%. Their content of pentosans make oat hulls an important raw material for the manufacture of furfural, a chemical intermediate and solvent. β-glucan is present in significant amounts. The fiber of oats is found mainly in the hulls and consists principally of cellulose, hemicellulose, and lignin. Dry oat hulls contain about 16.7% lignin (not a carbohydrate) and 29.4% α-cellulose. Oats generally contain a higher percentage of protein than other cereals, and this constituent has a higher biological value than the protein of any other common cereal. This situation is due, of course, to higher amounts of essential amino acids such as lysine, which are limiting in wheat, corn, etc. The protein of oats differs from the protein of other cereal grains in that its major (about 55%) protein is a globulin type rather than a glutelin (about 21 to 27%). These figures are subject to considerable uncertainty, varying substantially depending on the extraction method and subsequent technique, but probably not varying much with different cultivars. Albumin, which is the water-soluble fraction of the proteins, is thought to be composed almost entirely of enzymes, although many of the enzymes have not been identified or characterized. Albumin is present in amounts of 9-20% of the total protein.

Oat groats have the highest lipid concentration of all the cereal grains. The ether or petroleum extractables of oats can vary from about 4-10%, and are distributed among the parts of the grain as follows (percentages on dry basis): whole grain 5.4%, groats, 7.6%, hulls 0.62%, germ (hand-dissected) 11.2%, germ-free groats 5.8%, germ plus bran coats 7.5-9.1%, and endosperm 6.2%-6.7%. There have been relatively few reports on the proteolytic enzymes in oat groats. The endosperm is almost free of proteolytic activity when the grain is in a dormant state, but protein-digesting enzymes develop rapidly in the early stages of germination. Aleurone contains an active protease. A substance which inhibits trypsin activity is found in oats. It is, however, digested by pepsin and is thermolabile, so that is presumably not effective in reducing the nutritive properties of the grain.

Oat gums dissolve in hot water, but more readily in dilute alkalies to give highly viscous solutions that slowly lose viscosity on standing. This characteristic obviously leads to the idea that the material could be useful as a texture-enhancing ingredient for beverages and foods. The chief problem with this approach is that, according to Wood, no economically feasible commercial process exists for separating glucan from oats and purifying it. A patent has been granted for a process which calls for treating oat bran with enzymes to produce a white, tasteless powder that is rich in β-glucans. When heated with water and then allowed to cool, the powder changes to a gel capable of giving foods a creamy texture similar to that imparted by fat emulsions. The value of such a material would be the possibility of formulating low-calorie versions of food ordinarily containing high levels of fat, and of adding to them the presumed cholesterol-reducing value of the glucans.

The average composition per 100 g is: protein 13%, fat 7.6%; calcium 55 mg, iron 4.3 mg, vitamin B_1 0.6 mg, B_2 0.1 mg, nicotinic acid 0.9 mg; and food energy 1.62 MJ. The various forms in which oats are used include:

oatmeal;

ground oat;

oat flour- ground, and bean removed;

goats- husked oats;

Embden grouts- crushed groats;

Sussex ground oats- very finely ground oats;

Scotch oats- groats cut into granules of various sizes; and

rolled oats- crushed by rollers and partially precooked.

oat flour. A specially prepared oat product flour having antioxidant properties; it is used in ice cream and other dairy products to prevent oxidation of the fat, in countries whose dairy laws do not prevent its use.

occupational air. The name given to the air present inside plants, factories, offices, and heavily crowded places such as railway stations and service establishments. If air becomes heavily polluted, the food products are likely to be contaminated and spoiled.

odoratism. A kind of disease experimentally produced by feeding sweet pea seeds, *Lathyus odoratus,* to rats. It results in damage to the spine and aorta, caused by the presence of a toxic substance, known as BAPN (β-aminopropionnitrile). This is present both in the sweet pea and the Singletary pea (*L. pusillus*), but not in the chick pea, *L. sativus,* which causes lathyrism in man.

odorivectors. The . odoriferous substances. For a given substance to be an odorivector it must possess the following properties:

1. It must have a vapour pressure that is sufficient to supply a concentration exceeding the threshold for excitation of the olfactory receptors.
2. It must be water-soluble in order to dissolve in the mucous layer covering the olfactory epithelium.
3. It must bne capable of being adsorbed on to olfactory epitelium.
4. It must also be lipid-soluble in order to penetrate the membrane of the olfactory cell.
5. It must normally be absent from the olfactory epithelium because the sense of smell rapidly adapts.
6. It must be capable of exciting the olfactory receptors.

odour intensity index. In the test method of the American Society for Testing and Materials (ASTM), the number of times that an odorant must be diluted by a factor of 2 in order to reach the threshold concentration.

odour nuisance. Any distinctive, unpleasant odours resulting from manufacturing or natural process. Many food processing industries create odour nuisances as well as air and water pollution.

odour threshold. In principal, the lowest concentration of an odorant that can be detected by a human being. In practice, a panel of sniffers is nor-

mally used and the threshold taken as the concentration at which 50% of the panel can detect the odorant (although some workers have also used 100% thresholds).

oedema. Excess fluid in the body indicated by pitting of the subcutaneous tissues when pressure is applied with the finger. It may be caused by cardiac, renal or hepatic failure and by starvation (family oedema).

oenin. An anthocyanidin from the skin of purple grapes.

offal. A corruption of off-fall. In reference to meat, originally meant only the entrail; now used for all parts that are cut away when a carcass is dressed, including heart, liver, kidney, brain, spleen, pancreas, thymus, tripe, tongue. In reference to flour-milling means the bran and germ that are removed in the milling of white flour.

offensive industry. Any business which by reason of the process involved, or the methods of manufacture, or the nature of the raw materials or goods used, produced or stored, is likely, as a result of the inadequacy of the available means of control, to cause effluvia, fumes and odours of a character offensive to persons on adjacent land. Historically, the offensive trades have included those dealing in the by-products *e.g.*, blood, hides and bones, and the process for dealing with condemned meat and fish. Also known as noxious industry.

ogumoh. A relatively uncommon vegetable (*Solanum nigrum* var. guineense) cultivated mainly in some of the western African countries. Ogumoh normally grows to a height of about 0.6 m. Also grown for its fruit is the closely related plant, efodu. Both plants are usually grown from seeds which are sown broadcast and thinned later so that individual plants are left growing at a spacing 15-23 cm. apart. They can also be grown from cuttings although the seeds are generally produced in generous quantities. A reasonably fertile soil is required for these plants.

oidium lactis. A mold commonly found in sour milk, butter, cheese and other dairy products. The mold develops as a dull white, velvety layer, the greater part of the mycelium being submerged beneath the surface of the medium. It is characterized by dichotomus branching. It is thought necessary for the production of flavour in Camembert cheese. A member of a genus of fungi called Candida.

oils. A large group of fatty substances which are divided into three general classes: vegetable oils, animal oils, and mineral oils. The vegetable oils are either fixed or volatile oils. The fixed oils are present in the plant in combined form, and are largely glycerides of stearic, oleic, palmitic, and other acids, and they vary in consistency from light fluidity to solid fats. They all boil in the temperature range 260-316°C, decomposing into the compounds. The volatile, or essential, oils are present in uncombined form and bear distillation without chemical change. Seed oils, or oilseeds, obtained from various plant seeds, are fatty acids of varying chain lengths containing hydroxy, keto, epoxy, and other functional groups.

The seeds of the Chinese tallow tree are coated with a semisolid fat. An oil similar to linseed oil is inside the kernel. The oil can be used as a substitute for cocoa butter and for fatty acids in cosmetics.

Fish oils are thick, with a strong odour. Vegetable and animal oils are obtained by pressing, extraction, or distillation. Oils that absorb oxygen easily and become thick are known as drying oils and are valued for varnishes, because on drying they form a hard, elastic, waterproof film. Unsaturation is proportional to the number of double bonds, and in food oils these govern the cholesterol depressant effect of the oil. Oils and fats are distinguished by consistency only, but waxes are not oils.

Mineral oils are derived from petroleum or shale and are classified separately. The most prolific sources of vegetable oils are palm kernels and copra. About 1,134 kg of palm oil is produced per acre annually, and the yield of coconut oil per acre from plantation plantings is about 550 kg. This compares with 159 kg of oil per acre from peanuts and 91 kg per acre from soybeans. Under comparable aggressive plantation, from 10-20 times more palm and coconut oil can be produced per acre than peanut or soybean oil. Babassu oil is almost chemically identical with coconut oil, and vast quantities of babassu nuts grow wild in northeast Brazil.

The blown fish oils are used for paints, enamels, and printing inks, are peroxidized and destearinized, and have specific gravities about 0.98-1.025. Crystol oils are kettle-boiled fish oils used in the manufacture of paints. Blown oils are fatty oils that have been oxidized by blowing air through them while hot, thereby thickening the oil. They are mixed with mineral oils to form special heavy lubricating oils, such as marine engine oil, or are employed in cutting oils. They are also used in paints and varnishes. The flash point and the iodine value are both lowered by the blowing. The oils usually blown are rapeseed, cottonseed, linseed, fish, and whale oils.

oil equivalent. In principal, the mass of a standard oil that would on combustion produce the same quantity of heat as a given mass of a given oil. In practice certain arbitrary rules are applied in calculating oil equivalents and there differ from one country to another.

oil palm. A genus of palms, akin to the cocoanut palm, found chiefly in tropical Africa. One species produces fruit in large clusters, containing about 150 orange-colored drupes having an oily pulp. The oil from this pulp is exported and is much used in making candles and toilet soaps. When chilled, it hardens like butter, for which it is sometimes eaten as a substitute, when fresh.

oil seed. A wide variety of seeds which are grown as a source of oils, *e.g.,* cottonseed, sesame, groundnut, sunflower, soya, palm, etc. After extraction of the oil and residue is a valuable source of protein, and is called seed cake.

oiticica oil. A drying oil obtained from the kernels of the nuts of tree *Licania rigida* of northeastern Brazil. The oil contains about 80% licanic acid, which, like the eleostearic acid of tung oil and isano oil, gives a greater drying power than is apparent from the iodine value. Its specific gravity is 0.95, saponification value 186-193, and iodine number is between 142-155. Cicoil is the commercial name for a treated oiticica oil with improved qualities. Treatment generally involves heating to above 225°C. Phenolic resins attain greater body with oiticica oil than with tung oil.

The oiticica nuts are 2.5-5.1 cm long with the kernel about 60% of the nut, yielding about 60% oil. The average yield per tree is 159 kg of nuts, but a full-grown tree may yield 10 times that amount. Another species of the tree, *L. crassifolia,* of Surinam, yields a similar oil. Mexican oiticica is from the nuts of another species and is called cacahuanache oil. The kernels yield 69% of light-coloured heavy oil.

Oka cheese. A kind of soft cheese made by Trappist Monks in a monastery in Oka, Quebec, Canada, deriving its name from the location where it was first made. It is similar to Port du Salaut or La Trappe cheese.

okra. Family: *Malvaceae.* Genus: *Hibiscus.* Species: *Hibiscus esculentus.* An annual herb with a tall, erect stem that grows 1-2.5 metres high and is covered with small hairs. The leaves are cordate, 3- to 5-lobed and coarsely toothed, while the large flowers are yellow with crimson centres to them. There are two basic types of plants, depending upon the time span from planting to maturity. The long duration varieties mature in 3-4 months from sowing; the more rapidly growing types are ready for use in 6-8 weeks from sowing. Okra pods are anywhere from 10-30 cm long, hornlike in appearance, green or creamy green in colour and with ridges that are either smooth or hairy. The pods contain numerous seeds that are rounded, striate and hairy. The entire okra plant is aromatic emitting an order resembling clovers.

Okra has about the same degree of hardiness as cucumbers and tomatoes and may be grown under similar conditions. Okra has a heavy mucilaginous texture which provides body and texture to such preparations. The vegetable also is cooked, commonly with tomatoes, as a table vegetable also is cooked, commonly with tomatoes, as a table vegetable, as well as used in salads. Okra, also known as gumbo, okro, and lady's fingers, is a warm-weather vegetable. An unusual use for okra pods has been as blood plasma replacements. Small ridged mucilaginous pods resembling a small cucumber, grown in South America, West Indies and India; used in soups and stews. The average composition per 100 g is: carbohydrate 6%, protein 2%; iron 1 mg, vitamin A 250 mg, vitamin B_1 0.1 mg, vitamin B_2 0.1 mg, nicotinic acid 0.8 mg, and vitamin C 25 mg. Okra is extremely high in calcium and low in calories and because of and low in calories and because of the mucilage, is useful for stomach ulcers as well as sore throats, pleurisy and colitis. Currant findings suggests that it may also be useful for the treatment of diabetes. West Indians eat it when trying to lose weight. Also known as Gumbo; Bamya Bamies; Ladies' Fingers (*Hibiscus esculents*).

old yellow enzyme. A flavoprotein from yeast that catalyzes oxidation of NADPH.

oleandomycin. An antibiotic used as an addition to click feed to stimulate growth and improve feed efficiency; used in US at 1-2 g per ton but not permitted for laying hens. The tolerance for laying hens. The tolerance limit in uncooked edible tissues of chicken or turkey is zero.

oleic acid. $C_{18}H_{34}O_2$. Long-chain fatty acid with total of 18 carbon atoms; unsaturated with one double bond, 9-octadeacenoic acid occurring as the glyceride in oils and fats. Oleic acid occurs naturally in larger quantities than any other fatty acid. In many organisms oleic acid can be synthesized directly from stearic acid and further enzymatic paths exist for conversion to linoleic acid and linolenic acid. This pathway does not occur in man and the higher animals so plant sources are an essential dietary element. Oleic acid is the *cis*-form while the *trans*-form is called elaidic acid.

oleoresin garlic. A dark brown soft extract prepared by the vacuum concentration of the expressed juice and the aqueous extraction of the press-cake. It contains about 5 % garlic oil. The flavouring strength is about two to three times that of fresh garlic and eight times that of garlic powder, although the determination of these equivalents is very difficult other than directly in an end product.

oleoresins. In the preparation of some species such as pepper, ginger and capsicum, the aromatic material is extracted with solvents which are evaporated off leaving behind thick oily products known as oleoresins.

oligo dA. Homopolymer of deoxyriboadenylate that can be made as an artificial polymer *in vitro* and used as a synthetic template for polymerases.

oligodynamic. Sterilizing effect of trace of certain metals. For example, silver in concentration of 1 in 5 million will kill *Escheurchia coli* and staphylococci in 3 hours. Electrolytic method of getting silver into water is Katadyn process. Suggestions have been made for its use for the treatment of water, fruit juices and various foods.

oligomeric proteins. Proteins having two or more separate polypeptide chains. The polypeptides in oligomeric proteins may be identical or different. The number of polypeptide chains in an oligomeric protein can be found by determining the number of amino-terminal residues per molecule of protein. These proteins have high molecular masses and more complex functions than single-chain proteins. In oligomeric proteins each subunit polypeptide chain has its own characteristic secondary and tertiary conformation in space.

oligopeptide. An amino acid chain with less than 25 amino acid; *e.g.*, angiotensin II, vasopressin, oxytocin, bradykinin, gastrin, substance P, and endothelin.

oligosaccharide determinant. A small number (2-7) or 5, 6, or 7 carbon containing sugars (pentoses, hexoses, or heptoses) joined by glycoside linkages, that form the antigenic determinant site or epitope on a polysaccharide hapten.

oligosaccharides. Polysaccharides composed of two or more (arbitrarily up to about 10) monosaccharides, covalently bonded by glycosidic linkages. Some oligosaccharides occur naturally; these and many others may appear in partial hydrolysis of higher oligosaccharides or polysaccharides.

oligotroph. A low-nutrient environment or a microorganism that can survive and function in low nutrient environment.

olive. Family: *Oleaceae*. Genus: *Olea*. Species: *Olea europaea*.

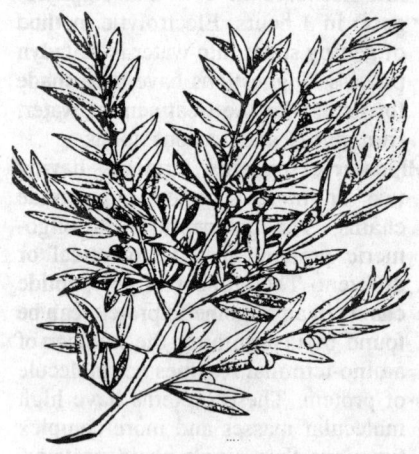

A fruit tree, of which there are several species. The common olive is a low, branching, evergreen tree 7-10 metres high, with stiff, narrow, dusky-green or bluish leaves. The small and white flowers appear from June to August. The fruit is a plumlike berry of greenish pulp, covered with a thin smooth skin and containing a hard stone. The tree is a native of Syria and it is cultivated in almost every warm, dry climate. The olive tree is an evergreen, commonly found in all of the Mediterranean countries, but widely cultivated in tropical climates as well. The hard, yellow wood of the gnarled trunk is covered by grey-green bark. The branches extend upwards to 8 metres or more. The leathery leaves are dark green on top and have silvery scales underneath. The tree yields fragrant white flowers and an oblong or nearly round type of fruit called a drupe that becomes shiny black when ripe. Other kinds of drupes would be plums, cherries, apricots and peaches. The oil which is produced from the fruit is quite valuable, having worldwide appeal for its excellent cooking and baking properties. The tree grows slowly and lives a long time. As its age increases the trunk becomes gnarled, and twisted into odd shapes, but it continues to produce great quantities of fruit even when it appears to be on the verge of decay. The wood is yellowish, beautifully streaked with dark lines, and can be brightly polished. It is serviceable in making boxes and small fancy articles.

From earliest times the olive tree has been held in veneration throughout the East. Among the Greeks it was sacred to Minerva, and olive wreaths were used by both Greeks and Romans to crown victors. The olive tree is associated with the garden of

Gethsemane and with many of the scenes described in both the Old and the New Testaments. To this day it is everywhere recognized as the symbol of peace.

Ripened black olives contain very little vitamin A, but have slightly more carbohydrate, fat and calories than green olives. The olives are high in minerals, especially sodium, calcium and potassium. They are fairly high in fat and fibre. Greek olives are generally black, salted and preserved in oil. Therefore they are saltier and richer than most other olives and consequently have more calories, protein, fat, carbohydrate and sodium. Olives are mildly purgative, antiseptic and weakly astringent. The oil is used as a laxative for chronic constipation, and as it reduces the flow of gastric secretions, it is still occasionally used to treat peptic ulcers. The leaves can be made into a strong decoction for wound treatment. In the old days they were used as an antipyretic and valued for their hypotensive activity. The oil stimulates bile secretion, facilitating the dumping of gallstones. Olive oil, obtained by pressing the ripe fruits, is used in cooking, as salad oil and for canning sardines. It is one of the few vegetable oils to contain only small amounts of polyunsaturated fatty acids. The average composition per 100 g is: 0.9 g protein; 11 g fat; 60 mg calcium; 1 mg iron; and 0.45 MJ food energy. It contains very little or no vitamins when pickled.

Olive family: *Oleaceae*. Characteristic in this family are flower parts in 2's with the anthers of the 2 stamens usually touching. The single pistil has a superior ovary of 2 fused carpels with, usually, 2 ovules in each. Plants in this family are shrubs, trees, and vines with opposite leaves, which may be simple or compound. Usually, the flowers are bisexual and have 4 sepals and 4 petals. Fruit types are berries, drupes, capsules and samaras.

The family include: *Olea* (olive); *Fraxinus* (ash); *Chionanthus* (fringe tree), *Forsythia* (golden bell), *Jasminum (jasmine),* Ligustrum (privet), *Osmanthus* (fragrant olive), *Syringa* (lilac).

olive oil. An oil extracted from the fruits of the olive tree. The olives are taken, as soon as picked, to a press, where they are run through a machine which crushes them into fine pulp. This is packed into short, open-mounted baskets of rushes, several of which are put together into a press, which squeezes out the oil into tubs half filled with water. The oil remains at the top, and the impurities sink through the water to the bottom. The pulp is gathered together after passing through the press the first time and is usually sent through three times more, each successive pressure producing oil of a different grade. The oil is filtered and clarified until it becomes a beautiful golden-yellow liquid, suitable for the table. The rich oleic content (80%) of olive oil makes it completely digestible, and increases the absorption of the fat-soluble vitamins A, D, E, and K. It is low in linoleic acid, so some nutritionists advise combining olive oil with another which is high in this acid such as safflower oil, to provide a well-balanced salad oil. Much oil that is sold as olive oil is peanut oil or cottonseed oil or badly adulterated olive oil.

Olivet cheese. A kind of soft, cow's milk cheese made in the Department of Loirte, France. The cheese has three types:

Unripened. It is made from whole milk plus the addition of cream and is similar to a cream cheese.

Half ripened or blue. It is made from whole or partly skimmed milk.

Ripened. It is made from the whole or partially skimmed milk. The cheese-making process is quite similar to the Camembert. To make the half-ripened, the cheese, after salting, is placed on straw covered shelves until a reddish smear develops on the surface. A bluish cast appears after two weeks when the cheese is ready to be marketed. Additional ripening is given to the half ripened cheese to make a ripened olivet.

Olla-podrida. A pot pourri made by the perfume manufacturers out of their waste materials, such as spent plant and animal materials, to which are added inexpensive herbs such as thyme, rosemary, together with lavender and rose petals.

Olmutzer quargel cheese. A variety of sour milk spiced hand cheese made in Austria and other parts of Europe. It is similar to Mainzer hand cheese. The small, formed, dried cheeses are soaked in salty whey, before packaging. It contains caraway seed.

omophagia. Eating of raw or uncooked food.

omphacium. An oil or juice used in Roman perfumes which was squeezed out of unripe olives or dates.

once-through cooling. The standard method for disposing of waste heat from the food industry or a power plant. Water is drawn from a lake, river, or estuary, passed through the steam condenser where its temperature is raised, and is then returned to the body of water from which it was drawn.

oncogenic. A term which describes the chemical, organism, or environmental factor that causes the development of cancer. Some viruses are oncogenic to vertebrates, including the *Rous sarcoma* virus of chickens, and some are suspected of being oncogenic (such as adenoviruses and papovaviruses). Many of these viruses contain genes that are responsible for the transformation of a normal host cell into a cancerous cell.

onion. Family: *Amaryllidaceae*. Genus: *Allium.* Species: *Allium cepa; Allium fistulosum* (green onion). A well-known plant, the bulbous root of which is much used as an article of food. It is a biennial herb, with long, narrow leaves and a swelling, pithy stalk. The peculiar flavor varies much according to the size of the bulb, the small reddish onions having much more pungency than the large ones. The onion may be grown from the tropics to the coldest regions of the temperate zone. There are at least twenty varieties of onion. Strassburg, Bermuda, Spanish and Portuguese onions are among the most esteemed varieties. In parts of the world, the onion forms a large portion of the food of the poorer classes. Egypt is believed to be the original home of the plant. The hollow tubular leaves die at the end of the growing season, leaving a hard-fleshed bulb with a thin outer scaly layer.

The shape may be oblong, flat, globe or oblate, and the colour brown, white or red depending on the variety and source. Onion is a biennial, although the common variety is grown as an annual propagated either from seed or from small bulbs called either from seed or from small bulbs called sets. The Egyptian onion. (*A. cepa* var. *vivaparum*) produces small bulbs or top-sets in the flower head. There are many varieties of A. *cepa,* which are classified according to their dry solids content and pungency. Many commercial crops are raised specially from cultivators to satisfy market requirements (*i.e.*, domestic use, pickling, canning, dehydration, etc.), with care being necessary during their husbandry as the plants are liable to be attacked by several diseases affecting quality and keeping properties. Onions have little smell until the tissues are cut or bruised. Once this takes place, the enzymatic reaction results in a complex mixture of sulphides that may be recovered as so-called oil of onion, by distillation. The amount recoverable depends on the variety and ripeness of the onions used, but averages 0.02-0.03 %.

The onion contains vitamin B, C and E, carotene, calcium, iron, phosphorus, potassium, sodium, sulphur and traces of copper. It is also rich in antimicrobial substances, fibre, glycosides, hormones similar to insulin, and volatile oil. In fact its constituents are similar to those of garlic and like garlic it contains a naturally antiseptic oil, ally disulphate, and cyclollin. It has been shown that cycloallin helps the walls of blood vessels to dissolve clots which form from inside. It seems that frying or boiling onions does not affect its efficacy in this area. The onion is reputed to be helpful for heart disorders and arthritis. The cycloallin also dissolves fibrin, which forms in inflamed joints as part of the inflammation process. Onions actively reduce the blood pressure and the blood sugar level. They are said to increase the flow of urine, to be slightly laxative and antiseptic, and to relieve sinus conditions. Used externally as a local stimulant, the juice can

be applied to cuts, and used to treat acne and promote hair growth. The onions are also helpful for the shine and growth of nails and hair. Crushed onion applied to the chest as a poultice relieves inflammation of the lungs and put between gauze bandages and applied over the ears, will relieve earache (although admittedly it looks very strange)! Boiled onions lose some of their calories and carbohydrates as well as a very small portion of their minerals. As one would expect, fried onions are high in calories; they increase in mineral content, and their vitamin content rises a little also. Spring onions contain traces of protein, carbohydrate, fibre and very little fat. They have more calcium and potassium and vitamin C than raw ordinary onions. They also have half the amount of sodium and just a trace of vitamin A. The average composition is per 100 g of onion is: protein 1.4%; fat 0.2%; calcium 31 mg; iron 0.4 mg; zinc 0.2 mg; vitamin B_2 0.05 mg; nicotinic acid 0.22 mg; vitamin C 8.4 mg; and food energy 0.15 MJ.

onion drying. 1. The common practice at harvest has been to place onions in crates and cure them in the field before moving to storage. With mechanical harvesting, however, onions can be moved in bulk or in pallets to storages and cured in bins with forced ventilation. The onions may be topped in the field before storage or may be stored with the tops on. Excess moisture is removed from the skin of the onions and tops during the curing operation. The use of heated air above 35°C has not been accomplished without the excessive shrinkage and is not generally recommended. Most successful results have been obtained with heated air by limiting the temperature rise to 11°C, with an air flow of 0.01-0.015 m³/m²s. The onions should be cooled after curing to about 10°C. The optimum storage condition for onions is 0°C without warming periods during storage. The dormancy of onions is easily broken if they are warmed after being cooled, and sprouting will result. To avoid bruising, the onions should not be stored more than 3.75 m deep.

2. Onions are prepared for tunnel drying by cutting into thin slices. A two-stage tunnel dryer, with the first stage at 71-87.8°C and the second stage at 54.4-60°C, is used to dry 90% product to 5-7% in 10-15 hours. Bin drying to 4% with 48.9°C air requires the tunnel dryer. More rapid drying is accomplished on a continuous stainless steel perforated belt, using air forced through the product with drying completed in 6 hours. Dried onion is sold as sliced, chopped, or powdered material.

onion flavours, encapsulated. Onion oil encapsulated by spray drying in gum acacia or a modified starch is available as a flavouring ingredient. The strength of these products depends on the manufacturer and may range from equal to ten times stronger than onion powder.

onion juice/extract. Onion juice carries all of the available flavour, actual and potential, and is a good basis for the preparation of a water-miscible onion flavouring. The juice is obtained by hydraulic pressing of the washed onions. This presents some difficulties, owing to the flat laminate cellular structure that tends to make the tissues slide rather than rupture. To obtain a good recovery it is usually necessary to employ multiple pressing with adequate water washing. Even when the expression is appar-

ently complete, the dry press-cake may still yield a further quantity of extractive after boiling with water. Normally, the freshly recovered juice is flash heated at 140°-160°C and immediately cooled down to about 40°C. This ensures its preservation until sufficient bulk is available for concentration in a vacuum falling-film evaporator to a product having a minimum of 75% dry solids. At this concentration, the concentrated juice is pale-brown in colour, has a strong fresh-onion odour, and a sweetish flavour free from the bitterness present in the unheated juice. The concentrated juice may further evaporated in a vacuum stirrer-pan until the dry solids content is 80-85%. The additional heat applied induces further non-enzymatic browning, the resulting product being a soft dark-brown extract having a markedly cooked/toasted onion character. For uniformity and ease of handling, this extract may be mixed with propylene glycol, lecithin and glucose to give a stable, semifluid, so called "oleoresin onion" that may be up to ten times stronger than the flavour of onion powder. By altering the base material, an oil-dispersible version is possible.

onion oil. The substance obtained by the distillation of crushed fresh onions that have been allowed to stand for some hours before distillation. As onion oil constituents are partially water-soluble, a special recovery technique is necessary to achieve a high-quality oil in a yield of about 0.02-0.03%, depending on the type of onion and the season. The chemical composition of onion oil, obtained either by direct distillation of crushed bulbs or from the expressed juice, has been the subject of many studies. Following compounds have been reported in the oil of onion: hydrogen sulphide, n-propyl mercaptan, ethanol, 1-propanol, 2-propanol, methyl disulphide, methyl n-propyl disulphide, n-propyl disulphide, methyl trisulphide, methyl n-propyl trisulphide, n-propyl trisulphide, acetaldehyde, propionaldehyde, n-butyraldehyde, acetone, methyl ethyl ketone.

More recent studies have identified following compounds in onion: methyl-1-propyl disulphide, cis-methyl-1-propenyl disulphide, transmethyl-1-propenyl disulphide, di-1-propyl disulphide, cis-1-propyl propenyl disulphide, trans-1-propyl propenyl disulphide, methyl-1-propyl trisulphide, and di-1-propyl trisulphide, and 3,4-dimethylthiophene.

onion salt. A mixture of onion powder and salt, often with an anticaking agent such as starch, tricalcium phosphate or silicon oxide, to maintain dry free-flowing properties. Standardized dispersions of onion oil, with or without onion extract, are available for use in blended seasonings. The flavouring strength of these products should be determined from the manufacturer.

onion, dehydrated. The dehydration of onions to produce onion powder and pieces of various sizes is now a major activity in California, Japan, Egypt and some central European countries. The onions are first flame peeled, washed to remove the burnt outer skin, and then mechanically sliced onto a perforated belt. The drying is carried out in a tunnel drier, the hot air circulating through the holes in the conveyor belt. Onions enter the system with a moisture content of about 80% and are dehydrated to about 4%. The dehydrated product may be sold as such, kibbled to various mesh sizes, or milled to a moderately fine powder. All of these products, particularly onion powder, absorb moisture and must be packed and retained in well-closed containers preferably having an impervious liner. Onions are dehydrated without blanching so that they retain their essential flavouring character. As a consequence of this, the products usually have a high microbiological count due to the presence of thermophilic spores that survive the drying temperature.

oomycetes. A collective name for members of the division *Oomycota*. Oomycetes resemble fungi in appearance, consisting of finely branched filaments called hyphae. However, oomycetes have cell walls of cellulose, whereas the wall of most fungi are made of chitin. Also known as water molds.

oospora. A group of molds in which the oospore or the egg cell is large and rich in food material. The male cell, very much smaller, penetrates and fertilizes the oospore which then develops into a thick-walled resting spore. The very destructive downy mildews belong to this group. It is one of the molds which adversely affect the dairy products.

ophthalmin. An obsolete name for vitamin A.

opiate. An analgesic drug derived from the opium poppy; *e.g.*, morphine, codeine. The term opiate also includes morphine derivatives, such as heroin (diacetylmorphine) which is prepared from morphine.

opioid. An analgesic drug with pharmacological similarities to opium (morphine). Includes both synthetic morphine-like drugs (*e.g.*, buprenorphine) and endogenous peptides (*e.g.*, met-enkephalin). More specifically, it refers to any directly acting opioid receptor agonist, not from opium, that is stereospecifically antagonized by naloxone. An opioid peptide is an opioid drug that is a polypeptide. Met-enkephalin is an exmple.

opium. The air dried milky latex obtained by incision from the unripe capsules of *Papaver somniferum* Linn. or its variety *P. album*. It is well known in many places as an ornamental garden plant. Commercially it is of more importance than any other drug. It is a powerful narcotic, and is used in medicine chiefly to procure sleep and to bring relief from pain. The juice, which is procured by making an incision in the green head or seed capsule of the flower, flows out in the form of a milky liquid; soon it hardens and turns black. It is then scraped off and dried thoroughly, and next goes through a kneading process and is molded into cakes or balls for the market. The agreeable effects produced on the system by opium have tempted many persons to form the opium habit. Evil effects as serious as those of excessive alcoholic drinking follow overindulgence in opium. The habitual use of opium was quite common in China in twentieth century, though it has decreased considerably in recent years owing to the influence of missionaries and general awareness.

Opium and morphine have narcotic, analgesic and sedative action and used to relieve pain, diarrhoea, dysentery and cough. Poppy capsules are astringent, somniferous, soporific, sedative and narcotic and used as anodyne and emollient. Opium is first stimulant, then narcotic, anodyne, antispasmodic, aphrodisiac, astringent and myotic. As astringent, opium checks haemorrhages, lessens bodily secretions and restrains the tissue changes. Generally opium is anodyne, hypnotic, antispasmodic, diaphoretic, narcotic, myotic, intoxicant and cerebral depressant. Morphine is an analgesic. Codeine is mild sedative and is employed in cough mixtures. Noscapine is not narcotic and also has cough suppressant action acting as a central antitussive drug. Papaverine has smooth muscle relaxant action and is used to cure muscular spasms. Opium, morphine and the diacetyl derivative heroin, cause drug addition. Abouse leads to habituation of addiction.

Opium contains about 25 alkaloids among which morphine (10-16%) is the most important base, The alkaloids are combined with meconic acid. The other alkaloids isolated from the drug are codeine (0.8-2.5%), narcotine, thebaine (0.5-2%)). noscapine (4-8%), narceine, and papaverine (0.5-2.5%). Morphine contains a phenanthrene nucleus. It also contains sugar, sulphates, albuminous compounds, colouring matter and moisture. In addition to these anisaldehyde, vanillin, vanillic acid, *p*-hydroxystyrene, fumaric acid, lactic acid, benzyl alcohol, 2-hydroxycinchonic acid, phthalic acid, hemipinic acid, meconin and an odourous compound have also been reported.

opium alkaloids. The alkaloids obtained from the dried exudate from the unripe seed capsules of the opium poppy Papaver somniferum. The alkaloids with medicinal use are morphine, codeine, papaverine and noscapine (narcotine). The alkaloids are traditionally divided into two chemical classes: phenanthrene derivatives such as morphine and codeine (analgesic action, antitutssive action) and benzylisoquinoline derivatives such as papaverine (smooth muscle relaxrit,

phosphodiesterase inhibitor, dopami-
nomimetric) and noscapine (cough
suppressant).

opsomania. Craving for special food.

opsseomucoid. A mucoid substance
forming part of the structure of bone.

optical activity. Certain substances such
as sugars and acids, possess the
ability to rotate polarized light and are
thus said to exhibit optical activity. If
the rotation is to the right the
substance is dextrorotatory, designated (+), if to the left it is levorotary
(-). (The old nomenclature used to be
d- and l-, not to be confused with
capital D- and L-,. Optical activity
depends upon the molecule being
non-symmetrical. A mixture of the (+)
and (-) forms, which results when the
compound is prepared by synthesis,
is optically inactivity and is termed
racemic. The degree of rotation under
standard conditions, measured in a
polarimeter, can serve as a measure of
the quantity or purity of an optically
active compound. Sucrose is dextrorotatory and yields on hydrolysis
glucose, which is (+) and fructose
which is more strongly (-). Thus on
hydrolysis the dextrorotation changes
to laevo and the hydrolysis of
sucrose is termed "inversion" and the
mixture of glucose and fructose are
the "invert sugars".

orange. *Citrus sinensis.* Most important
of the citrus fruits, the orange was
brought from Southern Asia to Spain
and Portugal during the sixteenth
century. Taken to South America by
the early explorers, it ran wild in the
tropical forests of the Amazon; about
the same time the sour orange was
brought into Florida by the Spaniards.
Here, until 1880, large wild groves
were to be found, usually on mounds
marking the former homes of the
natives. In more recent years the
stock of this class of oranges has
been utilized to graft the sweet orange
and the tangerine, which have since
been extensively cultivated.

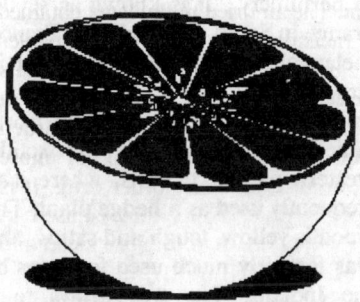

The orange tree is small and has
broad, green leaves. Under the most
favorable circumstances it seldom
exceeds 7-8 m in height, and in
cultivation it is kept much lower. The
branches are low, and the flowers are
white and waxlike; because of their
beauty and fragrance orange blossoms have long been worn in almost
all parts of the world by the bride on
her wedding day. The fruit is nearly
spheroid, bright yellow in colour, and
contains a pulp which consists of a
collection of oblong segments, filled
with a sugary and refreshing juice and
in most varieties containing several
seeds. Blood oranges are coloured
due to the presence of anthocyanins
(cyanidin-3-glucoside and delphinidin-
3-glucoside) in the juice vesicles.

In recent years, hybrids between
various species of citrus have acquired commercial importance, especially the tangors, which are hybrid
between tangerine and orange.

orange, bitter. *Citrus aurantium;* used
mainly as root stock because of its
resistance to the gummosis disease of
citrus. Fruit is too acidic to eat, and
is used in manufacture of marmalade;

the peel oil is used in manufacture of marmalade; the peel oil is used in the liqueur curacao; the peel and flower oils (neroli oil) and the oils from the green twigs (petit-grain oils) are used in perfumery. It is known as seville orange in Spain, Bigaradier in France, melangol in Italy, and khush-khash in Israel.

orange, osage. A tree native to North America, especially to the southwestern part of the US, where it is frequently used as a hedge plant. The wood is yellow, tough and satiny, and was formerly much used for bows by the Indians. The tree grows to a height of from 15-20 m. The fruit is large and round and has a pale yellow skin the texture of orange peel. It is not edible.

orange, Pera. A variety of orange. Some people believe the Pera sweet orange to be identical with Lamb's Summer. The variety was introduced into Brazil many years ago and is one of the important varieties grown in that country at present. The fruit is somewhat smaller and ripens earlier than the Valencia and is classified as a late midseason variety. The rind is medium-thin; colour is light-orange at maturity. The flesh is juicy and rich in flavor. The fruit is used in comparatively large quantities in Brazil for processing. Tristeza-induced stem pitting lowers productivity in Brazil.

orange, pineapple. A non-blood type sweet orange. This variety was first noticed in a Florida orange grove in about 1883. The name is indicative of the aroma of the fruit. The rind is glossy and a deep-orange colour. The flavor is described as vinous and sprightly. The seeds are large and rather numerous, ranging from 13-23 in number. The fruit ranges from nearly round to slightly oblate and the size from medium to large. When fully ripened, the fruit may display a reddish tinge. The flesh is of a medium-grain, orange-yellow in color. The Pineapple is considered to be the most highly colored variety in Florida. The fruit ripens in January and February, and is self-abscissing. The fruit has excellent processing qualities, with a juice content between 53 and 54%; total soluble solids content of about 10.5%. The pineapple orange is also grown in Mexico and South Africa.

orange, Salustiana. A variety of sweet orange of the non-blood or blanca type. A comparatively recent variety grown in Spain, Iran, and Morocco, the Salustiana is believed to have originated as a limb sport on a common sweet seedling tree. The fruit is of medium-size, well-colored at maturity. The flesh is juicy, with low acid content and sweet flavor. The variety is highly regarded because of its early maturing, its absence of seeds, and general good quality. The tree and fruit are essentially indistinguishable from those of Caderna, except that the fruit is flatter and somewhat later in maturing. The Salustiana tends to produce a poor juice color, low yield of soluble solids and a bitter aftertaste is harvested too early.

orange, Sanguinello comune. A variety of sweet orange, blood-type. It is described as a group of closely related clones and is one of the most important blood oranges in Italy. The color is orange at maturity, with some red blush. The flesh is deeply red pigmented. The fruit is juicy and of a pleasant flavour.

orange, Sanguinello Moscato. Sweet orange, blood-type and one of the most highly regarded blood oranges. This variety is grown in the Mount Etna region of Sicily. The fruit has few to no seeds, is orange in coloration; the apical portion is strongly red-blushed. The flesh is well flavoured, aromatic, blood-coloured, and very juicy. The fruit matures in mid-season and holds well on the tree. This variety is also grown in Iran.

orange, Shamouti. A variety of sweet orange that is completely orange-colored at maturity. A very attractive fruit, the juice content is generous and the rag content is low. As grown in the Mediterranean region, it is indistinguishable from the Jaffa or Joppa orange. In Israel, this variety constitutes about 75% of the country's total orange crop. For many years, the principal rootstock used was Palestine sweet lime, but this resulted in a fruit of low juice and soluble solids content. In recent years, sour orange rootstock has been used and quality has improved markedly. A campaign has been conducted in Israel for many years directed toward eradicating trees infected with tristeza. The fruit is medium-large, oval in shape, and seedless. The variety is also grown in Turkey and South Africa.

orange, sour. *Citrus aurantium L.* A variety of orange widely used as a rootstock to which sweet citrus varieties are budded. The sour orange tree also can be used effectively in landscape gardening. It was widely planted in the gardens of Moslem Spain during the period, AD 929-1031.

orange, Succari. A variety of non-blood type sweet orange. An exceptionally sweet orange that is almost devoid of acid. The sugar/acid ratio at maturity is 100/1. Thus, the fruit is not suitable for processing. It is called Sukkari in Egypt; the variety is of unknown origin. It is of medium-size, oblate to globose, and seedy, the variety has been well regarded in Egypt for many years and is of considerable commercial importance there.

orange, Tarocco. A variety of blood orange and a comparatively recent Italian variety. Flesh is medium-firm, fruit is juicy and usually well-pigmented. Its flavour is rich. The fruit ripens in midseason. Widely planted in the Mount Etna region of Sicily. Production is mainly for the fresh market.

orange, Temple. A tangelo, that is, a cross between a sweet orange and mandarin. The hybrid is distinguished by easily parted sections, an attraction for use as a dessert fruit. The fruit is oblate, tapering slightly to the stem. The size ranges from medium to large and the colour is a deep-orange red. The rind is smooth or pebbled, leathery, thin, and relatively easy to peel. The flavour is rich, vinous, spicy, and characteristic. Acidity and sweetness are well-blended. The Temple variety has about 20 seeds, and is less frost-resistant than most mandarins and more tender to cold than the sweet orange. Commercially, the Temple is generally considered and marketed as an orange and thus included in the table. It could equally well be considered a mandarin.

orange, Valencia. A variety of non-blood type sweet orange. It is believed that the Valencia was introduced into England from the Azores, but Spain or China have been suggested as its origin. The Valencia is grown widely in a number of citrus regions in the world, including Argentina, Australia, Brazil, Italy, Jamaica, Mexico, South Africa, Spain, and Tunisia, among others. The Valencia has superior processing qualities, having a juice content ranging from 55-59%; total soluble solids, 10.7-11.4%. Because of its extensive propagation, numerous bud mutations have appeared and have been exploited. These are virus-free and show increased yields. Popular varieties include Campbell, Cutter, Frost, and Olinda. The fruit of the Valencia is round or slightly oval; medium to large in size; slightly flattened, scarred; base is smooth, rounded; the calyx is small and sharp-pointed. The rind is smooth or slightly pebbled. The 9 sections (or more) of the orange are clearly marked. The flesh is orange and of medium-grain. The juice sacs are spindle-shaped and of medium size. The acidity and sweetness of the fruit blend well. The flavour of Valencia orange is quite rich, sprightly, and vinous. Its quality is usually excellent.

orange, Washington navel. The Washington Navel orange is rounded, somewhat tapering toward the apex which terminates in an umbilicus, the typical "navel" that gives the variety its name. Navel oranges are sometimes are large as 8.9-9.2 cm. The colour ranges from orange to orange-yellow. The base is rounded, sometimes flattened and frequently creased. The calyx is small; the rind is smooth, tough, and leathery, and from 0.3-0.6 cm. in thickness. The deep-orange flesh is rather coarse. The juice sacs are large and spindle-shaped. In well-cultured groves in good seasons, the juice is quite plentiful. The navel orange has been described as representing a pleasant blend of acidity and sweetness, with a rich, vinous flavor. The fruit is seedless and usually of excellent quality.

orange, Washington sanguine. A variety of blood-type sweet orange. This variety originated as a limb sport of Doblefina and was first found at Sagunto, Spain. Although the given name is Washington Sangre, the variety is much more important in Morocco-hence the use of the Moroccan spelling. In Algeria, the fruit is called *Doublefine Amelioree*. The fruit is oval shaped, large, somewhat lopsided, with medium-thick rind that does not adhere as tightly as that of the *Doblefina*. The fruit is acceptable as a table variety and it is an excellent shipper, but has not found to be suitable for juice processing.

Orange B. The colour component of Orange B is the disodium salt of 1-(4-sulphophenyl)3-ethylcarboxy-4-(4-sulphonaphthalzo)-5-hydroxypyrazole. This colour is approved only for the colouring of casings. The concentration of this colour cannot exceed 150 mg/kg in the finished food products.

Orange G. The name given to the edible colour, which is the disodium salt of phenylazo-2-naphthol-6,8-disulphonic acid. It is quite stable towards reducing agents.

Orange RN. The name given to the edible colour, which is the sodium salt of 1-sulpylazo-2-naphthol-6-phenhonic acid.

orange blossom. *Choysia ternata.* A flowering shrub growing up to a height of about 2 metres. The flowers, with a sweet scent reminiscent of the flowers of orange trees, provide an essential oil which is used in the manufacture of quality perfumes.

orange butter. Chopped whole orange is cooked, sweetened and homogenized.

orange colours. *See* Orange B; Orange G; and Orange RN.

orange flower water. Neroli oil is made from the flowers of the bitter orange by steam distillation. The condensed water layer from the distillation is orange-flower water. Also known as oil of Neroli water.

orange juice. A classical source of vitamin C and minerals. Commercially the juice is concentrated prior to marketing. It is an excellent food for patients and infants. The average composition per 100 g of the orange juice is: protein 0.5%; fat 0.1%; calcium 25 mg; iron 0.25 mg; zinc 0.18 mg; vitamin A 125 i.e.; vitamin B_1 0.05 mg; vitamin B_2 0.02 mg; nicotinic acid 0.1 mg; vitamin C 36 mg. It also contains sodium and potassium, and traces of manganese, nickel and cobalt. *See also* orange.

orange oil. The peel oil, containing about 90% limonene, main odoriferous constituent decanal, also linalool and nonylic alcohol. Oil of bitter orange is similar but contains a glucoside that confers the bitterness.

Orchid family: *Orchidaceae.* The orchid flower is so specialized that the illustrated species is needed for a structure by structure description. In general, the flower is usually bisexual, has 3 sepals that may resemble in color and form the 3 petals, a column of fused stamens and stigmas, and an inferior ovary of 3 carpels. Flower color vary widely. Nectar, odour, and form of the flower attract pollinators (specific in many cases). The fruit is a capsule with very tiny seeds. Seed food (endosperm) aborts, which necessitates a fungal relationship as a source of metabolites for seed germination. The plants are generally leafy, sometimes leafless. Leaves are alternate, very rarely opposite, whorled or reduced to scales. They are simple, thickened, whorled or reduced to scales. They are simple, thickened, usually linear, strap-shaped or round,

and basally sheathing the stem. These perennial herbs are distributed world-wide and comprise the largest plant family, with an estimated 30,000 species. They are terrestrial and saprophytic, deriving nutrients from soil and dead organic matter; or they are epiphytic, attached to the surface of another plant, where they obtain nutrients from the atmosphere and debris accumulations among the roots. Orchids have fungus-root (mycorrhizal) associations. Nutrient storage organs may be swollen stems (pseudobulbs) or swollen root-stem tubers, which the Greeks called "orchis" for their testiculate appearance; hence, the orchid name. Roots of most epiphytes are covered with a layer of dead corky cells called velamen.

The family include: *Anagrecum, Brassavola, Brassia, Cattleya, Cymbidium, Dendrobium, Epidendrum, Laelia, Miltonia, Odontoglossum, Oncidium, Paphiopedilum, Phalaenopsis, Stanhopea,* and *Vanda* are a few examples: *Vanilla* (extract from capsules); most wild orchids are considered to be endangered species and are legally protected. In the US, there are about 62 native genera.

orchid oil. A fragrant essential oil extracted by volatile solvents from an orchid, *Orchis militaris,* and related species.

orchil. Two closely related colorants are obtained from the lichens *Rocella tincotria* and *Licanora tartarea* by extraction with aqueous ammonia. These are: *Orchil* a thick reddish-purple liquid whose colouring principles are a mixture of red orcein $(C_{28}H_{24}O_7N_2)$, an amorphous yellow compound $(C_{21}H_{29}NO_5)$ and a compound related to litmus. The wine-red colour is only slightly soluble in water, but readily soluble in ethanol. It is pH sensitive, ranging from yellow in acid to blue in alkaline media. Orchil is permitted for use as a food colorant in several countries (not including the UK or US) and reference should be made to specific regulations.

oregano. *Origanum vulgare.* A very close relative of marjoram, so much so there is some confusion in the cross-pollination of their names: what is known as marjoram in UK turns up as oregano in Italy! This is the pungently aromatic herb of southern Italy, the one that is used, mainly in its dried form, to flavour pizzas and tomato sauces. Indeed, Greek cooks are convinced that dried oregano-rigani- is best used when dried. The fresh leaves are useful additions to salads, casseroles (towards the end of cooking), soups, sauces, pates, and poultry dishes. Dried oregano is especially good with beans, aubergines, courgettes, and rice, and in dishes such as pilaff and risotto.

organic. Pertaining or relating to a compound containing carbon as an essential constituent arranged in chains and/or rings; also containing hydrogen with or without oxygen, nitrogen, or other elements.

organic acid for grain storage. Certain organic acids are used for treating high moisture gains to prevent mold growth and deterioration. The organic acids used separately or in combination are propionic (CH_3CH_2COOH), acetic acid (CH_3COOH), and formic acid ($HCOOH$). Organic acids are sprayed on the wet grains, reduce the pH to 4, kill the mold organisms, and destroy the germinating capacity of the embryo. Organic acids are being used to control mold growth in cut forage in bales, wafers, and pellets. Application rates vary from 0.5-2.5 kg of organic acid per 100 kg of product, depending on the moisture content, product, and chemical used.

organoleptic. Technical term for taste and smell. Only four tastes can be distinguished on the tongue, bitter, sweet, acid and salt, all others are detected only by smell.

origanum oil. An essential oil with a thyme-like scent which is steam distilled from the leaves and tops of *Origannum heraleoticum.*

ornamental flowers. *Chrysanthemum.* An ornamental plant belonging to the aster family. The flowers are of various warm colours such as white, red or yellow, with dark green leaves; both of which taste somewhat like a mild cauliflower. The Japanese and Chinese have used both for centuries in their remedies and recipes.

Daffodil. There are several kinds. Some have a crimson or reddish-purple circle in the middle of the flower, while others have a yellow circle resembling a coronet or cup in the middle. The common daffodil gets about a foot high, with leaves that are long, narrow, grassy-looking and of a deep green. The single, large, yellow flower at the top of the stalk presses down a bit due to its weight.

Daisy. A low-growing European herb of the aster family which has small white or pink rays and yellow disks in its flower-heads. It grows to about 40 cm and has many broad leaves at its base with indented edges and finger-width size to them.

Day lily. This can be any plant of a genus of the lily family, which is characterized with long narrow basal leaves and showy yellow or tawny flowers in small clusters. Also any plant of a related genus (*Hosta*) bearing racemose white or violet flowers.

Geranium (Garden). A genus of South African plants, the species of which are widely cultivated in gardens everywhere on account of their very showy red or white flowers. There are also several kinds of scented geraniums as well, which some patients in the Russia who suffer from hypertension and headaches sniff for 20 minutes every day in order to obtain relief.

Hollyhock. A tall perennial Chinese herb belonging to the mallow family. This plant is cultivated in gardens as a biennial for its beautiful pastel flowers. Wee fairy folk were once thought to eat of its flowers a long time ago.

Iris (common). Cultivation has produced a great number of varieties, both among the bulbous or Spanish iris and the herbaceous or flag irises, which have fleshy, creeping rootstocks. The German or flat iris of modern American nurseries is a handsome plant with sword-like leaves of a bluish-green colour that are narrow and flat. Flower stems are nearly 1 metre high with large, deep-blue or purplish-blue flowers that have an agreeable scent reminiscent of orange blossoms a little.

Marigold. This can be any of several plants of the genus belonging to the aster family, especially African and French marigolds. A related species, marsh marigold, is known under the more familiar name of calendula for its marvellous skin-healing properties. All marigolds bear large yellow, orange or red terminal flower heads.

Nasturtium. This is an annual native to South America, but cultivated in gardens all over the world. The trailing or climbing stems grow 1 metre long and bear small, almost round, radially veined leaves and are adorned with either red, orange or yellow flowers larger than the leaves themselves.

Pansy. An annual plant widely cultivated as a garden ornamental but also occurs wild in fields and meadows and along the edges of forests. The angular, soft, hollow stem bears alternate, ovate to lanceolate, toothed leaves. The solitary, axillary flowers may be yellow, blue violet or two-coloured.

Peony. A perennial which grows wild and is cultivated elsewhere as a garden flower. The thick, knobby rootstock produces a green, juicy stem from 0.6-1.0 m high. The leaves are ternate or bi-ternate, with large, ovate-lanceolate leaflets. The large, solitary, red or purplish-red flowers resemble roses. This queen of all herbs was highly prized by ancient Greeks for its miraculous properties.

Petunia. Any of a genus of tropical American barbs with funnel-shaped or tubular-spreading petals or corollas. The common gardens petunia, as well as many forms and varieties, have all been derived from *P. axillaris* (with white flowers) and *P. violacea* (with violet flowers). Both are native to Argentina. Petunias belong to the same nightshade family (*Solanaceae*) that potatoes, tomatoes, tobacco and chilli peppers do.

Rose. There are over 100 species of rose in the genus *Rosa,* which consists of prickly shrubs found wild and widely cultivated in the temperate parts of the Northern Hemisphere. Their trailing, climbing or erect stems bear alternate, odd-pinnate leaves with familiar white to deep-red or, rarer still, black flowers that are single and five-petaled in wild species but mostly double in cultivated varieties.

They yield fruit-like, fleshy hips rich in vitamin C.

Snap Dragon. Any garden plant of the genus having snowy white, crimson, or yellow bilabiate flowers fancifully likened to the face of a dragon. The nightshade family (*Solanaceae*) to which petunias belong is closely related to the snapdragon order (*Scorphulariales*) and is a connecting link between it and the phlox family (*Polemoniaceae*), which is confined primarily to the western US.

Tulip. The name applies not only to any plant of this genus, but also to its flower or bulb as well. Tulips have been so long in cultivation that the common garden types cannot really be traced to any existing wild species to speak of. Holland is still the centre of tulip cultivation though bulbs for the market are now also raised in the US Horticulturally, tulips are classed under two main divisions: early-flowering and May-flowering tulips.

Violet. Not only does this name apply to any plant, flower, or species of the genus, but also it pertains to actual colours resembling some violets. The common purple or hooded violet is common to the some violets. Violet vary in hue from reddish-blue to blue-red, are of medium saturation and low to medium in brilliance of colour.

ornithine. $H_2N(CH_2)_3CH(NH_2)COOH$. An amino acid, that is not a constituent of proteins but is important in living organisms as an intermediate in the reactions of the urea cycle and in arginine. If arginase (from liver) is present when proteins are being hydrolyzed enzymatically, ornithine (along with urea) is produced from arginine. The exclusion of L-ornithine from the list of protein-derived amino acids is thus somewhat arbitrary. In Ornithine cycle (or arginine-urea cycle) in which the formation of urea from ammonia and carbon dioxide takes place, ornithine takes up ammonia, carbon dioxide and water to produce citrulline; this takes up ammonia (from aspartic acid) and loses water to form arginine which is then converted into urea and ornithine through the agency of the enzyme arginase. Ornithine formed can then repeat the cycle. Under appropriate conditions, ornithine acts in effect as a catalyst to promote the formation of urea from ammonia and carbon dioxide. In addition to its role in urea biosynthesis, ornithine serves as a precursor of the ubiquitous mammalian polyamines spermidine and spermine. Ornithine is not of nutritional importance since it is not found in protein foodstuffs.

Ornithine cycle. Cyclic series of biochemical reactions responsible for the conversion and detoxification of the nitrogenous products of protein metabolism. Ammonia and urea are derived from the metabolic pathway, ammonia being used to convert ornithine to citrulline and the innocuous urea being largely excreted. Some genetic mutants in the human have blocks in the cycle, resulting in, for example, the citrullinuria and ornithine transcarbamylase deficiency. Also known as urea cycle.

orotic acid. Uracil-4-carboxylic acid; an intermediate product in the synthesis of the pyrimidines which are present both in RNA's and DNA's. Pyrimidines are not included among the nutritional essentials for mammals, but they are essential for cell duplication and, hence, must be produced endogenously. This is accomplished by a condensation of carbamyl phosphate and aspartic acid to form carbamyl aspartic acid, followed by ring closure and oxidation.

orris root. *Iris germanica.* The root of several species of iris, especially of the European iris, which, on account of its pleasant odour, is employed in perfumery and in the manufacture of tooth powder. It was formerly used quite freely as medicine. Spectacular as the flowers are, it is the root or rhizome of the Florentine iris that is the valuable part of the plant. The name (orris) derives from the Greek work for rainbow, indicating the range of flower colours.

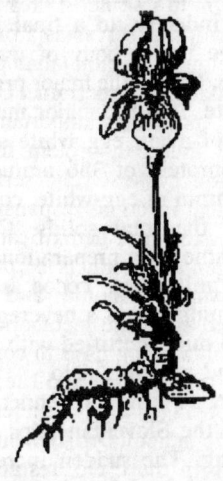

The orris powder made from the dried root, once formed the basis of most sachets, used as a fixative in pot pourri, in talcum powder, bath preparations, hair powders, and dry shampoos. A perfume was being made in 15th century comprising orris roots mixed with anise.

Ortanique mandarin. Citrus fruit; a variety of mandarin believed to be a unique orange-mandarin hybrid, probably from a chance seedling in Jamaica, where the variety is now produced commercially. The name was derived from ORange-TANgerine-unIQUE. The fruit ripens in mid-season, flesh is orange, rind is thin, rather tightly adherent. The flesh is of an orange colour and is juicy and flavorful.

oryzanin. Obsolete name for thiamin (vitamin B_1).

oryzenin. The major protein of rice; classed as one of the glutelins.

osage orange. *See* orange, osage.

osmanthus. A floral concentrate obtained by the extraction from flowers of Osmanthus fragrans, an evergreen tree that grows to a height of 5-7 metres. It has a jasmine-like fragrance. In China, the flowers, known as *Kwei Hwa* or *Mo Hsi* are used to scent tea and plums ans raisins.

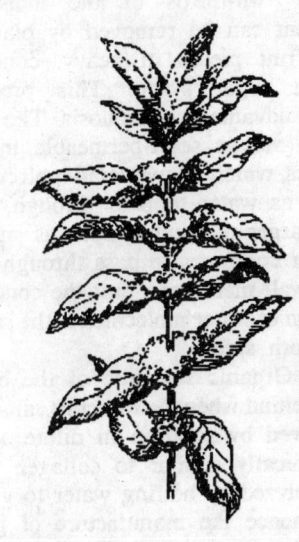

osmazone. Obsolete name given to an aqueous extract of meat that is soluble in alcohol regarded as the pure essence of meat.

osmophilic yeasts. Few organisms can grow in high concentrations of sugar or salts, e.g., in jams or brine pickles, due to the high osmotic pressure. Those few yeasts that are able to grow under these conditions are termed osmophilic. Zygosaccharomyes can tolerate up to 80% sugar and cause spoilage in honey, chocolate centres, sugar products.

osmotic agents. Agents used to raise the osmotic pressure of the tissue fluids in order to withdraw water from the CSF when there is high interacranial pressure, or from the eye in glaucoma. Hypertonic dextrose, urea, mannitol, sorbitol and glycerol may be u sed for these purposes.

Osmovac process. A method for partially dehydrating substances such as fruit pieces by osmosis then followed with vacuum drying. In this process, up to 50% of the weight of fruit or about two-thirds of the moisture content can be removed by placing the fruit pieces in heavy, concentrated sugar syrup. This process takes advantage of osmosis. The cell walls act as semi-permeable membranes, which allows small molecules, such as water to pass through, but not larger molecules, such as sugar. Water continues to pass through the cell-wall membrane unit the concentration of water molecules is the same on both sides.

ossein. Organic structure of the bone left behind when the minerals salts are removed by solution in dilute acid. Chemically similar to collagen and hydrolyzed by boiling water to gelatin, hence the manufacture of glue from bones- known as ossein gelatin.

Ossetin cheese. A kind of rennet cheese made from cows or sheep's milk in the Caucasus. After the curd is broken it is cooked until firm, kneaded together, and the whey is removed. The finished product is put into brine, where it may be kept for over a year. This long period in the brine produces a stronger, and harder cheese than the cheese produced by a brine period of less than three months.

osteomalacia. Bone disorder in adults equivalent to rickets in children; due to shortage of vitamin D leading to inadequate absorption of calcium and loss of calcium from the bones.

Ostermilk. Trade name for dried milk for infant feeding. Ostermilk No. 1 is half-cream; No. 2 is normal.

outfall sewer. A pipe or conduit used to transport either raw sewage, or treated effluent from the food processing industry, to a final point of discharge into a body of water.

ovalbumin. One of the major proteins of egg white. It is the major nutritional protein of avian egg white and is a phosphoprotein of 386 amino acids. The albumin of egg-white, comprises 55% of the total solids. Ovaltine. Trade name for a preparation of malt extract, milk, eggs, cocoa and soya, for consumption as a beverage when added to milk. Fortified with vitamin B_1, D and nicotinic acid.

Ovcji, Sir. A kind of rennet cheese made in the Slovenian Alps.

oven spring. The sudden increases in the volume of a dough during the first 10-12 minutes of baking- due to increase rate of fermentation and to expansion of gases.

overhead-fired. A direct fired dryer in which the oil or gas burner is installed above the drying tunnel usually done to save floor space.

overpack. An enclosure that is used by a single consignor to provide protection or convenience in handling of a package or to consolidate two or more packages.

over-run. Term used in ice-cream manufacture-the percentage increase in the volume of the mix caused by beating-in of air. Optimum overrun, 70-100%. To prevent excessive aeration US regulations state that ice-cream must weigh 4.5 lb per gallon.

ovoflavin. Name given to substance isolated from eggs, shown to be identical with riboflavin.

ovomucin. A carbohydrate-protein complex in egg-white, 1-3% of the total solids. Responsible for the firmness of egg-white.

ovomucoid. A protein of egg-white, 12% of the total solids. Acts as a specific inhibitor of the digestive enzyme trypsin, but is destroyed by the stomach enzyme pepsin.

oxalic acid. COOH-COOH. Lowest member of the dicarboxylic acid series. It is poisonous, but not in small doses; it is present in spinach, chocolate and rhubarb. The toxicity of rhubarb leaves is due to their high content of oxalic acid. Oxalic acid is normally excreted in human urine, 15-20 mg per day, increased in diabetes and liver disease.

oxidases. Enzymes that catalyze oxidation reactions in which the electron acceptor (oxidant) is oxygen, the product is water or hydrogen peroxide, and the oxygen atoms are not incorporated into the product of the reaction. For example, amino acid oxidases are flavoproteins that catalyze oxygen-requiring oxidation of amino acids to keto acids with the concomitant formation of hydrogen peroxide. Perhaps the most important example of an oxidase is the cytochrome oxidase which uses electrons from an electron transport chain plus protons from surrounding medium to reduce oxygen to water.

oxidation. In its original sense, oxidation meant simply combination with oxygen. Its use has, however, been considerably widened to cover a great many processes similar to oxidation, such as chlorination, and other processes of combination with strongly nonmetallic elements, which add electrons readily. In fact the term oxidation in its broadest sense means simply a chemical reaction whereby electrons are removed from one or more of the atoms of a substance. It is, most frequently accompanied by a simultaneous process, in the same reaction, whereby another substance or substances gain the electrons and thus undergo reduction; therefore, calling the process oxidation, under these circumstances, simply means that it is this part (*i.e.*, loss of electrons) of the particular process that is of greatest interest. The removal of hydrogen atoms from a hydrogencontaining organic compound (dehydrogenation) is a form of oxidation; it is effected by a catalytic reaction with air or oxygen, as in the oxidation of alcohols to aldehydes. Free radical chains play an important part in the oxidation of such organic compounds as rubber, drying oils.

oxidation ditch. A modified from of activated sludge process. In essence, it is an extended aeration process, capable of taking shock laidings without upset. The ditch is operated as a closed system.

oxidation pond. A shallow lagoon or basin, about 1.5 metres deep, within which waste water is purified, through sedimentation and both aerobic and anaerobic biochemical activity over a period of time; used in favourable climates.

oxidative fermentation. Decomposition of hexoses to compounds of simpler structure, occurring under action of bacteria, in which initial degradation of carbohydrate is similar to alcoholic fermentation; final stage leads, however, to products of higher oxidation number.

oxidative phosphorylation. The synthesis of ATP from ADP that is coupled to the operation of the mitochondrial electron transport system. This reaction occurs during the final stages of aerobic respiration, in which ATP is formed from ADP and phosphate coupled to electron transport in the electron transport chain. The reaction occurs in the mitochondria and takes place at three sites on the electron transport chain. The phosphorylation is controlled by proteins in the mitochondrial membrane, termed coupling factors, and is inhibited by uncoupling agents such as oligomycin and dinitrophenol.

oxidoreductases. Enzymes that catalyze oxidation/reduction reactions. Because all oxidizing reactions must be coupled to a reducing reaction the enzymes catalyzing such reactions (often called dehydrogenases or reductases) are more properly called oxidoreductases. For example, the enzyme that catalyzes the reversible oxidation of alcohol to acetaldehyde using NAD^+ as coenzyme may be called alcohol dehydrogenase, aldehyde reductase or alcohol: NAD^+ oxidoreductase.

oximetry. Continuous measurement of the amount of oxygen in the circulating blood.

Oxo. Trade name for a dried preparation of hydrolyzed meat, meat extract, salt and cereal in cube form, used as a drink or a gravy. The average composition per 100 g is: protein 9.5%; fat 3.5%; carbohydrate 12.5%; calcium 182 mg; iron 22 mg; and food energy 0.5 MJ.

oxygen. A gas comprising about 50% by weight of the earth's crust and oceans and thus is the most abundant terrestrial element. Gaseous oxygen constitutes 21% by volume of the air near the earth's surface, much of which is formed by photosynthesis of plants; water contains 88.8% oxygen by weight. It is vital to all animal and most plants as the supporter of the respiration-metabolism processes. The enclosed spaces such as vats, tanks, sewers, etc., may have insufficient oxygen present to support life due to replacement by other gases which may or may not be toxic by themselves, e.g., carbon monoxide is toxic and will kill. If the concentration of oxygen falls below 14% of the atmosphere, humans become irrational, dangerous to themselves and other people, and finally become unconscious and may die from asphyxia.

oxygen, absorbed. The amount of oxygen in parts per million absorbed by a sample of water from acidic potassium permanganate in 4 hrs. at 300 K.

oxygen debt. A physiological state that occurs when a normally aerobic animal is forced to respire anaerobically during temporary shortage of oxygen (anoxia), such as, due to violent muscular excretion. Pyruvate, a product of the first stage of internal respiration, is converted anaerobically to lactic acid, which is toxic and requires oxygen for its breakdown, thereby building up an oxygen is made available and allows oxidation of the lactic acid in the liver.

oxygen quotient. The rate of oxygen consumption of an organism or tissue. It is usually expressed in mL of oxygen per mg of dry weight per hour. Small organisms tend to have higher oxygen quotients than larger ones.

oxygen sag curves. Graphical curves which relate the dissolved oxygen content of water against time flow, within the context of the process of self-purification, following the discharge of pollutants into a stream **oxygenases.** The enzymes that are capable of catalyzing oxidation reactions (usually irreversible) in which oxygen is incorporated from molecular oxygen into the product. Oxygenase-catalyzed reactions are often the first oxidative step in metabolism of stable reduced compounds such as alkanes. Monoxygenases catalyze incorporation of a single atom of oxygen, the second atom being reduced in the same reaction to water by an electron donor (reductant) which is usually NAD(P)H. Monooxygenase reactions often involve a number of electron donor and the substrate: these components may include iron-sulphur proteins, flavoproteins or cytochromes. A typical example is the system occurring in mammalian liver for detoxification of foreign compounds; this contains a cytochrome called cytochrome P_{450}.

oxygenic photosynthesis. The photosynthesis that oxidizes water to form oxygen; the form of photosynthesis characteristic of the eucaryotic algae and cyanobacteria.

oxygenic photosynthetic bacteria. The two groups of bacteria namely *cyanobacteria* and the order *Prochlorales.* Because the latter is very small order with one genus, only the cyanobacteria are of interest to microbiologists.

oxyhaemoglobin. Form which oxygen is transported from the lungs to the tissues; a loose combination of oxygen with the haemoglobin, which is readily decomposed.

oxymyoglobin. Myoglobin is a coloured protein in muscle that serves as a store of oxygen; it takes up oxygen to form oxymyoglobin which is bright red, while myoglobin itself is purplish-

red. The surface of fresh meat which is exposed to oxygen is bright red from the oxymyoglobin, while the interior of the meat is darker in colour where the myoglobin is not oxygenated.

oxyntic cells. Or parietal cells; glands in the stomach that produce hydrochloric acid of the gastric juice.

oxytocin. A cyclic peptide hormone that consists of 9 amino acids, only 2 of which are different from those in vasopressin and that causes the contraction of smooth muscle.

oyster plant. A plant cultivated for its edible root, which has a flavour somewhat like that of oysters. The plant, a native of Europe, thrives in almost any temperate climate, though it has not the commercial importance of either carrots or parsnips. The second season it produces flower stalks three or four feet high, capped with purplish blossoms. The tapering roots are 20-30 cm long and about two inches in diameter at the top. Like parsnips, the roots are better if left in the ground in winter. Also known as salsify. *Compare* oysters.

oyster oil. An essential oil with a typical pine fragrance, distilled from the leaves of the bay pine tree, *Callitris rhomboides.*

oysters. Oysters (Osteridae) are found worldwide in a broad band between latitudes 64°N and 44°S. They are distributed from the inter-tidal zone down to approximately 39 m. Commercial edible oyster belong to two genera, Ostrea and Crassostrea. Some of the most common species include *Ostrea edulis* (the common or European oyster); *O. lurida*; *Crassostrea virginia* (the America oyster); *C. gigas, C. angulata, C. commercialis, C. cucullata*; and *C. chilensis.* The soft body of an oyster is covered by two shells or valves; the right or top valve is flat, and the left or bottom valve is heavier and cupped. An oyster attached and usually rests on its left valve. The two shells are joined together at the hinge by an elastic material known as the ligament. The shape of the shell is highly variable in *Crassostrea* and subcircular in *Ostrea*. More than 95% of the shell is calcium carbonate. Growth of shell depends directly upon water temperature. Oysters in northern water require about 5 years to reach market size (about 10 cm). Oyster meats contain about every element found in seawater. The amount of meat yielded varies with geographic location and time of year. The yield is usually greater in northern waters, particularly in winter. Meat quality drops during the spawning season. After spawning, oyster build up glycogen and are in their best condition at the height of this buildup. These seasonal changes are sometimes measured by the calculation of "percentage solids" (which is equal to the dry weight of meat multiplied by 100 divided by wet weight of meat). In the spring, glycogen is converted into sex products. The average composition per 100 g of raw oyster is: water 85%; protein 10.5%; fat 1%; calcium 192 mg; iron 5 mg; vitamin A 80 μg; vitamin B_1 0.1 mg; vitamin B_2 0.17 mg; food energy 0.21 MJ; with traces of carbohydrates, nickel and zinc.

ozone. A triatomic molecule of oxygen. Above minimal levels, it is an irritant to human beings and animals. In food industry, it is used as a powerful oxidising agent, as a bactericide in water purification and to kill algae and fungi. Higher concentrations of ozone cause headache, giddiness, pains in chest, difficulty in breathing, and finally unconsciousness. It is a natural constituent of the atmosphere occurring in concentration of about 0.01 mg/L; the toxicity threshold for workers is 0.1 mg/L. Ozone is found in the atmosphere at very high altitudes, and is responsible for absorbing sun's ultraviolet radiation, without this absorption by ozone the earth would have been subjected to a lethal amount of ultraviolet radiation. It is also produced by certain high voltage electrical equipment; it is also produced in certain circumstances when photochemical reactions occur in the atmosphere between ultraviolet light (sunlight) and the oxides of nitrogen and hydrocarbons emitted to the atmosphere by motor vehicles

Occupational exposure to ozone should be controlled in such a manner so that no employee is exposed to ozone at a concentration greater than 0.2 mg/m³ of air (0.1 ppm), determined as a time-weighted average (TWA) concentration limit for up to a 8-hour workshift in a 40-hour workweek, over a working lifetime.

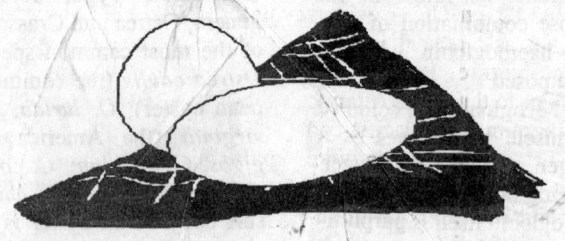

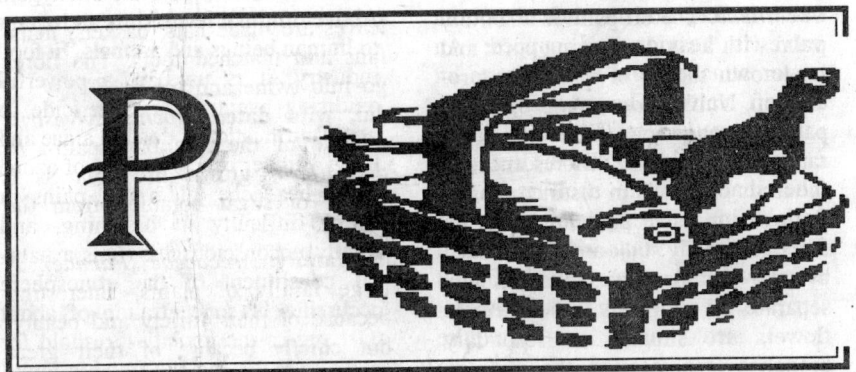

p.4000. A class of synthetic sweetening agents, chemically, they are nitro-aminoalkoxybenzenes. One member of this class, propoxyaminonitrobenzene is about 4,100 times as sweet as sugar and 8 times as sweet as saccharine but these compounds are considered harmful and are not permitted in foods.

P680. A form of chlorophyll that absorbs light optimally at 680 nm.

P700. A form of chlorophyll that absorbs light optimally at 700 nm.

PABA. Abbreviation for p-aminobenzoic acid.

pacemaker enzyme. An enzyme that catalyzes a reaction that is essentially irreversible in the chemical sense; such enzymes frequently catalyze either the initial, the final, or a branch point reaction of a metabolic pathway.

Pacific cod. Gadus macrocephalus. A kind of edible fish which achieves a length up to 1.2 m. It is widely distributed, but as a coastal inhabitant does not migrate. Its size and colour is similar to that of the Atlantic cod. The maximum age of Pacific cod is about 10-12 years. Its diet is quite diverse, but consist primarily of crustaceans and fishe. Sexual maturity is attained after 5-6 years. The spawning season is in late-winter. Eggs are laid in enormous numbers (similar to Atlantic cod), but instead of raising they sink to the floor, and adaptation to the more localized nature of these codfishes.

Pacific halibut Hippoglossus hippoglossus stenolepis. A subspecies of a Atlantic relative and is found in the North Pacific from the Bering Sea and Alaska to the Sea of Okhotsk and the California coast. It had been a favourite catch of the American Indians.

paddy. Rice in the husk after threshing. Also known as rough rice.

Paglia cheese. A kind of cheese, which is imitation of Gorgonzola cheese made in Switzerland. It is quite soft cheese and has very pleasant flavour.

Pago cheese. A variety of rennet cheese made in various sizes. It is made on the Island of Pago, Yugoslavia.

palm kernel oil. Oil extracted from the kernel of the nut of Elaeis guineensis. The oil from the pulp is termed palm oil; used for margarine and cooking fat. See also palm oil.

palm oil. Of the family Palmaceae (palm family), the oil palms are of the genus Elaesis. This genus has been classified with the genus Cocos in the tribe

Cocoineae. The oil palm is a solitary palm with a single growing point and no known means of vegetative production. Unlike *Cocs nucifera*, the oil palm is monoecious, producing separate male and female inflorescences in the axils of fronds in distinct phases. Both are massive panicles borne on compact woody stalk and surrounded by two fibrous bracts that usually separate at anthesis. The female flowers are situated on secondary branches (spadices) in the axils of spiny bracts and have a syncarpous trimerous ovary. Although at anthesis, all three ovules may be fertilized, usually only one develops. The fruit is produced as bunches of nuts; beneath the outer skin is a layer of fibrous pulp, the mesocarp or pericarp which is rich in oil called (red) palm oil. Inside is the seed from the inner kernel from which is obtained palm kernel oil. The palm oil is red in colour from the high content of β-carotene (up to 10 mg retinol equivalent) together with other carotenoids. Both palm oil and palm kernel oil are used for margarine and cooking fats.

palm, palmyra. A palm topped by a magnificent cluster of fan-shaped leaves, common in India, the Malay Archipelago and tropical West Africa. The trunk grows to be from 6-20 m high and the leaves attain a length of about 1.3 m, and have about seventy-five rays. This is one of the most valuable palms, its various parts being used in nearly 800 different ways.

In parts of India the natives depend almost entirely on this tree to supply all their wants. When the plant is young it is eaten as a vegetable; the fruit of the older tree also is edible. The trunks are used for building, the leaf stalks for making fences. From the leaves are made hats, baskets, mats, fans and thatched roofs. The fibres go into twine and rope.

palm, wild date. *Phoenix sylvestris,* relative of the true date palm, *P. dactylifera,* grown in India as a source of sugar obtained from the sap.

palm family. *Arecaceae (Palmae).* A large family of plants, interesting because of their variety and beauty, but chiefly because of their great value to man. Palms are second to the grasses in economic importance. The palms, numbering about 3,500 species, mostly consist of trees; shrubs and vines are also represented, most of them native to the tropics. Of these some are vines, slender as reeds; others are low, bushy plants with leaf stems springing directly from the ground; still others are trees with trunks from 1-1.5 m in diameter and reaching a height of about 30 m. This last is by far the largest group. The peculiarity of most palms is the tall, branches trunk, with its cluster of foliage, and in some species also fruit at the tip. As the trunk pushes upward in its growth and produces new foliage the old dies, and throughout its length its surface bears the scars and, in the case of some varieties, the dry, dead stumps of fallen leaves. The doum palm of Arabia is the only important species bearing branches. With the exception of grass, there is no plant in the whole vegetable kingdom so important economically as the palm. It has been put to a thousand or more uses. It has been made to supply the three fundamental necessities of man- food, shelter and clothing. The fruit of many palms constitute important food in many regions. Important among these are the date and coconut palms.

The Bacaba palm of Brazil, which produce clusters of berries yielding a valuable drink and an oil, and the sago palm, the trunk of which yields a starchy meal called sago. The trunks of some species of palms are converted into excellent timber suitable for houses, ships and other structures. The long stems of certain varieties are used for wicker furniture. The leaves of most of them are extensively used in the tropics as thatch for dwellings. The fibres of many palms are fine and strong and can be woven into cloth.

Among the other innumerable products of this group of plants are oil, from the oil palm, used for lubricating and illumination; vegetable ivory from the seed of the ivory palm, and wax, which exudes from the trunk of the wax palm. The spines which grow upon the trunks of certain species are used as needles and fishhooks. Mats, baskets, rope, twine, ship sails, rugs, screens, bedding, candles, wine, honey, resin and hammocks are a few of the articles made from palms. In desert regions where other vegetation is scarce the palm is regarded almost with veneration by the traveller, who finds refreshment in its shade and fruit.

Lodoiceae maldivica has the world's largest seed, a double coconut, made up of a 2-lobed drupe, and *Raphia fainifera* has the largest flowering plant leaf, about 20 m long. Palms have a single apical bud, called "heart of palm". When it dies or it is removed, the plant dies. Tree forms have an unbranched trunk with a terminal crown of leaves, commonly called "fronds," which emerge one at a time from the apical bud. Lignin, deposited in trunk tissues, provides sturdines. The leafy frond is made up of a blade, petiole, and a sheathing base. The blade types are: fan-shaped with feather-like (pinnate) veins, as in Lodoicea; fan-shaped with veins arising from one point (palmate), as in Sabal; feather-shaped (pinnately compound), as in Chamaedorea; or feather-shaped, twice-divided (bipinnately compound), as in Caryota Regardless of shape, the young leaf looks like a rod with a length-wise strip that peels down like a zipper, to free the 1 to many leaflets that unfold like a fan. The leaf petiole may be smooth or toothed on its margin. Small flowers are usually formed in loose clusters, called panicles, which have one or more bracts at the base.

Commonly, plants have separate male and female flowers (unisexual) on the same plant (monoecious) or on separate plants (dioecious), while others have flowers with both male and female parts within one flower (bisexual). Flower parts are usually in 3's, being separate or fused. Flowers are wind-, insect- or self-pollinated. Usually the fruit has one seed and is a berry or drupe type. The outside wall of the fruit can be fleshy, fibrous or leathery. Storage tissue (endosperm) within the seed is oily or fatty rather than starchy. In coconuts, it is a liquid.

The family include: *Areca catechu* (betel nut palm), *Calamus* and *Caemonorops* (rattan cane), *Cocos nucifera* (coconut palm), *Copernicia* (carnauba wax), *Elaeis guineensis* (oil palm), *Phoenix Dactylifera* (date palm), *Raphia pendunculata* (raffaia); *Arecastrum* (queen palm), *Arenga pinnata* (sugar palm), *Caryota mitis* (fishtail palm), *Chamaeodorea elegans* (parlor palm), *Chamaerops* (European fan palm), *Chrysalidocarpus* (Madagascar feather palm), *Cocothrinax argentea* (silver palm), *Erythea* spp. (Mexican fan palms), *Howeia* spp. (curly palm, sentry palm, flat palm), *Jubaea spectabilis* (coquitos palm), *Livistona spp.* (fan palms), *Metroxylon* (sago palm), *Rhapidophyllum* (needle palm), *Rhapis* (lady palm), *Roystonea regia* (royal palm), *Sabal palmetto* (cabbage palmetto), *Serenoa* (saw-palmetto), *Trachycarpus fortunei* (Chinese windmill palm), *Thrinax* (peaberry palm), *Washingtonia filifera (sentinel palm)*.

palma rosa oil. An essential oil with a rose-geranium like scent; it is steam distilled from the leaves of a variety of Rosha grass, locally called Motia (*Cymbopogon martinii*), which grows in dry regions of India, Pakistan, Afghanistan, and Indonesia. Also known as East Indian Geranium oil.

palytoxin. A neurotoxin isolated from a marine zoanthid *Palythoa toxica* and other *Palythoa* species. It is the most deadly non-protein toxin eer isolated. Its LD in mice is about 0.15 μg/kg by intravenous injection. It is therefore about 50 times more toxic than tetrodotoxin.

panada. A mixture of fat, flour and liquid (such as stock or milk) mixed to a thick paste; it is used to bind mixtures such as chopped meat and also as the basis of souffles and choux pastry.

pandanus oil. A honey-like essential oil extracted from the fresh male flowers of a water-loving tree resembling a date palm, mostly found near the sea beaches. The Indian name of the tree is Pandang, and is cultivated in Andaman Islands.

panary fermentation. Yeast fermentation of dough in bread-making.

pancreas. A gland in the abdomen with two functions; it secretes
(a) the hormone insulin, and
(b) the pancreatic juice.

pancreatic juice. The digestive juice that consists of the secretion of the pancreas and that is discharged into the small intestine; contains proteolytic enzymes, secreted as zymogens, nucleases, carbohydrases and lipase.

pancreatin. A preparation made from the pancreas of animals and therefore containing the enzymes of pancreatic juice; used as an aid to digestion.

pancreozymin. Hormone produced by the intestinal mucosa that stimulates the pancreas to secrete enzymes.

panettone. Popular name for the Italian, half bread-half cake. It is a kind of sourdough fruitcake traditionally consumed during the Christmas season, exhibits a number of unusual features that justifies its discussion here. The preparation process for panettone involves a fermentation process based on the yeast *S. exiguus* (the same organism found in San Francisco sourdough) and a heterofermentative lactic bacteria *L. brevis.* Other lactobacilli as well as *Enterobacter* and *Citrobacter* may also contribute to flavour development.

Panettone production begins with a 24 hour fermentation of a starter mixture composed for flour, water, and the necessary microorganisms. The ripened starter is used is inoculate a sour sponge composed of flour and water. The sour sponge is rebuilt two or three times to obtain a sufficient amount to make the "white dough." The latter composition is prepared by adding flour, butter oil, sugar, and water to the sour dough. The white dough is allowed to ferment for about 8-10 hours at 30°C, and then mixed with flour, water, egg yolk, butter oil, raisins, and candied fruit peels to make the "yellow dough." Yellow dough is divided, rounded, and molded before proofing for about 8-10 hours at 35°C and, finally it is baked for about an hour.

pangamic acid. N-di-isopropyl derivative of glucuronic acid. It is a very powerful methylating agent concerned with respiratory enzymes in cells. Also termed as vitamin B_{15}, but there is no evidence that it is a dietary essential.

Pannarone cheese. A fast-ripening Gorgonzola-type cheese with the blue mold. This unsalted cheese is cured at 25°C for the first week and the remainder of the curing (15-30 days) takes place at colder temperatures. Also known as Stracchino di Gorgonzola Bianco; Georgonzola Dolce.

pantothenic acid. One of the water-soluble B-group of vitamins. chemically β-alanine plus pantoic acid. Pantothenic acid is essential for several fundamental reactions in metabolism. It is part of the structure of Coenzyme A, needed for the transfer of acetyl groups and therefore essential for the metabolism of fats and carbohydrates. It is a water-soluble compound and is required in the diet of many vertebrates including the human. Dietary shortage never arises; universally distributed in all living cells. Sources of this vitamin include egg yolk, kidney, liver, and yeast, royal jelly and fresh vegetables. Deficiency symptoms in rats include greying of the hair, dermatitis, adrenal damage; in chicks, dermatitis; in dogs, gastrointestinal symptoms; but no definite pathological lesions in man. Based on needs, the human requirements would be about 6-8 mg/day. A deficiency results in symptoms affecting a wide range of tissues; the overall effects include fatigue, poor motor coordination, and muscle. cramps. Also termed as vitamin B_3.

pantoyltaurine. Similar to pantothenic acid but with the carboxyl group replaced by a sulphonic acid group; acts as an antagonist to the vitamin. When given to man, it leads to dizziness, postural hypotension, tachycardia, drowsiness and anorexia. Also called thiopanic acid.

papain. A protein-digesting enzyme occurring in the fruit of the West Indian papaya tree (*Carica papaya*). Papain is the dried and purified latex of the green fruits and leaves of *Carica papaya* L. (Fam. Caricaceae). The plant is cultivated in India, Sri Lanka, and many other parts of the world. The plant is about 5-6 metres in height bearing fruits of about 30 cm length and a weight up to 5 kg. The full-grown and unripe fruits are injured deeply at weekly intervals on four sides.

The latex comes out immediately and rapidly coagulates. It is collected, shredded and dried in sun or by heating. The crude papain is purified by dissolving it in water and precipitating with alcohol.

Papain contains several enzymes such as proteolytic enzymes peptidase I capable of converting proteins ino dipeptides and polypeptides, rennin-like enzyme, clotting enzyme similar to pectase and an enzyme having a feeble activity on fats. Papain is used to prevent adhesions; in sloughing and infected wounds; internally as protein digestant, as anthelmintic (nemotode), to relieve the symptoms of episiotomy (incision of vulva) and in meat industry for tenderizing beef. Rate of reaction slow at room temperature, increased at 55-75°C, maximum activity at 80°C and rapidly inactivated at temperatures higher than this, hence the papain continues to tenderize the meat during the early stages of cooking. Also known as arbuz; caroid; nematolyt; papayotin; Vegetable pepsin; Summetrin; Tromasin; Velardon; Vermizym.

papaveretum. A solution of the total pure alkaloids of opium as the hydrochlorides for oral use or for subcutaneous or intramuscular injection.

papaya. See pawpaw.

papovirus. One of a group of DNA-containing viruses that produce tumours in their hosts. Papilloma types produce nonmalignant tumours (such as warts) in all vertebrates; polyoma types produce malignant tumours in only certain classes of vertebrates (not including man).

paprika. A condiment prepared from the dried ripened pods of a species of capsicum. Paprika, while having the bright red colour of cayenne, is of very mild flavour. It is much used in salads.

para-. In chemical terminology, a prefix used to distinguish between isomers or nearly related compounds. Specifically;

(a) the derivatives of cyclic nuclei which contain substituents in the 1-4 position;

(b) some polymers are designated by the prefix para-, as paraldehyde;

(c) in certain acids which have several forms differing in water content, one of the forms may be designated by the prefix para-.

para-aminobenzoic acid. A compound classified in the Vitamin B-complex that exhibits growth-promoting effects from chicks and many bacteria. It may function as a precursor of folic acid. It is found in appreciable amounts in yeast, liver, wheat germ, etc. p-aminobenzoic acid is essential growth factor for microorganisms and therefore classed as a vitamin. No deficiency symptoms in higher animals except greying of the hair (achromotrichia) in rats. It is part of the molecule of folic acid and it is assumed that one of the functions of p-aminobenzoic acids is the formation of folic acid. Sulphanilamide is chemically very similar and kills bacteria by blocking access to the vitamin. It occurs in yeast, wheat germ; smaller amounts in meat, liver, vegetables. Also called the antigrey hair factor.

Paraben, methyl and propyl. Methyl and propyl p-hydroxybenzoates; used as preservatives at a concentration of 0.1%.

paracasein. The form of casein which is formed by rennin when milk is treated with rennet, as contrasted to an acid casein or hydrogen caseinate. Paracasein has twice the base-combining power of acid casein which has resulted in a number of theories.

Paraflow. Trade name for a plate heat exchanger used for pasteurizing liquids.

parakeratosis. Disease of swine characterized by cessation of growth, erythema, seborrhoea and hyperkeratosis of the skin; due to zinc deficiency, and essential fatty acids may be involved.

paralytic shellfish poisoning. Toxicity arising from eating clams or scallops that have been feeding on certain dino flagellates of Gonyaulax species in which saxitoxin or related substances are produced. The dinoflagellates are red in colour, and a high concentration in the sea gives rise to a so-called red tide.

parameter. A technical term originally coined to have precise meanings in various branches of mathematics. It is included here because it is frequently misused in many disciplines, including pharmacology and medical science generally, simply to mean any measured factor. An acceptable meaning in food science, arising through common usage, may be: a variable, the measurement of which is indicative of a function that cannot itself be precisely measured by the direct methods.

Paraquat. A bipyridyl-type herbicide which is widely used. Many cases of human poisoning have been reported. Toxic effects include damage to lungs, liver, kidneys and heart. The most striking toxic effect is a delayed (several days) and potentially lethal lung toxicity involving a widespread proliferation of cells in the lungs. It has been proposed that the paraquat undergoes a single-electron, cyclic reduction-oxidation with the formation of superoxide anion. Superoxide is spontaneously transferred to singlet oxygen which attacks polyunsaturated lipids of the cell membrane to form lipid hydroperoxides which decompose to lipid free radicals, which again attack the cell membranes so that a chain reaction occur.

parboil. A term denoting partially cook. Of special interest in nutrition is the par-boiling of brown rice, that is steaming of the rice in the husk before milling. The water-soluble B vitamins diffuse from the husk into the grain. When the rice is then polished the white rice contains far more of these vitamins than polished raw rice.

parillin. Highly toxic glycoside from sarsaparilla root; consists of glucose, rhamnose and parigenin. Also known as smilacin.

Parmesan cheese. Name of a kind of hard, Grana-type cheese such as Regina, Lodigiano, Lombardy, Lagazzo, Veneto or Venizia and Emiliano, made near Parma, Italy, hence the name. The above types are made in a similar manner. *S. thermophilus* is added as the culture, the curd is set, and cut into cubes, heated to 45°C and settled in the kettle. The curd is dipped, placed in a hoop and pressed. The curd is brine salted for 12-15 days and then dried. The cheese is cured at least a year (in the US 14 months) during which time it is washed frequently and may be coated with burnt umber, lamp black or grape-seed oil. This hard, grating cheese can be kept almost indefinitely. The average composition is: moisture, 30%, fat 28%, salt 4-5%. Federal Standards recommends that the moisture should not be more than 32%; and fat, not less than 32% in the solids.

Parmigiano cheese. A kind of cheese similar to Reggiano and is a variety of Grana cheese. The cheese is coated with oil, and may contain a few small eyes.

parsley drying. A green plant which is used as an herb and is harvested like hay and often dried. Drying to 4-5% is done in 30 minutes in a continuous belt three-stage drier. After drying the leaves are separated from the stems by air. The leaves are merchandised as flakes or granules. The leaves and stems are ground for powder.

parsley. Family: *Umbelliferae*. Genus: *Petroselinum*. Species: *Petroselinum crispum*.

A plant first known in Sardinia, but grown extensively throughout the world for two centuries. The plant is often cultivated as an annual for its foliage. There are numerous varieties. Parts used are the ripe fruits (seeds), the above-ground herb and the leaves. White or greenish-yellow flowers appear in compound umbels from June to August. Curiously enough, parsley is poisonous to most birds but is very good for animals, curing maladies such as foot-rot in sheep and goats.

The wild parasleys are closely allied to the celeries and were used by the Anglo-Saxons in ancient times to mend skulls broken in combat. One species, the common parsley, is a well-known garden vegetable, the leaves of which are used for seasoning and for the purpose of decorating table dishes. It is widely used in sauces, soups and salads and to decorate other dishes. Though in many textbooks it is described as a rich source of iron, vitamin C and carotene but the amounts eaten are insignificant its nutritive value cannot be taken seriously.

Parsley contains high levels of vitamins and minerals and particularly high in vitamins E, B and C, and iron, potassium, copper and magnesium. It is easily digested (in only 1.25 hours) and readily assimilated. All parts of the plant can be used but the leaves are used for bladder infections, especially combined with equal parts of echinacea and marshmallow. The root is particularly useful for treating chronic diseases and ailments of the liver and gall-bladder. It can be used with a small amount of licorice and marshmallow for the treatment of jaundice, asthma and coughs, and to relieve water retention. The leaves will cheer up depressed gastric digestive performance and relieve visceral and vascular spasms. Eating plenty of the fresh leaves will promote lactation, but heavy consumption of the herb, or ingestion of any of the seeds, must be avoided during pregnancy. The tea infused from the leaves tastes very bland.

Parsley is an invaluable addition to bouquets and *fines herbes* mixtures for grills and fish dishes. With its deep green, frilled or curly leaves, it is one of the best-known and most widely used herbs, as much for garnishing as for cooking. Neapolitan parsley, whose flat leaves are reminiscent of coriander, is less decorative, has a sharper flavour, and is easier to grow. Parsley has its culinary uses in nearly every savory category of food, not only in garnishing but in preparing soups, sauces, and casseroles, in marinades, and with meat, poultry, fish and vegetables. An infusion splashed on the skin is sad to lighten freckles and prevent thread veins, while the leaves provide a green or yellow dye.

parsnip. Family: *Umbelliferae*. Genus: *Pastinaca*. Species: *Pastinaca sativa*. Parsnips look like an anemic version of their cousin, the carrot. The parsnip's starchy root, however, is one of the most nourishing in the whole carrot family. This starch is converted to sugar whenever the root is exposed to the frost. Parsnip is not a common vegetable anymore, even though most of us have heard of it. Americans usually serve parsnips glazed with brown sugar and fruit juice only on special holidays like Thanksgiving or Christmas.

Refrigerated in a plastic bag, parsnips keep for nearly a month. Parsnips are a good source of vitamins A and C, carbohydrate, potassium, calcium and fibre. They are said to be useful to relieve the kidney of stones, as a diuretic, for various types of inflammation (gout, colitis, stomach ulcers) and for soothing diarrhoea. Average composition of *Patinaca sativa* per 100 g is: protein 1.0%; fat 0.28%; calcium 38 mg; iron 0.6 mg; vitamin B_1 0.06 mg; vitamin B_2 0.05 mg; nicotinic acid 0.1 mg; vitamin C 11 mg; and food energy 0.2 MJ.

parsnip oil. An oil steam-distilled from the fruit, flowers and roots of the parsnip, a vegetable plant. The oil is aromatic, with a suggestion of vetiver, and is occasionally used for spicy, herbal-type flavours.

Parson brown orange. A variety of sweet orange, nonblood type. The variety is planted principally in Florida, although the variety also performs satisfactorily in Arizona, Louisiana, and Texas. There are also plantings in Mexico. The Parson Brown is rounded, somewhat oblong, medium- to large size, yellow-orange to yellow skin; apex and base are rounded. The rind is smooth and bright and from 3-5 mm thick. The flesh is rather coarse-grained and yellow. The size of the juice sacs is medium to large. Juice is abundant and the variety has good processing quality and considered second only to Hamlin as an early-maturing variety.

partially fermented tea. *See* tea, partially fermented.

passion fruit. A fruit of the tropical American vine, *Passiflora* species. Purple or greenish-yellow when ripe, watery pulp containing small seeds; used in fruit drinks. The average composition per 100 g is: carbohydrate 16%; protein 1.2%; vitamin A 60 μg; vitamin C 20 mg. Also known as parchita, granadilla and water lemon.

passion, flower. A large genus of plants, native mostly of the warm regions of America. They are all twining plants, often spreading over trees to considerable length, and in many cases they are most beautiful objects, on account of their large, rich or gaily-coloured edible fruits called maypop. They received their name from the early Spanish missionaries, who believed that they saw in the beautiful flowers emblems of the crucifixion of Christ.

On account of their beauty, many of the species are cultivated in hothouses or even out of doors in mild climates.

passive immunity. Temporary but immediate specific acquired by injection of the appropriate antibody or of serum containing it. The material used in inducing passive immunity is serum, antiserum, or antitoxin. Antisera are obtained either from large-sized immunized animals, such as horse, or from human beings who have high antibody titers. The antiserum or antitoxin is standardized to contain a known antibody titer. Sometimes the γ-globulin fraction of pooled human serum is used as a source of antibodies. This contain a wide variety of antibodies that normal people have formed through the years by artificial or natural exposure to various antigens. Pooled sera are used when hyperimmune antisera are not available.

Antibody preparations used for producing passive immunity include botulinum antitoxin (animal sera containing antibodies to the toxins of *Clostridium botulinum* types A and B), diphtheria antitoxin (animal sera containing antibodies to the toxin of *Corynebacterium diphtheriae*) and tetanus antitoxin (immunoglobulin fraction of sera containing antibodies to the toxin of *Clostridium tetani*). Similar preparations are available for immunization against gas gangrene, leptospira, rabies, scarlet fever, and several venoms from snakes, spiders and scorpions.

passive transport. The movement of a solute across a biological membrane that is produced by diffusion, is directed downward in a concentration gradient, does not require carriers, and does not require the expenditure of energy.

pasta. Pastas are basically high-starch, low-protein foods with small amounts of vitamin enrichment to them. Pasta can be divided into two main groups; noodles and macaroni. Noodles are characterized by the addition of eggs to flour. This increases the protein, but also increases the fat content as well. Yoghurt may be substituted for eggs when making your own home-made noodles as the recipe below indicates. The macaroni group includes spaghetti, lasagne, macaroni, shells and other macaroni shapes. These are usually enriched with vitamins or wheat germ.

pasta filata. A name given to a number of Italian Cheese such as Caciocavallo, Provolone, Mozzarella, and Provatura, which are dipped in hot water or whey and are kneaded, stretched and molded while in a plastic condition, then placed in cold water to aid in retaining the desired shape. Also known as plastic curd.

Pasteur effect. The decrease in the rate of sugar catabolism and change to aerobic respiration that occurs when microorganisms are switched from anaerobic to aerobic conditions.

Pasteurella multocida. Facultatively an aerobic, nonmotile, oxidase-positive, Gram-negative rods that tend to stain in a bipolar manner. It inhibit the mouth and upper respiratory tract of healthy domestic animals, rats, and other animals. After an animal bite, it can cause soft tissue infection or osteomyelitis in humans. Most stains are sensitive to penicillin.

pasteurellosis. The general designation of all respiratory tract diseases of animals associated with *Pasteurella multocida* and *P. haemolytica*. The diseases are very contagious, and are associated with some type of stress placed on the animals during their transport from one place to another. Also known as shipping fever.

pasteurization. The partial sterilization of foodstuffs by heating to a temperature below boiling. This kills harmful microorganisms but retains the flavour. It is named after the pioneer of the method, Louis Pasteur, who used it to prevent spoilage of wine and beer.

Milk is pasteurized by heating at 62°C for 30 minutes. Vegetative forms of many bacteria can be killed by mild heat treatment, pasteurization, whereas total destruction of all bacteria and spores, sterilization, requires, higher temperatures for longer periods, often spoiling the product in the process. Pasteurization will prolong the storage life of foods but usually only for a limited period. Pasteurization of milk destroys all the pathogens, and although the milk will sour within a day or two it is not a source of disease.

Legally, pasteurization of milk means maintaining at 63-66°C for about 30 minutes, followed by immediate cooling, or so-called high-temperature short-time process, 72°C for atleast 15 seconds.

pasteurizer. Equipment used to pasteurize liquids such as milk, fruit juices, etc. They function, in effect, as heat-exchangers. The material to be pasteurized is passed continuously over heated plates, or through pipes, where it is heated to the required temperature, maintained at that temperature for the required time, then immediately cooled.

patchouli. An essential oil steam distilled from the dried and fermented leaves of a mint-like plant, called patchouli. The oil has a unique cidar-like odour with spicy undertones which improves with age. It is one of the most powerful of all the plant scents and one of the finest fixatives known. An inferior form of the oil called Khasia oil or oil of Assam is distilled from the leaves of a woody plant (*Microtonea cymosa*), which is native to Assam in India.

pathogenic organism. Any disease-producing agent; in common usage the term is restricted to a living organism (usually a micro-organism) that causes communicable diseases such as cholera, bacillary dysentery, typhoid fever, typhus fever, yellow fever, bacterial food poisoning, malaria, amoebic dysentery, infective hepatitis, and a number of other diseases. Wide varieties of pathogenic bacteria, viruses and parasites, are responsible for foodand water-borne diseases.

pathotoxin. A chemical of biological origin, other than an enzyme, that plays an important role in plant disease. Most pathotoxins are produced by plant pathogenic fungi or bacteria but some are produced by higher plants.

paunch. The partially digested material contained in the rumen of cattle, which is normally a waste product at time of slaughtering.

paunch drying. Cattle paunch products may be dried using a heated air rotary dryer. The dried paunch at 5-7% moisture may be pelletized and used for livestock or fish feed. A beef animal has about 20-25 kg of paunch with approximately 80% water.

Pavlov pouch. Surgical technique, introduced by Pavlov, in which a portion of the stomach is brought to the body wall. It is then possible to take a sample of the stomach contents directly from this pouch, as the secretion into the stomach contents directly from this pouch, as the secretion into the pouch is identical with that into the main part of the stomach.

pawpaw. Large green or yellow melon-like fruit of the *Carica papaya*, a tree similar to the palm.

It is the commonest tropical fruit second to the banana and is a rich source of vitamin A and C.

The average composition per 100 g is: water 89%; carbohydrate 9%; vitamin A 800 mg; vitamin C 80 mg; and food energy 0.16 MJ. The proteolytic enzyme, papain, is obtained as the dried latex of the skin of the fruit by scratching it while still on the tree, and collecting the flow. In the tropics meat is often tenderized by wrappings in pawpaw leaves. Also known as papaya.

pea. Family: *Leguminosae*. Genus: *Pisum sativum* (garden pea); *Pisum sativum* var. *arvense* (dried pea). A genus of plants belonging to the pulse family native to South-eastern Europe and South-western Asia.

The garden pea, one of the numerous species, is one of the most important of table vegetables, while the field pea is extensively grown as stock feed. Several species are extensively cultivated for their blossoms, which are almost unsurpassed for their pure and varied colours and delicate fragrance. The garden pea may grow as a vine or as a dwarf. It is a beautiful plant, crisp and light green. It produces small white blossoms, which are followed by plump, oblong pods bearing the edible seeds. There are two important varieties, one having smooth pods, the other bearing pods with wrinkled skin; the former usually a dwarf, the latter a climber. Peas have a high food value and are among the most satisfactory vegetables for canning purposes.

Besides garden or shell peas, there are two other edible-pod varieties: the small, flat, snow, or sugar peas often used in Chinese cooking and the plumper sugar snap peas that can be eaten raw or cooked and shelled when mature.

Young peas are high in protein, carbohydrates and vitamin B and E, whereas dried peas are rich in phosphorus, calcium, sodium and vitamin A and are valuable source of B-complex vitamins.

Peas contain as much protein as meat. Fresh peas are extremely nourishing and body-building. They help anaemia, low blood pressure and emaciation. They contain nicotinic acid, which is believed to reduce cholesterol in the blood. The average composition per 100 g of fresh pea is: protein 3%; fat 0.2%; calcium 10 mg; iron 0.95 mg; vitamin A 78 mg; vitamin B_1 0.15 mg; vitamin B_2 0.09 mg; nicotinic acid 1.0 mg; vitamin C 11 mg; and food energy 0.15 MJ.

Pea family. *Fabaceae (Leguminosae).* Members of this family are easily recognized by the usually alternate, compound leaves divided into leaflets, the typical pea flower, and the pea pod (legume) fruit. The form of plants ranges from small herbs to shrubs and trees. Pea family plants such as clover are often used in crop rotation because they increase soil nitrogen, a plant nutrient, by the presence of bacterial nitrogen-fixing nodules on the roots. Looking closely at the leaves, the base of each has a pair of leaf-like stipules. The leaf petiole has a swollen base (pulvinus) that has the ability to change the position of the leaf and leaflets when stimulated by light or gravity. When touched, *Mimosa,* the sensitive plant, demonstrates this ability, dramati-

cally. A pea flower has 5 fused sepals, with 5 separate petals or petals in 3 groups of 1 banner petal, 2 wing petals, and a keel of 2 fused petals which enclose the stamens and stigma. The 10 stamens may be held by their filaments in one or two bundles. There is one pistil whose superior ovary of a single carpel will enlarge into the pea pod after fertilization. The ovules are attached to the side of the carpel wall in 2 alternating rows. Some species have only 2 seeds per legume pod; others may have many. Pods may be straight such as in garden beans and peas, or straight and sectioned into compartments called a loment, or coiled in a spiral. When mature, the pod splits into halves.

The family include: *Arachis* (peanut), *Cicer* (chick pea), *Glycine* (soybean,) *Lens* (lentil), *Phaseolus* (bean), *Pisum* (pea), *Tamarindus* (tamarind); *Lupinus* (lupine), *Medicago* (alfalfa), *Melilotus* (sweet clover), *Trifolium* (clover), *Vicia* (vetch); *Acacia* (wattle), *Albizzia, Bauhinia* (orchid tree), *Cassis* (senna), *Cercis* (redbud), *Delonix* (poinciana), *Gleditsia* (honey locust), *Laburnum* (golden-chain tree), *Lathyrus* (sweet pea), *Lupinus* (lupine), Mimosa (sensitive plant), *Wisteria; Abrus precatorius* (precatory bean), *Astragalus* (locoweed), *Gymnocladus* (Kentucky coffee tree), *Lupinus argenteus* (silvery lupine), *Robinia* (locust); *Pueraria lobata* (kudzu vine).

pea drying. Peas that are dried may have the skin slit to provide more rapid drying and wetting, following a blanching operation. Slit peas may be dried in belt, cabinet, or tray dryers, using 88-94°C in initial stages of drying. The peas are dried to about 8%, then placed in a bin dryer with drying air at 49°C.

Dehydrofreezing, in which 70% of the water is removed from the raw pea, is also a procedure used to provide a product with good quality which is easily rehydrated. The moisture is removed on a belt trough dryer and them frozen.

pea, processed. Refers to peas that have been dried as distinct from fresh, garden, green, canned and frozen peas.

peach. *Prunus persica.* One of the most delicious fruits of temperate regions, closely allied to the plum and cherry, and in value second only to the apple among orchard products. A native of Persia, it is now grown extensively in many parts of the world, because of favourable conditions of soil and climate and the employment of up-to-date methods of cultivation. There are many varieties of peaches which are divided into two basic categories: freestones, with soft, juicy flesh that separates readily from the stone; and clingstones, with firmer flesh that adheres tightly to the stone. Clingstone varieties like the Red Haven are generally used for canning; freestones like the Rio Oso Gem are eaten fresh or frozen. Peaches originated in China several thousands years ago and were venerated as fruits of immorality.

Quince (Cydonoa cydonia). These yellow, pear-shaped fruits originated somewhere in Asia Minor and have been cultivated for some four millenniums. In medieval times most Europeans ate them fresh as well as cooking and preserving them. Quinces were once thought to be a type of pear, and in fact pears are often grown on quince rootstock, but the two fruits simply cannot be hybridized. Until the late 18th century, marmalade was usually made from quinces: the word "marmalade," in fact, derives from *marmelo,* which is Portuguese for quince.

peach drying. Peaches are halved, pitted, peeled (lye), and sulphured before drying. A countercurrent tunnel dryer, using incoming heated air at 68.3°C, requiring 25 to 30 hours for 13 kg/m^2, drying to 25% moisture content. Drying time may be reduced 30% if preceded by blanching.

peanut. Family. *Leguminosae.* Genus: *Arachis.* Species: *Arachis hypogaea.* Peanuts (groundnuts) are grown throughout the world mainly as an important oil seed crop. The edible portion of the peanut is a rounded kernel borne in a pale yellowish, wrinkled pod. There are one, two or three kernels to a pod, according to variety. A loamy soil finely pulverized is considered best for peanut culture. In the spring, when danger of frost is past, the kernels are planted in hills about a foot and a half apart. Two or three kernels, with skins left on, are placed in each hill. The plant takes the form of a hairy stem with numerous branches, bearing small, single, yellow flowers much like those of the garden pea. When a flower falls, the stalk supporting the undeveloped pod lengthens, and bending downward, pushes the fruit into the ground, where it ripens. Also known as groundnut, earth nut and monkey nut. Seed of the legume, *Arachis hypogaea;* Spanish and Virginia types have 2 kernels per pod, Valecia has 3-4. The nuts serve as an important source of protein in many tropical diets.

The oil, known as arachis oil, is used for cooking, as salad oil, for canning sardines and for margarine manufacture. The residue after oil extraction is a valuable source of protein for animal feed.

Peanuts are roasted and eaten as a delicacy, and they form the basis of many of the modern health foods. Its oil is used in making salads and as an ingredient of soaps is expressed from the seeds. Peanuts are highly nutritious but also very calorific. They contain tryptophan and methionine in low amounts and for this reason some nutritionists advise against eating peanuts as a complete protein. Average peanut butter is usually only 70% peanuts, the remaining 30% being hydrogenated fat and refined sugar in the form of dextrose. Buy peanut butter which is 100% peanuts and put it on whole grain bread to be assured of a complete protein.

Peanuts are rich in linoleic acid, which reduces the risk of cholesterol deposits in the arteries. They provide a higher proportion of pantothenic acid than any food except liver. Under certain conditions some substances in peanuts can combine with iodine and act as α-blocker so that it cannot reach the blood. So eat peanuts cautiously, certainly not daily and not in huge quantities.

Experiments with animals have found that peanut oil causes atheroma, and although it does not automatically follow that this happens in man, a question mark remains over it. However, when unrefined, it is a good source of linoleic acid and other polyunsaturates. The average composition per 100 g peanuts is: 25.6 g protein; 43 g fat; 1.9 mg iron; 9 mg vitamin A; 0.84 mg vitamin B_1; 0.12 mg vitamin B_2; 16 mg nicotinic acid; and food energy 2.3 MJ.

peanut butter. Peanut butter was first made in the US in about 1890. It is the food prepared by grinding one of the shelled and roasted peanut ingredients. 1. Blanched peanuts, in which the germ may or may not be included; 2. Unblanched peanuts, including the skins and germ, to which may be added seasoning and stabilizing ingredients, but such seasoning and stabilizing ingredients do not in the aggregate exceed 10% of the weight of the finished product. To the ground peanuts, cut or chopped, shelled, and roasted peanuts may be added. During processing, the oil content of the peanut ingredient may be adjusted by the addition or subtraction of peanut oil. The fat content of the finished food shall not exceed 55%. Seasoning and stabilizing ingredients that perform a useful function are regarded as suitable, except that artificial flavorings, artificial flavorings, artificial sweeteners, chemical preservatives, added vitamins, and colour additives, are not suitable ingredients of peanut butter. Oil products used as optional stabilizing ingredients shall be hydrogenated peanut oil or other vegetable oils in hydrogenated form, but the proportion of such other hydrogenated vegetable oils shall not exceed 3% by weight of the finished product. Where peanut butter is prepared from unbalanced peanuts (skins left on), a statement on the product label must so indicate. Peanut butter is available in three forms:

(a) A smooth product with an even texture and completely free of peanut particles;

(b) a so-called regular peanut butter, in which peanut particles do not exceed 1.5 m in their longest dimensions; and

(c) chunky peanut butter where peanut particles considerably larger may be present.

Early peanut butter processing encountered a number of problems, including a tendency for the oil and meal phases to separate; inconsistent flavor, resulting from variations in the blanching, cooling, and roasting processes; inconsistent shelf-life performance; and problems related to the effects of added materials, such as fats, carbohydrates, and stabilizers. These problems were largely overcome by experience, coupled with much improved control over the raw peanuts and processing throughout. Scaling up the size of the processing operations also contributed to greater product uniformity. The principal operations involved in peanut butter manufacture include:

(a) shelling,
(b) cleaning,
(c) roasting,
(d) cooling,
(e) blanching,
(f) picking and inspecting,
(g) grinding, and
(h) packaging.

peanut drying. The moisture content of peanuts at the time of digging is 36-60%. Peanuts can be dried to about 8% in field stacks in 4-8 weeks and to 9% in the windrow in 1-2 weeks. In an atmosphere of 64.4% relative humidity (approximately room temperature) the peanut kernels will be at 7% and the shells at 12.5% moisture. The major problem in drying peanuts is to prevent the splitting of the skin caused by rapid drying. Heated air, if properly managed, can be used for drying of peanuts. The air should not be heated above 43.3°C for peanuts which are to be used for table stock and temperatures up to 51.7°C can be used if the nuts are to be used for oil. When drying peanuts in piles, 3 sacks deep, 12 hours were required to dry peanuts in piles 3 sacks deep from 18-8% with 48.9% air. With heated air the shells lose more moisture than the nuts and during storage gain moisture from the nuts. It is advisable to stop drying when the peanuts are at 9% and the shells will pick up enough moisture to bring the peanuts down to 7%. On a continuous dryer with the peanuts on the vines placed 0.5 m deep the best drying and quality were obtained by using an air velocity of about 0.3 m/s at 29.4-32.2°C.

peanut flakes. A product made from peanuts to be used for a high protein food, similar to high protein soybean products. Peanut flakes are made from the whole peanut from which the shell and red skin have been removed. After processing of the peanut, the product is dried on a rotating drum dryer and removed in a thin sheet.

peanut flour. Within recent years, the popularity of peanut flours, as a source of protein and fat, coupled with good stability and solubility, has increased for use in prepared foods, such as bakery products, gravies, and sauces.

Peanut flour is being considered for extending meat, cheese, and other milk products. Peanut flavours are obtainable as a full-fat product, a partially defatted product, as a blended product with soy flour, and in roasted and unroasted forms. One full-fat, spray-dried peanut product contains 26.5% protein, 49% fat, 17.8% carbohydrate, 1.9% fibre, 2.3% ash, and 2.3% moisture. The product is used in breakfast cereals, snacks, meat extenders, sauces, gravies, and bakery products.

Both raw and toasted, partially defatted flours are obtainable. To produce these flours, about 55% of the original oil is removed by hydraulic pressing. Protein content of the unroasted product is 39.5 and 42.1% for the toasted product. Fat content ranges between 32.3-34.1% and carbohydrate content ranges between 18.7-20.2%.

peanut food products. The principal direct uses of peanuts in food products include:

(a) peanut butter, marketed separately, and as peanut butter sandwiches;

(b) salted peanuts; and

(c) peanut candies.

Peanut butter accounts for 55-57% of the peanuts shelled for direct food use. Of this amount, 3% is used for prepackaged peanut butter sandwiches, frequently marketed much as candy. Salted peanuts account for about 23% of the shelled peanut figure. Use of shelled peanuts in candies of various forms accounts for the remaining 20-22% of the total.

peanuts, salted. Roasted and salted peanuts (ground-nuts) are popular in many areas of the world and the roasting process may range from the very simple procedure of heating the peanuts in hot sand, ashes, or embers, to sophisticated and highly engineered roasters used for mass producing the product. Peanut flavor is determined mainly by the roasting process. A high percentage of salted-roasted peanuts in the US are the Virginia type (70-75%), with Spanish types making up most of the remainder. Only a small percentage of runner types is used.

In roasting, gases given off include carbon dioxide and traces of ammonia, hydrogen sulfide, and diacetyl. It has been concluded that the flavor of the product originates from the specific types of micromolecules rather than from general, macromolecular, cellular components, such as the large globulin proteins and starches. Peanuts for salting may be dry or oil roasted. Some dry-roasted peanuts are given a glaze of 1.5% to 2% of a formulated oil misted with 2.5% salt, without blanching, and roasted as in the process of making peanut butter. More commonly, the peanuts are blanched first, followed by oil-roasting or frying in oil. Where the drying process is used, the cooking temperature will range from 138-143°C and the time required will range from 3-10 minutes.

There is considerable flexibility that can be commanded by the processor to achieve flavour and product characteristics considered most desirable by the consumer. There is quite a range of market tastes and preferences. However, for any specific style or brand, all conditions must be maintained as uniformly as possible, with exacting quality control over raw peanut receipts. Good design of an oil roasted dictates that the heating elements be placed along the sides of the tank rather than at the bottom. As the peanuts are roasted, a certain amount of material (meal) collects on the bottom of the tank and, if this material becomes charred, it contributes a bitter flavor and dark colour to the oil and thence to the peanuts. Coconut and modified cottonseed oil may be used.

The oil requires constant filtration and testing to prevent peroxidation. Normally, about 10% of fresh oil will be added to the process daily. Peanuts are salted at a level of about 2% (weight). In salted peanuts, the taste of the salt is a major flavour constituent and, consequently, careful control must be exerted to keep calcium and magnesium impurities in the salt to a minimum. Calcium chloride, for example, contributes a harsh flavour to the product. Off-flavours also show up in frequently as the result of excessive use of insecticides and herbicides during the growth of the plants. Peanuts grown in excessively treated soils may develop a musty flavor, apparent after roasting and salting.

As with peanut butter, long shelf-life is an objective of the processor of salted peanut products. This requirement led to the development of antioxidants for treating the peanuts. The antioxidants may be applied to roasted peanuts by adding the chemicals to the cooking oil; to the salt; or sprayed or fogged onto the peanuts just prior to salting. The latter method is preferred by many processors. Antioxidants used include gum guaic, nordihydroguaia-uretic acid (NDGA), various tocopherols, lecithin, propyl gallate, butylate hydroxyanisole (BHA), and butylated hydroxytoluene (BHT). In the US, BHA, BHT, and propyl gallate are commonly used. In Europe, some of the higher gallates (ethyl, octyl, and dodecyl) are permitted.

The shelf-life of salted peanuts is also extended by care in packaging. Exclusion of light and air (vacuum packaging) is widely practiced. Deterioration of flavour and development of rancidity are directly related to oxidative breakdown of fats present. To further protect against this, packaging materials also are treated with antioxidants. Packaging materials may be coated with antioxidant-containing emulsions; or antioxidants may be added to the paraffin wax used for coating packaging materials. In the case of polyethylene films, the antioxidants may be added to the plastic

material just prior to film extrusion. Other developments have included the use of monosodium glutamate in the roasting oil to enhance the natural flavor, followed by vacuum packing. In another development, containers can be flushed with an inert gas (to remove oxygen) prior to sealing.

pear. *Pyrus communis.* This is a delicate, aristocratic, temperate-zone fruit that exists in thousands of varieties, with new ones being constantly produced. Few fruits vary so greatly in colour, texture, flavour, size and shape. Pears are also an exception to the usual rule that tree-ripened fruits are best, they are picked when full grown but still green, and attain their finest texture and flavour (soft on the inside but still firm on the outside) off the tree. America's most widely grown pear, the Bartlett, is bell-shaped, with yellow skin and a red blush when ripe. ً excellent for poaching, canning or eating raw in season, which is from July to mid-October.

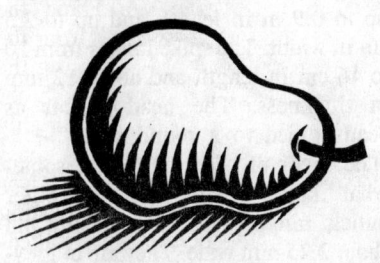

The average composition per 100 g is: 0.4 g protein; 0.3 g fat; food energy 0.2 MJ. It also contains small amounts of carotenoids, B vitamins and C.

pear drying. Pears are prepared for drying by halving, peeling, slicing, and sulphuring. Drying is done on trays in a countercurrent flow dryer with heated air in at 65.5°C.

pear, prickly. Fruit of the cactus *opuntia,* an important part of the diet in certain areas of Mexico. The average composition per 100 g is: water 81%; protein 1%; carbohydrate 26%; vitamin C 15 mg; and food energy 0.29 MJ). Also called Indian fig; barberry fig; and tuna.

pearl millet. *Pennisetum glaucum* or *P. typhoideum*. This is an annual, warm-weather grass that has been cultivated in Africa and Asia since antiquity. Pearl millet was probably domesticated somewhere in the dry savanna fringing the southern Sahara desert between western Sudan and Senegal-Mauritania. The plant is extremely drought-resistant and can be grown at the limits of agriculture near the deserts of Africa and India, where millions of people depend upon it for survival. It is one of the most nutritious cereals, containing food quantities of phosphorous, minerals, and vitamins A and E. Pearl millet has coarse, pithy stems that grow from 1.8 to 3.6 m in height. The stems are about 2.5 cm in thickness. Blades are up to 0.9 m in length and up to 2.5 cm in width. The spike ranges from 20 to 46 cm in length and about 12 mm in thickness. The head appear as beads glued to a round stick.

The seeds of pearl millet are somewhat larger than those of other millets, ranging from 3-4 mm long and about 2.25 mm wide. They are of grey-yellow colour and of an obovoid shape. The plant is cross-pollinated. Also known as cattail millet; penicillaria; and Mands forage plant (US); and as bullrush millet or Dukha (in Africa); as candle millet or dark millet (in Europe); and as bajra, cumbo, or sajja (in India).

peas. A general term for a wide variety of leguminous seeds. They are classed with beans and lentils; good source of protein (20-30%), moderate source of iron and vitamins B_1, B_2 and nicotinic acid. Peas form vitamin C on germination. Pigeon pea or red gram (*Cajanus indicus*); Chick pea or Bengal gram (Cicer *arietinum*); garden pea (*Pisum* sativum).

pecan. Family: *Juglandacea*. Genus: *Carya*. Species: *Carya olivaeformis*. The pecan is a native American tree. It will not survive severe winters and so is restricted to the milder climatic areas of the US. Nuts are harvested from both wild and cultivated trees. There is more variability in the pecan crop than in most other nut crops. Pecans are highly regarded as flavouring ingredients and decorative toppings for pies, cakes, cookies, and sweet rolls. Although their flavour is pleasant, it is mild and can easily be overpowered by species and other flavours. Because they are expensive, pecans are found mostly in premium goods, except when token amounts are used in chopped form to justify the claim of pecan flavor.

Pecan pieces are often mixed with chunks of walnuts or almonds to make toppings for doughnuts, cupcakes, and Danish pastry and for ingredients in cheap versions of pecan pies-particularly the small individual pies. Pecans can absorb up to 75% of their own weight in oil. They are a good nutritious food, recommended for people suffering from low blood pressure and emaciation, and help to build healthy teeth. In recent years, traders have started storing the nuts under refrigerated or freezing temperatures, so that they can be kept in good condition for longer periods of time and the year-to-year fluctuations in supply are reduced.

After harvesting, pecans are put in dry storage to undergo curing. During this holding period of about three weeks at room temperature, the moisture of the entire nut decreases to about 8.5-9.0%, and that of the meat to about 4.5%. Free fatty acid content and the peroxide value of the lipids increase, and the tannins of the seed coat oxidize with a resultant color change from pale to medium brown. The overall effects of these changes result in the development of a characteristic pecan flavor, appearance, aroma, and texture. The nuts will gradually develop staleness-both a loss of desirable flavour and the appearance of non-rancid flavours such as bitterness and, finally, rancidity will develop at a rate dependent on the temperature. Conditions of low temperature and 70-80% relative humidity are necessary if the fresh flavor is to be retained more than three months.

At -10°C the in-shell kernels will retain good quality for more than five years. Heating pecan meats to an internal temperature of 60°C in dry air or oil doubles the shelf-life by inactivating oxidative enzymes. Higher temperatures produce partially cooked flavour, while roasting for about 15 minutes by means of hot air or infrared radiation destroys natural antioxidants, accelerating rancidity development but increasing the flavour and aroma many times. This is a favourable condition for nuts that are to be consumed soon after roasting but has undesirable implications for products entering a long distribution system. Antioxidants such as BHA or BHT can be added to increase shelf life.

Development of the so-called amber colour is a kind of storage deterioration probably related to high temperature and high moisture content. If pecan meats are dried below about 3.5-4.0% moisture content, they become brittle and suffer excessive breakage during handling.

Pecorino cheese. This type of cheese are several in number and are made in Italy from cow's or ewe's milk. The most common is designated as Pecorino Romano (ewe's milk).

Vaccino Romano- cow's milk.

Caprino Romano- goat's milk.

Pecorino Dolce- coloured with annatto and highly pressed.

Pecorino Tuscani- smaller than Romano.

Other Percorino cheeses include Ancona, Cotrone, Puglia and Viterbo.

pectase. Enzyme in the pith of citrus fruits that removes the methoxyl groups from pectin to form water-insoluble pectic acid. The intermediate compounds with varying numbers of methoxy groups are pectinic acids.

pectate lyase. The enzyme that catalyzes the degradation of pectins whereby the glycosidic bonds between the monosaccharide residues are cleaved and water molecules are eliminated.

pectic substances. Polysaccharides that, together with hemicelluloses, form the matrix of plant cell walls. They are long-chain molecules, some forming the middle lamella of plant tissue; others, including the subgroup known as pectins, occur in ripening fruit. Since they form gels at low temperatures they are widely used in jam-making. They serve to cement the cellulose fibres together. Fruits are a rich source. They are principally made from the group sugar acids known as uronic acids. Pectic acids, the basis of the other pectic substances, are soluble unbranched chains of α-1,4 linked galacturonic acid units (derived from the sugar galactose).

pectin. A by-product of the apple and citrus fruit industries, used rather extensively in ices and sherbets but is not a very satisfactory stabilizer for ice cream. Chemically, it is a polymer consisting largely of galacturonic acid, galactose, and arabinose and is classified as a gum.

Purified sugar beet pectin forms a weaker and less brilliant gel than citrus pectin. Plant tissue contain protopectins (which are chemically hemicelluloses) cementing the cell walls together. As fruit ripens, there is maximum protopectin present, thereafter it breaks down to pectin, pectinic acid and finally pectic acid under the influence of enzymes, and the fruit loses its firmness and becomes soft as the adhesive between the cells breaks down.

Pectin is the setting agent in jam. Soft fruits, as strawberry, raspberry and cherry, are low in pectin; plum, apple and bitter orange are rich. Apple pulp and orange pith are the commercial source of pectin. It is added to confectionery, chocolate, ice-cream as an emulsifier and stabilizer instead of agar; it is also used in making jellies; and as anti-staling agent in cakes.

The pectin substances in foods of plant origin are important because the firmness and texture of many fruits and vegetables depends upon them. They also play a major role in canning and freezing processes. In the presence of over 50% sugar and a pH values below 3.6, pectins will form firm jellies. The proportion of sugar which pectin will form into a firm jelly determines the jelly grade of the pectin. This can be determined by a variety of methods, of which the measurement of the breaking strength of the jelly its elasticity modules, or the extent of sag attained in 2 minutes of the turned out jelly are most widely used. All of these tests must be performed under painstaking exactness and at standardized conditions. The jellification (gelling) in marmalades and jams is only partial, but is nevertheless important. In a jelly, jam, or marmalade, the proportion of total solids of sugars, the pH, and the proportion and nature of the pectin used will determine the extent of jellification obtained.

The use of added pectin in fruit jams, preserves, marmalades, and jellies is approved because the addition compensates for an incidental natural deficiency.

pectinase. Enzyme present in the pith (albedo) of citrus fruits, that hydrolyses pectins or pectic acids into smaller polygalacturonic acids, and finally glacturonic acid and its methyl ester. Also known as pectolase and polygalacturonase.

pectinesterase. Alternative name for pectase.

pectin promace. A term applied to citrus peel which has been carefully dried after leaching with water to lower the concentration of soluble sugars and acids. The leaching is normally done in a 2-step counter-current process using large volumes of water at ambient temperature. The dried pomace is used as raw material for pectin manufacture. The leach liquid is discharged and treated as waste.

pectolase. Alternative name for pectinase.

pectosinase. Alternative name for protopectinase.

Pekar test. A comparative test of flour colour. The flour is pressed on a board with a smooth applicator and colour comparisons are made immersed in water.

pelagic fish. Oily fish containing up to 20% fat; swim near the surface; pelagic fish include herring, mackerel, pilchards.

pellagra. Disease due to deficiency of nicotinic acid. Symptoms include characteristic symmetrical dermatitis on exposed surfaces such as face and back of hands, mental disturbances and digestive disorders.

pellitori. *Herba piretri.* An herb whose roots add flavour to cold foods, but causes thirst and remains on the stomach for a long time. If chewed, the root stimulates the flow of phlegm; mixed wth oil, it causes sweating. Some people claim it about it to be an effective treatment for prolonged trembling as well as for paralysis. Also known as pellitory of Spain.

pemmican. Indian word for meat prepared in such a way as to contain the greatest amount of nourishment in the most compact form. The Indians made it of lean parts of meat, deer, antelope, and buffalo, dried in the sun and pounded or shredded and mixed into a paste with melted fat. It is flavoured with acid berries. If kept dry, pemmican will keep for an indefinite time and is thus particularly serviceable in Arctic and Antarctic explorations. Pemmican, however, is not limited as emergency rations for explorers, but is preferred by hunters, canoers, and hikers. It is used as concentrated food source, such as on expeditions.

penicillinases. Enzymes that have the property of catalysing the hydrolysis of penicillin with the production of inactive penicilloic acid. The enzymes (also the known as β-lactamases) are both constitutive and inducible in bacteria; that is, the bacteria may already possess the enzymes or they may be induced after exposure to the drug. Penicillinases constitute the main mechanism through which bacteria are resistant to penicillins. How-

ever, a few are resistant because they possess the enzyme penicillin amidase. Penicillinases are elaborated by a range of different bacteria including penicillin-resistant *Staphylococci*, some strains of *E. coli*, *Klebsiella*, Proteus, Pseudomonas, Vibrio, Mycobacterium and Brucella. Certain partially synthetic pencillins (such as cloxacillin, oxacillin, nafcillin) are poor substrates for penicillinase and are hydrolysed only very slowly. They are called penicillinase-resistant penicillins. Partially synthetic penicillins and cephalosporins may act as inducers of penicillinase even though they are themselves resistant to, or poor substrates for, the enzyme.

penicillins. A series of β-lactam antibiotics whose molecules consist of a thiazolidine ring connected to a β-lactam ring to which is attached a side-chain.

They include, or are related to, benzyl-penicillin itself, originally obtained from the mould *Penicillium notatum*, but now, more productively, from an X-ray induced mutation of *P. chrysogenum*. Semisynthetic penicillins are prepared from 6-aminopenicillanic acid. They act on sensitive bacteria, mainly by inhibiting transpeptidase reaction that is part of the process of cell wall synthesis. Many penicillins are inactivated by penicillinase enzymes produced by resistant bacteria.

Those that are not (*e.g.*, methicillin nafcillin, oxacillin, floxacillin) are active against penicillinase-producing *Staph. aureus*. Their resistance to penicillinase is determined by the nature of the side-chain (R).

penicillium Roquefortii mold. Normally a blue-green mold which gives to Roquefort cheese its characteristic flavour. This mold grows best between 15°C with a relative humidity of 85-90%. and at pH 4.8-5. It is salt tolerant, growing at level as high as 4.5%.

The mold must have oxygen for growth hence the punching of the cheese. These characteristics are utilized during the making of blue-veined cheese.

pennyroyal. *Mentha pulegium.* Pennyroyal, a herbaceous perennial and a close relation of mint, has a strong, bitter, minty taste some people find unpleasant. It has a completely different growing habit than mint, its prostrate stems creeping along the ground and forming an effective, dense ground cover that can be used as a lawn.

It is a native of Europe where it grows freely in damp, shady places and is also found in North and South America. The leaves may be used sparingly in place of mint, but have more application medicinally and domestically. They can be used to relieve insect bites and stings, to ward off insect, as a moth repellent in drawers, for instance, and in the treatment of headaches, colds, and sickness.

The leaves have been used as a strewing herb, and in laundry rinsing water. Note that the herb pennyroyal should not be taken during the pregnancy.

pennyroyal oil. The oil obtained by the steam distillation of the herb *Mentha pulegium.* It has a minty, spicy, and slightly bitter fragrance. It is used in the manufacture of menthol and a number of medicines. Also known as oil of Pulegium.

pentosans. The complex carbohydrates widely distributed in plants, *e.g.*, fruit, wood, corncobs, oat hulls. They are not digested in the body but broken down by acid to yield the 5-carbon sugars or pentoses.

pentose phosphate pathway. This pathway, also referred to as the hexose monophosphate shunt, allows the oxidation of hexose to carbon dioxide and is important for the production of key metabolites. It is essentially a side pathway which begins and ends with the intermediates of Embden-Meyerhof glycolytic pathway.

The most important features to noted are:

(a) carbon-1 of hexose is rapidly lost as carbon dioxide in an early reaction, but carbon-6 is recycled, converted to trioses of the Embden-Meyerhof pathway, or incorporated in cellular constituents derived from intermediates in the pentose phosphate pathway;

(b) the oxidations of glucose-6-phosphate and of 6-phosphogluconate depend upon the availability of NADP (TPN) and readily furnish NADPH (TPNH) for the many biosynthetic reactions that require this reduced coenzyme;

(c) the ribose-5-phosphate in the cycle is formed both from direct glucose-6-phosphate oxidation and from non-oxidative transketolase-transaldolase catalyzed reactions beginning with fructose-6-phosphate and triose phosphate.

Intermediates used in biosyntheses are: ribose-5-phosphate to supply the pentoses found in nucleic acids, both RNA and DNA; ribulose-5-phosphate for conversion to ribulose-1,5-diphosphate, which reacts with carbon dioxide in photosynthetic organisms to form 3-phosphoglyceric acid and then sugars and other metabolites; erythrose-4-phosphate for the production of aromatic compounds in plants and microorganisms.

pentose. A monosaccharide with five carbon atoms. The importance of pentoses in metabolism derives from the fact that:

(a) D-ribose and D-2-deoxyribose are components of all cells, occurring particularly in nucleic acids and coenzymes,

(b) they are intermediates in important metabolic pathways such as the pentose phosphate pathway and the photosynthetic cycle, and

(c) the utilization of dietary pentoses and pentitols requires the existence of suitable metabolic reactions for the conversion of pentoses into useful products.

D-Ribose is found in many coenzymes and is a component of RNA. In the synthesis of nucleotides, ribose is usually attached to a nitrogenous substance *via* intermediate 5-phospho-ribosyl-1-pyrophosphate (PRPP), although ribose-1-phosphate may be a direct reactant in some transformations. 2-D-Deoxyribose found in DNA is formed directly from ribose after the latter pentose has become a component of nucleotides. For example, an enzymatic system from rat hepatoma and from *E. coli* converts cytidine diphosphate to deoxycytidine diphosphate.

Peony. *Paeonia foemina.* A plant which was believed in ancient times to shine during the niight, and driving away the evil spirts. The flowers are mildly fragrant and are used in sachets and pot pourri. Also spelled as Paeony.

pepato, Sicilano. *See* pepato.

Pepato cheese. A Romano-type spiced cheese made in Sicily and Southern Italy. Pepper is incorporated in the cheese as the curd is placed in the hoops. Also known as Sicilano pepato cheese.

pepper *(Nomenclature).* There is a lot of confusion about the use of the word `pepper' because of its multiple forms and meanings. There are two major categories of pepper of commerce. These are not related botanically or in any other way except that some forms in each category possess a tangy, pungent flavour.

1. Members of the family *Solanaceae* (nightshade or potato family): (A) Pepper with a sweet-fleshed fruit, commonly called *sweet peppers.*

(i) The familiar bell pepper, often simply called green pepper and sometimes called bullnose pepper because of its shape. In some regions, it is also called mango (not to be confused with the fruit of the mango tree, *Mangifera indica*). The term green pepper is not sufficiently definitive, however, because the color depends upon whether or not the sweet or bell pepper has been allowed to ripen before harvesting. The sweet pepper is green at maturity, but turns red as it ripens. It is marketed green or red.

(ii) The familiar pimiento pepper or simply pimento. This pepper is used only in the ripe, red stage of maturity, at which stage the pimiento retains its sweet flavor. (Some consumers mistakenly tend to association red color with pungency).

(iii) The paprika pepper, which is usually dehydrated and processed into paprika powder. This pepper has little or no pungency, but the flesh is of a dark-red color. Paprika is a relatively mild, bland condiment (not to be confused with red or cayenne pepper made from the chili pepper).

(B) Peppers with a hot- or pungent-flavoured fruit and sometimes called hot peppers. Even more commonly in recent years, these peppers are called chili peppers. They are used mainly for flavouring because they are too strong to be eaten alone. The condiment prepared from the dried and ground fruits of the chili pepper is known as red pepper or cayenne pepper.

2. Members of the family *Piperaceae* (pepper family).

(a) Black and white pepper prepared from the evergreen shrub or vine (Piper *nigrum*). The familiar condiment, black pepper, is prepared from the ground, dried, unripe fruit of the shrub. White pepper is prepared from the nearly ripe berries.

(b) Long pepper, often used in preserves and curries, is made from the fruits of the climbing *plant (P. retrofractum)*.

(c) Cubeb pepper, mainly used in medicines and some cigarettes, is obtained from the dried, unripe fruit of the climbing vine (*P. cubeba*).

(d) Kava, a Samoan beverage, is prepared by steeping the ground roots of a pepper plant (*P. methysticum*) in water.

(e) Ashanti pepper obtained from the vine (*P. guineese*).

Note : The term pepper appears in connection with other miscellaneous food substances. Guinea pepper, used as a medicinal and flavoring, is obtained from the seeds of the herb (*Aframomum melegueta*). Peppergrass, a potherb, is *Lepidium sativum*, also commonly called garden cress. Peppermint, a labiate herb (*Mentha piperita*), described under Mint. These uses of the world stem from the definition of peppery-sharp, pungent, stinging.

pepper (capsicum). Family: *Solanaceae*. Genus: *Capsicum*. Species: *Capsicum frutescens* and *Capsicum annuum*.

Bell peppers are most nutritious if eaten raw, and are valuable for liver disorders, obesity, constipation, high blood pressure and acidosis. It is used externally on serve cuts or grazes and taken internally as a tea, it should stop bleeding almost instantaneously by going immediately into the bloodstream and adjusting the blood pressure so that it is equalized throughout the body. This takes the high pressure which causes rapid bleeding away from the wound and clotting starts immediately. Cayenne is a great food for the circulatory system because it feeds the necessary elements into the cell structure of the arteries, veins and capillaries so that these regain the elasticity of youth, and the blood pressure adjusts itself to normal.

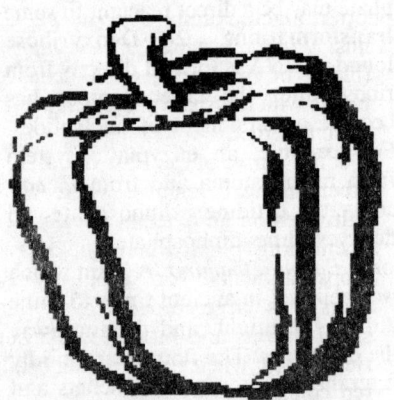

It rebuilds the tissue in the stomach and heals stomach and intestinal ulcers (astonishing though this may seem to the timid). It stimulates the peristaltic motion of the intestines and aids in assimilation and elimination. It is an excellent stimulant as well and can be used in plasters, poultices and ointments as a rubefacient where quick relief, as in the case of arthritis, rheumatism and sore muscles, is required. To stop a hemorrhage like nosebleed, one teaspoon of the powder in a cup of hot water to be drain as quickly as possible. Green sweet peppers are rich in fibre, potassium, folic acid, and vitamins C, B_1 and B_2, and are low in calories. Cayenne pepper is high in a variety of trace minerals and vitamin C. Red, yellow or brown fruits, often eaten raw in salads when green and unripe; very variable size and shape; some varieties can be spicy but mostly non-pungent. The average composition per 100 g is: 2 g protein, 0.45 g fat, 6.5 g carbohydrate, 38 kcal (0.16 MJ), 1 mg iron (green pepper (40 mg vitamin A, red pepper 310 mg), 0.05 mg B_1 0.07 mg B_2, 1 mg nicotinic acid 155 mg, vitamin C 50-300 mg.

pepper, black. Family: *Piperaceae.* Genus: *Piper.* Species: *Piper nigrum* (black, or true, pepper). A genus of plants which furnish the black pepper of commerce.

It is a native of the East Indies, and other tropical regions where it is cultivated on an extensive scale. It is a climbing plant which yields two crops annually for about twelve years, has large, broad leaves, very small flowers and little globular berries, which, when ripe, are of a bright red colour.

The black pepper consists of the dried berries. The berries are gathered when they begin to change colour, and are cleaned and dried in the sun or over a slow fire; in the process of drying the berries turn black.

White pepper is the seed freed from the external skin and fleshy part of the fruit.

Red pepper is obtained from the pods of the capsicum. The larger fruited peppers, green or ripe, are used for pickling, sauces, etc. Black and white pepper, fruit of climbing vine, *Piper nigrum,* grows in wet tropical conditions; fruits are peppercorns.

Black pepper is made from sun-dried unripe pepper corns when red outer skin turns black.

White pepper made by soaking ripe berries and rubbing off outer skin. Pungency is mainly due to alkaloid piperine, piperdine and chavicine. The average composition per 100 g is: 11 g protein; 7 g fat; 60 g carbohydrate; 5 g fibre; 0.05 mg vitamin B_1; 0.2 mg vitamin B_2, 1 mg nicotinic acid; and food energy 1.49 MJ.

Pepper is used medicinally to stimulate appetite and promote perspiration. It also stimulates the mucous membranes and the nervous system and raises the body temperature. It is therefore excellent at the beginning of a cold, but do not be timid about its use chew at least sixteen black peppercorns, one at a time and one immediately after another, if necessary with a glass of ice water on standby. It may be used as a gargle and externally as a ruberfacient.

Red pepper, chilli (or chili), is the small red fruit of *Capsicum frutescens,* bushy, perennial plant. Usually sun-dried therefore wrinkled; very pungent, ingredient of curry powder, pickles and Tabasco sauce.

Cayenne pepper is made from the powdered dried fruits. The average composition per 100 g (dried) is: 15 g protein; 11 g fat; 35 g carbohydrate; 23 g fibre; 9 mg iron; 200 mg vitamin A; 0.7 mg vitamin B_1; 0.6 mg vitamin B_2; 11 mg nicotinic acid; 10 mg vitamin C; and food energy 1.2 MJ.

pepper drying. Peppers which are used for spice and colour are dried with the sun and/or heated air drying. Whole or sliced pods are dried with heated air at 65.6-79.4°C, requiring 6 hours for slices and 12 hours for whole pods to dry to 7-8%. Drying may be with single or two-stage dryers. The final product may be whole, sliced, chunks, or powdered.

peppermint. A perennial herb, cultivated extensively for the pungent oil obtained by distillation from the leaves. It is easily distinguished from other kinds of mint by the leafy stalks and by the spike-like heads into which the flowers are grouped. The oil of the plant has a sharp, pleasant odour and taste, and is used medicinally and for flavouring. *See also* peppermint oil.

peppermint oil. The oil obtained by steam distilling the flowering plants of peppermint *(mentha piperata)*. A form of the oil known as Arvensis peppermint oil is distilled from varieties of field mint *(Mentha arvensis)* native to China and Japan. It has occasional use in perfumery, but is mostly employed in pharmaceuticals and toothpastes.

The yields are low, not exceeding 0.7% of weight of starting materials. The resulting oil is pale yellow with a characteristic order. The commercial oils are of three types, although much alike, depending upon their source: French, Italian, and North American. Before the oil can be used as a flavouring for foodstuffs, it must be rectified and is usually tri-rectified. Principal constituents of peppermint oil include a- and b-pinene, limonene, cineol, ethyl amylcarbinol, menthol, neomenthol, piperitone, among several other organic compounds. The oil is described as having fresh, strong, mainly odor and a sweet balsamic taste, with a characteristic cooling effect on tongue and mouth.

Pepsi. Trade name of a multinational soft drink; contains sugar, vanilla, essential oils, spices, phosphoric acid and extract of cola nut coloured with caramel.

pepsin. An enzyme that catalyzes the partial hydrolysis of proteins of polypeptides. It is secreted by the gastric glands in an inactive form, pepsinogen, and is activated by hydrogen ions. At pH values of 4.6 and less pepsin activates pepsinogen, *i.e.,* it is autocatalytic. Pepsin initiates the digestion of proteins, splitting them into smaller fragments. The extent of this action is proportional to the length of time the protein is in contact with the enzyme.

pepsin inhibitor. A polypeptide fragment that inhibits pepsin and that has a molecular weight of about 3000; it is removed, together with other peptides, from pepsinogen in the course of its activation to pepsin.

peptidases. The enzymes that are responsible for catalyzing the hydrolysis of certain peptide bonds. The peptidases help break down peptides into amino acids. They are divided into exopeptidases, which sequentially cleave single amino acids from one end of the peptide chain (such as the carboxypeptidase, aminopeptidase), and endopeptidases, which cleave peptides internally, often showing specificity for the adjacent amino acid (for example, chymotrypsin, pepsin, trypsin). Peptidases catalyze the digestion of protein in the alimentary tract, while within cells they convert proteins from one form (usually inactive) to another (active) form by limited proteolysis.

peptide. A molecule consisting of two or more amino acids joined by peptide bonds. The bond is hydrolysed by peptidases, enzymes that are important in the digestion of proteins. Dipeptides contain two amino acids, tripeptides three, and so on. Polypeptides contain more than ten and usually 100-300. Naturally occurring oligopeptides (of less than ten amin acids) include the tripeptide glutathione and the pituitary hormones vasopressin and oxytocin, which are octapeptides.

peptide antibiotic. An antibiotic, such as gramicidin or actinomycin-D, which consists largely or entirely of a peptide.

peptide bond. Joining of α-carboxyl group of one amino acid to α-amino group of another amino acid. Formation of the bond involves loss of a water molecule from the two amino acids, and the bond can be broken by hydrolysis. The equilibrium is in favor of hydrolysis; the reverse reaction, as in protein synthesis, requires an input of energy and information with respect to the sequence of amino acids. The orientation of the carbonyl group in the peptide is usually trans to the amino group, and because the bond has a partial double bond character (due to resonance) the bond is rigid and planar. This rigidity limits the number of configurations of a polypeptide chain and is a major determinant of the shape of proteins.

peptides. Compounds formed when amino acids are linked together through the -CO-NH- linkage. Two amino acids so linked form a dipeptide, three a tripeptide, etc. Long chains are polypeptides. Proteins are composed of multiple bundles of long chains of polypeptides joined by cross-linkages.

peptones. The partial degradation product of the protein, in the chain protein-proteoses-peptones-polypeptides-amino acids. It is distinguished from proteoses since they are not precipitated by ammonium sulphate. The name peptone is often given to a partial hydrolysate of protein of any type; thus bacteriological peptone is a bacterial medium produced by partial acid hydrolysis of the protein.

Pera orange. A variety of orange. Some people believe the Pera sweet orange to be identical with Lamb's Summer. The fruit is somewhat smaller and ripens earlier than the Valencia and is classified as a late midseason variety. The rind is medium-thin; colour is light-orange at maturity. The flesh is juicy and qute rich in flavour. The fruit is used in comparatively large quantities for processing.

perennial. A plant which extends its life cycle over many years. Two types of perennials can be classified, which are:
(a) the herbaceous perennials in which aearial shoots die back in autumn and the plant spends the climatically harsh part of the year hidden beneath the soil (often as a bulb, corm, rhizome or tuber); and
(b) the woody perennials which remain above ground at all times and survive unfavourable conditions through the construction of strong, resistant woody tissue in which lignin and cellulose have substantially strengthened the plant.

perfume. A concentrated essence of fragrant materials diluted in the minimum possible amount of a high-grade alcohol. Perfumes have been used since earliest times, not only for aesthetic value, but also for antiseptic value and for religious purposes. Simple perfumes usually take their name from the name of the plant, but the most esteemed perfumes are blends, and the blending is considered a high art. It is done by tones imparted by many ingredients. An ordinary perfume may contain more than 50 components, sometimes as high as 250, and the average perfume manufacturer employs about 2,500 components. Some of the chemicals are not odours, but give lasting qualities or enhance odour. Some are used as fixatives or blending agents. Since many of the odours come directly from esters, aldehydes, or ketones, they can be made synthetically from coal-tar hydrocarbons and alcohols. Synthetics are now most used in perfumes, although some natural odours have not yet been duplicated synthetically, and about 30,000 aromatics have been developed. As with jewellery, the use of perfumes, is generally classed as a luxury.

Fixatives are used in the manufacture of the finer perfumes. They are essential oils that are less volatile and thus delay evaporation. The animal oils, such as musk and civet, are of this class, and also the balsam oils. Some evil-smelling distillates from chemical manufacture may also be used as fixatives. *See also* perfume oil.

perfume families. The perfumes are generally classified under one of the seven family groups, called perfume families, or fragrance families, with the names indicative of the type of perfume they comprise. The families are: floral, green, aldehydic, chypre, oriental, tobacco/leather, and fougere.

perfume oils. Volatile oils obtained by distillation or solvent extraction from the leaves, flowers, gums, or woods of plant materials (although a few are of animal origin). Some oils with repungant odours have an attractive fragrance in extreme dilution and a persistence which is valued in blends and for stabilization. Some oils with heavy odours, such as coumarin, are used in diluted form. Hydroquinone dimethyl ether, $C_8H_{10}O_2$, has an odour of sweet clover but is used as a fixative in odour perfumes.

In general, the aldehyde odours are fugitive, and some become acid in the presence of light and/or atmospheric oxygen. Ketones in perfumes have been found to be more stable in comparison to aldehydes. Esters have been found to be usually stable, but some of them are easily saponified in hot solution, and thus cannot be used for perfuming soaps. Some esters, made from complex high alcohols, are used to give a fresh top note to floral perfumes. Linalyl acetate (obtained from citral) is an example of this type.

It may be noted that the acid perfumes neutralize free alkali and cannot be used for perfuming soaps. It has also been noticed that the phenolic odour alter the colour of soaps, and the odour may also become disagreeable in due course of time.

Some odours are never extracted from the flowers, but are compounded.

Crab apple has a sweet odour, and is compounded of 16 oils, including bois de rose, ylang-ylang, nutmet oil, nasmine, musk, heliotropin, coumarin, and many others.

Benzophenone, $C_6H_5(CO)C_6H_5$, is used for rose-geranium perfumes. It is a diphenyl ketone, melting at 47°C. This material is also used for making fine chemicals.

Geraniol, from citral, is a colourless liquid with a sweet, delicate rose odour.

Apple and peach odours are allyl cinnamate.

Synthetic rose is the ester of phenyl ethyl alcohol made from benzene and ethylene oxide. Although the natural rose odour is readily extracted, it is more expensive.

Attar (of rose) is one of the most ancient and popular perfume oils. The name is derived from the Persian *attar*, and is sometimes incorrectly given as *ottar* but with the same French pronunciation. The finest attar of rose is obtained from Bulgaria, where it is distilled from the flowers of the damask rose, *Rosa damascena*. The fresh oil is colourless, but turns yellowish green. About 1850 kg of flowers are needed to obtan 1 kg of essence, and it is so valuable that it is usually adulterated with geraniol or synthetic rose. In France the oil is distilled from the *R..centifolia*.

Rose water is the scented water left after distillation, or is made by dissolving attar in water.

The otto of baronia of Australia is a high-grade rose oil.

Bay oil, or myrcia oil, used in the toilet alcohol known as bay rum, and also in perfumes, is distilled from the leaves of the bay tree, *Pimenta acris*, of the West Indies. It contains eugenol, and has a spicy odour.

Musk (natural) is obtained from the male musk deer of Tibet. It is one of the most expensive materials used in making perfumes. Synthetic musk is as powerful as the natural. Astrolone is the trade name for a synthetic musk.

Musk ambrette is made from metacresol. Ambrette oil has a strong musk-like odour distilled from the musk seed, or amber seed, of the plant *Hibiscus abelmoschus* of India, Ecuador, and Egypt.

Civet is an odorous yellow fluid from the civet cat of tropical Asia and Ethiopia. Civettone is a liquid with a clean odour and easily soluble in alcohol, distilled from civet.

Patchouli oil is one of the best fixatives employed for preparing heavy perfumes. It is a powerfully odorous viscous liquid obtained by distilling and fermented leaves of the shrub *progostemon patchouli* of India, China, and the Philippines. The odour resembles sandalwood.

Cassie is one of the valuable oils with an odour similar to violet obtained by maceration in oil of the flowers of the shrub *Acacia farnesiana* of the Mediterranean countries and the West Indies. It is used to scent pomades and powders.

Oak moss was one of the perfumes of ancient Egypt. It is obtained from the lichen *Evernia prunastri* and *E. furfuracea* growing on oak and apruce trees of southern Europe. The resinous extract has the odour of musk and lavender. It is used as a fixative in poppy type perfumes.

Rue oil, used for sweet pea perfume, is distilled from the plants *Ruta graveolans* of France and *R. montana* of Algeria.

Mecca balsam is used in oriental types of perfume. It is a greenish oleoresin obtained from the plant *Commiphora opobalsamum* of Arabia. It has the odour of rosemary.

Rosemary is an oil distilled from the fresh flowering tops of the sweet-smelling evergreen shrub *Rosemarinus officinalis* of the Mediterranean countries. It is used in eau de cologne, soaps, and medicine.

Some oils such as lavender, from the flowers of the *Lavandula vera*, have no value when used alone but require skillful blending to develop the pleasant odour.

Versilide is a cyclic ketone synthetic musk that is very stable in soaps and cosmetics and does not discolour.

Geranium oil is obtained from the leaves or flowers of the *Pelargonium graveolens* of the Mediterranean countries and other species of geranium. It is used as an adulterant or substitute for rose oils in perfumes and soaps. Many geranium and rose oils are derived from geraniol obtained from citronella and other oils.

A synthetic rose-geranium is diphenyl methane, $(C_6H_5)_2CH_2$, a colourless solid melting at about 25°C.

Vetiver, a very sweet-scented oil used in high-grade perfumes and in medicine, is distilled from the roots of khuskhus plant, *Vetiveria zizamoides,* native to India but produced chiefly in Java, Reunion, and Haiti.

Opopanox, used in medicine, is an oleoresin from the roots of the *pastinaca opopanox* of the Orient and British Somaliland.

Frankincense, used in incense and perfumes, and in medicine under the name of olibanum, is a gum resin from the tree *Boswellia carterii* of the Sudan and Somaliland. It comes in hard yellow grains.

Orris is the dry root of the *Iris florentian,* and the powdered root is used in violet powders and as a flavour.

Kiounouk, used as a fixative, is a clear yellowish semiliquid obtained from olibanum.

Jasmine oil, a highly valued perfume material, is from the fragrant flowers of the shrub *Jasminus grandiflorum,* a species of jasmine grown in southern France especially for perfume. The oil is extracted from the fresh flowers by enfleurage.

A synthetic jasmine-rose oil, which also has a peach-apricot flavour and

a sweet taste, is benzyl propionate. It is liquid boiling at 220°C, and is used in perfumes and as a flavour.

Lavender oil is a mixture of the oil in water and alcohol, is obtained from the flowers of the shrub *Lavandula officinalis* of southern Europe. The dried flowers are fragrant and are used in sachets. It is used with rosemary in eau de cologne, and also as lavender water.

Spike lavender is the name of an inferior oil obtained from *L. latifolia* of France and Spain. It is used in perfumes and sometimes as a food flavour.

Herbandin is a synthetic ester made from petroleum and used as a replacement or extender for natural lavender oil. It has a pronounced lavender odour.

Espantone is a synthetic ketone with a spike lavender odour.

Carnation oil is obtained by solvent extraction or by enfleurage from the flowers of the *Dianthus caryophyllus,* of which there are more than 2,000 varieties grown in the Mediterranean countries. The less highly cultivated plants give the richest perfumes.

Violet oil is derived by solvents or maceration in hot oils from the flowers of the blue and purple varieties of *Viola odorata.*

Synthetic violet is the product obtained from ionone, derived from lemon-grass oil. The ionones are made synthetically by condensation of citral with acetone. They are monoenol and dinol butones.

Velvione is much like ionone with a powerful violet odour. The true violet odour is irone, which is a complex seven-ring compound. It can be obtained from the iris root and is one of the most odoriferous materials obtained from plants.

Wisteria has the honeylike odour of the mauve and white flowers of the climbing plant *Wisteria sinensis*. The oil is never extracted but is compounded from geranium, Peru balsam, benzoic, bois de rose, and synthetics.

Ylang-ylang, or *cananga oil*, is a valuable essential oil from the flowers of the tree *Canangium odorata*, cultivated in Indonesia, Malagasy, and the Philippines. About 240 kg are required to produce 1 kg of oil. It contains linalol and geraniol.

Another oil that rivals ylang-ylang in fragrance is champaca oil, from the flowers of the large tree *Michelia champaca*, of southern Asia.

Zdravetz oil is the name given to geranium oil obtained from *P. macnorhijum* of Cyprus. It is used in rose bouquet and lavender perfumes.

pericarp. In reference to cereal grain this consists of two to four fibrous layers next to the outer husk and outside the tests; of low digestibility and removed from grain during milling. It is the major constituent of bran.

perilla oil. An essential oil obtained by steam distillation from the leaves and flowers of perilla (*perilla frutescens*), a herb found in the Indo-China region, Japan, and Korea. It has a powerful spicy, cumin-like fragrance. An oil with the same name is distilled from the seeds of the same plant and has different uses.

perillartine. Non-nutritive sweetening agent derived from perillaldehyde, extracted from shiso oil (commercially available in Japan); it is about 2000 times as sweet as sugar.

periplasmic enzyme. A bacterial enzyme that exists either in free or in bound form in a region between the cell wall and the cell membane.

peristalsis. Method of movement along the intestine, peristaltic waves, caused

by counteraction of a ring of muscle, preceded by a wave of relaxation.

permeases. Bacterial enzymes present in the plasma membrane that facilitate the movement of specific substances into or out of the cell. In the lac operon of *E. coli*, the lac Y gene codes for a permease that transports lactose into the cell.

peroxidases. The enzymes which catalyze the reaction of hydrogen peroxide with a second compound, the latter serving as a hydrogen donor. Peroxidases are widely distributed in plants, and a number of different hydrogen donors have been used for their detection. The most commonly used tests utilize the enzyme-catalyzed reaction of hydrogen peroxide with aromatic polyphenols and polyamines. Peroxidases and catalases are predominantly protein in nature with an additional tightly bound compound (prosthetic group), which confers catalytic activity to the molecule.

In addition to protein and the prosthetic group, there is an appreciable amount of carbohydrate in some cases that appears to be an integral part of the molecule.

peroxide number. A measure of the oxidative rancidity of fats by determination of the peroxides present. Measured by the amount of iodine liberated from potassium iodide; peroxide value is the ml of 0.002 N sodium thiosulphate per gram sample. Also known as peroxide value.

peroxide value. *See* peroxide number.

Perrier water. Mildly alkaline, well-aerated natural water, containing sodium bicarbonate.

perry. Fermented pear juice analogous to cider from apples.

Persian berry (colour). Name given to yellow colour obtained from the berries of the buckthorn (*Rhamnus*) family; it is legally permitted in food in many countries. It contains the glucosides of two colouring matters, rhamnetin and rhamnazin.

persimmon. Fruit of the tree *Diospyros virginiana* (a variety of ebony). Egg-shaped fruit 3-5 cm in diameter; it is yellow in colour, and its astringency decreases as it ripens. Most of the persimmons grown are Oriental type, the tomato-shaped, bright-orange fruit known as "kaki." Many imagine them to be extremely sour, but in fact these fruits can be quite palatable somewhat stringent, but rich and sweet. Commercially grown persimmons are picked and marketed unripe because of their extreme perishability; they must be held at room temperature until quite soft for the flavour to develop. The average composition per 100 g is: water 80%; protein 0.5%; carbohydrate 18%; iron 0.4 mg; vitamin A 700 µg; vitamin B_1 0.02 mg; vitamin B_2 0.02 mg; nicotinic acid 0.02 mg; vitamin C 10 mg; and food energy 0.3 MJ.

Peruvita. Trade name for a protein-rich baby food developed in Peru. Sweet formulation contains about 30% protein, made from quinua and cotton-seed flour, with skim-milk powder, sugar, spices, vitamins A, B_1 and B_2 and calcium carbonate. The Savoury formulation contains about 35% protein, contains salt in place of sugar.

pervaporation. Evaporation from a colloidal suspension by heating in a collodion bag. If there are any crystalloids present they pass through the membrane and are deposited on the outside of the bag.

pesticides. Any toxic substance used to kill animals or plants that cause economic damage to crop or ornamental plants or are hazardous to the health of domestic animals or humans. All pesticides interfere with normal metabolic processes in the pest organisms and often are classified according to the type of organism they are intended to control, viz. fungicides, herbicides, insecticides, rodenticides, molluscacides, nematocides and fumigants. Methods of these pesticides employ similar toxic substances. The means of application, chemical nature, types of products, precautions to be observed, symptions of accidental poisoning, and immediate means of treatment are part of knowledge which must be known to the distributors and customers. The manufacturer must provide the efficacy of the product, its safety toward human beings, crops, livestock, wildlife and the general environment. The pesticide should not be deposited as residue on food or feed which causes such a hazard.

Chemicals are designated to be effective as rodenticide (against rats, mice, moles, etc), insecitides (against various insects and arthropods), herbicides (against weeds and undesirable plants) and fungicides (against all types of fungi). Particular chemical agents are used as poison baits, spray solutions, suspensions for spraying, aerosols, fumigants, residual poisons, stomach poisons, and repellents. They may be inorganic, or organic compounds obtained from natural sources, or synthetic organic complexes. The choice of chemicals employed is dependent on the type of pest. If the pest is a rat or mouse, the chemical used will differ according to the locating conditions of the pest. An insect pest may be a chewing or sucking type, a running or flying type, an indoor or outdoor type. Similarly, chemicals are selected properly to control weeds and parasitic fungi, herbicide or fungicide. Poisonous chemicals are put into poison baits to control rats and mice. The chemicals must be sufficiently toxic to kill in reasonably small amounts. A chemical known as Norbormide, which is 5-(α-hydroxy-α-2-pyridylbenzyl)-7-(α-2-pyridyl-benzylidene)-5-norbornene-2, 3-dicarboximide, is the most effective rodenticide. Norbormide consistently kills the laboratory rats but has no effect upon other test animals. The other most effective synthetic rodenticide is Warfarin, 3-(α-acetonylbenzyl)-4-hydroxycoumarin. It does not kill all rodents. Other chemicals are sodium fluoroacetate also known as 1080, 2-pivalyl-1, 3-indandione or Pival, a-naphthyl-thiourea or ANTU, thallium sulphate, zinc phosphide, arsenic trioxide and barium carbonate. Precautions must be taken that animal pets and small childern should not swallow any of these poisonous chemicals.

Salts of the alkaloid strychnine are used to control rodents. Such products are effective for small rodents, they are not commonly employed as rat poison. The toxicity of strychnine to other animals and its painful poisonous action do not make it a poison of choice.

petitgrain. An essential oil obtained by distillation of the leaves and small twigs of the bitter orange trees, *Citrus aurantium*, native to tropical Asia, but now grown in other countries. In Spain, it is known as the Seville orange. Paraguay is the chief producer of high-grade petitgrain, which is one of the best fixatives for fine perfumes and is also used in flavouring extracts. One kg of petitgrain is obtained from 90-120 kg of leaves. The fruits of the tropical bitter orange are large and of the finest golden appearance, but the pulp is very acid. The juice is used only for blending in orange drinks. It contains a dilactone, limonin, which gives it a bitter taste. The rind is used in marmalade and candied orange peel.

An essential oil distilled from the rind is known as curcao, and is used in perfumery and in curacao liqueur. The flowers are very fragrant, and from them neroli oil is distilled. Neroli is used in perfumery perfumery blends and for mixing with synthetic perfumes.

Neroli Portugal is inferior, and comes from the sweet orange *C. sinensis* by extraction.

Orange oil is obtained by expression from the ripe rind of the sweet orange, is a less valuable oil.

Bergamot oil is from the rind of the fruit of the small spiny tree *C. gamia* of Italy. It has a soft sweet odour, and is used in perfume blends and in soaps. The golden-yellow pear-shaped fruit has an acid inedible pulp.

The bioflavonoids used in cold remedies, are obtained from the white pulp, or albedo, of citrus fruits. They are alkaline-soluble crystalline compounds, variations of chrome, a benzpyrone, and flavone, the phenyl benzpyrone. The pressed product from the pulp is acidified, crystallized, and dried. More than 200 distinct chemicals have been produced from citrus fruits. The bioflavonoids are six-membered, double-ring compounds. Some are isolated and used directly, as the naringin from grapefruit peel, which is an effective substitute for quinine. Others are synthesized easily. The chromone and flavone are really the parent substances of many natural vegetable dyes, drugs, and tannins, and are readily convertible to these materials

Petit pois. Small peas; according to the code of practice for canned fruits and vegetables, up to and including 11/34 inch in diameter; medium up to 13/32 inch; large or standard, greater than 13/32 inch.

Petit Sirah grape. A red wine grape variety with extensive plantings in California. It is related to the Syrah of Hermitage, but is much more productive. Some authorities, however, believe that the Petit Sirah is actually the Duriff. It is used for the production of common red wines.

Petit suisse cheese. A small unripened cheese of France similar to Carre but having a slightly different shape and containing more fat.

Petit-grain oils. The oils prepared from twigs and leaves of the bitter orange by stead distillation; similar to neroli oil but less fragrant. Petigrain Portugal prepared from leaves of sweet orange. Mandarin petitgrain is prepared from tangerine tree leaves, and lemon petitgrain.

peucedan gum. A resin said to resemble ammoniacum obtained from the roots of the herb peucedan (*peucedanum officinale*). The roots have a strong odour of sulphur and the resin was once used in herbal remedies.

pFister cheese. An Emmentaler cheese made from fresh, skimmed, cow's milk. Thought to have been first made by pFister Hubber of Switzerland. The cheese is shaped like small rolls of Swiss cheese.

phagocytosis. The process whereby certain body cells, notably macrophages and neutrophils. engulf and destroy invading foreign particles. The cell membrane of the phagocytosing cell (phagocyte) invaginates to capture and engulf the particle. Pro-

teolytic and other enzymes are introduced into the vicinity of the particle to digest it. A potent feature of phagocytosis is the 'respiratory burst', a sudden acceleration glycolysis by the phagocyte with the production of oxygen metabolites, including hydrogen peroxide, that are highly active in destroying bacteria. However, microorganisms show widely varied susceptibility to phagocytosis. Free-living and parasitic amoeboid protozoa (*e.g.,* Entamoeba) feed by phagocytosis.

pharmacophore. A structural arrangement of atoms that is considered to impart pharmacological activity to a chemical substance.

pharmacopoeia. A book containing a list of all standard drugs (with a description of each, showing its standard strength and purity) and directions for their use. Such books are compiled by experts, most of them by government authorization. The first US pharmacopoeia was published in 1820. It was prepared at a convention of delegates from medical colleges and societies. Since then similar conventions have been held every ten years to revise the work. This book is a legal standard in the US, and registered pharmacists make use of it in their practice.

phase inversion. Milk is an emulsion of fat in water; butter is an emulsion of water in fat. the change from cream to butter is termed phase inversion.

phaseolin. Globulin protein in kidney bean.

phaseolunatin. A cyanogenetic glucoside found in certain legumes (such as lima bean, chick pea, common vetch), which hydrolyses to produce glucose, acetone and hydrocyanic acid; not proved harmful when present in the diet.

PHB ester. The ethyl and propyl esters of *p*-hydroxybenzoic acid and their sodium salts; mainly used as preservative in some countries.

phenol. C_6H_5OH. An organic compound which is employed as a strong and inexpensive disinfectant with a characteristic pine odour. At low concentrations it is bacteriostatic, but higher concentrations (1-2%) are bactericidal and fungicidal. Activity is lowered by cold, alkalinity, or the presence of lipids and soaps. It is thought to act by denaturing protein and is able to penetrate skin, causing inflammation and local precipitation of protein with necrosis. Also known as carbolic acid.

phenol oxidases. Enzymes that oxidize phenolic compounds to quinones; e.g., monophenol oxidase in mushrooms; polyphenol oxidases in potato and apple that are responsible for the development of the brown colour when the cut surface is exposed to air; tryosinase in plants and animals that is responsible for brown and black pigmentation.

phenylketonuria. Inherited metabolic defect wherein the essential amino acid, phenylalanine, is incompletely metabolized and the end-product, phenylpyruvic acid, is excreted in the urine. The product affects the brain and causes imbecility. The effect can be moderate by strict limitation of the phenylalanine intake.

pheromones. Substances generated and secreted by one individual that induce a physiological effect in another. They often act in extremely low concentrations and at large distances, and usually through the olfactory sense. Pheromones play an important role in the social behaviour of certain animals, especially insects and mammals. They are used to attract mates, to mark trails, and to promote social cohesion and coordination in colonies. Pheromones are usually highly volatile organic acids or alcohols and can be effective at minute concentrations. Certain members of the wild potato family secrete an air-borne substance that repels greenfly, and this substance also is described as a pheromone, even through, unusually, two different species are involved. Also known as ectohormone.

phitosite. High calorie food.

phlorrhizin. A glycoside of plant origin; abolishes the renal threshold for glucose, which therefore appears in the urine (glycosuria). This is known as renal diabetes or phlorhizin diabetes. It is used to examine formation of glucose from other ingredients of the diet. Also spelled phloridzin and phlorhizin.

phosphatases. Enzymes that catalyze the removal of phosphate groups. Acid phosphatase is particularly abundant in lysosomes.

phosphatase test for cheese. A test to determine if the milk used for making cheese or the cheese itself, has been pasteurized at appropriate temperature for not less than 30 minutes, or for a time and at a temperature equivalent thereto in phosphatase destruction. Different kinds of cheese and cheese of different ages have different buffering capacities and some of them require modifications of concentrations of the reagents. When phosphatases act on biological materials, as increase in inorganic phosphates occurs and the enzyme action can be followed analytically on this basis. Disodium phenyl-phosphate is used as the substrate in all of the variations of the phosphatase test. Phenol is liberated and it lends itself to accurate colorimetric measurements.

phosphate. One of several anionic forms of phosphoric acid (which is strictly termed o-phosphoric acid, and hence o-phosphate), often referred to as inorganic phosphate. The main physiologically important anions are $H_2PO_4^-$ and HPO_4^{2-}. These act as buffer in blood and other biological fluids. Most free phosphate in animals occurs as a component of hydroxyapatite in bones and teeth. Combined phosphate is found in many important esters phosphomonoesters (such as glucose-1-phosphate, glucose-6-phosphate, phosphoenolpyruvate), phosphodiesters (*e.g.*, phospholipids and nucleic acids), and anhydrides or pyrophosphates (*e.g.*, ATP, ADP). Some proteins, the phosphoproteins, have phosphate esterified to serine, threonine, or tyrosine amino acids, either in large amounts (such as caseinogen) or in small amounts (*e.g.*, glycogen phosphorylase). The addition of a phosphate group (phosphorylation) is important in controlling the activity of certain enzymes.

phosphatides. Fatty substances including phosphoric acid and a nitrogenous base in the molecule. They include lecithins, cephalins, sphingomyelins, and cerebrosides. Part of the structure of the brain and nervous tissue and involved in fat transport. Also combined with proteins as lipoproteins. Phosphatides are partly soluble in water as well as in fats and used in food technology is emulsifiers. From the dietary point of view they may be regarded as simple fats. Also known as phospholipins; phospholipids.

phosphatidic acid. A glyceride in which two of the three hydroxyl groups of glycerol are esterified with long-chain fatty acids while the third is esterified with phosphate. Phosphatidic acid is the parent compound of the phospholipids.

phosphatidyl choline. A major phosphoglyceride in higher plants and animals; consists of choline that is esterified to the phosphoric acid residue of phosphatidic acid. Also known as lecithin.

phosphatidylinositol. A phospholipid found in cell membranes in which the phosphatidic acid is esterified to inositol. The two fatty acids that are esterified to the glycerol of the phosphatidic acid are usually stearic and arachidonic in phosphatidylinostiol. Its importance in pharmacology is because of its role in certain second messenger system.

phosphatidylserine. A phospholipid containing the amino acid, serine.

phosphodiesterases. Enzymes that catalyze the hydrolysis of phosphodiesters such as cyclic nucleotides and phosphatidylinositol 4,5-diphosphate. Cyclic nucleotide phosphodiesterases occur as a number of isoenzymes, exhibiting distinct kinetic properties, substrate specificities and cellular localizations. Three basic forms of the enzyme occur in mammals. One is membrane-bound with a high affinity for cyclic AMP. The other two forms are cytosolic and are capable of hydrolyzing both cyclic AMP and cyclic GMP. One of these has about equal affinities for cyclic AMP and cyclic GMP, and cyclic GMP stimulates the hydrolysis of cyclic AMP. The other displays a higher affinity for cyclic GMP than for cyclic AMP, and is dependent upon calmodulin for activity.

phosphokinases. Enzymes that transfer the phosphate radical, together with its energy, to or from adenosine di- or triphosphate. Various other molecules can be involved but one of the pair of reactants is adenosine di- or triphosphate.

phospholipase. Any of a group of enzymes which catalyze the hydrolysis of a phospholipid. Phospholipase A releases one of the two fatty acids from the remaining lysophospholipid residue; phospholipase C yields a diglyceride and phosphorylated head group; and phospholipase D cleaves the head group to yield phosphatidic acid. These changes radically alter the properties of phospholipid and thus affect its role in cell membrane structure and function. A membrane-bound phospholipase C is involved in the action of certain hormones (*e.g.*, bradykinin) that bind to receptors on the cell membrane. They are present in lysosomes, in the cell membrane and in the outer membrane of mitochondria. Phospholipases A_1 and A_2 catalyze the removal, respectively, of the 1-acyl group and the 2-acyl group from glycerophospholipids; the products are known as lysophosphatides. These enzymes are concerned in the remodelling of membrane phospholipids. Phospholipase A2 (probably activated by a Ca-calmodulin complex) catalyzes the hydrolysis of phosphatidylinositol with the release of arachidonic acid and subsequent prostanoid synthesis. Phospholipase C catalyzes the breakdown of phosphatidylinositol 4,5-diphosphate in the so-called PI response.

phospholipids. A group of lipids having both a phosphate group and one or more fatty acids. Glycerophospholipids are based on glycerol; the three hydroxyl groups are esterified with two fatty acids and a phosphate group, which may itself be bound to one of a variety of simple organic groups (*e.g.*, in lecithin it is choline). Sphingophospholipids are based on the alcohol sphingosine and contain only one fatty acid linked to an amino group. With their hydrophilic polar phosphate groups and long hydrophobic hydrocarbon tails, phospholipids readily form membrane-like structures in water. They are important components of cell membranes and include the phosphoglycerides and sphingomyelins. Phospholipids are amphipathic molecules, the negative phosphate group and alcohol forming a polar head and the hydrophobic tail comprising the fatty acid chain. Also known as phosphatides.

photosynthesis. The synythesis of organic compounds using light energy absorbed by chlorophyll. With the exception of a small group of bacteria, organisms photosynthesize from inorganic materials. All green plants photosynthesize as well as certain prokaryotes (blue-green algae and some bacteria). In the green plants, photosynthesis takes place in chloroplasts, mainly in leaves. Directly or indirectly, photosynthesis is the source of carbon and energy for all except chemoautotrophic organisms. The mechanism is complex and involves two sets of stages: light reactions followed by dark reactions. The overall reaction in green plants can be summirized by the equation:

$$CO_2 + 4H_2O = (CH_2O) + 3H_2O + O_2$$

In the light reactions, light energy is absorbed by chlorophyll (and other pigments), setting off a chain of chemical reactions in which water is split and gaseous oxygen evolved. The hydrogen from the water is attached to other molecules, and used to reduce carbon dioxide to carbohydrates in the later dark reactions. The light reaction involves the conversion of ADP to ATP, a process known as phosphorylation. It is coupled to electron transfer reactions, which arise from two systems, pigment systems or photosystems I and II (PSI and II). Each system contains different forms of chlorophylls a, accessory pigments, and electron carriers in highly organized assemblies. Pigment molecules release electrons when energized by light and electrons from accessory pigments pass to special chlorophyll a molecules, which absorb light at longer wavelengths and act as energy traps. They are named according to the wavelength of the light they absorb (in nm), they are P680 in PSII and P700 in PSI. Electrons from these pass to electron acceptors. Photophosphorylation may be cyclic or noncylic. It is in noncyclic photophosphorylation that water acts as an electron donor and is split. The products are oxygen, ATP, and $NADPH_2$. Hydrogen ions from water ultimately combine with electrons to reduce NADP. Both pigments systems are involved. In the cyclic photophophorylation the only product is ATP and only PSI is involved. This may be used to generate extra ATP. During the dark reactions ATP and NADPH from the light reactions are used to reduce carbon dioxide to carbohydrate. The reactions take place in solution; in eukaryotes in the chloroplast stroma. Carbon dioxide is first fixed by combination with the 5-carbon sugar ribulose disphosphate (RUDP) to form two molecules of phophoglyceric acid (PGA), the first product of photosynthesis. PGA is then reduced to phosphoglyceraldehyde (triose phosphate) using the $NADPH_2$ and some of the ATP. Some of the triose phosphate and the rest of the ATP is used to regenerate the carbon dioxide acceptor RUDP in a complex cycle involving 3-,4-,5-,6-,

and 7-carbon sugar phosphates. The rest of the triose phosphate can be used in synthesis of carbodhydrates, fats, proteins, etc,.

photosynthetic bacteria. A group of bacteria able to photosynthesize through possession of a green pigment, bacteriochlorophyll, lightly different to the chlorophyll of plants. The do not use water as a hydrogen source, as do plants, and thus do not produce oxygen as a product of photosynthesis, but rather some oxidized by-product. Photosynthestic bacteria include the green sulphur bacteria, purple sulphur bacteria, and purple nonsulphur bacteria. They are unable to grow anaerobically in the dark, i.e., cannot grow by fermentation, but some species can grow aerobically in the dark, i.e., by aerobic respiration. In their natural habitats, it is probably that they all grow photosynthetically. Their pigment systems containing a number of carotenoids (which are, in most cases, responsible for their color) and a single chlorophyll, are particularly adapted to the absorption of light in the red region of the spectrum where green plant photosynthesis is inefficient. Consequently, photosynthetic bacteria may frequently be found on the under surface of leaves in stagnant waters.

The major groups of photosynthetic bacteria are:

(a) The green sulfur bacteria (*Chlorobacteriaceae*) includes the genus Chlorobium which is strictly anaerobic, strictly autotrophic, and strictly photosynthetic, using inorganic sulphur compounds as reductants for carbon dioxide fixation. Chlorobium species are non-motile, short bacilli. More recently, a motile green photosynthetic bacterium Chloropseudomonas ethylicum has been isolated which is also able to grow anaerobically in the presence of limited number of simple organic compounds including ethanol and acetate.

(b) The red sulphur bacteria (*Thiorhodaceae*) are a morphologically heterogeneous group which are strictly anaerobic and strictly photosynthetic, which can grow autotrophically or heterotrophically. Reduced sulphur compounds are commonly used as reductants for autotrophic growth, but hydrogen gas may be used. Chromatium species may be large motile bacilli, but motile spiral organisms (*Thiospirillum*) are known. These organisms accumulate elementary sulphur when grown with reduced sulphur compounds. Some species also require vitamin B_{12}.

(c) The non-sulphur purple and brown bacteria (*Athiorhodaceae*) include motile rods (Rhodopseudomonas) and spirilla (Rhodospirillum) most of which grow photosynthetically under anaerobic conditions in the presence of organic compounds, and also aerobically in the dark on the same organic compounds.

photosynthetic pigments. The plant pigments responsible for the capture of light energy during the light reactions of photosynthesis. The green pigment chlorophyll is the principal light receptor, absorbing blue and red light. However the carotenoids and various other pigments also absorb light energy and pass this on to the chlorophyll molecules. They are located either in the chloroplasts of plants or dispersed in the cytoplasm of prokaryotes. All photosynthetic organisms contain chlorophylls and carotenoids; some also contain phycobilins. Chlorophyll a is the primary pigment since energy absorbed by this is used directly to drive the light reactions of photosynthesis. Other pigments (chlorophyll b, c, and d, and the carotenoids and phycobilins) are accessory pigments that pass the energy they absorb on to chlorophyll a. They broaden the spectrum of light used in photosynthesis. They are divided into the principal pigments and accessory pigments. The former include various forms of chlorophyll, and the latter carotenoids (carotenes and xanthophylls) and phycobilins (phycocyanin and phycoerythrin).

photosynthetic quotient. A measure of the photosynthetic activity of a system that is equal to the number of moles of oxygen evolved divided by the number of moles of carbon dioxide taken up.

photosynthetic unit. The number of chlorophyll molecules that are required for the fixation of one molecule of carbon dioxide in photosynthesis.

phosphoproteins. Conjugated proteins containing phosphate other than as nucleic acid (nucleoproteins) or lecithin (lipoproteins), *e.g.*, casein from milk, ovovitellin from egg yolk.

phrynoderma. A follicular hyperkeratosis of the skin (blocked pores or toadskin) often encountered in malnourished people. Originally thought to be due to vitamin A deficiency but possibly due to other deficiencies, and occurs mildly in well-nourished people.

phycocolloid. Any of several colloidal macromolecular substance occurring in seaweeds; they are chemically classified as polysaccharides, or polymeric forms of certain sugars. They are strongly hydrophilic, forming gelatinous pastes by absorption of water.

physalin. Zeaxanthin dipalmitate; a carotenoid pigment found in the fruits of the Chinese lantern, *Physalis*.

physiological salt solutions. Solutions of salts containing essential ions such as Na^+, K^+, Mg^{2+}, Ca^{2+}, Cl^-, HCO_3^- and $H_2PO_4^-$ and glucose, and bubbled with air, oxygen or carbon dioxide (depending upon their buffering capacity). They are isotonic with extracellular fluid and of an appropriate pH. They may be used at room temperature or at any higher temperature up to and including normal body temperature. They are used to maintain isolated tissues by immersing, perfusing or superfusing them. They are of several different compositions usually denoted by the name of the scientist who first devised them.

physostigmatis. A plant of *Leguminosae* family. The seeds contains 0.15-0.3 % alkoloids. Physostigmine (0.15%) (eserine), eseridine, eseramine, isophysostigmine, physovenine, geneserine, N-8-norphysostigmine, calabatine and calabacine are the alkaoids isolated from the seeds. Exposure of the chief alkaloid, physostigmine, to heat light or air leads to oxidation and a red compound, rubreserine, is formed. Therefore, physostigmine should be protected from air and light. Physostigmine occurs as a white, odourless, finely crystalline powder. Physostigmine is cholinergic and miotic and used in atony of gastrointestinal tract. Its salicylate compound is used for contracting the pupil of the eye especially in mydriatics and glaucoma.

phyt-, phyto-. A prefix relating to plants, as phytosterol, phytase.

phytase. Phosphatase enzyme that hydrolyses phytin to inositol and phosphoric acid. It is present in yeast, liver, blood, malt and seeds. If a high level of yeast is used in baking with high-extraction flours, some of the phytin is broken down.

phytic acid. Inositol hexaphosphoric acid; present in the husk of cereals, dried peas and beans and some nuts. The phosphate is insoluble and not digested. Part of the phytic acid may be present as the calcium salt (phytin), but this is also unavailable to the consumer. Moreover, phytic acid can combine with calcium and also iron from other foods in the diet and render them insoluble and unavailable. For this reason it has been held responsible for rickets and iron-deficiency anaemia among people eating large amounts of whole-grain cereals. However, phytic acid is partially hydrolyzed by the enzymes of yeast (*e.g.*, in bread baking), and that present in peas and beans is partially hydrolyzed if these are soaked in water so the role of phytic acid in preventing the absorption of iron and calcium is not clear. It is not present in highly milled cereals since it is contained in the outer brany layers.

phytoalexins. An important class of antimicrobial compounds produced by a wide range of plants in response to bacterial of fungal infections or, less commonly, following chemical exposure or injury. Phytoalexins are a chemically heterogenous group of low-molecular mass aromatic compounds, a number of which are derived from isoflavonoids. Unlike toxic compounds which are produced by the plants in a nonspecific manner, phytoalexins are absent in healthy plants and are only produced in response to microbial invasion. More than 20 phytoalexins have been characterized. They include pisatin from pea (*Pisum sativum*), **phaseolin**

from the French bean (*phaseolus* spp.), and rishitin from the potato (*Solanum tuberosum*). Phytoalexin synthesis is induced by a variety of microbial components, including fungal β-glucans, glycoproteins, and acidic cell wall components. Phytoalexin synthesis is also elicited by pectin components released from the plant's own cell wall.

phytochemistry. That branch of chemistry which deals with the nutrition and metabolism of plants and with the chemical products obtained from them.

phytochrome. The protein-based plant pigment present in small quantities in many plant organs. It exists in two inter-convertible forms. P_R (or P_{660}) has an absorption peak at 660 nm (red light) and P_{FR} (or P_{730}) at 730 nm (far-red light). Natural white light favors formation of P_{FR}, the physiologically active form. The active form regulates many plant processes, such as seed germination and the initiation of flowering. Light intensities required for conversion are very low and it occurs within seconds. Phytochrome plays a vital role as a photoreceptor in a wide range of light-induced physiological processes: *e.g.,* photoperiodic responses; photomorphogenesis, including leaf expansion, leaf unrolling in grasses and cereals, and greening; and germination of light-sensitive seeds such as lettuce. P_{FR} is thought to induce changes in membrane permeability and the subsequent events often involve growth substances, particularly gibberellins, cytokinins, and possibly florigen.

phytosterol. General name given to sterols occurring in plants, the chief of which is sitosterol (structurally closely related to cholesterol).

pica. The tendency of eating earth, sand, clay, paper, etc.; quite common among young children.

piccalilli. Mixture of chopped, brine-preserved vegetables in mustard sauce (mustard and vinegar, thickened with tapioca starch, plus other spices, coloured with tartarine).

pickles, dill. Pickles that are fermented in a mixture of brine, cured dill weed, mixed spices and vinegar.

pickling. One of the classical methods of preserving vegetables. When vegetables are soaked in brine, they become dehydrated, because water leaks from the cells. This changes texture from crisp to soft. In addition, the brine inhibits the growth of many undesirable microbes while allowing lactic acid bacteria and certain yeasts to grow. These organisms convert the sugars in the vegetables primarily to lactic and acetic acids, which add to the tangy flavour of the product. Vegetables immersed in 5-10% brine undergo lactic acid fermentation, while the salt prevents the growth of undesirables. The sugars in the vegetables are broken down to lactic acid; at 25°C the process takes a few weeks, finishing at 1% acidity. Also called bringing.

pie cheese. The name applied to any kind of cheese which is used in making cheese pie, cheese cake or other bakery goods. Baker's cheese and Cottage cheese with or without a mixture of well-aged cheese, are typical examples.

pie crusts. One of the most important commercial type of unleavened bakery product. Leavening agents are not always absent from pie crust formulas; some recipes do call for small amounts of baking powder or sodium bicarbonate, but conventional and typical recipes omit such ingredients and they are not needed to obtain pie crusts having desirable eating qualities. There are several methods of merchandising pies and pie crusts, and they can determine which type of pie crust is the most desirable. Among these methods are:

(a) Raw pie crusts sold either as rolled out circles of dough or as trimmed dough fitted into foil pans. The dough-sans-pans is sold either as a frozen, refrigerated, or shelf-stable product and represents the smaller art of the market. Dough in foil pans is more convenient in some ways, but it causes inconveniences when two-crust pies are being made, because some hassle is involved in manually forming the top crust. The total amount of pie dough sold as unfilled raw crusts is though to be relatively small.

(b) Baked pie crusts. There is a low but consistent volume of sales of graham cracker and cookie crusts pressed into foil pans and offered for use available in small sizes for "tarts" and in large sizes for 20 or 25 cm pies. These crusts are not actually "baked," since the crusts themselves are merely pressure-formed from ground-up crackers or cookies which have been mixed with shortening and some other ingredients. There may be some regular unfilled backed crusts sold regionally in small amounts, but there are no brands marketed regularly on a national basis because these products are too fragile to withstand the transportation and warehousing abuse they would encounter in normal distribution channels.

(c) Unbaked pies. More crusts are sold as constituents of frozen unbaked pies than in any other form, except for crusts in bakery pies sold "fresh." The fillings in frozen pies are usually traditional pie fruits such as apple and cherry. Most frozen pies are probably sold through retail channels but there is a considerable foodservice market as well. There is also a comparatively small market for frozen unbaked "cobblers," which are deep dish, usually rectangular, fruit pies often with a top crust that is not attached to the bottom crust.

(d) Fresh baked pies. These pies are sold within a few days of baking by retail and wholesale bakeries, in bake-off sections of supermarkets, and in other outlets for purchase by consumers and foodservice customers. To reach the table in good condition, they should be sold within two or three days of baking, but many unquestionably exceed this shelf life before they are consumed.

(e) Frozen baked pies. An increasing volume of sales is developing for "thaw and eat" pies, especially cream topped pies. Some manufacturers are offering individually packaged, portion-sized slices for thawing and eating by people who do not wish to buy a whole pie. There is a considerable and increasing foodservice market for both whole and baked pies and prebaked slices in frozen form.

pilchard. Fatty fish, *Sardina (clupea) pilchardus;* young is the sardine. The average composition per 100 g is: 21.89 g protein; 10.8 g fat; 230 mg calcium; 3 mg iron; and 0.8 MJ food energy.

pilot plant. A small unit, larger than laboratory apparatus and smaller than the operating plant, of a drying, processing, or manufacturing activity. The design of a pilot plant is based on the best information available from bench, laboratory, or research results. Information from operating a pilot plant is used to evaluate the potential of a full-size operation and to provide basic information for design.

Pilsen. *See* Pilsener.

Pilsener. A kind of beer, known for its pale or light lagers. It is heavily hopped and hence has a slightly hoppy taste. It has a long-lasting head and has an alcohol content between 3.0-3.8%. It requires soft water for manufacture. Most of the beer made in India are of this type. Also known as Pilson.

pimento oil. An essential oil obtained by the steam distillation of leaves of pimento tree (pimenta officinalis). The oil has the scent resembling cloves with a touch of nutmeg and cubebs. It is an ingredient of bay rum. the dried leaves are used in sachets and pot pourri. Also known as pimenta oil; oil of allspice.

pin cherry. *Prunus penslyvanica* L.f. A kind of tree which is usually less than 9 m tall and 0.3 m in diameter. They may be shorter and look more like shrubs. The leaves range from 6-11 cm long and 2-3 cm wide. The bark is dark reddish-brown with orange marks. The leaves are shiny and yellowish-green on both sides. Color the flowers white and the cherries bright red. As the leaves appear on pin cherry trees, so do the showy flower clusters. Each flowers is attached to a long stalk and contains both male and female parts. After insect pollination, the flowers become small cherries that are eaten by many kinds of birds. This is to the tree's favour however, as the bird digests the pulpy fruit but not the inner, hard seed. Instead, many hours later and for away from the original tree, the seed is deposited unharmed on the ground and may grow into a new tree. Pin cherry trees need bright sunlight, so they are one of the first species to grow in a burned or cleared area. They prefer moist soil, but can survive in poorer soils. As fast-growing trees, pin cherries are used for fuel and pulpwood. They are also planted as nurse trees, to provide shade for younger trees.

Although the cherry tastes bitter when eaten from the tree, it can be made into tasty jelly. The red cherries are eaten by many species of birds such as grouse, pheasants, robins, waxwings, grosbeaks, and crossbills and mammals such as squirrels and chipmunks. White-tailed deer and moose eat the twigs and leaves. Fruit trees tree always useful for man and wildlife. Also known as red cherry; bird cherry; fire cherry.

pine nut. Family: *Pinaceae*. Genus: *Pinus*. Species: *Pinus pinea*. Pine nuts are a good source of protein, fats and carbohydrate and therefore excellent for body-building.

pine oil. An oil obtained from the wood of the *Pinus palustrics*, or longleaf pine, in the steam extraction of wood turpentine. It is used as a cold solvent for varnish gums and for nitrocellulose lacquers, and as a frothing agent in the floatation of ores. In paints and varnishes, it aids dispersion of metallic pigments and improves the flow. It is also used in metal polishes and in liquid and powder scrubbing soaps, as the oil is a powerful solvent of dirt and grease. When free from water, pine oil has a yellowish colour, but it is water-white when it contains dissolved water. It has an aromatic characteristic odour, and is distinct from the pine oils distilled from pine leaves and needles and used in medicine. It is used in the preparation of cleaning agent and insecticide, and is a constituent of standard gasolines for measuring detonation of engines. Pine oil is obtained mainly from old trunks and branches, and is a product formed by hydrolysis. Pine-oil disinfectants are made with steam-distilled pine oil.

Pine Power. Trade name for a preparation containing pine oil, with disinfectant properties.

pine-needle oil. An oil distilled from the Siberian fir tree, *Abies sibirica,* of northeastern Russia. It is also known as Siberian pine oil. It contains a high percentage of bornyl acetate and is used in soaps and perfumes.

pine-root oil. Pine oil derivative produced in Japan on a large scale for the manufacture of fuel oils. The terpenes of the pine oil are converted to aromatic and hydroaromatic compounds by catalytic reaction.

pine tree disinfectant cleaner 6. Trade name for a preparation containing pine oil, with disinfectant properties.

pineapple. A delicious, fragrant tropical fruit common in all markets. The pineapple is a native of South America and the West Indies and was introduced into Europe by the early Spanish explorers. It takes its name from pinya, the name of the edible nut of the Spanish pine, which it closely resembles in shape. Ordinarily the fruit is about the size of a coconut, but large specimens may weigh from sixteen to twenty pounds. The plants is a biennial. It has long pointed leaves, whose edges are in most species furnished with sharp spines. The leaves are thick and juicy. From the centre of the cluster a stem rises two or three feet and bears on its upper end a flower cluster, in the form of a conical spike. Each flower is placed in the axil of a bract, except those near the top, which develop into a cluster of small leaves, which crowns the ripened fruit. The fruit is the thickened fleshy flower stalk, and in this respect, as well as in its odour and flavour, the pineapple somewhat resembles the strawberry. The plant requires a warm climate and abundant moisture.

The fruit contains no sugar, but absorbs sugar from the stump in ripening, therefore the flavour of the fruit is greatly improved if it is allowed to ripen before picking. Its hard covering enables the pineapple to withstand more rough usage than any other tropical fruit. It will keep for a long time, and can be obtained throughout the year. These qualities, combined with its delicate flavour, make the pineapple a popular fruit. Most of the pineapples cultivated in the India are grown in southern India, where both soil and climate are especially favourable to their production. In the Philippines a beautiful fabric called pina muslin is woven of a fibre obtained from the leaves. The average composition per 100 g is: fat 0.1%; calcium 12 mg; iron 0.3 mg; vitamin A 18 mg; vitamin B_1 0.05 mg; vitamin B_2 0.12 mg; vitamin C 26 mg; and food energy 0.12 MJ.

pineapple cheese. A hard, rennet cheese, similar in shape to a pineapple, and originating in 1845 in Litchfield Country, Connecticut. It is very smooth and hard. The curd is prepared as a granular or stirred-curd cheese except that the curd is firmer. After pressing, heese is immersed in water at 45°C, after which it is hung up in loose-meshed bags to dry. While curing, the cheese may be rubbed with oil or shellacked to give a hard finish. The diagonal corrugations on its surface resemble the scales of a pineapple. **pineapple orange.** A non-blood type sweet orange. This variety was first noticed in a Florida orange grove in about 1883. The name is indicative of the aroma of the fruit. The rind is glossy and has deep-orange colour. The flavour is described as vinous and sprightly. The seeds are large and rather numerous, ranging from 13-23 in number. The fruit ranges from nearly round to slightly oblate and the size from medium to large. When fully ripened, the fruit may display a reddish tinge. Its flesh is of medium-grain, orange-yellow in colour. The Pineapple is considered to be the most highly coloured variety in Florida. The fruit has excellent processing qualities, with a juice content between 53-54%; total soluble solids content of about 10.5%. The pineapple orange is also grown in Mexico and South Africa.

pink. *Dianthus caryophyllus.* The garden pink or border carnation, romantically known as the gillyflower or July flower in Elizabethan and Victorian times, is a familiar and pretty cottage-garden plant. It grows wild in southern Europe and India, and has become naturalized in UK. The flowers may be single or double, and come in all shades of pink and red, from shell pink to carmine. The flowers have a sweet, spicy taste and are used to flavour syrups, especially for fruit salads, sauces, creams, jellies, butter, wine, fruit drinks, and salad dressings. They are candied to decorate cakes and desserts, and used to garnish salads. They may be used to scent toilet waters, and in pot pourri and herbal sleep pillows.

Pink family: *Caryophyllaceae.* Leaves of plants in this family are usually opposite and joined at the base on the stem. The flower's ovary has 2-5 carpels joined to form 1 chamber (locule) with the ovules usually in free-central placentation. This is one of the families in the subclass Carophyllidae that does not have betalain pigments. Instead there are anthocyanins. These temperate zone plants are mainly annual or perennial herbs or sometimes shrubs. The fruit is usually a one-chambered capsule with valves.

The family include: *Arenaria* (sandwort), *Dianthus* spp. (carnation, pink), *Gypsophila* (baby's-breath), *Lychnis* spp. (dusty miller, red/white campion, Maltese cross); *Cerastrium* (mouse-ear chickweed), *Scleranthus, Stellaria* (chickweed, starwort); *Dianthus armeria* (Deptford-pink); *Agrostemma githago* (corn cockle), *Drymaria pachyphylla, Saponaria vaccaria* (cow cockle), *S. officinalis* (bouncing Bet).

pink wintergreen. *Pyrola asarifolia.* Family: *Pyrolaceae.* A flowering plant. The flowers are about one cm wide, the stems are 15 cm high or more. It is common across North America. The sepals are red, the petals are rosy-pink, the style is red. The fruit is a round capsule containing innumerable tiny seeds. The plant also spreads by creeping underground stems. The leaves of this plant are similar to those of a pear tree and the generic name means "little pear." The plant grows in patches from underground stems where it is cool, damp, and shady.

Pinot Blanc grape. A variety of grape, planted mainly in Alsace, France, Germany, and Italy. It yields white wine of good quality.

Pinot Gris grape. A variety of grape related to the other members of Pinot varieties. The rose-gray grape yield white wines. Its plantings are rather widespread, including Alsace, California, France, Germany, Hungary, Italy, Luxembourg, and Rumania. It is called Rulander in Germany. Sometimes it is incorrectly referred to as Tokay.

Pinot Noir grape. A variety of grape, regarded by most authorities as one of the superior red wine grapes. It is the basis for excellent red wines and is also used in Champagnes. Its plantings are widespread and, in addition to France, are found in Alsace, Australia, California, Canada (hybrid is used), Hungary, and Italy.

pint, reputed. 13½ fluid oz.

Piora cheese. A kind of hard, cow's milk or goat's milk cheese with small eyes; made in the Swiss Alps.

pipe. Cask for wine of volume that varies with the type of wine, e.g., port, 115 gallons; Teneriffe, 100; Marsala, 93.

pipecolic acid. Piperidine-2-carboxylic acid. It occurs in fresh green beans, potatoes and mushrooms, in fresh fruit and the dried seed of legumes. Its pharmacological effects are still under investigation.

pistachio. Family: *Anarcardiaceae.* Genus: *Pistacia.* Species: *Pistacia vera.* Pistachio nuts are a good source of protein and contain several vitamins including A and B_1. They are fairly rich in potassium and phosphorus and have small amounts of iron and calcium.

Pitcher-plant family: *Sarraceniaceae.* Although three are only 3 genera in this family, these perennial herbs of the bog are of interest for their unusual insect-trap leaves. Forming in a basal rosette, the modified leaves digest insects for nutritional nitrogen. The bisexual flower consists of 4 to 5 sepals, 5 petals or none, numerous stamens, and 1 pistil. The style is lobed or expands into an umbrella-shape. A loculicidal capsule is formed from 3-5 carpels. The family include: *Darlingtonia, Heliamphora, Sarracenia.*

pits. Stones from cherries, plums, peach, and apricots. The oil is extracted from these pits and used in cosmetics, pharmaceuticals, canning sardines and as table oil. The press cake left behind contains the bitter amygdalin.

pizza. There are hundreds of pizza variations. Some are yeast-leavened, some are chemically leavened. Some are baked, some are fried. There are thick, thin, and medium pizzas, any of which can be found in rectangular or circular versions. The dough can be breadlike or crackerlike, spiced or plain. Fillings can be on top or inside. The kinds of toppings are limited only by the imagination: pizzas topped with tomato, meat, fish, shellfish, cheese, vegetables, the ever popular anchovy, even fruit-in every conceivable combination, are being sold.

pizza toppings. Most pizza toppings are based on a spicy tomato sauce and pieces of cheese. Nearly all pizzerias purchase the sauce already made, and many frozen pizza manufacturers purchase at least the basic sauces in bulk quantities from tomato canneries, although they may added other materials (such as spices and chopped vegetables) to the tomato product before applying the sauce to the pizza. Both pizzerias and mass producers often buy the topping ingredients in sliced or chopped form from specialized suppliers to the trade, though other go to the extreme of buying whole sausages, raw hamburger, fresh vegetables, and whole cheeses for further processing in their plant.

plansifter. A nest of sieves mounted together so that material being sieved is divided into a number of fractions of different size; widely used in flour milling.

plant conservation. There are numerous species of flowering plants in existence today. About a third of these are native to temperate regions, the rest are found in the tropics. A vast number of tropical plants are in danger of extinction in the wild within the next hundred years because the human populations of most tropical countries continue to double every 20-25 years and the forests are being cleared for wood and marginal cultivation. About 24% of the Amazon forest has been cleared by 1975, and at least 25 million additional acres are being cleared each year. We know so little of the plants of the tropics that many have not even been given a scientific name. Whatever samples of these plants are preserved may well be all we shall be able to pass on to our descendents in the 21st century and beyond.

In temperate regions, about 5% of the 85,000 native species are in current danger of extinction. Habitat destruction is only one problem. Overgrazing by domestic animals, use of fertilizers and herbicides, introduction of foreign plants without their natural controls, and destruction of insect, bird, and bat pollinators all can endanger plants. Of the approximately 20,000 species, subspecies, and varieties of native higher plants of the continental US, at least 10% are of much concern. About 100 species are recently (within the last 200 years) extinct or presumed extinct, about 750 endangered (currently in danger of extinction throughout all or a significant portion of their range), and more than 1200 threatened (likely to become endangered within the foreseeable future).

plant growth regulator. A chemical which modifies plant growth in a manner beneficial to the farmer. The natural plant growth-promoting substance, gibberellic acid, is obtained from the fungus *Gibberella fujikoroi* (Sawada). Six gibberellins, A_1, A_2, A_3, A_4, A_7 and A_9, have been isolated from filtrates of the fungus. Chemically gibberellins are the tetracyclic diterpenes. They are more highly functional than other groups of terpenoids. These compounds are produced in minute quantities within plants where they act as hormones of various developmental processes. Gibberellin-like compounds occur in higher plants. They are responsible for the development, maturation, budding, flower formation, fruit ripening and various other growth processes. Substances like 2,4-D and 2,4,5-T also possess auxin-like activity, but they are more effective as herbicides.

The plant growth regulators can be classified in three categories:

(a) Chemicals which have a direct visible effect which is of value to the farmer by reducing labour costs, facilitating cultivation and harvesting or producing some other economically advantageous effect. Such effects might include the promotion or retardation of vegetative growth, rapid crop establishment and shortening of the growing season, control of fruit fixing, setting, abscission and quality, defoliation and prevention of flowering.

(b) Chemicals which increase crop yields either by modifying the morphology or growth of the plant or by affecting the metabolism of the plant.

(c) Chemicals which affect morphology, growth or metabolism in such a way as to provide greater protection to the plant against environmental effects such as drought, heat, cold, soil salinity, vulnerability to weather damage, or susceptibility to atmospheric pollutants.

One reason why plant growth regulators have been the subject of less research effort than herbicides is that their screening and evaluation is much more difficult than that of herbicides. In herbicidal screening, selective toxic effects are sought by applying the chemical to a range of major crop plants and major weeds. In many cases, the results of such tests are clear and unambiguous and the precise pattern of selective toxicity which is observed indicates where the commercial opportunities are likely to be. For plant growth regulators, however, the botanist is being asked to observe any unusual effect of the chemical on the habit of growth or metabolism of any crop plant and then to equate those observations to a field situation in which such an effect could be of economic value to the grower. The difficulty is essentially of defining a manageable number of targets and of setting up a screening system which would be comprehensive for those targets yet not too large, expensive and resource-demanding. A further problem is that, at the moment, it is very difficult to predict from effects observed in the glasshouse exactly what effects will be produced in the field on the total crop, so that candidate plant growth regulators have to be field tested at an early stage, and this makes great demands on money, time and effects of skilled staff. Furthermore, plant growth regulators may have to be tested over a number of seasons

since a desirable effect produced in one season, e.g. increased yield of fruit, might possibly be offset by a swing back in the following seasons, or some long-term deleterious effects might be induced. Obviously, this is more of a problem with established perennial crops, such as orchards or vineyards, than with annual crops.

Toxicity and residue studies have to be far-reaching since a useful plant growth regulator, in order to produce a lasting effect, might be required to persist for some time within the plant. The cost of discovery and development of a plant growth regulator is, therefore, very high and it is likely to be economical to develop and sell a particular compound only if there is a large potential international market in a major crop. Because of the possibility of long-term effects, profitable markets are more likely to be in annuals than in perennials. There are a very large number of biological effects which might be the basis for commercially useful plant growth regulators. however, it must be remembered that, long before the idea of chemical plant growth regulators was conceived, man was attempting to produce plants which grow in the way most beneficial to him by plant breeding. This has been a highly successful approach and high-yielding crop varieties have been developed from poor-yielding natural species. Modern methods of plant breeding and the application of genetic engineering should increase the output of plant breeders and cut down the time scale for establishment of new varieties. Nevertheless, there will still be a place for plant growth regulators. It is very unlikely that all desirable qualities can be bred into one variety of a crop plant and, in practice, improvement in one aspect often induces of disadvantage in another. Thus many high-yielding crop varieties are much more susceptible to disease than the natural stock. The choice may therefore be between breeding for yield and using pesticides to control diseases or breeding for disease resistance and using plant growth regulators to increase yields.

plantain. A variety of banana with higher starch and lower sugar content than dessert bananas, picked when flesh is too hard to be eaten raw and used for cooking. Some varieties become sweet if left to ripen, others never develop a high sugar content. The average composition per 100 g of plantain is: 1 g protein; 0.2 g fat; 33 g carbohydrate; 0.05 mg iron; 31 µg vitamin A; 0.04 mg vitamin B_1; 0.06 mg vitamin B_2; 0.6 mg nicotinic acid; 20 mg vitamin C; and 0.05 MJ food energy.

plasma proteins. The proteins dissolved in blood plasma. In vertebrates such proteins include albumins, alpha-, beta-, and gamma-globulins (including immunoglobulins which constitute the majority of anti-bodies), transferrins, and proteins involved in blood clotting. The plasma proteins confer on the plasma a colloidal osmotic pressure which is important in osmoregulatory control. In solution in the blood plasma, main types are:
fibrinogen (0.2-0.4 g/100 ml);
albumin (4.4-5.3 g/100 ml); and
globulin (1.9-2.8 g/100 ml).

plasma, blood. Blood consists of red cells, white cells of platelets, suspended in a clear protein solution, the plasma. Plasma proteins include fibrinogen, albumins and globulins. Of the 9% total plasma solids, 7% are proteins.

plasmapheresis. Experimental method of reducing the serum proteins to a low level by removing part of the blood and returning only the red cells to the blood stream.

Plasmon. Trade name for a yellowish powder prepared by treatment of the curd precipitated from skim milk with sodium bicarbonate. The compound is kneaded in atmosphere of carbon dioxide and reduced to a soluble powder- the sodium salt of casein.

plastic cream. A highly concentrated cream containing about 80% fat. It is plastic in form, much the same as butter. In spite of its high fat concentration, the fat remains in substantially its original emulsion with the solids-not-fat present in the serum. Plastic cream is produced commercially by the use of a separator designed for skimming a very rich cream. Either whole sweet milk or sweet cream testing 40% fat or less may be used. After separating, the :am is quickly cooled and packed in butter tubs. Plastic Cream is used in the manufacture of butter, ice cream, coffee cream, cream cheese and other dairy products.

plastic curd. *See* pasta filata.

plate count. To estimate the number of bacteria in a sample it is poured on to an agar plate when each bacterial cell or group of cells multiplies to produce a colony which is visible to the naked eye. A count of the number of colonies gives the number of colonies gives the number of bacteria in that portion of the sample that was taken. Pasteurized milk contains about 100,000 bacteria/ml, good-quality raw milk contains less than 500,000/ml.

platelet. A small blood cell that is important in blood clotting (coagulation), thrombosis, and inflammation. The role of platelets in coagulation involves not only stopping bleeding after trauma, but also maintaining the general integrity of blood vessels in the face of wear imposed by blood pressure. Platelets are formed by the fragmentation of megakaryocyte cytoplasm in the bone marrow. They lack a nucleus, but possess granules containing a variety of enzymes, ADP, and 5-hydrozytryptamine (5-HT). Their cytoplasm also contains a contractile protein, thrombasthenin, and their cell membrane a phospholipid known as platelet factor 3. When platelets contact a damaged area in a blood vessel they first adhere to it and then initiate the so-called 'platelet release reaction', giving out ADP, 5-HT, and other cell contents. The formation of thrombin, a blood coagulation factor, also causes this release. ADP encourages the aggregation of platelets, during which further ADP is formed as part of a self-promoting response; the resultant aggregation is then irreversible. However, low concentrations of ADP can induce reversible adhesion without causing the platelet release reaction. The adhered platelets serve to plug the damaged blood vessel. At this stage the components of the blood coagulation systsem are activated by platelet factor 3, with the production of thrombin (and thus the further stimulation of platelet aggregation) and ultimately the formation of fibrin, the principal noncellular component of blood clots. Prostaglandins and thromboxane are also manufactured by activated platelets. In addition to mediating inflammation, these substances promote platelet release reactions and aggregation. Also known as thrombocyte.

platform dryer. A device for removal of moisture on which crops are placed over openings through which air is forced. The openings are provided in the top of a level platform. Products may be in bulk or placed in sacks or bags.

plenum. An air chamber maintained under pressure, either negative or positive, usually connected to one or more distributing ducts or false floor in a drying or aeration system. The term is also used to designate the air chamber under the perforated floor in a grain bin and the pressure chamber between grain columns in some types of batch or continuous dryers.

pluck. Butchers' term for heart, liver and lungs of an animal.

plums. Numerous species of *Prunus*. The common European plums are *P. domestica;* blackthorn or sloe is *P. spinosa;* bullace is *P. insititia;* damson is *P. damascena;* gages are *P. italica.* Plums are the most diverse and widely distributed of all stone fruits, with varieties suitable to almost any climatic condition; in fact, they are grown on every continent except Antarctica. Most commercially grown plums are descendants of either European or Japanese varieties. The European plums, oval or round in shape, include all the purple to black varieties as well as the smaller, greenish yellow, richly flavoured Green Gage. The small, bluish-black Damson is prized for jams and preserves. The larger, dark-purple Stanley is usually eaten as fresh fruit. The Japanese varieties are larger, with yellow to red skins and juicy flesh-like the crimson Santa Rosa. Prumes are the firm-fleshed variety of plums with a high enough sugar content to permit drying without fermentation around the pit. Plums contain small amounts of protein, carbohydrate and fat. The average composition per 100 g is: 100 µg vitamin A; 0.5 mg nicotinic acid, and 5 mg vitamin C.

pneumatic conveying. Transfer of material in powder form by means of air currents. Applied to flour, sugar, cements, etc.

pneumátic dryer. A device for removing moisture from products in which small particles, chopped, ground, or pulverized products, are conveyed by the drying heated air with temperatures up to 750°C. The material is dried almost instantaneously in a turbulent stream of hot air, which also acts as conveyor system. it is applicable to powdered, granular and flaky materials, and used for drying fine chemical powders, starch, fruit pulp, distilling wastes, and crops. Also known as pneumatic conveying dryer.

pneumatic ring dryer. A pneumatic dryer in which the product travels several times through a ring duct, impelled by hot air, and the drying time, temperature and rate of flow of the material can be controlled; used for starch, mashed potatoes, cereals, flour, powdered soups.

pod corn. A variety of corn which is the botanical curiosity, in which each kernel is contained within a pod or husk. A husk also covers the ear. The corn is classified as heterozygous. When planted is contained within a pod or husk. A husk also covers the ear. The corn is classified as heterozygous. When planted is segregates in a ratio of 1:2:1, namely, one normal type.

podophyllum. The dried rhizome and roots of *Podophyllum peltatum* Linn. Podophyllum contains resin (3.5-6%) whose active principles are lignans. The important lignans are podophyllotoxin (20%), β-peltatin (10%) and α-peltatin (5%) occurring in free state and as glucoside. In addition to these lignans, other closely related compounds like dimethyl podophyllotoxin and glucoside, desoxypodophyllotoxin and podophyllotoxone are present in the drug. All these compounds possess cytotoxic or antitumour activity. Treatment of lignans with alkali produces epimerization with formation of the stable *cis*-isomers which are physiologically inactive. Picropodophyllin, quercetin and peltatins are also present in podophyllum. Indian podophyllum contains excess amount of resin (6-12%) and the concentration of podophyllotoxin is up to 40%. No peltains are reported but the other constituents are almost the same as reported in American *Podophyllum*.

POEMS. Abbreviation for polyoxyethylene monostearate.

poikilotherms. Cold-blooded animals, those whose temperature varies with their environment.

polar lipids. The lipids present in the outer, or plasma, membrane of many cells, as well as in the membranes of intracellular organelles such as mitochondria and chloropiasts. All membranes contain polar lipids, which make up from 20-80% of the membrane mass, depending upon the type of membrane; the remainder is mostly protein. Like soaps, the polar lipids are amphipathic. In aqueous systems polar lipids spontaneously disperse to form micelles, in which the hydrocarbon tails of the lipids are hidden from the aqueous environment and the electrically charged hydrophilic heads are exposed on the surface, facing the aqueous medium. Such micelles may contain thousands of lipid molecules. Polar lipids readily form very thin bilayers separating two aqueous compartments.

pole bean. Any of the numerous varities of garden beans of the running, twining type (as contrasted with the bush types) that are cultivated by placing poles or wires in the field or garden to conserve space and add to the yield and convenience of picking. In some regions, the term is used to designate bean plants such as certain string and snap beans.

Polenske value. An expression used to designate the amount of volatile fatty acids, insoluble in water, that may be present in a fat or oil. It represents the number of cubic centimetres of 0.1 normal alkali required to neutralize the water insoluble, volatile fatty acids from 5 g of fat. Polenske value of butterfat is 1.5-3.5; other animal fats are much lower than this value, while vegetable oil like coconut oil are much higher.

polenta. Kind of porridge made from maize meal, common dish in Italy often with cheese added.

pollock *Pollachius virens.* A kind of fish which has about the same commercial significance as the haddock. In body shape, fin position and size it resembles the Atlantic cod, but other characteristics clearly distinguish it. The lower jaw protrudes somewhat and has a very small barb. The dark coloured mouth is also a distinctive feature. The pollock is a pelagic predator which, as a fast and skilled swimmer, feeds chiefly on schooling fishes, especially herring. However, its extensive migrations follow less well-established routes than those of other codfishes. Its inconstant, changing life habits making following its growth dynamics difficult, which adds to the difficulties of pollock fishermen. The fish can reach an age of 18-20 years. It attains sexual maturity in 4-5 years and thereafter spawns each spring in practically the same region as haddock. The eggs and larvae drift with the current and the young migrate into coastal waters after their pelagic development period. They spend their first year in coastal waters. Also known as the saithe or blister-back.

polrphyra. Red alga cultivated in Japan to make "Komba". In UK it is collected from the sea to make laverbread.

polyamines. Amines with more than two amino groups, such as spermidine and spermine. that were first found in semen (hence their names), but in fact they occur in most tissues. They are powerful growth stimulators of microorganisms and cultured mammalian cells. They exert several actions on nucleic acid metabolism which probably underlie their effects on growth. Spermidine and spermine are synthesized in the body from the amino acid ornithine.

polycythaemia. Increase in the number of red blood cells; results from hard and tough physical exercise, residence at high altitudes, administration of drugs or cobalt, and certain diseases.

polymyxins. A group of antibacterial polypeptide antibiotics produced by the growth of different strains of the soil bacterium *Bacillus polymyxa.* They are polypeptides, active against coliform bacteria; apart from clinical use they are of value in controlling infection in brewing. They are denoted by letters and numbers, *i.e.*, polymyxins A, B_1, B_2, C, D_1, D_2, E_1, E_2, M. Of these only polymyxin B (*i.e.*, B_1+B_2) and polymyxin E (*i.e.*, E_1+E_2, also called colistin) are sufficiently non-toxic for therapeutic use. Polymyxins are bactericidal on mot Gramnegative bacteria. They act by binding to the plasma membrane and causing leakage of essential small molecules.

polyols. Sugar alcohol such as glycerol sorbitol, inositol, etc.

polyose. Polysaccharide.

polyoxyethylene. The monoglycerides are soluble in fat, but by treatment with ethylene oxide the resulting polyoxyethylene derivatives become water-soluble to the desired limit. The compounds are polyoxyethylene esters, ethers, sorbitol esters,, etc. They are valuable as emulsifying agents in bakery. One of the best known is polyoxyethylene stearate, used as a crumb-softener.

polypeptide. A peptide comprising ten or more amino acids. Polypeptides that constitute proteins usually contain 100-300 amino acids. Shorter ones include certain antibiotics, such as, gramicidin, and some hormones, like ACTH, which has 39 amino acids. The properties of a polypeptide are determined by the type and sequence of its constituent amino acids.

polyphagia. Excessive or continuous eating.

polyphosphates. Complex phosphates added to foods, in particular to meat products; they prevent sausage discoloration, aid mixing of the fat, speed penetration of the brine in curing, cause protein fibres of meat to retain more water and swell, and thus improving the texture. They include pyrophosphate ($Na_4P_2O_7$), tripolyphosphate ($Na_5P_3O_{10}$), and longer phosphate chains of 100 phosphate units, polyphosphate glasses prepared by rapid quenching of $Na_2O-P_2O_5$ melts such as Calgon, which has 12 unit chain length.

polysaccharide. Any of a group of carbohydrates comprising long chains of monosaccharide (simple sugar) molecules. Homopolysaccharides consist of only one type of monosaccharide; heteropolysaccharides contain two or more different types. Polysaccharides may have molecular masses of up to several million and are often highly branched. Some important examples are starch, glycogen, and cellulose.

Polysaccharides are produced by a wide variety of microorganisms. Those of primary industrial interest are found on the outside of the microbial cell wall and membrane and are called exopolysaccharides. They occur in two distinct forms: attached to the microbial cells that synthesize them as discrete physical structures termed as capsules; or secreted from the cell into the surrounding environment in the form of soluble slime.

polytene. Describing the chromosomes condition caused by chromatids not separating after duplication. It leads to the formation of giant chromosomes consisting of numerous identical chromatids lying parallel to each other. Giant chromosomes have characteristic bands, which are thought to relate to the arrangement of genes along the chromosome, and they are used to study gene activity and make chromosomes maps. Polytene chromosomes are common in the salivary gland cells of dipterous insects, e.g., Drosophila.

pomace. Residue of crushed apple pulp after expressing juice; also applied to any pressed fruit pulp and to fish from which oil has been expressed.

pombe. African beer prepared from millet seed. The seed is sprouted to break down the starch to fermentable sugar, a process similar to malting in beer manufacture, and then allowed to ferment spontaneously.

pome. Botanical term for type of fruit, represented by apple, pear and quince.

pomegranate. Punica granatum. The pomegranate grows wild as a shrub in its native southern Asia and in hot areas of the world. Under cultivation, it's native southern Asia and in hot areas of the world. Under cultivation, it is trained as a tree to grow upward to 7 metres in height, being grown in Asia, the Mediterranean region, South America and the southern states of US. The slender, often spiny-tipped branches bear opposite, oblong or oval-lanceolate, shiny leaves about 2-5 cm long. 1-5 large, red or orange-red flowers grow together on the tips of the shoots. The brownish-yellow to red fruit about the size of an orange, is a thick-shinned, several celled, many-selled berry; each seed is surrounded by red, acid pulp. Juice contained in a pulpy sac surrounding each of a mass of seeds; outer skin contains tannin and therefore bitter. Sweet juice used to prepare grenadine syrup for alcoholic and fruit drinks. The average composition per 100 g is: water 81%; protein 1%; carbohydrate 17%; iron 0.7 mg; vitamin B$_1$ 0.02 mg; vitamin B$_2$ 0.02 mg; nicotinic acid 0.21 mg; vitamin C 9 mg; and food energy 0.3 MJ.

pomelo. Alternative name shadock; *Citrus grandis* from which the grapefruit is descended. Also spelled pomeloe; pummelo.

pomes. Botanical name for fruit formed by the enlargement of the receptacle which becomes fleshy and surrounds the carpels, *e.g.*, apple, pear.

Ponceau colours. A series of strawberry colours, used in food industry:

Ponceau MX is the disodium salt of 1-2(2,4- or mixed xylazo)-2-naphthol-3-disulphonic acid; also called Ponceau R and 2R and RS.

· Ponceau 4R is the trisodium salt of 1-(4-sulpho-1-naphthylazo)-2-naphthol-6,8-disulphonic acid; also called Cochineal red A. Ponceau SX is the

disodium salt of 2-(5-sulpho-2,4-xylyazo)-1-naphthol-4-sulphonic acid; called Red No. 4 in US.

Ponceau 3R is the disodium salt of 1-pseudocumylazo-2-naphthol-3,6-disulphonic acid. It is called Red No. 1 in US; Marachino cherry red colour.

Ponceau 6R is the tetra sodium salt of 2-(6'-sulpho-1'-*m*-xylylazo)-1-naphthol-5-sulphonic acid.

ponderal index. An index of adipose tissue; height divided by the cube root of the body weight; high for thin people, low for fat people.

ponderocrescive. Food tending to increase weight; easily gaining weight; opposite to pondoperditive, stimulating weight loss.

Ponkan mandarin. A variety of one of the ancient varieties of mandarin native to the Far East and mainly grown in the region-with plantings in China, India, and Pakistan. However, centuries ago, the variety extended west into various countries of the Near East and is also found elsewhere in the citrus belt. The fruit is rather large, globose, with a thin, loosely adherent and orange-colored rind. Maturity occurs in early mid-season. The fruit is juicy, with a fine flavor. A closely related variety (Indian) is found in Iraq. The Ponkan is somewhat less cold resistant than most mandarins and the fruit lose their quality and the rind puffs if they are not picked when ripe. The variety is self fruitful.

pont PEveque cheese. A kind of soft cheese made in Normandy, France. Mold ripened similar to camembert, but higher temperature, shorter coagulation, draining, and curing periods are used. Cheese is washed while curing, there is less growth of greyish-white surface mold and body is firmer and deeper yellow in colour than Camebert. The average composition is: moisture 45-50%; fat 25.3-28%.

Poona cheese. A kind of whole-milk, smear ripened, soft cheese said to have been made originally in New York State. The cheese has a Limburger like aroma, and a reddish smear on the surface. It is cured in 6 weeks.

poonac. The residue of coconut after the extraction of the oil.

popcorn. *Zea everta.* A variety of corn which has very hard, small, elongated oval grains which, when heated, explode into a white, fluffy, edible mass that requires no further cooking. Some corns of this type are cultivated for stock feeding and also as sources for starch and glucose. The American Indians considered popcorn an excellent foodstuff for use during long journeys.

popovers. A type of hot bread having typically an extremely coarse and irregular grain, the interior being formed of a few large cells. Water vapor contributes the greater part of the leavening action, although entrapped air also has some effect. Neither chemical leaveners nor yeast is used in these products.

Popover batters are made from a simple formula and procedure. In an average formula, about 85-130 parts by weight of liquid whole eggs and 200 parts of liquid whole milk will be used for each 100 parts of flour. Small amounts of shortening, salt, and flavorings constitute the remainder of the batter. Bread flour is generally used, and it should be sifted. Popover batter should be deposited in muffin tins or in specially designed pans. The cavities are filled about one-third full of batter. Before the batter is added, the pans are greased and placed in the oven to heat. These utensils should be heavy-walled to provide a good initial source of heat and should be transferred to the oven immediately after they are filled, as it is essential for the batter to undergo a rapid temperature increase if it is to expand properly.

poppy. Family: *Papaveraceae*. Genus: *Papaver*. Species. *Papaver somniferum* (opium poppy); *Papaver rhoeas* (corn poppy); *Papaver nudicaule* (Iceland poppy); *Papaver orientale* (oriental poppy). Although the part of the poppy most used for medicinal purposes is the petals of the corn (or red) poppy and the capsules of the opium poppy, the seeds have been used to treat intestinal disorders and to keep bowel movements regular.

The poppyseed is inappropriately classified as a nut. It is true that such a classification cannot be justified on a botanical basis. Many writers have included poppyseeds in their discussion of species, which makes even less sense. Poppyseeds are included in bakery products for their effects on appearance and texture. Their contribution to flavour is not particularly significant, which would seem to rule out their positioning as spices and quasi-spices. Poppyseeds are tiny (less than 1 mm diameter) seeds of a plant of the poppy family. They are used in bakery products both as the whole seed and crushed or ground with other ingredients to form pastes. The seeds are slightly crunchy and they have a somewhat nutty aroma and taste. Edible poppyseeds generally contain 6.8% moisture, 19.0 protein, 44.7% fat, 23.7% total carbohydrate (6.3% fiber), 6.8% ash.

Blue poppyseed, a type made famous by the Dutch, is considered the highest quality. There is a Federal Specification for poppy seed that describes it as the clean, dried, seed *of Papaver somniferum* L., having an agreeable nutty taste free from evidence of rancidity.

pork carcass. The average composition per 100 g of pork is:

Fat- protein 8.8%; fat 49%; iron 1.1 mg; vitamin B 0.31 mg; and food energy 2.0 MJ.

Medium- protein 10.4%; fat 39%; iron 1.2 mg; vitamin B_1 0.36 mg; vitamin B_2 0.10 mg; nicotinic acid 2.4 mg; and food energy 1.65 MJ.

Lean- protein 11.8%; fat 29%; kcal 312 (1.32 MJ), iron 1.4 mg; vitamin B_1 0.41 mg; vitamin B_2 0.12 mg; nicotinic acid 2.7 mg; and food energy 1.3MJ.

porphyrin. Any of a group of related organic compounds characterized by the possession of a cyclic group of four linked nitrogen-containing rings (a pyrrole nucleus). Porphyrins differ in the nature of their side-chain groups. Examples of such metalloporphyrins are the iron porphyrins (*e.g.,* haem in haemoglobin) and the magnesium porphyrin, chlorophyll, the photosynthetic pigment in plants. In nature, majority of metalloporphyrins are conjugated to proteins to form a number of very important molecules, *e.g.,* haemoglobin, myoglobin, and the cytochromes.

porphyropsin. Photosensitive pigment in the retinas of the eyes of freshwater fish, containing dehydroretinol that is analogous to rhodopsin in the eyes of marine fish, mammals, birds and amphibians.

port du Salut Cheese. A variety of cheese developed in 1865 by Trappist Monks a Port du Salut, Department of Mayenne, France. It is now made by Trappist monks in many countries who have kept the exact process secret. Similar cheese is made outside the monasteries. Port du Salut is similar to Pont Peveque with its Gouda-like or Limburger like flavour. The cheese is flat the cylindrical, being 25 cm in diameter and 5 cm thick. It is both brine salted and dry salted, and smear ripened.

Portugieser (Blauer) **grape.** A variety of blue grape which was introduced into Germany around 1800 from the Danube region. The grape is deep blue and the vine is modest in its demands of site and soil. It grows mainly in the Ahr, Rhenish Palatinate, Wurttemberg, and Rheinhessen wine-producing regions of Germany. The grape ripens early. Yields a pleasant "little wine" (Carafe wine); light, agreeable, mild. The wine is red. Of vineyard areas in Germany, this grape represents about 4.9% of total.

port wine. A type of wine manufactured in a closely specified area of the Upper Dour Valley in Northern Portugal. It is illegal in England to sell wine as 'Port' unless it comes from Portugal. However, it is no so in other countries like Germany, the US, Australia, Canada and South Africa where large amounts of 'Port' wines are manufactured. Fermentation of the grapes is continued for two days, and brandy is added to stop the fermentation. A sweet called 'Jeropiga' is added which gives the 'Port' wine its unique taste. Port wine, has a deep purple-red colour with about 20% alcohol and 6-8% of sugar.

portable dryer. An apparatus for moisture removal which can be readily moved on wheels or skids or can be easily carried. Commercial portable dryers may be moved from one location of another for use but are not commonly used for drying except in a stationary position. A hand-held hair dryer is portable but products are not moved through the dryer.

Porter wine. A dark brown ale with a heavy foam. It is less hoppy and slightly sweeter than pale ale. Its alcohol content is about 5%.

posset. A drink made from hot milk curdled with ale or wine, and is sometimes thickened with breadcrumbs and spiced. Formerly it was used as remedy for colds.

positive staining. A staining technique, used in electron microscopy, in which components of the sample are visualized through their binding of an electron-dense material; the staining of nucleic acids with uranyl acetate and the staining of antigens with ferritin-labeled antibodies are two examples.

positive supercoiling. Supercoiling of a DNA duplex in the same direction as the double helix itself is wound. Thus the normal b form of DNA is a right-handed double helix, and its further positive supercoiling will be right-handed.

Postum, instant. Trade name for a preparation of bran, wheat and molasses consumed as a beverage.

potassium. One of the essential elements in plants and animals. It is absorbed by plant roots as the potassium ion, K^+, and in plants is the most abundant electropositive ion in the cell sap. Potassium ions are required in high concentration in the cell for efficient protein synthesis, and for glycolysis in which they are an essential cofactor for the enzyme pyruvate kinase. In animals the gradient of potassium and sodium ions across the cell membrane is responsible for the potential difference across the membrane, which is important for the transmission of nerves impulses.

potato. English wine measure of half a gallon.

potato. Family: *Solanaceae.* Genus: *Solanum.* Species: *Solanum tuberosum.* White potatoes were first cultivated by South American Indians in the high Andes, and later taken to England in 1586 by Sir Francis Drake. From there their cultivation spread to Ireland, continental Europe and finally, in 1719 to the American colonies. Modern potatoes, the best of which are a far cry from the small, floury originals, fall into three general groups. New potatoes are the tender, thin-skinned ones usually harvested during late winter and early spring; they are used for boiling, creaming and potato salads. All-purpose potatoes like the Red Pontiac can be boiled, mashed, baked or fried. And the famous Idaho, or Russet, is a popular baking potato. Yams and sweet potatoes are often confused. Both are edible tubers, but they are from different plant families. Yams probably originated in West Africa; whereas, sweet potatoes, like squash, are native New World vegetables.

Contrary to public myth, potatoes need be neither boring nor fattening. Potatoes are super abundant in potassium and vitamin C (although this falls rapidly by spring if a potato is stored all winter). They are 80% water, 2% protein, wonderfully fibrous, and if the skins are left on, also very filling. It is the oil, milk or butter used to dress them that makes them so lethal for calorie-counters. Because potatoes are floury and moist and contain only 0.1% of fat they guzzle, fat as readily as spongy muffins and the modest amount of fat people usually put in mashed potatoes makes the calories rocket by 50%. The chip is three times more calorific than the boiled potato. Potato crisps are seven times more calorific, weight for weight.

Only by spooning neat butter straight into the mouth could one ingest more calories. They contain 250-290 calories per 100 grams, less than the same weight of dried toast (300 calories), water-biscuits (440 calories) and starched-reduced crispbread (380 calories). Baking a potato is the least calorific and most nourishing way to serve it. The skin as well because it harbors most of the nutrients, like iron, phosphorus, calcium, sodium, sulphur, potassium, vitamins B and C and traces of carotene. Add a tablespoon of yoghurt, sprinkle generously with fresh parsley, and you have a positive powerhouse of nourishing goodness.

Nutritionists recognize that all foods eaten in excess are fattening. Actually potatoes are less fattening, pound for pound, than most items in the daily Indian diet. For example, about 5 kg of potatoes are required to produce 0.45 kg of body fat, or about the same amount as milk, canned corn, canned peaches, or frozen peas. On the same basis, the "fattening" tendency of potatoes is about 10% that of margarine, 20% that of dry cereals, 33% that of bread, and 50% that of beef or hamburger. Potatoes alone actually are comparatively low in calories per unit of weight. Needless to say, the butter, fats, oils, etc. used in preparing potatoes, as with any other foods, greatly enhances the total of calories. A well-recognized fact in many parts of the world is that the potato provides a low-cost source of energy. It is also worth pointing out that some nutritionists often fail to stress the significant amounts of low-cost vitamins and minerals provided by the potato.

potato, sweet. Tubers of herbaceous climbing plant *Ipomea batatas.* The flesh may be white, yellow or pink (if carotene is present); the leaves are also edible. Sweet potatoes come in many varieties but are of two basic types; the dry fleshed, with pale-yellow flesh; and the moist fleshed, with deep-yellow to orange-red flesh (often incorrectly called a yam). The common name (*D. sativa*) and the 10 months yam (*D. alata*) are both widely cultivated throughout the South Pacific and have been known to reach weights of up to 25 kg. They can be baked, boiled, roasted and fried, or used raw in salads. The average composition per 100 g of sweet potato is: protein 1.1%; fat 0.3%; iron 0.8 mg; vitamin A 150 μg; vitamin B_1 0.08 mg; vitamin B_2 0.04 mg; nicotinic acid 0.5 mg; vitamin C 19 mg; and food energy 0.4 MJ.

potato, explosin-puffing. Explosion-puffing of potatoes is carried out after potato pieces have been reduced to about 25% moisture by conventional hot-air drying. During explosion-puffing at an elevated pressure and in a stream of superheated steam, the water within the partially dried pieces is rapidly brought to a temperature above its atmospheric boiling point. When the pieces are instantly brought to atmospheric pressure, a fraction of the water flashes into steam, creating a porous structure. After puffing, the potato pieces are dried by conventional means to 3-4% moisture.

potato, frozen French-fried. Frozen potato products consist largely of frozen French fries, but there are other frozen products, such as diced potatoes, mashed, hash brown, potato puffs, au gratin, rissole, cakes, shreds, and dehydrofrozen products (partial dehydration combined with freezing). Flavour is especially important in these products. Intensive research continues to improve the flavour and texture of these products after they have been thawed and cooked. In making frozen French fries, the potatoes are first peeled with lye or steam. Abrasion peeling results in excessive losses. Potatoes which have unpeeled area, black spots and decayed portions, are trimmed by hand or sorted out. Potatoes are then cut into strips, the most popular size having a cross-section of 9 x 9 mm; 12 x 12 mm. Prior to frying, the strips are blanched in hot water to give a more uniform color of fried product, to reduce fat absorption, reduced frying time, and improve texture. Two blanchers usually are used. The first blancher uses hot water; the second blench uses a dilute dextrose solution. Blanched strips are then moved to and through the fryer, using temperatures 177-190.5°C. Excess fat is then removed by passing the fries over a vibrating screen. After this, the product is frozen and packaged (or vice versa). Extrusion French fries are now being thoroughly researched.

potato, Irish. Tuber of *Solanum tuberosum*. Although commonly classed as a carbohydrate food, potato contains 80% water; its main contribution to the diet is vitamin C. The high vitamin C content of new potatoes falls during storage. The average composition per 100 g is: protein 1.6%; fat 0.1%; Ccalcium 6 mg; iron 0.7 mg; vitamin B_1 0.08 mg; vitamin B_2 0.04 mg; nicotinic acid 1.4 mg; vitamin C 9 mg; and food energy 0.3 MJ.

potato blight. A disease of the potato plants caused by the fungus *Phytophthora infestans*. The pathogen remains viable over the winter as a mycelium in infected potato tubers. These potatoes are often infected with *P. infestans*. If culled potatoes are left undisturbed until spring, the tubers will sprout and the fungus can sporulate and infect nearby fields.

potato bread. A kind of bread made by using a primary ferment that includes mashed cooked potatoes. This is the original method and it gives a sour dough type of flavour together with a moistening and softening effect arising from the potato starch. Some of the original potato flavour will carry through to the finished loaf if enough of the mashed vegetable is present. For many years, however, the potato breads has been made from a white bread formula with some potato flour added. Although this approach will not give the sourdough flavour that is obtained when a starter is used in the sponge, it does often cause an improvement in texture and a slight difference in flavour.

potato chips. Potatoes intended for chip-making must meet rather rigid specifications. Particular emphasis is placed on the use of cultural practices that produce tubers of maximum solids content. High solids content is especially important for chips because the yield of chips per initial quantity of potatoes is in direct proportion to their solids Potatoes for chip making are usually peeled by the abrasion method, after which they go through rotary or other slicers. The slices are washed in rotating reels with jets of water under high pressure to remove starch from the cut surface and to remove slivers of potato. Sometimes slices are leached with hot water or put through a chemical treatment to fix sugars and thus prevent browning reaction. Slices are then fried in automatic equipment with slices submerged most of the time in hot oil. As the chips are lifted from the fryer, they receive salt from a hopper at the rate of 0.7-0.9 kg/45 kg of chips. The chips then drop onto a cooling and inspection belt prior to going to packaging machines. Very significant trends have occurred during the past decade in some consumer acceptance of a "formed" potato chip, made from dried potatoes, cottonseed oil, salt, and dextrose. Genuine potato chips are difficult to pack because of slices variations and shape caused by the varying contours of the fresh potato. The "formed" chips are essentially identical and are easily stacked for sale in cylindrical containers.

potato drying. The handling and storing of potatoes may involve:
(a) curing period, including drying;
(b) cooling period;
(c) warming period; and
(d) the conditioning period.

During the curing period the potatoes heal after being injured or bruised during harvest. Potatoes are maintained at about 15.6°C with air at 90-95% relative humidity during the curing period with an air circulation of 0.001 m³/m³s for about 2 weeks. The heat of respiration from the potatoes will provide the necessary heat for maintaining the desirable temperature in the fall. A temperature of approximately 4.4°C and relative humidity of 95% are desirable for storage during the holding period. Excessive shrinkage and early sprouting occur depending on the variety if held at temperatures above 10°C. At temperatures below 4.4°C the sugar content may increase and the sprouting is retarded. The potatoes can be cooled down to 4.4°C by ventilation within one or two months after harvesting with air movement. If adequate insulation is used it is not necessary to supply artificial heat to maintain a temperature of 4.4°C in northern climates. If potatoes are graded and handled at 4.4°C, some injury may result. Before handling after storage it is desirable to warm the potatoes to about 10°C to reduce injury. Potatoes which are to be used for chipping are conditioned by heating to 15.6-21.1°C and to prevent shrinkage a humidity of about 85% is maintained. Either a gravity or forced air circulation system can be used. Air is distributed by shell- or through-circulation. Air is moved by gravity or is forced through slotted walls of the bins, which are about 4 m wide with shell-circulation. The shell system is satisfactory in the northern climates. With through-circulation, air is forced around each potato by a duct system or slatted floor arrangement such as is used for grain and hay drying. A slatted floor or side wall ports can be used to direct air through pallet boxes.

Potatoes can be dried for animal feed with equipment used for dehydration of hay in which an entering air temperature of 65°C is used. The steps involved in drying are:
(a) washing to remove stones and dirt;
(b) grinding in a hammer mill with 1 cm diameter holes in the screen;
(c) mixing some of the dried material with the entering wet material while keeping the entering moisture content to 40% to prevent formation of balls; and
(d) drying.

potato flour. A highly concentrated and nutritious flour, ground from the pulp of the cooked potato. The flour embodies all of the chemical constituents of the potato, retaining all of the mineral salts. The flour is heavy and thus comparatively small amounts are required in backed products. The flour is also used as a thickening agent in soups and stews and for breading meats and fish. Also known as potato meal.

potato meal. *See* potato flour.

potato spindle disease. A disease of the potatoes, caused by a viriod causing the potatoes to become gnarled.

potato starch. Starch prepared from potato tuber and widely used as a stabilizing agent when gelatinized. Large grains gelatinize very easily when heated. Also called farina.

pot-au-Feu. Traditional French dish made by stewing meat with vegetables. Soup is made from the liquor.

pot pourri. A mixture of fragrant materials placed in a bowl or jar and used for perfuming the rooms. Early pot pourri was usually made of fresh, moist ingredients, with rose petals and orange flowers predominating, which were left to infuse for a month or two with salt added as preservative, after which other powdered perfumes or essential oils were added before the composition was brought into use.

potted. Originating in the US, it is made by grinding well-ripened cheddar very fine and mixing it with butter, spices, etc. Better known now as Club Cheese.

pouch. To cook for a short time in shallow layer of liquid kept at a temperature just below the boiling point.

pound cake. Rich cake containing a pound, or equal quantities, of each of the major ingredients. It is an excellent example of product based on whole egg foams and containing shortening. It is always denser than good quality angel food cakes. Pound cakes were traditionally based on the very old formula of one pound each of flour, butter, whole eggs, and sugar. Modern formulas have departed considerably from this archetype. Most present-day commercial versions include at least some baking powder, although the amount is usually kept considerably less than in layer cakes so as to retain the relatively dense and firm but tender and somewhat crumbly texture expected in pound cake. Other changes often encountered in modern formulas are decreases in eggs and butter accompanied by an increase in sugar to give the sweeter, more tender cake preferred by many consumers. Very frequently, some or all of the butter is replaced by vegetable shortening to decrease the ingredient cost and improve shelf life. This change also improves the grain and increases the specific volume if the vegetable shortening is of the emulsifier type.

ppm. Abbreviation for parts per million; usually expressed as weight ratio; 1ppm is equivalent to 1mg/kg.

prairie crocus. *Anemone patens.* Family: Ranunculaceae. A flowering plant. Flowers are 5 cm across; plant grows close to the ground. The sepals are pale purple, the stamens golden yellow, and the pistils gray. The leaves are gray. The leaves are gray-green and the seed heads are gray. When the sepals wither and fall a head of gray seeds with long feathery tails appears. The wind scatters the seeds and those that fall on gravelly soil or unploughed land may grow in the spring. Petals are absent in this plant. The colored parts that resemble petals are sepals. The leaves are finely divided into many narrow segments. They have a soft hairy covering that gives them a silky feeling. Now that prairies have been ploughed for agriculture the crocus is scarce but preserves are being established so that everyone can still enjoy this dainty wildflower.

Praline. Trade name for a rich paste of ground nuts and suga;r used as chocolate centres.

Pratigu cheese. A variety of cheese, named from the valley in which it is made in Switzerland. It is made similar to Limburger. Skim milk is used in its preparation.

prawns. Shellfish of various tribes of suborder *Macrura*. Large fish of species of *Palaemonidae, Penaeidae* and *Pandalidae* are prawns smaller fish are shrimps.

In addition Deep-water prawn is *Pandalus borealis;* common pink shrimp is *Pandalus montagui,* brown shrimp is species of *Crangon.* Dublin Bay Prawn is Lobster.

The average composition per 100 g is: 20 g protein; 1.9 g fat; 148 mg calcium; 1 mg iron; and 0.45 Mj food energy.

preconcentration. In food technology, a process before drying or dehydration in which an appreciable amount of moisture is removed, such as with an evaporator or vacuum pan. Removal of water in an evaporator, where applicable, is less expensive than in a dryer.

precursor, enzyme. Some enzymes are secreted as an inactive precursor that has to undergo a reaction before it shows normal activity. Thus trypsin is secreted as inactive trypsinogen that must react with enterokinase before it becomes active; similarly pepsinogen and chymotrypsinogen.

preformers. Devices for placing products to be dried into uniform sizes of particles, aggregates, or granules, so that the products can be dried more or less uniformly. Paste must be partially dried before or as a part of preforming. Evaporation of moisture from liquid materials may be necessary before forming the paste. Various types of preformers include: groove drum, which may be heated and accomplish some drying; band, in which material is fed out of bottomless box onto a conveyor; mincing, pressing devices; reciprocating extruder, a trough-like die plate containing many holes over which a pair of heavy rubber rollers reciprocate; direct pressure extruders, with produce being forced out through a die with product under pressure behind the die; the pelleting. Rough grinding and screen classification of solids provide another means of getting aggregates.

premier jus. Best-quality suet prepared from the oxen and sheep kidneys. The fat is chilled, shredded and heated at moderate temperature. When pressed, premier jus, like rendered tallow, separates into a liquid fraction (oleo oil or liquid oleo) and a solid fraction (oleosterin or solid tallow).

preservation. During storage food can deteriorate under the influence of microorganisms, its own enzymes and chemically by oxidation. Preservation must stop these reactions, and the normally practised methods, such as refrigeration, sterilization, dehydration and addition of chemicals, control them to varying extents. Short-term preservation is achieved by pasteurization, salting, smoking and pickling. Some destruction of the vitamins, a small degree of leaching out of the minerals and vitamins, and under conditions of severe heating, some small degree of damage to proteins, can occur during preservation, In general, refrigeration and dehydration under vacuum or by freeze-drying, cause no nutritional loss. *See also* preservatives.

preservatives. The chemicals used to prevent oxidation, fermentation, or other deterioration of foodstuffs. The antioxidants, inhibitors, and stabilizers used to retard deterioration of industrial chemicals are not usually called preservatives. The most usual function of a preservative is to kill bacteria, and this may be accomplished by an acid, an alcohol, an aldehyde, or a salt. A legal requirement under the Food and Drug Act is that a preservative must be non-toxic in the quantities permitted.

The only permitted preservatives in UK are sulphur dioxide and benzoic acid, and, in specified case, methyl or propyl p-hydroxy-benzoate, sorbic acid and the antibiotic, nisin. The following are excluded from the regulations: salt, saltpeter, sugar, lactic and acetic acids, glycerine, alcohol, species, essential oils and herbs.

Sugar is a the most commonly used preservative for fruit products.

Sodium chloride is used for protein foods.

Sodium nitrate is reduced to sodium nitrite in curing meats, and the nitrite has an inhibitory action on bacterial growth, the effect being greatest in acid flesh.

Acetic acid is normally more toxic to bacteria than lactic acid, but when sugar is present the reverse is true, and citric acid then has little toxicity. The inhibitory action of inorganic acids is due mainly to the pH change which they produce.

Potassium sorbate, a white water-soluble powder, inhibits the growth of many molds, yeasts, and bacteria which cause food deterioration, and is used in cheese, syrups, pickles, and other prepared foods. The inhibitory effect of organic acids is due chiefly to the undissociated molecule.

Beverages containing fruit juices or little carbonation are preserved with less than 0.05% sodium benzoate.

Methyl, propyl, butyl, and ethyl parabens; potassium sorbate; sodium dihydroacetate; and imidazolidinyl urea are all industrial microbials used in the food, cosmetic, and pharmaceutical industries.

The antimicrobial effect of vanillic acid esters generally increases with increasing molecular mass. Only small quantities of such chemicals are usually needed for preservation.

Isobutyl vanillate, an ester of vanillic acid, is effective as a preserving agent in milk and some other foods when only 0.10-0.15% is used. Preservatives are also marketed for external application to food-stuffs in storage, though these are more properly classified as fumigants.

press drying. A method of drying by applying heat to opposite faces of a board using heated platens to remove moisture from the board. The heating is done by conduction heating provided by contact between heated platens and boards by using a platen pressure of 1.75-5.3 kg/cm^2 with temperatures in the range from 121-232°C. Ventilated openings are provided to carry and moisture away. Drying rates of 1.3-0.60 g H_2O/cm^3-min for temperatures of 104-137.8°C are representative.

pressed cheese. A hard cheese, such as Cheddar, that has been subjected to pressure to remove the whey, to produce physical conditions essential to ripening, and to put it in a convenient form for handling.

Prestost cheese. A variety of Swedish rennet cheese made from fresh cows' milk and resembling Gouda. It is cylindrical in shape. In Sweden it is also known as Salad Pfarr. After the whey is drawn off, the curd is put into a cloth and kneaded. Whisky is mixed with the curd, which is then packed in a basket and after salt is sprinkled on the surface it is put into a cool, moist cloth. The cloth is changed daily for 3 days, after which the cheese is washed in whisky.

Pretzels. Hard brittle German biscuits made from flour, water, shortening, yeast and salt. The dough is fermented and chopped into lengths and shaped; they are boiled in 0.3 sodium hydroxide, salted, baked and dried. Originally called bretzels and still made in the shape of the letter B.

prexia. Rise in body temperature.

prickly ash. *Zanthoxylum americanum.* A tall shrub, or rarely a small tree, can reach heights of over 7 metres. It is characterized by thorny stems and branches and leaves that are hairy young, smooth when older with resinous dots on them and emitting the smell of lemon when crushed. The greenish flowers, in clusters on last year's wood, appear before the leaves. They are followed by reddish-brown, rough capsules containing black seed or seeds, the taste of which is spicy. Prickly ash is found from Canada to Virginia and Nebraska.

prickly pear cactus. *Opuntia polyacantha.* Family: *Cactaceae.* A flowering plant whose flowers are 5-7.5 cm across. Each joint of the stem is 5-12 cm long. The stems are green, the spines are reddish-brown, the sepals and petals are lemon yellow, sometimes lined with pink. The stamens are yellow. The fruits are brownish when ripe. The flowers open in late spring and are followed by pear-like fruits with many seeds. Joints of the stem that break off may root and form new plants. The prickly near cactus has developed a fleshy, jointed, and flattened stem that stores any water that is available so it can be used by the plant during dry periods. Instead of leaves it has clusters of sharp, reddish-brown spines with barbed tips. These protect its water supply from grazing animals. The plants grow in clumps close to the ground.

Procea. Trade name of a white loaf with slightly increased protein content. The average composition per 100 g is: protein 10.8%; fat 2.3%; carbohydrate 50%; calcium 145 mg; iron 1.6 mg; and food energy 1.08 MJ.

processed cheese. The varieties of cheese made from a combination of one or more batches or kinds of natural cheeses which are heated to pasteurization temperatures and packaged. Essentially unknown in some parts of the world, process cheeses are a comparatively recent development in the centuries-old history of cheese manufacture. Basic patents were initially held by a few businesses, with a limited number of other manufacturers licensed to operate under these patents. The original objectives of process cheese manufacturing were to approximate natural cheese while extending the keeping quality uniformity, and slicing quality. Concentration has been maintained at this level by these early entrants, partially by effective brand differentiation and competitiveness at the retail level, making entry into the market by new brands difficult. Most of the firms in this business also package process cheeses under private labels for food chains as well as under their own labels.

process waste. The solid waste resulting from processing, disposed of by landfill or burial. In other words, the term process waste is referred to that portion of incineration or composting process that, winds up worthless end product in the form of ashes, slag, scrap, etc.

product standard. Derived standards or working levels of pollutants applied to products such as food or detergents. The maximum acceptable level or potential pollutants in the specified product is designed to ensure that under specified circumstances primary and secondary ambient quality protection standards are not exceeded.

proenzyme. The inactive form in which some enzymes are synthesized and secreted, particularly by the pancreas. This prevents self-digestion of tissues, which can happen in certain diseases, such as pancreatitis. Activation usually occurs by limited proteolysis of the proenzyme to yield the active form of the enzyme. For example, the proenzyme trypsinogen is converted to trypsin by the enzyme enterokinase.

profilin. The protein of molecular mass ~16000 that binds to unpolymerized actin, thereby retarding polymerization. It is thought to modulate the availability of free actin in cells and is particularly abundant in sperm and blood platelets.

profiteroles. Tiny rounds of choux pastry used to decorate cakes.

Proflo. Trade name for partially defatted, cooked, cottonseed flour. It is popular in many countries.

progressive dryer. A tunnel dryer, operated periodically or intermittently, in which the product moves through the unit, used for clay, pottery, and lumber. The tunnel is filled with products, the heat and air are turned on, the temperature is held constant, and the air flow is uniform. The hot air at about 93.9°C enters first, coming in contact with the nearly dry product leaving, and the air leaving the dryer comes in contact with green ware. The product then moves to the kiln for finishing.

prohormone. The inactive form of a hormone: the form in which it is stored. Activation usually involves enzymatic removal of some part of the prohormone; for example, removal of amino acids from the polypeptide prohormone, proinsulin, to form insulin. Biochemical alterations to a prohormone will result in the release of the more active metabolite; e.g., proinsulin.

proinsulin. Prohormone of the hormone insulin. It is synthesized in the β-cells of the islets of langerhans and consists of a polypeptide chain of about 80 amino acids. The central section of 30 amino acids is cleaved out by specific proteolytic action, leaving the two terminal peptides which, by association, form the active insulin molecule.

prolactin. A protein hormone, secreted by the anterior lobe of the pituitary gland, that is essential for the initiation of lactation in mammals. Prolactin also has a gonadotropic effect and stimulates progesterone secretion by the corpus luteum. In birds prolactin stimulates secretion of crop milk by the crop glands. This polypeptide hormone is produced by the mammalian pituitary gland and analogous tissue in other vertebrates. It stimulates lactation (milk production) and also encourages progesterone release by the corpus luteum. It is single chain polypeptide of 198 amino acids and is somewhat similar to growth hormone. In lower vertebrates, prolactin affects growth and osmotic regulation. Also known as lactogenic hormone; luteotrophic hormone.

prolamins. Proteins insoluble in water, neutral solvents and absolute alcohol, but soluble in 60-80% alcohol; e.g., wheat gliadin.

They are low in lysine, rich in proline and glutamic acid.

proline. Pyrrolidine carboxylic acid; a non-essential amino acid. One of the 20 common amino acids and one with a non-polar side-chain. It is a cyclic molecule and gives rise to a bend in a polypeptide chain where it occurs.

Prolo. Trade name for a protein-rich baby food containing 49% protein. It is made in UK from soya flour with methionine, minerals and vitamins A, B_1, B_2 and nicotinic acid, incorporated in it.

Pronutro. Trade name for a protein-rich baby food containing 22% protein. It was developed in South Africa, and made from maize, skim-milk powder, groundnut flour, soya flour and fish protein concentrate with yeast, wheat germ, vitamins A, B_1, B_2, and nicotinic acid, iodized salt and sugar.

proof spirit. By a British Parliament Act, "Proof Spirit" is defined to be a mixture of alcohol and water of such density that at 51°F, 13 volumes shall weigh the same as 12 volumes of water at the same temperature. This is equivalent to spirit containing 49.24% by weight of alcohol and specific gravity 0.9184 at 60°F. An entire system of alcohol measurement based on the above system of proof has come into existence where the strength of the spirit is expressed as percentage over a under proof.

In India, the excise departments and distillers use the British Proof for measurement of alcohol. American Proof is that alcoholic liquor which contains one-half its volume of alcohol of specific gravity 0.7939 at 60°F. According to this scale absolute alcohol is 200° proof where as per British scale absolute alcohol is 175.4 proof. More simply, under the American system the figure of proof is twice the alcoholic content by volume. The absolute alcohol is 175.25 degrees proof UK and 200 degrees proof US Spirits are described as under or over proof. A mixture 30 degrees over proof contains in 100 volumes as much alcohol as 130 volumes of proof spirit; 30 degrees under proof means that 100 volumes contain as much alcohol as 70 volumes of proof spirit. In Germany per cent alcohol by weight is used; while in Italy and France, it is per cent by volume. Proof spirit is a solution of alcohol of such strength that it will ignite when mixed with gunpowder; specifically at 10°C it weighs 12/13 parts of an equal volume of distilled water.

propionates. Salts of propionic acid, CH_3CH_2COOH. The free acid and its sodium and calcium salts are used as mould inhibitors, e.g., on cheese surfaces; also to inhibit rope in bread. Propionic acid is formed in the rumen of cattle together with acetic and butyric acids, and all three are converted into milk constituents. In the body it is metabolized to pyruvic acid, which is normally formed in the body, and thus considered harmless.

Propionibacteria. Members of the genus *Propionibacterium* are mostly anaerobes, or aerotolerant; they produce propionic acid as a fermentation product. One species, *Propionibacterium acnes*, universally inhabits the tiny oil glands of the human skin, while another *Propionibacterium freudenreichii* is responsible for the holes and flavor of Swiss cheese. Their action not only hastens the development of "eye" but also helps to produce the characteristic mild, nutlike flavour in the cheese.

propionic acid. One of the volatile fatty acids produced by the rumen microflora and absorbed directly from the rumen into the bloodstream of the animal. The propionate (propionate) is carried to the liver where it is converted to glucose; this represents a significant source of energy for ruminants.

propionic fermentation. The fermentation of glucose, and generally also of lactic acid, that yields propionic acid and other products and that is characteristic of propionic acid bacteria.

Propionigenium. A Gram-negative, strictly anaerobic bacterium that ferments succinate to propionate and carbon dioxide. The fermentation is unusual because of the role Na^+ plays in establishing an ion gradient that ultimately drives ATP synthesis. The free energy released during the fermentation of succinate is insufficient to drive substrate-level phosphorylation, thus an ion gradient is necessary to trap the available energy from the fermentation for eventual conversion to ATP. *Propionigenium* also grows on fumarate, malate, aspartate, oxaloacetate, and pyruvate as sole energy sources, but does not ferment sugars or carry out anaerobic respiration linked to nitrate, sulphate, or other potential electron acceptors.

proso millet. *Panicum milliaceum.* There are three main subspecies of the plant:

(1) *P. miliaceum* effusion (characterized by broad panicles that spread out in all directions;

(2) *P. miliaceum contractum* (one-sided panicles that have a limited spread); and

(3) *P. miliaceum compactum* (compact, thick, erect panicles).

Most varieties of proso millet grown in the Middle-Eastern countries are derived from southeastern Russian varieties. Varieties grown to a limited extent in North America include Early Fortune. Turghai, and Yellow Manitoba. There is a period of about 3.5 months from the time of planting to harvesting of proso millet. Seedlings are prone to damage by early frost. Thus, in the northern latitudes, the time of planting is critical.

The height of the mature proso plant ranges from 0.3-1.2 m. The inflorescence is an open panicle from 10-30 cm long. Seeds range from 2.25-2.5 mm in length and are about 2 mm wide. The plant is self-pollinating. Also known as broomcorn millet, hot millet, and Hershey millet (US); and as common millet (in Europe).

Prosparol. Trade name for an emulsion containing 50% vegetable fat. It is used as a concentrated source of energy.

prosthetic group. The non-protein component of a conjugated protein. Thus the haem group in haemoglobin is an example of a prosthetic group, as are the coenzyme components of a wide range of enzymes. The prosthetic group is at the active site of the enzyme and is changed during the course of the reaction. Prosthetic groups are tightly bound to the enzyme (sometimes covalently to form the holoenzyme). They differ from coenzymes in that regeneration of the prosthetic group occurs in situ; it does not need to dissociate from the enzyme for regeneration. Examples of prosthetic groups include FAD (in flavoproteins), thiamine pyrophosphate (in decarboxylases), biotin (in carboxylases) and pyridoxal phosphate (in amino acid aminotransferases). The part of the enzyme without the prosthetic group is the apoenzyme. Certain oxidizing enzymes have a prosthetic group that functions as a built-in hydrogen acceptor. Example, peroxidase contains haematin as its prosthetic group.

protamines. The simplest natural proteins containing only a limited number of amino acids, chiefly the basic ones, especially arginine. Soluble in water, not coagulated by heat, so basic that they from salts with strong mineral acids, e.g., salmine from salmon sperm, sturing from sturgeon sperm, clupeine from nerring sperm, clupeine from nerring sperm, scombrine from mackerel sperm.

protean. An insoluble, primary derived protein that is obtained by treatment of a protein with heat, acid, enzymes, or other agents. These are slightly altered proteins, probably an early stage of denaturation, which have become insoluble.

proteases. See proteinases.

proteins. Essential constituents of all living cells; distinguished from fats and carbohydrates in containing nitrogen; basically composed of carbon, hydrogen, oxygen, nitrogen, sulphur and sometimes phosphorus. All proteins are composed of large combinations of 20 amino acids (some bacterial proteins contain additional unusual amino acids). Meat, fish, eggs, cheese, hair, leather, fur, and many hormones are proteins. They serve as major structural component in animal tissues.

In the form of skin, hair, callus, cartilage, tendons, and ligaments, proteins hold together, protect, and provide structure to the body.

In the form of enzymes, hormones, antibodies, and globulins, they catalyze, regulate, and protect the body chemistry.

In the form of haemoglobin, myoglobin, and various lipoproteins, they affect the transport of oxygen and other substances within the body.

The large molecules of proteins (molecular mass usually range from 10,000-5,000,000) are composed largely of carbon, hydrogen, nitrogen, oxygen, and smaller amounts of sulphur (sometimes traces of other elements may also be present). The molecular masses of most proteins can be estimated only approximately by centrifugal sedimentation methods for soluble proteins, which vary from few thousand to many millions. Other methods are osmotic pressure measurements, X-ray diffraction, light scattering effects, gel filtration and chemical analysis.

Proteins are natural polymers usually consisting of long polyamide chains (a polypeptide) to which are attached various side chains or functional characteristic of each amino acid in the chain. The number of amino acid units comprising a given protein is usually large, hence the possible combinations of different amino acids is enormous.

Digestion of protein begins in the stomach. Hydrolysis of protein is initiated in the stomach by the enzyme pepsin and protease. Pepsin and protease are secreted by cells lining the walls of the stomach Gastric mucosa secretes hydrochloric acid and mucus also. The hydrochloric acid is responsible for low pH of gastric juice (pH 1-2). This acidic pH helps in the activity of pepsin in two ways:

(a) Pepsin is first secreted as pepsinogen. This pepsinogen is converted to pepsin by pepsin itself at acidic pH. Pepsin preferentially attacks peptide bonds involving residues of aromatic amino acid.

(b) Maximum pepsin activity occurs at pH 1-2. Pepsin helps in breaking of large protein molecule to smaller polypeptide chain.

Protein digestion in the small intestine is catalyzed by enzymes secreted by pancreas. Carboxypeptidase, chymotrypsin and trypsin convert polypeptides into small polypeptides and dipeptides. In the small intestine brush border area, smaller polypeptides and dipeptides are converted to free amino acids by peptidases. Amino acids produced from the protein are absorbed through the small intestine. Absorbed amino acids will be utilized for the biosynthesis of new protein according to the need of the individual cell. A portion of amino acid absorbed is concentrated by liver cell and the remaining portion pass into systemic circulation for other tissues. Amino acids which are in excess of hepatic needs are deaminated and the amino group is utilized for urea formation, and the ketoacids are oxidized to carbon dioxide and water. Vital proteins like plasma albumin, a,b-globulin and fibrinogen are synthesized in the liver.

Protein consumption is an index of a country's economic status, becaus quality protein is the most expensive food. Protein malnutrition leads to poor health, disease and even death. Proteins are very essential as building blocks of cells, and are required to make enzymes which play a vital role in various other metabolism. Ingested proteins are degraded in the GI tract to smaller units called amino acids.

protein efficiency ratio. A measure of the nutritive value of proteins carried out on young growing animals. Is defined as the gain in weight per gram of protein eaten. The maximum values, e.g., egg protein, are about 4.4. Zero values are obtained for those proteins which, when fed alone, do not permit growth, but may still have some limited value.

protein equivalent. A measure of the digestible nitrogen of an animal feeding stuff in terms of protein. It is measured by direct feeding or calculated from the digestible pure protein plus half the digestible non-protein nitrogen

protein factor. The factor 6.25 that, when multiplied by the weight of nitrogen (in grams) derived from a sample containing protein, gives the approximate weight (in grams) of the protein in the sample.

protein fractionation. The separation of a mixture of different proteins for the purpose of isolating one particular type of protein; it requires the use of one or more physical-chemical techniques such as precipitation, centrifugation, or electrophoresis.

protein kinases. Enzymes that phosphorylate proteins. Protein kinase A is cyclic AMP-dependent, while protein kinase G is cyclic GMP-dependent and protein kinase C is Ca^{2+}-dependent.

protein milk. Partially skimmed lactic acid milk plus milk curd (prepared from whole milk by rennet precipitation); richer in protein and poorer in fat than ordinary milk-supposed to be better tolerated in digestive disorders. Also known as albumin milk.

protein rating. A term used in Canadian Food Regulations to assess overall protein quality of a food. Protein efficiency ratio multiplied by protein content of food (per cent) multiplied by the amount of food that is reasonably consumed. Foods with rating above 40 may be designated excellent dietary sources; foods with rating below 20 are considered to be insignificant source; 20-40 may be described as good sources.

protein shift. Name applied in flour milling to the phenomenon in which the protein content of the smaller particles of flour (up to 15 microns) is higher, namely 15-20%, than the flour as a whole, 81-4%, while particles of intermediate size, 15-35 microns, have a lower protein content than the flour as a whole.

protein synthesis inhibition. Protein synthesis is characteristically inhibited by many different antibiotics. On of the most important inhibitory antibiotics is puromycin, which has a structure very similar to that of the 3' end of an aminoacyl-tRNA. It acts by interrupting peptide-chain elongation by virtue of its ability to replace an entering aminoacyl-tRNA, thus causing formation of a peptidyl-puromycin. No new amino acid residues can be added to a peptidyl-puromycin; hence it is discharged from the ribosome, thus terminating synthesis of the polypeptide. Tetracyclines, another class of antibiotics, inhibit protein synthesis by blocking the A site on the ribosome, rendering it incapable of binding amino-acyl-tRNAs. Streptomycin causes misreading of genetic code, and tunicamycin prevents attachment of oligosaccharide side chains to certain glycoproteins. Some other inhibitors of protein synthesis include chloramphenicol, cyclohexamide, diphtheria toxin, and ricin.

protein synthesis. The process by which living cells manufacture proteins from their constituent amino acids, in accordance with the genetic information carried in the DNA of the chromosomes. This information is encoded in messenger RNA, which is transcribed from DNA in the nucleus of the cell: the sequence of amino acids in a particular protein it deter-mined by the sequence of nucleotides in messenger RNA. At the ribosomes the information carried by messenger RNA is translated into the sequence of amino acids of the protein in the process of translation. There are five major stages in protein synthesis, each requiring a number of components. These are:

Stage 1. Activation of amino acids. This takes place in the cytosol, not on the ribosome, each of the 20 amino acids is covalently attached to a specific transfer RNA at the expense of ATP energy. These reactions are catalyzed by a group of $M'g^{2+}$ dependent activating enzymes, each specific for one amino acid for a corresponding tRNA.

Stage 2. Initiation of the polypeptide chain. In the second step, the messenger RNA bearing the code for the polypeptide to be made is bound to the smaller subunit of a ribosome followed by initiating amino acid, attached to the tRNA to form an initiation complex. The tRNA of the initiating amino acid base-pairs with a specific nucleotide triplet or codon on the mRNA that signals the beginning of the polypeptide chain. This process requires GTP and is promoted by three specific cytosolic proteins, called initiation factors.

Stage 3. Elongation. During this stage, the polypeptide chain is elongated by the covalent attachment of successive amino acid units, each carried to ribosome and put into its proper position by its corresponding tRNA, which is base-paired to its corresponding codon in the messenger RNA. This is promoted by cytosolic proteins called elongation factors.

Stage 4. Termination and release. The completion of the polypeptide chain, which is signaled by a termination codon in the mRNA, is followed by its release from the ribosome, promoted by releasing factors.

Stage 5. Folding and processing. A protein is not biologically reactive until it is in its native folded conformation, which is determined by the amino acid sequence. At some point during or after its synthesis, the polypeptide chain assumes its native conformation. In this way the linear or one-dimensional genetic message brought by the messenger RNA is converted into the three dimensional structure of the newly synthesized polypeptide. The newly made polypeptide chain does not attain its final biologically active conformation until it has been subjected to processing or covalent modification. Several kinds of processing may occur, depending upon the type and nature of the protein.

protein, alpha. Trade name for a protein isolated from soya-bean, used for paper coating, water-miscible paints, leather finishing, adhesives. 88.7% protein, 8.5% water.

protein, beta. Trade name for a protein isolated from soya-bean, mainly used to prepare adhesives for plywood.

protein, crude. Total nitrogen multiplied by the factor 6.25 (equal to 100 divided by 16). The nitrogen content of most pure proteins is 16% and determination of crude protein, in effect, assumes that all the nitrogen present is protein. The error involved in this assumption is not usually large unless there is an abundance of the purine nitrogen present. For milk, the protein factor is 6.38, while for cereals, it is 5.7.

protein, first class. First and second class proteins are obsolete terms indicating those of high or low nutritive value, generally, but not invariably, animal and plant protein respectively.

proteinases. Group of enzymes whose action is to split proteins into smaller peptides. Such enzymes are abundant in lysosomes, especially in liver. Proteinases are used widely to digest protein in the purification of nucleic acid from chromatin. Also known as endopeptidases; proteases.

protein-energy ratio. Protein content of a food or diet expressed as ratio of energy from protein to total energy. Previously termed protein calories per cent, being expressed as a percentage of total calories supplied by protein.

proteins, conjugated. The molecule contains protein and a non-protein prosthetic group; *e.g.*, nucleoproteins, glycoproteins, phosphoproteins, chromoproteins, lipoproteins.

Protenum. Trade name of concentrated food preparation containing 42% protein, 46% carbohydrate and 2% fat.

proteolysis. The hydrolysis of proteins to amino acids by alkali, acid or enzymes.

proteoses. A general term for the partial degradation products of proteins. The stages of breakdown are: protein-proteoses-peptones-polypeptides-amino acids. The proteoses are distinguished from peptones in that they are precipitated from solution by ammonium sulphate whereas peptones are not. Primary proteoses precipitated with half saturated ammonium sulphate, secondary proteoses require full saturation.

Proteus. The genus characterized by rapid motility an by production of the enzyme urease. By DNA homology it shows only a distant relationship to

E. coli. Proteus is a frequent cause of urinary tract infections in people and rarely may cause enteritis. Because of the urea splitting ability, *Proteus* has been implicated in several kidney infections. The species of *Proteus* probably do not form a homogeneous group, as is indicated by the fact that DNA base composition vary over a fair wide range (39-50% GC). Because of rapid motility of Proteus cells, colonies growing on agar plates often exhibit a characteristic swarming phenomenon. Cells at the edge of growing colony are more rapidly motile than are those in the centre of the colony. Although all enteric bacteria can use nitrate as alternate electron acceptor anaerobically, *Proteus* has the additional ability to use several sulphur compounds as electron acceptors for anaerobic growth; these include thiosulphate, tetrathionate, and dimethylsulphoxide.

prothrombin. Protein of the plasma involved in coagulation of the blood.

Protone. Trade name for a protein-rich baby food containing 24% protein. It is manufactured in UK from maize, skim-milk powder, yeast with added vitamins and minerals.

protopectinase. The enzyme in the pith of citrus fruits that converts protopectin into pectin with the resultant separation of the plant cells from one another. Also known as pectosinase and pectonase.

protoplasmic poison. An obsolete expression sometimes formerly used to describe a depressant drug whose mechanism of action was unknown: for example, quinidine was formerly described in the way with respect top its depressant action on the heart.

protozoa. The microorganism belonging to the *Protozoa* subkingdom, are unicellular or acellular eucaryotic protist whose organelles have the functional role of the organs and tissues in more complex forms. Protozoa vary greatly in size, morphology, nutrition, and life cycle. More than 66,000 protozoan species have been identified; over 31,00 are fossil, around 23,000 are free-living, and about 12,000 are symbiotic in or on animals or plants, even on other protozoa. These microorganisms are directly related only on the basis of a single negative characteristic- they are not multicellular. All, however, demonstrate the basic body plan of a single protistan eucaryotic cell. Protozoa play a significant role in the economy of nature. For example, some constitute a large part of plankton, small, free-floating aquatic organisms that serve as an important link in many food chains and food webs of aquatic environments. Protozoa are also useful in biochemical and molecular biological studies. Many biochemical pathways used by protozoa are employed by all eucaryotic cells. Because protozoa are eucaryotic cells, in many respects their morphology and physiology resemble those of multicellular animals. However, because all their functions must be performed within the individual protist, many morphological and physiological features are unique to protozoan cells. Some protozoa can secrete a resistant covering and go into a resting stage called a cyst. Cysts protect the organism against adverse environments, function as a site for nuclear reorganization, and serve as a means of transmission in parasitic species.

Providencia sp. Enterobacteria that resemble *Proteus* but are urease negative. It is an opportunistic pathogen found in human feces, and causes urinary tract infections and burn wound sepsis.

proving. In bread-making, fermentation of the dough at the stage just before it goes into the oven.

provirus. The state of a retrovirus after oncogenic transformation of its host cell. A DNA copy of the viral RNA, made with the aid of a reverse transcriptase enzyme, is integrated into the cell DNA, thus changing the cell's genetic constitution and causing it to become cancerous. This occurs, for example, with *Rous sarcoma* virus of chickens.

provitamin. A substance that is converted into a vitamin such as 7-dehydrocholesterol which is converted into vitamin D. In the old nomenclature carotene was termed provitamin A.

Provolone cheese. A Pasta Filata (plastic curd) type of cheese of Italian origin which is made in many shapes and sizes and usually smoked after drying. It is light coloured, mellow, smooth and has an agreeable flavour. Raw or pasteurized milk is put into a vat similar to the type used for making Cheddar cheese and then starters consisting of 1-2% *S. lactis*, 0.2% *S. thermophilus* and 0.1% *L. bulgaricus* are added. The milk is held until the acidity increases 0.01%. Rennet and a lipase enzyme extract are added to the milk in small quantities. After coagulation the curd is cut, cooked to 40°C and the whey is drained when the acid in the whey has increased 0.03% or when the pH of the curd is 6.1 The drained curd is handled like Cheddar until the acidity reaches 0.4-0.6% and when the pH of the curd is approximately 5.3. The curd is milled into thin strips and then placed in twice its weight of hot water. It is then stretched and kneaded into the desired shape and placed in cold water for hardening after which it placed in a salt brine for a time, depending upon cheese size. The cheese are then tried with rope string and hung in a smoke room (cold smoke for 2-4 hours). The average composition is: moisture 40%, fat 28%, salt 3%. Federal Standards recommends that the moisture should not be more than 45%; and fat, not less than 45%.

proximate analysis. Nearly complete analysis comprising protein, fat and ash, and, by subtracting these from the total, calculating "carbohydrate by difference". The last value may be corrected for crude fibre.

pseudoglobulin. Water-soluble globulin which is not precipitated from salt solutions by dialysis against distilled water. Pseudoglobulin fractions occur in blood serum, in animal tissues, and in milk.

psoralens. Naturally occurring constituents of certain plants. They are also called furocoumarins and they have the property of inducing pigmentation. They stimulate the melanocyte response to ultraviolet light.

psychrophile. A microorganism that grows well at 0°C and has an optimum growth temperature of 15°C or lower and a maximum temperature around 20°C. Psychrophiles are found in cold marine environments, glacial lakes, and in polar environments. The majority of psychrophiles are members of the genera *Pseudomonas, Flavobacterium,* and *Alcaligenes.*

psychrophilic bacteria. Prefer temperatures 15-20°C and will still grow at and below 0°C, that is, in cold stores. Bacteria of the genera *Achromobacter, flavobacterium, Pseudomonas,* and *Micrococcus. Torulopsis* yeasts, and moulds of the genera *Penicillium, Cladosporium, Mucor* and *Thamni-*

dium can all develop at low temperatures. Temperatures must be reduced to about -10°C before growth stops, but the organisms are not killed and will regrow when the temperature rises.

psychrotroph. A microorganism that grows at 0°C, but has a optimum between 20-25°C, and a maximum of about 30°C.

psyllium. *Plantago ovata.* A stemless or short-stemmed annual herb. Its leaves are in a rosette or alternate, clasping the stem strap-like, and average 5-20 cm in length and 5-10 mm in width. The flowers are white, minute, four-parted, in erect, ovoid or cylindrical spikes. The fruit is ovate with the top half separating when ripe, releasing smooth, dull ovate seeds that are either pinkish-grey-brown or pinkish-white with brown streaks on them. Each seed is encased in a thin, white, translucent hums which is odourless and tasteless. When soaked in water, the whole seeds expand considerably in size.

PTJ - pure lemon juice. Trade name for lemon juice containing about 53 mg of the vitamin C per 100 g of juice.

ptomines. Compounds produced during the decomposition of proteins; some are poisonous, hence lead to the so called ptomaine poisoning. Cadaverine (diaminopentane) formed by decarboxylation of lysine; muscarine (hydroxyethyl trimethylammonium hydroxide); putrescine (tetramethylenediamine) formed by the decarboxylation or arginine; and neurine (trimethylvinylammonium hydroxide).

ptyalin. Old name for salivary amylase.

pudding, black. Sausage made of suet, pearl barley, and oatmeal and sometimes including pig's blood.

pudding, hasty. Old dish made from oatmeal boiled with water for only 2-3 minutes; the finished dish is very low in water content.

puff drying. A method of drying generally used for removing moisture from a juice concentrate. The concentrate is expanded about 20 volumes in a vacuum of 2-6 mm of mercury to incorporate vapor bubbles. The expanded material is dried in a vacuum heated 93.3-60°C to remove water. Drying may be carried out in a vacuum shelf batch dryer or on a vacuum belt continuous dryer. Drying time varies from 1.5 to 5 hours. Juices are dried to about 3% moisture. The products formed from puff drying are readily reconstituted.

puffer fish poisoning. *See* tetraodontin poisoning.

puff pastry. The product obtained by the interleaving of thin layers of the fat with thin layers of dough so that, upon baking, a partial separation of dough strata occurs. During preparation continuous layers of fat are formed between layers of dough; upon baking steam accumulates between the dough layers and causes them to expand forming large spaces between thin layers of pastry. The individual dough layers contain no leavening and undergo very little expansion during baking. Water vapor is generated in the dough but quickly passes from the dough adhesions that have formed during the repeated sheeting operations. As a result, steam is trapped in the pockets formed by partial fusion of the dough layers. These vesicles or bubbles tend to be comparatively large and irregular; their greatest dimension is nearly always in the horizontal direction. The expanding water vapor can cause a very substantial puffing of the piece. Products made with puff pastry include turnovers and millefeulle pastries such as napoleons, vol-au-vents, and patty shells. Simulated strudel can also be made with puff pastry, although the genuine article is made from a single, very thin sheet of dough that is painted with oil or melted butter before it is wound around the filling in many layers.

pullulan. A homopolysaccharide compound composed of maltotriose units linked by β-1,6 bonds. It is produced by the fungus *Aureobasidium pullulans*. Films made by pullulan are claimed to have antioxidant properties and have been proposed as a biodegradable material for food packaging and coating.

pulque. Sour beer produced by the rapid natural fermentation of aquamiel, the sweet mucilaginous sap of the Agave (American aloe or century plant). It contains 6% alcohol by volume, common in Central and South America.

pulse. A term applied collectively to peas, beans, and lentils. Pulse may refer to the edible pod produced by these plants. Fresh peas and beans contain 65-90% water but the mature seeds contain only 10-13% water. Their protein content is higher than that of cereals (20% of dry weight); they are a good source of thiamin and nicotinic acid; although they do not contain any vitamin C this vitamin is formed during germination so that sprouted pulses are a valuable source.

Pulses constitute a valuable part of tropical and subtropical diets as an important source of protein. The problem with all pulses is the amount of intestinal disturbance they cause, embarrassingly sulphuric and antisocial without and uncomfortable within. Such flatulence is the result of two incompatible starches (stachyose and raffinose). They do not pass through the walls of the small intestine, and instead of their being converted into blood sugar intestinal bacteria go to work on them splitting them into carbon dioxide and hydrogen (an intestinal gas-bomb). Soaking the beans goes part way towards solving this problem but it is in the cooking that the job can really be done properly. Plenty of water is used to ensure soaking beans absorb all they can and the water still floating on the surface is thrown away. Soya beans are the only group that need to be refrigerated to stop fermentation while they are soaking. A quicker method than simply soaking them is to bring the beans gently to the boil, remove them from the heat and leave them to soak for an hour.

Cooking beans generally requires three quantities of water to one of soaked beans with the exception of soya beans and chick-peas which need five to one. Apple cider vinegar is added just before boiling to the cooking water will reduce the gas-producing activities of beans. At the beginning of the last half hour of cooking the saucepan is removed from the heat, a quarter of a cup of liquid is scooped out and is replaced with the same quantity of apple cider vinegar. The vinegar is stirred with a wooden spoon and flavouring substances such as herbs, spices, celery, carrots, onion, garlic, etc. are added at this stage. The saucepan is returned to the heat and simmered gently. If a bean squashes easily between thumb and forefinger it is well cooked. Interestingly, the more often you eat beans the less intestinal gas you create. Apparently the multiplication of the intestinal bacteria responsible for breaking down stachyose and raffinose is promoted by frequent bean eating. Sprouted

beans do not cause flatulence because the starch is partially converted
to sugar. Remember that long storage
of any pulses will harden them so
much that no amount of soaking or
boiling will tenderize them.

Adzuki, lentils, limas, mung beans
and split peas can all be cooked in the
same pot as grains, and happily all
pulses are rich in lysine which is the
essential amino acid generally deficient in grains. So grains and pulse
make an excellent, perfectly balanced
marriage as far as human nutrition is
concerned; a fact the world has long
unconsciously recognized with famous combinations such as beans on
toast, rice and soya, beans and
tortillas, and rice and dhal.

Always remember that *Leguminosae*
Group of plants, in common with the
Solanaceae are capable of producing
nasty surprises. The seeds of laburnum and lupin (both part of the former
group), can cause death if eaten in
large quantities. Favism was thought
to be the result of eating too many
broad beans; paralyzing lathyrism can
result from eating too many grass
peas.

It has been found that a toxic factor
in kidney beans called haemagglutinin
can result in acute gastroenteritis if it
is not completely destroyed by adequate cooking. The beans need first
to be well soaked and rinsed, which
will reduce the haemagglutinin to the
level found in other dried beans
(soaked or unsoaked). Then boil the
beans really vigorously for ten minutes. Reduce the heat and simmer
them till tender. This will remove any
residual danger. It is possible to use
a slow cooker provided the beans are
first boiled for ten minutes as in-
structed above. They can then be
decanted into the slow cooker.

pulse drying. Drying of pulse is concerned primarily with drying of the
pods, if wet, at time of harvest and
of drying products made from the
pods. Flour and soup are made from
these leguminous pods. Procedures
for handling pea beans are usually in
such a manner to avoid cracking or
checking.

Peas, on the other hand, may be
made into split pea soup. For soups
the product(s) are processed before
being either condensed lentil soup are
made the same way. Processing
before canning consists of soaking
followed by steam cooking for 30
minutes at 110°C in a retort.

Pultost cheese. A Norwegian cheese
made in small dairies in the mountain
section. It is usually made from sour
milk, although rennet may be used. It
is also known as Knoast or Romost.

pumpernickel. Bread made wholly from
rye, baked at rather low temperature
for up to 12 hours in steam. It is
brownish-black and has no crust.

pumpkin. Pumpkin is a variety of winter
squash recognized by its smooth,
round shape and hard-ribbed, orange-
coloured rind, For cooking purposes,
the small sugar pumpkins averaging 1
kg or so are best. Squashes originated
in the New World and were introduced to the conquistadors by early
Native Americans, who in turn carried
these food plants back to Europe with
them later on.

Squash is divided into two basic
groups: the quick-growing, tender-
skinned "summer" squashes, which
are harvested immature; and the
larger, slower growing, hard-shelled
"winter" squashes, harvested when
fully mature. Summer squashes like
yellow crooknecks, pattypans and
zucchini, are consumed whole. But
winter squashes such as Hubbards,

butternuts, aciorns and sugar pumpkins have inedible skins which must first be removed after cooking them before they can be eaten. However they are usually tastier and more nutritious than the summer varieties.

pumpkin drying. Pumpkin or squash may be made into flour. The flesh is removed and cut into 5 mm pieces. After steaming on trays the product is air-dried to 6% moisture. The dry material is reduced in size with a hammer mill.

pumpkin flake drying. Pumpkin may be used for making instant flakes. Pieces of the pumpkin are softened by exposure to 104-121°C for 15-45 minutes. The pumpkin is pureed in a pulper resulting in a product with about 20% solids. The puree is dried on a double-drum dryer, heated with steam. Sheets are removed from the drums which are passed through a grinder to make flakes.

punch. An ice in which fruit juices have been reinforced with an alcoholic beverage. Often rum or whiskey flavouring is used instead of liquor.

pure culture. A population of cells that are identical because they arise from a single cell.

purine. A simple nitrogenous organic molecule with a double ring structure. Members of the purine group include adenine and guanine, which are constituents of the nucleic acids, and certain plant alkaloids, *e.g.*, caffeine and theobromine.

purothionine. A sulphur-containing protein found in wheat flour; kills yeast at a concentration of 0.0001-0.005 mg per ml and may be the "yeast-poisonous" principle that has long been known by bakers and brewers to be present in wheat flour.

purpurogallin test. A test to determine peroxidase in milk. Place 2 ml of fresh skim milk in a test tube, add 10 ml of distilled water, 2 ml of freshly prepared 5% solution of pyrogallic acid, and 2 ml of 1% hydrogen peroxide solution. Shake the contents well, and pour paraffin oil on the surface to form a thin layer, so as to protect the solution from the air. A red precipitate of purpurogallin, which slowly increases on standing, indicates the presence of peroxidase in milk.

putrescible wastes. Wastes which consist mainly of plant or animal residues and which undergo degradation by bacteriological action; *e.g.*, animal residues, cannery wastes, fats, fish residues, fruit wastes, vegetable wastes.

putrescine. $NH_2(CH_2)_4NH_2$. The amine 1,4-butanediamine, derived from the decarboxylation of ornithine. It is found associated with DNA in certain species of bacteria and is the precursor of spermidine which exerts several actions on the control of nucleic acid metabolism.

Paygel. Trade name for a processed wheat starch, used in many food preparations.

pyrethrum flowers. The flowers collected from 2-6 years old plants by hand. They are dried and stored. The plant is widely grown in India, Kenya, Ecuador, Japan, Yugoslavia, east central Africa, and Brazil. The insecticidal activity of Pyrethrum arises from four esters, the pyrethrins I and II and the cinerins I and II. They are complex esters of chrysanthemum carboxylic acid and the monomethyl ester of chrysanthemum dicarboxylic acid with pyrethrolones and cinerolones. The pyrethroids (or rethroids) are synthetic compounds of a similar structure of the pyrethrins themselves. The most important pyrethroids are allethrin, furethrin and cyclethrin. The

Pyrethrum flowers are a contact poison for insects. They are largely used in the form of powder, but sprays in which the active principles are dissolved in kerosene or other organic solvent. It can cause severe allergic dermatitis and systemic allergic reactions.

Large amounts may cause nausea, vomiting, tinnitus, headaches and other CNS disturbances. Pyrethrum flower heads, or Insect Flowers, Dalmation insect powder; Persion insect powder; are the dried flower heads of *Chrysanthemum cinerariaefolium* or of *C. marschallii* (Fam. Compositae). Pyrethrum contains about 0.5% of total pyrethrins.

pyridoxine. A water soluble vitamin (Vitamin B_6) present in milk to the extent of about 0.7 mg/L. There are several metabolically active forms of Vitamin B_6 (pyridoxine, pyridoxal, and pyridoxamine). These compounds function biologically as constituents of enzyme systems which are concerned with protein metabolism. They may also function in fat metabolism. Deficiency of Vitamin B_6 is characterized in some species by the development of dermatitis, anemia, and impaired growth. Cereals, fish and meats are good sources of Vitamin B_6 and vegetables and milk are fair sources.

pyrithiamine. Pyridine analogue of thiamin; antagonistic to the vitamin.

pyrogens. Substances that cause a rise in body temperature. They may arise from microorganisms (viruses, bacteria, moulds, yeasts), especially Gram-negative bacteria, in which case they are high molecular mass lipopolysaccharides. That produced by certain strains of *Escherichia coli* is effective in raising body temperature in doses as low as 1 ng/kg. The bacterial pyrogens act by causing the release of an endogenous pyrogenic lipid-polypeptide complex from polymorphonuclear leucocytes and monocytes, and this in turn activates prostaglandin synthesis in the hyothalamic temperature-regulating centres. The steroid substance namely, aetiocholanolone (a stereoisomer of androsterone) is a potent pyrogen in man. It is a normal intermediary metabolite in man, but abnormally excessive production may be responsible for some fevers. It acts in a similar way to bacterial pyrogens.

pyruvic acid. An intermediate compound produced during glycolysis and converted to acetyl coenzyme A. It can be converted to lactate during anaerobic metabolism, to acetyl coenzyme A in order to enter Krebs cycle, and to oxaloacetate to initiate the process of glyconeogenesis. It also arises from the amino acid alanine by transamination or deamination. Also known as 2-oxopropanoic acid.

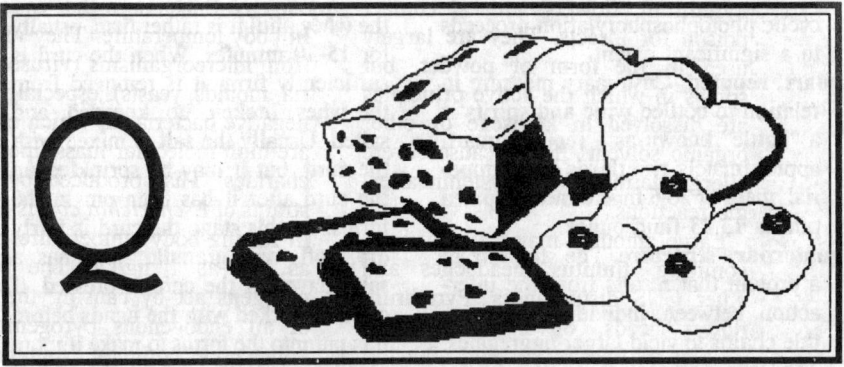

Q-enzyme. A factor isolated from the potatoes which catalyses the formation of branching linkages of the 1,6-α-type in starches; the reaction appears to be irreversible, *i.e.*, Q-enzyme cannot hydrolyze the 1,6-α-linkages.

Q_{O_2}. Symbol used in measuring cell respiration in the Warburg manometer; the number of μL of oxygen consumed (or carbon dioxide or other gas produced) per mg dry weight of tissue per hour.

Q notation. A method used in the past to denote enzyme activity, especially that of respiratory enzymes. The Q_g value of an enzyme was taken to be the number of microliters, at standard temperature and pressure, of the substrate used up per hour per milligram of enzyme.

Q-Tac starch, Trade name for an ammoniated starch. It is prepared by reacting the cornstarch with quaternary ammonium groups.

Quacheq cheese. A kind of sheep's milk cheese made in Macedonia; a small quantity of sour whey is added to the milk to coagulate the curd. It is eaten both fresh and ripened.

quadruple-effect. A multiple-effect unit, such as an evaporator, in which there are four stage. Each successive stage of an evaporator is at a higher vacuum.

quality class. QC. A general method of indicating the general growth performance of a strand of trees. The QC value is calculated from the relationship between the average height of 40 trees of the same type and their age. Generally, the faster the rate of growth the higher the quality class. Many QC calculations have been made for specific tree types and average growth rates. In the forestry system such calculations have been made for all the main commercial species and five QC divisions established ranging from QCI (best) to QCV (poorest). QC values are not comparable between different species and are of only limited use as indicators of future timber yield from a forest.

quantum requirement of photosynthesis. A quantity defined as the number of quanta necessary to evolve 1 molecule of molecular oxygen (O_2). Two quanta are required to raise one electron from the level of water to that of NADPH, and since the formation of one molecule of O_2 is a 4-electron process, a total of 8 quanta are required. This value will, of course, be greater, if in addition to O_2 production cyclic photophosphorylation proceeds to a significant extent.

quart, reputed. Customary measure in relation to bottled wine and spirits is a "bottle" known as a reputed quart, approximately two thirds of an imperial quart, or 26.6 fluid ounce. Reputed pint is 13.33 fluid ounce.

quaternary structure. The structure of a protein that results from the interaction between individual polypeptide chains to yield larger aggregates. The four polypeptide chains fit together in an approximately tetrahedral arrangement, to constitute the characteristic quaternary structure of haemoglobin.

QC. *See* quality class.

quebracho. The material obtained from the bark of *Aspidosperma quebracho-blanco*. It is used as source of tannins and alkaloids. Also known as aspidosperma.

queen substance. The material secreted by the queen bee which inhibits the ovaries of the worker bees and stops them constructing queen cells.

quenelle. A ball of chopped, spiced meat or fish.

quercetin. A flavone found in onion skins, tea, hops, horse chestnuts; the disaccharide derivative containing rhamnose and glucose is rutin.

queso blanco cheese. Name of the principal Latin American cheese. This kind of cheese is made from whole, partly skimmed or skim milk. The cheese may be eaten fresh or cured from two weeks to two months. The fresh, warm cow's milk is put into a wooden vat or tub, or in some instances a hollowed-out log, and it is curdled with rennet, sometimes after considerable acid has developed in the milk. After a coagulation period of 30-45 minutes, the curd is broken up by hand and gently squeezed in the whey until it is rather firm, usually for 15-30 minutes. When the curd is sufficiently firm, it is removed from the whey, broken, up, kneaded, and salted. Usually the salt is mixed with the curd, but it may be sprinkled on the curd after it has been put in the forms. At this stage the curd is fairly dry, soft, and granular, and has a salty flavor. If the curd is pressed, if often is worked with the hands before it is put into the forms to make it more pliable and plastic, and the cheese will be more compact.

The cloth liner is drawn up over the cheese and topped with a wooden cover, which is weighted down with a heavy rock or lever press. The pressed cheese is really hard, crumbly, matted rennet curd with a salty flavor and rather open texture.

The high salt content, usually 5% or more, retards or prevents curing; however, when the cheese is held it develops a strong flavour and odour and it dries and may be used as a grating cheese. Some of the skim-milk cheese is smoked for 2-3 days, which darkens the surface of the cheese and dries it somewhat in addition to giving it a smoked flavour.

Skim milk uncured cheese are named as: Queso de Puna Puerto Rico;

Queso Fresco- El Salvador and Venezuela; Panela- Mexico. Part skimmed pressed cheese are named as:

Queso de Penso- Mexico, El Salvador; Wueso del Pais- Puerto Rico;

Queso de la Tierra- Puerto Rico. Skim milk pressed not cured type of cheese are name as: Quesco

Descreamado- Costa Rica; Quesco Huloso- Costa Rica.

queso de cincho cheese. A kind of sour-milk cheese made in Venezuela and marketed in the form of balls, from 20-30 cm in diameter, wrapped in palm leaves. Also known as Queso de Palma Metida.

queso de crema cheese. A kind of popular Costa Rica cheese which resembles the soft Brick cheese. In Cuba, Venezuela and other Latin American countries, this term refers to a rich, unripened, cream-type cheese.

queso de hoja cheese. A variety of Peurto Rican cheese made from fresh cows' milk. Curd is drained and immersed in hot water or whey at 60°C to toughen curd. Each cheese is about 15 cm in diameter, 2-5 cm thick, and has slightly rounded top and bottom surfaces. When cut it appears to be in layers like leaves one on top of another, hence the name, signifying leaf cheese.

queso de mano cheese. A kind of sour-milk cheese resembling a hand cheese, made in Venezuela; it is about 18 cm in diameter.

queso de Prensa cheese. A variety of hard, Puerto Rican cheese made from cow's whole milk. In one method the milk is ripened, set with rennet and the coagulum is broken by hand. Part of the whey is removed and the curd is drained, salted and pressed. In second method, the milk is heated to 85°C, acetic acid is added to coagulate the milk and then sodium bicarbonate is added to neutralize the acid. The curd is cut into small pieces, salted and pressed. The cheese is eaten fresh or ripened.

queso de puna cheese. A puerto Rican cheese similar to the cottage or Dutch cheese of the US. The curd is put into a hoop 12 cm in diameter, where it remains without pressure for 2-3 days, till it retains its form; usually eaten fresh.

queso del pais cheese. A white, pressed, semisoft perishable cheese made in Puerto Rico. The cheese is usually eaten fresh in which case it resembles Cottage cheese in body. Also known as Quesco de la Tierra (native cheese).

questionnaire. A series of questions (in written form) designed to deduce useful information from an informant on a given topic. It may be administered by an enumerator or interviewer or self-administered. Answers are usually recorded on the questionnaire form itself. The nature of the questions is decided in relation to the subject of the survey and the type of answers required. The questions may be designed to educe opinion, factual, or knowledge responses and are set in a standardized form in order to increase comparability across respondents. The questions are arranged in a logical order and the questionnaire may have printed on it definitions and instructions to the interviewer or to the informant. The layout of the questionnaire is designed primarily to facilitate the task of this interviewer and/or respondent but also to help further processing such as coding and data entry. Questionnaires vary greatly in their structural complexity. The questions are generally phrased in everyday language with a special effort to achieve unambiguous wording. The construction of a questionnaire is often preceded by an exploratory pilot investigation and its efficacy may be ascertained by means of a field pre-test.

quetelet's index. Weight times 100 divided by height squared; index of adiposity.

quick breads. A term generally used for baked goods such as biscuits, muffins, griddles, cakes, waffles and dumplings in which no yeast is used, but the raising is carried out quickly with baking powder or other chemical agents.

quick freezing. As the term implies, a rapid freezing of food by exposure to a blast of air at a very low temperature. Unlike slow freezing, small crystals of ice are formed which do not rupture the cells of the food and so the structure is relatively undamaged. A quick-frozen food is commonly defined as one that has been cooled from a temperature of 0°C to -5°C or lower, in a period of not more than 2 hours, and then cooled to -18°C.

quillaja. The dried bark of *Quillaja saponaria* which contains sapotoxin, tannin and quillaja. It is used to produce foam in soft drinks and shampoos and fire extinguishers.

quince. Pear-shaped sour fruit of *Cydonia* species, with flesh similar to that of the apple; rich in pectin and used chiefly in jams and jellies; used to be known as apple and the vine.

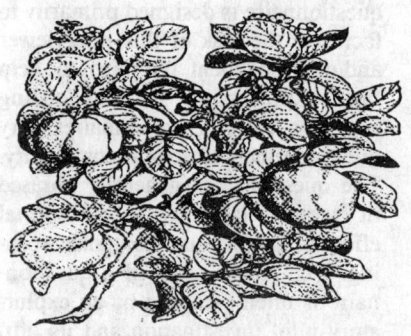

The average composition per 100 g is: water 82.5%; protein 0.5%; carbohydrate 6.5%; vitamin C 14 mg.; and food energy 0.1 MJ.

quinoa. Glutinous seeds of the plant *Chenopodium album*, grown in Chile. It is made into bread. The average composition per 100 g is: protein 11%; fat 5.5%; carbohydrate 62%,; fibre 6%; calcium 125 mg; iron 8 mg; vitamin B 0.5 mg; vitamin B_2 0.3 mg; and nicotinic acid 1.5 mg.

quinoline yellow. D&C yellow no. 10. The disodium salt of 2-(2-quinolyl-1,3-inadandionesulphonic acid. It is a yellow powder, which is soluble in water and glycerol to give a bright greenish yellow solution. Quinoline yellow has good light-resistance and is very stable in acid media and in the presence of sulphur dioxide; it is only poorly stable in alkaline media and fades with benzoic acid. It is permitted for use in the EEC countries. The colour is used widely throughout Europe and Central and South America. It is currently not permitted for use in foods in the US.

quinones. The cyclic diketones of such a structure that they are converted by reduction into hydroquinone. Since, quinones are highly conjugated, they are highly coloured. Their ready interconversion provides a very convenient oxidation-reduction system. Mitochondria contains a quinone called ubiquinone. The length of the side chain varies with the source of mitochondria. In animal tissues, the quinone possesses ten isoprenoid units in its side chain and is called coenzyme Q_{10} (CoQ_{10}). Because of its long aliphatic side chain, ubiquinone is lipid soluble, and together with cytochrome c, it is easily solubilized from inner mitochondrial membrane. When the quinone is extracted from mitochondria, the transport of electrons from substrates to oxygen is inhibited; the activity is restored when quinone is added back. Because it is readily reduced and oxidized, it serves an additional electron carrier between the flavin coenzymes and the cytochromes (quinone-hydroquinone system). The enzyme which transfers hydrogen from quinone system to cytochrome c, called ubihydroquinone-cytochrome C reductase.

radappertization. Treatment of food by radiation in doses sufficient to reduce the number of harmful organisms below the detection limit, *i.e.*, commercial sterility. This process is usually applicable to precooked (enzyme inactivated) foods that are hermetically sealed-in metal cans, flexible pouches, aluminium or plastic trays. A comparatively high dosage of irradiation is used and sometimes the process is called radiation sterilization. It has been found that the process is applicable to the precooked red meat, poultry, fin fish, and shellfish, as well as to dry foods, animals feeds, and spices. The resulting radappertized products are free of food spoilage microorganisms and organisms of public health significance, including the pathogens such as *Clostridium botulinum, Salmo-nellae, trichinae*, among others. The radappertized products can be stored without refrigeration for long periods (for years in some cases), the limiting factor being the integrity of the primary packaging material to avoid post-processing contamination. Although the radappertized products are ready to eat, they can also be warmed prior to table serving and additional culinary preparation, using a variety of recipes, can be applied to these foods.

Radener cheese. A variety of hard, rennet cheese made in Mecklenburg, Germany from skim milk. It is made similar to Emmentaler, except that it is pressed to a lesser extent. The rolls are 10 cm thick and 40 cm in diameter. Also known also as skim milk Rundkase.

radiation pollution. The pollution occurring as a result of radiations of any potentially harmful nature. In practice, the harm arises from a combination of intensity, wavelength, and time of exposure. Although the mutagenic effects of radiation have recognized for a long time, the exact mechanism of their action is not completely known. Various explanations have been offered, mainly on the basis of *in vitro* effects of radiation on DNA. Thus X-rays and other ionizing radiations are known to produce in aqueous solutions the free radicals such as OH, HO_2, and F, which are short-lived and highly reactive; these supposedly could react somehow with DNA, causing mutation and, in stronger doses, death of the cell.

radiation source. A term referring to usually, an artificial sealed source of radioactivity used in food or any other industry. According to some authors, accelerators radioisotopic generators, and natural radionuclides may also be considered as radiation sources.

radiation standards. The exposure standards, permissible concentrations, rules for safe handling, regulations for transportation, regulations for industrial control of radiation, and control of radiation exposure by legislative means. These are based on the rates of injury under certain known conditions.

radiation units. The units of measurement used to express the activity of a radionuclide and the dose of ionizing radiation.

The units curie, roentgen, rad, and rem are not coherent with SI units but their temporary use with SI units has been approved while the derived SI units becquerel, gray, and sievert have become familiar.

The becquerel (Bq), is the SI unit of activity, it corresponds to the activity of a radionuclide decaying at a rate, on average, of one spontaneous nuclear transition per second;

$$1 \text{ Bq} = 1 \text{ s}^{-1}$$

The former unit, the curie [Ci], is equal to 3.7×10^{10} Bq. The gray (Gy), the SI unit of absorbed dose, is the absorbed dose when the energy per unit mass imparted to matter by ionizing radiation is 1 joule per kilogram.

radicidation. Treatment of food by radiation in doses sufficient to reduce the number of viable specific non-spore-forming pathogens below detectable levels, i.e., doses lower than

radippertization, q.v. The term radiation pasteurization has recent been differentiated into radicidation and radurization.

radioactive contamination. The radiation released upon the disintegration of radioactive atomic nuclei takes the form of particulate or wave radiation of very high energy. When this radiation impinges on living cells, various interactions can result. The most important of these is the ionization of atoms. If this process of ionization of atoms takes place in living tissue, in certain circumstances a variety of damage may result.

radioactivity. Isotopes of various elements break down with the emission of ionizing radiation. Advantage is taken of this property to prepare substances of physiological interest with radioactive carbon or hydrogen or other element in the compound. When these are administered to the subject their metabolic fate can be observed. Also used therapeutically, i.e., radioactive iodine accumulates in the thyroid gland and is used to depress an overactive thyroid. Radioactive materials are also used to inhibit enzymes and microorganisms in foodstuffs and so effect a kind of cold sterilization.

radioimmunoassay. A radioimmunoassay technique that utilizes a purified radioisotope-labeled antigen or antibody to compete for antibody or antigen with unlabeled standard and samples to determine the concentration of a substance in the samples. It is used for assaying hormones, drugs, peptides, and other substances that are antigenic and present in very low concentration in biological tissues and fluids. It depends upon the ability of the unlabeled antigen to inhibit competitively the binding of radioactively labelled antigen to specific antibody. Protein hormone concentrations to 1 pg/ml can be measured accurately. Radioactive isotopes are used to label hormones which are then introduced, with specific antibodies, into the tissues or fluids that are being analyzed. The proportion of labelled hormone that becomes bound to the antibody is recorded.

radioisotopic enzyme assay. An enzyme assay based on the measurement of radioactivity in a product of the enzyme-catalyzed or other similar reaction when one of the reactants is radioactively labeled.

adiopasteurization. The sterilization of foods by ionizing radiation often confers unpleasant flavours on the food. This can be avoided by using a combination of heat with a lower dose of radiation (radiopasteurization). Doses of 200,000-300,000 rads plus heat can lengthen the shelf life of meat 5-10 times.

diophosphorus decay. The radioactive disintegration of P^{32}, particularly that in P^{32}-labeled phage nucleic acid. The disintegrations lead to breaks in the sugar-phosphate backbone of the nucleic acid. Single-stranded nucleic cid is inactivated when a chain break ccurs, but double-stranded nucleic cid is inactivated only when a break ccurs in both strands.

ish. Family: *Cruciferae*. Genus: *phanus*. Species: *Raphanus sativus*. dishes contain vitamins B and C, as ll as calcium, copper, iron, magnem, phosphorus, potassium, som, sulphur, fibre, volatile oil, and e of carotene. They are excellent relieving dyspepsia, and are used promote salivation (hence the om of serving them at the begin-; of meals). They were once loyed in the treatment of coughs

and bronchitis, and may be used with other remedies to treat liver conditions, especially where bile secretion is inadequate. They are good for the teeth, gums, hair and nails. They also relieve constipation and catarrh and improve the condition of fluids flushing through the mucous membranes. They have a mild diuretic effect. The average composition per 100 g is: fat 0.22%; protein 0.5%; calcium 21.3 mg; iron 0.5 mg; vitamin A 6 µg; vitamin B_1 0.02 mg; vitamin B_2 0.01 mg; nicotinic acid 0.21 mg; vitamin C 13.2 mg; and food energy 0.05 MJ.

Radolfzeller cream. A kind of cheese made near Lake Constance which is between Germany, Switzerland and Austria. This Mainauer-lime Munster-like cheese is made from cow's whole milk. During curing, the cheese is turned daily and later every 2-3 days. It is smear ripened.

radurization. Treatment of food by radiation in doses sufficient to enhance its keeping properties by reducing the number of spoilage organisms. The term radiation pasteurization has recently been differentiated into radicidation and redurization.

raffinade. Best quality refined sugar.

raffinose. A trisaccharide found in cotton seed and sugar-beet molasses. It hydrolyzes to give fructose and melibiose, which in turn hydrolyses to glucose and galactose; it possesses 23% sweetness of sucrose. Also known as meltose; melitriose.

raisin oil. The oily substance obtained from seeds of Muscat grapes, which are removed before drying the grapes for raisins. It is used primarily to coat the raisins to prevent them sticking together, render them soft and pliable, and less subject to insect infestation.

raisins. Dried seedless grapes of several kinds. Valencia raisins from Spanish grapes; fruit dipped in potash lye and dried on cane trays in the sun.

Ralston. Trade name for an American breakfast cereal; contains whole wheat plus added wheat germ.

ramekin.´ 1. Porcelain or earthenware mould in which mixture is baked and then brought to the table. Paper souffle cases nowadays called remekin cases. **2.** Formerly the name given to toasted cheese; now tarts filled with cream cheese are called remekins.

rancidity. 1. A term applied to any fat or oil that develops a disagreeable odor when left exposed to warm, moist air for certain period. Rancidity arises due to the presence of volatile, bad-smelling acids and aldehydes. These compounds result from attack by oxygen at reactive allylic positions in the fat molecules. It is thus autooxidation of lipids and is a chain reaction providing a continuous supply of the radicals that initiate further peroxidation. To control and reduce peroxidation, antioxidants are employed. Propyl gallate, butylated hydroxyanisole and butylated hydroxytoluene are some of the antioxidants used for this purpose. Naturally occurring oxidants include vitamin E (tocopherol), which is lipid soluble, and vitamin C (ascorbic acid), which is water soluble.

2. In dairy technology, the term rancidity refers to the flavour defect of dairy products resulting from the hydrolysis of butterfat with the subsequent liberation of fatty acids of low carbon content, particularly butyric acid. In milk, rancidity often accompanies odour problem and frequently appears in milk from cows well along in lactation. Dairy products which have been held in storage often have this defect as a result of the action of the enzyme lipase, or of acids, or iron and copper salts which act as catalysts. This rancidity is not always a defect as lipolytic enzymes or rennet paste are added to milk in the making of certain types of Italian cheese to promote rancidity. This defect is found in all dairy products.

Rangiport cheese. A kind of cheese which is very similar to Port du Salut cheese. It is about 15 cm in diameter and 6 cm thick. It is made in the Department of Seine-et-Oise, France.

rape. *Brassica napus.* A plant closely related to garden swede. Its seed are used as source of edible oil although its content of erucic acid has raised problems. Residual oilcake used for animal feed although it contains goitrogens. Also known as cole; coleseed.

rapeseed oil. An oil obtained from seeds of the mustard family, *Cruciferae.* The genus *Brassica,* a form of turnip, species of which are referred to as *B. campestris, B. rapa, B. napus,* and *B. hirta,* is grown in India, Pakistan Europe, and Canada. Also known as rapeseed oil, colza oil, and recently, canbra oil.

Rapeseed is one of the principal oil seeds of the world. It is widely used as an edible oil, and for mixing with lubricating and cutting oils and for quenching oils. The seeds contain 40% oil. The edible oil is cold-pressed and refined with caustic soda. The burning and lubricating oils are refined with sulphuric acid. The refined oil has a mustard-like odour which can be deodorized. Its iodine value is ~100, the specific gravity 0.915, and flash point is 235°C. The oil contains palmitic, oleic, linoleic, and stearic acids and 43-50% of the typical acid, erucic acid, also called brassidic acid, $C_{21}H_{41}COOH$. It occurs also in rapeseed oil. For edible oils, the erucic acid is reduced, generally to less than 5%; the high-erucic-acid oils are used industrially as lubricant additives. Genetic variants with no erucic acid have also been made.

Crambe seed oil is obtained from *Crambe abyssinica,* an Asiatic mustard, and contains about 55-60% erucic acid, which can be broken down to perlargonic acid. It is used as a substitute for dibasic acids such as azelaic acid and brassylic acid.

The name colza refers to any kind of refined rape oil. Colza oil is a rape oil extracted from French seed. It is used to mix. with mineral oils for making cutting oils.

Chinese colza oil, obtained from the *B. campestris chinoleifera,* contains mustard volatile oil. Its specific gravity is 0.91, saponification value 174, and iodine number 100.3. 15-20% of blown rapeseed oil is mixed with mineral oil for lubricating marine engines.

Cameline oil, called also doddar oil and German sesame oil, has the same used as rape oil. It is obtained from the plant *Camelina sativa.* The seeds contain 35% oil which contains oleic and palmitic acids and also erucic acid. The seed itself is high in mineral and protein content.

rapid sand filter. A filter bed used for the filtration of water. the bed comprises layers of coarse sand and graded gravel with an under-drainage system. Such filters are provided with backwashing arrangement. Also known as rapid gravity filter.

rare bases. The purine and pyrimidine nucleoside phosphates that occur in nucleic acids. They include compounds such as 1-methylguanosine, ribothymidine and 5-ribosyluracil which are found in the molecules of transfer RNA.

raspberry. (Red, Black) *Rubus idaeus, R. crataegifolius, R. occidentalis).* Red raspberry produces a spring and fall crop, with the latter being sweeter on account of the cooler weather (unless the spring is cool, too). The red raspberry has less seeds and is juicer than the black variety. The black is darker and its shape is more odd, being that of a skull cap rather than the ball shape of the red kind. Its season is only 4 weeks.

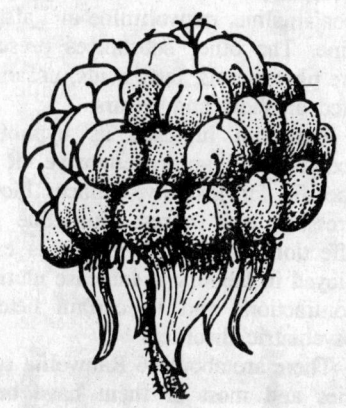

The average composition per 100 g of raspberry is: protein 1.4%; fat 1.2%; calcium 43 mg; iron 1 mg; vitamin A 35 mg; vitamin B_1 0.03 mg; vitamin B_2 0.07 mg; nicotinic acid 0.3 mg; and vitamin C 25 mg.

rastrello. Common name for a sharp-edged spoon used to cut out the pulp from halved oranges and other citrus fruits.

ratafia. Popular name for the flavouring essence made from bitter almonds; also a small light macaroon biscuit used in trifles; also a liqueur made from plum, peach and apricot kernels and bitter almonds.

Rauwolfia. The dried rhizome and roots of *Rauwolfia serpentina* Benth. It is one of the various Indian plant species that have been enlisted as endangered, threatened, or rare. Sometimes with piece of rhizome and aerial stem bases are attached. Rauwolfia contains about 0.7-2.4% total alkaloidal bases from which more than 50 alkaloids have been isolated. The prominent alkaloids isolated from the drug include reserpine, rescinnamine and deserpidine. The other alkaloidal components found are: ajmalinine, ajmaline (rauwolfine), ajmalicine serpentine, serpentinine, tetrahydro-reserpine, raubasine, reserpinine, isoajamaline, rauwolfinine and alstonine. The other substances present are phytosterols, fatty acids, unsaturated alcohols and sugars.

Rauwolfia in used as hypnotic, sedative and antihypertensive. It is specific for insanity, reduces blood pressure and cures pain due to affections of the bowels. It is employed in labours to increase uterine contractions and in certain neuropsychiatric disorders.

There are about 86 Rauwolfia species and most of them have been examined for reserpine and related alkaloids. *R. tetraphylla (R. canescens* Linn., *R. hirsuta)* is widely distributed in tropical areas of south America, Caribbean, India, and Australia. Its roots had been substituted for *R. serpentina.* It is recognized by its non-stratified cork, and sclereid groups in the phloem. The alkaloids reserpine and deserpidine are isolated on commercial scale from *R. tetraphylla. R. nitida* is found in West India. 33 indole alkaloids have been isolated from its root-bark.

raw feed. The product fed into the dryer which may be considered on the basis of the following physical and chemical properties: source of raw feed, number of products from same dryer, previous dewatering, raw feed storage, method of handling product to and from dryer, particle size distribution, physical characteristics for modulability, abrasiveness, odour, fire hazards, explosion hazards, temperature limitations, temperature effects, and corrosive effects.

raw milk. Milk which has not been subjected to any heat treatment such as pasteurization or processed in any other way. Therefore any objectionable bacteria which it may contain have not been destroyed.

raw sugar. Brown unrefined sugar, 96-98% pure; contaminated with mould spores, bacteria, cane fibre, and dirt.

Reblochon cheese. A soft French cheese, made from fresh whole milk and curdled with rennet.

read-through protein. A protein that is produced as a result of a failure in the termination of translation of a polycistronic messenger RNA; such a protein consists of the regular amino acid sequence specified by its cistron along with a sequence of amino acids that corresponds to a translated intercistronic region.

reciprocal ponderal index. Height divided by cube root of weight; index of adiposity.

Reckangel's phenomenon. Slight increase in the specific gravity of milk that may continue for up to 12 hours after milking; total effect may be equivalent to 0.15% solids-not-fat in the milk. The cause is not yet known.

recommended intake. As applied to food and nutrition, the amount thought to be needed to maintain health, and excludes any additional needs arising from disease, stress, etc. The recommended intake of the nutrients varies from person to person and according to the physical fitness and physical activity performed by person.

reconstituted milk. Whole milk powder or non-fat milk powder to which has been added the required amount of water (the amount of water to be used is stated on the package of milk powder). The mixture is placed in a container and shaken vigorously or mixed with an egg beater. If any undissolved lumps remain, the mixture should be strained. It should be chilled in the refrigerator, stirred well, and served as ordinary milk. Milk of fluid composition may also be reconstituted from plain condensed and evaporated milk, either whole or skim milk, by the addition of a proper quantity of water.

reconstructed cream. A product made by combining unsalted butter and fresh skim milk by passing them through a homogenizer or emulsifier at high temperature. This mixture is often sold as fresh cream, but such a practice should not be tolerated. Milk may also be reconstructed in similar fashion.

rectifying column. A distillation column so arranged that the vapour condenses and redistills many times before it finally condenses to form the distillate, and so is purified to greater degree than in simple distillation.

recycling. The return of discarded or waste materials to the production system for utilization in the manufacture of goods, with a view to the conservation as far as practicable of nonrenewable and scare resources. Recycling goes beyond the reuse of a product (such as glass milk bottles) and involves the return of salvaged materials, such as paper or metals or broken glass, to an early stage (pulping or melting stage) or of the manufacturing process. In many instances, recycling has always been profitable to certain industries, opin-ion now seems to favour an increased tempo and scale of recycling to conserve resources for the future of mankind beyond what may be profitable in the shorter term. The capacity of an industry to recycle is in many cases limited by technical as well as economic consideration.

red algae. A division *Rhodophyta*, including approximately 4,000 species of red algae, most of which are seaweeds. A few red algae are unicellular but most are filamentous and multicellular. Some are up to 1 metre long. The red algae contain the red pigment phycoerythrin, one of the two types of phycobilins that they possess. The other accessory pigment is the blue pigment phycocyanin. The presence of these pigments explains how the red algae can live at depths of 100 m or more. The wavelengths of light (green, violet, and blue) that penetrate these depths are not absorbed by chlorophyll a but, instead, by these phycobilins. The phycobilins, after absorbing the light energy, pass it on to chlorophyll a. The algae appears decidedly red when phycoerythrin undergoes photodestruction in bright light, other pigments predominate and the algae take on shades of blue, brown, and dark green. Because the red algae possess the same pigments as the cyanobacteria, it has been suggested that cyanobacteria become symbiotic in the cells of the heterotrophic ancestors of the red algae and developed into their chloroplasts. The life cycle of red algae are complex and usually involve an alternation of generations, like that of the brown algae. None of the reds have flagella or cilia at any stage in their life cycle; they also lack centrioles. The cell walls of the red algae include a rigid inner part composed of microfibrils and a mucilaginous matrix. The matrix is composed of the sulphated polymers of galactose called agar, funori, porphysan, and carrageenan. It is these four polymers that give the red algae their flexible, slippery texture. In addition, many red algae deposit calcium carbonate in their cell walls and play an important role in building coral reefs.

red clover. *Trifolium pratense.* Family: *Leguminosae.* A flowering plant whose flowers are about 10 mm long in a head up to 3 cm long. The plants are about 30 cm high. The flowers are rosy red and the leaves are dark green. Red clover flowers smell like honey and are attractive to both bumblebees and honey bees. Nectar is the reward these insects receive for spreading pollen from one plant to another. The fruit is a small pod. The flowers are tube shaped, small, and sweet smelling.

red colours. The frequently used red colours used in food industry. The use of some of them is not permitted in US and many other countries.

Red 10 B. The disodium salt of 8-amino-2-phenylazo-1-naphthol-3,6-disulphonic acid.

Red 2G. The disodium salt of 8-acetamido-2-phenylazo-1-naphthol-3,6-disulphonic acid.

Red 6B. The disodium salt of 8-acetamido-2-*p*-acetamide-phenylazo-1-naphthol-3,6-disulphonic acid.

Red FB. The disodium salt of 2-(4-(1-hydroxy-4-sulpho-2-naphthylazo)-3-sulphophenyl)-6-methylbenzothiazole.

Fast Red E. The disodium salt of 1-(4-sulpho-1-naphthylazo)-2-hydroxynaphthalene-6-sulphonic acid.

red herrings. Herrings that have been well salted and smoked for about 10 days. Bloaters are salted less and smoked for a shorter time; kippers lightly salted and smoked overnight. Also called Yarmouth bloaters.

red radish. *Raphanus sativus.* Daikon radish. *Raphanus sativus longipinnatus.* Radishes have been around since the days of Mosses. The Egyptian pharaohs included them as standard rations, along with garlic, leeks, onions and cucumbers, for the several hundred thousand Hebrew slaves who constructed their mighty pyramids for them. In US, the cherry-sized red reddish is the most common variety sold, but radishes come in all shapes, sizes and colours, including an intriguing black one. Popular varieties besides the Scarlet Globe and Cherry Belly (both globular red radishes), are French Breakfast (an elongated, white-tipped red radish), White Icicle (long and mild tasting) and the favorite of all Japanese, the Daikon (a long, sharp-tasting white radish).

reducer. A hetertrophic individual which utilizes the chemical energy of organic matter while breaking it down or reducing it to more simple substance.

reducing sugars. Sugars that contain the aldehydic or ketonic reducing group, such as glucose, fructose, lactose, pentoses. They are tested for by their ability to reduce reagents such as Fehling's solution, Benedict's solution.

reduction. 1. Addition of hydrogen to, or subtraction of oxygen from a substance. Though reduction can be regarded simply as the removal of oxygen, it also has a broader meaning; the acceptance of one or more electrons (or their equivalent) from another substance. Reduction can also be effected by the addition of hydrogen to a molecule.

2. Lowering the valence of an element in combination, as reducing ferric chloride to ferrous chloride.

3. Both the preceding processes, and the complete reactions of which they are a part, involve an interchange of electrons between atoms, where upon the atom gaining the electron(s) is reduced, and the atom losing the electron or electrons is oxidized.

reductones. Enediols which may be formed from sugars carrying a free carboxyl group by heating in alkaline solution. The simplest is hydroxyglycoaldehyde. Reductones may be formed in carbohydrate foods during heat processing, and as they have similar properties to vitamin C they interfere with its estimation.

reference man. An arbitrary physiological standard; defined as a man of 25 years, healthy, weight 65 kg, living in a temperate zone at a mean annual temperature of 10°C, assumed to require an average daily intake of 3,200 kcal (13.5 MJ).

reference protein. A theoretical concept of the perfect protein which is used with 100%, efficiency at whatever level it is fed in the diet; used as a means of expressing recommended intakes. The nearest approach to this theoretical protein are egg and human milk proteins which are used with 90-100% efficiency when fed at low levels in the diet (4%) but not when fed at high levels (10-15%).

reference woman. An arbitrary physiological standard; defined as 25 years of age, 55 kg weight, engaged in general household duties or light industry, using 2,300 kcal (9.7 MJ) per day, and as reference man, living in a temperate zone at a mean annual temperature of 10°C. .

refractive index. A measure of the bending or refraction of a beam of light on entering a denser medium; the ratio of the sine of the angle of incidence of the ray of light to the sine of the angle of refraction. It is constant for pure substances under standard conditions. It is used as a measure of sugar or total solids in solution, purity of oils, etc.

refractometer. Optical instrument used to measure the refractive index. The Abbe refractometer consists of two prisms between which is spread the substance under examination (jam, fruit juice, sugar syrup, etc.) and light is reflected through the solution. The immersion refractometer dips into the solution.

refrigerant. In general, any substance used to attain reduced temperatures. In specific sense, a fluid used for heat-transfer purposes in refrigerating equipment. The substances most frequently used for this purpose are fluorinated hydrocarbons, and they are also widely used as propellants in aerosol spray dispenser cans.

They should be referred to either by their chemical names or by their international designations, which consist of a number preceded by the letter R (for example, R12 is dichlorodifluoromethane, and R22 is chlorodifluoromethane). Fears have been expressed that the fluorinated hydrocarbon propellants released from spray cans, drifting upward in the atmosphere, might be responsible for reducing the amount of ozone in the ozone layer, thus permitting a greater proportion of the solar ultraviolet radiation to reach the earth's surface, with serious consequences for the life on the earth.

refuse. The complete range of unwanted or undesirable material generated in the course of producing, processing and consuming useful products.

regeneration. 1. Returning a changed material or natural product to its original state or condition after it has been chemically modified for processing purposes. Regeneration should not be confused with reclaiming, which only partially restores the original properties of a material.
2. Renewing or reactivating a catalyst, molecular sieve, or ion-exchangers by any of several recommended methods. Catalysts fouled with coke or other deposits are regenerated by treatment with hot reactive gases such as oxygen, hydrogen steam, etc.

Reggiano cheese. A variety of Grana cheese which is commonly called Parmesan or Reggiano Parmesan in US. This cheese was first made in Reggio Emilia region of Italy.

regulatory site. A site on a regulatory enzyme to which an effector binds, as distinct from a catalytic site to which the substrate binds. Also known as allosteric site.

regulon. A group of genes that are not associated as an operon but yet are responsible for the coordinate induction of a number of enzymes. Although these genes are scattered along the chromosome, they are apparently under the control of a single regulator gene.

Rehfuss tube. An instrument used for removing samples of food from the stomach after a test meal. It is a small-diameter tube with a slotted metal tip. Another type is the Ryle tube.

Reichert-Meissl value. Measure of the volatile fatty acids in fats. It is defined as number of ml of 0.1N sodium hydroxide required to neutralize the distillate from 5 g of fat. Also called Riechert-Meissl number.

relative biological effectiveness. RBE. The ratio of the biological effect produced by one ionizing radiation to that produced by an identical dose of a different ionizing radiation; also equal to the ratio of the doses of two different ionizing radiations that produce the same biological effect. For such calculations, the biological effect produced by X-rays, γ-rays, or β-particles is generally assigned a value of unity.

relative humidity. The ratio between the actual weight of water vapour in a given volume of air and the amount which would be present if the air was saturated at the same temperature, expressed as a percentage. The total amount of water vapour that a given volume of air contains (expressed in grams per cubic metre) is called the absolute humidity. The humidity measurements are of great significance for several reasons:

(a) the amount of water vapour present in a given volume of air is an indication of the atmosphere's potential capacity for precipitation;

(b) water vapour, in its power to absorb radiation, is a regulator of heat loss from the earth;

(c) the amount of water vapour present in the atmosphere decides the quantity of latent energy stored up in the atmosphere for the growth of storms; and

(d) the amount of water vapour present is an important factor affecting the human body's rate of cooling.

The relative humidity depends depends both upon the absolute humidity and the temperature; if the moisture content remains the same, then the relative humidity will decrease as the temperature rises and will increase as the temperature falls.

Relative humidity is very important in food preservation as microorganisms require moisture to live, but under some moist conditions, *e.g.*, in a high concentration of sugar solution, the moisture is not available. Moulds will not grow on jam, 30% water, but will grow on cereals, 10% water. Bacteria need more moisture than yeasts, therefore less of a hazard. Minimum relative humidity requirement for yeasts is 75%, increasing as temperature decreases.

release agents. Substances applied to tinned or enamelled surfaces or plastic films to prevent the food adhering; e.g., fatty acid amides, microcrystalline waxes, petrolatum, starch, methylcellulose.

renal threshold. Blood level of a particular substance at which it is excreted through the kidney; for example, renal threshold of glucose is about 180 mg/100 ml, and diabetics excrete glucose because this level is exceeded. Various drugs can reduced the renal threshold.

rendering. The process of liberating the fat cells that constitute the adipose tissue. Dry rendering orheating fat dry, when water is present.

renin. The enzyme that stimulates angiotensin formation from liver globulin and is synthesized in the kidney. It is released in increased amounts in humans suffering form high blood pressure.

rennet. An extract containing the enzyme rennin, or dried preparations of rennin. Commercial rennet is sold in clarified saline solution or in powdered form. It usually contains a certain amount of pepsin. It is widely used in curdling milk for the preparation of cheese and casein.

rennin. An enzyme found in gastric juices and responsible for the coagulation of casein in milk. It acts by hydrolyzing peptide links. At 37°C, rennin can coagulate 10^7 times its own weight of milk in ten minutes. It has

been crystallized out but is manufactured from the stomach of animals and sold under the name rennet. It is used in the manufacture of cheese and junkets. It is secreted in the stomachs of young mammals. The extract containing rennin is called rennet and its usual source is the inner lining of the fourth stomach of young calves, lambs, and goats, Rennin is one of the most powerful catalysts known and is widely used in coagulating the casein of milk in cheese manufacture. In the nourishment of young calves that are fed milk, rennin, by clotting the milk, retains it in the digestive tract where it can be acted upon by the digestive enzymes. This enzyme has only a weak proteolytic power at the pH of milk.

rentschlerizing. Sterilizing by treatment with ultraviolet light.

R-enzyme. Enzyme present in beans and potatoes that splits the 1,6-glucosidase found in muscle. Also known as the "de-branching" factor.

replication. The mechanism by which exact copies of genetic material are formed. Replicas of DNA are made when the double helix unzips and the separated strands serve as templates along which complementary nucleotides attach themselves by hydrogen bonding. The result is two new molecules of DNA each containing one strand of the original molecule, and the process is called semiconservative replication. In certain RNA viruses it has been demonstrated that the RNA is capable of replication. In replication, the strands of DNA will separate and new complementary strands of DNA will be assembled from the four available deoxyribonucleotide triphosphates from each of the two separate parent strands. Assuming the base pairing to be precise, the two new DNA molecules should be identical to the parent molecules. This type of replication has been called semiconservative.

Another possibility is that the final duplication product consists of a double helix of the original two strands and a second double helix consisting of newly synthesized chains. This process is called a conservative type of replication.

A third possibility, called dispersive, could take place if the nucleotides of the parent DNA are randomly scattered among the components of the daughter DNA material so that the new DNA consists of a mixture of old and new nucleotides scattered along the chains. Replication is discontinuous and always occurs in 5' to 3' direction on both strands of a duplex DNA. The process begins at several points along the duplex strands; however, for initiation to begin, the duplex strand must first be separated into single strands for the polymerases to function. Presumably at the several points, unique proteins of low molecular mass (~35,000), in both procaryotic and eucaryotic organisms, binds specifically to one of the two strands. The binding appears to relate to those regions of the duplex rich in A-T base pairing. Since A-T base pairs have a lower energy of hydrogen bonding than G-C base pairs, these regions appear to be more susceptible to melting or conversion from duplex to single-stranded DNA. These proteins called unwinding proteins, are essential for initiation as well as for the continuation of replication.

repressible enzyme. Enzyme formed in bacteria only when the cells are grown in the absence of its product (or the final product of the metabolic pathway of which the repressible enzyme is a component).

repressor protein. A protein coded for by a regulator gene that can bind to the operator and inhibit transcription; it may be active by itself or only when the corepressor is bound to it.

Requeijao cheese. A kind of cheese prepared in northern Brazil. Skim milk in held until coagulation takes place. This coagulum is heated to 80°C, drained, and pressed in bags. This curd is broken up and mixed with two parts of skim milk. The mixture is heated, and stirred as before. The draining, pressing and washing with skim milk take place once more. Hot butterfat or cream is added and the mixture is heated. The cheese is then molded into boxes.

residual chlorine. The amount of available chlorine present in industrial water at any given time after chlorine or hypochlorite has been added to it.

residual use. A use other than a beneficial use in of respect of water, e.g., the disposal of liquid effluents.

resin acids. The mixture of oxyacids, carboxylic acids and phenols. They are present in the free state or as esters. they are soluble in aqueous alkaline solutions which form soaplike froath on shaking. Abietic acid in Rosin or Colophony, copaivic acid and oxycopaivic acid in Copaiba, guaiaconic acid in Guaiac, pimaric (pimarinic) acid in Frankincense, sandaracolic acid in Sandarac, aleuritic acid in Shellac and commiphoric acid in Myrrh are the examples of resin acids.

resin alcohols. The complex molecules with high molecular mass. They are present in the free state or as esters of simple aromatic acids, e.g., benzoic acid, salicylic acid, cinnamic acid and umbellic acid. They are further sub-divided as:

Resinotannols. These are tannins and form blue colour with ferric chloride, such as aloeresinotannol from Aloe, amoresinotannol and galbaresinotannol from Ammoniac, peruresinotannol from Balsam of Peru, siaresinotannol and sumaresinotannol from Benzoin.

Resinols. Resinols do not contain tannins. Benzoresinol from Benzoin, storesinol from Storax and guaiacre-sinol from Guaiac resin are the examples of resinols.

resins. Solid or semisolid plant exudates formed in schizogenous or schizo-lysigenous ducts or cavities. They are complex mixtures of compounds like resin alcohols (resinols), resin acids, resinotannols, (resinphenols), esters and resenes. Some resins (*e.g.*, Ben-zoin and Balsam of Tolu) are formed when the plant is injured. These resins ae called as pathological resins.

Resins are classified on the basis of their occurrence in combination with another compounds as:

Balsams. The resinous substances which contain large proportions of benzoic or cinnamic acids either free or in combination or their esters. Tolu balsam contains 35-50% of balsamic acids (chiefly benzoic and cinnamic) which are present partly in the free state and partly in combination with complex 'resin alcohols'. Benzoin, Peru balsam and Storax, are another examples of balsams.

Oleoresins. When resins occur with volatile oils, the mixture is called as oleoresins. Turpentine, Capsicum, Ginger, Male fern, Canada Balsam and Copaiba are oleoresins.

Gum Resins. When resins are found in combination with gums, then such resins are known as gum resins.

These resins are purified by dissolv-ing the associated gum in water. Asafoetida, Gambage and Myrrh are gum-resins.

Oleo-gum resins. Oleo-gum resins are associated with gum and volatile oil both. Volatile oil is removed by steam distillation while gum is sepa-rated by dissoling in water.

Glycoresins. Some resins are found in combination with glycosides. These resins occur in Ipomoea, Scammony, Jalap and Podophyllum. On hydroly-sis they produce sugars and complex resin acids as aglycones.

resin composition. Purified resins are amorphous, brittle, transluscent, hard solids. On heating they are softened and then melt. They are practically insoluble in water but dissolve in organic solvents like alcohol, ether and chloroform. Varnish-like film is formed on evaporation of the solvent. They produce smoky flame on burn-ing. Chemically, resins are complex mixtures of many compounds includ-ing resin acids such as abietic acid, copaivic acid, and sandaracolic acid; resin alcohols and resenes. *see also* resin acids; resin alcohols.

resin formation. In many instances, a resin in plants is formed in special passages or tubes called resin ducts, which usually anastomose. Thus a single incision may drain the resin from a considerable area of the plant. The cells lining the ducts possess a layer (called the resinogenous layer) of slimy matter bounded by a fine cuticle and resin is secreted in this layer. It is excreted through the cuticle into the resin duct.

In some cases, such as Copaiba, numerous resin ducts are present. Tapping is necessary to drain the ducts. Such resin is called as normal or physiologically-produced resin. In other instances, *e.g.*, turpentine, only a few resin ducts are normally present, but following injury to the cambium the new or secondary wood subsequently formed contains very large number of ducts. The resin from these is called wound, traumatic or pathologically-produced resin.

Resin may continue to flow for a considerable period from wounding, or in some cases it may be necessary to inflict wounds at frequent intervals. Further, invasion of the wound by fungi and bacteria sometimes plays an important part in the composition of the resin exuded. For example, the simple wound resin of Styrax and Benzoin differs materially from the resin exuded after fungal invasion of the wound.

resonating drying. The process of moisture removal (also applicable to foods) which involves, in addition to conventional heated air drying, vibrating the product at a resonant frequency.

respiration. Although commonly used to mean breathing, more specifically related to the consumption of oxygen and the production of carbon dioxide. Thus respiratory enzymes are those involved in cell oxidations.

respiratory pigments. The coloured compounds that are capable of reversibly binding with oxygen at high oxygen concentrations and releasing them at low oxygen concentrations. Such pigments are present in the blood, transporting oxygen within the circulatory system from the respiratory organs to the tissues of the body. Haemoglobin is the blood pigment in all vertebrates and wide range of invertebrates. Other blood pigments such as haemoerythrin (containing iron) and haemocyanin (containing copper) are found in lower animals, and in many cases are dissolved in the plasma rather than present in cells. Their affinity for oxygen is comparable with haemoglobin, though oxygen capacity is generally lower.

respiratory quotient. RQ. The number of moles of carbon dioxide produced by a tissue or an organism divided by the number of moles of oxygen consumed during the same time. A theoretical RQ value can be calculated for the various foodstuffs used in respiration, giving a value of 1 for carbohydrates, 0.7 for fats, and 0.8 for proteins. However, in practice, more than one foodstuff is required at one time and other metabolic processes may produce carbon dioxide or use oxygen, so an RQ measurement for an organism gives unreliable information about the type of foodstuff respired.

response time. The time which elapses after a sudden change in the quantity being measured up to the point at which the measuring instrument given an indication which does not differ from the correct indication corresponding to the new value of the quantity by an amount greater than a given value. In order to determine the response time, it is necessary to calibrate instrument of each type:

(a) the initial value from which the change in the quantity measured must be made,

(b) the value of this change, and

(c) the difference between the current indication and the indication at the end of the period takes as being the response time.

The response time is therefore the time required for a readout device to reach a specified fraction of its final value in response to a step-function input to the detector. If this fraction is specified as 0.63 ($1^{-1/e}$), the response time is equal to the time constant; if, as is often the case, it is specified as 0.98, the response time is approximately equal to four time constants. The response time is of critical importance when components are assembled to form an analytical system, e.g., when a recorder is added to a detector and amplifier. A short response time is important in real-time measurements. (The response time is sometimes, particularly in US, referred to as the fall time when it follows a decrease, and the rise time when it follows an increase, in the quantity being measured.)

retardin. Substance secreted from the pancreas claimed to regulate the fat metabolism.

retention time. In food technology, the term refers to the duration of time necessary for the fermentation of a given quantity of substrate to an end product. In case of continuous or semicontinuous operation, a given amount of input feed is introduced into the vessel during the course of each day and equal amount of digester contents are withdrawn, so that once the fermentation is established, the rate of gas production remain steady. The retention time then equals the capacity of the digester divided by the feed rate (volume/time). The loading rate (concentration) is particularly important since at high loading rates the retention time is reduced. Thermophilic digestion at temperatures around 320K can reduce the retention time of mesophilic digestion by 50% or more.

reticulin. One of the structural elements (together with elastin and collagen) of skeletal muscle. Chemically it is identical with collagen but histologically it stains black with silver while collagen stains yellow or brown; it is

thought to be a precursor or a degraded form of collagen.

reticulocyte. Young form of the red blood cell (normocyte or erythrocyte) in which the remains of the nucleus is visible as a reticulum. Very few are seen in the normal blood, they are retained in the marrow until mature, but on remission of anaemia, when there is a high rate of production, reticulocytes appear in the bloodstream (reticulocytosis).

reticulo-endothelial system. A system of cells distributed throughout the body, with phagocytic properties. It is present in spleen, bone marrow, liver, and lymph nodes, and are also mobile in the tissues and blood stream. They are as scavengers of tissue debris and bacteria. The reticuloendothelial system also removes red blood cells when they have completed their life 120 days. The iron is recovered for further use, the rest of the haemoglobin is converted to bile pigments, stercobilin in the faeces and urobilin in the urine.

retinal. Aldehyde of retinol, formerly termed A aldehyde.

retinene. Obsolete name for retinal.

retinoic acid. Acid derived from retinol, formerly it was called vitamin A acid.

retinoids. Derivatives of vitamin A. Some authors include natural forms of vitamin A (retinol or vitamin A_1 and 3-dehydroretinol or vitamin A_2) in the definition. Retinol (vitamin A alcohol) may be converted in the body to retinal (vitamin A aldehyde) or retinoic acid (vitamin A acid). The synthetic analogues include etretinate and isotretinoin. Main use of these compounds is in dermatology, where they exert beneficial effects in a number of skin diseases.

retinol. Former name for alcohol derivative of vitamin A.

retorrefying. The redrying of barley or other grain, with hot air currents, generally restricted to the application of the hot air as in a rotary kiln.

retort. In connection with food technology, an autoclave.

retrogradation. A change in gelatinized starch occurring on storage which results in reduced solubility and a change of texture. It is important in products such as dehydrated potatoes and the baked products. In ungelatinized (raw starch the granules are in a definite pattern, which is lost when the starch is heated and gelatinized. On storage the granules slowly associate with each other to reform a pattern; gel is destroyed and amylose is precipitated as an insoluble flock. This crystallization is retrogradation. It is involved in the staling of bread crumb (not crust) and crumb-softeners such as polyoxyethylene and monoglyceride derivatives of the fatty acids function by slowing retrogradation.

reversible inhibition. The inhibition involving equilibrium between the enzyme and the inhibitor, the equilibrium constant being a measure of the affinity of the inhibitor for the enzyme. The different types of reversible inhibition are:
(a) competitive inhibition;
(b) noncompititive inhibition; and
(c) uncompititive inhibition.

reversible inhibitor. An inhibitor that binds to an enzyme in an equilibrium reaction so that the inhibition can be reversed by removal of the inhibitor from the enzyme by such processes as dialysis or ultrafiltration.

revertant. A strain in which the wild-type phenotype that was lost in the mutant is restored. Revertants can be of two types. In first-site (true) revertants, the mutation that restores activity occurs at the same site at which the original mutation occurred. In second-site revertants, the mutation occurs at some different site in the DNA.

reworked. 1. A former name for process cheese. 2. Also refers to cheese which is returned to be re-processed due to defective packaging, filling, or due to an undesirable moisture content.

rhamnose. A methylpentose sugar; having 33% sweetness of sucrose.

rheology. Science of deformation and flow of matter. In food technology it involves the study of brittleness and plasticity of fats, doughs, milk curds, grains, etc.

Rhesus antigen. Red cell antigen of Rhesus blood group system. A number of allelic genes govern the appearance of the Rhesus antigens.

Rhesus blood group system. A complex human blood group system involving various antigens. If the Rh antigen is present on a person's erythrocytes, he/she is Rh-positive, if it is lacking, the person is Rh-negative. The Rh-positive adult is generally not at risk for most Rh-blood group problems. As long as other antigens are compatible, such a person can receive either Rh-positive or Rh-negative blood transfusions, since Rh-positive blood is generally compatible with other Rh-positive blood, while Rh-negative cells lack the Rh antigen. Anti-Rh antibodies are formed by a pregnant woman may damage her offspring. The resulting disease is called hemolytic disease of the newborn, or simply Rh disease. While an Rh-negative mother is carrying an Rh-positive fetus, few fetal red blood cells generally enter the mother's circulation via placenta, usually not enough to provoke a primary antibody response. However, at the time of birth, enough of the baby's Rh-positive erythrocytes may enter the mother's circulation to incite a vigorous immune response.

rheumatoid factor. Antibody against slightly denatured IgG; présent frequently in serum of persons with rheumatoid arthritis in whom it can sometimes be shown to be an auto-antibody.

rhiotin. Unidentified urinary excretion product of biotin, together with miotin and triotin.

Rhizobium. A bacterium existing in symbiosis with leguminous plants such as lucerne and soybean. It can fix atmospheric nitrogen in the root nodules of the associated plants, the nitrogen compounds formed being utilized by the legume, which in turn supplies energy-rich sugars to the bacteria via photosynthesis. The efficiency of nitrogen fixing can often be improved by the inoculation of more effective strains than those naturally colonizing the plant.

rhodamine B. Hydrochloride of diethyl-m-aminophenolphthalein; until recently it was used as a red colour in meat paste and mint rock, but now not permitted in UK and many other countries.

rhubarb. Chinese rhubarb. *Rheum officinale.* Garden rhubarb. *Rheum rhaponticum.* Species of rhubarb are denoted by their large and sturdy sizes and large leaves borne on thick petioles. Leafstalks of perennial plant, *Rheum rhaponticum;* it contains only traces of protein and carbohydrate, 6 kcal/100 g, 10 mg vitamin C raw, 7 mg cooked. High content of oxalate, leaves are toxic for this reason. These hardy perennials grow between 2-3 metres high, are native to southern Siberia, China and India, and widely cultivated elsewhere. Chinese rhubarb is used more for medicinal purposes, while the garden variety is grown more for its edible stalks (petioles) and ornamental beauty.

Ribena. Trade name for a preparation of black currants juice and sugar syrup plus added vitamin C. It is a very rich source of vitamin C. The average composition per 100 g of Ribena is: 60% sugar and 206 mgvitamin C.

riboflavin. One of the water-soluble B-group of vitamins. Riboflavin is widely distributed in both plant and animal foods. Its rich sources are milk, liver, kidney, meat, eggs, cheese, peanuts, spinach, fresh peas, etc. It is present in milk to the extent of 1.5-2.0 mg/L. Riboflavin was formerly called Vitamin G, is an odourless, crystalline compound, orange-yellow in colour, and showing a yellow-green fluorescence in water solution. It is quite heat stable, especially in acid media, but deteriorates rapidly when exposed to light. Riboflavin is a constituent of several enzyme system (flavoproteins). Riboflavin acts as a coenzyme for hydrogen transfer in the reactions catalyzed by these enzymes. Two forms of phosphorylated riboflavin are known to exist in various enzyme systems: FMN (flavin mononucleotide) and FAD (flavin adenine dinucleotide). Riboflavin is an isoalloxazine derivative, *i.e.*, a pteridine ring with a benzene ring fused on to it. The side chain is a C-5 polyhydroxy group. The systematic name is 6,7-dimethyl-9-ribitylisoalloxazine. When a deficiency of this vitamin occurs, it is usually in conjugation with a deficiency of several other vitamins. A deficiency of riboflavin retards growth in young animals, produces dermatitis, affecting eyes, skin and hair; and causes inflammation of lips and impairment of nervous system.

ribonucleic acid. RNA. A complex organic compound (a nucleic acid) in living cells that is concerned with protein synthesis. In some viruses, RNA is also the hereditary material. Most RNA is synthesized in the nucleus and then distributed to various parts of the cytoplasm. An RNA molecule consists of a long chain of nucleotides in which the sugar is ribose and the bases are adenine, cytosine, guanine, and uracil (compare DNA). Messenger RNA (mRNA) is responsible for carrying the genetic code transcribed from DNA to specialized sites within the cell (known as ribosomes), where the information is translated into protein composition. Ribosomal RNA (rRNA) is present in ribosomes; it is single-stranded but helical regions are formed by base pairing within the strand. Transfer RNA (tRNA, soluble RNA, sRNA) is involved in the assembly of amino acids in a protein chain being synthesized at a ribosome. Each tRNA is specific for an amino acid and bears a triplet of bases complementary with a triplet on mRNA.

ribonucleotide. Compound consisting of a purine or pyrimidine base bound to a ribose sugar, which is itself bound to a phosphate group. RNA is a polymer of such units.

ribose. $C_5H_{10}O_5$. A pentose sugar of outstanding physiological importance; it is part of vitamin B_2, of coenzyme I and II, of adenylic acid, and in the nucleoproteins either as ribose or desoxyribose. It rarely occurs free in natural substances but it is important as a component of RNA (ribonucleic acid). Its derivative deoxyribose, is equally important as a constituent of DNA (deoxyribonucleic acid), which carries the genetic code in chromosomes.

ribosomal precursor RNA. A high-molecular mass RNA, having a sedimentation coefficient of 45S, that is synthesized in the nucleus of eucaryotic cells and that serves as the precursor of both the 18 and the 28S ribosomal RNA.

ribosomal protein. Protein used in the formation of ribosomes in which each molecule of RNA is associated with up to 30 molecules of small protein molecules.

ribosome. A small spherical body within a living cell that is the site of protein synthesis. Ribosomes consist of a type of RNA (called ribosomal RNA) and protein. Usually there are many ribosomes in a cell, either attached to the endoplasmic reticulum or free in the cytoplasm. During protein synthesis they are associated with messenger RNA in the process of translation. In most species they are composed of roughly equal amounts of protein and RNA. The ribosome consists of two unequally sized rounded sub-units which are arranged on top of each other like a cottage-roof. Eukaryotic cells have larger ribosomes than prokaryotic cells but the ribosomes in mitochondria and chloroplasts are about the same size as prokaryotic ribosomes. Ribosomes actively engaged in protein synthesis are linked together, probably by messenger RNA, in chains of about five ribosomes called polyribosomes. It is believed that the ribosomes move along the length of the mRNA molecule adding amino acids from transfer RNA molecules according to the code in mRNA. They are thus important in the build up of polypeptide chains during translation.

ribosome cycle. The set of reactions whereby ribosomal sununits combine to form the intact ribosome during the initiation of translation, travel along the messenger RNA as intact ribosomes, and dissociate back to the subunits during the termination of translation.

ribosubstitution. The replacement of some of the deoxyribonucleotides in a DNA by ribonucleotides; achieved by the in vitro synthesis of DNA under conditions that allow the incorporation of ribonucleotides from a mixture of ribo- and deoxyribonucleoside-5'-triphosphates. Ribosubsituted DNA can be used as an aid in the determination of the base sequence of the DNA.

Ribotite. Trade name for a mixture of disodium inosinate and disodium guanylate used as a flavour enhancer for savory dishes.

rice. Family: *Gramineae*. Genus: *Oryza*. Species: *Oryza sativa*. This species embraces many thousands of cultivars, which have been developed, since rice is self-fertilizing and for thousands of years the harvest has been carried out by hand, cutting off each individual panicle, selecting the best for the next crop. The most important groups are India and Japonica. Over 90% of the total world production is grown in Asia. The largest producers are China, India, Indonesia, Bangladesh, Thailand, and Japan.

Rice demands a high growing temeprature, during its growth, i.e., about 30-32°C, is optimal. The minimum temperature for germination is 18°C for tropical varities and 10-12°C for subtropical varities. It cannot endure frost at any stage of growth. It needs proper soil type, and grows in the pH range of 4.5-8, the optimum pH is 6-7. A heavy soil which can hold a lot of water is generally preferred.

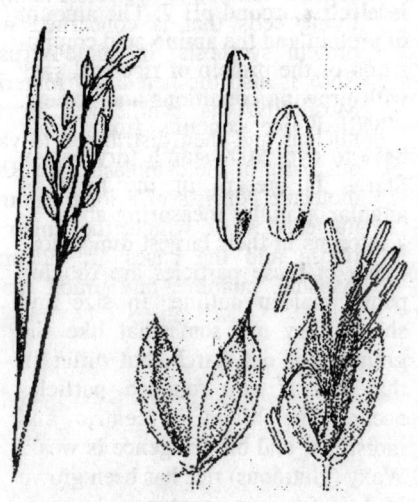

Rice is a major food in many parts of the world. Rice when threshed is known as paddy, and is covered with a fibrous husk comprising nearly 40% of the grain. When the husk has been removed brown rice is left. When the outer bran layers up to the endosperm and germ are removed the ordinary white rice of commerce of polished rice is obtained (usually polished with glucose and talc).

The nutritional quality cf rice protein is high relative to that of most other cereal proteins. This is due to rice's relatively high content of lysine, which is the first limiting amino acid. Most of the so-called storage proteins in rice kernels are found in discrete protein-rich bodies (aleurins) in the endosperm, similar to the situation in many other seeds. This protein is largely insoluble in water. Most of it 80% or more in milled rice, is the type called glutelin, soluble only in dilute acids or alkalies. The second most abundant type of protein is the salt-soluble globulin. Both of these are composed of a number of molecular species that are generally isoelectric around pH 7. The amount of protein and the amino acid composition of the protein of rice will vary with growing conditions and variety.

Milled rice contains from about 84% to over 90% starch (dry basis). Starch is present in the form of angular granules measuring about 2-7 microns in their largest dimension. Many of these particles are roughly pentagonal in outline. In size and shape, they are somewhat like the granules of oat starch, but differ in that few if any rounded particles occur. The hilum is centric and indistinct, and birefringence is weak. Waxy (glutinous) rice has been grown in Asia for many centuries. In some countries, most of the crop consists of these varieties. The principal differences between waxy and normal rice depends upon the starch. Typically, waxy rice will contain 2% or less of amylose. There is not much lipid material in milled rice, perhaps it is about 0.3-0.4% by acid hydrolysis could be considered average.

Rice bran contains a much higher percentage of lipids, perhaps 21%. Nearly all the studies of rice lipids have concentrated on rice bran oil, and there is a substantial trade in the fatty materials extracted from rice bran and refined. Fatty materials extracted from rice bran and refined. Fatty acids in the glycerides of the rice bran oil contain mostly even number of carbon atoms from 14-20 as well as odd-numbered fatty acids of chain length 11,13, and 15. These odd-numbered chains are present in small amounts of 0.2%, 0.6%, and 0.9%, respectively, in one sample. Gas-liquid chromatographic studies indicates that bran lipids have significantly higher mean contents of linoleic and linolenic

acids, but lower contents of myristic, palmitic palmitoleic, and stearic acids, than the lipids of milled rice. Only thiamin and niacin are important vitamins in rice. The following data are in mg per 100 g, first figure for raw, second for parboiled rice. Thiamin was present at levels of 0.13 and 0.15, niacin at levels of 1.54 and 3.2, pyridoxine at a level of 0.14 for raw, and riboflavin at 0.04 and 0.044.

When compared on an energy basis with the RDA for adult women and when rice is a large part of the diet (2,000 Kcal), brown rice would give more than sufficient niacin, thiamin, and phosphorus. Protein needs would be nearly enough 91%. but calcium and riboflavin needs would be low, both about 23% (zinc about 60%). Milled rice, however, would be deficient in all nutrients with only protein, niacin, and phosphorus supplying more than 50% of the RDA. Milled rice is not an important source of minerals.

The content of ash in a large series of samples ranged from 0.26% to 1.95%, dry basis, with a mean of about 0.65%. There is a considerably higher concentration of minerals in the bran, but the availability of at least some of these is adversely affected by the high concentration of phytin in the bran. Potassium and phosphorus are the most abundant mineral elements in rice (e.g., 88 mg and 140 mg/100 g DWB, respectively). Calcium, iron, sodium, silicon, magnesium, sulphur, and minor amounts of other elements have also been found in the ash. Appreciable amounts of silicon are found in the mature rice plant, and slight amounts in milled rice. Sodium, magnesium, and calcium were found at mean concentrations of 8.1, 28, and 25 mg, respectively, in whole kernels of six varieties of milled rice. Of the trace minerals, iron is present in brown rice and white rice at 1.8 and 0.9 mg per 100 g, dry weight basis, respectively, and zinc is present at 1.6 and 1.4 mg per 100 g, as is basis, respectively. Sugars, hemicellulose, nucleic acids, pigments, phytin, and numerous other substances have been found in small amounts in rice. Phytin, the principle phosphorus compound in rice, is said to constitute more than 8% of the bran in some samples. There is a small, but important, amount of sugars, brown rice containing about 0.8% to 1.4% total sugars. Reducing sugars are typically near 0.1%. Parboiled rice can be excepted to contain around 0.7% to 1.1% total sugars, and about 0.16% reducing sugars. Milled rice typically contains much lower amounts of total sugars, about 0.4%, and perhaps 0.06% reducing sugars. The amount of fiber varies greatly, depending on the method of analysis, the variety of rice and its growth conditions, the processing that has been applied to the rice, and other factors. Among reported values for fiber in brown, milled, and parboiled rice are 0.9%, 0.3%, and 0.2%, respectively.

Brown rice, including the germ, consists of (per 100 g): protein 7.5%, fat 1.8%; calcium 15 mg; iron 1.4 mg; vitamin B_1 0.3 mg; vitamin B_2 0.05 mg; nicotinic acid 4.6 mg; and food energy 1.5 MJ. In conversion to polished rice there is considerable loss of vitamin B_1 (and nicotinic acid), hence the widespread occurrence of beriberi among rice-eating people. The average composition 100 g of the white rice is: protein 6.7%; fat 0.7%: calcium 10 mg; iron 1 mg; vitamin B_1 0.08 mg; vitamin B_2 0.03 mg; and nicotinic acid 1.6 mg. Excessive milling removes all the vitamin-rich scutellum of the grain, particularly B_1, which is not crucial if the diet is varied but which can result in beriberi-disease marked by swelling of the body and paralysis, if it is not. Commercial milling (as opposed to the old-fashioned pestle-and-mortar method) is particularly culpable.

Washing rice also leaches out B_1, and in the East such water is usually saved for soups. Mulligatawny soup was originally based on rice water. During the colonial wars in Madras the British officers besieged at Trichinopoly were served rice by their faithfully sepoys while the sepoys themselves subsisted on the water in which it was cooked. The sepoys stayed healthy while the officers got beriberi! Brown rice is easily digested and provides all the essential nutrients for the body, so it is a complete food in itself. It also contains B_6 and vitamin K and is altogether richer in nutrients than its white cousin, which has to have B_1, niacin and iron added back into it after processing. It is bulky, satisfying, low in calories (123 per 100 grams when cooked), rich in minerals and so body building. Unpolished rice contains no purines whatsoever. (Purines are substances found in food which may be toxic and cannot be utilized but must be eliminated, which puts additional strain on the eliminative organs.) Rice or rice water is excellent for stopping diarrhoea, for flatulence, and for ulcers, and is helpful for chronic nephritis, anaemia, high blood pressure. It is also useful for dressing wounds, and being gluten free is valuable for coeliacs.

rice beverages. The beverages prepared by the fermentation of rice. Very large quantities of broken rice are used as a carbohydrate source by the brewing industry. Shaohsing wine is made in Taiwan from glutinous rice, wheat, and water. Two kinds of starters are used one made from wheat and the other from rice. Mold is grown on the grain to produce an enzyme preparation that can convert the starch of the raw materials to sugars that can be fermented by yeasts. Mash is prepared from the starters, water, steamed rice, and wheat. Sake, the rice wine of Japan, is a clear, pale yellow liquid with specific gravity of 1.0 and alcohol content of 15-16%. Brewing of sake involves using koji to enzymatically convert the starch of rice to fermentable sugars (and perform other changes), while simultaneously fermenting the mixture with sake yeast. Hong (red) wine of China is made from a rice mash which has been digested and fermented in a manner somewhat similar to the beverages previously discussed, but late in the fermentation the liquid is changed to a red colour by the addition of a Monascus culture. A number of distilled beverages are made from mashes consisting principally of rice. The mashes are generally treated with fungal preparations to hydrolyze the starch into fermentable sugars, although malt may also be used in some cases. For Taiwanese rice liquor, the most active molds are thought to be *Rhizopus* spp. and the yeast *Saccharomyces* spp., as *S. peka*.

rice cake. A wet product made from either glutinous or nonglutinous rice. The rice is milled, refined, washed, and soaked. It is then drained of excess moisture, kneaded, made into various forms, packed in a plastic film, heat pasteurized, and cooled. The cake is further manipulated and cooked by the consumer. Seasoning include various combinations of salt, pepper, reddish, monosodium gluconate, and sugar. There is a fermented version made in Taiwan from rice, sugar, and a biological leavener.

Japanese rice cakes are roughly classified into *namagashi* (pastry or unbaked cake) and *higashi* (dried cake). *Dango*, is dumpling of steamed rice, while *mochi* (rice paste) and *mochigashi*, are processed rice paste, and *uiro*, is a kind of rice pudding, are representative forms of namagashi.

rice drying. Combined rice normally contains about 4% excess moisture which needs to be removed before storage. Rice kernels are dense and the diffusion of moisture through the kernels is slow and limits the speed of drying. The capacity of a heated air dryer can be increased by removing the surface moisture and then storing the rice until the moisture is evenly distributed throughout the kernels and again using heated air drying. Heated air temperatures up to 54.4°C can be used if the grain temperature does not exceed 43.3°C and is forced through the rice at the rate of about 1.34 m³/m³s. The drying procedure for alternate drying with heated air is as follows:
First drying.
(a) It begins within 6 hours after combining.
(b) Dry for 30-45 minutes with air at 54.4°C.
Second drying.
(a) It begins 6-12 hours after completion of first drying period.
(b) Dry for 20 to 30 minutes at 54.4°C.
Third drying and additional drying as required to reduce the moisture to 14.5%.
(a) Begin 6 to 12 hours after completion of previous drying.
(b) Dry for 20 minutes at 54.4°C.

Last Drying.
(a) Begin within 24 hours after previous drying.
(b) Drying without artificial heat unless the relative humidity of the atmosphere is above 75%. Air temperatures up to 65.5°C might be used to reduce the drying time, but there is a noticeable effect on the milling qualities can be dried with unheated forced air using about 0.035 m³/m³s. Multipass dryers with crossflow of air are used for rice. The flow of grain and air and the temperature of air are controlled to minimize cracking of rice.

rice, red. West African species, *Oryza glaberrima*, with red bran layer.

rice, unpolished. Rice which has been under-milled in that the husk, germ and bran layers have been partially removed.

rice vinegar. *See* vinegar, rice.

rice, wild. *See* wild rice.

ricin. A toxic glycoprotein isolated from castor bean. Its molecule consists of a neutral chain (molecular mass 32000 daltons) connected by S-S bonds. The neutral chain inhibits protein synthesis and the acidic chain serves to bind the molecule to cells. Ricin has been proposed as a chemical warfare agent, and has been used for political assassinations.

ricing. A culinary term meaning cutting into small pieces about the size of rice grains.

rickets. Malformation of the bone in growing children due to shortage of vitamin D leading to poor absorption of calcium. In adults the equivalent is osteomalacia.

Ricotta cheese. A kind of cheese made of the coagulable material. It is composed mainly of whey albumin, from the whey of Cheddar, Swiss and Provolone. Sometimes called whey cheese, Ziger, Schottenziger, Recruit, Broccio, Brocotte. All the fat is left in the whey and from 5-10% of whole milk or skim is added. The sweet whey is heated to 80°C. The coagulated albumin rises to the surface and is dipped with a ladle. It is drained, pressed and salted. It is usually eaten fresh. The yield is about 5%.

Riesengebirge cheese. A kind of soft, rennet cheese made from goat milk in the mountains of Bohemia. About 18 kg of cheese is obtained from 100 litres of milk.

Riesling grape. A variety of grape, considered by many authorities as the noblest white wine grape known. It appears as small, insignificant-looking berries, and is very late ripening. It finds favorable growing conditions in all German regions, particularly in the Mosel-Saar-Ruwer region, Rheingau, Rhenish Palatinate, and the Nahe and Mittelrhein regions. Riesling wines are racy, usually of high quality, and delicately fragrant. It should not be confused with other vine species, such as the Welsch or Italian Riesling. However, the species has been extensively transplanted and is now found in Australia, Austria, California, Chile, Luxembourg, Rumania, South Africa, and Switzerland. Of vineyard areas in Germany, this grape represents about 21.5% of total.

riffle flumes. Washing equipment consisting of stepped channels along which the product being washed is carried in a flow of water; stones and grit are retained on the steps.

rigor mortis. Stiffening of muscle that occurs after death. At death muscle is soft and pliable, the cessation of blood flow causes the remaining metabolism of tissues to be anaerobic, with formation of lactic acid and a fall in pH. As the concentration of adenosine triphosphate decreases the muscles harden, this is rigor mortis and meat eaten at this stage would be tough. After hanging for a few days in cooler the muscles soften by some undefined mechanism and the meat becomes edible. Meat that has been kept in this way (conditioned) is preferable to freshly killed meat with regard to texture.

rind. The surface or outer coat of a hard cheese which is usually drier and harder than the interior portion of the cheese. There is no definition as to the depth of this rind. It has been shown that three is 6-10% difference in moisture between the first 2 mm layer and the second 2 mm layer. There is only 1-2% difference in moisture content between the second and third 2 mm layers. Therefore, in a cheese dried 2 mm layers. Therefore, in a cheese dried for 24 hours in a drying room at 15-20° C, the rind may be considered to be less than 2 mm in thickness.

rindless (natural) cheese. Rindless loaf cheese is natural (not processed) cheese that is packaged and marketed in a transparent, flexible wrapper. Much Cheddar, Brick and Swiss are now put up in this manner. There is no rind formation on such cheese and drying losses are small. This type of cheese may be packaged by manufacturer, wholesaler or by the retailer, either before or after it is cured.

rindless, Swiss cheese. A type of cheese that is wrapped and cured in a flexible stretchable film. This process is slightly different from the cheddar process in that the cheese is wrapped after it has been salted in the brine tank. A stretchable film must be used to allow for the normal production of gas when stored in the warm room.

Ringer solution. A physiological salt solution originally devised by Sidney Ringer for maintaining the beat of the frog's heart. It is commonly used for other amphibian tissues also, but is unsuitable for mammalian tissues. Its composition is: (mmol/L): NaCl, 103-111; KCl, 1-1.9; $CaCl_2$, 0.9-1.1; NaH_2PO_4, 0-0.1; $NaHCO_3$, 1.2-2.4; and glucose 0-11.1. It is bubbled with air.

Rinnen cheese. A kind of sour milk cheese which was known as early as the 18th century. It is made in Pomerania, Poland and derives its name from the wooden trough in which it is laid to drain. Caraway seed is usually added during its manufacture, to impart typical flavour.

Riola cheese. A kind of soft textured and strongly flavoured cheese, usually made from sheep's or goats' milk. It is made similar to Mont d'Or cheese but is ripened for 2-3 months.

RNA polymerases. A group of enzymes for catalyzing the synthesis of RNA from a DNA template (sense strand). Bacteria possess only a single type of RNA polymerase, but eukaryotic cells possess at least four. They are designated:
type I (pol, I), which is responsible for synthesis of ribosomal RNA (except 5S RNA);
type II (pol II), which is responsible for synthesis of messenger RNA (and its precursor, heterogeneous nuclear RNA);
type III (pol III), which is responsible for synthesis of transfer RNA and the small ribosomal 5S RNA;
type IV, which is the RNA polymerase of the mitochondria. RNA polymerases are sensitive to various antibiotics: for example, pol II is sensitive to a-amanitin and pol I to actinomycin-D.
Since a single species of RNA

polymerase is responsible for synthesis of all messenger RNA, the specificity of gene expression is clearly not determined by the polymerase enzyme, but since the promoter sequence upstream of the initiation site of the coding sequence is recognized by the enzyme, differences in the sequence of the promoter between different genes will affect transcription rates. RNA polymerases are complex proteins. The bacterial enzyme consists of a core enzyme comprising α-, β- and β'-subunits, and a sigma factor.

RNA primase. Enzyme that synthesizes the short primer RNA of about 10 nucleotides that is elongated by DNA polymerase to form Okazaki fragment of DNA during DNA replication. The leading strand of DNA is presumed also to be initiated by such a primer.

RNA replicase (RNA-dependent RNA polymerase). Enzyme found in certain RNA phages (*e.g.*, MS2).

RNases. Abbriviation for ribonucleases. Enzymes that degrade RNA. Distinct forms which are extensively used or analyzed include RNase A, which attacks the phosphate linkages of pyrimidines internally located in an RNA, RNase P which cleaves bacterial tRNA precursor to yield mature tRNA, and RNase T1 which specifically cleaves the phosphate groups of internal guanosine residue.

roasting. As applied to food technology, essentially, baking in a closed oven. Meat shrinks and squeezes out juices, but some of the juice evaporates before it has time to drip away. This leaves some of the meat extractives on the surface, improving flavour and reducing the losses. Only 20% of the extractive is lost during roasting, as compared to 50% losses in steaming or boiling. The loss of

vitamin B_1 is greater than that in boiling, and amount up to 35-50%; 10-20% loss of B_2 and nicotinic acid, same as boiling. Roasting suitable only for prime cuts as tough connective tissue is not broken down during roasting.

Robbiole cheese. A kind of soft, rich, fast-ripening Crescenza-like cheese made in the Italian Alps. The cheese is made from whole or partly skimmed milk. The milk is set, cut and placed in 20 cm diameter forms. After forming, the cheese is drained for 2-3 days and dry salted and left to ripen for 12-15 days.

Robbiolini cheese. A kind of soft Cresenza-like cheese made in Lombardy region of Italy. The milk used may be of cow, or a mixture of cow's, ewe's or goat's milk. About 10% acid whey is added to the milk before setting. After 24 hours the curd is cut into slices and kneaded into small rolls. Salt is added during kneading.

Robison ester. Name given to a mixture of glucose-6-phosphate and fructose-1-phosphate, which are intermediary stages in glucose metabolism.

Robinson mandarin. A variety of mandarin, that is a cross between a Clementine mandarin and the Orlando tangelo. (C. reticulata X [C. reticulata x C. paradisi)]. The Orlando tangelo is described in entry on Grapefruit. The juice of Robinson can be blended with orange juice concentrate for colour improvement.

rocambole. Similar to garlic.

Rochelle sat. Potassium sodium tartrate; used to combine with the copper in Fehling's test for reducing sugars.

roe. Hard roe is the eggs of the female fish; soft roe is from the male fish, also known as milt.

Roentgen. R. The amount of radiation which on passage through dry air

under standard condition, produces an electrostatic unit of ions, of either plus or minus charge, per cubic centimetre.
In SI system; 1 R = 0.258 mC/kg.

rokelax. A Scandinavian term for the smoked salmon.

roller dryer. The material to be dried is spread over the surface of internally heated rollers and drying is complete in a few seconds. The rollers rotate against a knife that scrapes off the dried film as soon as it forms. There is little damage by this method; for example, roller-dried milk is not scorched, but there is some loss of vitamins B_1 and C, more than in spray drying.

roller mill. Pairs of horizontal cylindrical rollers, separated by only small gap and revolving at different speeds. The materials is thus ground and crushed in the one operation. Used in flour milling.

roll-on closure. Aluminium or lacquered tin plate cap for sealing on the narrow-necked bottles with a threaded neck. The unthreaded cap is moulded on the neck of the bottle and forms an airtight seal.

Romadour cheese. A kind of cheese similar to Limburger cheese, and is prepared in southern Bavaria from sheep's and goat's or cow's milk. It is said to be a little finer variety than Limburger cheese and is sold for a slightly higher price. The cheese is cured a shorter time and with less surface smear than Limburger cheese. Also known as Remoudour cheese; Romatur cheese.

Romanello cheese. A variety of hard grating cheese made in north Italy. It is similar to Romano cheese, except that the curd is placed in a wicker basket to drain, the imprint of the woven basket remaining on its sur-face. It is about 25 cm in diameter and 12 cm high.

Romano cheese. A popular and very hard variety of cheese of Italian origin which is used for grating. A 2% fat milk, raw or pasteurized is warmed to 35°C and culture is added. The culture consists of *Streptococcus thermophilus* and *Lactobacillus bulgaricus* which should have an acidity of 1.2-1.3%. The milk is ripened for 10 minutes before the addition of rennet. Traditionally a rennet paste was used but now rennet plus a lipolytic enzyme may be added. The coagulated curd is cut with knives and is cooked in one half an hour to 40-45°C. The curd is stirred for 20 minutes after which one half of the whey is removed. Stirring is continued until the acidity has increased about 0.4%. The whey is drained and the curd is salted at the rate of 2%. The salted curd is their pressed. After pressing the cheese is usually brine salted for 36 hours. The cheese is removed and cured at 15-20°C. This cheese is cylindrical in shape, 25 cm in diameter and 15 cm thick and may be coloured black on the surface. Federal standards recommends that the moisture should not be more than 34%; and fat, not less than 38% in the solids.

root beer. Non-alcoholic carbonated beverage flavoured with oil of sassafras and oil of wintergreen.

roots. Roots are organs specialized for anchorage, absorption, storage, and conduction. Gymnosperms and dicots commonly produce taproot systems, monocots commonly produce fibrous root systems. The extent of the root system is dependent upon several factors, but the bulk of most feeding roots are found in the upper meter of soil. The apical meristems of most roots contain a quescent center; most meristematic activity, or cell division, occurs a short distance from the apical initials. During primary growth, the apical meristem gives rise to the three primary meristems, protoderm, ground meristem, and procambium, and the latter differentiate into epidermis, cortex, and vascular cylinder, respectively. In addition, the apical meristem produces the root cap, which serves to protect the meristem and aid the root in its penetration of the soil. Many epidermal cells of the root develop root hairs, which greatly increase the absorbing surface of the root. With the exception of the endodermis, the cortex contains numerous intercellular spaces. The compactly arranged endodermal cells contain Casparian strips on their anticlinal walls. Consequently, all substances moving between the cortex and vascular cylinder must pass through the protoplasts of the endodermal cells. The vascular cylinder consists of pericycle and the primary vascular tissues, which are completely surrounded by the pericycle. The primary xylem occupies the center of the vascular cylinder and has radiating ridges that alternate with strands of primary phloem. Branch roots originate in the pericycle and push their way to the outside through the cortex and epidermis.

Aerial roots are adventitious roots that may serve as prop roots and, in some trees that live in swampy habitats, provide aeration. Some roots, such as those of carrots, sweet potatoes, and beets, are specialized for storage. Such fleshy roots contain an abundance of storage parenchyma permeated by vascular tissue.

rope. Bacteria of the type *B. mesentericus* and *B. subtilis* occur on wheat and thence in flour. These organisms from spores that can survive baking and then are present in the bread. Under the right conditions of warmth and moisture the spores will germinate and the mass of bacteria convert the bread into sticky, yellowish patches which can be pulled out into rope-like threads, hence the term ropy bread. The bacteria growth is inhibited by acid substances. It can also occur in milk and carbonated beverages.

ropy milk. A kind of abnormal milk, characterized by a sliminess or ropiness varying in degree from a slightly increased viscosity to a ropiness so pronounced that the milk may be drawn out in threads several metres long. Ropiness is not present at milking time but develops only after the milk has been stored for sometime and is due to the formation of gums or mucins by bacteria. Many of the causative organisms are capsulated. Ropy milk is not harmful and its flavour is usually no different from that of normal milk. The organism responsible is usually picked up from improperly sanitized equipment, particularly on the farm.

Roquefort cheese. A kind of semi-soft to hard, rennet cheese made in southern France from sheep's milk and mold-ripened in caves from 1-5 months in order to develop a characteristic green mold throughout the centre of the cheese. The Roquefort type now made from cow's milk is ripened in refrigerators under controlled temperature and humidity and is known as Blue cheese. In appearance the cheese is white with a rumbly body streaked with green mold and possesses a rather sharp, spicy, "pigment" flavour. Federal Standards recommends that the moisture should not be more than 43%, and fat, not less than 50% in the solids.

Rose family. *Rosaceae.* Common features in this family are leaf stipules, usually present, flower parts in 5's, and a flower with a cuplike receptacle or floral tube, called a hypanthium, which develops around the ovary. Plants in the rose family range from herbs and shrubs to trees. Many have spines and a few are climbers. Usually, the leaves are alternate, simple or compound, and with toothed margins. The flower is usually bisexual and has an enlarged nectar cup that inflates the floral tube, stamens in whorls of 5, and a single compound pistil or many pistils together.

The family include: achene, drupe, follicle, and pome. Rose family plants have English common names for the edible fruits. In Strawberry *(Fragaria)* is an aggregate of achenes. Pear *(Pryus),* Apple *(Malus),* and quince *(Cydonia)* are pomes. Cherry, peach, plum, and apricot (all *Prunus* spp) are drupes, while blackberry, raspberry, and loganberry (all *Rubus* spp.) are aggregates or drupelets. The fleshy fruit of the almond (*Prunus dulcis*) is not eaten; the common name represents the seed inside the drupe's pit, while is similar appearing seed in the peach drupe contains a poison, cyanide, as do the pome seeds of apple *(Malus).*

rose hip syrup. Extract of rose hip with added sugar, used as source of vitamin C, about 150 mg/100 g.

Rose-Gottlieb test. A test for fat in milk; it involves a very accurate gravimetric method, by extracting the fat in appropriate solvent.

rosemary. Family: *Labiatae.* Genus: *Rosmarinus.* Species: *Rosmarinus officinalis.* An evergreen shrub, rosemary is available fresh year-round. This is just as well because, once dried, it loses much of its flavour, and its pine-needle-like leaves become unpalatable spiky. The dried leaves are used to flavour soups, sauces and meat. It is a pretty herb, with trusses of pale or bright blue flowers lasting, in the right climate, right through spring and summer. It is native to the countries bordering the Mediterranean, where it grows in profusion, its slightly camphoric scent far more pronounced than it can ever be in cooler climatic conditions. It is cultivated commercially for its essential oil, used in medicine and perfumery.

Rosemary and lamb go together in many ways. Make slits in lamb for roasting and tuck in sprigs of the herb, place larger sprigs over chops for grilling, and include them in casseroles and stews. The many branches have an ash-coloured, scaly bark and bear opposite, leathery thick leaves which are lustrous and dark green above and downy white underneath. They have a prominent vein in the middle and margins which are rolled down. Rosemary is used in bouquets garnish, sparingly with fish, and in rice dishes. Medicinally, a tisane of the leaves is taken as a tonic for calming nerves, and is also used as an antiseptic. Rosemary leaves contain about 5% protein, 15% fat, 64% carbohydrates, minerals (including calcium, iron and magnesium), vitamins (including A and C), and 0.5% volatile oil, increasing to 2% in very hot climates. They also contain saponoside, heterosides and tannin.

Rosemary oil kills various types of bacteria but it is also toxic to humans and can be fatal if taken in large doses. On a minor level, it can cause skin problems and contact dermatitis, as well as eye irritations to certain individuals, but on a much more serious level, it can cause abortion, convulsions and even death. So, if the oil is to be used internally, it should always be taken under the close supervision of a qualified consultant medical herbalist.

Rosemary may be employed as tonic, stimulant and carminative in treating indigestion, stomach pains, headaches, head colds and nervous tension. Externally, it is useful for rheumatism, eczema, bruises and wounds. An infusion will help to prevent baldness, dry scaly skin and dandruff. Rosemary is excellent for vasoconstrictory types of headaches and migraines, meaning those that improve if a heated pad is laid on the forehead or the neck. It is also useful for palpitations and other signs of nervous tension affecting the circulation. It is useful for malfunctioning liver. It is an excellent memory specific helping to get blood circulating into the brain and easing depression and debility linked with nervous tension. The rich fragrance of rosemary also controls cabbage moths, bean beetles, carrot flies, and mosquitoes.

Rose wine. A pink wine made from black grapes or form a blend of black and red grapes in a process which permits the skins to be in contact with the must for only a limited period, just long enough to extract a pleasant pink coloration. (The colouring matter of the grape resides in the skin.) Control of colour is accomplished by drawing off the fermenting grape juice after about the first 24 hours of fermentation. This is done when the winemaker observes just the right color. The entire mass is transferred to a wine press where the partially fermented grape juice is separated from the skins and other residues. Production from this point is essentially that followed in the making of white wines.

Travel is prepared from a mixture or blend of several varieties of white and black grapes which are known from many years of experience to yield the desired characteristics, including color. Nearly all countries produce some type of rose wine. A number of high-quality roses are produced from the Cabernet Franc, Gamay, Grenache, or Pinot Noir grape varieties, as well as some Italian varieties.

rotary burner. A device which uses centrifugal force in which oil to be burned moves from the center of a rotary cup and is thrown to the outside into the air where it ignites and burns.

rotary drum dryer. A device for removing moisture from products in which the product is conveyed internally through a slowly rotating drum through which heated air is forced. Direct- or indirect-heated rotary dryers may be used.

rotary dryer. The general designation of a device for removing moisture from products in which the active drying occurs in or through a rotating chamber. Rotary dryer is the most common designation for a revolving horizontal drum, through which the product and drying air are moved, using either countercurrent or concurrent flow. The external drum dryer, with internal heating and external product drying, is more commonly designated as a drum or roller dryer.

roughage. A general term for the undigestible (mainly carbohydrate) material in plant foodstuffs, such as cellulose (flesh, skin and seeds), bran (in cereals). As the material is not digested, it passes through the intestine unchanged, but absorbs and holds water and acts as laxative.

rough fish. A general term for the fish undesirable as food, or for other activities such as sports. Most destructive of all rough fish is the carp; it may uproot extensive quantities of vegetation.

rough lemon. A variety of lemon sometimes used as rootstock for other citrus fruits. It is widely used as a rootstock for oranges. It is postulated that Vasco da Gama originally found the variety in India and took it to America and Africa. The rough lemon is highly polyembryonic and is readily propagated by the seeds. Because of its importance is a rootstock, research into improving it continues. Within the last several years, varieties that exhibit a tolerance or resistance to the burrowing nematode have been developed.

Roux. Trade name for a preparation of flour and butte for thickening gravies and sauces.

Rovimix. Trade name for retinol stabilized in beadlet form in a gelatin-sugar-starch base.

Royal jelly. The food on which bee larvae are fed and which causes them to develop into queen bees. Richest known source of pantothenic acid (500 μg/g dry weight); also contains vitamin B_6 and 2% of its dry weight is 10-hydroxy-δ-2-decenoic acid.

rubber. A gum resin exudation of a wide variety of trees and plants, but especially from tree *Hevea brasiliensis* and several other species of *Hevea* growing in all tropical countries and cultivated on plantation in southern Asia, Indonesia, Sri Lanka, Zaire, and Liberia. The gum resin was formerly referred to as India rubber.

rubble reel. Machine for cleaning materials such as wheat. The material is fed into a long inclined reel made of perforated metal that rotates inside a frame. The perforations become larger nearer the bottom so that there is a graded sieving of the material as it passes down the reel.

Rubner factors. Factors used to calculate the energy content of foods in kilocalories after allowing for losses of urinary nitrogen but not allowing for incomplete absorption, therefore greater than Atwater factors; protein 4.1, fat 9.3, carbohydrates 4.1.

rue. *Ruta graveolens.* Most herbs have retained their popularity over the centuries not only because of their culinary and medicinal properties, but also their pleasant scent. That cannot be said to rue, a herb whose aroma has been likened, not unfairly, to the smell to tomcats. Accordingly, its culinary applications have not been enthusiastically handed down from one generation to the next, while even its medicinal applications need approaching with care. Rue, a sub-shrub known as the herb of grace, is a native of southern Europe, where it will flourish in the poorest of soils. It will easily take to poor garden soil, as well, where it makes a compact and decorative bush. The plant is not now used in the kitchen, and should be approached with extreme care for medicinal purposes. The tisane, which was once taken for rheumatism, and used, much diluted, as an eye bath, is not now recommended. Sprays of the leaves may be hung indoors to repel insects. The seed heads are particularly attractive, and can be used in dried flower arrangements.

Rue family: *Rutaceae.* Aromatic oils are produced in glands that appear as dots on the leaves. Another characteristic feature of this family is that within the usually bisexual flower, the pistil has a superior, usually lobed ovary situated on a nectar disc. Rue family plants include trees, shrubs, and herbs, with many fruit types represented. They include capsules, leathery-rind berries (hesperidia), drupes, and samaras.

The family include: about 60 *citrus* species, with many hybrids between these species- *C. sinesis* (sweet orange), *C. limon* (lemon), *C. paradisi* (grapefruit), *C. aurantifolia* (lime), *C. reticulata* (tangerine), *C. medica* (citron); *Fortunella* (kumquat); *Calodendrum* (cape chestnut), *Dictamus* (gasplant, fraxinella, dittany), *Murraya* (orange jessamine), *Phellodendron* (cork tree), *Poncirus* (trifoliate orange), *Ptelea* (hop tree, wafer ash), *Ruta* (common rue), *Zanthoxylum americanum* (prickly ash); *Z. flavum* (West Indian silk-wood); *Dictamnus, Ruta graveolens, Ptelea.*

Rulander grape. German variety of the Grauer Burgunder (Pinot Gris). The grape is of medium-size, heavy, and strong. The vine prefers a rich, deep soil. It ripens relatively early, but may extend late into the season. The species favours the growing conditions found in the Baden, Rhenish Palatinate, Rheinhessen, and Hesische Bergstrasse wine-producing regions of Germany. The wine is fiery, full-bodied and of uniquely delicate bouquet. Its Spatlese and Auslese belong to the range of German high quality wines.

rum. A spirit distilled directly from sugarcane product. Although rum can be produced directly from sugarcane juice, it is traditionally and principally made from molasses (blackstrap), a by-product of the cane sugar industry. In the olden days, 'Rum' was considered a 'low' drink socially and its consumption was popular only amongst the sailors. When cocktails became popular, rum became an important ingredient to it. It is now drunk with soda, lemon or other fruit juices, milk, coca-cola or bitters. It is used in the preparation of 'Punch'.

Rum is an alcoholic distillate or mixture of distillates from the fermented juice of sugarcanes, molasses or other sugarcane by-product, distilled at less than 190° proof in such a manner that the distillate possess the taste, aroma and characteristics generally attributed to rum. There are many varieties of sugarcane, but on an average 72% of their weight is water, 16.5% sucrose and 9.5% cellulose. Although rum is produced in most sugar growing countries of the world like India, Cuba, Australia, US, and South Africa for local consumption, the world demand for rum is mainly supplied by the West Indies where it originated.

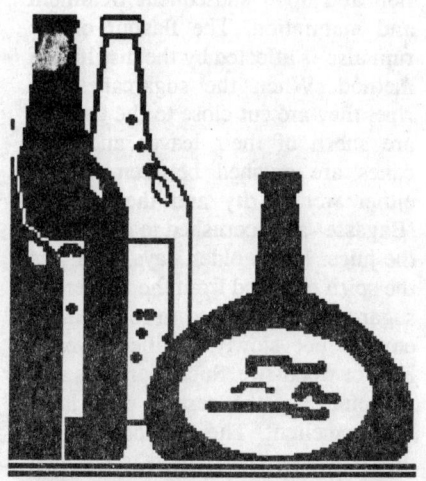

Rums can be classified in a number of ways, possibly the most meaningful being the light rum and full-bodied rum categories.

Light rums such as those produced in Puerto Rico and Cuba, are distilled to a proof range of 160-180° proof. Continuous stills are used. Ageing is not required. They are also widely used for preparing cocktails. Bacardi rum, once exclusively Cuban, is now produced elsewhere as well.

Heavy, or full-bodied rums, such as those produced in Jamaica, are usually preferred in western Europe and in the United Kingdom, particularly in the Midlands and northern England. These rums are of good quality and pungent. They are distilled to a proof range of 140°-160° proof in pot stills.

So-called "Continental Flavor" rum is particularly favored in Germany. It is highly flavored and aromatic substances.

Types of rum depend upon the quality of the ingredients, upon the method of fermentation and distillation and upon subsequent treatment and maturation. The flavour of the rum also is affected by the distillation method. When the sugarcanes are ripe, they are cut close to the ground, are shorn of their leaves and bare canes are crushed between rollers, either wet or dry and the residual 'Bagasse' again crushed to extract all the juice. In the olden days, rum was the spirit obtained from the fermented sugarcane juice placed in some earthenware pot slowly distilled over a bark or wood-fire. Such a process was wasteful, but the results may have been excellent. The method is quite different now. The liquid is warmed almost to boiling point and then cooled and separated from the sludge that settles down. The dark sugar solution is treated with lime and heated again. The thick scum which forms is removed and used for making rum. The liquid is evaporated further to obtain more sugar and as it becomes very difficult for the sugar

to crystallize out, the molasses obtained is used for fermentation to make alcohol for industrial purposes and to make rum. The thick liquid molasses is diluted with water and mixed with the scum and 'dunder' which is the residue left in the still. This mixture is allowed to ferment for a few days. The methods vary widely.

In some distilleries, the mash is allowed to sour by itself with the aid of natural yeasts. In this case, 'bagasse' is added to the vat. In other places, yeast is supplied and in more modern factories, a pure culture yeast is used. Pure culture yeasts are supposed to give a better flavoured rum. Before fermenting, a little acid is added, to counteract the effect of the liming of the juice. The substances which give rise to the aroma and the flavour of the rum are known as 'Congenerics', that is, substances formed along with alcohol. Those which cause the characteristic odour and flavour and esters, acids and higher alcohols. The distillation is carried out in spot-stills in the olden factories. In the modern ones, different methods are used. Different firms distilled to different strengths, from just over proof (57% in the UK, 50% in the US) to almost pure alcohol. It is nearly water-white because the colouring matter of the molasses do not leave the still. The type of yeast, fermentation environment, distillation techniques and systems, the maturation conditions and not least the blending skill are important in determining the final character and quality of rum. Fictitious rums, however, are made from alcohol flavoured with essential oils (Rum Essence). In general, top fermenting yeasts are employed in rum distilleries, in spite of the fact that most other distilleries employ bottom-fermenting yeasts.

While there appears to be no definite optimum temperature at which a yeast thrives best, there is a fairly narrow range over which reasonably good results can be obtained. For the production of rum, it is unusual to allow the maximum temperature of the wash to exceed 35°C and temperatures above 37.5°C should most certainly be avoided if reasonable yields are to be expected. However, lower the temperature, slower will be the fermentation, but the quality of the rum be the fermentation, but the quality of the rum produced will be better. For good quality rum, the temperature should be maintained at about 27°C.

The products of metabolism of yeasts have the effect of regarding the metabolism and may also cause the formation of involution forms which are usually associated with old cultures where there are accumulations of waste products. Next to alcohol, the organic acids constitute the most important components of rum and they are found in the final product, not only in the free state but also combined with alcohols as esters. Of the free acids, some 97% - 98% is acetic acid, the remainder being butyric acid, formic acid, caproic acid, pelargonic acid, capric acid and other aliphatic acids. The acids may be produced by the direct fermentation of sugars by means of bacteria and by the bacterial oxidation of the products of alcohol fermentation. The majority of these acids are to be found in traces in rum, and in view of their high boiling points as compared with alcohol and probably distilled in steam towards the end of the distillation. They should, therefore, be more concentrated in the retort lees, a fact which is borne out

by the use of these less for the preparation of *Lime Salts* used in the preparation of *High Ether rums*. The ageing of rum is very important. The best rums are kept in casks for three years or more.

The quality of rum is considered to continue to improve in good oak casks for twenty years or more. Colour is taken up from the casks and due to some changes between the various constituents of rum, the taste improves. Sometimes, ageing is hastened by adding charred oak chips. Caramel is sometimes added to give it a better colour. Where sugarcane is grown, rum, is made. It is a profitable outlet for products which would otherwise be wasted. For every hundred weight of sugar made, three gallons of rum can be produced and rum is a more valuable product.

rumen. Ruminating animals such as the cow, sheep and goat, possess four stomachs in distinction from monogastric animals such as man, pig, dog and rat. These four are: the rumen, or first stomach, where bacterial fermentation produces lower fatty acids, and from whence the food is returned to mouth for further mastication (chewing the cud); the reticulum, where further bacterial fermentation produces lower fatty acids; the omasum; and the abomasum or true stomach. The bacterial fermentation allows ruminants to obtain nourishment from grass and hay which cannot be digested by monogastric animals.

runner bean. Family: *Leguminosae.* Genus: *Phaseolus.* Species: *Phaseolus coccineus.* Runner beans contain a variety of vitamins and minerals, including vitamins A and C, iron, potassium and calcium.

rutabaga. *Brassica campestris rutabaga, B. campestris.* Rutabaga is thought to have originated in Sweden somewhere during the Middle Ages. It is larger, coarser and more emphatically flavoured than the turnip, of which it may be a mutant form. Rutabaga is more elongated than a turnip is and usually adorned with a slightly purple top. Most have yellow or orange flesh, but a few are white. Throughout much of recorded history, turnip has occupied a lowly position on the gastronomic scale being considered only as a food for peasants and livestock. Turnips come in many different varieties, but those grown here in America are generally the white-fleshed kind, with purple or green tops. This distinct-tasting vegetable goes well with braised beef or roast pork.

rutin. A disaccharide (rhamnose and glucose) derivative of quercetin; found in grains, tomato stalk, elderberry blossom.

rye. Family: *Gramineae*. Genus: *Secale*. Species: *Secale cereale*. Grain of the predominant cereal in some parts of Europe; very hardy and withstands adverse conditions better than wheat. Rye flour is dark and the dough lacks elasticity; rye bread is usually made with sour made with sour dough or leaven rather than yeast. Rye has long been valued for its blood-cleansing properties as it helps stimulate the circulation and prevents hardening of the arteries. It is also good for regulating glandular activity and stopping constipation. It is rich in iron and B-complex vitamins and so is helpful in cases of anaemia. It is high in fluorine, which encourages the formation of tooth enamel. It has the highest sodium, potassium, calcium and iodine content of all the cereals.

The rye kernel, like other cereal grains, is a caryopsis, a small, dry, indehiscent, one-seeded fruit varying to as much as 6-8 mm in length and 2-3 mm in width. Ripe grain is free-threshing and of various colours, but commonly grayish yellow. The seed consists of an embryo attached through a scutellum to the endosperm and aleurone tissues. The endosperm and aleurone are enclosed by the remnants of the nuclear epidermis and the testa or seed coat. The pericarp or fruit coat surrounds the whole seed and adheres closely to it. A crease or furrow extends the full length of the grain on the ventral side. The outline of the embryo can be seen at the base of the dorsal side. Mature kernels often have a shriveled appearance. Developing kernels are served by four vascular traces emanating from a basal vascular bundle.

Protein content of the rye kernel ranges from 6.5-14.5%; samples near the latter figure apparently originated from fields given very high levels of nitrogen fertilizer. In general, rye is lower in protein content than in wheat. There is about 1.5-2.0% crude fat in rye, not far different from the amount found in wheat and barley, but considerably lower than the fat contents of oats. Rye lipids differ from those of most other cereals by having a slightly greater proportion of the unsaturated linoleic acid. Because with fatty acids are very susceptible to oxidation, rancidity development tends to be the factor limiting the storage life of rye flour, assuming the product is protected against insect infestation and is not of sufficiently high moisture content to encourage mold growth. The nitrogen-free extract consists primarily of starch. Rye starch granules have a mean particle diameter greater than those of other cereals, and the size distribution covers a wider range. The granules fall into two classes depending on shape, one type being lenticular and the other being smaller and approximately spherical. Like other cereal starches, rye granules show birefringence in transmitted polarized light and, as usual, this birefringence disappears when the starch gelatinizes. The birefringence endpoint temperature and gelatinization temperature range of rye starch granules are similar to those of wheat starch. Rye flour suspensions give very low peak amylograph viscosities as compared to wheat, but this is due to high alpha-amylase activity in the former. Although there is some dispute about the amylopectin: amylose ratio in rye starch, most authorities seem to think that, in most cultivars, it is about the same as in wheat starch. In rye the nonstarchy polysaccharides are more important than protein in determining the quality of bread. This is the principal reason that rye bread has larger pores and seems moisture than wheat bread. These substances, predominantly pentosans, are present at evens of about 8% in rye, compared to about 3% in wheat. Crude fibre content is similar to wheat kernels, perhaps slightly less, depending on the cultivar and the method used for determining fiber. Rye has a significant content of a few micronutrients such as thiamin, nicotinic acid, riboflavin, pyridoxine, pantothenic, and tocopherol. These substances are present mainly in the embryo, scutellum, and aleurone. Typical figures on content in the whole kernel, per 100 g dry basis, are thiamin 0.44 mg; riboflavin 0.18 mg, niacin 1.5 mg; pantothenic acid 0.77 mg; and pyridoxine 0.33 mg. Rye is essentially devoid of vitamin C and vitamin A.

Typical mineral content of rye grain per kg includes calcium 60 mg; iron 10 mg; magnesium 120 mg; phosphorus 340 mg; potassium 460 mg; sodium 1 mg; copper 0.78 mg; manganese 6.7 mg; and zinc 3.0 mg.

There are of course, many enzymes in fresh rye kernels (*i.e.*, those not damaged by heat or long storage). Many of these enzymes are substantially inactive in mature dry grain. Some of the enzymes that have received a great deal of researcher's attention are α-amylase, proteases, esterases, and beta glucosidases.

rye bread. The characterizing ingredient in all rye breads is, of course, some type of processed rye grain. Most of the possibilities are enumerated and described in the chapter on ingredients from "other" cereal grains. Commercially available rye products are white rye flour, medium rye flour, dark rye flour, rye meal, cracked rye, and rye flakes. Other commonly used ingredients, the characteristics of which have a significant effect on rye bread quality are wheat flour, salt, sours or cultures, sweeteners, malt, shortening, and flavors (species, etc.). Caraway is a spice that is found in the majority of rye breads, and most consumers regard it as an essential part of rye bread flavor. A strong wheat flour must be included in rye doughs. Because rye flour is nearly inert so far as providing an effective gluten structure is concerned, this function must be taken over by the wheat flour if good machining properties are to be had in the dough and good volume and texture obtained in the bread. Most rye breads contain a fairly high percentage of salt, 2% (FWB) is not unusual and 3% can be found in some samples. Sweeteners may or may not be included. Many bakers prefer to add about 1% diastatic malt syrup instead of regular sweeteners; this material not only has its own sweetening effect but produces sugars from the rye starch through its saccharifying action. For the lighter types of rye bread, from 5% to as much as 10% of sweeteners can be added. Caramel colour is an indispensable ingredient in darker forms of rye bread. Even with 100% rye flour processed by any practical baking method, it is impossible to obtain the very dark loaves desired by some consumers. Some formulas call for as much as 10% (FWB) of caramel color. Shortening is used at zero to 2% in the darker and sour types of rye bread, and at somewhat higher levels in light hearth and pan rye breads. More shortening leads to a softer crust, and this can be a detriment in some types of rye breads. There are many different kinds of rye breads. They differ from one another in the type of rye meal used, in acidity of the crumb, and in the flavoring adjuncts such as species that are included in the formula. A typical formula for American-style rye bread will include about 30-40 parts white or light rye flour and 60-70 parts of high-protein spring wheat clear flour in addition to salt, malt extract or sugar, yeast food, shortening, caramel color, and yeast. It can be made by either the straight dough or the sponge method. Processing is similar to the procedure used for wheat bread, with care being taken to avoid over-mixing and over-development. Sour or Jewish rye breads will be made with a sourdough or a commercial culture or a flavoring composition that includes citric or lactic acid. Each of these options will respond in different to changes in processing conditions, and each will yield a product having features that may appeal to a specific market. At one end of the organoleptic spectrum are such items as Westphalian pumpernickel, which undergoes virtually no leaving action and contains 100% whole rye in the form of slightly broken kernels. It is baked for hours in a slow oven with steam applied (often throughout the baking) to prevent drying. Westphalian pumpernickel is a very dense, dark, and chewy loaf with a flavor strongly reminiscent of wet hay. The flavors are affected by enzymic and other reactions occurring during the long, slow bake. The breads sold as pumpernickel or even Westphalian pumpernickel being merely darker versions of the regular rye formulas, usually strongly colored with caramel. Westphalian pumpernickel rarely, if ever, contains caraway.

Ryle tube. Instrument for removing samples of the contents from the stomach at intervals after a test meal. It is a narrow rubber tube with a blind end containing a lead weight, with holes above this level. Another instrument used for similar purpose is Rehfuss tube.

Ryvita. Trade name for a crisp bread. The average composition per 100 g is: protein 7%; fat 2%; carbohydrate 77%; calcium 40 mg; iron 3.7 mg; phytic acid phosphorus 54% of total P (295 mg/100 g); and food energy 1.45 MJ.

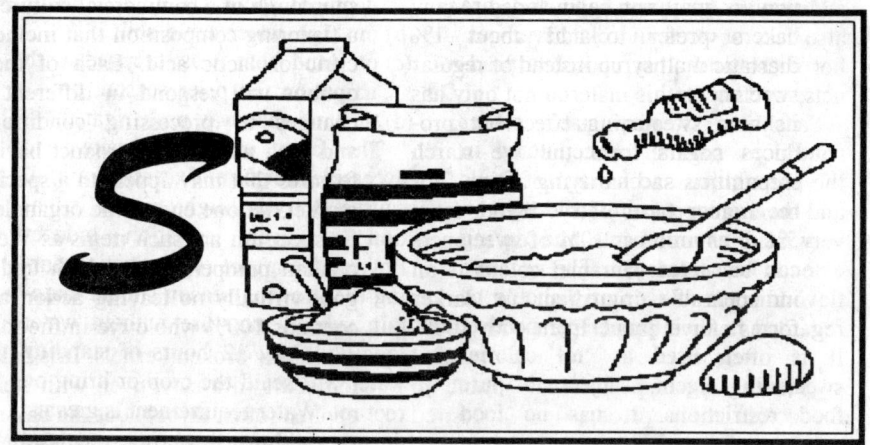

S-100 protein. An acidic brain-specific protein that has been implicated in neurophysiological functions; the protein has a molecular mass of about 20,000 and is rich in aspartic and glutamic acids.

Saanen cheese. A kind of Emmentaler cheese made in Switzerland. It is prepared from cows' milk. It has been made since the 16th century and is exported in limited amounts to many European countries. It is sold for a higher price than regular Emmentaler, but the process of manufacture is identical with that of Emmentaler, except that it is cooked much drier, takes longer to cure, and keeps longer, and the eyes are few and small. This type of cheese has traditional values as well. For example, it is often made at the birth of a child and portions are eaten on feast days during his life and at the time of his burial.

saccharases. A group of enzymes that attack sugars to liberate glucose or fructose depending on the type of saccharase.

saccharic acid. A dibasic acid derived from glucose.

saccharin. 2,3,-Dihydro-3-oxobenzisosulfonazole. An artificial sweetener derived from coal tar and is about 500 times sweeter than sucrose when the two substance are compared in dilute aqueous solutions. Federal food laws generally prohibit its use in food products. According to National Academy of Sciences, US, saccharin is a weak carcinogen in animals and a potential human carcinogen. Therefore, the products containing saccharin must have a warning label. Its name has also been included in the list of Carcinogen Assessment Group of Environmental Protection Agency. However, special permission is sometimes granted for its use in making so-called diabetic ice cream. An exact match to sucrose cannot be obtained because saccharin has flavour notes that are not present in sugar, and vice versa. Many people find that saccharin has bitter, astringent or metallic tastes, especially at high concentrations. These off-flavours tend to be particularly objectionable in delicately flavored fruit products, but may be partially concealed in foods that contain sucrose or corn sweeteners in addition to saccharin, and they are also less obvious in cola beverages, hot cocoa and other chocolate products, coffee, etc.

Saccharin is very stable under conditions normally encountered in the preparation and storage of foods and beverages retaining its identity in very acid environments and during extends heat treatment. The negative flavour notes of saccharin should be regarded in their proper perspective. It is often used as 'nil calorie' sweetening agent, subject to pure food restrictions. It has no food value; useful as a sweetening agent for diabetics and simmers.

safe concentration. The concentration of the material to which prolonged exposure will cause no adverse effect.

safflower oil. Oil of the seeds of the family Compositae, the safflower plant, *Carthamus tinctorius* L., It is a low, thistle-like annual plant with yellowish-red flower which have tubular corollas. Safflower is cultivated mainly because of its seeds which are a source of polyunsaturated oil. From the standpoint of chemical constituents, safflower oil is probably the simplest of the vegetable oils, 91% of its content being made up by compounds of linoleic acid (78%) and oleic acid (13%). The seeds are processed by conventional screw press and solvent extraction methods. After pressing, the seeds contain from 10-20% oil and after the pressings are extracted with hexane, the residual oil cake contains about 1% oil. The cake is ground to protein meal, which contains from 20-42% protein, depending upon growing and processing condition variables. Safflower is successfully grown on:

(a) dry land on followed soil when there is adequate moisture to a depth of about 1.2 m;
(b) on high water table soil;
(c) on land that was cropped with irrigation the prior season; or
(d) on land that was pre-irrigated.

The crop is very sensitive to excessive moisture. Excessive rainfall causes Botrytis blight. Flood irrigation or over irrigation induces Phytophthera root rot. Irrigation during the growing season should maintain subsoil moisture without water logging. Only 12 hours of standing water will scald the crop or bring on root rot. Water requirement is greatest during budding, flowering and seed development. Safflower should be irrigated three to four times after flowering begins, with irrigation at 10- to 14-day intervals, depending upon temperature, wind, and soil type. The last irrigation should be timed so it is applied about 1 week after flowering has finished. Safflower does best on deep, fertile, well-drained soils with a neutral pH. an outstanding feature of safflower is its tolerance to salt. A salt concentration at about 7 millimhos/cm will reduce yield only by about 10%, but will about double the time required for seedling emergence. Few crops demonstrate this tolerance. Safflower seeds must be placed in most soil for germination, and emergence is improved if crusting over the seed is broken up. Refined, bleached, and deodorized safflower oil is attractive to many nutritionists because it is highly polyunsaturated for use as a frying medium as well as being a component of "health" foods. A special high oleic safflower oil is available, particularly where high-stability is required.

saffron. The dried stigma of *Crocus sativus* (related to garden crocus). It contains glycoside picrocrocin, and colouring principles crocin and crocetin. It is a very expensive. One acre of these plants will yield about 2 kg of dried saffron.

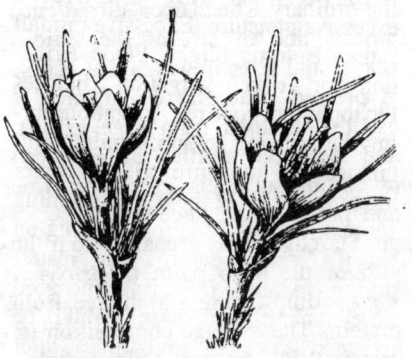

Three varieties are produced, a light colored (yellow-orange) saffron that is also light in flavour, an orange colored saffron that is stronger in flavour, and a darker coloured (red-dish-orange) saffron that is strongest in flavour. An important characteristic of this ingredient is its ability to colour the products in which it is used. In many cases, the colour may be more noticeable than the flavour, which has been described as being a spicy, sweet, floral aroma with an earthy, bitter, fatty, herbaceous taste. It is used for colouring as well as flavouring a large number of Indian food dishes. Saffron buns have been made for centuries, but are seldom seen nowadays. The spice can also be used in cakes and other products having a mild background flavour and light colour, but the flavour of saffron is easily overwhelmed and other spices and essences must be used with care when formulating such combinations.

Safi. A herbal remedy for skin diseases such as acne vulgaris, boils, skin rashes, blemishes, etc. It is also claimed to check nose bleeding, cures constipation, corrects indigestion, and improves complexion.

sage. Family: *Labiatae.* Genus: *Salvia.* Species: *Salvia officinalis.* A perennial shrub that grows wild in southern Europe and the Mediterranean area of the world, but is cultivated in many other places as a valued culinary spice. A strongly branched root system produces square, finely hairy stems which are woody at the base and bear oblong leaves. The floral leaves are ovate to ovate-lanceolate. The purple, blue or white flowers are two-lipped and grown in whorls. Sage is a decorative evergreen subshrub, though its leaves are not necessarily green. Some varieties have grey or grey-green downy leaves, and one has deep purple leaves and exceptionally pretty mauve-blue flowers. The flavour, which has faint overtones of camphor, is very strong in some types, so making sage a herb to use little and often. The plant is a native of the Mediterranean region, where it thrives on poor, dry soil, and is especially important in Yugoslavia.

Sage is traditionally used in sauces and stuffing for fatty meats such as goose, duck, and pork, in bouquets grains, and in sausages. In Italy the fresh leaves are lightly fried with liver, and rolled up with ham and veal in *salitmbocca.* In Germany and Belgium they are added to eel and other oily fish dishes, while in some Middle Eastern countries they are liberally used in salads. Medicinally, the leaves are used as an antiseptic and an astringent, while the tea is taken for sore throats and to calm the nerves. Sage leaves are strewn in bath water, and in the rinsing water when washing hair to st engthen dark colouring. Dried sage leaves are a frequent pot pourri ingredient. Dried leaf of the Dalmatian sage fragrant and spicy and is the most important herb used in the kitchen for flavouring meat and fish dishes and in poultry stuffing. Other sages (Greek, Spanish, English) differ in flavour from the Dalmatian variety. Also sage oil from the same source by steam distillation. It contains the essential oil thujone together with a-pinene, cineol, borneol and D-camphor.

Sage contains a hydrocarbon known as salvina, as well as other essential oils, such as boneol, pinene, cineol and thujone. It is also rich in oestrogenic substances and contains flavonoids, saponins, tannin and resin as well as various minerals. It is astringent, healing and antiseptic on mucosal surfaces. It is a peripheral vasodilator and stops perspiration, and in this respect it is particularly useful for night-sweats, and also for excessive salivation and lactation. It regulates hormonal problems in the menopause. The patients have been treated, particularly successfully for night sweats, during the menopause by administering three drops of sage oil three times a day in honey water. It acts as an excellent mouthwash and gargle for infections of the throat and it restores digestive and circulatory function during convalescence. The tea is useful in liver disease and in nervous conditions like anxiety and depression. It may be used as a douche in leucorrhoea and in baths to treat skin problems.

It has also been used traditionally to treat female infertility because of its high oestrogen content. It is reputed to retard ageing and enhance the memory, to prevent hand trembling and eyes dimming. It may be noted that it is a very powerful herb and particularly when used in its oil from should be taken under the close supervision of a qualified consultant medical herbalist.

Sage cheese. A kind of cheese made by the ordinary Cheddar or stirred curd process and of any of the various shapes and sizes in which that cheese is pressed. The flavour of sage is usually obtained from sage extract, and the green mottles are produced by cutting succulent green corn fine and pressing the juice out.

sago. Starchy grains prepared from the pith of the sago palm (*Metroxylan sago*); almost pure starch free from protein. The average composition is: protein 0.5%; fat negligible, carbohydrate 88%; and trace of B vitamins.

saithe. *Polachius virens.* A kind of edible fish. Apart from being eaten cooked, it is smoked, salted and dyed red, when it is similar to smoked salmon. Also known as coley and coal fish.

Sake. Japanese beer made from rice. Cooked whole rice grains are fermented with a yeast-like fungus culture for 10-14 days and stored in wooden barrels. Contains about 17% alcohol, by volume. Also known as rice wine.

salad burnet. *Poterium sanguisorba.* A popular herb in English cottage gardens, salad brunet was taken to North America by the early colonists. It is native to Europe, where it grows on chalky soil, and particularly on the chalk downs of southern England. With their mild, cucumber-like flavour, the young leaves are useful in salads and, like borage, in ice-cold summer drinks. It is mainly used in France and Italy, where it is frequently included in bunches of mixed salad leaves and herbs sold in markets. Fresh leaves may be used in salads, sauces, soups, and pates; in softened butter known as *ravigote;* steeped in vinegar for salad dressing; as a garnish; and in fruit salads and drinks. Medicinally, the fresh leaves act as a digestive. In self-help medicine, a decoction of the roots was used to stop bleeding, and an infusion of leaves to cool sunburn.

salad cream. Oil-in-water emulsion made from vegetable oil, vinegar, salt, spices, emulsified with egg yolk and thickened. Legally, in UK must contain not less than 25% by weight of vegetable oil and not less than 1.35% egg-yolk solids. Mayonnaise usually contains more oil, less carbohydrate and less water. By US regulations salad dressing contains 30% vegetable oil and 4% egg yolk; mayonnaise contains 65% oil plus egg yolk.

salamagundi. An old English dish consisting of diced fresh and salt meats mixed with hard-boiled eggs, pickled vegetables and spices, dressed on a bed of salad.

Salamana cheese. A kind of soft sheep's milk cheese made in southern Europe. It is eaten as spread on bread or mixed with corn meal. It is filled into bladders and allowed to ripen. It has a very pronounced flavour.

salicylates. Drugs that are derivatives of salicylic acid. Aspirin (acetylsalicylic acid) is the prototype. Aspirin and related drugs inhibit cyclo-oxygenase and thereby reduce prostaglandin synthesis. Salicylates are anti-inflammatory, antipyretic and analgesic drugs. In small doses they inhibit platelet stickiness because they inhibit thromboxane synthesis before prostacyclin synthesis.

saline agglutinin. Antibody which produces agglutination of cells in physiological salt solutions without addition of proteins, enzymes or other substrates.

saline purgatives. The soluble inorganic compounds, or the salts of inorganic cations, which are barely if at all absorbed from gut and which therefore, stimulate defaecation through their osmotic effect, which increases the bulk of the colon contents byretaining water. Examples include magnesium sulphate and sodium phosphate.

salinity. The total content of dissolved mineral constituents, of all kinds, in water. Natural sources of salinity include springs passing through rock formations which contain soluble salts. Other sources of salinity include domestic and industrial wastes, oil-well brines, and mine water. The use and re-use of water, particularity where irrigation is carried out, increases the threat of excessive salinity which makes water unsuitable for public supply and for further irrigation. Water containing more than 500 ppm of dissolved solids is not considered desirable for domestic supplies. Water containing more than about 2,000 ppm is considered to be unsuitable for irrigation under average conditions, in the long term. High levels of salinity in soil water in many countries, is a major environmental hazard associated with agriculture, and particularly with irrigation. In many areas the groundwater is naturally saline. Average salinities in most of the rivers are generally less than 400 g/m^3 of total dissolved solids. Factors contributing to this salinity include flows from tributary catchments, ground water inflow, surface drainage, and sub-surface drain effluents from irrigated areas. The salinity problem of the polluted rivers is particularly important because of the number of agricultural and urban users who are supplied from it.

Salisbury cure. Exclusive protein diet, supposed to cure or alleviate a number of diseases.

Salisbury steak. Similar to hamburger, minced lean beef mixed with bread, eggs, milk and seasoning, shaped into cakes and fried.

saliva. Secretion of the salivary glands in the mouth. There are three pairs of glands, parotid, submandibular and submaxillary. Dilute solution of the protein, mucin, and the enzyme, amylase, with small quantities of urea, potassium thiocyanate, sodium chloride and bicarbonate. 1.0-1.5 L/day secreted of solution of 0.5% solids. The mucin lubricates the food, and the amylase hydrolyses starch to maltose.

salmonella food poisoning. See salmonellosis.

salmonella. A genus of Gram-negative, motile, non-spore-forming bacilli that are found in the intestinal tract of animals and humans. *Salmonella* and *Escherichia* are quite closely related; the two genera have about 45 to 50% of their DNA sequences in common. However, in contrast to *Escherichia*, members of the genus *Salmonella* are usually pathogenic. The infection they cause are called salmonellosis. The majority of infections result in gastroenteritis, but a more severe infection called typhoid fever occurs when the organism penetrates the intestinal tract and invades the blood stream. Animals such as turkeys, chickens, swine and cattle are the primary reservoirs of the major pathogenic species. Infections in humans occur when products from these animals are cooked inadequately and are left at room temperature. These conditions support the rapid growth of salmonella organisms, and when enough are ingested, gastroenteritis

results. The *Salmonella* are characterized immunologically on the basis of three cell-surface antigens, the O, or cell wall (somatic) antigen; the H, or flagellar antigen; and the Vi (outer polysaccharide layer) antigen, found primarily in strains of *Salmonella* causing typhoid fever. The O antigens are complex lipopolysaccharides that are part of the endotoxin structure of these organisms. The genus *Salmonella* contains over 1000 distinct types having different antigenic specificities in their O antigens. Additional antigenic subdivisions are based on the antigenic specificities of the flagellar (H) antigens. There is hardly any correlation between the antigenic type of a *Salmonella* and the disease symptoms elicited, but antigenic typing permits tracing a single strain involved in an epidemic.

salmonellosis. A disorder caused by *Salmonella serovars*. The most frequently reported one for humans is S. serovar *typhimurium*. The initial source of the bacterium is the intestinal tract of animals. Humans acquire the bacteria from contaminated foodstuffs such as beef products, poultry, and eggs. Once the bacteria are in the body, the incubation time is only 8-48 hours. The disease results from a true food infectious because the bacteria multiply and invade the intestinal mucosa. Also known as salmonella food poisoning; salmonella gastroenteritis.

salmon. A valuable food fish that is extensively canned. There are five commercial species of north Pacific salmon of the genus *Oncorhynchus;* steelhead trout, or salmon trout, *Salmo gairdneri,* is of the Atlantic. The Atlantic salmon, caught off Newfoundland, is *S. salar.* Red salmon, or sockeye salmon, *O. nerka;*

the pink salmon is *O. gorbuscha;* and the Chinook, or king salmon, is *O. tschawytscha.* The catch is in the rivers on both sides of the Alaska peninsula and in the Columbia River where the fish enter the rivers to spawn. Australian salmon, which is the chief fish canned in Australia, is of a different genus, *Arripis trutta.*

salmon oil. A pale-yellow oil obtained as by-product in the salmon-canning industry, and employed as a drying oil for finishes and also used in soaps. There are different classes of the oil, depending upon the type of salmon. The oil contains about 23.5% arachidonic acid, 16.2% clupanodonic acid, 11.5% linoleic acid, 17.1% oleic acid, 15% palmitic acid, 10.6% palmitoleic acid, 4% myristic acid, and 2% stearic acid. The specific gravity is 0.926. It has a high iodine number, up to 160, but does not form an elastic skin on drying, and is not a good varnish oil untreated. It is, however, a valuable source of fatty acids for paint-oil blends and for plastics.

Saloio cheese. A hand cheese made in the farming district around Lesbian, Portugal, from cows skim milk.

salsify. Plant of the family *Chicoriaceae* (chicory family), salsify (*Tragopogon porrifolius*) is raised for its spindle-shaped root Which possesses an oyster-like flavour when cooked. The roots are white and large, ranging from 20-30 cm in length and about 2.5 cm in diameter. The plant is a biennial herb and native to the Mediterranean region. Its roots also are used in stews and soups and sometimes deep fried in much the same way as real oysters. Salsify, also known as vegetable oyster or oyster plant, may be grown in particularly any area with a temperate climate and reasonably good soil. The plant is similar to parsnip in its requirements, but requires a slightly longer growing season. Thus, it does not thrive in areas as far north as parsnip. The plant is hardy, however, and can be sown earlier than the parsnip in the spring. The soil is prepared to a depth of at least 0.3 m. Very heavy soil should be lightened by the addition of sand or some other soil amendment. The uptake of nutrients by salsify is high and thus generous application of plant food should be practiced. One of the better known varieties is Sandwich Island.

salt. In food terminology, the term salt commonly refers to sodium chloride, unless and otherwise stated; it keeps the body fluids in balance. In the body there is a fine balance of sodium and potassium and these act together to maintain the osmotic pressure in a state of equilibrium inside and outside the cells and ensure the proper functioning of the neuromuscular system. The concentration of sodium salts in the body is vital. The kidneys act as the basic regulator, excreting water and salt as necessary. However, an imbalance of the sodium and potassium due to the intake of excess sodium can lead to high blood pressure, arthritis, water retention, hormone imbalance and other problems. A deficiency of sodium causes muscular shrinkage and weakness, nausea, loss of appetite, and flatulence.

No matter where the salt is from, sodium and chlorine are vital minerals for the body. Deficiency of chlorine causes hair and tooth loss, weak muscles and poor digestion. Chlorine regulates our acid-alkaline balance, it enhances osmosis, stimulates production of hydrochloric acid and helps maintain healthy joints and tendons.

The two minerals are bound, as sodium chloride, in a variety of foods including tea vegetables, carrots, celery, beets, lentils, olives, cheese, pickles and soya sauce. Sea vegetables are a particularly good source of natural sodium chloride because the salt is accompanied by the abundant trace minerals, including iodine, held in solution in sea-water. Because sodium and chloride are so widely distributed in natural foods, it is almost never nutritionally essential to add salt to food.

Salt with food is an acquired not an inborn taste. The only circumstance in which it is necessary to add salt to your diet in when you do long strenuous exercise in extremely hot weather to which you have not had a chance to acclimatize. Remember that nearly 90% of the salt you eat is actually hidden in food. The amount of salt needed daily by an adult in a temperate climate is 4 g and this can always be obtained from natural foods. Most people add so much salt to their diet that their intake can be as much as 20 g a day. Canned and processed foods invariably have added salt, and the additives in them, including monosodium glutamate, sodium bicarbonate, sodium nitrite, sodium benzoate, sodium propionate and sodium citrate, also contain salt. Foods containing salt include some surprising examples like hard cheeses, dried, evaporated or condensed milk, baking powder and breakfast cereals. It is important to realize that all salt, whether it be rock or plain table salt, has virtually the same chemical composition and sodium content; so there is no point in just switching to another kind because it sounds healthier. There are various salt substitutes on the market, some of which contain mostly potassium chloride, and others of which are mostly a mixture of potassium chloride and ordinary salt. Unfortunately it is often not very clear from the label whether a product is very-low-sodium (mostly potassium chloride) or merely sodium-reduced (a mixture with ordinary salt). If cooking with these substitutes you can replace salt in exactly the same quantities although some manufacturers recommend that those which contain mostly potassium chloride should be added towards the end of the cooking time as prolonged heating can accentuate a bitter aftertaste. Because it is not yet established whether the substitutes have the same preservative properties as salt, it is probably best not to use them in foods like pickles. Used in bread, where salt normally helps to control the development of yeast and strengthen the gluten, all give good results with little effect of texture or appearance.

Our taste for salt seems to be largely acquired so in theory it should be possible to unlearn it and cut down progressively without too much difficulty. It is worth experimenting with herbs and salty foods at a very early age. A good salt substitute is two parts kelp powder mixed with one part parsley, one part marjoram, one part garlic powder and one part cayenne pepper.

salted butter. Butter to which salt has been added. It is salted to improve keeping quality, to season it, and to suit the requirements of the trade. The amount added, averages from 1.5-3% by weight of the butter. Nearly all butter for household use is salted.

salted peanuts. *See* peanuts, salted.

salt-free diets. More correctly these are diets low in (never completely free from) sodium, but as most of the sodium chloride or salt, they are referred to as low-salt diets. Sodium controls the retention of fluid in the body and reduced retention, aided by low-sodium diets, is required in cardiac insufficiency accompanied by edema, in certain kidney diseases, toxemia of pregnancy and hypertension. The average sodium intake is 1,000-2,000 mg per day and restricted diets are usually about 500 mg and can be as low as 150 mg. To improve the palatability of such diets salt mixtures are available containing potassium and ammonium chloride together with citrates, formates, phosphates, gluta-mates, as well as herbs and spices. Foods low in salt- (0-20 mg/100 g): flour, fruit, green vegetables, macaroni, nuts; medium salt- (50-100 mg/100 g) chicken, fish, eggs, meat, milk; high salt (500-2,000 mg/100 g), corned beef, bread, ham, bacon, kippers, sausages, cheese.

salting in. The increase in the solubility of a protein that is produced in solutions of low ionic strength by an increase of the concentrations of neutral salts; due to a stabilization of the charged groups on the protein as a result of a decrease in the activity coefficients of these groups.

salting out. The decrease in the solubility of a protein that is produced in solutions of high ionic strength by an increase of the concentrations of neutral salts; believed to be due to a partial dehydration of the protein as a result of the competition between the protein and the salt ions for solvating water molecules.

saltlicks. An adequate intake of sodium chloride is necessary to all including the grazing animals. Grass is relatively poor in sodium, and its high potassium content induces excretion of sodium in the urine. This loss causes a craving for sodium which is satisfied by natural or artificial saltlicks.

saltpetre. Potassium nitrate, used together with salt in the curing of meat. The salt restrains the growth of unwanted organisms; the nitrate is converted to nitrite which combines with muscle pigment to give the red colour of pickled meat. Also known as Bengal saltpetre.

Salustiana orange. A variety of sweet orange of the non-blood or blanca type. A comparatively recent variety grown in Spain, Iran, and Morocco, the Salustiana is believed to have originated as a limb sport on a common sweet seedling tree. The fruit is of medium-size, well-colored at maturity. The flesh is juicy, with low acid content and sweet flavor. The variety is highly regarded because of its early maturing, its absence of seeds, and general good quality. The tree and fruit are essentially indistinguishable from those of Caderna, except that the fruit is flatter and somewhat later in maturing. The Salustiana tends to produce a poor juice color, low yield of soluble solids and a bitter aftertaste is harvested too early.

salt-rising bread. This product is a specially brad that owes its unusual texture and distinctive pungent aroma to a combined yeast and bacterial fermentation. It was formerly prepared by a natural sour dough method that used a high concentration of salt at one point in the process to guide the survival and growth of the types of organisms needed to give the typical flavor. Practically all of the commercial salt-rising bread now being made in this country contains a dry "yeast" preparation or culture. As is the case with many strong-flavoured products, it exhibits a dichotomous distribution of acceptance, many people finding it very desirable while others dislike it extremely. The odour is said to be suggestive of cheese, since cheese can be prepared with a wide variety of flavours, most of which are due to bacterial action, this description is neither unexpected nor particularly helpful. The interior, or crumb, of salt-rising bread is close-grained and firm so that its specific volume will be three-fourths, or less, that of ordinary bread. The loaves have a tendency to crack on the sides, so it is customary to mold the loaf in two parts or to pan as a double loaf so that the split comes in the middle. It must be emphasized that true salt-rising bread cannot be made with ordinary bakers' yeast, either compressed or dry. There is a hot water reconstitution step for the special culture which would completely inactivate any preparation of *S. cerevisiae.*

salvage metabolic pathway. A pathway that utilizes compounds formed in catabolism for biosynthetic purposes, even though these compounds are not true intermediates of the corresponding normal biosynthetic pathway. Thus free purines may be salvaged from the hydrolysis of nucleotides and then used for the biosynthesis of nucleotides; likewise, free choline may be salvaged from the degradation of phosphatidyl choline and then used for the biosynthesis of phosphoglycerides.

sambhar. Name given to a spicy curry in southern India; equally popular in parts of northern India. It is prepared by boiling a number of chopped vegetables, pulses along with chilli and other spices. It has characteristic flavour and taste. It is generally taken along with *Dosa* and *Vada.*

sambol. Name given to a curry of fairly solid consistency in India and other parts of the south-east Asia.

sami. Socially acceptable monitoring instrument. A small, heart-rate counting apparatus used to estimate energy expenditure of human subjects.

samma. A butter oil produced in Egypt somewhat similar to the ghee, which is an Indian product.

samp. Coarsely cut portions of maize with bran and germ partly removed.

Samsoe cheese. A Danish cheese 50 cm in diameter. It has a small amount of uniform eye formation. The curd is drained, brine-salted and cured at 20-25° C for 3-5 weeks to produce the desired eye formation. Then curing is completed at lower temperatures.

Sanatogen. Trade name for a preparation of casein and sodium glycerophosphate for consumption as a beverage when added to milk.

sandwich nut cheese. A cheese made by mixing chopped nuts with Cream or fresh Neufchatel cheese.

San Francisco sourdough. This product, sometimes called Pacific Slope sourdough French bread, generated tremendous interest in the trade, probably more interest than the consuming public showed. Typical examples have a rather pungent aroma, a definitely acidic taste, a thick crust, and a dense chewy crumb. Many elaborate fermentation and proofing schemes and many formulations were proposed to solve the "secret" of San Franciso sourdough bread. None were, or could be, completely successful unless the doughs were inoculated with sours containing the mixed culture of microorganisms developed in the originating shops. The predominant yeast in this culture (*Saccharomyces exiguus*), is a different species from standard bakers' yeast.

A major difference is that it does not ferment maltose, so this sugar can provide more nutrient for the bacteria that are present. A luxuriant growth of a specific bacteria generates many of the substances that contribute unique flavor notes to this bread. Commercial cultures in frozen form are now available for bakers.

sanguinaria. A herb consisting of dried rhizome of *Sanguinaria canadensis* Linn. (Fam. Papaveraceae). It is a low perennial herb with horizontal branching rhizome. The plant is found in Canada. Alkaloids of protopine series have been isolated from Sanguinaria in addition to sanguinarine, chelerythrine, protopine, allocryptopine, homochelidonine and resin. Sanguinaria has stimulating and emetic properties. An extract of Sanguinaria is used as toothpaste base, in gingivitis and in periodical diseases.

Sanguinello comune orange. A variety of sweet orange, blood-type. It is described as a group of closely related clones and is one of the most important blood oranges in Italy. The color is orange at maturity, with some red blush. The flesh is deeply red pigmented. The fruit is juicy and of a pleasant flavor.

Sanguinello Moscato orange. A variety of sweet, blood-type orange, and one of the most highly regarded blood oranges. This variety is grown in the Mount Etna region of Sicily. The fruit has few to no seeds, is orange in coloration; the apical portion is strongly red-blushed. The flesh is well flavored, aromatic, blood-coloured, and very juicy. The fruit matures in mid-season and holds well on the tree. Sanguinello Moscato orange is also grown in Iran.

Sanka. Trade name for a decaffeinated instant coffee.

sapodilla. Fruit of the tree of the same name. This edible fruit is also sometimes called the Sapodilla Plum and is of the genus (*Achras*) and of the family Sapotaceae. Some botanists consider the sapodilla, *Achras sapota*, Linn, as one of the better fruits that are indigenous to the American tropics. The tree is now extensively cultivated in Asia, notably in southern India. The tree can withstand temperatures down to -2.2°C for short periods. Chicle, the basis of chewing gum, is made from the latex of the same tree. The average composition per 100 g is: water 75%; protein 0.5%; fat 1%; carbohydrate 21%; iron 0.8 mg; zinc 0.5 mg; vitamin B_2 0.03 mg; nicotinic acid 0.2 mg; vitamin C 14 mg; and food energy 0.41 MJ.

saponification value. A term used with reference to fats as an indication of the nature (molecular weight) of the fatty acids present. Defined as the number of milligrams of potassium hydroxide required to saponify 1 g of fat. Values greater than 200 are short chain fatty acids, below 190 are of high molecular weight.

saponin. The plant glycosides that have the characteristic of forming colloidal aqueous solutions which normally forms lather on shaking; saponins are powerful hemolytic agents that either have a tri-terpenoid structure or are steroid glycosides. Saponins are extracted commercially from soapwort or soap bark and used as foam producer in beverages, fine extinguishers, as detergent and for emulsifying oils. Bitter in flavour. There is a second group, the steroid saponins, that are cardiac active and are used as a starting material for the synthesis of sex hormones. It is often added to anthrax vaccines for veterinary use. Saponin is believed to act by causing a local reaction that retards loss of antigen from the inoculation site and attracts antibody forming cells.

Sapsago cheese. A kind of cheese made principally in Glarus, Switzerland, from the skim milk of cows. It is also known as Schabzieger, Glarnerkase, Grunerkase, and Krauterkase. It is said to have been made as early as the 13th century. This small, hard, green cheese, is flavoured with the leaves of a species of aromatic clover, and is shaped like a truncated cone, 10 cm high, 8 cm at the top. Federal Standards recommends that the moisture should not be more than 38% and the fat, 5-9.4%. The milk is put into a round kettle and stirred while it is heated to boiling temperature. Cold buttermilk is added slowly as heating and stirring are continued. The coagulum that appears on the surface is removed, set aside, and added to the curd when it is put into the forms. Then enough sour whey is added to precipitate the casein, as in making Ricotta, and stirring is stopped. If too little whey is added, the curd will be too soft and moist; if too much or too sour whey is added, the curd will be too firm and dry. The curd is collected in a cloth or strainer and spread out to cool as the whey is drained off. Then the coagulum that was set aside is mixed with the curd, salt may be added, and it is placed in perforated wooden forms, covered with a press lid, and pressed under heavy pressure at a temperature 15.6°C. The curd is ripened (cured) under low pressure at this temperature for at least 5 weeks. At this stage, it is ready for use in making the cheese.

Saran. Trade name for thermoplastic materials made from polymers of vinylidene chloride and vinyl chloride. They are clear transparent films used for wrapping food, resistant to oils and chemicals, can be heat-shrunk on the product.

Sarcina. The genus Sarcina contains two species of bacteria that divide in three perpendicular planes to yield packets of eight cells or more. Sarcina are obligate anaerobes and are extremely acid tolerant, being able to ferment sugars and grow down to pH 2. Cells of one species, *S. ventriculi*, contain a thick fibrous layer of cellulose surrounding the cell wall. The cellulose layers of adjacent cells become attached and this functions as a cementing material to hold together packets of *S. ventriculi* cells. Sarcina can be isolated from mud, soil, fees, and stomach contents.

Sarcodina. The organisms such as Amoeba which are always naked in vegetative phase, and organisms which secrete a shell during vegetative growth. Sarcodina do not have rigid cell walls and the cytoplasmic streaming within the cell results in ameboid movement. During ameboid movement, the cytoplasm moves in the direction in which there is least resistance. A wide variety of naked amoebas are parasites of man and other vertebrates, and their usual habitat is the oral cavity or the intestinal tract. Shelled sarcodines present a wide variety of interesting morphological forms. The best known of the shelled forms are the *foraminifera*, which are exclusively marine organisms, living primarily in coastal waters. The shells, called tests, of different species show distinctive characteristics.

sarcolactic acid. Old name for the form of lactic acid which turns the plane of polarized light to the right, *i.e.*, (+) lactic acid; found in muscle, as distinct from the inactive lactic acid (mixture of + and -) found in sour milk. Also known as paralactic acid.

sardine. Young pilchard, *Sardina (Clupea) pilchardus.* Composition of canned product per 100 g is: 20.5 g protein; 22.5 g fat; 200 mg calcium; 4 mg iron; 30 µg vitamin A; 8 µg vitamin D; 0.3 mg vitamin B_2; 6 mg nicotinic acid; and 1.25 MJ food energy.

sardo Romano. A grating Romano type cheese made on the island of Sardinia from cow's and ewe's milk. Pecorino Sardo is made solely from ewe's milk. Sardo made also in US and Argentina.

Saridele. Trade name of a protein-rich baby food (26-30%) protein) developed in Indonesia; contains extract of soya bean with sugar, calcium carbonate, vitamins B_1, B_{12} and C.

sarsaparilla. *Smilax officinalis.* This tropical American perennial plant produces a long, tuberous rootstock, from which grows a ground-trailing vine that climbs by means of tendrils coming in pairs from the petioles of the ovate, evergreen leaves. The small, greenish flowers grow in axillary umbels. Flavour is prepared from oil of sassafras and oil of wintergreen or oil of sweet birch; used in a carbonated beverage.

sassafras oil. An oil used to flavour root beer and similar beverages. Its main component is safrole; believed to be a weak hepatic carcinogen and banned in some countries.

saturated fatty acids. The compounds of the type RCOOH, where, R is a saturated alkyl group. Long chain saturated fatty acids are synthesized from acetyl-CoA by a cytosolic complex of enzymes including acyl carrier protein (ACP), which contains phosphopantetheine as its prosthetic group. ACP contains two types of -SH groups, one furnished by the phosphopantetheine (Pn) and the other by a cysteine (Cys) residue. ACP functions as the carrier of the fatty acyl intermediates. Acetyl-S-Cys-ACP, which is formed from acetyl-CoA and carbon dioxide, reacts with malonyl-S-ACP, formed from malonyl-CoA, to yield acetoacetyl-S-ACP with release of carbon dioxide. Reduction to the D-3-hydroxy derivative and its hydration to trans-D^2-unsaturated acyl-S-ACP is followed by reduction to the latter to butryl-S-ACP at the expense of NADPH. Six more molecules of malonyl-S-ACP react successively at the carboxyl end of the growing fatty acid chain to form palmitoyl-S-Cys-ACP, the end product of the fatty acid synthase complex. Free palmitic acid is then released by hydrolysis. Palmitic acid may be elongated to yield the 18-carbon stearic acid. Palmitic and stearic acids in turn can be desaturated to yield palmitoleic and oleic acid, respectively, by the action of mixed function oxygenases.

saturated solution. Solution remaining in equilibrium with another phase (solid, liquid or gaseous) which contains dissolved constituent. A solution that contains the highest possible concentration of a solute at a given temperature without becoming unstable.

Sauerkraut. Prepared by lactic fermentation of shredded cabbage. In the presence of 2-3% salt, acid-forming bacteria thrive and convert sugars in the cabbage into acetic and lactic acids which then act as preservatives.

Saurine poisoning. *See* Scomberoid poisoning.

sausage. Chopped meat, mostly beef or pork, seasoned with salt and spices, mixed with cereal (usually wheat rusk prepared from crumbled unleavened biscuits) and packed into casings of animal intestines or cellulose. There are six main types namely, fresh, smoked, cooked, smoked and cooked, semi-dry and dry. Frankfurt, Bologna, Polish and Berlin sausages are made from cured meat and are often smoked and cooked. Thuringer, soft salami, mortadella and soft cervelat are semi-dry sausages. Pepperoni, chorizos, dry salami, dry cervelat are slowly dried to a hard texture.

saute. Toss in hot fat without browning (saute potatoes usually cooked first and browned).

sauvagine. A linear polypeptide (40 amino acids) isolated from the skin of the South American frog *Phyllomedusa sauvagei*. It produces pronounced vasodilatiation in some vsscular beds and a consequent fall in blood pressure. It also stimulates the release of corticotrophin and β-endorphin from the pituitary but inhibits therelase of prolactin, GH and TSH.

Sauvignon Blanc grape. A variety of wine grape. Some times only the word Sauvignon is used to identify this outstanding white wine grape. Some authorities believe that this variety is only second in quality to the Chardonnay or true Riesling. It is extensively planted in the Graves region of France. The variety is also planted in California, Chile, South Africa, and the USSR

saveloy. Highly seasoned smoked sausage; the addition of saltpetre gives rise to the bright red colour. Originally a sausage made from pig's brains.

savory. Family: *Labiatae*. Genus: *Satureja*. Species: *Satureja hortensis* (summer savory); *Satureja montana* (winter savory). A plant with strongly flavoured leaves used as seasoning in sauces, soups, salad dishes. This annual herb grows wild in the Medi-

terranean area and is widely cultivated elsewhere in the world as a nice culinary spice. Its branching root produces a bushy, hairy stem which grows over a food high, often taking on a purple hue as it matures. The small, oblong-linear leaves are sessile and usually have hairy margins to them. The pink or white, two-lipped flowers grow in whorl-like cymes.

Summer savory is annual, *Satureja hortensis,* winter savory is perennial, *Satureja montana.* The plants are cut down at flowering time and dried for later use. Summer savory contains essential oils (carvacrol and cymene), as well as phenolic substances, resins, tannins and mucilage. It is antiseptic, expectorant, carminative, stomachic, stimulant and diuretic and protects against worms. Its main use is in gastric complaints to help the digestion and to stimulate the appetite. It is an excellent antiseptic gargle. Its old reputation as an aphrodisiac was probably due only to its stimulating effect. Winter savory contains almost the same constituents as summer savory and medicinally is used in much the same way.

Saxifrage family: *Saxifragaceae*. Distinctive characteristics to identify this family are lacking. The flower parts tend to be in 4's or 5's with stamens one or two times the number of sepals and with a pistil of 2-5 united carpels having numerous ovules. Leaves are mostly without stipules and usually alternate on these commonly perennial herbs and deciduous shrubs. the fruit type is a capsule or berry.

The family include: *Ribes* spp. (gooseberry, currant); *Astilbe* (false goat's-beard), *Deutzia, Heuchera* (coral bells), *Hydrangea, Philadelphus* (mock (orange), *Saxifraga* spp. (saxifrages), *Mitella* (bishop's-cap).

Saxin. Trade name for saccharine.

saxitoxin. A potent non-protein toxin. Its name is derived from the fact that it was first isolated from the Alaskan butterclam, *Saxidomus giganteus,* but in fact it originates not in the claim but in the dinoflagellates, *Gonyaulax catanella,* that a variety of clams and mussels may ingest when climatic conditions are such that they occur in vast numbers. Saxitoin gives rise to paralytic shellfish poisoning. It acts to block voltage-dependent Na^+ channels in the nerve fibre membranes by a mechanism resembling that of tetrodotoxin. In addition, it has a weak neuromuscular blocking action, possibly related to the fact that its molecule possesses two positively charged nitrogens. Tetrodotoxin contains one guanine group, whereas saxitoxin contains two.

scald. Defect occurring in stored apples consisting of formation of brown patches on the skin with browning and softening of the tissues underneath. Due to accumulation of gases given off during ripening.

scale. 1. A deposited layer or incrustation of calcium carbonate or calcium sulphate (or any other water insoluble substance) on the lining of boilers or in water pipes, resulting from prolonged contact with hard water.

2. A type of paraffin wax which retains several percent of liquid distillate; scale wax has a lower melting point, 325 K, than fully pressed and refined wax and is type commonly used for packaging, candles, etc.

scale-up dryer. The general term applied to design of larger dryers based on experience with smaller units. Typical scaleup involves small oven sample testing, laboratory scale, pilot plant, semi-commercial unit, and full-sized plant. The oven test may be used to evaluate the effect of basic phenomena such as heat or circulation rates on drying rates. The pilot plant is the first unit which uses equipment and materials similar to those expected to be suitable for the finished plant. Good pilot plant testing usually allows skipping the semi-works state for design parameters, limiting its use to cases where developing markets preclude major investment at once. Scaleup magnitudes from 2 to 1 to 5 to 1 have been replaced by values approaching 100 to 1 with increasing knowledge of the fundamental factors affecting processes. Computer simulation has been very helpful in studying the effect of various design parameters. Parameters of major significance in drying include: air circulation rate, moisture content of air in and out, average temperature of air and material being dried, state of subdivision of the material being dried, effect of depth of bed or layer, pattern of air circulation, etc.

scamorze. *See* scarmorze.

Scanno cheese. A kind of sheep's milk cheese, made in Abruzzi, Italy. The rennet curd is collected in a linen cloth and dipped in a 0.25% solution of iron oxide in sulphuric acid. The curd is left in this solution for 24 hours. The outside of the cheese is black, with a deep yellow interior. It has a buttery consistency, a burnt taste, and is eaten usually with fruits.

scarlet runner bean. *Phaseolus coccineus, or multiflorus).* A vine that is frequently grown for ornamental purposes, in which case it may be identified as the Flowering Bean or Painted Lady. The Dutch case-knife variety is a vegetable-garden plant cultivated for its beans. Beans of the multiflorus species are particularly favoured in Mexico and Latin America as food. In this group are also the prehistoric beans grown by the Aztec Indians of Mexico. The scarlet runner bean plant is also cultivated in Europe for its flowers. The pods sometimes are used for forage.

Scarmorze cheese. A small, soft, mild pasta filata type of cheese first made from buffaloes' milk in southern Italy. Now also made from cow's milk. It is made similarly to Caciocavallo except that it is not cured. The cheese is formed into an oval shape with an indentation and lappets at the top for handling. Also spelled as scamorze.

scented-leaved geranium. A pot of scented-leafed geranium in the kitchen is one of the most useful of herbs. You can put a couple of leaves in the base of a cake pan when making sponge cakes or other baked goods, add a leaf or two to sauces, syrups, salads, and fruit salads, and use the pretty, sometimes variegated leaves for decorating and garnishing dishes of all kinds. The pelargonium species originate in South Africa, and are ideal for growing indoors. Outside, they are half-hardy perennials that collapse at the first touch of frost.

Different varieties have different aromas. One may choose between lemon scented, *P. crispum minor;* apple scented, *P. odoratissimum;* oak-leaf scented, *P. quercifoliuml;* rose scented, *P. graveolens* and *P. radens;* nutmet scented, *P. fragrans;* peppermint scented, *P. tomentosum,* and many others. The flowers, which may be white, pink, mauve, or red, are small and insignificant, and most have no smell. The fresh leaves may be infused in milk, cream, and syrups for desserts, sorbets, and ices; chopped into softened butter for sandwiches and cake fillings; and used extensively for garnishing. The dried leaves are a fragrant addition to pot pourri and sachets to sent clothes and linens; the fresh leaves can be infused in bath water or rinsing water for hair.

Schardinger dextrin. A group of oligosaccharides that are formed by the action of amylase on starch from Bacillus macerans; includes α-dextrins, which contain six glucose residues per molecule, and β-dextrins, which contain seven glucose residues per molecule.

Schardinger's enzyme. The same as xanthine oxidase which oxidizes a whole range of aldehydes to acids, and also xanthine and hypoxanthine to uric acid.

Scheurebe wine grape. A relatively new variety of grapes that is breeding cross between Silvaner and Riesling. The grape grows well in Rheinhessen, Rhenish Palatinate, and Franconia regions of Germany and ripens quite late. Produces full-bodied, flowery wines of Riesling character. Its bouquet is strongly aromatic, reminiscent of black currants. Of vineyard areas in Germany, this grape represents 2.7% of total.

Schiff's reagent. A reagent used for testing for aldehydes and ketones; it consists of a solution of fuchsin dye that has been decolorized by sulphur dioxide. Aliphatic aldehydes restore the pink colour immediately, where as aromatic ketones have no effect on the reagent. Aromatic aldehydes and aliphatic ketones restore the colour slowly.

Schloss cheese. A Limburger type soft-cured, rennet cheese made in northern Austria and Germany; it is similar to Romadur cheese. Schloss cheese is wrapped in tin foils prior to marketing. Also known as Schlosskase cheese; Castle cheese.

Schordinger dextrin. A group of oligosaccharides that are formed by the action of amylase on starch from *Bacillus macerans*; includes α-dextrins, which contain six glucose residues per molecule, and β-dextrins, which contain seven glucose residues per molecule.

Schuetz-Borrisow rule. An empirical rule that states that the velocity of an enzymatic reaction is proportional to the square root of the enzyme concentration; the rule was developed for pepsin and applies, under limited conditions, to pepsin and other proteolytic enzymes.

Schwarzenberger. A Limburger-type part skim, rennet cheese made in southern Bohemia and western Hungary. During the 2-3 months ripening period it is washed daily with salt water. The cubes of cheese weigh approximately 0.45 kg.

scleroprotein. Any of a group of proteins found in the exoskeletons of some invertebrates, notably insects. Scleroproteins are formed by conversion of the relatively soft elastic larval protein by a natural tanning process (sclerotization) involving the orthoquinones. These are secreted and form cross linkages between polypeptides of the proteins, producing a hard rigid covering.

Scomberoid poisoning. A food-borne disease comprising aspect of seafood poisoning. It is caused by products of microbial spoilage of one group if fish, scomberoid fish, including tunny, mackerel, sardines, pike-mackerel. The etiologic agents are histamine-like substances. Histidine in flesh is broken down by action of *Proteus morganii* or other organisms. It is thermostable and can withstand boiling for at least 1 hour. Histmaine is a capillary dilator. Symptoms of the poisoning are evident from a few minutes after ingestion to about 1 hour. There is intense headache, dizziness, nausea, vomiting, metallic or peppery taste, diarrhea, facial swelling and flushing, epigastric pain, throbbing of carotid and temporal vessels, rapid and weak pulse, burning of throat, thirst, difficulty in swallowing, edema, and itching of skin. Although an illness of great discomfort, recovery usually occurs within 12 hours. Likely sources of this poison are scombroid fishes, such as tuna, bonito, mackerel, and skipjack. Good prevention requires refrigeration of fish immediately after they are killed. The fish should be consumed promptly, if not immediately refrigerated. Also known as Scomberotoxism; Saurine poisoning.

Scomberotoxism. *See* Scomberoid poisoning.

scone. A variety of tea cake originally made from oatmeal and sour milk, in Scone, Scotland.

scoop. A device used to cut the curd horizontally in the manufacture of Swiss cheese.

scrapple. Meat dish prepared from pork carcass trimmings, maize meal, flour, salt and spices, cooked to a thick consistency.

screen analysis. The classification of material by size, accomplished by shaking it on screens of successively smaller sizes, and collecting separately the portions that fail to pass through the various screens.

screw conveyor dryer. A conveyor in which the trough is heated with steam, hot water, or electricity, and the screw shaft can also be heated for drying. The product may be heated with electric or gas heated infrared units located above the conveyor. The unit is used for drying pastes and granular materials. The unit is operated in a vacuum chamber for some applications.

scuppernong. Name of the most widely cultivated of the muscadine grapes, used chiefly in wine rather than as a dessert grape.

scurvy grass. *Cochleria officinalis.* A variety of grass which grows along the seashores; it is a good source of vitamin C.

scutellum. Area surrounding the embryo of the cereal grain; scutellum plus embryo is the germ. Rich in vitamins.

SDS. Abbreviation for sucrose distearate.

seal oil. An oil resembling sperm oil obtained from the blubber of the oil seal, *Phoca vitulina,* a sea mammal native to the Atlantic Ocean. The oil has a saponification value as high as 195, and an iodine value up to 150. In the nineteenth century as many as 400 ships at a time operated from Newfoundland in seal catching, but the unrestricted catch resulted in the destruction of the herds, and North Atlantic sealing was reduced to three ships by the middle of the twentieth century. The industry now centres around South Georgia in the South Atlantic as an adjunct to the whale industry, but considerable oil and seal meal come as by-products of the Alaskan fur-seal industry. Some seal oil is obtained from Steller's sea lion, a large-eared seal occurring from southern California to the Bering Sea. The adult male weighs up to 998 kg. The blubber is about 75% oil, with an iodine value of 143 and saponification value of 190. From 40 to 50% of the carcass is a dense, dark-red, edible meat, but in the US seal meat is used only in animal foods.

seaside clover. *Trifolium wildenovii.* A variety of clover native to the US, this perennial is commonly found in several of the western states, sometimes near saline water. The plant features creeping rootstocks that are quite tolerant of soil salinity. Some authorities believe that it will increase in popularity for hay and pasture. The plant is palatable to livestock and competes with the salt grasses and sedges.

seaweed. A substance used as a mineral supplement for cattle as it contains 15-20% ash on dry weight, including about 60 minerals. It also contains carotene, vitamin B_1, folic acid, vitamin E, and is said to be the only vegetable source of vitamin B_{12}. Occasionally incorrectly claimed as a source of protein but most seaweeds are low in protein and of very low biological value.

Seckel pear. A variety of pear. Fruit is quite small unless heavily thinned. Shape is obovate-pyriform in shape, usually symmetrical. Skin is dull brownish-yellow, usually overlaid with russet and blushed dull red. Flesh is somewhat granular, with some grit at center. Buttery and very juicy. Noted for sweet, aromatic, spicy flavor and rates among the best of the dessert quality pears. It is susceptible to core breakdown if held on tree too long. It does not ripen properly if harvested prematurely, and responds well to cold storage. Tree is moderately vigorous, sturdy, very productive, with a tendency to overbear. Somewhat resistant to blight. The Seckel does not lose much in quality of allowed to ripen on tree.

secondary metabolites. The products of metabolism that are synthesized after growth has been completed. Most secondary metabolites are complex organic molecules that require a large number of specific enzymatic reactions for synthesis. For instance, it is known that at least 72 separate enzymatic steps are involved in the synthesis of antibiotic tetracycline and over 25 steps are involved in the synthesis of erythromycin, none of which are reactions occurring during primary metabolism. The characteristics of secondary metabolites are:

(a) Each secondary metabolite is only formed by a relatively few organisms.

(b) Secondary metabolites are seemingly not essential for growth and reproduction.

(c) The formation of secondary metabolites is extremely dependent upon the growth conditions, especially on the composition of the medium. Repression of secondary metabolite formation frequently occurs.

(d) Secondary metabolites are often produced as a group of closely related structures. For instance, a single strain of a species of Streptomyces has been found to produce 32 different anthracycline antibiotics.

(e) It is often possible to get dramatic overproduction of secondary metabolites, whereas primary metabolism, can usually not be overproduced in such a dramatic manner.

secondary treatment. A series of biochemical, chemical and mechanical processes used in sewage treatment which remove, oxidize, or stabilize non-settleable, colloidal, and dissolved organic materials found in sewage, following primary treatment. The two techniques most commonly used are either treatment on trickling filters or the activated sludge process. These carry out in a controlled manner, the biological assimilation and degradation processes that occur in nature. Trickling filters; also known as biological filters, consist of beds of coarse material over which the sewage is sprinkled at a uniform ate; they are generally not less than 2 m deep and circular in plan. The activated sludge process of sewage treatment is in effect an artificially accelerated self-purification process, promoted by oxidation. As in the case of the trickling filter, the impurities in the sewage are oxidized mainly by the action of aerobic bacteria. The most common methods of introducing oxygen into the sewage in the activated sludge process is to blow compressed air through porous plates placed in the bottom of the tanks; underwater paddles assist in the distribution of air and help to keep the sludge in suspension. The sewage, after passing through the activated sludge tanks, is allowed to settle in secondary sedimentation tanks; after a suitable retention time the activated sludge (other than that mixed with fresh sewage) is pumped to sludge digestion chambers.

secretin. A hormone, secreted by the intestinal mucosa, which travels via the bloodstream to the pancreas and stimulates this organ to secrete. Is a small, basic polypeptide, destroyed by pepsin and trypsin, and therefore ineffective when given by mouth. This polypeptide hormone comprises 27 amino acids, produced by the anterior part of the small intestine (the duodenum and jejunum) in response to the presence of hydrochloric acid from the stomach. It causes the pancreas to secrete alkaline pancreatic juice and stimulates bile production in the liver. Secretin was the first substance to be described as a hormone.

Sedge family. *Cyperaceae.* Distinguished from grasses, which have hollow, round stems, sedges have solid-pitched, often 3-sided, stems. Sedge leaves usually emerge from a stem area in three directions (3-ranked), each with blade and a closed sheath. The flower is subtended by one bract or scale. Sedges are usually bog or marsh plants and grow in clumps or extend from creeping, underground, rhizome-like stems. Minute flowers are arranged in spikelets. Sepals and petals are reduced to bristles, hairs, or scales or are absent. Usually there are 3 stamens and 1 pistil with a superior ovary consisting of 2-3 carpels fused to form 1 chamber with 1 ovule. The pistil's style sometimes forms a beak on the achene-type fruit.

The family include: *Cyperus papyrus* (pith used to make paper), *Cyperus* spp. (mat grass, hay grass, roof thatching), *Eleocharis* spp. (basket making), *Scirpus* spp. (bulrushes-basket-work, mats, chair seats); *Eleocharis tuberosa* (Chinese water chestnut: tubers); *Cyperus alternifolius* (umbrella plant); *Carex* spp. (sedges).

sedoheptulose. A seven carbon sugar. Also called sedoheptose.

seepage pit. A buried perforated tank or gravel-filled cavity allowing effluent, *e.g.*, from a septic tank, to seep into the surrounding soil.

Seitz filter. Asbestos disc with pores so fine that they will not permit passage of bacteria, thus solutions filtered through a Seitz filter emerge sterile.

selection of drying system. The selection of a system of drying considers the cost of operation as related to the quality of product, value of product, safety considerations, effect on the environment, and ease of installation. Factors to be considered include: installed cost, operating cost, loss of materials, safety, putting product in a desirable form if not already (such as grinding, pelleting), changes of size of load, control of drying operation as compared to effect on the product, and versatility.

selenium. Highly toxic element, placed in group VIA of the periodic table; classed as a nonmetal. In terms of abundance, selenium ranks 34th among the elements occurring in the earth's crust. Its high levels in the soil can accumulate in plants and render them toxic. Acts synergistically with vitamin E. Selenium in much smaller amounts is required in the diet of animals. It has been shown that selenium is an essential component of the prosthetic groups of several enzymes, particularly glutathione peroxidase, which functions together with the peptide glutathione to protect cells against the destructive effects of hydrogen peroxide. In red blood cells the iron of haemoglobin is normally in the ferrous form but it is readily oxidized to the ferric form by hydrogen peroxide to yield methemoglobin, which is inactive in carrying oxygen. Glutathione peroxidase protects against formation of methaemoglobin by consuming hydrogen peroxide in the reaction. The active site of glutathione peroxidase contains a residue of the unusual amino acid selenocysteine, in which the sulphur atom of cysteine is replaced by a selenium atom. Presumably, the -SeH group of this residue has advantageous properties in the mechanism of this and other selenium enzymes.

Dietary intake of selenium depends on food consumption patterns and selenium levels in foodstuffs, the latter being determined mainly by the character of the foodstuff and by geochemical conditions. Vegetables and fruits generally represent a poor dietary source of selenium levels in contrast to grain, grain products meat (particularly internal organ meat) and seafood, which contain substantial selenium levels, usually well above 0.2 µg/kg on a wet weight basis. The chemical composition of the soil and its selenium content have a marked influence on the selenium content in grain from different countries, ranging from about 0.04 µg/kg to 21 µg/kg. Its compounds are toxic, and may cause severe burns of the skin and eyes and intense pain around finger nails. Sudden inhalation of a large amount of selenium dioxide fume causes severe lung irritation.

Soluble selenium salts, such as sodium selenite, are readily absorbed in the gastrointestinal tract of rats. Absorption exceed 95% whether the diet contained 20 µg or 4000 µg of selenium per kg. About 93% of selenium was absorbed by man when milligram doses of sodium selenite were administered in aqueous solutions. Thus humans, like rats exhibit no homeostatic control limiting gastrointestinal absorption of large amounts of selenite.

Absorbed selenium is widely distributed in organs and tissues, with high levels present in the liver and kidneys. Selenium penetrates through the placenta and also into the milk the extent depending on the chemical form. Within the body, two primary metabolic pathways predominate. One is direct incorporation into or binding by proteins. The other, reduction followed by methylation is responsible for the production of dimethylselenide and trimethylselenonium ions.

When its rate of formation exceeds the rate of further methylation to a urinary metabolite trimethylselenonium ion, the volatile dimethylselenide is exhaled. Under the conditions of exposure prevailing in the general population urinary selenium excretion predominates.

The rate of selenium elimination depends on the chemical form in which selenium is administered and on the selenium nutritional status. Available human data indicate that selenium administered as selenite is excreted more rapidly from the body than when given in organic form, such as selenomethionine. In rats, the biological half-time of selenium decreased dietary selenium levels.

For total recoverable inorganic selenite the criterion to protect freshwater aquatic life is 35 µg/L as a 24-hour average and the concentration should not exceed 260 mg/L at any time. The available data for inorganic selenite indicate that acute toxicity to freshwater aquatic life occur at concentrations as low as 760 µg/L, and would occur at even lower concentrations among the species that are more sensitive than those tested. No data are available concerning the chronic toxicity of inorganic selenite to sensitive freshwater aquatic life. For total recoverabie inorganic selenite the criterion to protect saltwater aqua-tic life is 54 µg/L as a 24-hour average and the concentration should not exceed 410 µg/L at any time. The ambient water quality criterion for selenium is recommended to be identical to the existing drinking water standard whicn is 10 µg/L.

self-purification. The general tendency of a water body to recover naturally from contamination by organic wastes; thus when a river receives, continuously or intermittently, quantities of organic wastes it will tend to purify itself and recover naturally in the course of time. The process of self-purification depends very largely upon biochemical reaction in which bacteria (and other microorganisms) in the presence of sufficient dissolved oxygen use the organic matter as food, breaking down complex compounds into simpler and relatively harmless products. Other factors such as dilution, sedimentation and sunlight also play an important part in the self-purification process. However, the dominant requirement is a sufficient quantity of dissolved oxygen. If this is used up, that is the rate of absorption of oxygen exceeds the rate of replenishment, self-purification will cease and a septic condition will prevail. Septic conditions are associated with offensive odours, floating masses of black sludge and the termination of aquatic life. The organisms contributing to the process of self-purification include fungi, algae, bacteria, protozoa, crustaceans, shellfish, worms, insect larvae, snails, fish, dig predatory animals and waterfowl. The last two are the terminal members of the biological self-purification chain in the water.

In water and sewage, the bacteria, algae and fungi absorbed dissolved and dispersed organic and inorganic constituents. In the metabolism of the organisms, these substances are incorporated into the body matter or ultimately broken down into water and carbon dioxide for the purpose of providing energy. In order to sustain these processes, dissolved oxygen is absorbed from the water. Owing to their autotrophic manner of feeding, the algae containing chlorophyll are in a position by day to return the

oxygen so absorbed. If the water is quite rich in nutrients, *i.e.*, overloaded with plant nutrients such as nitrogen or phosphorus, these can well be an explosive proliferation of algae. This will result in a shortage of oxygen as, owing to the limited absorptive capacity of the water, once saturation points is reached the oxygen produced by day will by give off in the form of gas.

The absorptive capacity depends largely on the water temperature. At higher temperatures, the saturation point is reached more rapidly. If algae are present in the water in over abundance, the oxygen requirements at night will lead to a severe oxygen deficiency. The protozoa, which absorb bacteria and algae as nutrients, are also able to utilize dissolved organic substances to some extent. Crustaceans, snails and worms feed on undissolved, deposited or suspended matter. They also ingest protozoa. Bigger cursaceans and insect larvae, for their part, feed on small curstaceans, worms and also on protozoa. Fish and waterfowl, which are also liable to fall victims to predatory animals in their turn, often prey on curstaceans and worms. The intensity of self-purification is determined not only by optimum functioning of the living communities but also by the conformation of the riverbed. In naturally formed river-beds, that is to say, in waters with large surfaces and strong turbulence (irregular strong water currents of high turbulence), the higher input of oxygen makes for more favourable living conditions for the organisms than are found in corrected or dammed river courses. Even minor changes in one or another of the determining biological, chemical or physical factors can completely upset self-purification capacity of the waters. The oxidation of organic matter during self-purification is effected in two stages:

(a) Carbonaceous oxidation stage, in which most of the organic carbon is oxidized to carbon dioxide. Water and ammonia are also formed from the hydrogen and nitrogen of organic matter.

(b) Nitrification stage, in which biochemical oxidation of ammonia to nitrous and ultimately nitric acid occurs, and the residual organic carbon is consumed.

Finally, a dark brown or almost black complex organic material remains, known as humus. Deposited by the river bed, it is very resistant to further decomposition by microorganisms. Humus contain carbon, hydrogen, oxygen and nitrogen with a C:N ratio of about 10:1. A shallow, fast-flowing watercourse will purify itself in a much shorter period of time than a watercourse which is deep and sluggish, through a higher rate of re-aeration. The speed of chemical or biochemical reactions increases with a rise in temperature; hence the process of self purification will tend to be more rapid in the summer months than in the winter months. The speeding up of the process will increase the amount of dissolved oxygen required in any given length of river or stream. However, since warm water contains much less dissolved oxygen than cold water, a heavy pollution load has a greater likelihood of deoxygenating a river or stream in the summer than in the winter, thereby creating septic conditions.

Seliwanoff's test. A biochemical test to identify the presence of ketonic sugars. such as fructose, in solution. A few drops of the reagent, consist-ing of resorcinol crystals dissolved in equal amounts of water and hydrochloric acid, are heated with the test solution and the formation of red precipitate indicates a positive result.

semi-indirect fired dryer. A type of rotary dryer in which the heat from the fire box and burner (a) is used for heating the exterior of the rotating cylinder; and (b) is moved through the inside of the rotary kiln in contact with and in the opposite direction as the incoming product, such as for coal drying.

semipermeable membrane. A membrane or septum through which a solvent but not certain dissolved or colloidal substances may pass through; used in osmotic pressure determinations. Many natural membranes are semipermeable. Also known as semipermeable diaphragm.

semolina. The granular starchy product obtained from the endosperm of hard wheat; the fine floury part of the endosperm is semolina flour. Soft wheat give endosperm that does not hold together in granules during cooking. It is used for the preparation of alimentary pastes (macaroni, spaghetti, etc.) and as a milk pudding. In US farina is defined as the purified middling of hard wheat other than Durum wheat.

senna bean. *Cassia occidentalis.* Any of a number of plants, members of Leguminosae, but of the subfamily Caesalpiniaceae (senna). The senna bean is cultivated mainly for its leaves which, when dried, can be used for laxatives and other medicines.

sensitive volume. 1. The volume of a biological specimen in which an ionization must occur to produce a particular effect. 2. The volume of an ionization chamber through which the radiation must pass in order to be detected.

sensitivity. 1. In sensory analysis, the ability to perceive, identify, and/or differentiate, qualitatively and/or quantitatively, one or more stimuli by means of the sense organs. 2. The sensitivity of a procedure is (for a simple procedure) the slope of the calibration curve, *i.e.*, the differential of the measure with respect to concentration, *dx/dc*. It is not the smallest amount, or lowest concentration, that the procedure will detect; the correct name for the latter quantity is limit of detection.

septic. A biochemical condition depending on anaerobic bacterial activity, characterized by putrefaction.

Septmoncel cheese. A hard, blue-mold rennet cheese made from cows' milk plus a little goats milk. It is similar to Gex and Sassenage, and its manufacture is nearly identical with that of Roquefort. It is made almost exclusively on isolated farms. Also known as tura bleu.

sequestering agent. A type of chelating or coordination compound which immobilizes (sequesters) the metal ions by binding them into complexes that are both stable and soluble. As a result, the ions are prevented from acting as oxidation catalysts and from forming insoluble precipitates. Ethylenediaminetetracetic acid (EDTA) is an example of this type. Also known as a metalion deactivator.

Sequestrene. Trade name for disodium salt of ethylenediaminetetraacetic acid.

Serbian cheese. A kind of rennet cheese made by warming the milk in a kettle over fire or in a tub by immersing hot stones. After the rennet is added, the milk is allowed to stand 1 hour, when the curd is lifted in a cloth and the whey allowed to drain. It is then placed in a wooden vessel, salted, and covered with whey for 8 days or so, and with milk for about 6 days.

serendipity berry. *Dioscoreophyllum cumminsii.* West African fruit with an extremely sweet taste.

series-parallel trickling filter. A process of treatment of sewage by two-stage trickling filters with series-parallel arrangement; Its biological oxygen demand. Its removal efficiency is about 90-95%.

serine. Amino-hydroxypropionic acid. A non-essential amino acid;

serosal. In reference to the intestine means the outer side of the intestinal wall as distinct from the inner or mucosal side.

serotonin. 5-Hydroxytryptamine. A derivative of the amino acid tryptophan that is widely distributed in tissues, particularly in blood platelets, the intestinal wall, and central nervous system. It is pharmacologically active mediator of immediate-type hypersensitivity. Serotonin is formed from tryptophan and is released from mast cells during the allergic response; it has hormone-like properties and causes vasodilation, increased capillary permeability, and contraction of smooth muscle.

serra da estrella. The highly prized of the Portuguese cheeses. The name is derived from the mountainous regions where it is produced. It is a soft goats and ewe's milk cheese with a pleasant, acid taste. A similar cheese, made in another part of Portugal, is called Castello Branco. Usually the milk is coagulated with the flower extract of a thistle.

Serratia marcescens. Enterobacteria that characteristically produce pink or red pigment at room temperature; it is found widely in nature and as an opportunistic pathogen in nosocomial infections. It causes endocarditis, osteomyelitis, septicemia, and wound, urinary tract, and respiratory tract infections. Most strains are resistant to several antibiotics because of the presence of R factors.

serum. The fluid expressed from a blood clot as it contracts after coagulation of the blood. The essential difference between plasma serum is that the latter does not contain fibrinogen.

serum, albumin. The major protein component of serum in higher species. It is soluble in water and in salt solutions such as 50% saturated ammonium sulphate. It readily migrates to anode on electrophoresis relative to globulins.

serum, blood. Blood plasma without the fibrinogen. When blood clots, the fibrinogen is converted to fibrin which is deposited in strands that trap the red cells and form the clot. The clear liquid that is exuded is the serum.

serum blocking power. The capacity of an immunoadsorbent to adsorb antibodies from a serum and to decrease the antibody titer of the serum.

serum thymic factor. A nonapeptide secreted by thymus epithelical cells and found in the peripheral circulation, that partially restores T-lymphocyte function in thymectomized animals.

sesame. Family: *Pedaliaceae*. Genus: *Sesamum*. Species: *Sesamum indicum*. The meal remaining after oil extraction is a rich source of protein, especially the amino-acid methionine as well as calcium, phosphorus and niacin. Sesame seeds contain little carbohydrate. The lecithin content lowers blood cholesterol leaves and the seeds have mucilaginous (soothing) properties.

Seville orange. A Spanish term for the bitter orange.

sewage. The contents of sewers carrying the waterborne wastes of a community. Sometimes the term foul sewage is used to distinguish between sewage, as defined here, and the contents of sewers carrying surface or storm water only.

sewage accelerator. A device that combines air diffusion and agitation. The impeller of the accelator is placed close to the bottom of the tank. Air is mixed with the settled sewage entering at the bottom of the tank.

sewage fungus. Unsightly slimes resulting sometimes from the pollution of rivers discharges of organic matter.

sewage gas. The highly poisonous gas, generally methane (or a mixture of methane (CH_4) and hydrogen sulphide (H_2S)), formed during the anaerobic bacterial decomposition of sewage and sludge.

sewage goals. The proper sewage goals should contain at least the following aims:
(a) removal of sewage from houses and industries;
(b) collection and disposable of waste waters in a safe manner;
(c) proper protection of freshwater sources; and
(d) proper prevention of unsafe and unaesthetic pollution.

sewage lift station. A pumping station installed in sewer network to lift the sewage from a lower level to a higher level, with a view to avoiding too deep excavation for laying sewers. Such a lift station is required to be installed when a sewer invert reaches 6 metres or more below the ground surface.

sewage pump house. A pump house close to a sewage treatment plant or outfall to pump the sewage from a lower level to a higher level. This may be a dry well type or wet well type.

sewage purification. Until relatively recent times, the self-purification capacity of static running waters was still sufficient to reduce the contaminants contained in them. Loading the waters with sewage from different sources has proliferated, however; and owing to the accretion of these contaminants, the reduction processes in the waterways have either come to a standstill by the extermination of micro-organisms or been intensified by the increase in nutrients. With the multiplication of organisms, more oxygen has been extracted from the waters. The self-purification capacity of the waters has been overloaded, and the regenerative powers of the waters have been disrupted. The immediate consequences of such pollution have been the extermination of fish life, deposition of mud, and putrefaction processes. The most serious loading of the waters stems from domestic and industrial waste disposal.

The water purified by the primary and secondary treatment, passes finally to the biological stage, which comprises a restoration basin (percolating filter) and a second filter, or final sedimentation tank. In the restoration basin, bacteria and other microorganisms convert the suspended and dissolved matter into removable sludge by absorbing the parti-cles and dissolved matter as a nutritive substratum and by forming cell lumps as they proliferate, which, owing to their increase in weight, sink to the bottom. The whole process, is facilitated and intensified by artificial induction of air by means of bellows, rotors and cylinder pumps. In order to ensure that the microorganisms required for decomposition are present in sufficient quantities, parts of the microorganisms sludge deposited on the floor of the secondary filter tank are returned to the restoration basin. The purified water on the surface of the secondary filter tank is fed in to the receiving stream. The sludge from the primary and secondary settlers is digested in septic towers with the aid of anaerobic bacteria. By this process, methane gas is formed which can be used to provide energy for the plant. Earlier the digested sludge was usually dried out in beds to compact it. In new plants, the preference is for mechanical dehydration plants, such as centrifuges and presses, because of the smaller space they take up. The dehydrated sludge can then be further processed together with household refuse. Under optimum conditions the mechanical-biological sludge drying plant can achieve a purification performance of over 90%. For future purposes, however, this performance level is still too low, so that a further stage, the chemical stage, needs to be added. The chemical precipitation process employed serves to eliminate phosphates and other (especially industrial) pollution. With the aid of microsieves and similar technical appliances, organic resides can be further reduced. In addition, a hygienic improvement in the sewage may be achieved by means of the chlorination, radiation, heating or ozonization.

sewage sludge composting. A method of composting undigested sewage sludge without using admixtures. The raw sewage is spread over a drying bed, which is subsequently ploughed, harrowed, and rototilled, and then set up in windrows. Ripe, usable, hygienic compost, with excellent fertilizer values, is produced by this process in about 4-5 months.

sewage sludge composting. A method of composting undigested sewage sludge without using admixtures. The raw sewage is spread over a drying bed, which is subsequently ploughed, harrowed, and rototilled, and then set up in windrows. Ripe, usable, hygienic compost, with excellent fertilizer values, is produced by this process in about 4-5 months.

sewage treatment. The modification of sewage to make it more acceptable to the environment. Sewage treatment may be divided into four main stages:
(a) *Primary treatment*. The removal of suspended matter by physical and mechanical means, *e.g.*, screening, grinding, flocculation or sedimentation.
(b) *Secondary treatment*. The removal of finely suspended solids and colloidal matter, and the stabilization and oxidation of these substances and the dissolved organic matter by means of air and the activity of living organisms.
(c) *Tertiary treatment*. The attainment of higher effluent standards for many purposes.
(d) *Sludge disposal*. The disposal of the suspended matter removed.

A decision as to the stages of treatment to be adopted depends on what is to become of the final effluent. For example, an industrial house, especially food processing industry situated close to the sea may discharge its sewage without pretreatment at a suitable distance out to sea; this approach is known as disposal by dilution. Where conditions are not satisfactory for this method of disposal, the final effluent which will be discharged into a watercourse undergoes at least two stages of treatment.

sewer pill. A ball-shaped skeleton frame almost of same diameter of sewer is allowed to pass through the sewer along with the flow of sewage. During its travel it cleans the sewer walls.

sfumatrice. Machine for obtaining the oil from the peel of citrus fruit. Based on the principle that the natural turgor of the oil sacs forces out the oil when the peel is folded.

shad. A food fish of the family of herrings, including two species, the common, or allice, shad, and the white shad. The common shad inhabits the sea near mouths of large rivers, and in the spring ascends them for the purposes of depositing its spawn. The form of the shad is the same as that of other herrings, but it is of larger size, and in some places receives the name of herring king. Its colour is a dark blue above, with brown and greenish lustre, the under parts being white. An American species, varying in weight from 2 to kg, is highly esteemed for food and is consumed in great quantities in the fresh state. Shad are found along the coast from New England to the Gulf of Mexico, and have been successfully introduced on the Pacific coast.

shaddock. Alternative name for pomelo, *Citrus grandis*, from which grapefruit is descended (named after Captain Shaddock who introduced it into West Indies).

shade-grown tobacco drying. During the first five weeks of curing heat is required about one-fifth of the time to provide the proper environment. The storage temperature is maintained at about 8-11°C above the outside temperature, with 29.4-37.8°C being most desirable. Heat is usually supplied the major part of the first week of curing, and for one or two periods of 8-24 hours a week until cured.

shallot. Family: *Amaryllidaceae*. Species: *Allium ascalonicum*. A plant species related to a great number of other species of the genus of similar odor and taste. Closely related species are chive, garlic, leek, onion, and Welsh or Japanese onion. The shallot is a small onion of the multiplier-type. Its bulbs have a more delicate flavor than most onions. Shallots seldom form seed and are propagated by means of the small cloves or divisions, into which the plant splits during growth. The plant is hardy and may be left in the ground from year to year, but best results are obtained by lifting the clusters of bulbs at the end of the growing season and replacing the smaller ones at the desired time.

Shamouti orange. A variety of sweet orange that is completely orange-colored at maturity. A very attractive fruit, the juice content is generous and the rag content is low. As grown in the Mediterranean region, it is indistinguishable from the Jaffa or Joppa orange. In Israel, this variety constitutes about 75% of the country's total orange crop. For many years, the principal rootstock used was Palestine sweet lime, but this resulted in a fruit of low juice and soluble solids content. In recent years, sour orange rootstock has been used and quality has improved markedly. A campaign has been conducted in Israel for many years directed toward eradicating trees infected with tristeza. The fruit is medium-large, oval in shape, and seedless. The variety is also grown in Turkey and South Africa.

Shamser cheese. A rennet cheese made in the Canton of Graubunden, Switzerland, from the skim milk of cows.

sharp-lobed hepatica. *Hepatica acutiloba.* Family: Ranunculaceae. A flowering plant whose stems are 5-15 cm long and the flowers are 12-25 mm wide. The bracts are light green and the leaves are dark green, some with brownish-red blotches near the edges. Hepaticas are insect pollinated. After fertilization, seeds are produced which germinate readily. Hepaticas have 5 or more colored parts which may be pink, blue, mauve, or white. The new leaves develop after the flowers. They grow in a clump and are divided into 3 pointed lobes. The flowers open in the sunshine and close at night or in cloudy weather. They are one of the earliest spring flowers to bloom in the eastern half of North America.

shashlik. Similar to shishkebab, steeping the meat in wine. According to some recipes shashlik is the same as shishkebab.

sheepshead. The name of a fish abundant on the Atlantic coast of the United States, highly esteemed as a food. It receives its name from the resemblance of its head to that of a sheep. It is a stout and deep-bodied, of a greyish colour, with eight vertical bands and dark fins. It is rarely more than thirty inches in length.

shelf-life. This refers to the length of time any edible product may be kept on a retailer's shelf without developing any defects. For instance, a cheese product may develop mold, become bleached in colour or dried out before it is sold to the consumer. Most cheese products are tested in the laboratory for shelf, under the adverse conditions of temperature humidity and light which might be expected in a retail store.

shellfish, edible. A general term that include prawns, shrimps, lobsters, crayfish and crabs. Zoologically they are of the order *Decapoda*, suborder *Macrura* (prawns, shrimps, lobsters, crayfish) and suborder *Brachyrura* (crabs).

shepherd's purse. *Capsella bursa-pastoris.* This ubiquitous annual plant is found in field and waste places and beside roads everywhere in the US and Canada. Its erect, simple or branching stem grows from half a foot to a foot and a half tall; above it is a rosette of basal, grey-green, pinnatifid leaves. The small white flowers grow in terminal cymes, in many places blooming all year. The fruit can be flat, heart-shaped or triangular, notched pods.

sherbet. A frozen mixture of water, sugar, flavouring, stabilizer, and sometimes milk product (milk, cream, or ice cream mix).

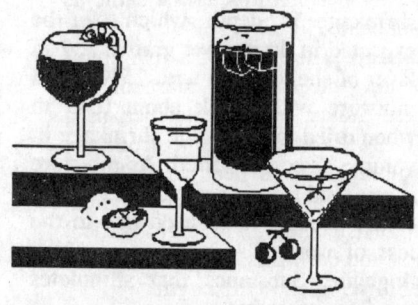

It differs from an ice in that it contains a milk product, and from an ice cream in its much higher sugar content, more pronounced acid and fruit flavour, much smaller amount of fat and serum solids, and much lower over-run, usually between 35-45%.

Sherry. The most popular of the fortified wines; a Spanish wine, made in the neighborhood of Jerez, in the province of Andalusia, near Cadiz, the location of the choicest vineyards of Spain. Dry sherry is the most highly prized. It is a strong wine, esteemed for its delicate flavour. Sherry is more largely imitated and adulterated than any other wine. True Sherry, is made only in a restricted area in the Spanish province of Cadiz. Sherry is made from dried grapes. The ripened grapes are gathered and dried out under the sun. If they are intended for dry sherries, they are dried for twenty four hours, but if for the sweeter sherries, they are left for longer time.

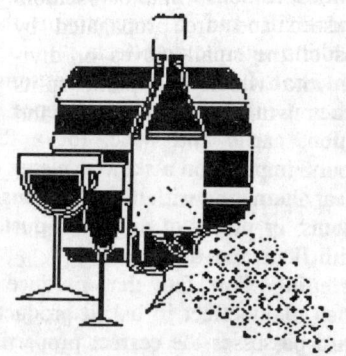

The dried grapes are next trodden out to express the juice and fermented in big casks after being slightly sulphured. After cellar practices and racking (as previously described), the wine begins to turn itself into Sherry. At some stage the fermentation is arrested by the addition of brandy obtained from the distillation of a previous sherry sample. The resulting beverage with the residual sugar will be sweet. This is then matured. If all the sugar present in the juice is fermented, dry sherry is formed.

Shigella. A Gram-negative, non-spore-forming bacillus, but unlike *Salmonella* is nonmotile. The shigellas are genetically very closely related to *Escherichia*; in fact they are so similar that they are able to undergo genetic recombination with each other and are susceptible to some of the same bacteriophages. The test for DNA homology show strains of Shigella having 70 to almost 100% homology with *E.coli*. In contrast to

Escherichia, however, Shigella is commonly pathogenic to humans, causing a rather severe gastroenteritis usually called bacillary dysentery. *S. dysenteriae* is transmitted by food and waterborne routes and is capable of invading intestinal epithelial cells. Once established, it produces both an endotoxin and a neurotoxin that exhibits enterotoxic effects.

shishkebab. Lamb (although beef sometimes used) cut into cubes steeped in onion, garlic and wine, for a few hours, impaled on a skewer; pieces of meat alternating with tomatoes, mushrooms, or pieces of eggplant, dusted with flour and then broiled.

shortening. Soft fats that produce a crisp, flaky effect in baked products. Lard possesses the correct properties to a greater extent than any other single fat. Unlike oils, shortenings are plastic and disperse as a film through the batter and prevent the formation of a hard, tough mass. Shortenings are compounded from mixtures of fats or prepared by hydrogenation and are still called lard compounds or lard substitutes.

shrimp. A genus of small crustaceans, closely allied to the crawfish. The common shrimp, found in the North Atlantic on both the European and American coasts, and in the Pacific, is about two inches long, greenish-grey in colour, with brown dots; on the Pacific coast it is pink. Shrimps are caught in nets and are marketed in canned form. The pink shrimp commonly sold at fishmongers is *Pandalus montagui*. The average composition per 100 g (without shell) is: protein 22.5%; fat 2.3%; carbohydrate almost nil; calcium 325 mg; iron 1.8 mg; zinc 0.7 mg; vitamin B_1 0.03 mg; vitamin B_2 0.03 mg; nicotinic acid 2.5 mg; and food energy 0.5 MJ.

shrinkage. 1. In cheese industry, loss of weight of cheese during curing. The amount of shrinkage is depends upon the temperature of curing, relative humidity, the use of paraffin on the cheese and the moisture content of the cheese. Paraffined cheese under normal curing conditions undergo about 2% shrinkage in six months.

2. The agricultural products such as food grain shrinks in both weight and volume when dried. Volume of shrinkage for shelled corn is relatively high when compared to other grain. Knowing the volume of shrinkage is important in the operation of drying systems to determine the amount of shrinkage in depth which can be expected in drying wet grains. A 2 m layer of shelled corn with 25% initial moisture will shrink about 0.43 m when dried to 12%. The shrinkage in volume as corn is dried. As moisture is removed from a product, the weight of the product is reduced due to the loss of water.

sialogogue. Substance that stimulates the flow of saliva.

siderophilin. Or transferrin, an iron-carbonate-protein complex, the form in which iron is transported in the blood plasma.

siderosis. Accumulation of haemosiderin, an iron-protein complex, in the liver, spleen and bone marrow, in cases of excessive blood destruction, and on poor diets relatively rich in iron. Said to be a common disorder among the Bantu people, who cook their maize in iron pots and consume up to 100 mg of iron per day.

Sierra leone bologi. *Crassocephalum biafrae*. A climbing plant with arrow-shaped succulent leaves. The tips of the shoots are often removed in order to encourage leaf production, but when allowed to flower, small clustres of cream and white flowers are produced at the ends of the shoots. Propagation is by cuttings or seeds. The seedlings or rooted cuttings are planted in a well-prepared soil at a distance of 0.6-0.8 m apart, and since the plant occupies soil for a relatively long period, the planting holes should be treated with liberal dressings of compost. The native growers usually train the young shoots to grow over a wooden table or trellis made of sticks, although upright poles are equally suitable to support this strongly growing plant.

sieving. The process of separating a mixture of particles according to their size by one or more sieves. Size analysis by sieving, the division of a sample by sieving into size fractions, and the reporting of results. The International Standard nominal aperture for test sieves are 128 in number, ranging from 22μm to 12μm.

silage. Any green fodder preserved by excluding air from the storage site. After cutting, plant material continues respiration and loses much of its nutritional value unless kept from the air. Under proper storage conditions in silos or bunkers, silatge made from green fodder crops, for example, maize, legumes, grasses, kale and rape, ferments slightly and keeps for several months. Silage is best with 50-65% moisture content and sufficient packing. Some crops, notably grass, oats, peas, beans and vetch may be treated with treacle and water.

sild. Young herring, *clupea harengus.*

Silesian cheese. A variety of cheese made from cows' skim milk, made similar to a 'hand cheese'. Flavouring substances, such as onions or caraway seed, may be added. It is eaten while fresh.

Silvaner grape. A well-regarded, productive white wine grape that originated either in Austria or Germany. Although most extensively planted in Germany, where it represents 17.2% of total vineyard area, the Silvaner is also found in Austria, California, and Chile. In Germany, the Silvaner is grown predominantly in Rheinhessen, Rhenish Palatinate, the Nahe and Franconia regions. The grape is of medium-size, very juicy, producing a pleasant, milk wine with a pleasing low-acid content.

silver. A white metal, softer than copper and harder than gold. Silver is present in the earth's crust at a concentration of about 0.1 mg/kg. It has antiseptic properties which are utilized in medicine and dentistry, and it plays an essential part in the formation of photographic images. The light-sensitive halides are used in photography; the iodide is effective in atmospheric nucleation for rain-making.

The conventional water-treatment practices have been shown to be effective in removing silver from water and, consequently, many treated waters contain very low levels of silver. However, because some metals (such as lead and zinc) used in distribution systems may contain traces of silver and also because in some countries silver oxide is used to disinfect water supplies silver levels in tap-water may sometimes be elevated. Levels exceeding 50 mg/L have been recorded on rare occasions, particularly when silver-containing point-of-use water purifiers have been employed to obtain drinking-water. The average levels in tap-water are low and certainly less than 1 mg/L. Assuming a consumption of 2 litres per day the average daily exposure from drinking-water would thus not be likely to exceed 2 mg.

Relatively, little is known about the absorption and metabolism of silver in humans except that individuals absorb the metal selectively. Animals seem to absorb about 10% of any ingested silver. Silver can be detected in various organs; the liver and spleen especially seem to concentrate the metal. In humans, more than 50% of the body burden can be found in the liver 16 days after exposure. Inhaled silver is also absorbed to a slight extent. Silver combines with the sulfhydryl component of some enzyme systems and other biologically important chemical groups, thus influencing the precipitation of proteins and inactivating some enzyme systems. Animal experiments have also shown that silver interacts metabolically with copper and selenium. Most of the absorbed silver is excreted almost exclusively with the faeces, and only small quantities are permanently retained by the tissues the exception being the skin, where larger amounts of silver can accumulate. Silver that is available for excretion has a biological lifetime in the body ranging from a few days to a few weeks.

There is no evidence that silver is essential to the human organism. Cases of fatal poisoning have been recorded but only with extremely high doses. The main effect of silver is discoloration of skin, hair, and fingernails (argyria). This has been detected when silver arsphenamine has been administered as medication. A single dose of 1 g of silver, injected as silver arsphenamine can produce this effect. The effect has also been observed in workers industrially exposed to silver, the condition is rarely encountered, however. It is possible that argyria may occasionally mask some mild systemic effects. There is no evidence that ingested silver is carcinogenic.

The available data indicate that chronic toxicity to freshwater aqu-atic life may occur at a concentration as low as 0.12 mg/L. For saltwater aquatic life the concentration of total recoverable silver should not exceed 2.3 mg/L at any time. The ambient water quality criterion for silver has been re-commended to be identical to the existing drinking water standard which is 50.0mg/L.

silvicide. Nonselective herbicides which kill or defoliate woody plants, bushes and small trees. Ammonium sulphamate has been used effectively for this purpose. Defoliants such as picloram may also be classed as silvicides if the trees die as a result of its application.

single cell protein. Name given to bacteria, algae and yeasts grown in mass culture as a source of dietary proteins.

sippet. A small piece of bread, fried or toasted, served as a garnish to a mince or hash.

Sippy diet. For peptic ulcer patients; hourly feeds of small quantities, 150-200 ml of milk, cream or other milky food.

Siraz cheese. A kind of Serbian semi-soft mellow cheese made from whole milk. It is smooth and has no holes. The small flat cakes are sun dried after which they are salted an placed in wooden containers to ripen.

Sister Laura's food. Trade name for an infant food comprising wheat flour, sugar and salt. No vitamins are claimed.

sitapophasis. Refusal to eat as expression of mental disorder.

sitology. The scientific study of foods.

sitomania. Mania for eating.

sitophobia. Fear of food; also known as phagophobia.

sitosterol. The main sterol found in vegetable oils, similar in structure of cholesterol with an extra ethyl group.

Skanausia suria. A soft Lithuanian cheese made from partly skimmed milk. The curd is pressed in bags and is marketed in one to two weeks. This cheese is made in Michigan and Wisconsin. Also known as Michigan farm cheese.

skate. A broad, flat-bodied fish belonging to the ray family, usually found on sandy bottoms near the shore. The chief portion of the body is made up of the expanded pectoral, fins, which are concealed under the skin. The tail is long and slender; the snout is pointed, with a prominent ridge, or keel. Most species are edible.

skim milk. Milk from which most of the fat has been removed. Legally the removal of any of the fat from milk results in a product which is skim milk, often called fat free milk. US Standards recommends that the portion of milk which remains after removal of the cream in whole or in part. The products made from skim milk include acid precipitated casein, bakers cheese, bakery products, bristles, buttermilk cultured, chocolate milk, concentrated sour skim milk, condensed milk, plain and sweetened, confections, cottage cheese, dried skim milk, dry mixes, feed for animals, fibre, glue, ice cream, low lactose skim milk, paint, paper-coating, plastics, pot cheese, rennet casein, skim milk cheddar cheese.

skin factor. Obsolete name for biotin.

skorup. A fermented milk used in Serbia and Montenegro. Similar to yoghurt or leben except that cream or boiled milk is used instead of whole milk. Skorup is of a creamy consistency and has an agreeable sour taste. Foods such as potato with a little salt are often added to the skorup.

skullcap. *Scutellaria lateriflora.* A North American perennial which grows in wet places throughout Canada and the northern and eastern US as well as in other parts of the world, such as Southeast Asia. The fibrous, yellow rootstock produces a branching stem from 0.2-1.0 metre high, with opposite, ovate, serrate leaves that come to a point. The axillary, two-lipped flowers are pale purple or blue.

slime mold. A common term for member of the division *Acrasiomycota*. Slime molds are nonphototrophic eucaryotic microorganisms that have some similarity to both fungi and protozoa. They can be divided into two groups, the cellular slime molds, whose vegetative forms are composed of single amoeba-like cells, and the acellular slime molds, whose vegetative forms are naked masses of protoplasm of indefinite size and shape called plasmodia. They live primarily on decaying plant matter, such as leaf litter, logs and soil. Their food consists mainly of the other microorganisms, especially bacteria, which they ingest by phagocytosis.

slipcote. A soft, unripened rennet cheese made from cow's milk in UK. It is an old variety, having been well known in the middle of the 19th century. When ripe the surface loosens and has a tendency to slip off. The cheese is ripened between leaves of cabbage for 3 days to a week after which it is ready to eat.

sliwowitz. Plum brandy, originating in Yugoslavia. Some of the stones are included with the fruit and produce a characteristic bitter flavour from the hydrocyanic acid (0.008%), which is present in the finished brandy.

sloe. Wild sour plum of the blackthorn (*Prunus spinosa*), used for the manufacture of sloe gin.

sludge. 1. A soft or muddy bottom deposit as on tideland or in a stream bed. It consists of large amounts of organic matter mixed with silt, clay, and sand, and with enough water content to remain in a semisolid state. 2. The solid material removed from the streams of sewage by a sewage treatment plant. It consists primarily of fecal matter, but may also contain food matter from garbage disposals, silt, sand, bits of leaves etc., living micro-organisms, especially algae and bacteria, that have entered the sewage at various points along its path; and chemical precipitates of industrial effluents.

sludge volume index. SVI. An empirical measurement index defined as the volume in ml. occupied by 1 g of mixed liquor solids (activated sludge) by dry weight after settling in 1000 ml. cylinder for 30 minutes. On this basis, the rate of sludge return and plant operation are controlled. In practice, it is the percentage volume occupied by the sludge in a mixed liquor after 30 minutes settling.

sludge volume ratio. SVI. The volume of sludge blanket maintained at the bottom of a thickener divided by the volume of thickened sludge removed daily. The SVR normally ranges between 0.5 and 2 days. The lower values are required in hot climates.

slurry. 1. A dilute suspension of particulate solids in water, for example, the aqueous dispersions of clay, fibre particles, or metal powders. 2. A semi-fluid mixture of faeces and urine, often containing rain water and washing down water from livestocks. It is sometimes mixed with litter to produce farmyard manure. It may also be stored in a lagoon or tank, where it is diluted with water and is then piped on to the fields. It contains valuable nitrogen, phosphate, and potash; but its composition varies according to the type of livestock, diet, dilution, etc.

SM. Trade name for a protein-rich baby food (15% protein) made in Ethiopia from teff, peas, chick peas, lentils and skim-milk powder.

SMA. Trade name for a milk preparation for infant feeding modified to resemble the composition of human milk.

smear ripened. The ripening action of the slimy, reddish or reddish-brown, surface growth which is found on cheese such as Brick and Limburger when held in a humid room. Yeasts develop first on the cheese surface followed by *Bact. linens* in 6 or 7 days. The yeasts raise the *p*H to a point where *Bact. linens* can grow. This organism apparently plays a role in the ripening, aids in protein breakdown and flavour development and aids in production of colour at cheese surfaces.

smell. The sense of smell originates in the olfactory lobes of the brain, and the olfactory nerves coming from these centres are distributed to the mucous membrane of the upper part of the nasal cavities. In order that odour may be detected, air must pass through the nostrils; hence a person sniffs when he desires to scent an odour more keenly. The sense of smell in man is not nearly so keen as in many of the lower animals, though he can probably detect more odours than any of these animals. Odours are numerous and difficult to classify, and they are named from the substance from which they arise, as the odour of musk and the perfume of violets. The nerves of smell are stimulated by an odour when it first acts upon them, but if long continued, this is lost, and the person fails to recognize it at all. The nature of odour is not well understood. That it arises from gaseous or volatile matter all agree, and some authorities consider that it can arise from matter in a gaseous state alone; others disagree, and in support of their theory point to the fact that substances like musk can fill a large space which odour for weeks and not diminish perceptibly in weight. The sense of smell is closely allied to the sense of taste, which it undoubtedly aids.

smelling salts. A preparation of ammonium carbonate, usually scented with lavender, sometimes with bergamot; used as a stimulant and restorative in cases of faintness. It is put up in small, fancy bottles which may easily be carried in a pocket or handbag.

smilax. A group of plants belonging to the lily family. Most of them are climbing or trailing, and numerous species are found in Asia and America. Sarsaparilla is obtained from the roots of several species, and the roots of others are edible. The species known as green brier and the carrion flower are found in the US. The cultivated plant known to gardeners as smilax is really an asparagus.

Smithco RT. Trade name for tall oil esterified with glycerine; used for varnishes and paints.

Smithco PE. Trade name for tall oil esterified with pentaerythritol; used for varnishes and paints.

smoke point. A term used with reference to frying oils; the temperature at which the decomposition products become visible (bluish smoke). The temperature varies with different fats and range between 160 and 260°C.

smoking. Meat and fish are often smoked after pickling to assist preservation and improve the flavour. Hard woods, oak, elm, and ash, produce a smoke containing aldehydes, phenols and acids with a preservative action, a surface dehydration also helps preservation. The flavour may be obtained from:
(a) a chemical liquid smoke added to the milk or curd;
(b) a so-called smoked salt may be used for salting; and
(c) cheeses may be hung on racks and smoked like meat, preferably by use of hickory wood smoke.

Only good quality cheese should be smoked. Some pasta filata type cheeses are smoked as are also some Process cheese, cheese foods and spreads.

smorgasbord. Scandinavian; table laden with delicacies such as fish, meat and cheese, as traditional gesture of hospitality.

smorrebord. Danish open sandwiches; literally means smeared bread.

SMS. Abbreviation for the sucrose monostearate.

smut. A group of fungi that attack wheat; includes loose or common smut (*Ustilago tricti*) and stinking smut or bunt (*Tilletia tricti*). Small fungi which live in certain plants as parasites. Wheat, oats and barley smuts attack the seeds, and can be destroyed be treating the seeds before planting. Wheat seeds soaked for five minutes in a solution of one pound of copper sulphate to a gallon of water are rendered immune; and oat seeds are treated by spreading them on the floor and sprinkling them with a formalin solution. Another remedy consists in soaking the seeds in water above 45°C. As corn smuts do not attack the seeds, they require a different treatment. Rotation of crops is the safest cure for corn smut, as the spores cannot live in the soil more than one season. Infected ears should never be used for planting, but should be destroyed by burning.

snail, edible. *Helix pomatia.* Family: Helicidae. Commonly referred to as escargot, it inhabits vineyards and all regions which are not too moist, particularly bush. With the onset of winter, the edible snail burrows into loose soil to a depth of up to nearly 30 cm. The shell aperture becomes covered by an epiphragm, and thus the snail survives the cold season. *Helix pomatia* becomes active again with the warmth of spring, recuperates, and above all equalizes its loss of water content. Edible snails produce sperm throughout the entire warm season, but eggs for only a limited time. Even in ancient times, the Helix snail was a favorite food item, and the edible snail also played a role in folk medicine. Napoleon's soldiers carried canned edible snails as emergency rations during their campaigns. Aside from the fastidious French, people in southwestern Germany and many other regions of the world also consider edible snails in a herb sauce a great delicacy. These snails are especially bred for the food industry.

snowberry. The popular name of a tropical American shrub which bears snow white berries.

Snowflake oil, Trade name for a heavy-bodied oxidized soybean oil. It has a specific gravity of 0.986-0.989 and iodine number from 64-95.

Snow Flake starch. Trade name for a processed corn-starch.

snuff. A powder made from the tobacco plant. The dry leaves and stems of the plant are ground in mortars and then scented. Snuff is inhaled through the nostrils, or is rubbed on the gums as an indulgence, like tobacco chewing.

soaked curd. This is a modification of the cheddar process which results in a milk Cheddar. Cheddar cheese, after milling, is covered with cold water for a period of 5-30 minutes. This results in a high moisture, quick ripening, soft-bodied, open textured cheese. The average composition is: moisture, not more than 42%; Fat, not less than 50% in the dry matter. Also known as washed curd cheese.

soapstock. In the refining of crude edible oils the free fatty acids are removed by agitation with alkali. The fatty acids settle to the bottom as alkali soaps and are known as soapstock or 'foots'.

soda bread. Made from flour and whey, or butter milk, using sodium bicarbonate and acid in place of yeast.

soda water. A popular summer beverage in almost all parts of the world. It is made of water charged with carbon dioxide and fruit flavouring. It contains no soda.

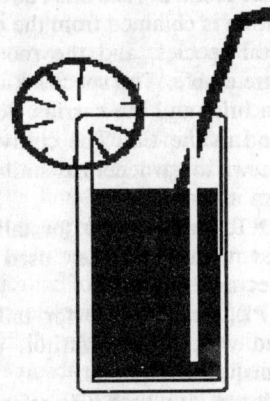

It is called soda water because bicarbonate of soda was formerly used in making it. The liquid carbon dioxide is stored in a steel container under heavy pressure; when released by means of a faucet it permeates the water as carbonic acid gas, causing it to effervesces and imparting to it a pungent taste. Pop, ginger ale and other similar drink consist of water flavoured with various extracts and charged with carbonic acid gas, which is kept under pressure in the bottle. When the cork is removed the gas escapes rapidly and causes the effervescence.

sodium caseinate. A hydrated casein product made by the addition of sodium salts to calcium caseinate or cottage cheese curd; used in ice cream manufacture as a source of lactose-free serum solids and in some cases to improve whipping ability of the cream.

sodium. A dietary essential which is almost invariably satisfied by the normal diet.

sodium. A metallic element and one of the major minerals required in animal diets. Sodium ions (Na^+) are the principal cations in blood serum and other extracellular body fluids, but occur at relatively low concentrations inside cells. Their concentration is thus the main factor in determining the osmostic pressure and hence volume of body fluids, and also plays a role in maintaining the acid-base balance. Moreover, the movement of sodium ions into and out of cells, closely linked with a counter-flow of potassium ions, is vital in maintaining the electrical potential of cells and the ability of nerve and muscle cells to transmit nerve impulses. Sodium is also required for the absorption of sugars and amino acids.

Sodium levels in blood are regulated by the kidneys under the influence of corticosteroid hormones, notably aldosterone. However, defi-

ciency of sodium in the diet may lead to retarded growth, impaired egg production, and other clinical signs. Excessive sodium in the blood (hypernatraemia) also has various pathological consequences; the commonest cause is salt poisoning. The body contains about 100 g of sodium, and the average diet contains 3-6 g, equivalent to 10 g of sodium chloride. The intake varies enormously in different individuals and the excretion varies accordingly. Vegetables are relatively poor in sodium and rich in potassium. Animal foods are rich in sodium. Sodium ions are the principal cations in blood serum and other extracellular body fluids, but occur at relatively low concentrations inside cells. Their concentration is thus the main factor in determining the osmotic pressure and hence volume of body fluids, and also plays a role in maintaining the acid-base balance. Moreover, the movement of sodium ions into and out of cells, closely linked with a counter-flow of potassium ions, is vital in maintaining the electrical potential of cells and the ability of nerve and muscle cells to transmit nerve impulses. Sodium is also required for the absorption of sugars and amino acids.

sodium-potassium ratio. The body contains about three times as much potassium as sodium. Vegetables and fruits contain a great excess of potassium, e.g., potatoes 80:1; boiling with salt reduces this ratio to about 3:1.

soft Corn. *Zea saccharata.* A variety of corn which display little if any denting and have soft kernels. These types also have variegated coloring of the kernels. Also known as flour corn.

soft cheese. A class of cheese characterized by a soft physical appearance as contrasted with the hard cheese such as Cheddar, etc. Some of the more common soft cheeses are cottage, cream, Neufchatel, Limburger and Camembert.

soft drink. Legal standards for fruit content (ready-to-drink without dilution) -citrus-and-barley, like juice and soda, 47 fluid ounce per 10 gallon; other types, 80 fluid ounce per 10 gallon.

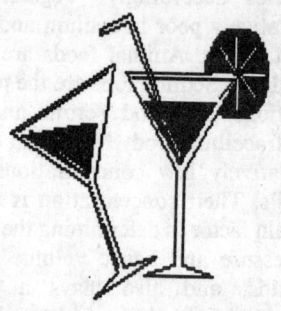

Drinks requiring dilution, squash, crush, cordial or concentrate: citrus-and-barley, 1.5 gallon per 10 gallon; citrus fruit, 2.5 gallon per 10 gallon (25%); other fruits, 1 gallon per 10 gallon. Comminuted whole orange: ready-to-drink, 5.5 pounds orange per 10 gallon; for dilution, 27.5 pounds per 10 gallon.

Essentially any beverage that is not alcoholic, with a water base and that is chilled before serving. The two principal categories are:

(a) still (uncarbonated) drinks, such as natural fruit juices diluted with water or artificially flavored and colored still beverages, which are frequently prepared from powdered ingredients at the point of consumption; and

(b) carbonated beverages, sometimes referred to as "pop" or soda pop" and which include the various cola-type drinks, ginger ale, root beer, and many others. For the mass market, carbonated soft drinks widely use synthetic flavouring and colouring agents. The sugar-sweetened drinks provide a source of calories. One-hundred grams of a sweetened quinine soda water, for example, will contain about 31 food calories, as derived from a sugar content of about 8% (weight).

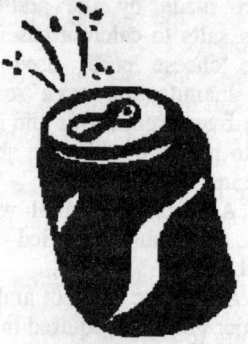

A cola-type drink will provide about 39 calories per 100 grams; a cream soda drink (about 43 calories); and a fruit-flavored (citrus, cherry, grape, strawberry, etc.) soft drink (about 46 calories, derived from a sugar content of from 10 to 13% by weight). In the last few decades, diet soft drinks, containing 1 or 2 calories or less, have been available.

softener. This term is widely used in chemical technology in its common meaning to denote a material or agent which is added to a product or process to increase the pliability or plasticity of any substance. A special usage is in the treatment of water in which the term 'water softener' is applied to a substance used to remove undesirable salts.

sogo ice cream. A sorghum-flavoured ice cream developed at the University of Tennessee. The flavour is produced by the addition of 1 pound of especially prepared sorghum syrup to 5 gallons of regular ice cream mix in the freezer. A flavour similar to caramel and butterscotch is produced.

solanine. Toxic glycoside found in potato and especially the sprouts; consisting of glucose, galactose and rhamnose plus the alkaloid solanidine. A considerable portion is removed with the peel and some is leached out on cooking.

solar drying. Open air solar drying of products-building, food, crops, aggregates, etc. is the oldest method of drying, in which the product is placed on platforms, pavement, trays which may or may not have means of coverings (mobile roof, mobile tray, canvas) for preventing wetting from rain. The product may be stirred periodically to provide uniform heating. Down-draft of air over solar heated beds increases drying rate. Solar air collectors may be used to supply warm air, with a fan and air distribution for drying products. To dry a 5 cm depth of grain from 20 to 15% requires about 7-8 hours with a down-draft air flow 0.005 m^3/m^2s. To dry the same grain without forced circulation, but with occasional stirring, requires at least twice as long, or two days of drying. Various devices are used for collecting the solar energy from the sun called solar energy collectors. For drying the sun is used for heating air which is circulated through the product to be dried. The solar collector consists of three basic parts: the cover plate (except the bare plate collector), the absorber, and the back plate. Collectors may have one or two air channels. Solar energy collectors are: (a) flat plate; or (b) concentrator type. With the former the area of the absorber and the cover plate are equal; with the latter the energy is collected on a large area and absorbed on a small area, usually to get a higher temperature than that obtained with the flat plate. During sunny days, 17,000 kJ/m^2 day, and for cloudy but not overcast days, 10,225 kJ/m^2 day can be collected. An air flow of 0.04-0.06 m^3/m^2s over the collector surface is used for drying, which will give a temperature rise of approximately 8-15°C. For higher air flows over the collector, a higher efficiency is obtained, but with a lower temperature rise. The collector efficiency is the useful energy collected by a solar energy collector divided by the amount of energy arriving at the face of the collector. The solar collector efficiencies of various types of collectors at the noon hour and for the full day. Passive solar energy collection refers to the design to the design of structures and other devices to make maximum use of the solar energy for drying without a separate collector.

solids-not-fat. SNF. Refers to the solids of milk excluding the fat, i.e., protein, lactose and salts. SNF serves as an index of milk quality and is determined by measuring the specific gravity in the lactometer. Normal specific gravity is 1.032 at 15.5°C. The per cent total solids is equal to

0.25 X S.G. + 1.2 X % fat + 0.14.

solid waste management. A planned system of effectively controlling the production, storage, collection, transportation, processing and disposal or utilization of solid wastes in a sanitary, aesthetically acceptable, and economical manner. It include all administrative, financial, legal, and planning functions, as well as physical aspects of solid waste handling.

solid wastes. All material of a solid or semi-solid character that the possess or no longer considers of sufficient value to retain.

soluble coffee. *See* coffee, soluble.

somatomedin. A protein hormone, produced by the liver in response to stimulation by somatotrophin, that stimulates protein synthesis and promotes growth. It is biochemically similar to insulin and has some actions similar to insulin; it is therefore sometimes said to have insulin-like activity (ILA) or is referred to as insulin-like growth factor.

somatostatin. Peptide hormone, released by the hypothalamus, that inhibits the production of growth hormone (somatotrophin) by the anterior lobe of the pituitary gland. It also inhibits insulin and glucagon production by the pancreas. The somatostatin gene has been isolated from the human and cloned in E. coli, active somatostatin being recovered form the clone. Both growth-hormone releasing factor and somatostatin are controlled by complex neural mechanisms related to sleep rhythms, stress, neurotransmitters, blood glucose, and exercise.

somatotrophin. A hormone, synthesized and stored in the adenohypophysis, that promotes bone growth and stimulates protein synthesis (via somatomedin). Its release is controlled by the opposing actions of growth-hormone releasing factor and somatostatin.

sorbet. 1. A semi-frozen water ice flavoured with liquor. In a large-scale dinner sorbet is served before the roast to clear the palate.

2. A superior sherbet of fine texture. It is made by scalding the milk and sometimes adding whipped egg whites.

sorbic acid. CH_3-CH=CH-CH=CH-COOH. An organic acid used to inhibit selectively growth of yeasts and moulds (not bacteria). Metabolized in the same way as the naturally occurring caproic acid (of butter) and so generally held to be harmless; used in margarine (0.05%), fruit juice (0.02%), sauces, cheese, jam, flour confectionery (0.1%). Permitted in UK in flour confectionery and cheese. Potassium sorbate is more soluble in water. It occurs in certain berries as the free acid and the delta-lactone. It is active as the undissociated acid and therefore the concentration for preservation is related to the acidity of the food; effective at pH 5.0-7.0.

Sorbistat. Sorbistat K. Trade names for sorbic acid, and its potassium salt.

sorbitol. A six-carbon sugar alcohol formed by the reduction of fructose. Although it is metabolized in the body it appears to be tolerated by diabetics and is therefore used to sweeten diabetic foods. 6-0-% as sweet as sucrose. Found in plum, apricot, cherry and apple but in raspberry, black currant, strawberry or currant.

sorghum. Family: *Gramineae*. Genus: *Sorghum*. Species: *Sorghum vulgare*. A cereal that thrives in semi-arid regions; important humans food for humans and animals in tropical Africa, central and north India and China. Sorghum produced in US and Australia is used for animal feed. Also known as kaffir corn (in South Africa), guinea corn (in West Africa), jowar (in India) and millo maize. The white grain variety is eaten as meal, red grained has a bitter taste and is used for beer; sugar syrup is obtained from the crushed stems of the sweet sorghum. Sorghum has good body-building properties and is easily digested. The composition of the sorghum grain is similar to that of corn in many respects. This similarity extends to characteristics of the starch and protein, as well as to some of the other components. A typical mature sorghum seed of the common hybrids contains about 15% protein, of which around half would be prolamines, or alcohol soluble proteins, about a third would be glutelin type proteins, perhaps 7-9% would be globulins, and the remainder, usually near 5-6%, would be albumins.

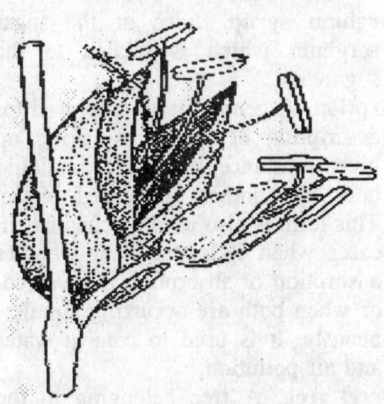

The tissues differ in their percentage contents of protein, and in the types of proteins which make up the total. There is very little prolamine in the germ and hull, while they predominate in the endosperm. The aleurone layer is rich in albumins and globulins. A major factor affecting the amino acid composition of the proteins is the cultivar-variety and hybrid. Carbohydrates other than starch are present only in small amounts. Both waxy and regular types average 1.20% total sugars composed of approximately 0.85% sucrose, 0.09%

glucose, 0.09% D-fructose, and 0.11% raffinose. Sweet varieties contain about 2.8% of these sugars. Starch granules from grain sorghum are very similar to those from corn, but the diameter may reach 35 μm as opposed to a top of about 30 μm for corn starch. Sorghum starch usually appears to have more of the large granules. Waxy sorghum starch granules are much the same as those from regular starch, but they have a maximum diameter somewhat larger than regular sorghum starch granules. Fatty acid composition of a typical crude and dewaxed oil was reported to be myristic acid 0.2%, palmitic acid 8.3%, stearic acid 5.8% hexedecenoic acid 0.1%, oleic acid 36.2%, and linoleic acid 49.4%. Bran contains a relatively high amount of iron, but a lower percentage of non-haem iron absorption with increased content of bran in the diet has been reported. Some plant phenols, particularly those occurring as non-hydrolysable tannins, are potent inhibitors of iron absorption. Polyphenols are more potent than phytic acid as inhibitors of iron absorption. Sorghum can contain large amounts of these substances. Most varieties of sorghum contain no vitamin A activity. As compared to corn, sorghum contains about the same concentrations of riboflavin and pyridoxine and higher levels of pantothenic acid, niacin, choline, folic acid, and biotin. The bioavailability of some of these appears to be at low level. The average composition per 100 g is: 10 g protein, 2. 4 g fat; 68 g carbohydrate; 2 g fibre; 4.6 mg iron; 0.6 mg vitamin B_1; 0.11 mg vitamin B_2; and 3.6 mg nicotinic acid.

The toxic factors and nutritional inhibitors found in sorghums fall into two broad categories:

(a) Substances which occur naturally in the plant as a result of its physiological reactions. These include polyphenols, phytates, cyanogenic glycosides, and possibly other not yet identified. Even though symptoms of acute or chronic toxicity may not be observed, the presence of nutritional inhibitors may be evidence by such phenomena as lower than expected rates of weight gain in test animals, and

(b) substances produced by microbial or other parasites living on the grain under certain conditions. Aflatoxin is an obvious example.

It appears that most cultivars of sorghum contain higher concentrations of these undesirable substances than does corn, wheat, oats, or barley. Some of the preparation methods, including simple ones such as pearling, tend to make the grain not only more palatable but also less harmful.

There are a number of industrial uses for sorghum. A considerable amount is used as a source of starch. High quality for such processing would depend on a high starch content, low fiber and protein content, and, usually, light colour. A fair amount of waxy sorghum starch is used in foods. The starch is separated by a wet milling process similar to that used in making cornstarch, and this procedure removes most, if not all, of the undesirable flavors. It is important that the grain so processed be free of off-flavors, light in colour, and with minimal amylase activity. Of course, the starch fraction should be as near as possible to 100% amylopectin. An outlet of large potential volume is the use of sorghum grits as a carbohydrate source by brewers. This material would be much cheaper than the broken rice now used in such large quantities. Beer made with sorghum grits takes on a bitter flavour due to the anthocyanogens present in the grain. Light-coloured grain with a minimum of colour staining would also be required for this application. Sorghum flours are used as strengthening additives in building materials made of wood fiber, mineral wool, or gypsum. Crude flours are used as flocculating agents in aluminium ore refining. Gelatinized and ungelatinized sorghum flours have been used as binders in charcoal briquettes.

sorghum syrup. Juice of the sugar sorghum which is related to the sugarcane.

sorption. A general term employed for description of ability of taking up given substance (sorptive) from liquid bulk by another condensed phase. This term is also used by chemists in cases when it is not clear whether adsorption or absorption is involved, or when both are occurring simultaneously. It is used to combat water and air pollution.

sorrel tree. A tree belonging to the heath family, found in the southeastern part of the United States as far north as Pennsylvania. The leaves are long and toothed and strongly acid, and from them a cooling drink may be prepared. Clusters of small, white, ball-shaped flowers are produced in summer, and after these, tiny egg-shaped berries covered with down. The sorrel tree some times grows to be sixty feet high. The wood is hard and fine-grained, and is used for making such articles as tool handles. *Rumex scutatus* is French sorrel, as it is known, is similar to spinach with lemony overtones, and so makes a distinctive and useful herb and vegetable. A herbaceous perennial, it is easy to grow, is always on hand, and has a variety of uses. And with its green-tipped-with-red flower spikes, it is decorative, too. In short, it earns its keep in any decorative or kitchen border. The leaves may be cooked as a vegetable, drained well and dressed with oil and vinegar, cream, yoghurt, or a dash of lemon juice. They are very good as salad, and make an unusual and delicious soup garnished with swirls of cream and garlic croutons. They are also used in lamb and beef casseroles, and to curdle milk and make junket.

souffle. An icy product made from water, eggs, sugar, and flavouring material.

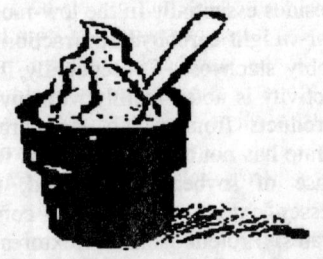

It differs from a sherbet mainly in that it contains the whole egg instead of just the egg white. Also a souffle is usually frozen with a high overrun to obtain a fluffy product.

soup drying. Soup is made from a wide variety of materials from which can be made dry soup. Dry soup mix is made from either a mixture of dry ingredients or by drying a complete cooked soup. Atmospheric and vacuum drum dryers, freeze dryers, or spray dryers are commonly used for drying. Fluidized bed drying is used for pieces of soup. Continuous belt drying in a vacuum may also be employed for this purpose. The final moisture content of dry soup is about 3-4%.

sour milk. Milk in which the acidity has increased so as to be detected by smell or taste. There are varying degrees of sourness from approximately 0.15% lactic acid to the thick sour milk, clotting at room temperature containing approximately 0.6% or more lactic acid. The souring process is due chiefly to the growth of bacteria, usually *lactic streptococci* and *coliform,* in the milk.

sour orange. *Citrus aurantium L.* A variety of orange widely used as a rootstock to which sweet citrus varieties are budded. The sour orange tree also can be used effectively in landscape gardening.

souse. A cooked meat product treated with vinegar.

southernwood. *Artemisia abrotanum.* With the delightful popular names of lady's love and old man, southernwood, a bushy shrub, is grown in many cottage gardens and herbaceous borders as a decorative and strongly aromatic plant, which is, however, said to be repellent to bees. The French called it *grade-robe* because they used it in wardrobes to ward off moths. The pungent leaves were used in Italy as a flavouring for meat and poultry stuffing, and for cakes, but have few culinary uses now.

Medicinally, the dried plant may be used as an antiseptic and a stimulant. An infusion of the leaves may be used as a hair rinse to combat dandruff, while dried leaves can be used in linen bags to repel insects, and also in pot pourri. A yellow dye is extracted from the stems.

Soyalene. Trade name for the alkali-refined soybean oil for varnishes. Its specific gravity is 0.924, and iodine number is 130.

soybean. Family: *Leguminosae.* Genus: *Glycine.* Species: *Glycine max.* A bushy plant from 0.5-1.5 metres in height, native to China, but now grown on an increasingly large scale in many parts of the world. It is a plant of economic importance, and an expanding source of profit to agriculture. 18% of the mature bean consists of oil. More than half of this oil is utilized in paints, where it is supplanting linseed oil, and in varnishes, enamels, and lacquers; the remainder finds uses in salads, breakfast cereals, flour, canned products, etc. In paints soybean oil holds its original colour longer than linseed oil. The automotive industry purchases this oil in great quantities now for body-finishing; the demand is in excess of the supply. Before the economic importance of the soy bean was realized, it was a forage crop only, the seed being sown broadcast and the plant cut while in bloom. When intended for bean harvest, the plant is cut as the pods mature.

Soybean is of importance as a source of both oil and protein. The protein is of high biological value, higher than many other vegetable proteins and is of great value for animal and human food. When raw it contains a trypsin inhibitor destroyed by heat. The original variety was 20% protein with no fat but modern varieties contain 40% protein and 20% fat. As a food the soybean is extremely rich in both protein and oil, in the form of unsaturated fat. It contains as much protein as steak, and is rich in lecithin and all the essential amino acids, plus, iron, calcium and phosphorus. Soya beans are a valuable food for diabetics and the high lecithin content is excellent as protection against cholesterol deposits and to fight fatigue.

In their native state, soybeans are known to contain several factors which cause an adverse physiological response in laboratory animals. These include trypsin inhibitor, hemagglutinins, saponins, estrogens, phytate, goitrogens, antivitamin factors, flatulence factors, and lysinoalanine. Heat treatment of soybean products destroys most of these factors, particularly the trypsin inhibitor, the hemagglutinins, phytate, goitrogens, and antivitamin factors. Like most leguminous plants, the ingestion of soybeans leads to the formation in many individuals of gastrointestinal gas which, in turn, can cause nausea, cramps, diarrhea, and general social discomfort. The gas-producing factor resides essentially in the low-molecular-weight carbohydrate fraction, notably stachyose. Consequently, flatus activity is noted mainly with soybean products from which the carbohydrate has not been removed, as in the case of soybean flours and, to a lesser extent, soy protein concentrates. Protein isolates, textures soy protein products, and fermented soy foods, such as tempeh, are essentially free of flatus activity.

soybean curd. Precipitate from soybean milk. Tofu is an Oriental preparation. Tofu does not differ significantly from the protein found in most other soybean products. The average composition per 100 g is: water 86%; protein 6%; fat 5%; carbohydrate 2%; fibre 0.1%; iron 2 mg, vitamin B_1 0.04 mg; vitamin B_2 0.05 mg; nicotinic acid 0.4 mg; and food energy 0.32 MJ.

The biological evaluation of the nutritive value of soybean curd using animals or human subjects has given values which are comparable to properly heated soybean flour. Tofu has been tested as a source of protein in the solid diet of weaning infants and its performance evaluated with respect to acceptability, weight gain, nitrogen balance, and serum level. On the basis of these criteria, tofu was judged to be nutritionally equivalent to the protein derived from a mixture of eggs, fish, and liver.

Soybean flour. Meal produced by heat processing averages 40% protein and 20% fats, while meal from solvent extraction has 42-50% protein and a maximum of 2.5% fats. Further processing of the meal to remove sugars and other material varies the final protein content of the flour, and meal from different types of beans vary in content. The protein content can be increased by removing the soy hulls before (front-end dehulling) or after (tail-end dehulling) solvent extraction. A processed soybean flour has about 40% protein and 20% fats with the sugars that give easily solubility for blending. It is used as a partial replacement for milk powder and wheat flour in baked goods. The average composition per 100 g of full fat: protein 40%; fat 22%; calcium 200 mg; iron 6.3 mg; vitamin A 40 mg; vitamin B_1 0.75 mg; vitamin B_2 0.3 mg; nicotinic acid 2.5 mg; and food energy 1.5 MJ.

The average composition per 100 g for defatted product is: protein 45%; fat 5%; calcium 250 mg; iron 7.6 mg; vitamin A 31 mg; vitamin B_1 0.6 mg; vitamin B_2 0.5 mg; nicotinic acid 3 mg; and food energy 1.1 MJ.

There is about 25% carbohydrate in the bean, of which 12% is polysaccharide (dextrins, galactans and pentosans) and 12.6% sugars (6% sucrose, 5% stachyose and 1.5% raffinose). This food product used in the human diet in several ways:

(a) as a separate item of the diet, although problems of acceptability frequently limit its use in this fashion;

(b) as an ingredient of a wide variety of common dishes, such as soups, stews, beverages and desserts;

(c) in the formulation of bakery and cereal products or as a meat extender;

(d) as starting material for the preparation of infant formulas, protein concentrates, or isolates; and

(e) as a protein supplement to cereal grains and other foods.

Experiments in the use of soybean flour as the sole source of protein diets have been quite limited. Toasted full-fat soy flour (known in Japan as *kinako*), when fed as a main source of protein of weaning infants, has been well accepted and is known to support good growth and nitrogen retention. In a study with African children, it has been found that soybean flour when used as a protein supplement to a basal rice diet had reasonably good nutritive value although its biological value was somewhat less than that of milk. In a similar study with Indian children on a basal rice diet, it was found that defatted soybean flour when fortified with methionine was as good a protein supplement as that of skim milk. Other uses of soybean flour in processed foods are described later.

soybean meal. The product obtained by grinding the soybean chips from the expeller process, or the soybean oil cake from the hydraulic process. The meal is marketed as stock feed or fertilizer. It is chiefly used as a protein feed for dairy cattle, but it is inferior to fish meal for poultry, as it lacks the mineral salts and vitamins of fish meal. Soybean meal hardened with formaldehyde is used as a filler with wood flour in plastics to give better flow in molding.

soybean milk. Traditionally, soybean milk is an aqueous extract of whole soybeans and has been of considerable interest to nutritionists as a possible substitute for cow or human milk, particularly in the feeding of infants who are allergic to the natural milks. Soybean milk and cow's milk have approximately the same protein content (3.5-4%), and a comparison of the amino acid composition shows a good correspondence. The main deficiency of soybean milk is that of the sulfur-containing amino acids, notably methionine. Animal experiments have shown that the nutritive value of soybean milk ranges between 60-90% of that of cow's milk, but with methionine supplementation it can be raised to essentially the same level as that of cow's milk. As impairment of soybean milk occurs as the result of cooking at high temperatures for long periods. A number of studies have shown that, in general, there is comparatively little superiority of cow's or human milk over suitably fortified soybean milk for human consumption. The average composition per 100 g is: water 92%; protein 3.5%; fat 1.6%; carbohydrate 1%; fibre 0.4%; iron 0.5 mg; vitamin B_1 0.09 mg; vitamin B_2 0.05 mg; nicotinic acid 0.2 mg; and food energy 0.14 MJ.

soybean oil. A pale-yellow oil obtained by expression from the seeds of the plant *Glycine soya,* native to Manchuria but grown in the US. Soybean oil is a linolenic acid oil; in contrast, the other three major oilseed oils, cottonseed, peanut, and sunflower, are oleic-linolenic acid oils, because they contain more than 50% of these fatty acids. It is primarily a food oil but has an undesirable off-flavour unless highly purified. It is also used as a drying oil for linoleum, paints, and varnishes, or for mixing with linseed oil. It is also used in core oils and in soaps. The bean contains up to 20% oil. The average yield factor is 15%, but by trichlorethylene extraction a bushel of beans will yield 5 kg of oil and 21 kg of high-protein meal containing less than 1% oil. The oil content decreases in warm climates. Southern-grown soybeans contain 2-5% less oil and 22 kg of meal per bushel of beans.

The oil is easy to bleach, has good consistency as a food oil, and does not become rancid easily, but has less flavour stability than many other oils. There are 280 varieties of the bean grown in the United States and 2,500 varieties listed. The pods contain two or three beans which range in colour from light straw through gray and brown to nearly black. Most varieties are straw-coloured or greenish yellow. The stalks and leaves of the plant contain much nitrogen, and about half of the crop is usually plowed under for fertilizer. The specific gravity of the oil is about 0.925, iodine value 134, and it should have a maximum of not more than 1.5% free fatty acids and not more than 0.3% moisture and volatile matter. The fractionated oil yield 15% cut soybean oil of an iodine value of 70-90, used for soaps, lubricants, and rubber compounding. Also known as soya bean oil.

soybean-wheat protein blends. Because of the complementary effect which soybean proteins exert on lysine-deficient wheat protein, much attention has been given to the use of soybean flour or soybean concentrates in bread formulations. Bread makes an excellent vehicle for protein fortification because it is a staple food in many areas of the world, not requiring drastic changes in taste and dietary habits. When soy proteins are considered for a baking application, important factors include: water-holding capacity; enzyme activity; water-soluble protein; and fiber, carbohydrate, and lipid contents. Flavour, particle size, and whether or not lecithin is required, also must be considered. When the continuous baking process was introduced, it was found that nonfat dry milk had a deleterious effect on dough-handling characteristics and the use of that additive was largely discontinued. It was soon found that certain types of soy flour with whey and other ingredients made a satisfactory replacement for nonfat dry milk.

Soyolk. Trade name for full fat soya flour.

Soy protein. Trade name for a product used in canned soups and meat products. It is roasted to eliminate all enzyme activity. It contains about 50% protein with 2% lecithin and 3% lysine.

soy sauce. A product of the fermentation of soybeans, is traditionally made by mixing salt, soybeans, and wheat with the mold *Aspergillus oryzae*. This mixture, called Koji, is allowed to stand for 3-4 days which results in the production of large amounts of fermentable sugars, peptides, and amino acids. After this first step, the mixture is put into a large container with 18% NaCl solution together with the bacterium *Pediococcus soyae* and the yeasts *Saccharomyces rouxii* and a *Torulopsis* sp. This mixture is allowed to ferment for 8-12 months, after which the liquid is drained off and sold as soy sauce. The modern process is carried out at high temperature or in an autoclave for a short time. Average composition per 100 g is: water 65%; protein 6%; fat 3%; carbohydrate 5%; calcium 100 mg; iron 5 mg; vitamin B_1 0.03 mg; vitamin B_2 0.05 mg; nicotinic acid 0.3 mg; and food energy 0.2 MJ.

Spans. Trade name for a group of compounds made by reacting sorbitol with fatty acids; are surface active or emulsifying agents and have been used, for example, as crumb softeners in bread.

sparkling wine. The wine that has more than 1.5 atmospheres pressure 10°C. It is estimated that the amount of dissolved carbon dioxide at this temperature and pressure is about 3.9 grams/liter.

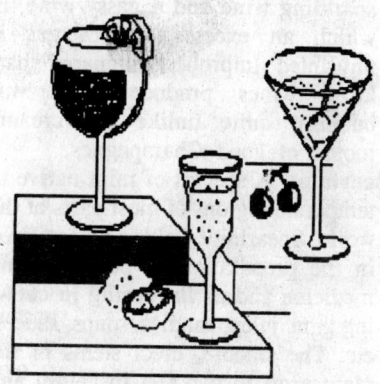

At a temperature 26.7°C, the internal pressure will rise to about 2.4 atmospheres. French authorities have suggested a pressure of 4 atmospheres at 20°C. The standards set by various countries cover a rather wide range. Considering the carbon dioxide present, this may come from:

(1) An excess of the gas resulting from fermentation. This is the principal source of Alsatian, Ger-

man, French (Loire), and Italian sparkling wines, including some California wines.

(2) An excess of gas resulting from a malo-lactic fermentation. There are numerous examples of wines carbonated in this way, notably the *Vinho Verde* wines (northern Portugal) and several others found in Italy and many other European countries.

(3) An excess of gas from the fermentation of sugar added to the process after fermentation. Many of the sparkling wines made worldwide fall into this category. With variations, this is the process used in making Champagne.

(4) An excess of gas created by adding the gas by way of a carbonation process.

Authorities distinguish between the sparkling wine and a gassy wine, in which an excess (any of gas is unwanted. Improperly prepared sparkling wines produce large was bubbles, quite unlike the creamy mouse of good Champagnes.

spearmint. A species of mint native to temperate regions of most parts of the world. Spearmint yields an oil utilized in the preparation of perfumes and medicine and as flavouring in chewing gum, julep, candies, soups, sauces, etc. The smooth, erect stems of the plant grow to two feet in height and bear at the top whorls of pale purple or white flowers.

species. A category used in the classification of organisms that consists of a group of similar individuals that can usually breed among themselves and produce fertile off-spring. Similar or related species are grouped into a genus. Within a species are grouped into a genus. Within a specis groupes of individuals may become reproduc-

tively isolated because of geographical or behavioural factors. Such populations may, because of different characteristics from the main populatin and so form a distinct subspecies.

specific dynamic action. SDA. The name given to the increase in metabolism that follows the ingestion of foods, normally amounting to 5-7% of the food intake. The reason for specific dynamic action (SDA) is not known, but it is suggested that it is partly the result of flooding the cells with metabolites and partly the heat of deamination of amino acids. In practice it means that 5-7% should be added to calculated calorie requirements (called thermic effect).

specificity. 1. In relation to enzymes refers to the ability of an enzyme to catalyse only a limited range of reactions, or, in some cases a single reactions, or, in some cases a single reaction. Specificity is the main distinction between enzymes and catalysts, as the latter are non-specific. Examples, arginase will hydrolyze L-arginine only not even the D-isomer; esterase will hydrolyze the whole group of compounds containing the ester linkages, but no others.

2. The degree of selectivity shown by an antibody with respect to the number and types of antigens with which the antibody combines, as well as with respect to the rates and the extents of these reactions.

3. The degree of selectivity shown by a membrane, or a membrane component, with respect to the type and the degree of permeability to substances transported across the membrane in mediated transport.

spectrometric analysis. Emission spectral analysis using photoelectric detectors for direct measurement of intensity of spectral lines.

spectrophotometry. An analytical technique based on the investigation of dependence between intensity of electromagnetic radiation interacting with matter (emission, absorption, reflection, scattering) and radiation wavelength; this term usually refers to ultraviolet, visible and infrared region.

spectropolarimetry. Analytical method based on measurement of dispersion of optical rotation; used for determination of optically active compounds, structural research and for identification of some optically active group.

spectroscopy. The branch of analytical chemistry that deals with the determination of the structure of atoms and the chemical composition of molecules by measuring the radiant energy they absorb or emit in any of the wavelengths of the electromagnetic spectrum. When atoms or molecules are excited by energy input from an arc, spark, or flame, they respond in a characteristic manner; their identity and composition are signaled by the wavelengths of incident light they absorb or emit, the emission spectra being in the form of lines (atoms) of distinctive colour, such as the yellow sodium D-line, or bands (molecules). The intensity of these varies with the amount of an element present and thus affords a basis for quantitative analysis of the sample.

spelt. Coarse type of wheat, mainly used as cattle feed.

spent wash. Liquor remaining in the whisky still after distilling the spirit. A source of unidentified growth factors detected by chick growth. When dried is known as distillers' dried solubles.

Sperm 42. Trade name for a sperm oil with carbon chains of C_{10} to C_{22}. It is emulsifiable in cold or warm water.

sperm oil. The waxy oil extracted from the head cavity of the sperm whale, *Physeter breviceps* and *P. catadon,* and Bottlenose whale, *P. macrocephalus.* In composition it differs but slightly from common whale oil. which is separated from the spermaceti and the blubber. The spermaceti is first separated out, leaving a clear yellow oil. It is purified by being pressed at a Low temperature. It is grade according to the temperature of pressing. A good grade of sperm oil has a specific gravity of 0.875-0.885, and a flash point above 227°C. Oils from other whale species, such as the humpback, fin, and sulphurbottom, have specific gravities ranging from 0.91-0.93. Inferior grades of sperm oil may be from sperm-whale blubber. Commercial sperm oil is likely to be one-third head oil and two-thirds body oil.

Sperm oil differs from fish oil and whale oil in consisting chiefly of liquid waxes of the higher fatty alcohol esters and not fats. Sperm oil absorbs very little oxygen from the atmosphere and resists decomposition even at temperatures above 204°C, and it will pour below its cloud point of 3-7°C.

spermaceti. The white crystalline flakes of fatty substance, or wax, that separate out from sperm oil on cooling after boiling. It is cetyl palmitate, a true wax, and does not yield glycerine when saponified. It is purified by pressing, and the triple-refined is snow white. It is also separated out from dolphin-head oil. Spermaceti is odourless and tasteless, has a melting point of 43°C, and is insoluble in water, but soluble in hot alcohol. It burns with a bright flame. It was formerly used for candles but now is employed chiefly as a fine wax for ointments and compounds. Sperm oil and spermaceti are inedible and indigestible. Cetyl alcohol, $C_{16}H_{33}OH$, originally obtained from spermaceti, is now made synthetically from ethyl palmitate.

sphingolipids. The second large class of membrane lipids, having a polar head and two nonpolar tails, but contain no glycerol. Sphingolipids are composed of one molecule of a long chain fatty acid, one molecule of a long chain amino alcohol (sphingosine or one of its derivatives), and a polar head alcohol.

sphingomyelins. The phospholipids containing a fatty acid, phosphate, choline, and a complex amino alcohol, sphingosine. Sphingomyelins are the simplest and the most abundant sphingolipids. Because the sphingomyelins contain phosphorus, they may also be classed as phospholipids, together with phosphoglycerides. Indeed, sphingomyelins closely resemble phosphoglycerides phosphatidylethanolamine and phosphatidylcholine in their general properties, and they have similar electric charges. Sphingomyelins are present in most membranes of animal cells; the myelin sheath surrounding certain nerve cells is very rich in sphingomyelins.

spice. The name given to a group of vegetable seasonings, including pepper, mace, nutmeg, cloves, ginger, allspice, cinnamon, capsicum and mustard. Some are produced from seeds, as mustard; some from bark, as cinnamon; some from root, as ginger, and some from fruit, as nutmeg. Spices contain a very small percentage of nourishment; they are valuable for food only because of their stimulating effect on the digestive organs. Employed in moderation they are wholesome, but are injurious if used in excess. Distinguished from herbs only that part instead of the whole of the aromatic plant is meant, such as root, stem, seeds. Originally used to mask putrefactive flavours. Some have preservative effect because of their essential oils, e.g., cloves, cinnamon and mustard. Consumed in too small a quantity to provide any nutrients except possibly for curry powder which contains 65 mg iron per 100 g.

spiced cheese. Cheese flavoured with spices such as anise, caraway, cloves cumin, pepper and sage. Sometimes an oil extract of a spice is added to impart the flavour. The cheese is usually of the hard type, the spice added with the salt. Spiced cheese is made in many countries, but is especially popular in Scandinavian under such names as Kumin or Kommenost, Noekkelost, Christian IX (Denmark). Friesian Clove, Pepato, Sage, and Bondost (Swedish) which is also made in Wisconsin, US. Federal definitions and standards for spiced cheese specify that it must either be made from pasteurized milk or be cured for not less than 60 days at a temperature not lower than 8°C, and that if it is made from whole milk it must contain not less than 50% of fat in the solids, and if it is made from partly skimmed milk not less than 20% of fat in the solids.

Spiderwort family: *Commelinaceae*. Popular as houseplants, these annual or perennial herbs are from tropical and subtropical regions. Closed sheathing leaf petioles and flower parts in 3's are characteristic. The alternate leaves have entire margins and parallel venation. Leaf-like bracts sometimes partially enclose flower clusters. The bisexual flower can also occur singly. Parts of the flower include 3 sepals, 3 petals, 6 stamens and 1 pistil. The stamens' filaments often have hair. The pistil has a superior ovary of 3 fused carpels, 1 style, and 1 stigma. There are no nectar glands. A loculicidal capsule is usually the fruit type.

The family include: *Callisia* (striped inch plant), *Commelina* (dayflower), *Cyanotis, Dichorisandra, Gibasis* (Tahitian bridal veil), *Rhoeo* (Moses-in-the-cradle), *Tradescantia* spp. (spiderwort, wandering Jew, inch plant), *Zebrina* (wandering Jew).

spinach. Family: *Chenopodiaceae.* Genus: *Spinacia.* Species: *Spinacia oleracea.* As a cultivated plant, spinach originated in or near Persia and later reached Spain by way of the invading Moors around 1100-1200 AD Spinach can be either smooth-leafed or, more commonly, of the crinkle-leafed "Savoy" type. It can also be round-seeded or prickly-seeded. Fresh, young, tender leaves are delicious in salads or can be steamed with a little water until tender.

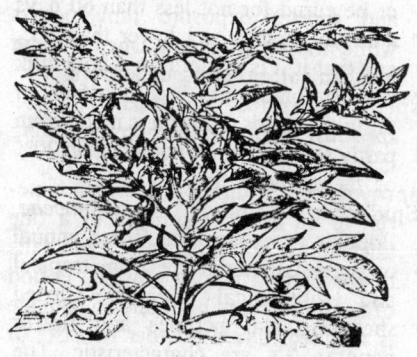

Spinach has long been considered extremely healthy although the iron content has been over-rated (perhaps because of Popeye's avid promotion of it). It contains plenty of vitamins C, A and B and some vitamin K, as well as potassium, calcium, magnesium, iron, iodine and phosphorus, and it is low in calories. Drained canned spinach has more calcium and salt and less vitamin C than fresh spinach, and defrosted and cooked leaf spinach has approximately the same nutrients as when fresh and cooked, though if it is finely chopped it loses some of its vitamins C and A. Cooked spinach yields up oxalic acid that binds up the trace minerals in it just as phytic acid does in grain, with the result that the high calcium and iron content cannot be properly utilized. So it is not a good idea for pregnant women or the elderly to eat copious quantities of it. Its oxalic acid can be particularly neutralized by cooking in milk, but it's best to eat raw. Spinach is recommended for constipation (it has noticeable laxative properties), for anemia and for all sorts of nerve deficiencies, for hypertension, bronchitis and dyspepsia and the vitamin K in it makes it useful in promoting blood clotting. The average composition per 100 g is: protein 1.9%; fat 0.18%; calcium 65 mg; iron 2.5 mg; vitamin A 2.5 mg; vitamin B_1 1 mg; vitamin B_2 0.15 mg; nicotinic acid 0.5 mg; vitamin C 50 mg; and food energy 0.08 MJ.

spingomyelins. Complex phosphatides found in brain and nerve tissue and as part of cell structure; composed of the base sphingosine plus fatty acids, phosphoric acid and choline.

spiraea. A class of herbs and shrubs of the rose family, found in the north temperate zone. There are about sixty species, adapted to a wide range of soil and conditions. The well-known varieties are drop-wort, meadow-sweet, hardhack, saxifrage and shadbush. The flowers grow in clusters of various forms and may be white or pink. Several species are among the showiest of shrubs. The steeplebush, with its spiral-like clusters of tiny white flowers; the bridal wreath, with its dainty, graceful, downward curving stems covered with little leaves and bearing profusely drooping clusters of tiny feathery white flowers.

spiral dryer. An internal power driven rotor, from 0.15-2 m diameter, having spiral guide plates, inside a heating jacket, which is used for drying heat-sensitive products. The moist product is fed into the dryer in a fluidized state at the bottom of the dryer. The product moves around the spiral air guides. The revolving rotor, moving at 1-10 rpm, moves the product to the heated section for drying. The dry product leaves the top of the dryer and is removed in a cyclone separator.

spirit, silent. Highly purified alcohol, or neutral spirit, distilled from any fermentable material.

spirulina. Blue-green alga which can make use of atmospheric nitrogen; eaten for centuries round Lake Chad in N. Africa and in Mexico.

spitz. A small, rennet cheese made from cows' milk. It is cylindrical in shape, 10 cm high, and 3 cm in diameter.

Spitzkase cheese. A variety of small, spiced, Limburger-type cheese made in Germany from cow's milk. It is similar to backsteiner as to the making procedure, except that caraway seed is added to the curd.

spores. In relation to bacteria they are the resting state; thick-walled, highly resistant to damage by heat. Under suitable conditions they germinate to produce bacteria. Not all bacteria can form spores; the so-called spore-bearers are a hazard in pasteurization and sterilization as the spores can remain undamaged in the processing and the material is consequently not sterile.

sporozoa. A large group of protozoa, all of which are obligate parasites. They are characterized by lack of motile adult stages and by a nutritional mode of life in which food is generally not ingested but instead is absorbed in soluble form through the outer wall, such as occurs in bacteria and fungi. Although the name sporozoa implies the formation of spores, these organisms do not form true resting spores, like those of bacteria, algae, and fungi, but instead produce analogous structures called sporozoites, which are involved in transmission to a new host. The most important members of the sporozoa are the *coccidia*, usually parasites of birds, and the plasmodia, which infect birds and mammals, including humans.

spouted bed dryer. A special fluidized bed dryer for removing moisture from particulates in which there is a convective flow of drying fluid and products being dried. As compared to stationary bed dryers, faster drying and shorter exposure time occurs while mixing is accomplished without mechanical agitators or stirrers.

sprat. *Sprattus sprattus (Clupea sprattus)* related to the herring; young is brisling.

spray dryer. Equipment in which material to be dried is sprayed as a fine mist into a hot-air chamber and falls to the bottom as dry powder. Period of heating is very brief and so damage is avoided. Dried powder consists of hollow particles of low density. Spray drying is widely applied to many foods (such as milk) and pharmaceuticals. A high moisture product, which may first be condensed in a vacuum pan or an evaporator, is pumped through an atomizing nozzle with atomization taking place inside the chamber of the dryer. The product is dried quickly by moving air, usually filtered it for food, over small droplets formed by atomization. The dried product must be removed from the dryer quickly to avoid heat damage. The inlet air temperature varies from 93.3-760°C, depending upon the type of product, moisture content, and rate of drying. The usual inlet temperatures are from 500-550°C with an outlet temperature of 65-70°C. Steam heated spray dryers have an overall thermal efficiency of 35-40%, while direct fuel fired units have an efficiency of 80-85%. For spray drying, 1.2-1.8 kg of steam per kg of moisture evaporated are required. Units are rated in terms of production of dried product which may reach 38 kg/s or more or in terms of evaporation rate of 115 kg/s or more or in terms of evaporation rate of 115 kg/s or more. Spray dryers are characterized by continuous operation, minimal labor to operate, ability to handle many different products, short time of heat contact during drying, operational efficiency depending on large surface area produced by different atomization methods, separation of product and air after drying and a lower thermal efficiency as compared to drum dryers.

S-protein. A long fragment of the enzyme ribonuclease that is obtained by a subtilis in catalyzed cleavage of the molecule between amino acid residues 20 and 21.

sprouted seeds. Seeds are high in protein, containing about 35%, but like other vegetable proteins they need to be combined with foods higher in amino-acids, in which they are low. Seeds are best complemented by nuts and dairy produce. They are added to pulse dishes, sauces, and grain dishes, to make more protein available, add are also added to bread, soups and salads. Seeds seal in their goodness, so the rich level of B vitamins keeps longer than B vitamins in vegetables, which decrease soon after harvesting. Seeds are also a good source of vitamins E and A, phosphorus and magnesium, and contain some iron and zinc. All seeds store energy in the form of starch. When they begin to sprout, enzymes which hitherto have lain dormant, become active and begin to break don the stored starch into simple sugars and to split long-chain proteins into free amino acids, as well as converting saturated fats into free fatty acids. In fact this enzymatic activity is so intense at this early stage of sprouting that it stimulates the body's own enzymes into greater activity and so accelerates the body's innate healing activity. Sprouts are in effect predigested and so have many times the nutritional efficiency of the seeds from which they grew. They provide more nutrients than any other natural food. Within a few hours of germination vitamin C develops and continues increasing for some days. The vitamin C in soya beans, for example, multiplies five times in three days of germination. Most importantly, as far as vegetarians are concerned, vitamin B_{12} is found in most sprouted seeds and can provide the body's daily requirement in one large helping. The body can only assimilate minerals properly if they are part of organic molecules. The calcium, zinc and iron in peas and beans and some grains are bound to phytic acid, making them unavailable for absorption. Phytin is an important ingredient of many seeds and in certain varieties it accounts for up to 80% of the phosphorus they contain. However, sprouting greatly reduces the phytin content of seeds, so liberating the minerals bound to phytin for use. Simultaneously it increases their level of desirable phosphorus compounds like lecithin (necessary for healthy nerves and brain function). Lecithin also helps to break up and transport fats and fatty acids round the body and encourages the transportation of nutrients through cell walls, stimulating the secretion of hormones at the same times.

Spumoni. A fancy ice cream made in cup-shaped form. The outside is usually vanilla ice cream, and the inside is usually chocolate mochas and tutti-frutti mouse. It is severed in wedge-shaped portions.

Spurge family: *Euphorbiaceae.* A large family of 283 genera, often have a poisonous, milky, latex sap. Very diverse forms are represented. There are weedy herbs, commonly called spurges, showy ornamental herbs, and trees, and cactus-like succulents. Most of them have a biting, milky juice, which is of high commercial value, being the source of castor oil, croton oil, cassava and rubber. The plants have small, inconspicuous flowers, but some of them, notably the poinsettia, have brightly coloured bracts. Some of the plants resemble cacti. The fruit, which is three-lobed, is dry and rather fleshy. Most of the tropical species are known as Euphorbias. Most are tropical. Stems usually have stipules that take the form of hairs, glands, or spines false flowers, often with petal-like appendages, have unisexual, male and female flowers aggregated in a structure called a cyathium. Male flowers, of 1 stamen each, may number 1 to many in a cyathium. The female flower is 1 pistil composed of a superior ovary with usually 3 fused carpels, 3 styles, and 3 or 6 stigmas. The fruit is usually a schizocarp in which the 3 carpels, bearing seeds, break apart.

The family include: *Aleurites fordii* (tung oil), *Hevea brasiliensis* (para rubber), *Manihot esculenta* (tapioca), *M. glaziovii* (ceara rubber), *Ricinus communis* (castor oil); *Acalypha hispida* (chenille plant), *Codiaeum* (croton), *Euphorbia*-1550 species (poinsettia, crown-of-thorns, spurges, etc.), *Phyllanthus* (Otaheite gooseberry), *Ricinus communis* (castorbean); *Euphorbia* spp., *Mercurialis* (mercury), *Ricinus communis.*

squalene. A hydrocarbon, $C_{30}H_{50}$, found in liver of shark and rat; suggested as a possible intermediate in the synthesis of cholesterol in the body.

squaw vine. *Mitchella repens.* A perennial, evergreen herb. Its creeping or trailing stems grow up to a foot long, rooting at various points, and bear opposite, orbicular-ovate leaves that are dark green and shining on top and are often streaked with white. The funnel-shaped white flowers grow in pairs and the fruit is a scarlet berry-like drupe up to 7-8 mm in diameter.

St. Benoit cheese. A soft, rennet cheese similar to Olivert, made in the Department of Loiret, France. Charcoal is added to the salt which is applied to the exterior of the cheese. Ripening requires from 12-20 days, depending upon the season. Each cheese is about 15 cm in diameter.

St. Claude cheese. A small square cheese made around Saint Claude, France, from goats' milk.

St. Johnswort. *Hypericum perforatum.* This shrubby perennial occurs in dry, gravely soils, fields and sunny places throughout the world. A woody, branched root produced many round stems which put out runners from the base. The opposite, oblong to linear leaves are covered with transparent oil glands that look like holes. The yellow flowers have petals dotted with black along their margins.

St. Marcellin cheese. A goats' milk cheese made in France. It is about 8 cm in diameter, 15 mm thick. The cheese making procedure is similar to that of Brie. Blue mold is cultivated on the surface only.

St. Remy cheese. A kind of soft, rennet cheese that is quite similar to Pont Peveque. It is made in Haute-Saone region of France.

stabilizer. A protective colloid used to make a stable emulsion with two immiscible liquids. As applied to the dairyand food industry, a substance such as gelatin used to give stability or firmness to the food products. Stabilizers find numerous applications in food processing industry, as they:

(a) prevent the breaking up, as it were, of the ingredients of an ice cream mix when frozen;

(b) help prevent churning of the fat during the freezing operation;

(c) give a certain amount of firmness and smoothness and thereby preventing excessive ice-crystal formation;

(d) in processed cheese, salt stabilizers are used for the prevention of fat separation;

(e) in evaporated milk or coffee cream they prevent feathering.

Common stabilizer used in chocolate milk and ice cream include gelatin and sodium alginate (Dariloid); salt or mineral stabilizers are usually citrate and phosphate; or Krageleen (modified Irish Moss). They help make finished products smooth. For evaporated milk, disodium phosphate stabilizer is permissible for commercial practice to control the heat stability.

The legally permitted list includes superglycerinated fats, propylene glycol alginate and stearate, methyl-, methylethyl- and sodium carboxymethylcellulose, stearyl tartrate, sorbitan esters of fatty acids.

stachyase. Enzyme that hydrolyses the tetrasaccharide stachyose to fructose and a mannosaccharide consisting of glucose and two molecules of galactose. It is found in the digestive juices of crustaceans and molluscs.

stachyose. A non-reducing tetrasaccharide composed of one unit of fructose, two of galactose and one of glucose. Hydrolysis yields fructose and manninotriose; believed to be used to a limited extent by animals. Present in many foods such as soybeans, lupins, tubers of *Stachys tuberifera*, etc. Also called mannotetrose and lupeose.

stackburn. Name given to heat retention within stack of cans when stored after sterilization without being cooled. A high temperature is maintained in the centre of the stack for long periods and causes deterioration of the contents and accelerates internal corrosion.

Staff-tree family. *Celastraceae*. The most obvious characteristic of this family is the pulpy orange or red aril usually covering the seed. Small clusters of green flowers usually have flower parts in 4's or 5's. And there is 1 pistil with a superior ovary surrounded by a nectar disc. Plants in this family are woody shrubs, trees, and twining vines. Fruit types are capsules, berries, samaras, and drupes.

The family include: *Catha* (cafta), *Celastrus* (bittersweet), *Elaeodendron*, *Euonymus alatus* (burning bush), *Gymnosporia*, *Maytenus*,

Pachystima, Tripterygium; Euonymus europaeus (european spindle-tree).

staling. As applied to backed products such as bread, is thought to be due to the slow passage of water from the starch to other components of the bread. It is suggested that anti-staling agents function by forming an insoluble coating round the starch granules, which slows down the passage of water.

standard. Levels of exposure to pollutants which should not be exceeded; standards may be statutory or presumptive. Two levels have been adopted by the US Environmental Protection Agency. 1. Primary levels judged necessary to protect health with an adequate margin of safety. 2. Secondary levels judged necessary to protect public welfare from any known or anticipated adverse effects. These are essentially environmental quality standards. Standards may also prescribe the contents of products, *e.g.*, the amount of phosphates in detergents, or pesticide residues in foodstuffs. They may also take the form of emission standards, *e.g.*, the upper limits of what may be emitted from the exhausts of motor vehicles or from the chimneys of industrial plants. *See* product standard.

staphylococci. The catalase-positive, Gram-positive, facultative-anaerobic bacteria that grow as clusters of spherical cells. These bacteria are highly resistant to drying, withstand heat of 330K for 30 minutes, and grow in the presence of 7.5% NaCl solution. *Staphylococcus aureus* and *S. epidermidis* are common inhabitants of skin, respiratory tract, mucous membrane, and intestine. The bacteria produce heat-stable enterotoxin that accumulates in the food. Staphylococcal infections require rapid and effective treatment because the bacteria readily become resistant to the penicillins. Their resistance to penicillin is carried on a plasmid and mediated by extracellular penicillinase. Infections caused by penicillinase-resistant Staphylococcus can be treated with methicillin which is not hydrolyzed by penicillinase.

staple food. The principal food, *e.g.*, wheat, rice, maize, etc.

Starbake starch. Trade name for a processed wheat starch.

starch. A polysaccharide consisting of variours proportions of two glucose polymers, amylose and amylopectin. It occurs widely in plants, especially in roots, tubers, seeds, and fruits, as a carbohydrate energy store. The common cereal grains contain from 55 to 75% starch, and potatoes contain about 18%. Starch is a major energy source for animals and is a basic need of all people. Much of it is employed in its natural form, but it is also easily converted to other forms and more than, 1,000 different varieties of starch are available in the market.

In general, starch is a white, amorphous powder having a specific gravity from 0.5-0.52. It is insoluble in cold water but can be converted to soluble starch by treating with a dilute acid. When cooked in water, starch produces an adhesive paste. Starch is easily distinguished from dextrins as it gives a blue colour with iodine while dextrins give violet and red. The starch molecule is often described as a chain of glucose units, with the adhesive waxy starches as those with coiled chains. But starch is a complex member of the great group of natural plant compounds consisting of starches, sugars, and cellulose, and originally named carbohydrates because the molecular formula could be written as $C_n(H_2O)_x$, but not all now-known carbohydrates can be classified in this form, and many now-known acids and aldehydes can be indicated by this formula. Starch can be fractionated into two polymers of high molecular weight. Amylose is a straight-chain fraction having high adhesive properties for coatings and sizings, and amylopectin is a branched-chain fraction best known as a suspending agent for foodstuffs. Amylose is chemically identical with cellulose, but the chain units of the molecule have an alpha linkage and are coiled, while the cellulose molecule is rigid. It has a molecular mass of about 150,000, while amylopectin has a molecular mass more than 1 million. The 1-4 alpha linkage of amylopectin with random branches at the 6-carbon position makes the material easily dispersible in cold water but resistant to gelling. Amylopectin is thus best suited for thickening, but, since it can be combined and cross-linked with synthetic resins and is highly resistant to deterioration, it is used with resins for water-resistant coatings for paper and textiles.

Most of the commercial starch comes from corn, potatoes, and mandioca. Starches from different plants have similar chemical reactions, but all have different granular structure, and the difference sin size and shape of the grain have much to do with the physical properties.

It may be noted that Alant starch, or inulin, $(C_6H_{10}O_5)_6 \cdot H_2O$, is not a starch in the ordinary sense, but is an insoluble sugar which occurs as the reserve polysaccharide in many plants. It is obtained from the roots of the artichoke, *Helianthus tuberosis*. Unlike starch, the molecule has fructose units held in glucoside linkage, and hydrolysis converts it to fructose.

Arrowroot starch is obtained from the tubers of *Maranta arundinacea* of the West Indies. It is easily digested, and is used in cookies and other food products, especially baby foods. Florida arrowroot is from the *Zamia floridana*.

East Indian arrowroot is from the plant *Curcuma angustifolia,* which belongs to the ginger family. Arrowroot from St. Vincent, used in instant-pudding mixes and icings, is marketed as a precooked powder of about 200 mesh. It swells in cold water, and does not add flavour. The starches do not crystallize like sugar, and they may be added to some confections to minimize crystallization. They are also used a binders in candies and in tablet sugar, but any considerable quantity in such products is considered as an adulterant. Metabolism of starch in the human system requires conversion to sugars, and the taking in of excessive quantities of uncooked starch is undesirable.

Cornstarch is the chief food starch in the Europe, although sweet-potato starch is used where high gelatinization is desired, and tapioca starch is used to give quick tack and high adhesion in glues.

Rice starch is polygonal and lamellar, and has very small particles. It makes an opaque stiff gel and is also valued as a dusting starch for bakery products, although it is expensive for this purpose.

Sweet-potato starch is from the tuber *Opomoea batata*. An average of 4.5 kg of starch is produced per bushel. The root has poor shipping qualities, and the starch is expensive, but it has excellent colloidal qualities and gelatinizes completely at 74°C. It is used in some foodstuffs. It has a pleasant sweetish flavour, and in Latin countries great quantities are marketed in the form of a stiff gel as a dessert sweet known as *dulce de batata.*

Tapioca starch has rounded grains truncated on one side and is of lamellar structure. It produces gels of clarity and flexibility, and, since it has no cereal flavour, it can be used directly for thickening foodstuffs.

Wheat starch is a fine white starch made by separating out the gluten of wheat flour by wash floatation. It is used in prepared mixes for foam-type cakes and pie crusts to improve texture, add volume, and reduce the amount of shortening needed. It replaces up to 30% of the wheat-flour content of the mix.

White-potato starch has conchoidal or ellipsoidal grains of lamellar structure. When cooked, it forms clear solutions easily controlled in viscosity, and gives tough resilient films for coating paper and fabrics. Prolonged grinding of grain starches reduces the molecular chain, and the lower weight then gives greater solubility in cold water. Green fruits, especially bananas, often contain much starch, but the ripening process changes the starch to sugars.

Pregelatinized starches are preheat-treated starches that require no cooking for use in dry food mixes or adhesives.

Laundry starches are usually ordinary starches, but silicone resin emulsions may be added to starches to permit higher ironizing temperatures, improve slipperiness, and improve the hand of the starched fabric. The so-called permanent starches, for household use, that are not removed by washing, are not starch, but are emulsions of polyvinyl acetate.

starch, arum. From root of the arum lily; similar to sago.

starch, modified. Starch with the molecule altered by chemical treatment to give characteristics suitable for particular industrial requirements. Such kinds of starch have special importance in food processing, because of the desired change in gel strength, flow properties, colour, clarity, stability of the paste. The modified starches and especially prepared starches are usually sold under trade names.

Acid-modified starch. Acid treatment reduces the viscosity of the paste (used in sugar confectionery, e.g. gum drops, jelly beans.)

Oxidized starch. Peroxide, permanganate, chlorine, etc., alter viscosity, clarity and stability of the paste (major use is outside the food industry).

Derived starch. Chemical derivatives such as ethers and esters show properties such as reduced gelatinization in hot water and greater stability to acids and alkalies (inhibited starch), it is useful where food has to withstand heat treatment as in canning or in acid foods. Further degrees of treatment can result in starch being unaffected by boiling water and losing its gel-forming properties.

Pregelatinized starch. Raw starch does not form a paste with cold water and therefore requires cooking if it is to be used as a food thickening agent. Pregelatinized starch, mostly maize starch, has been cooked and dried. Used in instant puddings, pie-fillings, soup mixes, salad dressings, sugar confectionery, as binder in meat products. Nutritional value the same as the original starch.

Waxy starch. The starch containing a high percentage of amylopectin;

such kind of starch does not form rigid gels when gelatinized.

starch drying. The starch granules in vegetables determine to a large extent their texture. During dehydration of products high in starch, such as potatoes, the moisture diffuses through the starch gel, which controls the drying and heating rates.

starch equivalent. S.E. A measure of the energy value of animal feeding stuffs; the number of parts of pure starch that would be equivalent to 100 parts of the ration as a source of energy. It is determined by direct feeding experiments. Protein has S.E. 0.94, crude fibre 1.0, ether extract of oilseeds 2.4.

starter. Culture of bacteria used to inoculate or start growth, such as in milk for cheese production, or butter to develop the flavour, or any fermentation.

stassanising. A regenerative enclosed method of pasteurizing milk in order to kill harmful organisms and preserve the quality of the milk. The milk is heated to 70°C under slight pressure in a thin layer between two heated surfaces in order that all the carbonic acid may be retained. It is claimed that there is practically no milk stone formation, less destruction of vitamins, no evaporation of milk, and more economy in steam utilization than in the more recognized methods of pasteurization.

steam baking. In baking an even temperature is maintained in the oven by means of closed pipes through which steam circulates. This is sometimes erroneously believed to mean that the bread is baked in live steam.

steam dryer. One of several types of dryers which uses steam, either direct or indirect, as a source of heat for drying. More commonly, the designation is used for units in which steam is used directly for drying, such as for lumber, sawdust, coal, etc.

stearic acid. $CH_3\text{-}(CH_2)_{16}COOH$. Long-chain fatty acid with a total of 18 carbon atoms; present in most animal and vegetable fats as the triglyceride; used in pharmacy and cosmetics. Also known as octadecanoic acid.

stearin. The chief ingredient of suet and tallow, or the harder ingredient of animal fats, olein being the softer one. It is prepared for practical use from beef suet and cottonseed oil, and it yields an oil used in the manufacture of butterine. Sterin has a pearly lustre and is soft to the touch, but not greasy. It is insoluble in water, but soluble in hot alcohol and ether. When treated with superheated steam, it is separated into stearic acid and glycerine, and when boiled with alkalis the stearic acid combines with the alkali and forms soap and glycerine. When melted, stearin resembles wax.

steatorrhoea. Excess of fat in the stools. May be due to lack of bile, lack of lipase in the digestive juices, or defective absorption of fat. Treatment by feeding low-fat diet.

steer. Bull castrated when very young; if castrated after reaching maturity known as a stag.

Steinbuscher cheese. A kind of soft cheese made first in Steinbusch Germany. The cheese has a yellow surface and a buttery consistency and is similar to Romadur cheese. The milk is set, the curd is cut, cooked and dipped into Limburer-type forms. The cheese is dry salted and placed in a humid curing room during which time a white mold develops on the surface. After sufficient mold growths, the cheese is rubbed dry and wrapped in parchment.

stepsin. Obsolete name for pancreatic lipase.

sterile. Free from all micro-organisms-bacteria, moulds and yeasts. When foods are sterilized, as in canning, they are preserved indefinitely as they are protected from recontamination in the can, and also from chemical and enzymatic deterioration.

sterilization, cold. A term generally applied to preservation with sulphur dioxide, but more particular to sterilization with radioactive materials. Very large doses of ionizing radiation are required to inhibit enzyme activity and the growth of microorganisms, and some foods develop unpleasant flavours on such treatment.

sterilized milk. In general, this term is given to milk that has been heated to a temperature of 70°C or higher for a length of time sufficient to kill organisms present. Theoretically this is not accurate for some germs will survive this treatment.

sterocobilin. One of the brown pigments of the faeces; formed from the bile pigments, which, in turn, are formed as breakdown products of the haemoglobin of obsolete red blood cells.

steroid. Any of a group of lipids derived from a saturated compound called cyclopentanoperhydrophenanthrene, which has a nucleus of four rings. Some of the most important steroid derivatives are the steroid alcohols, or sterols. Other steroids include the bile acids, which aid digestion of fats in the intestine; the sex hormones (androgens and oestrogens); and the corticosteroid hormones, produced by the adrenal cortex.

Cholesterol is the major sterol in animal tissues. Cholesterol and its esters with long chain fatty acids are important components of plasma lipo-proteins and of the outer cell membrane. Plant cell membranes contain four kind of sterols, particularly stigmasterol, which differs from cholesterol only in having a double bond between the carbon atoms 22 and 23. The cholesterol molecule has a polar head group, the hydroxyl group at position 3.

steroidal alkaloids. The alkaloids possessing a cyclopentenophenanthrene nucleus. Alkaloids with C_{27} group are known as *Solanum* alkaloids, *e.g.,* solanidine, and tomatidine. The alkaloids found in the Apocynaceae *(Holarrhena* and *Funtumia* sps) and in the Buxaceae, possess 21 carbon atoms.

sterols. Alcohols derived from the steroids; include cholesterol, widely distributed in animal tissue including brain and egg yolk, coprosterol in faces, ergosterol in yeast which is the precursor for the synthetic vitamin D_2, and sitosterol and stigmasterol in plants.

stevioside. Naturally occurring, non-nutritive sweetening agent, 300 times as sweet as sucrose, thus the sweetest natural compounds. It is a glucoside of steviol, which has a steroid structure, and is present in the leaves of a Paraguayan shrub, *Stevia rebaudiana.* It has not been accepted for use in foodstuffs.

stickleback. The popular name for certain small fishes, so called because of their dorsal spines. These fishes are found in both salt and fresh waters, are very active and voracious and live upon aquatic insects and worms. The sticklebacks are among the very few fishes which build nest for their young. The nests is composed of straw, sticks and similar materials, and is shaped like a muff. In it the eggs, yellow in colour and about the size of poppy seeds, are deposited.

stickwater. The aqueous fraction from pressing cooked fish in the manufacture of fish meal. It contains amino acids, vitamins, and minerals and is added to animal feed or mixed back with the fish meal and dried. Also known as fish solubles.

stilboestrol. Synthetic substance with potent activity as female sex hormone; they are widely used clinically and for food production (such as for chemical caponization of cockerels and to stimulate the growth of cattle).

Stilton cheese. A kind of hard, blue-veined, cows' milk cheese. An English cheese first made in Leicestershire, England and thought to be the finest English cheese. It is rich and mellow, and has a peculiar flavour which is milder than Roquefort. This kind of cheese has veins of blue-mold throughout the interior and a wrinkled rind resulting from molds and bacteria that grow on the surface. The open flaky texture provides aeration for *Penicillium roqueforttii*, so the cheese does not have to be pierced. The cheese measures about 20 cm in diameter.

stiparogenic. Foods that tend to cause constipation.

stiparolytic. Foods that tend to prevent or relieve constipation.

stirred curd method. A method of making cheddar cheese, exclusively used for many years in US. It is also called the granular process. It differs from the cheddar method in that:
(a) the curd remains longer in the whey to develop more acidity and firmness;
(b) after separation from the whey the curd is transferred to a curd sink and stirred frequently to keep the small pieces separate instead of being packed and cheddared;
(c) the time between removal of whey and salting is much shorter; and
(d) the time between salting and pressing the curd is much longer.

It is much more difficult to make cheese of perfect texture with the stirred curd method, and while this method may produce cheese which has moisture content; the undesirable fermentation are less easily controlled than in cheddar process.

Stixie. A registered trade name for a frozen confection on a stick consisting of sherbet and water-ice in contrasting colours, one being an inner core and the other being an outer coating.

stock. Liquid in which the meat or bone or vegetable, or a mixture of these, has been boiled until most of the water-soluble matter has been extracted. Meat and bone contains collagen, which is converted into gelatin by prolonged boiling, hence the stock may set to a gel on cooling. The main nutritive value of stock is due to the mineral content.

stockfish. Unsalted fish that has been dried naturally in air and sunshine; mostly prepared in Norway. It contains 12-15% water, and 1 kg is made from 4.5 kg of fresh fish. The average composition per 100 g after boiling is: protein 31%; fat 1%; calcium 20 mg; iron 1.6 mg; zinc 0.7 mg; and food energy 0.59 mJ.

Stork process. The name given to the process of ultrahigh temperature sterilization of milk followed by sterilization again inside the bottle.

Stout. A very dark ale with a sweet, slightly burnt taste due to the addition of about 7 to 10% of roasted malt. It is heavily hopped but the resultant bitter taste is slightly masked by the addition of small quantities of sugar as the brewing stage. The taste is improved due to post-fermentation by long storage in the bottles. Alkaline water containing magnesium sulphate and sodium bicarbonate as well as water with higher concentration of chlorides are suitable for some stouts.

STP. Conventional abbreviation for standard temperature and pressure. The standard temperature is 273.16 K and the pressure is 1 atmosphere, equal to (1.01325 X 10^{-1} MPa).

stracchino. A generic name applied to several forms of soft, whole milk, Italian cheese, such as Stracchino de Milano, Fresco, Quardo, Quartirola, Crescenza, Salame, Formaggio Salame.

strandin. A substance isolated from brain tissue which dries in long strands; composed of fatty acid, sphingosine, carbohydrate and a small proportion of neutraminic acid.

strawberry. Fruit of genus *Fragaria*. A small plant of the rose family which produces a delicious red fruit also called strawberry.

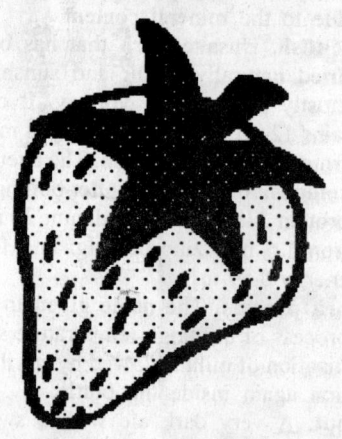

In the technical sense, the strawberry cannot be classified as a berry, for, unlike the currant and the gooseberry, it has no outer skin enclosing pulp and seed, the tiny yellow seeds lying in little pits on the surface. It is heart-shaped and juicy, with a delicate perfume and rich flavour. It is a favourite fruit in many countries and is widely cultivated. The plant is hardy. The cultivation of the strawberry is not difficult, if a few essentials are regarded. The plants, which are small, seldom more than 15 cm high, send out runners or vines, which creep along the ground and at intervals take root. The young plants obtained from the rooted runners are the most productive. They are transplanted in the late autumn or spring in rows or hills three or four feet apart, with 50 cm separating the plants. As they grow they send out runners, which may be cut off or allowed to mat, the former treatment resulting in less numerous berries but larger ones. The richer the soil the better, and it should have been under cultivation at least two seasons. Success with strawberries means crop rotation, and when the bearing season is over the beds should be plowed under and planted to something else for two or three years before strawberries are again planted. When the plants are set out in the fall they should be mulched with straw. This should be raked between the rows but left around the plants, as it keeps the berries off the ground. To prepare soil for spring planting, drain thoroughly and cover with manure. In the spring rake off all trash and work the soil until it is light to a depth of six inches. A good fertilizer, such as nitrate of soda, applied just before the blossoming, increases the crop. The plants must have a great deal of moisture, and sometimes may require irrigation. The average composition per 100 g is: protein 0.8%; fat 0.6%; calcium 25 mg;

iron 0.7 mg; vitamin A 18 mg; vitamin B$_1$ 0.04 mg; vitamin B$_2$ 0.05 mg; nicotinic acid 0.4 mg; vitamin C 65 mg; and food energy 0.15 MJ.

strepogenin. Name given to a peptide-like fraction from natural sources, claimed to be essential for microorganisms and higher animals. The needed for special peptides for the latter has not been confirmed.

streptococci. The Gram-positive, spherical, nonmotile cells that grow in pairs or chains by fermenting glucose under anaerobic or micro-aerophilic conditions. The streptococci are one of the few groups of air tolerant bacteria unable to make catalase. The absence of catalase is a key marker for differentiating between the streptococci and the catalase positive staphylococci. Only a few of the many species of streptococci cause disease in humans. Most of the pathogenic species produce either an α- or β-hemolysin that is easily detected when isolates grow on blood agar plates. Other characteristics by which the pathogenic streptococci can be differentiated include the antigenic serotype, sensitivity to bacitracin or optochin (an inhibitory chemical), presence of capsules, and bile solubility. Many non-pathogenic species are found in natural environments and some have industrial applications.

streptococcus lactis factor. A fermentation product of the mould *Rhizopus nigricans,* Known as rhizopterin, which is essential to *S. lactis* R. Related to folic acid.

streptococcus pyogenes. The most important species of the genus, is an opportunistic pathogen associated with humans that cause both cutaneous and systemic infections. It is the main cause of acute bacterial pharyngitis. The ability of the microorganism to adhere to the respiratory epithelium is correlated with the presence of a protein called M protein and lipoteichoic acid on the cell envelope. These two components form a fibrous network on the surface of the streptococcus in which the lipid moiety of lipoteichoic acid serves as binding factor to the host cell. The receptor on the host cell is believed to be albumin-like protein. Antiserum to lipoteichoic acid but not other surface components inhibits adherence of the streptococci.

streptokinase. Proteolytic enzyme prepared from haemolytic streptococci; used clinically to liquefy thick pus in empyemata and to remove the fibrin clot covering wounds. Streptodornase is a similar enzyme preparation that attacks pus cells.

stress. The non-specific response of a body or organism to any demand made up on it, primarily preparing the organism for physical activity. Stress is one of the mechanisms suspected of leading to disease in modern life.

string bean. Common name for fresh garden beans which are raised for their young, green, immature pods. The word string, still widely used, arose from the tough fibre that holds the two halves of the pod together and which, unless the bean is tender, tends to come apart longitudinally, thus producing undesirable strings. New varieties are much improved, making the word stringless now more appropriate. Generally, string beans, stringless beans, and snap beans are synonyms. Yellow-coloured string beans are usually called wax beans.

stringy milk. A term often used to describe milk from in infected udder. The condition is due to the presence of masses of leucocytes and fibrin. Unlike ropy milk, stringy milk is recognized as such when drawn from the cow. This is also spoken of as flaky or gargety milk.

strudels. A food product made by wrapping fillings in many layers of very thin dough. The dough usually is made up of flour, egg, water, salt, and oil. There is no leavening and the method of preparation discourages incorporation of bubbles. The home methods of preparation, which involve hand stretching of the dough while brushing it with oil, are time consuming and tedious. Commercial methods have been developed to prepare strudel dough leaves that are distributed in frozen form.

struvite. Small crystals of magnetism ammonium phosphate which occasionally form in canned fish; resemble broken glass.

strychnine. A poisonous drug obtained from the seeds of *nux vomica* and certain other plants. It is prepared in the form of crystals, which are odourless but intensely bitter. One-eight of a grain of strychnine will kill a large dog; three-eight of a grain will produce spasms in man. A half grain is sometimes fatal to man, a whole grain almost always so. In very small doses-from one-fifteenth to one-fiftieth of a grain-strychnine is valuable as a tonic.

sturgeon. A group of fishes of the order Chondrostei, family *Ac enseridae,* comprising numerous species, found in both fresh and salt waters of the north temperate zone. Their chiefly external characteristic is the series of bony plates arranged in rows along the back and sides, separated by wide spaces containing only small hard elements. Some of them are very large. The body of sturgeon is long and slender, terminating in a forked tail, and covered with rows of bony plates. The mouth is comparatively small, funnel-shaped and toothless, and the food, consisting of small marine animals and vegetable growths, is sucked in whole through the thick lips under the long, pointed snout. The sturgeon is important in the fishing industry. The flesh, which is well flavoured, is usually smoked for the market; the eggs are used in the preparation of caviar, and the bladder of the Russian sturgeon is used in making isinglass. The sturgeons are considered excellent food fishes and are the source of caviar. There are about fifteen European species and nine North American species. Sturgeon have poor vision, but this is partly compensated by fleshy whiskers which trail in the sand and assist in locating food at the bottom. Rare among the fishes, the sturgeons have taste buds external of the mouth. It is believed that these also assist in locating a food supply. Also quite rare among fishes is the fact that sturgeons eat quite slowly. The diet includes crawfish, insect larvae, snails and some small fish.

substrate. In relation to enzymes refers to the substance on which the enzyme acts. Thus the substrate for the enzyme amylase is starch, which is hydrolyzed to maltose. Substrate can also mean the medium on which microorganisms grow.

subtilin. Antibiotic isolated from a strain of *B. subtilis* grown on a medium containing asparagine; used as a food preservative (not permitted in Great Britain) as it reduces the thermal resistance of spores and is effective against thermophilic flat source; thus subtilin permits a reduction in the processing time.

Sucaryl. Trade name for sodium or calcium salt of cyclohexyl sulphamate.

Succari orange. A variety of non-blood type sweet orange. It is an exceptionally sweet orange that is almost devoid of acid. The sugar/acid ratio at maturity is almost 100/1. Thus, the fruit is not suitable for processing. It is called Sukkari in Egypt, the variety is of unknown origin. Succari orange is of medium-size, oblate to globose, and seedy, the variety has been well regarded in Egypt for many years and is of considerable commercial importance there.

succory. Another name for chicory.

succotash. Stew of green maize and lima beans (butter beans), an American-Indian dish.

suchar. A type of activated carbon, used to decolorize solutions.

sucralose. 4,1',6'-trichloro-4,1,6'-trideoxy-galactosucrose. A chlorine-containing compound approximatley 600 times sweeter than sucrose, is under FDA review for use in 15 food categories, including baked goods. It appears to have good stability, maintaining its integrity throughout baking. This as yet unapproved sweetener is said to have synergistic sweetening effects with other artificial sweeteners, especially cyclamate.

Sucron. Trade name for mixture of saccharine and sucrose, four times as sweet as sucrose alone.

sucrose esters. Di- and trilaurates and mono- and distearates of sucrose; used as emulsifiers, wetting agents and surface active agents, e.g., for washing fruits and vegetables, as anti-spattering agents, anti-foam agents and anti-staling or crumb-softening agents.

sucrose. A sugar comprising one molecule of glucose linked to a fructose molecule. It occurs widely in plants and is particularly abundant in sugar cane and sugar beet (15-20%), from which is it extracted and refined for table sugar. If heated to 200°C sucrose becomes caramel. The average composition per 100 g of crude brown sugar is: 97% carbohydrate; and contains 1% water; 0.2% protein; 2 mg iron; 0.02 mg vitamin B_1; 0.01 mg vitamin B_2; 0.3 mg nicotinic acid. Refined white sugar is close to 100% pure and contains no minerals or vitamins. Also known as Cane sugar; beet sugar.

suet. Fat prepared from the kidneys of oxen and sheep.

sugar acid. An acid formed from a monosaccharide by oxidation. Oxidation of the aldehyde group (-CHO) of the aldose monosaccharides to a carboxyl group (-COOH) gives an aldonic acid; oxidation of the primary alcohol group (-CH_2OH) to -COOH yields uronic acid; oxidation of both the primary alcohol and carboxyl groups gives an aldaric acid. The uronic acids are biologically important, being components of many polysaccharides, for example glucuronic acid (from glucose) is a major component of gums and cell walls, while galacturonic acid (from galactose) makes up pectin. Ascorbic acid or vitamin C is an important sugar acid found universally in plant tissues, particularly in citrus fruits.

sugar alcohol. An alcohol derived from a monosaccharide by reduction of its carbonyl group (C=O) so that each carbon atom of the sugar has an alcohol group (-OH). For example, glucose yields sorbitol, common in fruits, and mannose yields mannitol.

sugar beet. *Beta vulgaris* subsp. *cicla,* the most important source of sugar (sucrose) in temperate countries; contains 15-20% sugar; biennial related to the garden beet root but with white, conical roots.

sugar beet drying. The loss of sugar in sugar beets occurs in storage when the temperature is above 18.3°C, with approximately 0.1-0.5 kg loss per day per ton. The use of mechanical harvesting equipment has made the potential heating losses of sugar beets significant because the beets can be harvested much faster than they can be processed. Air can be blown into the pile when the air is 2.7 to 3.3°C colder than the hot test spot in the beets. In the initial cooling of the beets it is desirable to use from 1.0 to 1.5 X 10⁻⁶ m³/kgs, followed with approximately 0.5 m³/kgs to maintain the temperature of the pile. One air distribution system for cooling sugar beet piles consists of using 200 litres drums with the ends removed and the drums welded together with strips of iron maintaining a space of about 1.2 cm between the drums. The fan is then placed on one end of the tunnel. The optimum relative humidity of air forced into the piles is 80%.

sugar beet seed drying. To decorticate sugar beet seeds, it is necessary that the moisture content be 11% or below. Moisture can be reduced to almost 11% with unheated forced air if the temperature is above 15.6°C and relative humidity below 40%. Heated air can be used at 43.3°C if the seed is exposed to the heat for over one hour, which would occur in deep bin drying with heated air, or 43.9°C if a thin layer of 1.6 cm is dried so that the seeds will not be heated for more than an hour. The static pressure at a given air flow through the whole seeds is slightly less than for shelled corn.

sugar cane. *Saccarum officinarum.* A plant of the grass family from which about one-half of the sugar of commerce is obtained. Sugar cane is supposed to be a native of the tropical regions in Asia, but it is not at present found in the wild state. In general appearance sugar cane resembles maize or Indian corn. It grows to heights varying from 2-6 metres, according to soil, climate and cultivation. The stalks vary from one to two inches in diameter, and are jointed like corn stalks. At each joint there is a bud or eye, which, when the cane is planted, sprouts and produces a new plant. The leaves grow to about three feet in length and are about two inches wide at the base, tapering gracefully to a point; they resemble leaves of corn. When young the plant presents a fresh, green appearance, but as it matures some of the leaves turn a purplish blue, and those at the bottom turn yellow, wither and fall off.

sugar doctors. To prevent the crystallization or "graining of sugar in sugar confectionery, a substance called the sugar doctor or candy doctor is added. This may be a weak acid, such as cream of tartar, which "inverts" part of the cane sugar during the boiling, or invert sugar or starch syrup.

sugar drying. The production of dry sugar from the juice of sugar cane by pressing or beet sugar by diffusion is similar. The juice from sugar cane is obtained by pressing between rolls with a fibrous material, bagasse, remaining. The juice is purified, concentrated in a multiple stage (two to five) evaporator, then boiled in a single stage vacuum unit and seeded with sugar crystals. The product is then centrifuged and dried. Sugar is removed from slices of beet sugar in a battery of diffusers. The beet pulp remains, which is not as fibrous as bagasse, and is often dried. Beet pulp and bagasse are dried from 75-85%

moisture to 5-15% in a direct-fired, parallel flow, forced draft rotating drum (internal with baffles) dryer. The heated air may enter the drum at about 538°C and leave at 93.3-137.8°C, the beet pulp or bagasse approaching 100°C upon drying. The crystallized product is first mechanically dried with a centrifugal device, reducing the moisture content to 1%. Crystal sugar has a very low equilibrium moisture content compared to many other food products which are dried and is very hygroscopic. Sugar is one of the food products which are dried and is very hygroscopic. Sugar is dried to 0.1% to get a free flowing product. Above 0.2-0.3% the sugar is tacky or sticky. The most common dryer is an internally heated rotary drum with internal flights. The drum is mounted at an angle to assist in moving the sugar through. The drum is mounted at an angle to assist in moving the sugar through. Counter-current flow of sugar and air is used. The flights pick up the sugar on the bottom and drop the sugar through the air moving at about 1 m/s, the air entering at 32.2-43.3°C, with a residence time of the product of 5-10 minutes. The residence time in the dryer varies greatly depending on the diameter and length of drum, temperature and speed of air flow, original and final moisture content of the product, etc. Air is drawn rather than pushed through the dryer to minimize escape of dust into the room in which the dryer is located. Vertical dryers, with discs mounted on a rotating shaft, are also used. The wet sugar enters on top, is thrown out centrifugally, and moves down to the next tray, as air moves up through the dryer removing moisture. Fixed trays may also be used in which the sugar is scarped from one tray and falls to the next in the heated air, which removes moisture from the product. Upon leaving the dryer the sugar is passed through a screen to break/remove lumps.

sugar maple. *Acer saccharum* Marsh. Family: *Aceraceae*. A kind of tree often growing 21-30 m tall and 0.6-0.9 m in diameter. Maple sugar trees may grow up to 40 m high and 1.5 m in diameter. During summer, the leaves acquire a deep yellowish-green on the top and paler beneath. They change to bright red, yellow, or orange in the fall. The bark is dark gray and the twigs are reddish-brown. At the same time as the new spring leaves are unfolding, flowers appear in hanging clusters. The paired seeds of sugar maples are made in the fall and each seed has a long wing (2-2.5 cm). The wind catches the seed-wing and carries it through the air. Hopefully, it will land in a good spot for growing. Sugar maples prefer the rich, moist, well-drained soil of valleys and uplands, but they can also grow in poorer soils. The industry relies upon the boiled spring sap to make all kinds of maple treats, including maple syrup. It would take about 32 bottles of sap to make 1 bottle of syrup. Many kinds of wildlife need this tree. In the winter, white-tailed deer browse on the twigs and the buds are nipped off by grouse. chipmunks, squirrels, deer mice, and grosbeaks eat the large seeds. The soft, shapely leaves provide shade as you stroll along, and a pebbly brook usually running through the hardwood stand offers coolness. In autumn the woods seem almost afire with the brilliant reds, yellows, and oranges of frost-nipped sugar maple leaves. Also known as hard maple; rock maple.

sugar palm. *Arenga saccharifera,* grows

wild in Malaysia and Indonesia; sugar (sucrose) is obtained from the sap.

sugar, caster. Ordinary sugar (sucrose) crystallized in small crystals.

sugar, icing. Popular name for powdered 'sucrose.

sugar. Usually refers to sucrose or table sugar obtained from the sugar can or sugar beet. May also refer to any of the sugars such as milk sugar (lactose) fruit sugar (fructose), grape sugar (glucose), malt sugar (maltose).

The simplest carbohydrates are classified as sugars, subdivided into monosaccharides, disaccharides and polysaccharides. The health implication of sugar that everybody knows about is its drastic effect on the teeth. Statistically dental disease is the number one health problem in India and many other countries, and sugar is the universally recognized culprit where dental decay is concerned.

Sugar reacts with saliva to form acids that dissolve the enamel of the teeth, forming an ideal environment for the bacteria that cause decay. Sugar in its refined state is only 'empty calories'; it is 99.96% sucrose and totally devoid of vitamins, minerals and enzymes. Vitamins, minerals and enzymes are essential for the digestion, assimilation and utilization of sugar, but analysis of molasses, the by-product of sugar-refining, shows six B vitamins and eight minerals which have been detached from the sugar, and these are just a portion of the nutrients your system must somehow provide to metabolize the sugar. The missing elements must be stolen from the 'real food' in a diet, from nutrients in your blood that are intended for other functions, even from the reserves stored in your very bones. Only in this way can a simple carbohydrate (such as refined sugar) imitate a complex one and act like a real food. By contrast, a complex carbohydrate which is a real food has its sugars accompanied by fibre, vitamins, minerals, enzymes, protein and fat; in other words everything necessary to complete the metabolic activities that will be fired by sugar. Complex carbohydrates supply the body with a slow, steady, stream of blood sugar and none of the essential companions are missing. This is natural sugar metabolism. Eating refined sugar causes the blood sugar level to leap and plunge dramatically. Sugar also inhibits the ability of the white blood cells to destroy bacteria. Test shows that a couple of teaspoons of sugar can undermine the strength of white blood cells by 25%. Sugar can reduce your resistance to everything from colds to cancer. Many members of the medical establishment fail to recognize the relationship between sugar consumption and adult- onset diabetes. It seems they are waiting for proof positive; eventually they will get it, if only because what goes up always comes down and as the sugar consumption comes down among the enlightened in the western world, so will the incidence of diabetes. Bearing all of this in mind, for those who suffer hunger pains between meals, or from the symptoms of hypoglycemia (low blood sugar) it is far better to eat small amounts of proteins between meals (a few spoonfuls of yoghurt or a small handful of sunflower seeds) than to seek a boost from sugar. Various advantages for those who eliminate or curtail sugar consumption including reduction of dental decay, particularly in children, helping weight control (an indirect link to coronary disease), improvement or correction of various blood abnormalities involving fats, uric acid, glucose, the stickiness of blood platelets and the concentration of insulin and cortisol. All this can be summarized as follows. The darker in colour the higher the proportion of health-protecting elements and structural information it contains. Though, that brown sugars generally contain a thin film of molasses surrounding the sucrose crystal which contains some 200 organic nutrients which are useful in themselves and also essential for the correct break down of sugar in the body. Bearing all this in mind it is far preferable that you use a small amount of honey or black strap molasses as sweetening. The following sweeteners do not depend on sucrose for their sweetening power. Of the above only date sugar is solid and it is the only one that is a whole food. It consists of dates that have been pitted, dried and ground. It is suitable for sprinkling on foods but does not mix well or dissolve easily and therefore can be a problem if used for baking and cooking.

The liquids are easier to work with in baking and cooking, but all recipes that are being converted from solid-form sucrose need to have their liquid content appropriately adjusted to compensate for the liquid of the syrup and/or honey. Use 3/4 cup honey to replace 1 cup sugar and at the same time decrease the amount of liquid in the recipe by up to 1/4 cup of each 3/4 cup honey used. Note the more delicate the flavour of the recipe, the lighter the honey should be. The darker the honey the higher the mineral content and the stronger the flavour. Honey can also be mixed half and half with molasses or malt syrup but this should only be done where the molasses or malt flavour is compatible with the other ingredients in the recipe.

All artificial sweeteners have to be approved for safety by the Food Advisory Committee before they can be used by the food industry or sold over the counter. The committee on Toxicity of Chemicals in Food, Consumer products and the Environment reports to the FAC, and the government is advised if there is a need to withdraw a product on grounds of uncertainty. At one time saccharine was thought to induce bladder cancer in rats, but no such link has been shown in humans. Although aspartame was recently the subject of investigation about its effect on blood pressure and behaviour, the Food Advisory Committee remains satisfied as to its safety. These types of sugars are as suspect as any other artificial additives and therefore would not advise their use. Note also that substances like thaumatin, acesulame K, mannitol, xylitol, hydrogenated glucose syrup, isomol and sorbitol are increasingly being added to manufactured foods instead of ordinary sugar.

sugaring of dried fruits. A type of deterioration of dried fruit on storage, most frequently on prunes and figs. A sugary substance appears on the surface or under the skin, consisting of glucose and fructose with traces of citric and malic acids, lysine, asparagine and aspartic acid. When occurring under the skin of prunes it is called "red sugar".

sugar baby watermelon. An early maturing variety of watermelon that takes 75-80 days from planting. The melon is small, weight 3.6-4.5 kg and is from 17.5-20 cm in diameter. It is frequently called an "icebox" melon because of its small size. The rind is thin, hard and tough, and can be either dark green with indistinct darker veining, or medium-green with darker veining. The flesh is medium red, firm, crisp, sweet and of fine texture. There are relatively few seeds, which are small, dark tan and mottled with black. This variety is free of whiteheart.

suicide substrate. An enzyme substrate that is converted by the enzyme into an irreversible inhibitor of that enzyme. The enzyme may therefore be thought of as having committed suicide. The advantage of the required sites. Suicide substrates have been designed and developed for GABA transaminase (*e.g.*, vinyl GABA and 4-aminohex-5-ynoic acid), for peripheral DOPA decarboxylase (*e.g.*, difluoromethyldopa), for monoamine oxidase A and monoamine oxidase B (for example, pargyline and segyline), and for a number of other enzymes including formlglycinamide ribonucleotide aminotransferase, 5a-reductase, serine proteases and hydroxylases.

Suines. Pigs, boars, hogs, and peccaries (*Suines*) comprise one of the more primitive groups of the order *Artiodactyla* (even-toed hoofed animals). The group is not large in terms of identifiable species in the wild as contrasted, for example, with the antelopines and even the bovines, but because they are so highly valued in terms of the domestic breeds, they do comprise an extremely large population of mammals.

Pigs, unlike cattle and sheep, are not ruminants, that is, they do not chew their cuds. They all dig with their muzzles and have a preference in nature for vegetable matter. They are characterized by having large litters. There are certain misconceptions concerning pigs that should be clarified. By nature, swine are not dirty. When in the wild and left to their own habits, these animals are exceptionally orderly and clean. It is true that most species of Suines enjoy mud wallows where they go to cool off, to remove external parasites from their bodies, and to cleanse themselves. Mud, as some beauticians acclaim, is an excellent cleaner, containing helpful antibiotics. The pig in captivity that wallows in mud that is littered with excrement, rotting garbage, etc., does not do this out of choice. In the wild, these animals never excrete in their mud wallows.

The terms pig and swine are generally considered synonymous in most parts of the world. Some producers refer to pigs as animals that are under about 3 months of age. Adult animals are commonly called hogs, particularly the marketable and commercial animals.

Hog also refers to a castrated boar. A gilt is a young female pig, usually unbred, but sometimes refers to an animal with its first litter.

A sow is an adult female pig, after she has produced her first litter.

A boar is a well-developed male animal used for breeding service.

A boar pig is a male animal under breeding age (usually less than 6 months old).

A stag is a male animal that has been castrated in maturity-after the tusks, shields, enlarged sheath, crest, and other characteristics have developed.

A barrow is a male animal that has been castrated before sexual characteristics have developed.

A shote is an immature animal of either sex.

The meat from swine is referred to as pigmeat, pork, viande de porc (French), or carne de cerdo (Spanish).

The word porcine is frequently

used in English literature to describe a part of the hog carcass, such as porcine muscle.

Whereas a large percentage of beef and lamb meat is sold fresh (or frozen), only about 30% of pork is sold fresh, the remainder being curd by a number of methods, such as pickling, smoking, etc.

sulfuring. See sulphuring.

sulpha drugs. Group of synthetic drugs derived from sulphanilamide (or amino-benzensulphonamide) used to combat bacterial infection. Sulphanilamide itself functions as an antivitamin to bacteria, as it inhibits the uptake of p-aminobenzoic acid, an essential nutrient.

sulphate. The ion formed as a result of ionization of sulphuric acid. It occurs in foods and in the body in two main forms, (a) as sulphate salts of sulphuric acid, and (b) in the amino acids methionine and cystine.

sulphite, fixed. A term used when referring to sulphite as a preservative. Sulphites can combine with aldehydes, ketones, simple sugars, and possibly other food constituents, and such combined or fixed sulphite has no preservative action, only the undissociated acid is effective.

sulphur. An element that is part of the amino acids cystine and methionine and is therefore present in all proteins. It is also part of the molecules of vitamin B_1 and biotin. Apart from its presence as part of these compounds there appears to be no dietary need for sulphur in any other form and no deficiency has ever been observed, although it is essential for plants. The old-fashioned remedy of sulphur and molasses was not only quite unnecessary but elemental sulphur is probably not used by the body.

sulphuring. The treatment of fruits and/ or vegetables with sulphur dioxide gas or sulphite to control browning.

sultanas. Made by drying the golden sultana grapes (Turkey, Greece, Australia, and S. Africa); the bunches are dipped in alkali, washed, sulphured and dried. Sultanas of the European type produced in the US are termed seedless raisins.

suma. *Pfaffia paniculata.* A shrub growing prolifically in the Goias area south of the Amazon Basin in Brazil. Here much of the soil is very red, signifying large amounts of iron oxide and aluminium hydroxides but very little of other nutrients. In this rocky, laterite soil, this member of the pig weed (amaranthacene) family grows. Its top part is rather fragile, but the below-ground rhizome is usually quite thick. Even with limited amounts of rainfall, suma has adapted quite nicely. Also known as Brazilian ginseng; Brazilian carrots.

sumac leaf drying. The leaves of sumac contain about 25% tannin which is used for processing leather and preparing ink. The seed of the sumac are undesirable for processing purposes. Sumac has about 60% moisture when cut. It is important that the leaves do not get wet during drying because the tannin will be lost through leaching. Unheated forced air can be used for drying in much the same procedure as for hay. Air heated about 5 to 7°C above atmospheric is better than natural air, even though more expensive, as long as the leaves are not heated above 60°C.

summer savory. *Satureja hortensis.* Winter savory. *S. montana.* Summer savory, a half-hardy annual that self-sows freely, has a strong, hot and slightly bitter flavour reminiscent of thyme, and retains a particular affinity with peas and beans, broad beans especially. Winter savory is a shrubby perennial with a similar, though somewhat stronger, flavour that was at one time frequently used with trout and other oily fish. Summer savory is used with pork and game, in soups, sausages, pates, and stuffing, in bouquets grains, and with vegetables, particularly fresh and dried peas and beans. Winter savory has similar uses, but its stronger flavour is considered inferior. Both herbs may be used as a tonic and a digestive, and are said to ease insect bites and stings.

Sumstar 190. Trade name for a diallyl starch made by acid oxidation of cornstarch. Small amounts of the powder added to kraft, tissue, or towelling pulp increase the wet and dry strengths.

sun curing tobacco. Developed as a cottage industry in many areas of the world in which leaves of the tobacco are strung on rocks, placed in open fields, along roads and streets, so that the tobacco is exposed to the sun to heat. The exposure is provided for about 1 month until the tobacco leaves turn a golden yellow.

sunfish. A name applied to several groups of widely varying fishes, both marine and freshwater. The North American freshwater sunfish, never more than ten inches long, is brightly coloured. The common sunfish, which is orange-coloured and about 20 cm long. It delights the amateur angler by its energetic manner of biting. The ocean sunfish, which attains a length of several feet, is of grotesque appearance. This variety is unfit for the table.

sunflower. Family: *Compositae.* Genus: *Helianthus.* Species: *Helianthus annuus* (common annual); *Helianthus orgyalis* and *Helianthus decapetalus* (perennial); so called because the blossoms with their large seed disks and long radiating yellow petals bore an ideal resemblance to the sun with its golden rays. The flowers are 5-8 cm across and the plant is 1-2 m tall, which are nearly hidden by large, heart-shaped leaves. The surrounding bracts are dark green, as are the stems and leaves. Pollinating insects land on the broad ray flowers and search for nectar in the central tubular flowers. Birds eat the seeds and disperse them in their droppings. The plants are easily grown from seeds, though the roots are perennial. The species are numerous, but almost all are found in North America. The gigantic sunflower common in gardens is a native of Peru. The seeds form an excellent food for poultry and for cage birds; and an edible oil has also been expressed from them.

Sunflower seeds are remarkably rich in the B-complex vitamins and are an excellent source of phosphorus, magnesium, iron, calcium, potassium, protein and vitamin E. A combination of equal quantities of pumpkin seeds, sunflower seeds and sesame seeds is a perfectly balanced protein - and the three seeds combined sprinkled over cereals taste delicious. Seeds are used as source of edible oil, rich in polyunsaturated fatty acids; residual oil cake used for animal feed. Seeds also eaten raw. The average composition per 100 g is: 25 g protein; 38 g fat; 21 g carbohydrate; 100 mg calcium; 8 mg iron; 2 mg vitamin B_1; 0.2 mg vitamin B_2; 5.6 mg nicotinic acid; and 2.3 MJ food energy.

sunlight flavour. Name given to unpleasant flavours developing in foods after exposure to sunlight. In milk it is said to be due to the breakdown of methionine in the presence of vitamin B_2; in beer due to a change in the bitter principles from the hops.

sunset yellow FCF. FD&C yellow no. 6. The disodium salt of 1-(p-sulpho)-phenylazo-2-naphthol-6-sul-phonic acid. It is an orange powder, readily soluble in water and glycerol (both 19% at 25°C) to give an orange-yellow solution. It is poorly soluble in the glycols (2% at 25°C) and almost insoluble in ethanol (95%). The colour is light-fast and has good stability in both acid and alkaline media, but fades in the presence of SO_2. It has good stability with benzoic acid and is a widely permitted food colorant.

superglycinerated fats. Normal fats are triglycerides, *i.e.*, three molecules of fatty acid to each molecule of glycerol. The mono and diglycerides are known as superglycerinated. Glyceryl monostearate (GMS) is solid at room temperature, flexible and non-greasy; used as a protective coating for foods, as plasticizer for softening the crumb of bread, to reduce spattering in frying fats, as emulsifier and stabilizer. Glyceryl mono oleate (GMO) is semi-liquid at room temperature.

superheated steam. Steam to which heat has been added to increase the temperature above that temperature corresponding to the temperature of boiling for the pressure of the vapor. By adding sensible heat to dry saturated steam, while maintaining the same pressure, superheated steam is obtained. Heaters for vapour heat transfer, known as superheaters, are used. The greater the degree of superheat, the greater the amount of heat that can be removed without condensation.

Superlose. Trade name for amylose obtained from cornstarch. Auperlose is is the name of amylose obtained

from potato starch.

Supro. Trade name for a protein-rich baby food (24% protein) made in East Africa from maize or barley flour with torula yeast, skin-milk powder and flavouring.

Supro 610. Trade name for a spray-dried powder having up to 95% protein, with a light cream colour and no bitter flavour.

Surati cheese. A buffalo's milk cheese made in India. It was first made in Surat of Maharashtra, India. The curd is placed in bamboo baskets lined with salt to drain. The cheese is kept in whey while curing. Lactic starter is added to fresh, whole fresh, whole milk (preferably pasteurized), and rennet is added at a temperature of about 35°C. An hour later the curd is ladled in thin slices into small, clean bamboo baskets that are dressed on the inside with salt. Additional salt is mixed with the curd. The baskets of urd are placed on a draining rack to drain (and shrink) for about an hour, and the cheeses are inverted in the baskets. The whey that drains from the cheeses is strained, and the cheeses are removed from the baskets and ripened by floating them in the whey, at a temperature of 23.9-26.7°C for 12-36 hours. Then they are ready for consumption or shipment. Each cheese weighs about 113 g. About 38% (weight) of cheese is obtained from buffalo's milk containing 6% of fat. Also known as Surati paneer.

Surati paneer. *See* Surati cheese.

surfactants. Basically the same as emulsifiers, i.e., substances that lower the surface tension. When this effect occurs between two liquids or between a liquid and a solid the surfactant aids emulsification and wetting of powders. Examples are mono and diglycerides, polyethylene derivatives, pectins, alginates, gums, gelatin, lecithin. Also retard hardening rate of jellies, and reduced stickiness of caramels.

surf clam. The Atlantic surf clam (*Spisula solidissima* Dillwyn) is estimated to have lived on the earth for many millions of years. The oldest known fossils are from deposits of the upper Miocene age in North Carolina. Surf clams are the largest bivalve mollusks in the region; some have a maximum length of over 20.3 cm. Their shells are a familiar sight along ocean beaches after storms. Many names are in common use for the surf clam, such as bar clam (Canada); hen clam (Maine); sea clam (Massachusetts) and beach clam or skimmer clam (middle Atlantic states). The surf clam fishery is considerably more recent than the soft-shell clam operations, most of the growth taking place since World War II. The industry has gained considerably importance since the 1950s. Surf clam meats are processed into canned chowder, canned minced meats for home-made chowder, canned minced meats for home-made chowders and party dips, and products for restaurants. The perishable surface clam is processed rapidly under careful hygienic conditions. They are not marketed in the shell, as in the case of oysters or hard-shell clams.

suspended solids. Solids in a liquid that can be removed through sedimentation or filtration.

suspension. Disperse system in which particles of solid dispersed phase have dimensions greater than 500 nm.

Sustagen. Trade name of food concentrate in powder form, also usable for tube feeding; mixture of whole and skim milk, casein, maltose, dextrins and glucose. The approximate composition is: protein 24%; fat 8%; carbohydrate 68%; along with requisite amounts of vitamins A, B_1, B_2, nicotinic acid, C, D, E, B_{12}, calcium pantothenate, pyridoxine plus choline, calcium and iron.

Sveciaost cheese. A kind of Swedish, cow's milk cheese made for domestic consumption from whole or skim milk. The cheese is made in much the same way as Gouda and resembles Gouda except that it has a more open texture.

swallowing. A muscular act, beginning in the mouth. The tongue is raised against the front part of the hard palate, the uvula takes a horizontal position to close the opening into the nostrils, the epiglottis is pressed down upon the glottis, or opening into the larynx, and when the food reaches the back of the throat it is seized by the involuntary muscles, carried quickly through the pharynx, slowly through the esophagus to the cardiac orifices, which opens to allow the food to enter the stomach. A juggler can drink while standing on his head, because swallowing is a muscular act.

sweat. Solution of salt (about 0.3%), urea 0.03%, lactate 0.07%. It varies in composition but is hypotonic to blood plasma.

sweating. The procedure of holding products in large bins for a time after drying to equalize the moisture content throughout the product.

swede (or rutabaga). Family: *Cruciferae.* Genus: *Brassica.* Species: *Brassica napus* var. *rapobrassica.* Root of *Brassica rutabaga* or Swedish turnip. The average composition per 100 g is: protein 1.2%; carbohydrate 4.4%; calcium 55 mg; iron 0.4 mg; vitamin A 3 µg; vitamin B_1 0.5 mg; vitamin B_2 0.05 mg; nicotinic acid 0.7 mg; vitamin C 29 mg; and food energy 0.09 MJ.

The tall, soft sprouts of the Swede that grow after it has been lifted and stored can be boiled and served with butter like asparagus and are very rich in vitamins A, B and C.

sweet basil. *Ocimum basilicum.* With a pot of basil on the windowsill and a tomato plant in a window box outside, you have the perfect partnership for many summer salads, sauces and casseroles, for basil and tomatoes go together in any combination you care to mention. The herb is a half-hardy annual emanating from warm climates and is therefore a sun-lover. With care and adequate heat, a plant will stay in leaf indoors right through to midwinter, a luxury for those who love to use their herbs fresh. In Italy and France, basil is used to make, respectively, *pesto* or *pistou* sauce, in which it is crushed with garlic and pine kernels. The sauce may be served with spaghetti or stirred into soup. Basil is good not only with tomatoes, but with sweet peppers, aubergines, and corrugates; with chicken, eggs, and steak (when it is pounded with softened butter and drizzled over the meat). Medicinally, it may be used as a mild sedative and to relieve stomach pains and sickness. A pot of basil in the kitchen is said to discourage flies.

sweet bay. *See* bay laurel.

sweet birch oil. An oil distilled from the bark of the sweet birch tree (*Betula lenta*) found in N. America. The oil is almost identical with Gaultheria oil.

sweet cicely. *Myrrhis odorata.* Sweet cicely grows wild in northern Europe, and provides good visual value in a border or herb garden, With its large, bright-green, lacy leaves and mass of creamy-white flowers borne on huge umbel-like clusters, it makes a perfect back-of-the-border plant. It is in full leaf from very early spring until midwinter, after most herbs have died back, and is therefore especially useful. The whole plant of this herbaceous perennial is fragrant, with a mildly aniseed aroma that complements fruit dishes and fruit salads. The leaves do not dry well and are best used fresh. The leaves may be used fresh in salads and fruit salads, and chopped into other fruit dishes such as pies and compotes. The peeled roots can be boiled and eaten as a vegetable, accompanied by a white sauce or vinaigrette dressing. The seeds are used in the making of the well-known Chartreuse liqueur.

sweet corn. *Zea saccharata.* A variety of corn which is frequently considered apart from other types of corn and treated along with vegetables. However, there are but few differences. The proportion of sugar to starch in sweet corn exceeds that . oportion of sugar to starch in sweet corn exceeds that of other types. This characteristic is conditioned by a single recessive gene, termed sugary-1, with the symbol su_1. Other less pronounced differences from other types of corn are the tenderness of the sweet corn kernels when mature, wrinkled seeds when dried, a tendency to produce suckers at the base of the plant, and what is considered by many to be a more refined taste. In recent years, a new kind of sweet corn has been developed that is sweeter than the traditional variety. The sweetness is not conditioned by sugary-1 gene, but by similar genetic factor designated as shrunken-2. This gene conditions an even higher level in sugar in the kernels, giving them a sweeter taste and prolonging the edible taste by 3-4 days. Sometimes it is called sugar corn.

sweet corn drying. Kernels which are

somewhat soft are removed from the cob of sweet corn and blanched before drying. The corn kernels can be frozen and stored before drying. Sweet corn is dried on trays in a tunnel dryer or continuously on a belt dryer. A two-stage tunnel dryer, with air entering the first at 82.2°C and the second stage at 73.9°C. The tunnel dryer may be followed by a bin dryer to dry to 5% moisture or less. Single stage drying can be carried out in trays placed in a tunnel or cabinet dryer, using air at 82.2°C. The temperature may be reduced as drying occurs until the sweet corn is 5 to 6%.

sweet cream butter. Butter made from fresh, sweet cream which at no time before or during manufacture shows more than 0.2% acidity. The cream is produced without the use of a butter culture and without cream ripening. Sweet cream butter lacks the typical flavour and aroma of ripened cream butter, but its keeping qualities are better. This butter generally contains from 2-2.5% salt.

sweet cream. That portion of milk, rich in milk fat, which rises to the surface of milk on standing, or is separated from it by centrifugal force. It is fresh and clean containing not less than 18% of milk fat and not more than 0.2% of acid-reacting substances, calculated in terms of lactic acid.

sweet curd cheese. A variety of hard rennet cheese, which closely resembles Cheddar cheese. Cow's milk is set while it is sweet. Cutting of the curd and cooking are done rapidly without regard to development of acidity and the cheese is put to press immediately. Sweet curd Cheddar Cheese is generally considered to be a defective cheese. It can be easily subjected to spoilage by organisms which usually are suppressed by larger amount of acid. On the other hand, Gouda and Edam are also typed as sweet curd cheese, but in this case no inferior cheese is implied.

sweetening agents, non-nutritive. Refers to sweetening agents which are not sugars and have no food value, such as saccharin and cyclamate. Also known as sweeteners.

sweetening agents. The sugars of which the commonest is sucrose. Fructose has 173% of the sweetness of sucrose, glucose, 74%, maltose, 33% and lactose, 16%. The common synthetic non-nutritive sweeteners include saccharine (550 times as sweet as sucrose), dulcin (250 times), sucaryl (30 times), and P4000 (4,000 times).

Sweetex. Trade name for saccharine.

sweet flat. A rush-like plant of the arum family, found in marshy places throughout the northern hemisphere. The leaves are all long and sword-shaped, and the slender, green stem bears a spike of greenish flowers. The root, which is long, cylindrical and knotted, has a strong aromatic odour and a pungent, bitter taste. It has been employed in medicine since the time of Hippocrates. It is also used by confectioners in making candy and in the preparation of aromatic vinegar and other articles.

sweet hoof. A fragrant material which is obtained from operculum, or plate, over the entrance to the shell of certain marine snails (such as *Strombus lentigenosus, Ungues odorati,* and others) found on sea coasts of India to the Red sea. Sometimes it is known as Onycha.

sweet marjoram. *Origanum majorana.* Sweet or knotted marjoram is highly perfumed and has thick trusses of dainty white, pale mauve, or purple flowers, which make it one of the most decorative plants in the herb garden.

It also represents good value since the leaves dry or freeze well for culinary use, and the flowers may be dried for long-lasting arrangements or pot pourri. In warm climates, where it originates, sweet marjoram is a perennial, but it must be treated as half-hardy annual in colder conditions, since it will not survive severe winters. Fresh leaves are added to casseroles just before serving to retain the full flavour. They can also be used in sauces, stuffing, sparingly in salads, in egg and cheese dishes, and in fruit salads. Medicinally, the plant may be taken as a digestive, and it is useful in the home as an insect repellent. With their sweet, pungent aroma, the dried leaves and flowers are good in pot pourri and herbal sleep pillows. Hang the flower stems upside down in a warm, airy place to dry them for arranging.

sweet orange. An essential oil extracted from the peel of the fruit of the sweet orange tree (citrus sinensis). It is used both as a flavouring and in modern quality perfumes. Also known as oil of Portugal.

Sweetose. A trade-name for an enzyme-converted colourless corn syrup of the following composition: moisture 17.0%; dextrose equivalent 64.5% carbohydrate; solids composition: dextrose 43.0%; maltose 23.0%; dextrin 34.0%. In ice cream manufacture, this type sugar is used to replace some of the sucrose, to impart definite qualities to the body and texture of the ice cream.

sweet pea. One of the most popular of all garden plants, related to the vegetable of the same name. There are about 150 varieties, belonging either to the climbing or the dwarf type. The flowers, which have a delicate fragrance, are white, pink, blue red, purple and variegated. Sweet peas require a rich, well drained soil, plenty of sunlight and a free circulation of air.

The seeds are planted in April in a trench which should be gradually filled as the plant grows in order to give the roots the necessary depth.

sweet pea oil. An essential oil extracted by enfleurage from the flowers of the seet pea (*Lathyrus odoratus*), possibly native to southern Europe and now cultivated widely in many parts of the world. Its odour suggests orange blossom and hyacinth with a hint of rose.

sweet potato. *Ipomoea batatas.* A plant of the convolvulus family, a native of the tropics, but now cultivated in all the warmer parts of the world, and in some areas it is the major source of nourishment.

Columbus carried sweet potatoes to Spain as a gift to Queen Isabella, and by the middle of the sixteenth century they were in general cultivation in the country. Sweet potato has smooth, creeping stems, heart-shaped leaves and a flower that some what resembles the morning-glory. The large root constitutes one of the chief American vegetables. The roots can be stored for several weeks, with special treatment for many months.

sweet potato curing. Low temperatures, especially those below 4.4°C, will injure sweet potatoes. To heal after harvest sweet potatoes should be cured using air at a temperature of 29.4°C and a relative humidity of 85%, requiring about 10 days. If the relative humidity is too low healing will not take place even though the temperature is high. The curing period, for which heat is required in most areas of the US, will takes from 10-20 days. If the curing period is too long excessive sprouting will occur. The optimum temperature for storage is 10-12.8°C, whereas the relative humidity should be maintained at about 80-85%. Ventilation is required during storage to provide the proper uniform temperature and to prevent condensation. A heater with an output of about 105-180 kJ/m³ storage capacity is adequate for most installations.

sweet potato drying. Sweet potatoes are peeled, diced, blanched, and sulfited before drying. Sweet potatoes are dried on a conveyor with heated air at 121°C forced through the product or tunnel dryer, first stage at 79.4 to 100°C and second stage at 60 to 71°C, to provide 10 to 12% moisture content product. Bin drying using 60 to 71°C can be used for final drying to 4% moisture content after conveyor or tunnel drying.

sweet potato flake drying. Sweet potatoes for flaking are peeled, cut, and blanched. The pieces, which are about 2.5 cm thick, are pureed and adjusted to 20% solids with hot water. The slurry is drum dryer, heated with steam at 516 to 585 kN/m². A sheet of dried product is stripped from the drums which is ground to produce flakes.

Sweet William. *Dianthus barbatus.* A garden plant native to eastern Europe. The clove scented flowers are dried for use in pot pourri.

swells. A term generally applied to the infected canned foods when gases produced by fermentation inside the can cause the ends to swell. A hard swell has permanently extended ends. If the ends can be moved under pressure, but not forced back to the original position, they are soft swells. Springers can be forced back, but the opposite end bulges. A flipper is a can of normal appearance in which the end flips out when the can is struck. Hydrogen swells are harmless, and due to acid fruits attacking the can.

swill. The name given to waste food from kitchens used for feeding pigs. It should be sterilized before feeding by through boiling, for at least 1 hour, to prevent the transmission of infectious diseases.

Swiss cheese. This product can be made from raw or unpasteurized milk. After adjusting the milk temperature to 31.1°-34.4°C, a number of bacterial cultures are added to the vat. These include *Streptococcus lactis* or *S. cremoris*, plus *S. thermophilus*, *Lactobacillus bulgaricus* or *L. helveticus*, and *Propionibacterium shermanii*. Separate pure culture or mixed cultures may be used. After a relatively short period for incubation, rennet is added. The developed curds are cut into small sizes (about size of a wheat kernel). Over about a 30 minute period, the curd-whey mixture is brought up to a temperature of about 52.2°C, with stirring until a firm curd is formed. Hooping and pressing follows, after which the cheese is cooled. Both cooling and salting are accomplished by immersing the cheese in a brine tank, a process which requires up to 3 days. After salting, the cheese is aged for 5-10 days at a temperature of 10-15.6°C followed by another holding period at a temperature of 21.1-23.9°C. During these holding periods, the familiar eyes or holes form in the cheese. The operator judges the extent of eye formation by swelling of the cheese. After eye formation is complete, the cheese is held at a lower temperature in readiness for cutting and packaging. Use of *S. thermophilus* and *L. bulgaricus* promote the production of lactic acid at higher temperatures and also inhibit various fermentation that may be objectionable.

The primary role of *P. shermanii* is that of accomplishing the 2-step fermentation of lactose of lactic acid and then to propionic acid. The latter combines with calcium in the cheese to form calcium propionate, the substance that gives the cheese its characteristic sweet flavor. During this fermentation, acetic acid, carbon dioxide, and water also are formed. The eyes in the cheese are formed as the carbon dioxide gas finds avenues of escape. Several Swiss-type cheeses are manufactured. Processing conditions are altered such that *S. thermophilus* and *L. bulgaricus* are not required to produce acid at relatively high temperatures.

sycamore. The frut of the plant sycamore, which is similar to mulberry tree. It bears sweet-flavoured frut with pulp similar to that of true fig. The best frut is large and black coloured. In the spring, before the fruit appears, a sap is obtained from the bark.

It is diluted with water, and applied as an ointment on wounds.

syllabub. Name of an Elizabethan dish made of milk or cream, mixed with wine or brandy, sweetened and whipped. Also spelled as sillabub.

symbiotic algae. Green algae, most resembling the genus Chlorella, are found in many freshwater protozoa, sponges, hydra, and some flatworms. Most of these algae reproduce by simple cell division and are found within the host cell's vacuoles, which divide when the alga divides. Another green alga, Platymonas convolutae, is found mostly in the subepidermal cells of the marine flatworm. Within the flatworm, Platymonas has no cell wall and an irregular shape; its plasma membrane, greatly increased in surface area by fingerlike projections, is more or less in direct contact with the vacuole membrane of the host cell. When removed from the flatworm and cultured, Platymonas has a cell wall, four flagella and an eyespot, all lacking when it is symbiotic.

The most direct relationship between green algae and invertebrates involves certain nudibranchs, which are marine molluscs, and the chloroplasts of some siphonaceous green algae, such as Codium. The chloroplasts, which are presumably acquired when nudibranchs eat the algae, are found in cells that line their entire respiratory chamber. In the presence of light these chloroplasts carry on photosynthesis so efficiently that individuals of the nudibranch *Placobranchus ocellatus* are reported to evolve oxygen more rapidly than it its consumed. Certain dinoflagellates (division Pyrrophyta), which resemble the nonflagellated cells of Chlorella when they occur as symbionts, inhabit the cells of various marine sponges, coelenterates, molluscs, flatworms, and protozoa. In the giant clams of the family, *Tridachnidae,* the dorsal surface of the inner lobes of the mantle may appears chocolate-brown as a result of the presence of symbiotic algae of this group, which are found in the blood sinuses and probably occur mainly within amoeboid blood cells. Dinoflagellates are also important symbionts in reef-building corals. Coral tissues may contain as many as 30,000 microscopic algae/ml. The exact role of these algal symbionts in the coral economy is not known, but tracer studies using radioactive carbon have shown that organic substances pass from the algae to the coral, and it has also been shown that the reef grows much more rapidly when the algae are present. Even though the coral animals are heterotrophic, the reef as a whole is autotrophic.

syneresis. The shrinking of a gel with the expulsion of a free liquid stand (e.g., jelly or baked custard or cheese-making). In cheese-making, after cutting the curd and with an increase in acidity and temperature, the para-casein fibrils become more and more dehydrated and whey is expelled. This shrinking is an example of syneresis. Also known as weeping.

Syrah grape. A very high-quality red wine grape and is the red variety used in the production of Hermitage, renowned wine of the Rhone Valley. The variety also has been transplanted in Australia and California.

syringa. A group of hardy shrubs belonging to the olive and, according to early botanists, including the syringa, the lilac and the jasmines. The syringa, which is a favourite garden shrub, bears an abundance of single white flowers, noted for their fragrance.

syrup. A solution of sugar which may be from a variety of sources such as maple, corn, sorghum, and stage in refining such as top syrup, refiners syrup and sugar syrup. The product of refining is called golden syrup. Its average composition per 100 g is: water 20%; sugar 79%; protein 0.3%; 1.25 MJ, iron 1.5 mg; and food energy 1.25 MJ. The sugar solutions used for canning fruit are also syrups; light syrup - 15° Brix, syrup 20 or 30° Brix, heavy syrup - 30 or 40° Brix, extra heavy syrup - 40 or 50° Brix. (Degrees Brix = per cent sugar.)

systemic poison. A poison that is spread throughout the body of a living organism. The term is used both for poisons that act systemically (*i.e.*, that affect all parts of an organism) and for compounds that spread systemically without harming an organism but happen to be poisonous to the organism's enemies. Systemic poisons are useful as pesticides for ornamental plants but their use on fodder and food plants is not recommended.

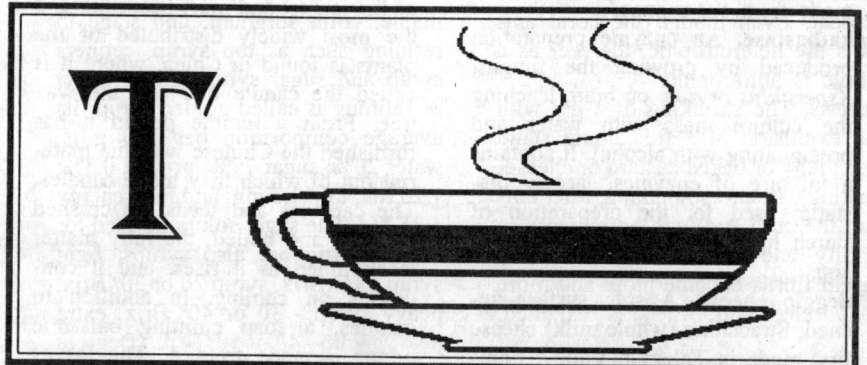

table beets. Table beets are grown in a wide range of soils and climates. Since beets produce their best colour and quality in a cool climate, they are grown in mild climates as fall, winter, and spring crops; in relatively mild, temperature climates as early-summer or late-fall crops; and in colder climates as summer and early-fall crops. For processing and where quick maturity is not important, Detroit Dark Red, Perfected Detroit, and Ruby Queen varities are most commonly grown. Certain varieties, such as Crosby green Top, are grown for beets greens, but other varieties can be used if harvested at the proper time. Monogerm varieties with superior quality and uniformity, such as Pacemaker, Mono-King, Explorer, and Monogerm, have been introduced in recent years. The ability to match the growing season with the prevailing climate enables the grower to achieve maximum yields.

Table beets are classified according to the shape of the root and the time of maturing. For example, Crosby's Egyptian, Green Top Bunching, Ruby Queen, and Early Wonder are flat or globular early-maturing varieties. Detroit Dark Red and Perfected Detroit are globular and medium-early-maturing varieties. Long Dark Blood, or Long Smooth Blood are late-maturing varieties. The root of most table beets are dark red or purplish. The dark red colour arises due to the presence of anthocyanins. However, when beets are grown in hot weather, the roots may develop light-coloured zones. In cool weather, these zones are less conspicuous. The light-coloured zones tend to disappear when the beets are cooked. Sugar content in the root is highest when beets are grown in cool temperatures and good sunlight. Crosby Egyptian and Early Wonder varieties are generally recommended when rapid growth to market size is desired. Both are slightly flattened and have alternate zones of purplish flesh in warm weather. Plantings that reach harvest stage in cool weather have darker flesh and less prominent differences in color zones.

tachysterol. One of the compounds produced (along with vitamin D_2 or calciferol) by ultraviolet irradiation of ergosterol. It has no antirachitic activity until it has been reduced to dihydrotachysterol, also called AT-10. It is also used for the treatment of deficiency thyroid functions.

tafia. An alcoholic spirit similar to rum; made from sugar cane.

takadiastase. An enzyme preparation produced by growing the fungus, *Aspergillus oryzae,* on bran, leaching the culture mass with water and precipitating with alcohol. It contains a mixture of enzymes, largely diastatic; used for the preparation of starch hydrolysates. Also known as koji.

Taleggio cheese. A soft, surface-ripened, Stracchino (whole milk) cheese first made in Taleggio Valley, Lombardy, Italy.

tall oil. An oily resinous liquid obtained as a by-product of the sulphite paper-pulp mills. The alkali saponifies the acids, and the resulting soap is skimmed off and treated with sulphuric acid to produce tall oil. The name comes from the Swedish talloel, meaning pine oil. The crude oil is brown, but the refined oil is reddish yellow and nearly odourless. It has a specific gravity of 0.98, flash point of 182°C, and acid number about 165. The oil from Florida contains 41-45% rosin, 10-15% pitch, and the balance chiefly fatty acids. The fatty acids can be obtained separately by fractionating the crude whole oil. The oil also contains up to 10% of the phytosterol sitosterol, used in making the drug cortisone. Tall oil is used in scouring soaps, asphalt emulsions, cutting oils insecticides, animal dips, in plastics and paint oils. It is marketed in processed and concentrated form.

Detergents are made by reacting tall oil with ethylene oxide. Saturated alcohols are produced by high-pressure hydrogenation of tall oil. The high linoleic acid content makes tall oil suitable for making drying oils.

tallow tree. The name of several trees which produce a tallow-like substance, used for making candles. One of the largest and most beautiful, and the most widely distributed of the plants is found in China, where it is called the candle tree and the wax tree. From a remote period it has furnished the Chinese with the material out of which they make candles. The capsules and seeds are crushed together and boiled; the fatty matter is skimmed as it rises, and it condenses on cooling. In addition to candles, a soap emitting balsamic odour is made from it. The leaves furnish a black dye; the stem yields a resinous substance, called copal, an ingredient in the making of varnishes

tallow. A solid fat, obtained from animals, especially cattle and sheep, by subjecting the carcasses to steam heat in closed kettles. Beef tallow of the best quality comes from the fat around the kidneys; that of a cheaper grade is obtained from the caul and other tissues. Tallow is purified by heating to a high temperature and then straining. When cold, it is white and hard, resembling lard, except that it is somewhat whiter. The most extensive use of tallow is in the manufacture of soap, candles, lubricants, and in dressing leather. A specially prepared tallow is used in making oleomargarine. A substance similar to animal tallow is obtained from certain trees.

tallow, rendered. Beef or mutton fat prepared from parts other than the kidney, by heating with water in an autoclave; used for soap and candles. When pressed separates to a liquid fraction, oleo oil, used in margarine, and a solid fraction, oleosterin, used for soap and candles.

tamales. Mixture of meat, spices and maize meal wrapped in corn husks or special paper.

tamarack. *Larix laricina.* Family: *Pinaceae.* A medium-sized tree of the Pine Family, usually 12-24 m tall and 0.3-0.6 m in diameter. The soft, flexible needles (leaves) are usually 2-2.5 cm long and 1 mm wide. they grow in clusters on the main, stubby branches of the tree, and singly on longer branchlets. Young bark to tamaracks is gray and darkens to a reddish-brown with age. The inner bark is dark reddish-purple. The twigs are orange-brown. Cones, rose red when young, darken to brown. The needles are light blue-green, turning to yellow in autumn. Each tamarack has both male and female reproductive parts, but they occur in separate cones. The tree depends on wind to carry pollen to female cones. Female cones are located higher up in the trees than the male cones, so pollen must be carried upward to the female cones of another tamarack. Tucked away between each closely packed scale of the female cones is a minute opening, waiting to receive pollen. Tiny, winged seeds develop in the summer and are released in the fall. The cones stay attached to the branches until the following summer. This species is common in wetlands such as bogs and swamps, but also grows well in moist, well-drained, light soils. It prefers unshaded areas, so it often grows alone or in association with other finely branched trees such as trembling aspen and white birch. Unlike most trees, the roots of the tamarack have special uses. The slender, fibre-like roots were used by Indians to sew together birch bark strips for canoes and to stitch wounds from wars and hunts. Thicker roots, bent at right angles, were prized by ship-builders for joining a ship's ribs to the deck timbers. The durable lumber is used for railroad ties, framing material for houses, poles and posts, boxes and crates, and pulpwood.

Tannin for tanning leather can be taken from the bark. The larch sawfly feeds on the needles, leading to damage or death to the tree. As unfortunate as this may seem, sawflies are an important food for insectivorous birds and the role tamaracks play in supporting sawflies is important in nature's complex food web. This unique tree is a popular ornamental choice in cooler climates. Also known as hackmatack; eastern larch.

tamarind. *Tamarindus indica.* A large, beautiful tree, native of the East and West Indies. Its pods are filled with a sweet, delicately flavored pulp, which, together with the seeds it contains, is preserved in sugar, packed in layers in casts. The seeds are used to make yellow and red dyes and eaten fresh and used in seasonings and curries. The wood, especially in the roots, is beautiful, but it is so hard that it is difficult to work. This is an evergreen tree which grows in tropical climates. The tree may achieve a height of over 24 metres when fully grown. The tree is cultivated for its acid fruits (sometimes called Indian dates) which find numerous uses. The alternate even-pinnate leaves have from 20-40 small, opposite, oblong leaflets and the pale yellow flowers have petals with red veins, growing in racemes at the ends of the branches. The fruit is a cinnamon-coloured oblong pod, from 10-20 cm long, within a thin, brittle shell enclosing a soft, brownish, acidulous pulp. The fruit is black with a sweet-sour taste. Commercial quantities of tamarind are produced in India, Egypt, Malaysia, and Sri Lanka. The aqueous concentrated extract (so-called) is concentrated juice and pulp and is used as a flavoring agent. It is frequently used in the preparation of beverages, curry powders, and many kinds of syrups. The average composition of tamarind (raw) per 100 g is: water 31.4%; protein 2.8 g; fat 0.6 g; carbohydrates (total) 62.5 g; fibre 5.1 g; ash 2.7 g; calcium 7.4 mg; phosphorus 113 mg; iron 2.8 mg; sodium 51 mg; potassium 781 mg; vitamin A (Intl. Units) 30; thiamine 0.34 mg; riboflavin 0.14 mg; niacin 1.2 mg; ascorbic acid 2 mg; food energy about 240 calories.

Tamie cheese. A kind of whole milk, rennet cheese made by the Trappists in Savoy, France. The method of manufacture is, to a large extent, a trade secret. It is similar to Tome de Beaumont.

tammy. A cookery term meaning to strain through a fine woolen cloth; a tammy cloth.

tangelo. A fruit which is hybrid between tangerine and grapefruit.

tangerine. A variety of orange, so named from Tangier, Morocco, where the first specimens were found. It is flatter and deeper in colour than the orange. The peel is easily removed from the pulp, which is sweet, juicy, and highly prized because of its flavour.

tankage. Ground, dried residue from slaughter house excluding all the useful tissues.

tannin. One of a mixed group of substances which, as defined by industry, combine with hide to form leather. Tannins are also used in dyeing and ink manufacture. Many plants accumulate tannins particularly in leaves, fruits, seed coats, bark, and heartwood. Tannins precipiate proteins and hence inactivate enzymes; they are therefore segrated in cell vacuoles, organelles, or cell walls. Chemically they are polymers derived either from carbohydrates and phenolic acids by condensation reactions, or from flavonoids.

tanners' greases. Trade name for various mixtures of waxes, sulfonated oils, and soaps; used for sponging or milling onto the leather.

tannia. Corm of *Xanthosoma sagittifolium;* known of new cocoyam in W. Africa; same family as taro. The average composition per 100 g of tannia is: 2 g protein; 0.4 g fat; 30 g carbohydrate; 1 mg iron; 0.1 mg vitamin B_1; 0.02 mg vitamin B_2; 0.6 mg nicotinic acid; 11 mg vitamin C; and 0.57 MJ food energy. Also known as tanier.

tansy. *Tanacetum vulgare.* A well-known plant of the Composite family, abundant in Europe, and naturalized in many parts of the world. It is a tall plant, with divided leaves and button-like heads of yellow flowers. Every part of the plant is bitter. Tansy tea is an old popular medicine, believed to be a fine tonic. Tansy is now cultivated in gardens, and grows along roadsides. The young leaves were formerly used for flavouring cakes, puddings, etc. It was a common cottage-garden herb in medieval times, when it was used as an insect repellent, a strewing herb, and as a source of orange dye. The use of tansy leaves in deserts was once so widespread that 'tansy' became the generic name for baked or boiled egg custard flavoured by infusion the leaves. It may be used in salads, egg dishes, and casseroles, but only in small quantities, In self-help medicine, the leaves were used as a digestive. Leaves and young shoots are used for flavouring food articles such as puddings and omelettes. Tansy cakes made with eggs and young leaves used to be eaten at Easter. Tansy tea made by infusing the herb formerly used as tonic and for intestinal worms. Root, preserved in honey or sugar, was used for gout.The flowers may be hung in a dry, airy place and used in dried flower arrangements. The dried leaves act as a powerful insect repellent, and were 'put up in bags' for this purpose. It may be noted that the herb should not be taken during pregnancy.

tapioca. *Manihot esculenta.* A starch food prepared from the roots of the cassava, a plant found in the tropics. It is called cassava in southern Asia, manioc in Brazil, mandioca in Paraguay, and yuca in Cuba. This perennial vegetatively propagated shrub was cultivated as far back as 2,500 years ago, and there is some indirect evidence that it has been grown for 4,000 years in the Americas. Its fresh roots contain 30-40% dry matter and have a starch content of approximately 85% of the dry matter. It is used in enormous quantities for food in some countries, and in some areas much is used for the production of alcohol. In the US it is valued for adhesives and coatings, and only a small proportion in globules and flakes, known as pearl tapioca, is used in foodstuffs.

Tapioca is used chiefly in the preparation of a nutritious pudding; it is also used in thickening soups, as when boiled it swells and forms a jelly-like mass. In preparing the substance for the market the roots are washed and ground to a pulp, and the mass is strained until the fibres are eliminated. The tapioca is then dried on hot iron plates, which causes the starch grains to form into small lumps.

The term is also used of starch in general as in manioc tapioca and potato flour tapioca. The commercial tapioca pearls commonly used in puddings comes from the starchy long, thick, tuberous roots of a half-woody shrub that grows anywhere from 1-4 metres high. These dark, brown, fat roots contain not only solid white starchy insides as potatoes do, but also considerable milky latex as well.

tapioca-macaroni. A mixture of 80-90 parts tapioca flour, with 10-12 parts of peanut flour, or tape, peanut, semolina, 60:15:25, baked into shapes resembling rice grains or macaroni shapes; developed in India. Also referred to as synthetic rice.

tare. The common name of different species of the pea family, known also by the name of vetch. There are numerous species and varieties of tares, but that which is found best adapted for agricultural purposes is the common tare, which flourishes in poor soils, and of which there are two principal varieties, the summer tare and the winter tare.

taro. Several perennial herbaceous plants of the genus *Colocasia* of the *Arum* family are commonly referred to as *taro* and, in some parts of the world, by the name *cocco* or *cocoyam.* These large and leafy plans are cultivated for their fleshy roots, which comprise a main foodstuff in parts of Polynesia and in southeast Asian countries. In some areas, the roots are called eddoes. The tubers contain a high percentage of starch, but considerably more protein than another common starchy vegetable, the potato. The leaves of taro plants are large and heart-shaped, resulting in one variety being called the elephant's ear. The plant is characterized by greenish flowers that resemble a call, without petals, a floral envelope, stamens, or pistils. The fruit of the plant is a berry. Many varieties and forms of taro are known to the natives of the Pacific islands. *Colocasia esculenta* is the principal and most commonly known form of taro. This is the main form of taro, cultivated in Hawaii, for example, and is the basis of poi. This paste-like material is prepared by steaming or boiling the tubers, after which they are peeled and pounded to form a mash. This mash is then permitted to ferment for several days. The average composition per 100 g is: 2 g protein; 25 g carbohydrate; 1 mg iron; 0.1 mg vitamin B_1; 0.04 mg vitamin B_2; 1 mg nicotinic acid; 4 mg vitamin C; and 0.5 MJ food energy. The taro is also eaten much as the potato, usually parboiled after which it is baked. The tender leaves of the taro plant, sometimes termed luau, are used as greens.

Tarocco orange. An Italian variety of blood orange. Flesh is medium-firm, fruit is juicy and usually well-pigmented. Flavour is rich and sprightly. The fruit ripens in midseason; widely planted in the Mount Etna region of Sicily. Production is mainly for the fresh market.

tarpon. A large game fish of giant strength. The tarpon is shaped something like the salmon. It attains a length of about 2 m. Tarpon fishing is a favourite sport, for this fish is a skilful fighter. Its flesh it too coarse for food; but its large, tough, silvery scales are used in ornamental work.

tarragon. Family: *Compositae.* Genus: *Artemisia.* Species: *Artemisia dracunculus.* Dried leaves and flowering tops of the bushy perennial plant has an antise-like flavour and is used to flavour vinegar, and pickles, and is one of the ingredients of *fines herbes.* In Europe it is cultivated for its aromatic leaves that impart a licorice-anise flavour to sauces salads and vinegary foods. It grows about 60 cm high and has long, narrow leaves, which, unlike other members of its genus, are undivided. Tarragon is closely allied to wormwood and has long, fibrous roots spreading everywhere by runners and small flowers in round, yellow-black heads that are seldom fully opened. Tarragon vinegar is made by steeping the fresh herb in white wine vinegar and is used in making sauce tartare and French mustard. Tarragon produce produces a volatile oil, estragon, which is used as a flavouring in liqueurs and in perfumery. Chemically the oil is the same as anise oil. These promotes digestion, and stimulates the appetite, heart and liver. Indeed the ancient herbalists used to call tarragon 'a friend to head, heart and liver'. It was formerly used for toothache and to promote appetite.

A distinction must be made between the true French tarragon or estragon and its Russian counterpart, *A. dracun-culoides,* which is much coarser, and is one of the four ingredients of the *fines herbes* mixture. It is one of the great culinary herbs of France, and has a battery of dishes created around it *poulet a letragon* and *oeufs engelle a lestragon,* to name just two. Tarragon has a strong and distinctive flavour, and must be used sparingly, especially as it is usually associated with delicate dishes such as chicken, white fish, creamy sauces, and egg and cheese recipes. Fresh springs of the herb are used to flavour vinegar for use in salad dressings and sauces.

tartar. Name given by the alchemists to animal and vegetable concretions, such as wine lees, stone, gravel and deposits on teeth, as they were all attributed to the same cause.

tartar emetic. Potassium antimonyl tartrate, produces inflammation of the gastrointestinal mucosa and used to be used as an emetic.

tartaric acid. COOH-CHOH-CHOH-COOH. Dihydroxysuccinic acid. It occurs in fruits, the chief source is grapes; used in preparing lemonade, added to jams when the fruit is not sufficiently acidic.

tartrazine. FD&C yellow no. 5. The trisodium salt of 3-carboxy-5-hydroxy-1-sulphophenyl-4-p-sulphophenyl-azopyrazole. It is an orange-yellow powder, which is very soluble in water 20% at 25°C) and glycerol (15% at 25°C) but much less soluble in the glycols (7% at 25°C). It is almost insoluble in ethanol (95 %). The solutions are golden-yellow and have good light stability. Tartrazine is very stable in acid and weakly alkaline media, but in the presence of strong alkalis it acquires a deeper reddish hue. It has been necessary to label the presence of this colour specifically, since it is structurally related to aspirin and a small segment of the population is allergic to it.

tartronate. Salt of tartronic (hydroxy-malonic) acid; suggested as coenzyme in the decarboxylation of oxalosuccinic acid in the citric acid cycle and also claimed as a dietary essential for the rat but not confirmed.

taste buds. Situated mostly on the tongue; about 9,000 elongated cells ending in minute hair-like processes, the gustatory hairs.

taurine. 2-aminoethyl sulphonic acid. A component of bile, in which it occurs combined with cholic acid to form taurocholic acid, a bile salt. It is formed from cysteine by oxidation and decarboxylation. There is some evidence that taurine may function as an inhibitory transmitter or modulator in the brain. It is a central depressant with antiepileptic activity and attempts to make analogues that might serve as useful antiepileptic drugs are underway. Taurine may also be involved in the control of Ca^{2+} fluxes in cardiac muscle cells.

tea. Family: *Ternstroemiaceae*. Genus: *Thea*. Species: *Thea sinensis*. The name applied to an oriental evergreen tree, to the leaves, a commercial article, and to the highly-regarded beverage prepared from them. In its natural state the trees is widely branching and attains a height up to 10 metres or more; under cultivation it is constantly pruned and kept at heights between 0.8-2 metres to increase the number of leaves. The leaves are dark green, shaped somewhat like those of the willow, and grow to be four inches long. The small, fragrant flowers are cream-coloured and are shaped like a double rose. It is not known where the plant originated. The beverage was drunk by the Chinese are early as the sixth century. It was introduced into Europe in the seventeenth century. Today the chief sources of supply are India, China, Ceylon, Japan, Java. In India, Java and Ceylon tea is grown on large plantations several hundred acres in extent; in the other tea growing countries it is cultivated on small pieces of ground and in gardens. The plants are grown from seeds under cover, and when four or five inches high are set out in rows, there being about ,1500 plants to an acre. The plants are commercially profitable when tree years old and reach full productivity at the age of five years. The crop is gathered three times a year, the second harvest yielding tea of the finest quality. The leaves are picked mostly by women and girl. They are then dried and withered and afterwards.

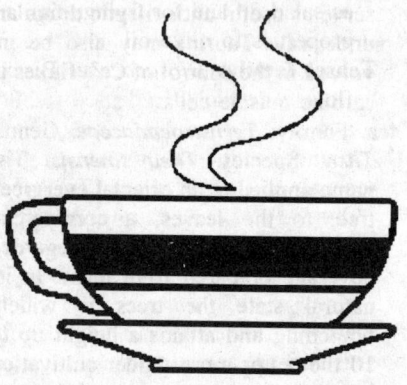

Different grades of tea are prepared from leaves of the same plant. They are all divided into two classes, green tea and black tea. To prepare what is commercially known as green tea, the leaves are roasted almost immediately after they are picked, rolled by hand to crack the veins and set the acids, and are then dried quickly to preserve the colour. Black teas go through a longer process of drying the roasting, and this causes them to turn black. The cheaper grades of green tea are often coloured with Prussian blue, powdered talc or some other colouring substance. In India and Ceylon the leaves are machine rolled (the more delicate leaves of the Chinese tea are not successfully prepared by machine-rolling, but are treated by hand). After the leaves are roasted, cutting machines break up the rolled leaves into small pieces. The leaves are then sifted and packed for shipment. Chinese green-tea brews do not contain the same deleterious sprays (like salts of copper) found in the usual imported varieties which cause our imported tea's bad effects, and in China this green tea is valued for its digestive properties, its ability to assist the circulation and regulate body temperature.

Black tea contains twice the amount of caffeine (2-4%) in coffee and apparently coffee got its bogus name of caffeine poisoner because people tended to brew it very strongly and so imbibe more caffeine. The theine in tea, like caffeine, makes it a very strong stimulant which excites the nervous system and can over secretion of gastric juices. The tannin in black tea inhibits the proper absorption of iron and can result in indigestion and lack of energy.

tea, partially fermented. A kind of tea prepared with the order of processing slightly changed. After moderate withering of the freshly picked leaves, they are modestly fermented, after which they are dried. Then the leaves are rolled, followed by a moderate steaming to halt fermentation action. Some authorities observe the oolong teas tend to combine the qualities of both black and green teas, but nevertheless have their own distinctions. Lapsang Souchong, grown near Star Village in the Wu-I Mountains of northern Fukien, is an oolong tea with a strong, mellow taste and an elusive smoky flavor. Oolong teas are sometimes scented and/or compressed. Formosa Oolong is considered to be a superior-quality oolong tea.

tea, unfermented. A kind of processed tea. The first step in the processing is steaming rather than withering the freshly picked leaves. Steaming, in addition to preventing fermentation, also makes the leaves quite pliable.

After rolling, as in the case of black tea, leaves pass through firing processes which kills any microorganisms that otherwise might discolor the leaves or commence fermentation.

Commercial grades of green tea include Hyson, Young Hyson, Imperial Hyson, gunpowder or pearl, and Twankay, among others. Specifically Chinese green tea include Chunmee and Sowmee, to mention a few.

Different kinds of green tea are produced mainly in China, Japan, India, and Indonesia.

The Hyson tea shrub has exceptionally large leaves. For Imperial Hyson, large round rolled leave are used.

Gunpowder or pearl tea consists of small, round, rolled leaves. Firing of the leaves can be accomplished in baskets or pans. Long leaves are fired in baskets, whereas the shorter leaves are fired in pans. Sometimes these designations are included in the name or specifications of these kinds of tea.

A less-mentioned category of tea is sometimes called white tea. These are unfermented tea leaves that require no rolling. This type of tea is a specialty of Fukien Province of China. Among the best of these is Flowery Pekoe. This is selected buds and tender leaves that are gathered from varieties of shrubs that have large leaves. The brewed tea has a pleasant, mild taste, is pale yellow in color, and has a relatively high tannin content. Another tea of this type is called Paimutan White. Also known as green tea.

tea drying. Leaves from the tea plant are at 88% moisture content when harvested which is followed by drying. Tea leaves are fermented from which an extract is made. The liquid extract may be concentrated to 25-30% solids

with a falling film evaporator from which the volatiles may be recovered. Drying of the concentrate may also be done with a vacuum continuous belt dryer or vertical spray dryer tower using air at 190°C.

teaseed oil. Oil from the seed of *Thea sasangua,* cultivated in China; used as salad oil and for frying; similar in properties to olive oil.

Teasel family: *Dipsacaceae.* Bisexual flowers develop in a dense head or on a spike. Individual flowers are surrounded at the base by a bract. Small sepals are jointed into a cup-shape or divided into 5-10 hairy or bristle-like segments. Petals are united into a tube with 4-2 stamens attached. The single pistil's ovary develops into a achene fruit. Plants in this small family usually are annual, biennial, or perennial herbs.

The family include: *Cephalaria, Morina, Pterocephalus, Scabiosa* (pincushion flower); *Dipsacus* (teasel, used in dry flower arrangements).

technical name. A recognized chemical name currently used in scientific and technical handbooks, journals, and texts. Generic descriptions authorized for use as technical names are organic phosphate compounds, organic phosphorus compound mixtures, methyl parathion, and parathion.

teff. Millet-like cereal grain; major protein of the diet of Ethiopia.

teichoic acids. The acessory polymers found specifically in bacterial cell membranes of gram-positive bacteria (as glycerol teichoic acids) or cell walls of Gram-positive bacteria (as ribitol techoic acid). They are linear polymers of glycerol phosphate or ribitol phosphate, respectively, with phosphodiester linkages.

Teleme cheese. A kind of peculiar pickled cheese made in Rumania,

Bulgaria, Greece and Turkey, from sheep's or goat's milk; sometimes known as Branza de Braila. It is cured for 8-10 days either in dilute salt brine or packed between layers of salt. The cheese, which is marketed in 8-10 days, is white and creamy.

tempeh. An Indonesian dish composed of soybeans which have been cooked and then fermented by the mold *Rhizopus oryzae.* The protein content of tempeh is about 20% on a wet basis and 50% when dried. It is very seldom eaten raw, but is usually roasted, cooked in soup, or fried in oil. The amino acid composition of the protein is not grossly altered by the fermentation process, although decreases in lysine and methionine have been reported. Steaming of the fermented product had little effect on its amino acid content, but as much as 20% of the cystine and lysine content was destroyed by deep-fat frying. Although tempeh is a research into its nutritive values has been conducted. One advantage of the product appears to be the elimination of some of the oligosaccharides during the cooking in water, which is believed to be cause of flatulence and indigestibility.

Tempetin. Trade name for textured vegetable protein.

Temple orange. A tangelo, that is, a hybrid between a sweet orange and mandarin. The hybrid is distinguished by easily parted sections, an attraction for use as a dessert fruit. The fruit is oblate, tapering slightly to the stem. The size ranges from medium to large and the colour is a deep-orange red. The rind is smooth or pebbled, leathery, thin, and relatively easy to peel. Its flavour is rich, vinous, spicy, and characteristic. Acidity and sweetness are well-blended. The Temple variety has about 20 seeds and is less frost-resistant than most mandarins and more tender to cold than the sweet orange. Commercially, Temple variety is generally considered and marketed as an orange and thus included in the table. It could equally well be considered a mandarin.

tenderizer. In food technology, a term that usually refers to the enzyme papain, when used to tenderize meat. Weak acids such as vinegar and lemon juice and 2% sodium chloride also tenderize meat.

tepary bean. *Phaseolus acutifolius.* A small bush when grown on dry soil, but a spreading, twining plant when in richer soil. The pods are from 5-10 cm long and contain about 4-6 seeds, ranging from white to black and having a prominent beak. The plant has been cultivated by American and Mexican Indians for at least a few centuries, but only comparatively recently has it received the serious attention of agronomists as an attractive, drought-resistant crop. Farmers in Arizona and New Mexico have recognized the value of the tepary as an excellent dry shell bean and as a good crop for soil restoration.

tequila. Distilled liquor obtained from a fermented mash made from the cultivated cactus *Agave tequilane;* 90-100 degrees proof; common in Mexico. Mescal is similar but made from the mescal Agave, which grows wild, and is much cheaper.

terminal enzyme. An enzyme that catalyzes the addition of nucleotides to the terminal of a nucleic acid strand in the absence of a template, with nucleoside triphosphates serving as substrates.

terpenes. The class of organic compounds characterized by the presence of the repeating units of isoprene. The name terpene used properly refers to the hydrocarbons which are exact multiples of the skeletal isoprene unit. However the name terpene, sometimes used loosely include not only hydrocarbons but also other functional types of naturally occurring organic compounds which contain the reoccurring isoprene skeletal. In strictest sense, the name terpenoid or isoprenoid should be used instead of the more loosely applied usage of terpene. Terpenoids are divided into subclasses namely: hemiterpenoids, monoterpenoids, sesquiterpenoids, diterpenoids, sesterterpenoids, triterpenoids, Tetraterpenoids, and polyterpenoids.

Although terpenes constitute about 90-95% of citrus oils they are not responsible for the characteristic flavour, and as they readily oxidize and polymerize to produce unpleasant flavours they are removed from citrus oils by distillation or solvent extraction leaving the so-called terpeneless oils. Further, the terpenes are not very soluble so that unless they are removed the oils cannot be used for flavouring beverages and clear jellies.

tertiary structure. The irregular three-dimensional folding of the polypeptide chain upon itself, as in a globular protein, that results from the interaction of amino acid side chains which are either close or far apart along the chain; the arrangement in space of all the atoms of protein or of a subunit without regard to the relationship of the atoms to neigbouring of the atoms to neigbouring molecules or subunits. The term may likewise be applied to the three-dimensional structure of a polynucleotide strand.

tertiary treatment. Any sewage purification process which is capable or removing over 98% of the pollutants from sewage, following a secondary treatment plant. During the past few years several methods by which effluents from percolating filters may be improved or 'polished' have been examined. These methods have included the use of microstrainers for the treatment of effluent direct from the filters and the treatment of humus tank effluents by irrigation over land and by passage through slow sand filters, lagoons, or pebble-bed clariers. Polishing is also described as advanced water treatment or tertiary treatment.

Using a polishing process, a effluent may be much improved, both the BOD and the suspended solids beings less than 10 ppm. For example, treatment by addition of ferric alum, followed by filtration and chlorination will yield a clear colourless water free from bacteria contamination suitable for many industrial purposes. Rapid sand filters are also used in tertiary treatment. Most of the straining is effected by the top layers of sand. Rapid filters are easier to clean in comparison to the slow sand filters and the area required is much less. About a 40-70% reduction in BOD and a 70-90% reduction of suspended solids is achieved by this method. A considerable amount of interest has recently been shown in the application of upflow filtration techniques for the tertiary treatment of sewage works effluent.

Terzolo cheese. The Italian term used to differentiate between Grana type cheese made in winter and Maggengo (April to September) and Quartirolo (September to November).

testa. In reference to cereal grains the test is a fibrous layer between the pericarp and the inner aleurone layer.

testosterone. A naturally occuring androgen secreted by the testis under the influence of luteinizing hormone. Its secretion during adult life is responsible for the development, function, and maintainance of secondary male sexual characteristics, male sex organs, and spermatogenesis. Testosterone is also secreted from the adrenal cortex and the ovaries. It is metabolized in the liver, its metabolites (*e.g.,* androsterone) being excreted in the urine. The most significant metabolic product of testosterone is dihydrotestosterone (DHT). The reaction is catalyzed by 5α-reductase, an NADPH-dependent enzyme. Testosterone can thus be considered a phoromone, since it is converted into a much more potent compound. A small fraction of testosterone is also converted into estradiol by aromatization. Androstanediol, another potent androgen, is also produced from testosterone.

tetanus. A bacterial disease of livestock and man which enters the body *via* wounds, particularly from the soil. Muscles become stiff, spasms may occur, and the muscles which close the jaws may become continuously contracted. Also known as lockjaw.

tetany. Over-sensitivity of motor nerves to stimuli, particularly affects face, hands and feet; caused by reduction in the level of ionized calcium in the bloodstream and can accompany severe rickets.

Tete de Moine. *See* Bellelay cheese.

tetracyclines. A group of broad-spectrum antibiotics that inhibit the binding of aminoacyl transfer RNA to 70S ribosomes. Chemically they are based on the tetracycline nucleus, and various substituent groups are introduced to produce chlorotetracycline, dimethylchlorotetracycline, doxycycline, methacycline, minocycline, oxytetracycline, and tetracycline. The

first tetracyclines (chlorotetracycline, oxytetracycline and demeclocycline) were obtained from Streptomyces species. The remaining members of the group (tetracycline, methacycline, doxycycline, clomocycline, minocycline) are either prepared from the naturally occurring compounds or are totally synthetic.

Tetracyclines are bacteriostatic, with activity against Gram-positive and Gram-negative bacteria, mycoplasmas, ricketisiae, and chlamydias. Their activity against Gram-positive organisms is less than that of penicillins. Tetracyclines inhibit protein synthesis in microorganims by binding to ribosomes and preventing peptide binding. Microorganisms can develop side-resistances to other members of the group, and there may be cross-resistance with chloramphenicol. They act by binding to the 30 S subunit of the bacterial ribosomes and to mRNA.

They are used in some countries for preserving food and, when added to animal feed at the rate of a few mg per ton, improve growth. Of special use for poultry; the bird is dipped in solution of 10 mg/L and, when stored at 5°C, shelf life is extended from 10-14 to about 17-21 days. It has been noticed that about 2 mg/L of the antibiotic is left in the poultry, and is much reduced on cooking. Tetracyclines are also of great value in extending the storage life of fresh fish by 2-3 days, by adding 5 mg/L antibiotic to the ice or chilled water, or by dipping fillets into water containing 5-20 mg/L.

tetraodontin poisoning. The food poisoning caused by consuming fish of *Tetraodontidae* family (puffer fish) and amphibia of *Salamandridae* family due to toxins in the entrails. There are about 90 toxic species of puffer fish (fugu, blowfish, globefish, porcupine fish, molas, burrfish, balloonfish, and toadfish). The etiologic agent is tetradotoxin (tetraodontoxin.) It is a neurotoxin (paralysis of central nervous system and peripheral nerves). The toxin is stable to boiling except in alkaline solution. Toxin is water-soluble. The toxin mainly attacks nerve endings by blocking movements of all monovalent cations. Onset of illness usually occur within 10-45 minutes after ingestion, although it may be delayed up to 3 hours. Symptoms including tingling or prickly sensation of fingers and toes, malaise, dizziness, pallor; numbness of lips, tongue, extremities; ataxia, nausea, vomiting, diarrhea, epigastric pain, dryness of skin, subcutaneous hemorrhages and desquamation; eyes fixed, reflexes lost, respiratory distress; muscular twitching, tremor, incoordination, muscular paralysis, intense cyanosis. Case fatality rates s close to 60%. Best prevention is complete avoidance of eating puffers. The sale of puffers in Japan is governed by regulation. Puffer cooks and restaurants must be licensed. Proof of experience in preparing puffers is required.

Possibly, the most common of the food-borne diseases of fungal origin is that caused by the mycotoxins present in certain variety of mushroom. There are however, a number of mycotoxicosis diseases emanating from other fungal sources. Also known as puffer fish poisoning.

tetrapack. Tetrahedral cartons used to pack milk, oils, and beverages; used widely in India and many other countries where milk solid in self-service stores; it is more expensive than reusable glass bottles.

tewfikose. A sugar once claimed as distinct from lactose obtained from the milk of the Egyptian buffalo.

Texatrein. Trade name for textured vegetable protein made by extrusion.

Texgran. Trade name for textured vegetable protein.

textured vegetable protein. Spun or extruded vegetable protein made to simulate meat.

theine. Alternative name for caffeine.

Thenay cheese. A kind of soft, whole-milk cheese resembling Camembert and Vendome varities, made around Thenay, France. It is of comparatively recent origin and its consumption is limited practically to the region where it is produced. It is about 12 cm in diameter and 10 cm in height. The cheese is placed in well ventilated rooms for 20 days during which time it becomes covered with mold. The mold is removed and the cheese is cured for another 15 days.

therapeutic diets. The diets formulated to treat disease or metabolic disorders.

thermal death point. The lowest temperature required for the sterilization of a standard suspension of bacteria in 10 minutes.

thermal death time. The minimum time required for the sterilization of a standard suspension of bacteria at a given temperature.

thermization. Heat treatment, less severe than pasteurization, e.g., heat treatment of milk for cheese-making whereby the number of organisms is diminished.

thermoduric. Bacteria that are heat resistant but not thermophilic. Such kind of bacteria are found in milk. They survive pasteurization temperatures but do not develop at them. Usually not pathogens but indicative of insanitary conditions.

thermolysin. A proteolytic enzyme from the thermophilic bacterium *Bacillus termoproteolyticus Rokko*.

thermopeeling. A method of peeling tough-skinned fruits in which the fruit is rapidly passed through an electric furnace at about 900° C then sprayed with water.

thiamine. A water soluble, white, crystalline compound of yeasty odour and salty-nutlike flavour. It is not easily destroyed by oxidation, nor by heat if it is in acid solution, but deteriorates rapidly in alkaline or neutral media. It is essential for complete carbohydrate metabolism; and is a factor in prevention and cure of beriberi and polyneuritie; stimulates appetite; promotes good muscular tone in the intestinal tract and general good health. Rich sources of thiamine are dry brewers' yeast, husks and germs of grains such as wheat, barley, oats, rice, etc., and in whole grain or enriched food products made from grains. It is found in milk to the extent of about 0.4 mg/L and in fruits and is also produced synthetically.

The unusual features of thiamine include:

(a) blood contains most cocorboxylase in leukocytes.

(b) exerts a hormonal function in plants, controlling root growth;

(c) easily poisoned by heavy metals, acetyl iodide;

(d) aids phosphorylation in liver; dephosphorylation in kidney;

(e) not available from intestinal bacteria,

(f) plant and animal cocarboxylases are identical;

(g) exerts a diuretic effects and is constipative; and

(h) can be allergenic on injection.

Factors which contribute to a lessening of thiamine bioavailability include:

(a) Cooking, inasmuch as the vitamin is heat labile and water soluble;

(b) presence of certain enzymes in food, such as thiaminase for vitamin breakdown;

(c) presence of live yeast and alkalis;

(d) destruction by nitrites and sulfites;

(e) destruction by calcium carbonate, dibasic potassium phosphate, and manganous sulphate; and

(f) diuresis and gastrointestinal diseases.

An increase in availability can result from:

(a) presence of cellulose in diet which increases intestinal synthesis;

(b) storage capacity in heart, liver, and kidney;

(c) simulation of bacterial synthesis in intestine.

Antagonists of thiamine include pyrithiamine, oxythiamine, and 2-n-butyl homologue. Synergists include vitamins B_2, B_6 B_{12}, and niacin, pantothenic acid, and somatotrophin (growth hormone).

thiaminase. An enzyme present in many species of fish that hydrolyses thiamine and can therefore cause vitamin B_1 deficiency.

thiochrome. Compound to which vitamin B_1, can be oxidized (for example, by potassium ferricyanide) and which gives a strong blue fluorescence in ultraviolet light. This is caused as an assay of the vitamin.

threshold limit value. TLV. The quantity referring to the airborne concentrations of substances and represent conditions under which it is believed that nearly all workers may be repeatedly exposed day after day without any adverse effect. Because of wide variation in individual susceptibility, however, a small percentage of workers may experience discomfort from other substances at concentrations at or below the threshold limit; a smaller percentage may be affected more seriously by aggravation of a preexisting condition or by development of an occupational illness.

thrombin. A proteolytic enzyme that converts the soluble protein fibrinogen into the fibrous fibrin during blood clotting. It is formed from prothrombin under the influence of thromboplastin, calcium ions, and other factors, which are activated when blood is removed from the circulation, usually by injury. Thrombin is not normally found in circulating blood, but instead is repressed by its inactive precursor prothrombin. The conversion of prothombin to thrombin requires the presence of blood platelets, calcium ions, and thromboplastin.

thrombokinase. A substance liberated from damaged tissue and blood platelets; converts prothrombin to thrombin in the coagulation of the blood. Also known as thromboplastin.

thromboplastin. *See* thrombokinase.

thumping. An act performed by a grader of Swiss cheese. Thumping is done to locate the eyes or absence of eyes in the cheese. This is done by rapping the cheese with the fingers. The presence of eyes in the interior of the cheese produces a hollow sound. A blind cheese will not emit the same sound.

Thunberg tube. A test-tube carrying a curved hollow stopper that is used to hold one of the reactants; the whole tube can be evacuated through a sidearm. It is used to study oxidation reactions where it is necessary to keep reactants separate until oxygen has been removed from the system.

thuricide. Name given to a living culture of *Bacillus thuringiensis* which is harmless to man but kills off insect pests. Known as a microbial insecticide; it is used to treat certain foods and fodder crops to destroy pests such as corn earworm, flour moth, tomato fruit worm, cabbage looper, etc. The bacillus is mass-produced and stored like a chemical.

thyme. Family *Labiatae*. Genus. *Thymus*. Species: *Thymus vulgaris* (common or garden thyme). Thyme is the general name for the many herbs of the *Thymus* species, all of which are small, perennial plants native to Europe and Asia. Common or garden thyme is considered the principal type and is utilized commercially for flowering and ornamental purposes. This low-growing, woody shrub has grey-green leaves and white, pink or purple flowers. Thyme is produced and collected in most European countries, including France, Spain, Portugal, and Greece.

The three principal varieties of thyme are English, French and German, and they differ in leaf shape, leaf colour and essential oil composition. Dried leaves and flavouring tops of *Thymus vulgaris* are used in sausage and as flavouring in soup, meat, fish and poultry dressing. Garden thyme contains 1% of volatile oil that is composed mainly of thymol and carvacrol, along with minor amounts of many other aroma chemical constituents include tannins, flavonoids, phenolic acids such as caffeic acid and chlorogenic acid and triterpene acids.

Much of the cultivated garden thyme both in Europe and in the US is used in the production of thyme oil. This oil is used as a flavouring agent in processed foods, as well as in pharmaceutical and cosmetic products. It is also used as an antiseptic, anti-spasmodic, carminative and counterirritant or rubefacient, and in commercial products like cough drops, ear drops, mouthwashes and some feminine hygiene products.

The biological effect of garden thyme is due to thymol and/or carvacrol. Both of these have antibacterial and antifungal properties, as well as antispasmodic, carminative and expectorant properties, thymol being the most dominant. They also have anti-parasitic effects particularly against hookworms. Both are irritant to the skin and when ingested by accident can cause nausea, vomiting, stomach ache, headache, dizziness and even convulsions and coma if taken in large quantity, as well as subsequent cardiac and respiratory collapse.

In China, wild thyme has been used for treating arthritis and rheumatoid arthritis. In Western countries, it is used to treat asthma, and children's respiratory conditions as well as bedwetting and diarrhoea. It is also recommended for chronic gastric inflammations and is an excellent mouthwash for periodonthritis as well as a superb gargle for throat infections. It can also be used externally for itchy eczema as long as the skin is not broken. Occasionally, a wild thyme wine is used for treating traumatic injuries that make the whole body ache. It is taken internally. The wine is easily made by soaking 65 g of dried thyme in 1 litre of white wine for 24 hours and then straining.

thymic hormones. Hormones synthesized within the epithelial cells of the thymus gland and released into the general circulation, affecting the development and maintenance of the immune response. The hormones include thymosin, facteur thymique serique (FTS), and the thymic humoral factors.

thyroglobulin. The protein-bound form in which thyroxine and tri-idothyronine exist in the thyroid gland; it is broken down under the influence of the thyroid-stimulating hormone of the pituitary gland to liberate the free hormones which pass into the blood stream. Here they travel in combination with plasma protein as the so-called protein-bound iodine (PBI). The concentration of PBI in the blood is thus an index of thyroid activity.

thyroid-stimulating hormone. TSH. A hormone, synthesized and secreted by the adenohypophysis, that stimulates the thyroid gland to produce the hormones thyroxine and triiodothyronine. The production of TSH is itself controlled by negative feedback from the thyroid hormones. Also known as thyrotrophin.

thyroxine. An iodine-containing polypeptide hormone that is secreted by the thyroid gland and is essential for normal cell metabolism. Its effects include increasing oxygen consumption and energy production. It is used therapeutically to treat hypothyroidism (cretinism and myxoedema.

tichiniasis. *See* trichinosis.

Tillmans-Luckenbach test. A test for the detection of neutralizers in cream. This method is based on the difference in buffer action, while passing through a given pH range, of the serum from a normal cream which may or may not be sour and that of a cream to which a neutralizer has been added.

Tilsit, ragnit cheese. A variety of hard, rennet cheese made in East Persia from the whole milk of cows. The cheese is from 15-30 cm in diameter, 8-10 cm in height. It is a medium-firm, slightly yellow cheese; it is similar to brick, with mechanical openings and in some cases round eyes and has a medium to sharp piquant flavour similar to a mild Limburger. Sometimes caraway is added.

tin. Tin, one of the ancient metals, was known before 3500 BC. Bronze is an alloy of tin and copper. The general importance of the metal need not be stressed. Though used widely, lasting harmful effects from exposure to tin and its compunds in industrial applications or via the food chain have not been much reported. Inorganic tin is poorly absorbed from mucous membranes and the gastrointestinal tract. Containers for food and liquid are plated with the metal because of its corrosion-resistant qualities and the ease with which it can be soldered. Electrical, radio, and automobile parts are coated with tin. A benign respiratory disease, stannosis, resulting from exposure to dust or fumes of tin or tin oxide has been described. Stannic chloride (tin tetrachloride) used in weighting silks and as a stabilizer for colours in soaps and fabrics among others, can be highly irritating to the mucous membranes and eyes.

In earlier days, there was a traditional belief in parts of France that tin and its compounds were of value in controlling furunculosis (boils). The basis of the use of tin powder probably stemmed from the observation that the tin workers in Beauve never seemed to suffer from boils. Ingestion of stannous oxide did little good, butter neither did it do any harm. However, the dispensing of alkyl tin compounds led to a tragedy. A proprietary preparation, 'Stalinon', containing diethyl tin, traces of triethyl tin and linoleic acid was sold throughout France prior to 1960 for treating furuncles, other skin infections due to staphylococci, and osteomyelitis.

Foods, standing in contact with the tin plating of a can, accumulate large quantities of tin. As with other metals higher levels are leached by acidic foods such as tomato soups and ketchup. Fresh tomatoes were found to contain 0.02 µg/g of tin, while tomato soup contained about 1 µg/g. Coating the tins with a lacquer or resin will inhibit leaching of tin. A study comparing tin contents of foods packed in resin-coated and non-coated tin-plated cans indicated that while the resin coating remained intact, the quantity of tin leached out by foods in the former was reduced by a factor of 50. As expected, tin contents of foods packed in non-tin containers is considerably less. It has been demonstrated that tin is an essential nutrient for the growth of rats. The mechanism of biochemical activity of tin is not fully understood. It may act as an oxidation-reduction catalyst. Specific biochemical lesions associated with tin deficiency have not been described.

tisane. A French term for a kind of medicinal tea or infusion made from herbs (camomile, lime blossoms, fennel seeds, etc.)

titanium dioxide. TiO_2. An inorganic colouring pigment , which is a dense white, tasteless, odourless, infusible powder. It is insoluble in either cold or hot water or dilute acids. The purified food grade is used in the panning of sugar confectionery. Although it disperses readily in liquids, it tends to settle out unless the liquid is viscous (*e.g.*, sugar syrup).

tobacco. A plant of the nightshade family, extensively cultivated for its leaves, which are used for smoking and chewing and for snuff. There are several species, but that known botanically as *Nicotiana tobacum* is the one most extensively cultivated. It has an erect stem, that grows from 1.2-2.5 metres high and produces at the top a cluster of small, rose-colored flowers. The leaves are the important part of the plant. They are oblong and pointed and grow directly from the stalk, often attaining a length of 50-70 cm and a breadth of 20-25 cm. The plant is slightly poisonous, owing to the presence of nicotine.

tobacco curing. The process of using heat to reduce the moisture content of the leaves from 80-20%. Tobacco is harvested when some leaves begin to yellow. The heat used in drying is also the first step in fermenting. Without fermentation, tobacco smoking would be like smoking cabbage. Four general methods are used for curing, depending on the weather, region, type of tobacco, and use fire, flue, air and sun curing.

tobasco sauce. Tobasco peppers are macerated, fermented and left to cure for periods up to three years, then bottled with vinegar.

tocopheronic acid. A water soluble degradation product of α-tocopherol (vitamin E) isolated from the urine of animals fed tocopherol, together with tocopheronolactone, the lactone of tocopheronic acid, which is highly vitamin-E active.

toffee. A sweetmeat that is essentially a dispersion of minute globules of fat in a supersaturated sugar solution.

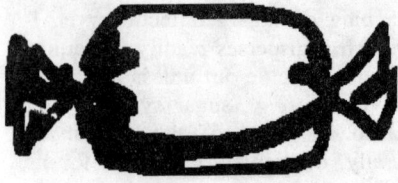

It is made from fat, milk, sugar and confectioners glucose. No real distinction between toffees and caramels except that toffees are boiled at a slightly higher temperature, 260-270°C compared with 250-255°C for caramels. Toffees contain water 5%, sugars 65%, protein 3%, fat 20%, along with traces of vitamins and other nutrients.

tofu. A Japanese product, soybean curd. It contains 5-8% protein, 3-4% fat, 2-4% carbohydrate and 84-90% water.

tomatine. An antifungal substance isolated from wilt-resistant tomatoes.

tomato. Family: *Solanaceae*. Genus: *Lycopersicum*. Species: *Lycopersicum esculentum*. A plant belonging to the nightshade family, same family as the potato and the egg plant. It is a native to the Andes region of South America and has been introduced into most warm or temperate countries. Is cultivated for its fruit, which is fleshy, usually scarlet or orange in colour and irregular in shape. Tomatoes are eaten raw or cooked, are used in salads, and the juice is a refreshing drink. For a long time after it was brought from Peru, the tomato was known as the love apple, and was considered poisonous. The earliest tomatoes were harvested by the Incus of the Andes, but later carried to Europe by the Spanish conquistadores. These small, yellow fruits were about the size of today's cherry tomatoes. But fear and ignorance, to a certain extent, kept them from becoming very popular, especially in France and UK. Even when reintroduced to America, they were still thought of as being poisonous, just like other members of the deadly nightshade group happen to be. The Ceroles in New Orleans finally brought tomatoes into the kitchen in 1812, but another half a century had to pass before other sections of the country got up enough courage and curiosity to try them. But even then the tomato's troubles were not over.

Botanically, they are really fruits, which confused many people because they are most often used like vegetables. Finally, it took a ruling by the Supreme Court in 1893 to reclassify the tomato as an official vegetable. Varieties of tomatoes available today include the large, all-purpose beefsteak types; the oval plum variety, used chiefly for cooking purposes; the small, tasty cherry tomato, often served in salads and the large, yellow or orange, low-acid tomatoes.

Tomatoes are an excellent source of vitamins A and C, have a high sugar and water content, and are also high in fibre, potassium and folic acid. The citric, malic and oxalic acids in them will stir up the activity of silicon in the body, loosening stiffs joints and so eventually relieving chronic arthritis. Tomatoes are often picked green and ripened during transportation, these are less nutritious than vine-ripened tomatoes. The green parts of the plant contain poisonous alkaloids and should not be eaten. The tomato is believed to be a natural antiseptic and protects against infection. Copious consumption of tomatoes would help the skin by purifying the blood, and help with gout, rheumatism, TB, hypertension and sinus troubles. There are also indications that tomato is good for cases of congestion of the liver, for dissolving gallstones, for relieving gas in the stomach, and for colds and obesity. A poultice applied to a troubled skin externally is also helpful. The nicotinic acid in tomatoes is believed to reduce cholesterol in the blood, and the vitamin K is an anti-haemorrhage. Summer tomatoes have more vitamin C than winter ones and those staked high as especially rich in this vitamin. Green, unripe tomatoes have slightly more calories, carbohydrate and vitamin A than ripe tomatoes. Boiled tomatoes are nutritionally similar to ripe tomatoes but have a fractionally higher vitamin A content (1000 IU for 100 g compared to 900 IU for the same fresh weight). Canned tomatoes are similar to fresh tomatoes but have less calcium, more sodium and less potassium. Diet canned tomatoes have a very low sodium content. Canned or bottled tomato juice is nutritionally similar to canned tomatoes, but has less fibre, less vitamin A and slightly fewer calories. Tomato puree has more calories, carbohydrate, sodium and vitamins than ripe tomatoes. The average composition per 100 g is: protein 1.1%; fat 0.3%; calcium 10 mg; iron 0.6 mg; vitamin A 200 mg; vitamin B_1 0.05 mg; vitamin B_2 0.03 mg; nicotinic acid 0.5 mg; vitamin C 25 mg; and food energy 0.08 MJ.

tomato drying. Sliced tomatoes may be dried on trays to make flakes. Two-stage tunnel dryers are generally employed to dry upto 4% moisture content. The slices are made into flakes or powder. A more popular procedure is to make a tomato puree, adjusted to 20% moisture content, and dried on a double drum dryer. Sulphur dioxide is used as a means of reducing scorching of particles and flavor deterioration. The product is dried to 2% moisture content to minimize caking.

tomato ketchup. Preparation of tomato puree, sugar, vinegar, salt and spices. Legally in UK, it must contain not less than 6% by weight of tomato solids excluding seeds and other coarse substances. No fruit other than tomato may be used except onion, garlic and spices. "Ketchup" or "catsup" derived from Chinese "koechiap" or "kitsiap" which is the brine of pickled fish, and now applied to a thick sauce made from pulp of fruits such as tomato or green walnuts. Also known as catsup; catchup; tomato sauce.

tomato seed oil. The oil obtained from the seeds of the tomato, *Lycopersicon esculentum,* the seeds being byproducts of the manufacture of tomato juice and tomato puree, vast quantities of which are produced in the US from the pulp. The seeds yield 17% oil by cold pressing, or 33% by solvent extraction. The cold-pressed oil is a clear liquid of 0.920 specific gravity, with an agreeable odour and bland taste. The iodine number is 113, and saponification value 192. It is used in salad oils, margarine, soaps, and as a semidrying oil for paints.

tome de Beaumont. A variety of French cheese made from cow's whole milk. The fine-cut curd is placed in cloth lined molds 18 cm in diameter and is pressed for 6-8 hours. The cheese is salted and cured for 5-6 weeks.

Tonkan mandarin. A variety of mandarin. Like the Ponkan, this is very old variety of mandarin native to the Far East and mainly grown in that region. The variety is intimately associated with ancient Chinese citriculture. The fruit is pyriform-shaped and somewhat smaller in size than the Ponkan. The rind is thick and rough, somewhat brittle, and adheres moderately. Many strains have developed from the Tonkan and have been commercially produced in the Far East and some other regions of the world. The internal color of the fruit is a deeporange. Maturity is medium to late. Shipping quality is considered good.

The tree has all of the characteristics of a mandarin, but the fruit exhibits some of the qualities of sweet orange and thus some authorities believe that the Tonkan may have arisen as a cross: Sweet orange x Mandarin hybrid.

Topfen cheese. A variety of sour-milk cheese manufactured in Germany from skim milk and eaten while fresh. It is packed in small packages.

Topfer's reagent. Dimethylaminoazobenzene; an indicator with a pH range 2.9-4.0, changing red to yellow. It is often used in titration of the acidity of gastric contents as it changes colour only in the presence of free hydrochloric acid.

toppings. During as last several years, there has been a strong trend toward the replacement of whipping cream with various substitute toppings. These usually are marketed in a prewhipped form, often in an aerosol dispenser. A representative formula would include the following:

Vegetable fat, ranging from 24 to 35%; protein, 1-6%; sugar, 6-15% (unless low-calorie type); corn (maize) syrup solids, about 0.05%; gum stabilizers, 0.01%; stabilizing salts, from 0-0.15%; with the remaining content being water.

tortillas. Flat circular cakes made from whole maize that has been soaked in water containing lime, boiled, ground and cooked; eaten in Central America. The lime appears to add considerable amounts of calcium to diet. There are two major kinds of tortillas, the older type developed by American Indians and made from the wheat flour tortilla. The corn tortilla is almost always unleavened, while some flour tortillas include a small amount of baking powder. Tortillas are used not only as a staple food (as rice, bread, pasta, and potatoes are used in other areas of the world) but also as a base for tacos, enchiladas, burritos, envueltos, flautas, and other items of Mexican cuisine. In these applications, tortillas may be baked, fried, used as a soup ingredient, etc. In a commercially significant development, they also form the basis of some of the fried snack chips sold in very large mounts in the US the masa tortilla is always made from alkali-treated corn dough. The method for tortilla preparation varies between geographical areas and ethnic groups. The description that follows is generalization of most of the home processes. Preparation starts with the addition of one part of whole dry corn kernels to two parts of a solution containing about 1% (corn weight basis) hydrated lime. This mixture is heated for 50-90 minutes and then allowed to stand for about 12-14 hours. The liquid is decanted, and the remainder, consisting of gelatinized corn kernels called nixtamal, is washed two or three times with water. The germs are usually not removed by the washing procedure, and parts of the skins also remain. The nixtamal is ground to a smooth dough, called masa. About 35-50 g of masa are hand patted into a disc about 15-20 cm in diameter and 2 mm to 3 mm thick. This cake is cooked or toasted on a heated flat surface for about 1-2 minutes. When it swells, the cake is turned over the cooked on the other side for about 30 seconds.

torularhodin. Carotenoid pigment in red yeast, *Torula rubra,* with vitamin A activity.

torulin. Antibiotic produced during aerobic culture of *Torula utilis.*

total bacteria count method. An important method by which the total number of bacteria is counted which are present in 1 ml of water. In this method, usually 1 ml of diluted water (1 ml of sample water is diluted to 100 ml, if required) is mixed with 10 ml of gelatine and then kept in incubator at 37°C for about 24 hours. The sample is taken out from the incubator and the bacterial colonies are counted; the dilution factor and number of colonies usually give the total number of bacteria present in every mililitre of water sample which is undiluted.

Touareg cheese. A kind of skim-milk cheese made by the Berber tribes, from the Barbary States to Lake Chad in Africa. It is a very hard, dry, unsalted cheese. To curdle the milk, some of the natives use the leaves of a Korouroutree.

Touloumisio cheese. A kind of Greek, Feta-like, cheese made in skin bags. The drained, salted curd is placed in wooden barrels until firm, then washed thoroughly and cut into small pieces, which are put in skin bags and covered with milk or whey to cure. During curing the bags are opened to permit the gas, formed by fermentation, to escape.

tous-les-mois. A variety of arrowroot, used as a source of starch.

tower spray dryer. A device for removing moisture having a chamber in the shape of a vertical tower in which the product is atomized, usually at the top of the tower, with the dry product removed at the bottom.

toxicant. An agent that can produce an adverse response (effect) in a biological system, seriously damaging its structure or function or producing death. The adverse response may be defined in terms of a measurement that is outside the normal range for healthy organisms. A toxicant or foreign substance may be introduced deliberately or accidetly into the foodstuffs or ecosystem, impairing the quality of environment and making it unfavourable for organisms.

toxicity tests. The test used to evaluate the concentrations of the chemicals and the duration of exposure required to produce the criterion effect. Toxicity tests are also used to detect and evaluate the potential toxicological effects of chemicals on organisms. Since these effects are not necessarily harmful, a principal function of the tests is to identify chemicals that can have adverse effects on organisms. These tests provide a data base that can be used to assess the risk associated with a situation in which the chemical agent, the organism, and the expo-sure conditions are defined.

toxigenicity. The production of a toxin, particularly the production of a toxin by bacteria.

toxins. Generally means poisons produced by bacteria. They are antigenic and stimulate the body tissues to produce specific neutralizing substances (antibiotics). Exotoxins are liberated by bacteria, are unstable to heat, e.g., destroyed by heating at 60°C for 1 hour, and include toxins responsible for botulism, tetanus and diphtheria. Endotoxins, inside the cell, more stable to heat.

toxohormone. A toxic substance that inhibits the activity of the enzyme catalase; apparently a polypeptide that can be extracted from cancer cells and that may also occur in normal cells.

toxoid. A toxin that has lost its toxic properties as a result of denaturation or chemical modification but that has retained its antigenic properties.

trace elements. The term mainly referring to five elements necessary for plant nutrition which are present in the soil in minute concentrations (less than 1000 parts per million). These are generally considered to be boron, copper, zinc, manganese, and molybdenum, Trace elements should not be confused with tracer elements.

tragacanth gum. A gum obtained from *Astragulus gummifer* Labilliardiere, or other Asiatic species of *Astragulus* (family Leguminosae). The plants are found in the eastern Mediterranean region. Unground tragacanth is comprised of flattened, lamellated, frequently curved fragments, or straight or spirally twisted linear pieces 0.5-2.5 mm thick. The material is a white to weak-yellow in color, translucent, and horny in texture. The material can be pulverized if heated to a temperature of 50°C. The gum also is available in powdered form with similar coloration. One gram of the gum dissolved in 50 ml of water will swell to form a smooth, stiff, opalescent mucilage free from cellular fragments. In addition to numerous technical and industrial applications, tragacanth finds wide use in food products as a stabilizer, thickener, and emulsifier. The chief constituent of the gum is galactan.

trade wastes. Wastes of organic as well as inorganic origin discharged by industrial and commercial enterprises. Organic wastes are discharged on a considerable scale by the food industries such as canneries, dairies, breweries, and fishmeat factories. Other contributors include paper-mills, tanneries, petrochemical industries, textile industry, and laundries, Inorganic wastes include acids, alkalies, cyanides, sulphide, sulphates, nitrates, chlorides and the numerous compounds of lead, arsenic, iron, nickel, copper, chromium, and zinc.

transferases. Enzymes responsible for catalysing the transfer of functional groups such as phosphate or amino groups from one molecule to another. Hexokinase catalyses the transfer of a high energy terminal phosphate group from ATP to glucose to give glucose-6-phosphate and ADP.

transferrin. An iron-carbonate-protein complex, the form in which iron is transported in the blood plasma. Also known as siderophilin.

transpiration. The loss of water vapour from the surface of a plant. Most is lost through stomata when they are open for gaseous exchange. Typically, about 5% is lost directly from epidermal cells through the cuticle (cuticular transpiration) and a minute proportion through lenticels. A continuous flow of water, the transpiration stream, is thus maintained through the plant from the soil via root hairs, root cortex, xylem, and tissues such as leaf mesophyll served by xylem. Water evaporates from wet cell walls into intercellular spaces and diffuses out through stomata. It may be useful in maintaining a flow of solutes through the plant and in helping to cool leaves through evaporation, but is often detrimental under conditions of water shortage, when wilting may occur. Transpiration is favoured by low humidity, high temperatures, and moving air, Compare guttation.

Trappist cheese. A kind of mild, semi-soft, whole-milk cheese originating with the Trappist in 1885 in a monastery near Banjaluka, in Yugoslavia. It is pale yellow in colour and is mild in flavour. The cheese is exported in large quantities to Austria and Hungary. Similar to the Port du Salaut of France and the Oka cheese of Canada.

Travnik cheese. A kind of soft, rennet cheese usually made from sheep's milk to which a small amount of goats' milk has been added. It originated in Albania, in northwestern Turkey, in Europe, and has been made for over a century. The cured is put in woolen sacks for whey drainage, then removed and hand pressed into flattened balls, and air dried. It is then packed in kegs. This soft, white, mild cheese may be eaten fresh or kept for several months. Also known as Arnaeten cheese.

trefoil. A genus of plants belonging to the bean family. There are numerous species, all having compound leaves in three division, like clover, Bird's-foot trefoil, so called because the pod clusters somewhat resemble a bird's foot, is a plant similar to the Irish shamrock. It grows on the European continent and in the southern part of the US. The name trefoil is also applied to a small three-part architectural ornament.

trehalose. A non-reducing disaccharide of glucose that occurs in the hemolymph of many insects. Almost 30% of the cocoon of the parasitic beetle Larinus maculates consists of the carbohydrate trehalose; on acid hydrolysis, trehalose gives D-glucose as the only product.

trembling aspen. *Populus tremuloides* Michx. Family: Salicaceae. A tree of the Willow Family. The average height is 12-21 m and the diameter is 0.3-0.5 m. The heart-shaped leaves are about 3.0-7.5 cm long. The bark is grayish-green, with white on the outer side where the fungus grows. In summer, the leaves are bright green on top and dull green beneath. The leaves turn golden in autumn. The trembling aspen reproduces in two ways. Seeds form when pollen from trees with male flowers is blown by the wind or carried by insects to trees with female flowers. New trees are also produced by suckering. "Suckers", or young trees, sprout from the shallow, wide-spread root system. This method of reproduction is especially common when abandoned field are colonized and in logged or burned areas. Trembling aspens grow in many types of soil, preferring a well-drained, but moist and sandy or gravelly base. They do not tolerate shade well so their growth is fast as they compete their neighbors for sunlight. The soft wood of trembling aspen is mainly employed for making pulpwood. Wildlife make good use of its offerings. Wintering deer, moose, and elk nibble at the twigs while rabbits, beavers, muskrats, and hardy birds including grouse and quail, eat its buds. The foliage or greenery is important to herbivores in summer. Also known as polar; quaking aspen; golden aspen; woman's tongue.

trichinosis. Disease due to infection with *Trichenella spiralis,* a worm that is a parasite in pork muscle. Destroyed by heat and by freezing. The infection is caused by eating undercooked pork or sausage meat. Also spelled as trichiniasis.

trickling filter process. An aerobic process used in secondary treatment plants for the processing of sewage. Trickling filters consist of beds of coarse material (generally 50-100 mm crushed stone) over which the sewage is sprinkled at a uniform rate; they are generally not less than two metres deep and circular in plan. Settled sewage may be applied to the bed either by mechanical distributors or by fixed nozzles so designed and spaced as to ensure proper distribution of the sewage over the whole area of the bed. The use of plastics (such as polyvinyl chloride) the beds of trickling filters roughly doubles the surface area on which the biological process takes place. The efficiency of standard trickling filters varies from 85-95% BOD reduction, 90-95% suspended solids removal, and from 80 - 98% bacteria removal. This secondary stage may be followed by tertiary treatment. Also known as biological filter process.

triglyceride. An ester of glycerol (propane-1,2,3-triol) in which all three hydroxyl groups are esterified with a fatty acid. Triglycerides are the major constituent of fats and oils and provide a concentrated food energy store in living organisms as well as cooking fats and oils, margarines, soaps, etc. Their physical and chemical properties depend on the nature of their constituent fatty acids. In simple triglycerides all three fatty acids are identical; in mixed triglycerides two or three different fatty acids are present. Triglycerides are nonpolar, hydrophobic molecules. Simple triglycerides are named after the fatty acids they contain. Most natural fats, such as those in olive oil and butter, are complex mixtures simple and mixed triglycerides containing a variety of fatty acids differing in chain length and degree of saturation. Naturally occurring triglycerides are insoluble in water, but solubel in nonpolar solvents, which are often used to extract fats from tissues. Triglycerides undergo hydrolysis when boiled with acids or alkalies, or when acted upon by enzymetically by the enzyme lipase. Also known as triacylglycerol.

triotin. Unidentified urinary excretion product of biotin, together with miotin and rhiotin.

tripe. Lining of the stomach of ruminant; usually ox. There are various kinds such as blanket, honeycomb, book, monk's food and reed according to which part of the stomach is used; contains a large amount of connective tissue which is converted into gelatin on prolonged boiling; water 75%, protein 16%, fat 8.5%.

triticale. Cross between wheat and rye; under investigation as a potential crop; some lines rich in protein.

trommel. A large rotating drum-like device which looks like a cement mixer and is used by the Australians to separate the curd from the whey during the cheddaring operation. This device also performs the stirring out operation.

tropical fruits. Some of the fruits grown in tropical region include:

Guava. Guavas are small, thin-skinned tropical fruits. They are often processed into jellies, jams and preserves, but they can also be consumed fresh. The fruits are round to pear-shaped, usually less than 5-10 cm in diameter, with green or bright-yellow skins; some have a reddish blush. Ripe guavas have a musky, pungent odour. They contain small, hard seeds that may irritate the throat, but some of the newer varieties are relatively free from seeds. Guavas are sensitive to frost, which explains why the majority of them grown in this country are found only in California and Florida.

Mango. These are the most luscious of all tropical fruits. However when they are not of good quality, the flesh can be disagreeably fibrous, with a flavour of turpentine. These highly perishable fruits also vary greatly in size, anywhere from 50 g to 2 kg; they can be round, oval, pear or kidney shaped, or even long and thin. The tough skin is usually dull green, with red and yellow areas that broaden as the fruit ripens. Some people have an allergic skin reaction to the fluid beneath the peel and must wear protective gloves when peeling the fruit. India still produces 80% of the world's crop of mangoes.

Papaya. A native of the Caribbean, the papaya now grows abundantly throughout tropical America. The fruit is usually pear-sized and has a central cavity filled with edible, pea-sized black seeds; the sweet, juicy flesh is rather bland, with a slight muskiness and a melon-like texture. Unripe papayas can be backed or boiled as vegetables, and the leaves, if attached, are often cooked as greens. Like mangoes, papayas also secrete a fluid that usually causes an allergic skin reaction in some people, thereby necessitating the wearing of rubber gloves while peeling the fruit.

Pineapple. These plump, heavy fruits wit fresh, green crown leaves, emit a fragrant aroma and have a very slight separation of the eyes or pips. Though the shell turns yellow as the fruit matures, pineapples do not ripen after harvest as some are inclined to think is the case. Columbus encountered the first pineapples on his second voyage to the New World on the tiny island of Guadelopue. These fruits were not introduced to Hawaii until 1790 and it took until the early part of the 20th century for Hawaiian plantations to dominate the world market in this delicious fruit.

trough dryer. A containers to hold the product for drying, shaped in a U or V, in which the product is moved by a spiral conveyor, spiral ribbon, or chain-driven paddles which may be operated under vacuum or atmospheric pressure. The heat is transferred primarily by conduction for steam or electric heated walls to the product and air is moved over or through the product to carry away moisture.

trout. The common name of a group of fishes belonging to the salmon family and living in streams and freshwater lakes. The common trout may be found in Northern Europe and North America, in rivers and lakes and even in small streams. The speckled brook trout, most highly prized of food fishes. Fish commissions have restocked waters of those states, and the angling season for brook trout is now strictly limited by law. There are several species of lake trout in America, among the finest and largest of which is the Mackinaw trout. The North American lake trout attains a weight of more than sixty pounds, but specimens of this size are rare. All species of trout are valuable food fish, and laws in many states protect them.

tree seed drying. Seeds trees falls into three groups as related to extraction involving drying:

(a) Tree seeds readily extracted from dry fruits, such as cones (cypresses, firs, larches, pines, spruces, white-cedars); conelike clusters (yellow-poplar); pods (Kentucky coffee-tree, honeylocust, locust); or capsules (aspens, cottonwoods, poplars, willows).

(b) Dry fruits with seeds surrounded by a tightly adhering fruit wall, such as the nuts (chestnuts, oaks), and omars (ashes, elms, maples, yellow-poplar).

(c) Seeds of fleshy fruits, such as dupes (cherries, dogwoods, plums, walnuts), and multiple or collective fruits (mulberries, Osage-orange), and berrylike conelets (junipers). Seeds of the second group are seldom extracted from the fruits because that is either unnecessary or very difficult. Those of the first and third groups are separated from the fruits by drying, threshing, tumbling, depulping, fanning, or sieving.

The simplest method of drying is to spread the fruits in shallow layers so that there is free circulation of air around each fruit. Where the climate is dry, drying may be done in the open. Where the climate is damp or the amount of fruit is great, drying is usually done under a roof. Protection from rodents and birds often is necessary to prevent serious seed losses during drying. Some cones do not open readily and must be heated artificially in special kilns. These kilns provide the highest dry heat (usually between 37.8 and 65.6°C that the seeds can stand without injury, and these predetermined safe limits must not be exceeded.

Two general types of kilns are used in extracting seeds from cones, simple convection and forced-air kilns. The first is the oldest, least expensive and simplest to operate. The second is more complicated and expensive but more efficient. Recommended temperatures and schedules in convection kilns for several pines are: Jack pine, 2-4 hours at 62.8 to 65.6°C; loblolly and slash pines, 6-48 hours (usually 8-10 hours) at 48.9°C; longleaf pine, 12-72 hours at 48.9°C; ponderosa pine, 3 hours at 48.9°C or less; red pine, 24-72 hours at 54.4 to 60°C; and Scotch pine, 5 to 24 hours at 54.4°C. In forced-air kilns, comparable schedules are 8-16 hours at 46.1°C for long leaf pine, 5 hours at 76.6°C for Scotch pine. Seeds of the following genera and species usually are extracted by air or kiln drying: Aspens, baldcypresses, chestnuts, cottonwoods, cypresses, Douglas-firs, elms, hemlocks, incense-cedar, larches, the pines, poplar:, sequoias, spruces, sweet-gum, sycamores, thujas, white-cedars, and yellow-poplar. Normally kilns are necessary for the hard to-open cones of these pines: Bishop, jack, knobcone, lodgepole, Monterey, pond, and sand. After drying, the cones are tumbled in revolving screened cages or drums to shake out and separate the seeds. The separation of the seeds of many dry fruits from the bunches, pods, or capsules in which they grow requires failing, treading under foot, or treatment in agricultural threshing machinery or special apparatus, such as a macerator, hammer mill, or mixer. Threshing or screening commonly is required to extract seeds of the alders, American beech Kentucky coffee-tree, firs, hickories, honeylocust, black locust, Siberian pea-tree, eastern redbud, and walnut. Some small fleshy fruits are dried whole, but the seeds of most fleshy or pulpy fruits must be extracted promptly to improve germination and to prevent spoilage. Small lots can be cleaned by hand methods, but larger lots should be processed by machine.

truffle. A fungus which grows underground, without visible root. Several species are highly flavoured and are used in cookery. The common truffle grows in loose soils, in woods and in pastures. The size ranges from one inch to several inches. It is black or brown and has a rough, warty surface. Truffles have a strong and pleasing odour, and dogs and pigs are trained to locate them by the scent. These fungi are not found in North America. Edible fungus that grows underground; the best varieties are found in France and Italy. Black or Perigord truffle (*Tuber melanospermum*) and white truffle (*T.*

album and *T. niveum*) which is held in lower regard. They contain about 75% water, 9% protein and 0.3% fat. It is used as a savory and for garnishing.

Trusoy. Trade name for full fat soya flour, which is heat-treated at appropriate temperature.

trypsin. Proteolytic enzyme of the pancreatic juice that attacks parts of the protein molecule left un-attacked by pepsin. Functions at alkaline pH, 8-11. Secreted as the inactive precursor, trypsinogen, liberated by enterokinase.

Tschil cheese. A variety of skim milk cheese made in Armenia from the milk of cows or sheep, for which the curd is kneaded by hand and the cakes are packed in skins.

TSP. Trade name for textured soya protein in extruded form.

tuber. Underground storage organ of some plants, for example potato, Jerusalem artichoke, sweet potato, yam.

tuberin. The protein of potato, a globulin.

tube settler. A device used for sludge treatment; based on the principle of shallow depth settling of suspended particles in water. In an inclined tube settler, the tubes are inclined at an angle of 45-60° to the horizontal. A flow pattern is established in which the settling solids are trapped in a downward flowing stream of concentrated solids. The capacities of the existing basin can be increased by 50-150% with improved effluent qua-lity by providing striply inclined tubes with the clarifiers or horizontal sedimentation tanks.

tumble dryer. A apparatus for removing moisture from clothes, consisting of a perforated cylinder which is rotated while heated air is moved through the cylinder. Heating is done by steam, gas, or electricity.

tumbleweed. The popular name for plants of low, bunchy growth, and in the fall when dry and crisp, they become more or less ball-like, break from the stem and are rolled about over the ground by the wind. This is nature's way of distributing the seeds; the plant is a nuisance to farmers.

tun. A vat containing 210 imperial gallons.

Tuna cheese. A kind of Mexican cheese which has been important from an early date. It is really a confection rather than a cheese, being made from the fruit of the *Tuna cardona,* to which nuts and flavours are added. It is chocolate in colour, wholesome, and pleasant to the taste. It will keep for a long time.

tuna (fish). The largest fish of the mackerel family. Tuna differs so much in their skeletal structure and circulatory system that they wee once classified in their own order. They body is similar to that of typical mackerel. Only the pectoral fins and the part of the body posterior to them are covered with small scales. A corselet extends from the back to beneath the rear end of the dorsal fin, and on the belly to behind the pelvic fins. The tail shaft has a median keel. The back is blue-black; the sides are silver-gray, and the belly is white. The front fins are smoky black, and the rear ones are lighter. The finlets behind the second dorsal fin and anal fin are light-yellow with a dark edge. The eyes are enclosed in bony capsules. There are a pair of deep depressions in front of the bones of the rear aspect of the head. A well-developed subcutaneous circulatory system is connected to the vessels of the lacteal musculature. Parts of the laternal muscles located on both sides of the vertebral column have a dark-red coloration. Another unusual vessel system is located on the inside of the liver and in the tail. This system is responsible for the "warm boldness" of tuna; when excited, tuna can have a body temperature of 6° to 12°C higher than that of their surroundings. The largest specimens attain a length of 3.5 metres, but fish of this size are seldom found. Tuna inhabit all warm seas. The bluefin tuna is the largest species of tuba, with lengths ranging up to 5 m and weighing up to 820 kg. Its diet consists of herring, mackerels, and gar, which are usually pursued in small schools for great distances near the surface of the water. The killer whale is the tuna's chief enemy. During the spawning period, tuna migrate to the Mediterranean coasts; then they retire again to their feeding grounds. Their small (1-1.2 mm) eggs develop quickly. The young (about 4 mm in length) hatch after 2 days, and they grow quite rapidly. In the fall of the same year, a great many of these juveniles migrate away from the coastal regions and begin feeding in the open sea. Since the main catch period corresponds with the tuna spawning period (when they are near the coast in greatest numbers), there has been a danger of over-fishing them. The yellow-fin tuna is found only in the warmer parts of the ocean. It achieves a length up to 2.5 m or more and weighs up to 225 kg. The species is characterized by a narrow, elongated second dorsal fin, and a similar anal fin. Both fins, plus the gill cover and front of the belly, are brilliant yellow. In one year, a single yellowfin tuna can gain up to nearly 25 kg. The flesh, even of the largest fish, is good, and tuna fisheries constitute an important industry in India, Southern Europe, and in Southern California, where the fish are found in large numbers. The flesh has a slight chicken flavour, and from this characteristic the tuna is sometimes called the chicken of the sea. Also known as tunny. It is also called the horse mackerel and the great albacore. The big-eye tuna is a very similar species, but it has shorter pectoral fins and larger eyes. Furthermore, it typically inhabits deeper water levels. The skipjack tuna achieves a length of about 1 m and a weight 20 kg. It is an important commercial species which belongs to a tuna group having stripes instead of spots. It grows very rapidly, but does not live longer than 4 years. The skipjack is especially prevalent in the Pacific, accounting for a high percentage of the total catch in some years. During the summer, skipjack may be found in the North Sea and Baltic Sea. It is recognized by the four to seven dark longitudinal bands on the sides of the body. Skipjack tuna lack a swim bladder.

Another member of this group, the bonito (*Sarda sarda*) has eight or nine longitudinal and dark stripes on its back, extending from the middle of the body upward. Bonitos are widely distributed in the Atlantic. A very similar species, *S. orientalis*, occurs in the Indo-Pacific, while in the northeastern and southeastern Pacific, *S. Chiliensis* is caught in California and Chili.

tunnel dryer. A type of dryer wherein the product being dried is conveyed through a tunnel-like chamber which may be continuous or batch type.

turbot. The most valuable of all flatfish. It is shorter and broader than most flatfish and sometimes weighs nearly a hundred pounds, though the average weight is twenty pounds. The upper surface is brown and studded with tubercles. These fish live in the ocean depths along the banks. The eggs-from five million to ten million to a fish, float upon the surface. The American spotted turbot is common on the North Atlantic coast, and is one of the most highly valued of food fishes.

turmeric. *Curcuma longa or C. domestica.* A perennial herb of the ginger family with a thick rhizome from which arise large, oblong and long-petioled leaves. Turmeric grows to almost a yard high and is extensively cultivated in India, China, Indonesia, Jamaica, Haiti, Philippines and other tropical countries. The part used is the cured (boiled, cleaned and sun-dried) and polished rhizome. India is the major producer of turmeric. The plant has been valued, notably in India for its various claimed medicinal values. The flavour has been described as aromatic and somewhat bitter. The dried powder is widely used as a major ingredient of curry powders, to which it contributes an orangish-yellow to lemonish-yellow coloration. It is valued by food processors as much for its colour as its flavor. It is a major ingredient of curry powder and is also used in prepared mustard. Some food preparations to which turmeric may be added include pickles, condiments, fish and seafoods, and egg preparations.

turnip. Family: *Cruciferae*. Genus: *Brassica*. Species: *Brassica rapa*. Turnips are 90% water so they have little nutrition in them, but their redeeming virtues are their taste and paucity of calories. They do have trace of vitamin and minerals but if you want nutrition eat the young tops. Because of their high water content cook with care, as they tend to quickly degenerate into a water mass.

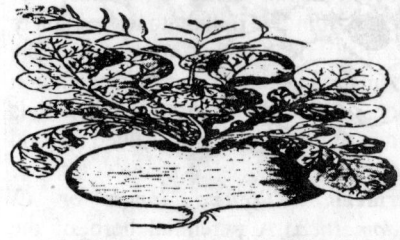

Raw young turnips, which taste deliciously sweet and crisp and make excellent crudites, are good for cleaning the teeth and strengthening the gums. In the old days turnip water was used to treat coughs, hoarseness and asthma. The average composition per 100 g is: protein 0.8%; carbohydrate 3.6%; calcium 60 mg; iron 0.5 mg; vitamin A 10 i.u.; vitamin B_1 0.04 mg; vitamin B_2 0.05 mg; nicotinic acid 0.7 mg; vitamin C 30 mg; and food energy 0.8 MJ.

TVP. Abbreviation for Textured Vegetable Protein.

Twdr, sir cheese. A variety of Serbian skim milk cheese made from sheep's and set with rennet at about 40°C. The curd is cut and is lifted from the whey with a cloth, salted lightly and pressed in forms 30-35 cm in diameter and 5 cm high. This cheese has small holes, a sharp flavour, and is similar to Brick but contains less fat.

Tweens. Trade name of a group of compounds formed of a group of compounds formed by reaction between a sorbitate ester of a fatty acid and ethylene oxide; they are surface active or emulsifying agents.

twinflower. *Linnaea borealis.* Family *Caprifoliaceae.* A flowering plant whose flowers are 10-15 mm long, on a stalk 10 cm tall. The flowers are pale pink and the leaves are dark green. Insects are attracted to the flowers by their fragrance. Inside the corolla darker lines guide them to the plant's nectar and they pollinate the stigma on the way. The ovary develops into a capsule containing a single seed. All the members of this plant family have leaves opposite each other on the stem. The leaves of twinflowers are ever green, retaining their color all winter under the snow.

Tworog cheese. A kind of sour milk cheese made in Russia. The sour milk is kept in Russia. The sour milk is kept in a warm place for 24 hours, after which the whey is removed and the curd put into wooden forms and pressed. This cheese is used in making a bread known as Notruschki.

tyrosinase. Enzyme that oxidizes tyrosine and other phenolic compounds with the ultimate production of brown and black pigments. Absent in albinos, and from the white areas of piebald animals. It is present in the potato and is responsible for the dark colour produced when raw potatoes or the juice are allowed to autoxidize in air.

tyrosine. Aminohydroxyphenylpropionic acid. One of the 20 common amino acids. It carries an uncharged polar side-chain and is an important precursor of melanin, adrenaline, thyroid hormones and some plant alkaloids. Tyrosine is formed from phenylalanine by the reaction catalyzed by phenylalanine hydrolase. Tyrosine is the starting material for the formation of melanin, the pigment in the hair and skin, increased after sunburn.

tyrosinosis. Inborn error of metabolism in which the administration of the amino acid phenyl alanine results in the excretion of tyrosine.

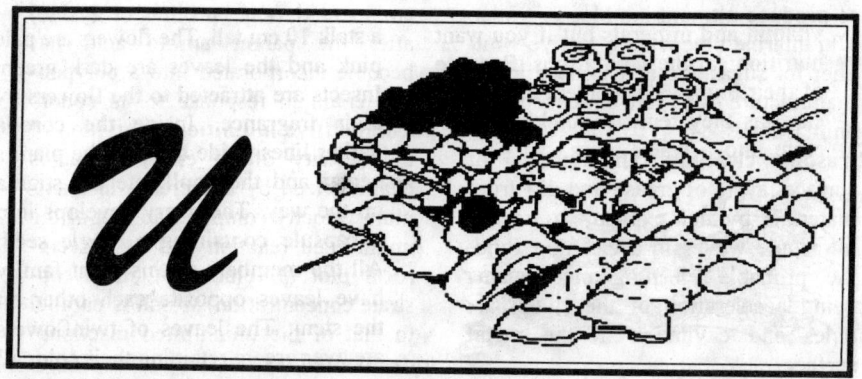

ubiquinone. General name given to a group of pigments widely distributed in nature, and first found in the livers of rats deficient in vitamin A. It is not considered as a dietary essential. Chemically it is a derivative of benzoquinone with polyisoprene side chains which differ in length and are distinguished by the number of carbons in the chain, e.g. ubiquinone 50, 45, etc.; identical with coenzyme-Q.

uncompetitive inhibition. The inhibition of the activity of an enzyme that is characterized by a decrease in the maximum velocity compared to that of the uninhibited reaction and by a reciprocal plot which is parallel to that of the uninhibited reaction.

Uffelmann's test. Add 10 per cent. ferric chloride solution drop by drop to a 1 per cent. solution of phenol in water until a bluish colour is produced. It is essential to prepare immediately before use. Mix equal volumes of this reagent and of filtered gastric contents. A yellow of greenish colour is given by lactic acid. Tests for lactic acid are not always very satisfactory, particularly when only small amounts are present.

ugli. A citrus fruit which is hybrid between grapefruit and tangerine.

ullage. Liquid left in cask or bottle after some has been removed to lost through defective container.

ultimate median tolerance limit. The concentration of a chemical at which acute toxicity ceases. Also known as incipient lethal level; lethal threshold concentration; and symptotic LC_{50}.

ultracentrifuge. A centrifuge system operating at very high speeds; will separate particles of different size in a colloidal suspension. It is used to separate the different fractions of cells. ultra-centrifuged milk has been treated for a few second at 15,000-16,000 rpm when spore-forming bacteria are sedimented.

ultra high temperature sterilization. UHTS. Treatment of milk at a very high temperature but for a short time, so causing very little flavour or nutritive damage. It is equivalent to pasteurized milk in nutritive value, flavour, and colour and superior bacteriologically; it is sterile and must be bottled aseptically.

ultramarine. Polysulphide of sodium (or potassium, lithium or silver) aluminosilicate. Its constitution is complex and unknown. The initial reaction produces ultramarine green, which may then be treated in various ways to produce ultramarine blue or violet. Ultramarine blue is an effective whitener for sugar and is also used in the manufacture of salt intended for animal feeds.

ultrasonic cleaning. The removal of surface layers of grease and dirt from materials, by their exposure to intense ultrasonic waves in a cleaning fluid, the probable cleaning mechanisms being ·acceleration of the fluid particles and cavitation at the metal surface.

ultrasonic coagulation. The formation of clusters of particles from individual solid particles suspended in a liquid or gaseous medium, when the medium is irradiated with intense ultrasound.

ultraviolet curing. The use of intense ultraviolet energy to treat certain solvent-free resin formulations applied paint, to make a hard surface coating, which will dry in a couple of minutes. A high pressure mercury vapor lamp may be used as an energy source. Whereas conventional paints may release 50-60% of their weight during curing the drying, about 2% of the weight of the coating is released with ultraviolet-cured resin. The curing process consists of converting the monomers of an ultraviolet-sensitive coating to a polymer.

umbles. Edible entrails of any animal which used to be made into pie umble pie or humble pie.

umbrella separator. In air-lift pumping of water, an umbrella-shaped plate placed at the top of the eductor pipe, against which the rising stream of mixed water and air strikes, and water gets collected in a tank.

uncoded amino acid. An amino acid, such as hydroxyproline or hydroxylysine, for which no codon exists. Such as amino acid is derived by enzymatic modification of the parent amino acid (*e.g.,* proline or lysine) after the parent amino acid has become incorporated into a polypeptide chain in response to its codon.

uncompetitive inhibition. Inhibition of the activity of an enzyme that is characterized by a decrease in maximum velocity compared to that of the uninhibited reaction and by a reciprocal plot (1/velocity *versus* 1/substrate concentration) which is parallel to that of the uninhibited reaction.

unfermented tea. *See* tea, unfermented.

universal donor. An individual of the O-type in the ABO blood group system, who can donate blood to any recipient.

universal recipient. An individual of the AB type in the ABO blood group system, who can receive blood from any donor.

unsalted butter. Butter containing no added salt. This butter is popular with many consumers and, in addition, it offers a convenient means of storing surplus butterfat for later use in dairy manufacturing. Unsalted butter is next to sweet cream in importance as a source of fat for ice cream making.

unwinding protein. Protein that untwists the DNA double helix before the replicating fork reaches that region during DNA synthesis. Such a protein, discovered in phage T4, has been termed the gene 32 protein.

upas. A tree belonging to the same family as the mulberry and breadfruit, common in the forests of Java and the Philippine Islands. The exaggerated stories formerly current concerning the deadly exhalations of this plant are now believed to have their origin in the presence of volcanic gases in the Japanese valleys. The sap, however, is poisonous and forms the principal element in a mixture used by the natives for tipping their arrowheads. The fibre of the bark is made into a kind of cloth.

uperization. A method of sterilizing milk by injecting steam under pressure to raise the temperature to 150°C. The added water is evaporated off.

uracil. A pyrimidine derivative and one of the major component bases of nucleotides and the nucleic acid RNA.

urea. $CO(NH_2)_2$ The waste nitrogen of most mammals is excreted in the urine as urea. It is formed in the liver by the urea cycle and excreted by the kidneys. A major end product of nitrogen excretion in mammals, being synthesized industrially from ammonia and carbon dioxide for use in urea-formaldehyde resins and pharmaceuticals, as a source of non-protein nitrogen for ruminant livestock, and as a nitrogen fertilizer. It is the main nitrogenous excretory end-product of most domestic animals. In pure form it is a white crystalline deliquescent solid, widely used as a cheap source of nonprotein nitrogen in feeds for ruminants. Urea is suitable for its role in excretion because of its high solubility and, compared to ammonia (the immediate product of much nitrogen catabolism), its low toxicity. It is produced by a series of reactions, the urea cycle, which involves the amino acids ornithine, citrulline, and arginine. The two nitrogen atoms of urea are derived from the amino acids aspartate and glutamate, and the whole process requires energy in the form of ATP. In birds and terrestrial reptiles, uric acid is the principal excretory nitrogenous compound.

ureotelic. Animals that excrete their waste nitrogen as urea, *e.g.*, the mammals.

uric acid. End-product of nitrogen metabolism in birds and reptiles and of purine metabolism in man and the anthropoid apes. Other mammals possess the enzyme uricase, which converts the uric acid to allantoin.

uricotelic. Animal that excrete their waste nitrogen as uric acid, e.g., birds and reptiles.

uridine diphosphate galactose. UDP-Gal. Nucleoside diphosphate sugar, found as an intermediate in the metabolism of galactose, and formed in a reaction between uridine triphosphate (UTP) and galactose-1-phosphate catalyzed by the enzyme UDP-Gal pyrophosphorylase.

uridine diphosphate glucose. UDPG. Nucleoside diphosphate sugar formed in a reaction between uridine triphosphate (UTP) and glucose-1-phosphate; catalyzed by UDPG pyrophosphorylase.

uridine. The ribonucleoside of uracil. Uridine mono-, di-, and triphosphate are abbreviated, respectively, as UMP, UDP, and UTP. The abbreviations refer to the 5'-nucleoside phosphates unless otherwise indicated.

urinary steroids. The 17-oxysteroids (previously known as ketosteroids) represent the main excretory products of adrenal (and to a lesser extent, testicular and ovarian) androgens. The 17-oxo and 17-oxogenic steroids are produced mainly in the liver by oxidative and other processes involving biotransformations brought about largely by inductible microsoml enzymes. They occur naturally in the urine largely as glucuronides or sulphates, and their exretion, like the secretion of their precursor adrenocortical steroids, varies throughout the day; also with age, sex, height, weight, and racial origin as well as with disease status.

urobilinogen. Pigment in urine derived from the bile pigments, which, in turn, are formed from haemoglobin. When urine is left to stand, the urobilinogen is oxidized in air to urobilin.

urogastrone. Hormone similar to gastrin found in urine; little known of its function.

uronic acid pathway. The reaction involving conversion of glucose in to glucuronic acid, which is necessary for the biosynthesis of the glycoproteins and proteoglycans. Like the pentose pathway, the uronic acid pathway does not directly produce ATP, but it does generates reducing equivalents, which can yield ATP by means of the electron transport chain. In the uronic acid pathway, glucuronic acid is formed from glucose in various steps. Glucose 6-phosphate is converted to glucose 1-phosphate which then reacts with uridine diphosphate glucose. This reaction is catalyzed by the enzyme UDPGlc pyrophosphorylase.

uronic acids. The product obtained on the oxidation of sugars at the $-CH_2OH$ group (not at the aldehyde group).

uropepsin. Proteolytic enzyme in urine; produced by acidification of uropepsinogen, which is identical with gastric pepsinogen. Urinary output serves as a measure of the amount of peptic glandular tissue.

U.S.P. unit. A unit is defined by the US Pharmacopoeia; the amount of a given drug, serum, vitamin, or the like, necessary to produce a certain effect upon a particular animal or animal tissue.

UV radiation. Electromagnetic radiation range of wavelength between 1 nm to about 400 nm. Most UV radiation for practical use is produced by various types of mercury-vapor lamps. The ordinary glass absorbs UV radiation and therefore lenses and prisms for use in the UV are made from quartz. Certain wavelengths of UV radiation are much more effective antimicrobial agents than those with immediately shorter or longer wavelengths. An important example of this is the band of wavelengths from 200-310 nm in the ultraviolet zone. The electromagnetic zone of enhanced killing includes the wavelengths that are optimally absorbed by the nucleic acids, with resulting damage to structure and function. The absorbed energy causes this damage by promoting the formation of thymine dimers in the DNA strand. Some organisms killed by ultraviolet radiation can recover because of the cells have mechanism to repair the damage. Furthermore, recovery of damaged viruses may also occur if they infect cells containing repair enzymes. The growth phase of microorganisms influences the effectiveness of UV radiation. Actively multiplying organisms are most easily killed while bacterial endospores are the most resistant. The use of UV radiation is limited to killing microorganisms in air and on clean surfaces.

uva ursi. *Arctostaphylos uva ursi.* A small, evergreen shrub found in the northern US and in Europe, especially in dry, sandy or gravely soils. A single long, fibrous main root send out several prostate or buried stems from which grow erect, branching stems 10-15 cm high. The bark is dark brown or slightly reddish. The small leathery obovate to spatulate leaves are rounded at the apex, 2-3 cm long, and slightly rolled down at the edges. Fall is the best time to pick the leaves. Also known as bearberry.

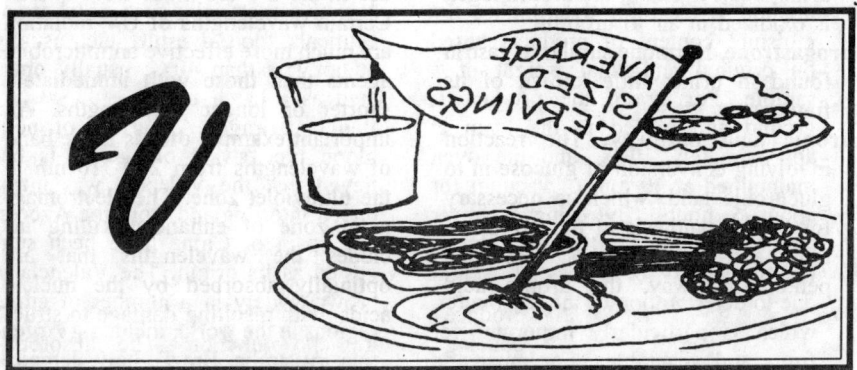

vac-ice process. An alternative name for freeze-drying.

vacreated cream. Cream that has been subjected to vaceration, which consists of:

(a) flash pasteurization by direct contact of the cream particles with steam of adjusted temperature in low vacuum;

(b) removal of extraneous objectionable flavour by steam distillation in Intermediate vacuum; and

(c) cooling and toning of the cream in high vacuum. A special type of pasteurizer known as a Vacerator is used, and cream thus treated is said by the manufacturers to make butter of a quality superior to that made from cream which has not been subjected to such treatment.

vacreation. Deodorization of cream by steam distillation under reduced pressure; developed in New Zealand.

vacuum contact dehydration. VCD. Drying carried out in a vacuum (absolute pressure of 10-15 mm) in which heating plates are moved in contact with opposite sides of the product.

vacuum contact plate process. Method of dehydrating food in a vacuum oven in which material is heated by hot plats both above and below. As the material shrinks due to water losses, continuous contact is maintained by closing of the plates. Has the advantage over a simple vacuum oven of supplying heat more effectively to the food.

vacuum desiccator. An apparatus for removing moisture from products under a vacuum. Often refers specifically to a laboratory unit of approximately one-fourth liter capacity, 23 cm diameter with a tray for holding the product to be dried. The unit can also with a tray for holding the product to be dried. The unit can also be used as lyophilizing chamber for freeze-drying small samples.

vacuum dryer. A device for removing moisture from products in which evaporation takes place in an environment at a pressure below atmospheric pressure.

vacuum filter. A cylindrical drum filter having a filter medium of synthetic fibre-woven cloth of wiremesh fabric enveloping the drum. The drum is dipped into the vat of sludge, and slowly rotates, a part of the circumference is subjected to an internal vacuum by which the sludge is drawn to the filter medium. This type of pumps are used for dewatering sludge.

vacuum oven method. The vacuum oven method is used for determining the moisture content of products based on original and final weight of a sample. For grain, the product is ground and placed in the oven at approximately 100°C and the oven maintained at 40 mm of vacuum for about 5 hours. By using a lower temperature or a shorter time, there is less possibility of a loss of weight due to deterioration of the dry matter, which is particularly important for fruits and vegetables. For meat and meat products, a sample representing 2 grams of materials dried in a vacuum oven to consider weight at 95-100°C under an absolute pressure not greater than 100 mm of mercury for about 5 hours. This method should not be used for high flat products for which an air drying method should be used. For accurate moisture content determinations it is necessary to prevent the sample from gaining moisture after the moisture has been removed from the sample. Moisture adsorption can be prevented by placing the sample in an alumina desiccator and weighing after the sample and container have cooled.

vacuum pan. Condensed or evaporated milk is produced by evaporating part of the moisture from skim or whole milk, usually 2:1 or 3:1 volume ratio before and after evaporation in a vacuum pan. Evaporation takes place at approximately 99 kPa of vacuum. The product is preheated to about 93.3°C before entering the evaporator. For a 1 metre diameter pan, 180-400 kW of steam is needed to provide a pan output of 56.7-453 kg/hr.

vacuum tray dryer. A device for moisture removal in which trays of product are placed on heated shelves in a vacuum chamber. The vacuum tray dryer is used for drying heat-sensitive materials, such as pharmaceuticals, food, dyestuff, etc., usually at not less than 40°C; usually operated as a batch unit.

Valencia orange. A variety of non-blood type sweet orange. It is believed that the Valencia was introduced into England from the Azores, but Spain or China have been suggested as its origin. The Valencia is grown widely in a number of citrus regions in the world, including Argentina, Australia, Brazil, Italy, Jamaica, Mexico, South Africa, Spain, and Tunisia, among others. The Valencia has superior processing qualities, having a juice content ranging from 55-59%; total soluble solids, 10.7-11.4%. Because of its extensive propagation, numerous bud mutations have appeared and have been exploited. These are virus-free and show increased yields. Popular varieties include Campbell, Cutter, Frost, and Olinda. The fruit of the Valencia is round or slightly oval; medium to large in size; slightly flattened, scarred; base is smooth, rounded; the calyx is small and sharp-pointed. The rind is smooth or slightly pebbled. The 9 sections (or more) of the orange are clearly marked. The flesh is orange and of medium-grain. The juice sacs are spindle-shaped and of medium size. The acidity and sweetness of the fruit blend well. The flavor is rich, sprightly, and vinous. Quality is usually excellent.

valerian. *Valeriana officinalis.* A perennial plant, about 1-1.5 m high. It is very common all over Europe. The yellow-brown, tuberous leaves each bearing 7-10 pairs of lance-shaped leaflets. The resulting smell of the dried, powdered rootstock is reminiscent of dirty socks or unwashed underwear. Various constituents within the root account for the peculiar smell and the strong sedative properties. The butyl isovalerate present has been used in a systemic, fermented egg product to attract coyotes and repel deer, while eremophilene has also been detected in ripe African mangoes. The valepotriates exert strong tranquilizing actions on the central nervous system.

valine. An essential amino acid, rarely, if ever, limiting in foods. Chemically amino isovaleric acid.

Vanaspati. Purified and hydrogenated mixture of vegetable oils, mainly mustard and ground nut; contains unsaturated fatty acids and vitamins A and D. It is used as cooking medium in India, Pakistan and Bngladesh in large quantities; similar to margarine; fortified with vitamin A and D.

vanilla. *Vanilla planifolia.* A genus of plants belonging to the orchid family, source of the well known vanilla of commerce. The plants are common in Mexico, and are also found in Central and South America and the East Indies. The vanilla plant climbs by means of aerial roots and has large white, red or greenish flowers. The fruit is a long, brown, shiny bean filled with a dark, oily, odorous pulp. This bean is gathered before it is fully ripe, and the oil is extracted by a slow process which brings out its peculiar odour and flavour. Vanilla comes from the fruit of an orchid cultivated in tropical and semi-tropical countries. Pollination is all done artificially, except in Mexico where it is partly performed artificially and partly by certain hummingbirds and butterflies not found anywhere else in the world. These pods, much like long string beans in appearance, are without desirable odour and flavor until they are cured in special ways to develop the characteristic aroma and taste of vanilla. The following method is said to be followed in Mexican curing of vanilla beans:

(a) the pods are stored in sheds until the pods are shriveled;

(b) the pods have shriveled, they are transferred to large wooden seating boxes;

(c) the boxes are surrounded with mats that help to maintain the sweating temperature until the desired enzymatic reactions are completed;

(d) the processes is repeated daily until the pods acquire a dark brown color;

(e) the frequency of the "sunning/ seating" is reduced of lower the moisture content; and

(f) the pods are placed in aging boxes in the warehouse for to o three months.

Vanillin is a major flavouring component, but at least 170 other volatile compounds are present in cured vanilla beans. Many of these, such as p-hydroxybenzaldehyde, *p*-hydroxybenzyl methyl ether, acetic acid, and diasteroisomeric vitispiranes, are important factors in the characteristic vanilla flavor and aroma. Vanilla is used in medicine as a stimulant, but its chief use is in the preparation of liquors and perfumery and in flavouring candy and other confections. Vanilla is produced artificially by several methods; the artificial product is very common. It is not only a very desirable flavor by itself, but is also an essential note in chocolate goods and many other compound flavors.

Chief flavouring principle present in vanilla is vanillin or methyl protocatechuic aldehyde, but other substances present aid the flavour, and synthetic vanillin has not the true flavour.

Although the ground pod is sometimes added directly to foods as an ingredient, it is far more common to use alcoholic extracts which incorporate nearly all of the desirable flavour notes present in the plant material. Pods are sliced into pieces about one-half inch in length, then immersed in dilute ethanol until extraction is deemed to be complete. Some manufacturers use a cold extraction, said to preserve ore of the delicate top notes, while others use warm or hot alcohol. The alcohol is usually circulated constantly through the mass of chopped beans. The extract is clarified by centrifugation and filtration and then aged in glass or stainless steel containers until the reactions that lead to an optimal aroma have taken place.

vanilla imitations. Preparations containing no extract of vanilla beans, but consisting entirely of various combinations of chemical compounds such as vanillin, coumarin, heliotropine, anisyl alcohol, aldehyde, etc. To imitate the colour of natural vanilla extract, burnt sugar or caramel is usually added.

vanilla sugar. Ground vanilla bean mixed with sugar.

vardoflavin. Name given to a substance isolated from grass, latter shown to be riboflavin.

vasoconstriction. Constriction of the blood vessels; the reverse of vasodilation.

vasodilatation. Dilation of the blood vessels; the reverse is vasoconstriction. Caused by a rise in body temperature and serves to lose heat from the body.

vassoura oil. An oil with a spicy, some-what grassy fragrance; obtained by steam distillation of the fresh leaves of a shrub, *Baccharis dracunculifolia.*

vastogotaost cheese. A Herrgardost-type cheese made in Vastergotland, Sweden. The making procedure is similar to herrgardsost except that the curd is broken up after the whey is removed from the heated curd. This results in irregular mechanical openings instead of the customary eyes.

VCD. *See* vacuum contact dehydration.

veal. Meat of the young calf, not less than three weeks old. The average composition per 100 g is: protein 15%; fat 10%; iron 1.9 mg; vitamin A 7 µg; vitamin B_1 0.1 mg; vitamin B_2 0.2 mg; nicotinic acid 5 mg; and food energy 0.7 MJ.

vegetable butters. Naturally occurring fats that melt rather sharply because they contain a preponderance of a single triglyceride. Cocoa butter from *Theoroma cacao,* Cocoa bean, used in chocolate.

Borneo tallow or green butter, is obtained from Malaya and E. Indian plant, *Shorea stenoplera,* resembles cocoa butter.

Shea butter, is the butter obtained from African plant, *Butyrospermum parkii,* softer than cocoa butter.

Mowarh fat or illipe butter, is obtained from Indian plant, *Bassia longifolia,* used for soap and candles.

vegetable casein. Name once used for wheat gluten.

vegetable drying. Geneally vegetables are prepared for drying by washing, chopping or dicing, blanching, and often sulphiting. A common method of drying is to place the prepared wet product on trays at 6-7.3 kg/m^2 through which heated air is forced. For a two-stage tunnel dryer temperatures of 71-93.3°C entering the first stage and 54.4-73.9°C entering the second stage. The moisture content of the product is reduced from 80-90% to 15-35% in the first stage and 6-10% in the second stage. From 5-15 hours are required for drying, except for leafy products. Drying is completed in a batch bin using 37.8-60°C air for 7-40 hours, drying to 3-5%. Some products are dried in a tunnel on a tray in a single stage dryer or in a cabinet dryer. Continuous flow perforated belt dryers, with higher temperatures than for tunnel dryers, with carefully controlled air flow may be used. Granules, particles, or powder can be produced. Some vegetable products are pureed and dried on a drum dryer (steam heated at 240 kPa to produce flakes or powder, or in a spray dryer in which air heated to about 176.6°C to produce powder.

vegetable juice drying. Tomato is the principal vegetable juice dried. For beverage quality tomato powder, the juice is first concentrated in an evaporator, then dried in a spray dryer. Puff drying, foam-mat drying, and foam-spray drying offers other approaches with minimum effect on the product. Drum drying is less expensive but gives a product with evidence of heat effect on flavor. Thus, drum drying is used for vegetable juices to be used for food manufacture or animal food. A product is pureed ahead of the dryer. Flaked product is produced which can be forced through a screen or put through a hammer mill to get a more uniform particle size.

vegetable oils. A class of oils obtained from plants, used as cooking medium and as drying oils, lubricants, cutting oils, and for many other purposes. Linseed, cottonseed, palm, olive, and castor beans are examples of these, and the oils are obtained by crushing.

The chief distinction between vegetable oils and fats is a physical one, oils being fluid at ordinary temperatures. Food oils used for cooking, are chosen by their content of essential fatty acids, but taste is an important factor. Linseed oil is not used for food in the US and many other countries although it has high food value and contains both linoleic and linolenic acids. In some cases the oil-bearing material, copra or soybean, may be dehydrated before crushing, making it simpler to extract the oil, and giving a better residue meal for animal feed.

Cherry kernel oil is obtained from cherry pits which contain 30 to 38% oil. The cold-pressed oil is yellow and has a pleasant flavour. It is used in salad oils and in cosmetics. The hot-pressed oil is used in soaps. The oil contains about 46% oleic acid, 40% linoleic acid, 4% palmitic acid, 3% stearic acid, and small amounts of arachidic and myristic acids.

Grapeseed oil is obtained by pressing the by-product grape seeds from the wine industry. The seeds contain 10-15% oil. It is valued in Europe as an edible oil, but used in the US mostly for paints and soaps. The oil contains about 52% linoleic acid, 32% oleic acid, and palmitic, stearic, and arachidic acids. The hot-pressed oil is dark green and not sweet, but the cold-pressed refined oil is colourless and has a nutlike taste. Another name for grapeseed oil is raisin seed oil.

Safflower oil is high in linoleic acid, ranks high as a food oil, only 1.35 g of oil being required to provide 1 g of essential fatty acids.

Olive oil, high in oleic acid with only one double bond, requires 14.2 g of oil for 1 g of essential acid. But olive oil requires less linoleic acid to counteract its effect than an equivalent amount of a saturated acid with no double bond.

Soybean, corn, and cottonseed oils used in margarine, rank high as food oils. Considerable oil is extracted from the kernels of the stones or pits of cherries, apricots, and other fruits as a by-product of the canning and drying of fruits.

vegetative reproduction. The forms of vegetative reproduction in plants are many and varied. Some plants reproduce by means of runners, long slender stems that grow along the surface of the soil. In strawberry, for instance, leaves, flowers, and roots are produced at every other node of the runner. Just beyond the second node, the tip of the runner turns up and becomes thickened. This thickened portion first produces adventitious roots and then a new shoot, which continues the runner. Rhizomes, or underground stems, are also important reproductive structures, particularly in grasses, in which the rhizomes produce stems bearing leaves and flowers. During growth, the underground stems or rhizomes are capable of invading areas adjacent to the parent plant. Each new node can give rise to a new plant, so that the species is not dependent solely upon seeds for survival. The noxious character of many weeds results from this type of growth pattern. Many garden plants, such as irises, are propagated almost entirely from rhizomes. Corms, bulbs, and tubers, all different kinds of underground stems, are structures specialized for storage and reproduction from which new individuals arise. The roots of some plants, for example, cherry, apple, raspberry, and blackberry, produce "sucker" or sprouts which give rise to new plants. When the root of a dandelion is injured, as by a grazing animal or a spade, each root fragment gives rise to another entire plant. In some few species, even the leaves are reproductive. One example is the genus Kalanchoe. Kalanchoe daigremontiana is familiar to many people as the *maternity plant* or *mother of thousands*, so-called because numerous pantalets arise from meristematic tissue located in notches along the margins of the leaves. The maternity plant is propagated primarily from these small plants. Another example is walking fern, *Asplenium rhizophyllum*, in which young plants form where the ends of the attenuated leaf tips touch the ground. Many crop plants and ornamentals are reproduced vegetatively; asexual reproduction ensures the preservation of the most desirable combinations of characteristics. Potatoes are propagated artificially from segments of the tuber, each with one or more eyes. It is the eyes of the seed pieces that give rise to the new plant. Propagation of sweet potatoes generally is accomplished with whole small roots. New shoots arise from adventitious buds. Commercial varieties of banana do not produce seeds and are propagated by suckers that develop from buds on the corm. In other kinds of seed plants, including many kinds of citrus, some grasses, and also dandelions, the embryos in their seeds may be produced asexually from the parent plant. Such seeds give rise to individuals that are genetically identical to their parents and therefore provide another instance of asexual reproduction.

velvet bean. *Stizolobium deeringianum.* Allied to the soybean (Glycine), some species of velvet beans are grown for ornamental purposes, but most are cultivated as a for ornamental purposes, but most are cultivated as a winter pasture crop. Commonly, the velvet bean is planted along with corn, and the crop is not cut because the long vines tangle easily and are difficult to handle. The vines are left on the field for grazing because frost and rain cause little or no damage to the vines, leaves, and seeds.

Vendome cheese. A kind of soft-ripened cheese resembling Camembert and Thenay varities, made in the region of Vendome, France. This variety of cheese is cured in cool moist cellars, and sometimes buried in ashes.

venison. The meat of deer (elk, etc.). It has always been a staple article of diet among numerous cultures, a favourite with hunters and epicures. The meat is covered with white, scented fat, which connoisseurs greatly appreciate. Many people regard venison as an excellent substitute for beef and mutton, which meats is resembles in texture, colour, and general characteristics. The flavour is distinctive, suggestive of beef rather than mutton. Venison becomes more tender and palatable when allowed to age for a short time. When conditions permit, it way be allowed to hang from 2-3 weeks before being processed into various cuts. It has the same chemical composition as beef and mutton, but is not nearly so fat as meat from well-fed cattle.

verbena. A genus of tropical and subtropical American plants of the *vervain* family, several species of which are cultivated for the beauty of their flowers. The cultivated varities have creeping or spreading stems and bear their blossoms in dense spikes, of almost every colour except yellow. The wild varieties are often troublesome as weeds. The verbena of the perfumeries is the lemon grass, from which the oil of verbena is extracted.

verbena oil. An oil obtained from the leaves of lemon verbena.

Verdot grape. A highly regarded red wine grape of France (Bordeaux district). It is often grown with Cabernets, Merlot, and Malbec.

verjuice. Extracted juice of green or unripe fruit, usually applied to apple and grape which have a green tint when unripe; in earlier days used as a drink but now only for culinary purposes.

Vermouth. A fortified herb wine and its constituents are wine, fortification spirit, sugar and extracts of various herbs, with a little caramel for colouring. Both sweet and dry Vermouths are made in France, Italy, UK, US, and a number of other countries. It is not a wine which allows of any great delicacy of flavour, and this is implicit in the fact that wines of a most ordinary type are employed. Although commonly associated with Martini cocktails in some countries, Vermouths are popular apertifs, either straight or with sparkling water. The basic ingredient of Vermouth is always a white wine, and usually one of very good quality. Barks, herbs, flowers, seeds, spices, and other essences may become part of the wine through infusion, by maceration to produce juices which are added, or by distillation (akin to the process of making gin. It is, however, the flavor of the wormwood flowers that predominates in most Vermouths. Some Italian Vermouths use a wide variety of aromatic ingredients, including coriander seed, cascarilla, angelica, orris root, cinnamon, dittany, thyme, sage, and , of course, the wormwood flowers. Not all ingredients are always used together, however. Infusions of ingredients are usually made in distilled spirits, using small casks as containers. After infusion for about 2 weeks, the infusion is transferred to the base wine, where it is allowed to blend for a month or so, racked, and left again for another period to blend and mature. There are two types of vermouth; Italian, which is sweet, and French, which is dry, though far from being as dry as an ordinary beverage wine.

There is little difference between the percentage of alcohol in each, but the Italian Vermouth contains four or five times as much sugar as the French Vermouth. Italian Vermouth contains about 15-16% alcohol and rather more sugar than alcohol. The wine used is a white one, which has been fermented to give only a few per cent of alcohol, leaving most of the sugar undisturbed. A blend with other wines is used as a base for dissolving out the essential principles from the herbs. About 40 or 50 herbs are used and the composition of the herbal mixture is a top trade secret. Some of the essential constituents are wormwood, ginger, coriander, gentian, cinnamon and so on. It is important not to use too much nor to allow them to infuse too long, or the vermouth will be too strong. The amount of herbs used is in any case between one and four ounces to a gallon of winebase.

Versene. Trade name for ethylenediaminetetraacetic acid.

vertical chamber dryer. The name applied to dryer in which the product is dried in a vertical or upright container. Most commonly applied to a classification of spray dryers, in which the drying air and product may enter together at either end or may enter at opposite ends.

vertical column dryer. A device for drying granular material with heated air in which the wet product enters at the top and moves vertically downward by gravity. Heated air is directed horizontally through the product.

vertical tube evaporator. A device having tubes for heating in a vertical position; used for removing water from liquids. In a short tube batch unit, the heating medium, usually steam, is contained in tubes which heats the product in a vessel, usually closed and under vacuum. In a continuous operating vertical tube evaporator, long tubes are used, with the product inside the tubes and heating medium external to the tubes.

Verv. Trade name for calcium stearyl-2-lactate; mainly used to reduce baking variations in flour. It produces a more extensible dough, more easily machined, and gives a loaf with better keeping properties and more uniform structure.

vervain. *Verbena officinalis.* A native of the Mediterranean region, vervain now grows wild on waste ground and by the wayside in Europe and North America. Although it has no culinary uses, it has a long history of medicinal applications, particularly in the treatment of nervous disorders. The tisane made from the fresh or dried leaves is a mild sedative, a soothing bedtime drink. The infusion may be taken to alleviate nervous conditions and depression, and to aid digestion. A diluted infusion was used as an eye bath to soothe inflamed and sore eyes.

vetch. A common name, rather loosely applied to several genera of climbing plants that are natives of the temperate zones. Many of them have been cultivated as forage plants for ages, and some yield edible seeds. The hairy vetch makes a good crop yielding from two to four tons of hay an acre. In Europe spring vetch, or tare, is more common. The plant has bluish-pink flowers resembling those of the pea, and compound leaves composed of twenty of thirty leaflets.

vicilin. Globulin protein in pea and lentil.

Vienna bread. A loaf with a very crisp, thin, highly glazed crust, with cuts on the upper surface, coarser than ordinary bread and with gas holes. It is baked in an oven which retains the steam.

viet. A food supplement having the same base as Cerophyl but differing from it in that certain vitamins have been added to make the quantity of the various vitamins conform more nearly to the quantity in which they are needed by the human being. It is considered very satisfactory for use as a supplement to an ordinary diet for the purpose of insuring that one receives an adequate amount of various nutrients.

Vieth's ratio. With reference to milk is the ratio of anhydrous lactose: protein: ash which is normally 13:9:2.

villi, intestinal. Small, finger-like processes covering the surface of the small intestine in large numbers. They provide an enormous surface area for the absorption of digested food from the small intestine.

vinasses. The residual liquor from sugar-beet molasses; contain appreciable quantities of betanine.

vinegar. This term may lawfully be applied only to a product of double fermentation. (The term "non-brewed vinegar", usually a coloured solution of acetic acid, is not permitted.) It is made from malt, wine, cider or spirits. The first fermentation produces alcohol; the second fermentation, for which the organism *Acetobacter* is added, converts the alcohol to acetic acid, and also produces the characteristic flavour due to esters and higher alcohols. The acetic acid content is 5%. *Acetobacter* grows as a film on the surface known as "mother of vinegar".

All kinds of vinegar except apple cider vinegar increases the acidity of the blood. Apple cider vinegar is rich in potassium and phosphorus and contains trace of iron, chlorine, sodium, magnesium, sulphur, fluoride, silicon and other trace minerals. Good brands contain about 120 mg of potassium in each 100 ml. The patients suffering from acid diseases have been advised to take apple cider vinegar and honey on a regular basis.

Apple cider vinegar has been recommended as a gargle for sore throats and, in diluted form, to help troubled skin. For the face it can be used in proportions of one part apple cider vinegar to one part of water and for the body it can be added to the bath in proportions of one part apple cider vinegar to ten parts of water.

vinegar, rice. Rice vinegar is an ancient and common product in the Far East. Rice vinegar is made by a series of steps which include saccharification of the starch to give fermentable sugars, fermentation of the sugars to yield alcohol, and conversion of the alcohol to acetic acid by other microbial reactions. The rice which is used as the main ingredient can be low quality rice, broken rice, etc. In Japan, the aqueous extract from rice wine fermentation is sometimes mixed with alcohol from other sources to form the substrate for the acetic acid fermentation. In traditional methods, the rice is first steamed to gelatinize the starch and denature the protein. An inculum of *Aspergillus* is then used to hydrolyze the starch, yielding primarily glucose. The inoculum is generally the preparation known as "koji," which consists of the fungus as grown on steamed rice. This material will contain very many different kinds of enzymes, but it is a particularly potent source of amylases. The yeast used for the alcoholic fermentation is Saccharomyces sake, which is evidently prepared in the factory from a culture medium consisting of steamed rice, koji, water, lactic acid, and phosphates which has been inoculated with an impure source of the yeast and then fermented for 15-20 days. The wine mash is pressed and filtered, then inoculated with seed vinegar from a previous batch to provide the necessary microorganisms for the acetic acid fermentation. Completion of this step can take about 1-3 months. The raw vinegar is stored in a separate tank for 2-3 months for ripening, then filtered through diatomaceous earth (or the like) before being pasteurized at 45°C for 30 minutes. The rice vinegar is then ready for bottling.

violet BNP. Sodium salt of 4:4'-di-(dimethylamino)-4"-di-(p-sulphobenzylamino) triphenyl-methanol anhydride.

violet no. 1. FD&C violet no. 1. Violet No. 1 is sometimes known as Wool Violet 5BN. It is a triarylmethane dye and has a structural formula similar to that of Fast Green, except that hydroxyl group is replaced by -N(CH$_3$)$_2$ group.

Chemically, it is the monosodium salt of 4-{[4-(N-ethyl-p-sulphobenzylamino)-phenyl]-4-(N-ethyl-sulphoniumbenzylamino)-phenyl]-methylene}-N,N-dimethyl-δ,2,5-cyclohexadieneimine). It is bright violet powder, which is very soluble in water,

glycerol and the glycols (at 20% 25°C), and is slightly soluble in a wide range of pH. It fades critically in the presence of sulphur dioxide, but is stable in sodium benzoate solution.

viosterol. Irradiated ergosterol, i.e., vitamin D$_2$.

Virol. Trade name for a vitamin preparation composed of malt extract, starch syrup and egg with added vitamins. The average composition per 100 g is: protein 3.5%; fat 11%; carbohydrate 60%; calcium 110 mg; iron 25 mg; and food energy 1.5 MJ.

viruses. The existence of viruses was first recognized when it was found that the causative agents of certain diseases could pass through the porcelain filters commonly used to trap bacteria. In size, they range from about 17 to more than 300 nm. Thus viruses are comparable to molecules in size, a hydrogen atom being about 0.1 nm in diameter and a large protein molecule being a few hundred nanometers in its greatest dimension. Large viruses are about three times as large (0.3 micrometer) as the smallest cellular organism (0.1 micrometer). Viruses are parasites that can multiply only within a host cell and are highly specific with regard to the type of cell in which they can multiply. In the host cell, they essentially "take over" the direction of the metabolism using their own nucleic acids to "command" the host cytoplasm to produce more virus particles. They compete with the genetic material of the host cell, which is similar to their own, in regulating cell functions. Cold viruses multiply in the mucous membranes of the respiratory tract, breaking down tissue and producing the all-too-familiar cold symptoms. Measles viruses and other rash-causing viruses multiply in the cells of the skin. The polio virus-

only about 28 nm in diameter-multi-
plies in the intestinal tract and
sometimes in the nerve cells. Even
bacterial cells have their own set of
viral parasites; indeed, one of the
techniques for rapid identification of
unknown bacteria is to expose them
to a spectrum of known bacterial
viruses. Plant cells that are completely
free of viruses may actually be
exceptional, and the implications of
this statement for agriculture may be
profound. Many plants may have
chromic infections of viruses, which
lower their general vigor but only
rarely becomes acute. A number of
cultivated plant with variegated foliage owe this characteristic to a viral
infection. It has been suggested that
every species of organism, including
the prokaryotes, may have at least
one specific virus associated with it,
in which case there may be literally
millions of species of viruses in
existence.

In past, viruses were considered to
be extremely small bacteria. Evidence
against this point of view began to
accumulate in 1933, when Wendell
Stanley prepared from infected plants
an extract of a common virus, the
tobacco mosaic virus, and purified it.
The purified virus precipitated in the
form a crystals. Crystallization is one
of the chief tests for the presence of
a single, uncontaminated chemical
compound, and so, clearly, viruses
were not composed of the complex
variety of organic compounds that
characterizes even so small a living
thing as a bacterial cell. But when
these needle-like crystals were put
back into the solution and reapplied
to a tobacco leaf, the infection
characteristic of tobacco mosaic virus
was produced. The tobacco mosaic
virus was subsequently identified as

a large nucleoprotein (about 300 nm
long), that is, a protein in combination
with a nuclei acid. In the case of
tobacco mosaic viruses, as well as
some others, the nucleic acid, which
is the genetic material, is RNA instead
of DNA. In other viruses, DNA
serves as the genetic material, again
combined with a protein. Viruses are
the only organisms that do not
contain both DNA and RNA.

Replication of viruses. The mode of
replication of particular viruses depends on their genetic construction.
The protein coat of viruses determines their attachment to host plasma
membrane and their entry into the cell.
But all viruses shed this coat before
they begin to replicate themselves. In
some, such as the bacteriophages, it
is left outside the host cell; in some,
it is shed within; and in others, it is
digested by the enzymes of the host
cell. When this has been accomplished, one of two things happens:
(a) A reaction may occur within the
cell that prevents virus multiplication, and the viral DNA may be
inserted in a linear fashion into the
bacterial chromosomes. In such a
state, the virus is called a *prophage.* Phages that are capable of
existing in prophage from are
called *temperate* phages. The viruses involved in trasduction are
temperate phages. Temperate phages do not destroy their host
cells unless they escape from the
host chromosome, and they are in
turn virtually unassailable by the
host's immune defense systems.
This phenomenon has been de-
monstrable only in DNA bacteriophages.
(b) The virus may multiply. Virus
multiplication takes place in three
steps. First, the virus nucleic acids

direct the host cells to produce new viral enzymes. Viral nucleic acids and structural proteins are then synthesized, each in its appropriate amount. Finally, these materials are assembled into virus particles. These steps generally overlap in time, often involve extensive genetic regulation, and lead to the production of many, often thousands, of new virus particles per cell. When the process of viral multiplication is complete, the particles escape from the host cell, which is generally dead by that time.

In viruses that contain DNA-such as the vaccinia virus, an organism that causes a pox-like disease in cattle-the viral DNA simply directs the synthesis of a series of different messenger RNA molecules which direct the production of different proteins. The DNA is usually double-standed, but single-stranded DNA occur in some very small bacterial viruses. In most RNA viruses, such as the tobacco mosaic virus, the RNA is single-stranded. This viral RNA replicates itself, presumably by directing the formation of a complementary strand which then serves as the template for new viral RNA molecules. The viral RNA also takes over the ribosomes of the host cell and acts as messenger RNA. In this role, it is responsible for the synthesis of enzymes and virus coat proteins. Viral activity may profoundly affect the metabolism of the host cell. In the bacterium *Clostridium,* it has been shown for some strains that the production of the lethal toxins associated with botulism takes place only with the active and continued participation of specific bacteriophages. Noninfected bacterial cells do not produce the toxin. Even more surprisingly, infection by other specific bacteriophages cause the same bacterial strain to produces the toxins associated with gas gangrene and many other diseases in animals. The causative organisms associated with botulism and gas gangrene had hitherto been considered to be different species of Clostridium, but they are, at least in part, the same species infected by different bacteriophages.

viscogen. A substance which enhances the whipping quality of cream. It is prepared by mixing a concentrated solution of cane sugar with freshly slaked lime. After the mixture has stood for some time, the clear liquid, Viscogen, is poured off. One part of Viscogen in 100-150 parts of milk or cream will give the desired effect. It reunites into clusters the fat globules which were broken up by heat. Sometimes used in neutralizing high acid cream, but its neutralizing strength is too low to make it of much value. Most often used to reduce acid in slightly sour cream and restore sugar sweetness previously lost by conversion of lactose into acid. Its use is not legal in some states. Also known as sucrate of lime.

viscous liquid. A liquid material that has a measured viscosity in excess of 2.500 centistokes at 25°C, when determined in accordance with the procedures specified in ASTM Method D 445-72 Kinematic Viscosity of Transparent and Opaque Liquids (and the Calculation of Dynamic Viscosity) or ASTM Method D 1200-70 Viscosity of Paints, Varnishes, and Lacquers by Ford Viscosity Corp.

vitamers. Substances structurally related to vitamins, possessing some biological activity through often less than the true vitamin.

vitamin A. $C_{20}H_{30}O$. A fat soluble vitamin produced by oxidation of such carotenoids as β-carotene. The term includes both retinol (previously called preformed vitamin A) and carotene previously termed vitamin A precursor). It is essential for formation of glycoproteins of the mucous tissue by acting as a carrier for the monosaccharides involved; thus maintains normal condition of moist epithelial tissues lining mouth, respiratory and urinary tract; essential for growth. The aldehyde, retinal, is needed for vision in dim light in combination with protein to form visual purple. Deficiency leads to night blindness, xerophthalmia (drying of tear ducts) and kerato malacia (ulceration of the cornea), blindness and stunting of growth. It occurs as retinol in fish liver oils (cod), milk and butter, and as carotene in green vegetables, carrots and palm oil. It is an important factor in maintaining the integrity of epithelial (skin) tissue and in preventing night blindness. Milk contains about 0.1-0.5 mg of Vitamin A per litre. A severe deficiency of Vitamin A results in xerophthalmia of the eyes; retarded growth; interference with regeneration of visual purple in the eye, thus causing night blindness. Reliable sources of Vitamin A are foods of animal origin, including butter-fat and all dairy products containing butterfat, egg yolk and fish liver oils. Green and yellow vegetables and fruit are excellent sources of β-carotene or Provitamin A. According to current literature, the normal daily requirement of vitamin A for adults is 5,000 I.U.; lactation period 8,000 I.U.; children up to 12 yr. 1500 to 4500 I.U.; youths 13 to 20, 5000 to 6000 I.U.

vitamin A₂. Old name for dehydroretinol, the form found in livers of freshwater fish; has 40% of biological activity of retinol.

vitamin B complex. These vitamins occur together in cereal germ, liver and yeast; are all coenzymes; and historically were discovered by separation from what was known originally as vitamin B: hence they are grouped together as the B complex. The vitamin B₂ complex is of purely historical origin and includes all except B₁.

vitamin B₁. Thiamin, Thiamin pyrophosphate is the coenzyme, cocarboxylase, needed in oxidative decarboxylation, e.g., the conversion of ketoglutarate to succinate and of pyruvic acid to acetyl. A deficiency of the vitamin leads to impaired metabolism of carbohydrate and clinically results in the disease beriberi in which pyruvate accumulates in the blood. The daily requirement is related to the amount of carbohydrate oxidized (the non-fat calories)- 0.6 mg/1,000 non-fat calories or 0.4 mg/1,000 total Calories (daily total approximately. 1 mg). Thiamin is water-soluble and there is little storage in the body. It occurs in cereal grains (little in white flour and white rice but these are enriched with added thiamin in many countries), in yeast, meat, especially pork, pulses, egg. It is one of the more labile of the vitamins and is destroyed by heat under alkaline conditions, by sulphur dioxide, and is lost by leaching into the cooking water. The baking of bread can lead to 15-30% loss; up to half can be lost in cooked meat and fish, depending on the conditions.

vitamin B₂. Riboflavin. In combination with a number of different proteins it forms a group of coenzymes called flavoproteins, essential for the oxidation of carbohydrates. It occurs in yeast, liver, milk, eggs, cheese and pulses. Processing losses are partly due to leaching into the water and partly to exposure to light. 50% of the riboflavin of milk can be destroyed in 2 hours by exposure to bright sunlight, and even on a dull day the losses can be 20%. Flavoproteins act as intermediary hydrogen carriers and include flavin mononucleotide, flavin adenine dinucleotide, cytochrome c reductase, etc. A deficiency of riboflavin impairs cell oxidation and results clinically in a set of symptoms known as ariboflavinosis. These include cracking of the skin at the corners of the mouth (angular stomatitis) fissuring of the lips (cheilosis) and tongue changes glossitis); seborrhoeic accumulations appear around the nose and eyes. Recommended intake is 0.55 mg/1,000 kcal or an average of 1.5 mg per day. The products of phenotoxidation of the vitamin B_2 destroy the vitamin C.

vitamin B_3. Name given to substance that was probably pantothenic acid.

vitamin B_4. Name given to a mixture of arginine, glycine and cystine.

vitamin B_5. Name given to a substance later presumed to be identical with vitamin B_6 or possibly nicotinic acid.

vitamin B_6. Generic descriptor for three derivatives of 2-methylpyridine, namely the hydroxy compound, pyridoxine, the aldehyde, pyridoxal, and the amine, pyridoxamine; all equally active. Deficiency causes convulsions and acrodynia (skin disorder) in rats, abnormal red cells in dairy cattle, anemia in dogs and epileptiform seizures in human babies. Functions as coenzyme for specific amino acid decarboxylases and deaminases, transminases and transmethylases. Rarely deficient in human diets; recommended intake thought to be about 2 mg per day; occurs in nuts, meat, fish, whole grain. Obsolete names adermin, yeast eluate factor, factor I and factor Y.

vitamin B_7. When a new factor was discovered that was claimed to be essential for chick growth and feathering, the claimant stated that as nine factors were known the new factors should be called vitamins B_{10} and B_{11}. In fact the B vitamins had been numbered only up to B_6, hence B_7, B_8 and B_9 have never existed.

vitamin B_{10}. The names B_{10} and B_{11} were given to two factors claimed to be essential for chick growth and feathering, they were later shown to be a mixture of vitamin B_{12} and folic acid.

vitamin B_{12}. Essential for nucleic acid synthesis and so essential for formation of red blood cells. Its deficiency gives rise to pernicious anaemia. Although a dietary essential, cases of dietary deficiency have been observed in very rare instances only, in individuals living solely on fruits and vegetables, i.e., Vegans, since it is found, apart from some seaweeds, only in animal foods. Pernicious anaemia is usually due to an inability to absorb the vitamin through lack of the "intrinsic factor" normally present in the gastric mucosa. Richest sources meat, liver and kidney; recommended intake not given in UK tables but 5 μg in US tables. Vitamin B_{12} is the generic descriptor; specific compounds are cyanocoblamin (formerly B_{12a}) hydroxocobalamin (formerly B_{12b}) and nitritocobalamin. Essential growth factors for animals were variously termed Animal Protein Factor (APF), Cow Manure Factor and Zoopherin before they were shown to be identical with vitamin B_{12}.

vitamin B_{14}. Not an established vitamin; a substance found in human urine which increases the rate of cell-proliferation in bone-marrow culture.

vitamin B₁₅. Pangamic acid; no evidence that it is a dietary essential.

vitamin B_p. Called the antiperosis factor for chicks, but can be replaced by manganese and choline.

vitamin B_T. An essential dietary factor for the mealworm, *Tenebrio molitor,* and certain related species; now known to be identical with carnitidine. In higher animals carnitine plays a part in fat synthesis by transferrin acetyl across the mitochondrial membrane but it is not a dietary essential.

vitamin B_w. Or Factor W; probably identical with biotin.

vitamin B_x. Obsolete name for para-aminobenzoic acid.

vitamin C. L-xyloascorbic acid (The isomer, D-araboscorbic acid, or isoascorbic acid or erythrobic acid has only slight biological activity, about 1/20th, but is used as an antioxidant in foods). It occurs in fruits and vegetables; and is used as an antioxidant and bread improver. The D-xylosarcorbic acid and L-araboascorbic have zero biological activity. It controls the production of intercellular cementing substances because it is essential for the hydroxylation of proline to hydroxyproline, a step in the synthesis of collagen. Breakdown of this matrix allows seepage of blood from capillaries, subcutaneous bleeding, weakness of muscles, soft, spongy gums leading to loss of teeth; in other words scurvy. Vitamin C is easily oxidized, especially in foods kept hot, and leached into cooking water. Its recommended intake is 30 mg/day according to UK and FAO authorities; 45 mg according to US authorities.

vitamin D. A group of fat soluble substances including calciferol and activated (irradiated) 7-dehydrocholesterol which function as antirachitic factors. Since the content of Vitamin D in normal milk is very low, much milk is enriched by adding performed Vitamin D. Richest sources of this fat-soluble vitamin are the fish liver oils such as halibut, cod, tuna, sword fish and others. It is also found in limited supply in the flesh of most food fish, and in smaller amounts in egg yolk and milk fat.

It is popularly called the "Sunshine Vitamin" because it is normally produced in the body by the process of irradiation, i.e., the direct action of the ultraviolet rays of the sun upon the Provitamin D (a form of cholesterol) in the skin and hair, and in the fur and feathers of birds and animals. It is very essential for proper growth, and for the formation of sound tooth and bone structure in young children and all young animals, for without it the body cannot utilize the calcium and phosphorus supplied in the diet, and the disease called rickets develops. Vitamin D not only prevents rickets but is effective as a cure, and is widely used in the form of fish liver oil, and irradiated products as Viosterol (irradiated ergosterol) and Vitamin D milk, to supplement the natural supply, especially in northern winter climates where efficient sunshine is limited.

vitamin D milk. Milk in which the normal concentration of vitamin D has been raised, usually to 400 I.U. per quart, by one of the accepted methods of fortification.

vitamin E. α-tocopherol. The antisterility vitamin which is a fat-soluble. It is generic descriptor for group of fat-soluble compounds essential for reproduction in animals. Essential for man (not for reproduction so far as is known) but rarely, if ever, deficient in the diet. It is derived from the oils of grains and seed such as wheat germ, cottonseed, palm, rice, and also from whole grain cereals. Lettuce and other greens are good source; it is also found in liver, pancreas, heart tissues, and milk, and is produced artificially. Deficiency of vitamin E in rats leads to abortion or to resorption of the fetus in females and to sterility in males. It has been proven that Vitamin E is essential in muscle nutrition in many species of animals, both fowls and mammals. The deficiency symptoms vary considerably in different animal species - sterility in mouse, rat, rabbit, sheep and turkey; muscular dystrophy in several species; capillary permeability in chick and turkey; anaemia in monkey. Many substances have vitamin E-like activity, eight in particular, (old names in brackets): 5,7,8-trimethyltocol (α-tocopherol); 5,8-dimethyltocol (beta) 7, 8-dimethyltocotrienol (gamma) and 8-methyl tocotrienol (delta). All expressed as α-tocopherol equivalents. These compounds are antioxidants with varying potencies and their natural occurrence in vegetable oils protects the latter against rancidity.

vitamin G. Obsolete name for vitamin B_2.

vitamin K. Fat-soluble vitamin essential for the production by the liver of prothrombin and several other factors involved in the blood clotting system. There is a discrepancy between the nomenclature of the International Union of Pure and Applied Chemistry and that of the International Union of Nutritional Sciences (given in brackets).

Genetic description: Menaqui-none, 2-methyl-1,4-naphthoquinone. Specific compounds such as phylloquinone (phytylmenaquinone), 3-phytyl de-

rivative, formerly called vitamin K_1, has been used therapeutically. Compounds with prenyl side chains are menaquinone-n (multi-prenyl-quinones) such as menaquinone-6 (prenyl-menaquinone-6). Potency expressed as phylloquinone (phytylmenaquinone) equivalents. The old designation vitamin K_2 (naturally occurring) was given to 2-methyl-difarnesyl-1,4-naphthoquinone. Synthetic analogues were termed K_3 (menaquinone); K_4 or menadiol, the hydroquinone form; K_5, 4-amino-2-methyl-1-naphthol (used as a food preservative); K_6, 2-methyl-1,4-naphthalene diamine (toxic); widely distributed in greenstuffs and synthesized by bacteria in the intestine but not known how much is absorbed; dietary deficiency is not encountered (except in newborn infants with a sterile intestine) only failure of absorption. It is used to prevent severe hemorrhage in many surgical operations, especially those connected with obstructive jaundice and other liver diseases. It is also used to prevent fatal bleeding in newborn infants.

The proper absorption and utilization of natural vitamin K requires the presence of normal bile in the intestinal tract. Small quantities of vitamin K probably are stored in the liver. All green plant material is rich in vitamin K. It has been found that a synthetic compound, 2-methyl-1-,4-naphthoquinone (menadione) has higher antihaemorrhage potency than the natural vitamin.

vitamin L. Vitamins L_1 and L_2 are factors in yeast said to be essential for lactation; they have not become established.

vitamin P. Name formerly given to a group of plant flavonoid substances that affect the strength of the walls of the blood capillaries, namely, rutin (in buckwheat), hesperidin, eriodictin and citrin (in the pith of citrus fruits). (Citrin is a mixture of hesperidin and eriodictin.) Now considered that the effect is pharmacological and that they are not dietary essentials; sometimes called "bioflavonoids". Called vitamin P from "permeabilitats vitamin". Once claimed as a cure for the common cold.

vitamins T. A factor found in insect cuticle, mould mycelia and yeast fermentation liquor, claimed to accelerate maturation and promote protein synthesis. Also known as torulitine. Said to be a mixture of folic acid, vitamin B_{12} and desoxyribosides and not a new factor.

vitamins. Naturally occurring organic substance essential in very small amounts for the normal functioning of the living cell. Thus a factor essential for an animal or microorganism and not essential for man is, nevertheless, termed a vitamin. It is now questionable whether it is desirable to group together substances as varied in function as for example, the B vitamins that function as coenzymes, and substances like vitamin D that appears to function as a hormone. For vitamins there is agreement between the two recommendations as follows: A generic descriptor indicates a group of substances with the specific biological activity; thus "vitamin A" is used in terms of vitamin A deficiency; otherwise specific chemical names are used, as retinol (old name vitamin A alcohol), dehydroretinol (vitamin A_2). carotene. Riboflavin and thiamin spelled without the final "e". Niacin is a generic descriptor, specific terms are nicotinic acid and nicotinamide. Vitamin B_6 is the generic descriptor, specific chemical

substances are pyridoxine, pyridoxal and pyridoxamine.

According to the Code of Practice no claims for the presence of a vitamin or mineral in a food should be made unless the amount ordinarily consumed in a food should be made unless the amount ordinarily consumed in the day contains one-sixth of the daily requirements. No claim should be made that the food is a rich or excellent source unless half of the daily source unless half of the daily requirement is present; no reference to the prevention of disease unless the full day's requirement is present. For this purpose the requirements are taken to be: vitamin A 900 mg; vitamin B_1 1 mg; vitamin B_2 1.7 mg; nicotinic acid 11 mg; vitamin C 25 mg; vitamin D 10 mg; calcium 0.8 g; iron 10 mg; iodine 0.1 mg; and phosphate 0.8 g.

Vita-wheat. Trade name for a crisp bread, popular in European countries. The average composition per 100 g is: protein 8.5%; fat 10.5%; carbohydrate 78%; calcium 45 mg; iron 3.5 mg; and food energy 1.9 MJ. Phytic acid phosphorus 59% of total phosphorus (772 mg per 100 g).

vitellin. One of the proteins of egg yolk; approximately four - fifths of the total protein; is a phosphoprotein and accounts for one-third of the phosphorus of egg yolk.

Vitis labrusca. The grapes originally used by the wine industry in the northeastern US were of *Vitis labrusca*. In recent years, cultivars of the original labruscans and of the European *Vitis vinifera* have been developed. The pure labruscans are high in fruity flavors. Changes in nonvolatile acids and other chemical constituents of New York State grapes and wines during maturation and fermentation have been investigated.

voanalakoly. Name of an aromatic shrub (*Rhinacanthus osmospermum*) found in Madagascar.

Vodka. An alcoholic liquor distilled from corn, rye, or potatoes, or from barley mixed with potatoes and oats, or from potatoes and molasses.

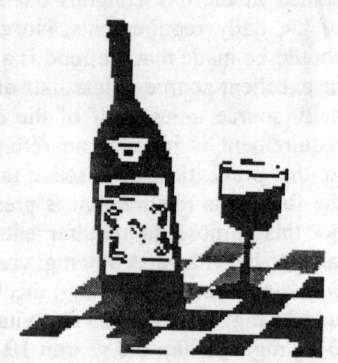

It is "hard liquor" of a most potent sort, for its natural alcoholic content varies from 60-90%; before it is retailed the amount of alcohol is reduced by dilution to about 40%; before it is retailed the amount of alcohol is reduced by dilution to about 40%. Vodka is strictly a Russian drink, and is the national beverage with little or no acid present so that there is no ester formation and hence no flavour.

Vol. Trade name for commercial ammonium carbonate, a mixture of ammonium bicarbonate and carbamate. It is used as an aerating agent in baking as it breaks down when heated to give carbon dioxide, ammonia and steam, without leaving any residue.

volatile organic compounds. The organic (or inorganic) compounds which evaporate easily. Technically, such compounds are defined as organic compounds with a vapour pressure of 1,300 pascals (about 1% of atmospheric pressure at sea-level). Compounds that fit this description are often considered in the same category for regulatory purposes due to their similar physical behaviour in the atmosphere.

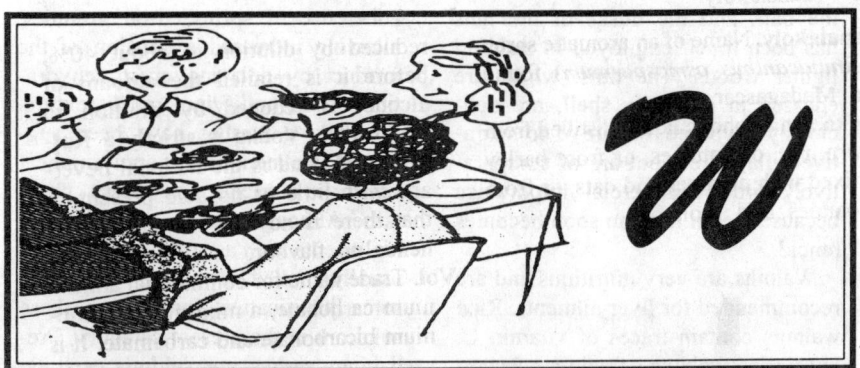

wagon. A equipment normally used for transporting products designed and equipped for drying with heated air.

wagon dryer. The dryers generally used for drying forages and nuts. Product handling is minimized with a wag on dryer. It may be necessary to place a cover over the top of the wagon, if an upflow system is used, to prevent excessive condensation on the product at the outlet. A cover may be placed over the top of the wagon to form a plenum to force the heated air downward.

wail. One of the most important aspects of all wine-making, is the careful inspection and testing of grapes as received. Tests include a determination of sugar concentration (usually by a hydrometer calibrated in Balling degrees), determination of total acidity by titration, and measurement of the pH of test juice prepared by using laboratory-type crushers. In some instances, particularly for table wines, if the acidity is too low, tartaric acid can be added, but preferably before fermentation and no later than when the wine is transferred from the fermenting vat to the storage tank. For very high quality wines, newly harvested grapes will be sorted and picked over by hand to eliminate damaged or defective berries and, in some cases, to sort out the well ripened, sweeter grapes. The French word for this operation is triage.

walnut. Family: *Juglandaceae*. Genus: *Juglans*. Species: *Juglans regia* (English walnut); *Juglans nigra* (black walnut); *Juglans cinerea* (white or butter nut walnut). The genus including about twelve species of beautiful trees, mostly natives of North America and Asia. The three best-known species in America are the English, or Persian walnut, the black walnut and the white walnut, or butternut. The English, or Persian walnut is a native of Persia and the Himalayan region. It is a handsome tree, attaining a height of from 20-30 metres. It yields a sweet sap, somewhat like that of the sugar maple. These nuts grow in a thin, wrinkled, two-valved shell, and have a high food value, being greater heat producer than almost any kind of meat. The unripe nuts are much used for making pickles and ketchup. The wood called Circassian walnut is valuable for cabinet work. It has been much used for interior finishing and for furniture, but is becoming rare. A beautiful brown dye obtained from the bark and the husks of the nuts has been much employed in staining lighter woods. The nuts, which are encased in a woody shell, are deliciously flavoured, but are of comparatively flavoured, but are of comparatively little commercial importance because the oil in them soon becomes rancid.

Walnuts are very nutritious and are recommended for liver ailments. Ripe walnuts contain traces of vitamin C, but unripe walnuts contain a substantial quantity. They are said to be good for constipation as they have a definite laxative effect. The leaves of the walnut tree, used both internally and externally are of benefit in a wide range of eruptive skin conditions. A tea made from the leaves is weakly hypoglycemic.

Warburg's yellow enzyme. A flavoprotein that is part of the cell oxidation chain; passes on the hydrogen from reduced Coenzyme I to cytochrome.

washed curd method. A method of manufacturing cheddar cheese in which the excess acid is washed out of the curd with a limited amount of water. This is done after milling and if not carefully controlled will lower the quality of the cheese. Also known as soaked curd.

washer. A general term for a dust collector, a droplet separator, or a gas purifier operating with a liquid as the collecting medium.

washes. The simplest kind of adjunct, often as simple as an aqueous solution of sugar or skim milk, or a brushed-on film of melted butter. They are applied to the surface of bakery products, either before or after these items are cooked, to modify the appearance (color, gloss, etc.) of the finished food. Washes may have other functions as well-improving the adherence of sprinkled-on granules, allowing increased expansion of the product by delaying crust dehydration, and modifying crust texture. Post-baking washes have been suggested as a medium for applying heat sensitive nutrients to bakery products. Although sprays of antimicrobial agents such as sorbic acid are not usually called "washes," there is some justification for putting these solutions in the present category. Pre-baking washes are seldom used on batters or very soft doughs because the added moisture can have destructive effects on the surface layer and result in collapse of the piece in the oven. They are of greatest value on bread and rolls where a fairly tough and slightly dry surface layer can support the wash and delay its absorption; also, they are traditionally used on the top crusts of certain types of pies. Their uses have been advocated on cookies and crackers to improve the gloss. Perhaps the main objection to their application is that the treatment sometimes lead to irregular patches of colour, which many consumers do not like. Also known as washovers.

Washington navel orange. A variety of orange, that is rounded, somewhat tapering toward the apex which terminates in an umbilicus, the typical "navel" that gives the variety its name. Navel oranges are sometimes as large as 8.9 to 9.2 cm. The colour ranges from orange to orange-yellow. The base is rounded, sometimes flattened and frequently creased. The calyx is small; the rind is smooth, tough, and leathery, and from 0.3 to 0.6 cm. in thickness. The deep-orange flesh is rather coarse. The juice sacs are large and spindle-shaped. In well-cultured groves in good seasons, the juice is quite plentiful. The navel orange has been described as representing a pleasant blend of acidity and sweetness, with a rich, vinous flavor. The fruit is seedless and usually of excellent quality.

Washington sanguine orange. A variety of blood-type sweet orange. This variety originated as a limb sport of Doblefina and was first found at Sagunto, Spain. Although the given name is Washington Sangre, the variety is much more important in Morocco-hence the use of the Moroccan spelling. In Algeria, the fruit is called *Doublefine Amelioree*. The fruit is oval shaped, large, somewhat lopsided, with medium-thick rind that does not adhere as tightly as that of the *Doblefina*. The fruit is acceptable as a table variety and it is an excellent shipper, but not suitable for juice processing.

waste. Any matter, whether liquid, solid, gaseous, or radioactive, which is discharged, emitted, or deposited in the environment in such volume, constituency or manner as to cause an alteration of the environment. The concept of a waste embraces all unwanted and economically unusable by-products at any given place and time, and any other matter which may be discharged, accidentally or otherwise, to the environment.

waste anesthetic gases. Gases and vapours that are released into work areas associated with, and adjacent to, the administration of a gas or volatile liquid used for anesthetic purposes. At present, six most commonly used anesthetic agents are: nitrous oxide, halo-thane, enflurane, methoxyflurane, diethyl ether, and cyclopropane.

waste disposal unit. A unit to dispose off wastes; For easy disposal of rubbish, garbage, etc. except papers, tins and glasses down the drain, a grinder driven elecrically is installed near the kitchen into which all sorts of rubbish, garbage, etc. are ground and drained out through the drain.

waste management. A term describing a comprehensive, integ-rated, and rational systems appr-oach towards the achievement and maintenance of acceptable environmental quality. It involves the preparation of policies; determination of environmental standards; fixation of emission rates; enforcement of regulations; monitoring air, water, and soil quality, and noise emissions; and offering advice to government, industry, land developers and public.

waste water. A genereal term for water containing biodegradable or foul matter.

water balance. The balance between intake and excretion. Intake as drinks averages 1-1.5 litres per day, as aqueous part of food, and formed in the body by oxidation of foodstuffs, 300-500 ml, in faeces 80-100 ml, in urine 1-=1.8 litre. Total body water 40-44 litres as blood plasma (2-3 litres) extracellular water (10 litres) and intracellular water 27-30 litres). The kidney controls the volume of extracellular water by excreting water. Ingestion of sodium chloride raised the osmotic pressure of the extracellular water causing thirst.

waterborne bacterial pathogens. Faecal pollution of drinking-water may introduce a variety of intestinal pathogens-bacterial viral and parasitic-their presence being related to microbial disease and carries, present at that moment in the community. Intestinal bacterial pathogens are widely distributed throughout the world. Those know to have occurred in contaminated drinking-water include the stains of *Salmonella, Shigella, enterotoxigenic Escherichia coil, Vibrio cholerae, Yersinia enterocolitica and Campylobacter* fetus. These organisms may cause diseases that vary in severity from mild gastroenteritis to severe and sometimes fatal dysentery cholera or typhoid. Other organisms naturally present in the environment and not regarded as pathogens may also cause occasional opportunist disease. Such organisms in drinking-water may cause infection predominantly among people whose local or general natural defence mechanisms are impaired; this is most likely to the case in the very old the very young and patients in hospitals for example with burns or on immunosuppressive therapy. Potable water used for drinking and bathing if it contains excessive numbers of organisms such as pseudomonas, *Flavobacterium, Acinetobacter, Klebsiella,* and *Serratia* may produce a variety of infections involving the skin and mucous membranes of the eye, ear, nose, and throat.

The modes of transmission of bacterial pathogens include ingestion of contaminated water and food contact with infected persons or animals and exposure to aerosols. The significance of the water route in the spread of intestinal bacterial infections varies considerably, both with the disease and with local circumstances. Although *Shigella* may be waterborne, but water is not usually the main route for the spread of shigellosis, but rather person-to-person contact in crowded living conditions in contrast cholera is usually waterborne and salmonellosis is food-borne. Among the various waterborne pathogens there exists a wide range

of minimum infectious dose levels necessary to cause a human infection. With *Salmonella typhi* ingestion of relatively few organisms can cause disease; with *Shigella flexneri* several hundred cells may be needed whereas many millions of cells of *Salmonella* serotypes are usually required to cause gastroenteritis. Similarly with toxigenic organisms such as enteropatho-genic *E. coli* and *V. cholerae* as many as 10^8 organisms may be necessary to cause illness. The size of the infective dose also varies in different persons with age, nutritional status, and general health at the time of exposure. The significance of routes of transmission other than drinking-water should not be underestimated as the provision of a safe potable supply by itself will not necessarily prevent infection without acco-mpanying improvements in sanitation and personal habits.

water hardness. Soap-precipitating power of water due to the formation of insoluble calcium and magnesium salts of the soap. Temporary hardness is removed by boiling, permanent hardness is not. May be measured in degrees Clarke; one degree is equal to 1 part of calcium carbonate per 100,000 parts of water.

water, demineralized. Water that has been purified by passage through a bed of ion-exchange resin which removes mineral salts. Demineralized or deionized water is as pure as, and can be purer than, distilled water.

water. Out water supply is purified and filtered by the addition of many chemicals, including chlorine and fluorine, the latter in an attempt to reduce tooth decay in children. Chlorine certainly· kills germs but significant research has linked chlorine to high blood pressure, anaemia and diabetes and it has even been indicated as a contributor to heart disease. Even in minute quantities, chlorine can undermine the body's defences against atherosclerosis. Additionally, free radicals can damage the lining of blood vessels and so create an ideal environment for the formation of plaque. The addition of fluoride to our water has caused a storm of controversy. On the positive side, it has been established that when it is taken before the formation of permanent teeth by children fluoride protects against tooth decay. Although it cannot be proved, it appears to provide similar protection for adults. It may also help protect them against osteoporosis and heart attacks. However, it must be remembered that fluoride is one of the trace minerals and therefore needs to be used in really minute quantities.

Fluoride is one of the most powerful compounds which inhibit enzymes by binding up the metal ions they need in order to function properly. Fluoride has been proved to be both mutagenic and carcinogenic. It would be wise for us to remember that the fluoridization of water is a massive medical experiment that is already banned in ten European countries. Wherever the hardness of hard water is due to calcium and magnesium, its drinkers have a significantly lower rate of death from heart disease.

Calcium is used by the heart muscles for contraction, and magnesium is used to produce the relaxation of the heart muscles between beats.

Magnesium can actually act as a preventative, rather than a cause of kidney stones. Soft water is generally proportionately higher in sodium, which can upset the balance between sodium and potassium, interfering with the electrical impulse responsible for a regular heartbeat. It is therefore wise for soft-water drinkers to supplement their diets with calcium and magnesium. If you cannot decide whether your water is soft or hard, make ice-cubes from it. Hard water will make clear cubes with a small white spot in the centre where the minerals concentrate, while soft water will make consistently cloudy ice-cubes.

Distilled water does not exist in nature. It is really dead water which lacks not only the minerals which have been extracted from it, but the electromagnetism. The one thing that can be said in its flavour is that it is absolutely pure and, contrary to popular belief, will not leach minerals out of the bones and blood.

As far as nutritional value goes, some bottled mineral waters contain certain minerals, but seldom in significant amounts. These do affect the flavour, and waters with a high mineral content taste quite distinctive. For making tea and coffee, bottled still water is flavored by the purists who dislike the taste of tap water or object to the surface scum produced by hard water. Over two-thirds of the bottled water sold in different countries is sparkling, either artificially carbonated or naturally sparkling as the result of carbon dioxide given off by rocks over which the water flows. Still waters occur naturally but some are produced by removing carbon dioxide from sparkling water. All sparkling waters are artificially carbonated. Bottled waters have been subject to strict regulations regarding composition, purity and labelling.

Hypertension, nervous and immune disorders and cancer have all been linked to contaminants leached from pipes made with materials such as galvanized iron, plastic, copper, lead, zinc and asbestos-containing cement. The effects tend to be more drastic when the water is soft, because soft water is more acidic than hard. Nitrates are seldom present in our drinking water in really significant amounts but in some areas the supply contains more than the maximum limit 50 mg/L recommended by the EEC guidelines. Water with over 100 mg/L is withdrawn from public consumption and the Department of Environment is currently considering whether or not to lower the acceptable limit to 50 mg/L. Water filters, which work out more cheaply than buying bottled mineral water, do not, however, filter out added fluoride from the water. Most water filters will remove up to 90% of the chlorine, 70-98% of the lead, 95-98% of the mercury, and 50-90% of the cadmium. One successful and safe filters is finely divided carbon, in the form of charcoal which absorbs and attracts the pollutants.

waterborne diseases. Diseases such as cholera, typhoid fever, dysentery, gastroenteritis, hepati-tis and bilharziasis, which are commonly transmitted through contaminated water supplies. While the classical water-borne diseases have been virtually eradicated from many of the developed countries, these diseases are still endemic in other parts of the world. Bilharziasis (caused by schistosomes or blood flukes) is commonly transmitted in tropical countries by bathing in polluted canal water. Urban filariasis (caused by filariae or nematode worms and associated, inter alia, with that breeds in polluted water. Although water transmission is thought to cause only a very small fraction of the disease hepatitis, nevertheless a major epidemic of infectious hepatitis did occur in Delhi, India, in 1955 and 1988, in circumstances suggesting that the treatment of highly polluted water had been successful in controlling bacteria, but not the hepatitus virus. There are Some common water-borne diseases are:

Cholera. This water-borne disease is mainly caused by bacteria. It is often fatal if it is not treated well. There are various symptons, of the this disease the most common symptoms are severe vomiting, diarrhoea, dehydration etc.

Bacterial dysentery. This disease is mainly caused by the several species of becteria. Diarrhoea is the most common symptom of this water. borne disease.

Typhoid. It is on of the most common water-borne disease caused by the bacteria.

Para typhoid fever. This disease is usually caused by the attack of several species of bacteria. The main symptoms of the is disease are severe vomiting, diarrhoea etc. in man.

Ameobic dysentery. The most common organisms to cuase Amelobic dysentery are protozoa. The main symptom of this disease is also diarrhoea, but prolonged diarrhoea in man in most possible way of detection of a patient suffering from Ameobic dysentery.

Infectious hepatitis. The organaism involved to cuase this disease is virus. It is the most common in most of this diseae are when man has yellow jaundice skin, enlarged liver, vomitting and often the apdminal pain. More readily identificable group of vacteria, which are generally known by us as cothfrom. Since these microorganisms are normally present in the intestinal tract of human and animals. The large number of collifoms in water acts as an indicator of contamination of water by untreated sewage. Chlorination of drinking water to protect the humans and animals from the attack of various diseases are usually applied. Recent studies show that though chlorination of drinking water is done to save the population from various disease but chlorination itself usually gave rise to other pollution problems.

water content. The quantity of water present in a system (or substance). It is usually expressed as percent; the weight of water in a wet mass divided by the dry mass and multiplied by 100. Also known as moisture content.

watercress. Family: *Cruciferae*. Genus: *Nasturtium*. Species: *Nasturtium officinale*. Watercress is a perennial plant which thrives in clear, cold water and is found in ditches and steams everywhere. It's cultivated for its leaves, which are principally used as salad greens or garnishes. Connected to a creeping rootstock, the hollow, branching stem generally extends with its leaves above the water. The smooth, somewhat fleshy, a dark green leaves are odd-pinnate with 1-4 pairs of small, oblong or roundish leaflets. Watercress is rich in vitamins A, B_2, C, D and E and contains nicotinamide, as well as various trace minerals, including manganese, iron, phosphorus, iodine, calcium, potassium, sodium and lots of sulphur. Its numerous medicinal attributes from countries all over the world include its use as an aphrodisiac, purgative and asthma remedy. It is also used for eye disorders, bleeding gums, arthritis and rheumatism, hardening of the arteries, kidney and liver cleansing and dropsy. It has antibiotic properties similar to those of the onion family and so makes useful preventive medicine against chronic congestive illnesses. It is also highly alkaline. The leaves of *Nasturtium officinale* have been recommended as cure for scurvy; not cultivated commercially until early 19th century. The average composition per 100 g is: 3 g protein; 0.6 g carbohydrate; 220 mg calcium; 1.5 mg iron; 1,800 µg vitamin A; 0.1 mg vitamin B_1; 0.5 mg nicotinic acid 60 mg vitamin C; and 0.06 MJ food energy.

waterglass. Sodium silicate; used to preserve eggs, a layer of insoluble calcium silicate is formed around the shell which scales the pores. Eggs coated with waterglass may be stored well for many months.

watermelon. A creeping variety of gourd. The rind of the fruit is smooth and dark green when ripe; the inside of the melon is a coarse red or yellowish pulp, ninety per cent of which is water. Its native home was Africa, but it has been widely cultivated from remote times. Most melons weigh from 4-10 kg. The watermelons of commercial importance assume three basic forms namely:

(a) The traditional long, oblate or oval form, which may range up to nearly 0.6 m. in length and 0.3 m. in diameter, and weigh from 9-18 and 22.5 kg, although in record growth situations, these dimensions may be exceeded.

(b) The small, sometimes called "icebox" melons that essentially are round and weigh from 1.8-4.5 kg or more.

(c) The seedless watermelons, which usually resemble large, round types, but of small dimensions, the weight usually ranging from 3.6-4.5 kg. Depending upon the breeding strategy used, some seedless watermelons may be considerably larger. Frequently a seedless melon will contain some seeds. The small citron melon, used for making preserves and also a member of *Citrullus*, should not be confused with the citron (*Citrus medica*), related to lemon.

watermelon, seedless. Several seedless varieties of watermelon have been developed. Generally, such melons are round and weigh from 3.5-4.5 kg. Their rind is thin, fairly tough, and striped. They have a deep-red flesh which is sweet, crisp, and of excellent texture. Yield of the seedless varieties is about 50% that of standard commercial varieties. Thus far, seedless varieties have not shown any particular resistance to any of the common watermelon diseases. The complex process involved in producing triploid seeds makes their cost quite high. The melons are usually sprouted indoors at rather elevated temperatures. The seedlings are held in hotbeds or in greenhouses until they have two or three well-developed levels. Seedless watermelons are not widely available on the market because of their high cost and difficulty in cultivating, mainly because of lack of disease resistance. The normal watermelon (diploid number) has 22 chromosomes. Triploids (3n or 33 chromosomes) and tetraploids (4n or 44 chromosomes) have been developed in an effort to produce seedless melons. Diploids, triploids, and tetraploids can be recognized by distinctive rind patterns characteristic of their chromosomal number. Seedless watermelon are produced by crossing a tetraploid melon with a diploid melon. The hybrid resulting from this cross is triploid, which is characteristically sterile. When a triploid is fertilized with pollen from regular seeded melons (diploid), the resulting fruits are seedless.

water polluting agents. Bacteria or viruses present in such concentrations or numbers as to impair the quality of the water rendering it less suitable or unsuitable for its intended use and presenting a hazard to man or to his environment. Pollution may be caused by:

(a) Bacteria, viruses and other organisms that can cause disease, *e.g.*, cholera, typhoid fever, and dysentery.

(b) Inorganic salts that cannot be removed by any simple conventional treatment process, making the water less suitable for drinking, for irrigation and for many industries.

(c) Plant nutrients such as potassium, phosphates, and nitrates which, while largely inorganic salt, have the added effect of increasing weed growth, promoting algal blooms and producing, by photosynthesis, organic matter which may settle to the a lake.

(d) Oily materials that may be harmful to fish and other forms of aquatic life, cause unsightliness, screen the river surface from the air thus reducing re-oxygenation, accumulate in troublesome quantities, or have high oxygen demand.

(e) Specific toxic agents, ranging from metal salts to complex synthetic chemicals.

(f) Waste heat that may render the river less suitable for certain purposes.

(g) Silt that may enter a river in large quantities causing changes in the character of the river bed.

water-soluble vitamins. All the members of the B complex (thiamin, riboflavin, nicotinic acid, panthothenic acid, pyridoxine, biotin, folic acid, *p*-amino-benzoic acid choline, inositol and B_{12}) and vitamin C. Unlike the storage of vitamins A and D in the liver, there is no specific site for storage of the water-soluble vitamins, they are merely dispersed in solution through the blood and tissues.

water treatment. The treatment of water differs withe the raw water quality and the desired qua-lity of treated water. In general, the process involves the removal of taste, colour, odour, tur-bidity, hardness and disease-causing orga-nisms. For use in boilers, com-plete removal of hardness is required. For preparation of medicines, distilled water and deminerlized water are to be produced.

wax apple. Peel wax contains triacontane, heptaconsanol and malol.

wax. Any of various solid or semisolid substances. There are two main types. Mineral waxes are mixtures of hydrocarbons with high molecular weights. Paraffin wax, obtained from petroleum, is an example. Wax are the esters of fatty acids with long-chain monohydric alcohols (fats are esters of fatty acids with the three-carbon trihydric alcohol, glycerol), such as beeswax, ester of palmitic acid with myricyl alcohol, spermaceti, cetyl palmitate. Animal waxes are often esters of the steroid alcohol, choles-terol.

Waxes secreted by plants or ani-mals are mainly esters of fatty acids and usually have a protective func-tion. Examples are the beeswax form-ing part of a honeycomb and the wax coating on some leaves, fruits, and . seed coats, which acts as a protective water-impermeable layer supplement-ing the functions of the cuticle. The seeds of a few plants contain wax as a food reserve.

waxy corn. A variety of corn in which the starch is comparable with the root starches. The type is frequently the raw material for wet-milling processes and for the production of cornstarch, corn oil (or maize oil). Corn oil meal is used as livestock feed.

weeds. A term applied to plants that are out of places, not wanted, and in most cases every troublesome. Many plants when grown and cultivated in gar-dens, as the goldenrod and the dandelion, are classed as flowers, while the same plants, running wild in uncultivated ground, are considered as weeds. The chief ways in which weeds are injurious are:

(a) they increase the labour necessary to cultivate the soil;

(b) they take up food from the soil, which should go to useful plants;

(c) their foliage smothers the young plants;

(d) they sometimes are poisonous to cattle.

Care should be taken to eradicate them as soon as they begin to grow. There are various ways to prevent their growth, different weeds requir-ing different methods. Planting of pure seed, diligent tillage of the soil, rotation of crops, cultivation of all open land with crops, are some of the means used. Some weeds while young can be destroyed without injury to the crop, by spraying the field with certain chemicals, called herbicides. Weeds are often of service to a farmer, in aiding him to know the needs of his land, since many kinds grow only where the conditions are peculiarly adapted to them.

Weetabix. Trade name for a breakfast cereal prepared from wheat flakes. It is popular in many European coun-tries. The average composition per 100 g is: protein 11%; fat 2%;

carbohydrate 76.0%; calcium 35 mg; iron 5 mg; vitamin B_1 0.6 mg; vitamin B_2 1.0 mg; nicotinic acid 8 mg; and nicotinic acid 7 mg.

Weisslacker cheese. A Bavarian, white, smeary, soft, cow's milk cheese similar to Limburger and Backsteiner with a lustrous surface. The curd is handled in the same way as Limburger except that the larger cubes of curd are not so well drained.

Wensleydale cheese. A variety of medium hard, blue-veined, cow's milk cheese made in Wensleydale, Yorkshire, England. It is similar to Stilton cheese, except that the melon-like outward appearance of Stilton is lacking. The cheese is white with blue veins and has a firm, smooth body, a rich creamy flavour, stronger than Stilton.

Werder cheese. A semisoft, cow's milk cheese made in West Prussia. This Gouda-shaped cheese is ripened initially by a white surface mold and later initially by a white surface mold and later by bacteria which produce a red colour on the surface. Werder is ripened the same way as Tilsiter but is softer and not as sharp. The cheese is dry salted, and is cured for a month at 20°C during which time the white mold grows; then curing is completed at 15°C. The cheese is ripened in 10 weeks. Also known as Elbinger cheese; Niederungkase cheese.

West friesian cheese. A kind of rennet cheese made from the cow's skim milk. The milk is coagulated in a copper kettle, in one hour. The curd is broken up, kneaded in a wooden tub and salted after several hours. It is pressed for 3 hours, washed in hot water, wrapped in a fine cloth and again pressed for 12 hours. The cheese is ready be eaten atleast after 1 week.

Westphalia cheese. A variety of hand cheese made in Westphalia, Germany. The sour milk is stirred while heating to 37°C; curd is placed in a sack; salt, butter and caraway seed or pepper are added. It is then molded by hand, dried for a few hours, and ripened in a cool cellar.

wetting agents. Chemicals used in making solutions, emulsions, or compounded mixtures, such as cosmetics, starch pastes, oil emulsions, dentifrice, and detergents, to reduce the surface tension and give greater ease of mixing and stability to the solution. In the food industries chemical wetting agents are added to the solutions for washing fruits and vegetables to produce a cleaner and bacteria-free product. Wetting agents are described in general as chemical having a large hydrophilic group associated with a smaller hydrophilic group. Some liquids naturally wet pigments, oils, or waxes, but others require a proportion of a wetting agent to give mordant or wetting properties. Pine oil is a common wetting agent, but many are complex chemicals. They should be powerful enough not to be precipitated out of solutions in the form of salts, and they should be free of odour or any characteristic that would affect the solution.

whalebones. The elastic, hornlike strips in the upper jaw of the Greenland whale and some other species. The strips are generally from 2-3 m long and number up to 600. Those from the bowhead whale of the Arctic Ocean are the longest slabs, measuring up to 4 m in length to 25-30 cm wide at the bottom. Finback whalebone is less than 1 m in length. See also whale, humback.

whale, humback. Megaptera longimana. The whale of the northern Pacific, a baleen whale with no teeth and with plates of baleen in the mouth to act as a sieve. It grows to a length of about 15 m. Whalebone is lightweight, very flexible, elastic, tough, and durable. It consists of a conglomeration of hairy fibres covered with an enamel-like fibrous tissue. It is easily split and when softened in hot water is easily carved. Whalebone has a variety of uses in making whips, helmet frames, ribs, and brush fibres. Baleen is a trade name for strips of whalebone used for whips, and for products where great flexibility and elasticity are required.

whale liver oil. The oil extracted from the liver of whales. It is used in medicine for its high vitamin A content. It also contains kitol, which has properties similar to vitamin A but is not absorbed in animal metabolism. *See also* whale oil.

whale meat. The meat of whale used for food in Japan, and in dog food in the United States. When cured in the air, the outside is hard and black, but the inside is soft. In young animals the flesh is pale; in older animals it is dark red. It has a slight fishy flavour, but when cooked with vegetables is almost indistinguishable from beef. It contains 15 to 18% proteins.

whale-meat extract. It is used in bouillon cubes and dehydrated soups. It is 25% weaker than beef extract.

whale oil. An oil extracted by boiling and steaming the blubber of several species of whale that are found chiefly in the cold waters of the extreme north and south. Whales are mammals, and are predaceous, living on animal food. The blubber blanket of fat protects the body, and the tissues and organs also contain deposits of fat. Most whale oil is true fat, namely, the glycerides of fatty

acids, but the head contains a waxy fat. In the larger animals the meat and bones yield fat than the blubber. Both the whalebone whales and the toothed whales produce whale oil. The bluehead whales of the south, *Silbaldus musculus,* are the largest and also yield most oil per weight. The whaling industry is blue whale units averaging 18 metric tons of oil each. The blue whale is about 8 m long at birth and reaches 21 m in 2 years. This species often reaches 30 m with a weight of about 136 metric tons and will yield about 24 metric tons of oil.

The gray whale, or California whale, of the northern Pacific, is a small 15 m species. The greenland whale of the north, *Balaena mysticetus,* and the finback whale of the south, *Balaenoptera physalus,* produce much oil.

The beluga, or white whale, *Delphinapterus leucas,* and the narwhal, *Monodon monoceros,* of the North Polar seas, produce porpoise oil. Both species of porpoise measure up to 6 m in length.

Whale oil is sold according to grade, which depends upon its color keeping qualities. The latter in turn depends largely upon proper cooking at extraction.

No. 0 and 1- fine pale-yellow oils

No. 2- amber

No. 3- pale brown, and

No. 4- is the darkest oil.

Grade 1 has less than 1% free fatty acids, while grade 4 has from 15 to 60% with a strong fishy odour. The specific gravity is 0.920-0.927, saponification value 180-197, and iodine value 105-135.

Whale oil contains oleic, stearic, palmitic, and other acids in varying amounts. But whales are now so scarce that the former uses of the oils and meat are restricted, particularly in the US. Whale oils of the lower grades were used for quenching baths for heat-treating steels, and also in lubricating oils. The best oils are used in soaps and candles, or for preparing textile fibres for spinning, or for treating leather. In Europe whale oil is favoured for making margarine because it requires less hydrogen than other oils for hardening, and the grouping of 16 to 22 carbon atom acids gives the hardened product greater plasticity over a wider temperature range.

Sod oil is oil recovered from the treatment of leather in which whale or other marine mammal oil was used. It contains some of the tannins and nitrogenous matter which make it more emulsifiable and more penetrant than the original oil.

wheat, Puffed. Trade name of breakfast cereal prepared by heating wheat grains under pressure and then rapidly releasing the pressure when the superheated steam in the grain suddenly expands so puffing or "exploding" the grain. It is popular in many countries. The average composition per 100 g of the puffed wheat is: protein 14%; fat 2%; carbohydrate 75%; iron 3.5 mg; vitamin B_1 1.2 mg; and food energy 1.5 MJ.

wheat bread. *See* bread.

wheat. Like all grasses, wheat (*Triticum aestivum*) is a monocot, and its fruit, the grain, or kernel, is one-seeded. Wheat is one of the most valuable and widely-known cereal crops, has constituted the staple food of civilized nations for countless centuries. It grows readily in all climates, except the hottest parts of tropical regions and the extreme cold portions of the frigid zones. However, it is best adapted to the temperate regions, and

within these regions the greater part of the world's crop is produced. It requires a rich clay soil or heavy loam, and clear, bright days while it is ripening. Wheat is supposed to be a native of Western Asia, but it has been cultivated so many centuries that the place of its origin is not fully known. It was introduced into North America in the sixteenth century.

The uniqueness of wheat among cereal grains depends mostly upon the characteristics of its protein content. In wheat, as in other plants, protein is developed from simpler substances extracted from the environment. As a plant develops from a seed, two metabolic processes take place in the cells, photosynthesis and nitrogen fixation. Photosynthesis involves formation of carbohydrates from carbon dioxide, water, and energy while nitrogen fixation is the conversion of nitrogen gas into chemically combined nitrogen that can readily assimilated by the plant. Nitrogen fixation can be carried out by legumes which bear root nodules containing certain kinds of bacteria, by some algae, by chemical syntheses, or by electrical discharges in the atmosphere (lightning).

The proteins of wheat are complex, and the there is no simple explanation of their constitution or biological function. Neither differences in the amounts of the various classes of proteins nor differences in the amount or kind of amino acids account for the wide variations in rheological and baking properties of flours. From a practical viewpoint, the great weakness in the multitude of ingenious approaches to the characterization of wheat proteins has been lack of proof of their direct association with quality. The storage proteins in wheat kernels are the source of gluten, which is the complex of nitrogenous compounds that give wheat flour doughs their cohesive and elastic properties. Gluten can be separated from wheat flour by making a stiff dough from a mixture of flour and water, then washing (manually or mechanically) this dough in an excess of water (as in a stream of water) until the starch granules and all soluble materials have been removed. Gluten appears to be a mixture of two major components called glutenin and gliadin. The gliadin fraction is soluble in neutral 70% aqueous ethanol. It consists mainly of monomeric proteins that associate by non-covalent hydrogen bonding and by hydrophobic interactions, but also contains polymeric proteins that are related structurally to some glutenin subunits. The glutenins are essentially insoluble in 70% ethanol, and appear to consist of proteins or subunits that are aggregated into high molecular weight polymers by covalent disulfide bonds. The protein content of wheat kernels is affected both by the genetic constitution of the plant and by environmental conditions during growth of the plant and development of the seed. Typically, hard red spring wheat and durum will analyze about 13-17% protein. Hard red winter wheat will test out at 11-15% protein, in most cases. Soft winter wheat and club wheat would ordinarily fall in the range of 7-11% protein. Of course, in the normal course of events, many samples will be found that fall outside this range because of unusual weather events, heavy fertilizer applications, disease, or characteristics of a particular variety. The total protein of the wheat kernel is not a well balanced nutrient so far as the human diet is concerned. It has a PER far below that of egg or milk, for example, although its protein quality is within the same range as most other cereals. The limiting amino acid is lysine, as is the case with most cereal proteins.

Starch is the carbohydrate present in the greatest in the mature wheat kernel; in fact, it exceeds all other types of compounds, being several times larger than the next largest classes of substances. It is formed out of carbon dioxide and water by the process of photosynthesis and is deposited in plant cells as microscopic particles of varying size and conformation. Many genes are involved in determining the shape, crystalline pattern, and chemical properties of starch granules. Developments in the carbohydrate field are too numerous, but the starch-protein matrix and the size of the starch granules in the wheat kernel are important considerations in flour milling and bakery processes. Starch is a polymer of D-glucose, most of the hexose units being joined together by α-(1-4) bonds. There are varying proportions of amylose and amylopectin, the former being virtually a straight chain, but with a few branch points, while the latter contains numerous side chains attached by 4-5% α(1-6)-D-glucosidic linkages and has a molecular weight greater than about 10^8. The starch granules grow in the developing endosperm as single entities in amyloplasts. In wheat starch, they have a bimodal size distribution, with about 3-4% (50-75% by weight) being lenticular and 15-40 μm in size and the remainder being small, approximately spherical, granules ranging in size from about 1-10 μm.

In accordance with their method of growth wheat are divided into bearded wheat and bald wheat. The first has glumes attached to the seeds, while the second has none. In regard to the colour of the kernel, the varieties are divided into light-coloured and dark-coloured, or white and red wheat. It is classified according to the time of planting all wheat are grouped under winter wheat and spring wheat. In each of these classes we find hard and soft wheat. The winter wheat is planted in the fall and is harvested early the following summer. It is well suited to warm temperate climates that have mild winters. The spring wheat is planted early in spring and matures the same season. It is adapted to the short season of the cool temperate regions. It is usually a hard wheat and of better quality than any of the varieties of winter wheat.

More than 80% of the bulk of the wheat kernel and 70-75% of its protein is in the endosperm. White flour is made from the endosperm. The embryo (wheat germ) forms about 3% of the kernel; it is usually removed as wheat is processed because it contains oil, which makes the grain more likely to spoil. The bran is the seed coat plus the aleurone layer (outer part of endosperm); it constitutes about 14% of the kernel. The bran is also removed when wheat is milled to make white flour. Actually, the bran somewhat decreases the nutritional value of the wheat kernel. Because it is mostly cellulose, it cannot be digested by man and tends to speed the passage of food through the intestinal tract, resulting in a lower absorption. The wheat germ and the bran are sometimes used for human consumption but more often are fed to livestock. Wheat is about 9-14% protein, most of which is contained in the endosperm. Its protein value is

diminished, however, by its lack of certain essential amino acids, notably lysine. Most of the vitamins are in the bran and wheat germ.

Among the enemies of wheat, those most dreaded are the chinch bug, the Hessian fly and the wheat midge, a small, yellowish insect, with a dark black, related to the Hessian fly, Hut differing in habits. The wheat midge, which is now common in the Mississippi Valley, probably came from Europe and has occasioned a great deal of damage to wheat, especially in warm and moist seasons. The damage is done by the little orange-yellow larvae, which destroy the embryos of the grain and prevent the heads from filling. As the larvae can live for several months without either moisture or food, they are carried about in the wheat heads, and so that species is distributed. The chinch bug and Hessian fly are described under their titles.

Many thousand varieties are known but there are three main types;

Tricitum vulgare - used mainly for bread,

Tricitum durum (Durum wheat) - largely used for macroni, and

Tricitum compactum (Club wheat) - which is too soft for ordinary bread. The berry is composed of outer branny husk, 13% of the grain, the germ or embryo (rich in nutrients) 2%, and the central endosperm (mainly starch) 85%. The average composition per 100 g is: (FAO figures) *hard wheat*- protein 12.2%; fat 2%; calcium 37 mg, iron 4 mg; calories 332, vitamin B_1 0.45 mg; vitamin B_2 0.13 mg; nicotinic acid 5.4 mg.

Soft wheat- protein 10.5%; fat 1.9%; vitamin B_1 0.38 mg; vitamin B_2 0.08 mg; nicotinic acid 4.3 mg; other values are almost same as hard wheat.

wheatfeed. Residue from the milling of wheat to produce flour, also known as millers' offal and wheat offals. Bran itself consists of the husk of the grain with some adhering endosperm. Particles with less husk and more endosperm are variously known as middlings, sharps, toppings. Very coarse middlings are known as pollards. These various designations have been dropped and the two categories weating and superfine weatings used.

Weatings- middlings or sharps containing not more than 5.75% fibre;

Superfine weatings- richer type of middlings containing not more than 4.5% fibre.

Coarse bran contains about 10% fibre. All three fractions containing about 15% protein, 3-4% fat and 60-70% carbohydrate.

wheatgerm. A supplemental food, which is an extraordinarily concentrated source of vitamin E. Taking the oil from the germ one may have an even greater concentration since all the E is in the oil. It can be further concentrated by isolating the E from the oil. Of course the further you go in steps of concentration, the more you leave behind in variety and balance. Wheatgerm oil is also a good source of vitamin F. It is an excellent source of B vitamins and protein. In the case of wheatgerm much of what is available is rancid. Rancidity occurs because most wheatgerm is rolled into flakes, which breaks the sac containing the wheatgerm oil. Exposed to air, oxygen begins to work on the work and make it rancid. It is almost certain that if the wheatgerm flakes are not vacuum packed within the day they are rolled, they will be rancid. So never buy wheatgerm flakes that have not been vacuum packed. They should have a sweet smell; if rancid they have an acrid odour. After opening, store them in the refrigerator. The burst way of all to guarantee wheatgerm oil will not be rancid is not to buy it in the flake form at all, but unrolled. Unrolled wheatgerm is variously known as embryo, chunk or unflaked wheatgerm. This is, however, harder to find than ordinary wheatgerm. Octacosanol is the active ingredient in wheatgerm responsible for its proven ability to increase vigor, stamina and endurance. It may also quicken reflexes, increase fertility, prevent miscarriages, lessen the severity of muscular dystrophy and multiple sclerosis, cure pregnancy toxaemia, and strengthen the heart muscles.

wheat flakes. Plump kernels of soft wheat are frequently used as the raw material for wheat flakes. After cleaning and sorting according to size, the kernels are tempered in steel bins of small diameter by adding moisture and holding about 25°C for about 24 hours. The wheat may be transferred one or more times during this period if such a procedure is necessary in order to keep the temperature within reasonable limits. After tempering, the wheat is steamed at atmospheric pressure until it reaches 95°C and 21%. The steamed wheat is bumped between smooth steel rollers set considerably rather apart than are flaking rollers. This treatment flattens the grain slightly, and ruptures the bran coat in several places making the kernel more permeable to the moisture which will be added during the cooking step. Next, the flattened kernels are transferred to pressure cookers, which are similar to those used for corn flakes, and the other ingredients are added. These ingredients normally include sugars, salt, malt, and sometimes a coloring substance such as caramel.

wheat-soybean blends. *See* soybean-wheat protein blends.

whey butter. A butter made from the cream obtained by running the cheese whey through a separator. It is comparable in composition and, in most instances, in flavour, in composition and, in most instances, in flavour, to ordinary butter but does not have the keeping quality of butter. It must be legally marked "whey butter" in many states.

whey, condensed. A product made by concentrating whey in a vacuum pan. The product has excellent nutritional properties because it is high in milk sugar and protein and in riboflavin which also is important nutritionally. It is used mostly for cooking purposes. Its approximate composition is; water 49%; protein 7.5%; fat 2.4%; lactose 21.5%; and ash 5.6%.

whey starter. A culture which is made from whey instead of milk or skim milk. Whey starters were formerly used to a large extent in Swiss Cheese operations. Often this starter was just a sample of whey incubated from the previous day's make.

whey products. Acetone, acrylic plastics, bakery products, butyl alcohol, candy, cheese and processed cheese, cheese spreads, coating, ethyl alcohol, feed, food acidulant; *foods*-infant, hydrolyzed lactose syrup, lactic acid, lactose, penicillin, pills, protein hydrolyzates, resins, riboflavin concentrates, soups, spirit vinegar, tanning, whey butter, whey cream, whey dried, whey drinks, whey condensed- plain, whey condensed-sweetened, whey pasteurized-sweet, and whey protein.

whey. 1. The residue from milk after removal of the casein and most of the fat (as in cheese-making); also known as lacto-serum. It contains about 1% protein (lactalbumin and lactoglobulin) together with all the lactose, water-soluble vitamins and minerals and therefore has some food value although it is 92% water. Whey cheese can be made by heat coagulation of the protein, and whey butter from the small amount (0.25%) fat. Dried whey is added to processed cheese; most whey is fed in liquid form to pigs.

2. In cheese-making, the serum which is separated from the curd after coagulation. Whey composition varies with different types of cheese, for instance, Cheddar, Swiss or Cottage cheese whey.

Because of its food value, large quantities of it are now used in candies and special cheese products; large quantities are also used in dry and concentrated form to be mixed with food and feeds, used in many human foods and as feed for poultry and livestock. Much of the whey is also condensed and spray dried by the roller process.

whipping aids. Substances added to influence the whipping quality of cream. If cream has been properly processed and has sufficient fat, whipping aids are usually unnecessary when the correct whipping procedure is followed. Viscogen, sodium alginate, gelatin, nonfat dry milks, and other substances will influence the time required to whip cream and also the stability of the whipped product. The addition of such materials is illegal is many cities and states. Formerly called thickeners.

whisky. The most popular of distilled liquors of commerce and is known all over the world. The word 'Whisky' is derived from the phrase for 'Water of Life' 'Visegebeatha'. In this respect, the Scots resemble the French who call brandy "cau-de-vie" or "Water of Life'. Most brands of whisky are a blend of pure malt whisky with spirit distilled from grain.

Scotch whisky, like Vodka and certain other liquors such as Kombranntwein, Tiquira and Kava, is a spirit made from starch. Among them, it is the universally acclaimed aristocrat and indeed its position in the world of liquor is : Whisky and Cognac first-with the rest nowhere. Just as Cognac is inimitable, no imitation of Scotch Whisky would deceive anyone - even a teetotaller. Soon after the war in 1947, attempts were made by different countries, to produce brands of whisky to match the glory of Scotch whisky, but none achieved any success. Australia for instance, and even Denmark made efforts, and did produce a sort of whisky which unfortunately did not bear even the slightest resemblance to Scotch whisky and so was not acclaimed by the people. The uniqueness of Scotch whisky which is unquestioned is still something of a mystery. whisky experts from all over the world attribute it to the peculiarities of the barley or of the bran water, used in its making, or to the virtues of the peat used to provide the fuel for the drying of the germinating grain, or to the shape of the pot-stills used to distil the spirit, or, in their more romantic moods, to the very air, which, as no one would think of denying to a Scotsman, is unique, in short to anything that is Scotch.

Unlike the making of wine, which involves only fermentation, or the production of brandy, which has two processes, the making of whisky is a multistage stage affair. Six principal operations are involved in the production of whiskey include:
(a) Selection and preparation of raw materials;
(b) fermenting;
(c) distilling;
(d) maturing and aging;
(e) blending (in most cases); and
(f) containerizing (usually bottles).

There are important variations in these operations from one country to the next and from one type of whiskey to the next. Grain, which is the raw material for whisky, contain starch which must be converted to sugar before fermentation to give the alcoholic liquid which is distilled because starch will not ferment with yeast. The production of whisky is a long and tedious process. Whisky is a spirit obtained by the distillation of mash of cereal grains saccharified by the diastase of barley malt. The cereals employed are barley, maize, rye and malted barley. Though certain substances such as potatoes, rice, sugar and molasses are used in the making of spirit in different parts of the world, they are not utilized in the making of whisky. The substances are subjected to the processes of mashing, pitching and fermenting, and the resulting liquid, called the "wash" undergoes distillation. In Scotland and Ireland, the distillation is carried out in fire-heated pot stills (pot stills are large copper kettles or pots having a pear shaped head and connected to a receiver by a copper worm which runs through a tub of cold water). The Scotch pot-still whisky is entirely malt whisky. Irish pot-still whisky is made from a mixed grist of barley, oats, maize and malt. In pot-still whisky, the secondary constituents, chiefly higher alcohols are present to the extent of about 0.2%. The cause of the improved flavour of whisky is in part due to the interaction of the spirit with the substances absorbed by the casks from the wine that they previously contained. Whisky may also be made in a patent still where rapid steam distillation gives a more highly rectified and stronger spirit. Whisky is generally blended when in bond. Whisky, straight from the still, is colourless, and the colouring of the various brands is carried out by storage in wine casks and by addition of a small quantity of sugar caramel. Pot-still whisky varies in strength from 15° to 25° overproof, when distilled. For use as a beverage, the patent still whisky is matured in casks for several years and carefully blended with matured pot-still whisky to produce blended Scotch.

Whisky contains acetic, valeric and propionic acids, and their ethyl and amyl esters, aldehydes such as furfural and acetaldehyde, and fusel oils.

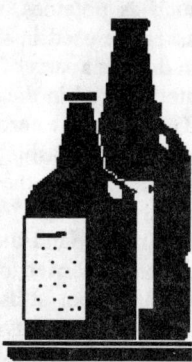

Scotch whisky, prepared from barley malt alone, is characterized by a smoky odour, traceable to the use of peat for firing malt drying kilns.

Irish whisky is prepared from barley malt to which wheat, oats, and rye are added.

Commercial whiskies are often blended with small amounts of additives, such as peach juice, glycerine, caramel, tea, coumarin, orris root, dried prunes, sherry wine, vanilla, caraway seed, cinnamon and cloves for improving the flavour. Imitation whisky is made from ethyl alcohol by colouring and flavouring.

white clover. *Trifolium repens.* A variety of clover and common perennial with low-growing profile and pink flowers. The plant is native to Europe and Siberia and some authorities believe it may be native to northeastern US as well. White clover is commonly used in the US as pasture plant and for lawns. Because of generally low yields, it is not attractive for hay-making, but is often mixed with other legumes and grasses. It is an excellent crop for honeybees. Today, white clover is found throughout the world, with a wide adaptability to climate, ranging from those of high altitudes and beyond the Arctic Circle to equatorial regions. The seeding characteristics of white clover still are not well understood. The plant will frequently appear in areas without prior planned seeding. The plant does best in clay and silt soils of humid areas and is excellent under irrigation.

whizzer. A term applied to centrifugal devices for drying (hydroextractors), especially those used for grains.

whole-wheat meal. Flour or meal prepared by milling the whole wheat grain, *i.e.*, 100% extraction rate.

wild oregon grape. *Berberis vulgaris or Mahonia aquifolium.* An evergreen shrub found in mountain areas; it was introduced to Europe as a cultivated plant and has become naturalized. Its irregular, knotty rootstock has a brownish bark with yellow wood underneath. This yellow pigment is the antibiotic alkaloid, berberine-the same constituent found in golden seal root. Its branched stems have 10 or more spiny, sessile leaflets adorning them.

wild rice. *Zizania aquatica.* A plant classified in the tribe Oryzeae. In appearance the plant does not greatly resemble rice, and the grain itself has few similarities.

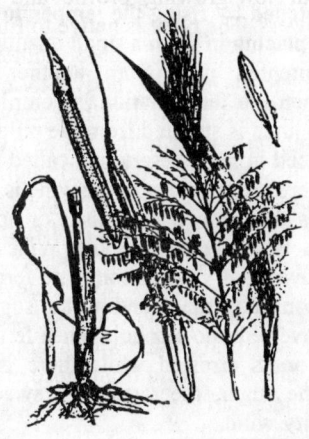

It is an annual grass, usually growing 2-3 metres. It bears 4-6 leaves, 1-4 cm in width and upto 60 cm long. The seeds are covered with palea and lemma when they fall from the penicle. It is said that the seeds of wild rice are sometimes planted in marshes and on green preserves, but the stands which are of the greatest economic importance have become established spontaneously. Except in cases heavy attacks by parastes occur, ample natural reseeding keeps the wild beds establshed year after year, even when most of the grain is harvested. Wild rice was traditionally harvested by Indians, mostly by the members of the Chippewa tribe. When harvested the grain may have as much as 40-80% moisture. This is unsuitable level for storing the grain, so it is dried for 2-3 days in open air. Then it is parched and the hulls are removed by pounding. Parching is often done with crude equipment, frequently a make shift container supported over a woodfire. Large processors pass the grain through rotating cylinders situated over heated units. the control of processing time and temperature is a skill which is dependent upon the accurate judgement of the texture and colour of the product. Excessive heat causes popping of rice.

Wills factor. A factor in autolyzed yeast effective in promoting red blood cell formation, probably folic acid.

Wilstermarsch cheese. The varieties of cow's milk cheese similar to Tilsiter made in Schleswig-Holstein, Germany. This cheese is classed as follows:

Rahm - a whole milk cheese with added cream.

Sussmilk - a whole milk cheese.

Zweizetige - a cheese made with a mixture of morning whole milk and evening skim milk.

Dreizetige - a cheese made from 12 and 24 hour old skim milk and fresh whole milk.

Herbst - a cheese made from a mixture of 12, 24, 36 and 48 hour old skim milk and fresh whole milk.

The milk is set in a copper kettle, and rennet is added to it. Curd is cut with scoop or ladle and some of the whey is removed. The curd is transferred to a cloth-lined type of curd sink where it is mixed and squeezed until firm. Salt is added, and the curd kneaded by hand and then transferred to cloth-lined, Tilsiter-like molds to be pressed heavily for 8-12 hours. After forms are removed, this soft cheese may be bandaged to control flattening. The cheese is turned daily a week or more, then curing is completed in a dry room. It is ready for market in 3-4 weeks. Also known as Holsteiner-Marsch cheese.

wilting. The decrease in strength and rigidity of plants, particularly leaves, due to lack of moisture as a result of droughty conditions or to cutting of the stem or other part of the plant. The moisture load on the dryer for grasses and hays and forages is often reduced by wilting the plants and field drying before drying on the dryer.

Wiltshire cheese. A kind of hard and sweet-curd cheese similar to Derby cheese, first made in Wiltshire, England. The milled, salted curd is pressed over night in a press vat. The following day the cheese is removed from the press, salted on the surface, dressed in cloth, dressed in cloth and pressed again. This process may be repeated once or twice after which the cheese is pressed for a week. The cheese is cured in the same manner as Derby cheese.

Windsor bean. Synonym for broad bean. Because of variations in terminology among countries and within regions of any given country, the names listed here may be at variance with some local customs. Several additional food substances are termed beans because of their general physiology. Beans such as coffee, cola, and vanilla beans are not included in this list because they are not related to the leguminous beans.

wine. Essentially a fermentation of sugar by yeast to produce alcohol, together with flavouring agent supplied by the fruit or vegetable. The grape sugar contained in grape juice is readily changed through fermentation into alcohol. The process of manufacture is simple. To separate the juice the grapes are placed in a crushing machine having two corrugated cylinders which crush the grapes without crushing the seeds. The must, as the resulting mass of pulp is called, is then forced by pumps through hose to large wooden vats or tanks, where the fermentation takes place, usually slowly. The fermentation is watched with the greatest care, for upon it depends the quality of the wine. It is hastened by rising the temperature or by placing in them a small quantity of fermented pulp from another vat. When the fermentation is completed, the juice is strained from the pulp and placed in large reservoirs, called tuns, where it remains until the wine is ripe. It is then drawn into casks or bottles and is ready for market. Wines are known as dry when complete fermentation takes place and all the sugar is converted into alcohol. When fermentation is arrested while there is yet some sugar, the result is a sweet or fruity wine.

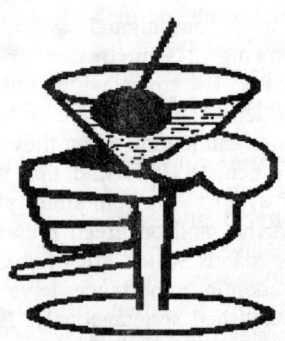

A sparkling wine is one which effervesces when the bottles are uncorked. Champagne is a good example. In such wines fermentation has been arrested before all the carbonic acid has escaped. In colour, wines are known as red or white. Red wines are produced by allowing the skins of the grapes to remain in the vat during fermentation. The amount of alcohol in wine varies from 16 to 25 parts in 100. In light wines it may be from 7 to 12 parts in 100.

Wines are manufactured in almost endless varieties, and many of them are named from the locality in which they are made, such as Port, Burgundy, Bordellais and Rhenish wines. The leading countries in the world in the manufacture of wine are France, Spain and Italy. Table wines are produced from grapes with sugar content such that the alcohol produced is not more than 11-14% by volume, dessert wines from grapes with higher sugar content and fortified by addition of brandy distilled from grape wine, to 17-21% alcohol.

wineberry. *Rubus phoenicolasius;* similar to raspberry, orange coloured.

wintergreen. A small plant, several inches high, which grows in the woods of the northern hemisphere. Glossy, oval leaves, green all winter, grow on the ends of reddish stems. Small white or pink flowers spring from the base of the leaf stems and scarlet berries follow them. The leaves yield an oil which is used for flavoring and for medicinal purposes.

winterization. Applied to edible oils, meaning the removal of the more saturated glycerides so that the oil remains bright and clear at low temperatures. The oil is simply chilled and the solidified palmitates and stearates filtered off.

Winter nelis pear. A variety of pear. Popular at one time, the variety has progressively declined in commercial flavor because of small size, unattractive appearance, and tendency to decay in storage. Fruit is small to medium in size. Shape is roundish-obovate to obtuse-obovate-pyriform.

Skin is fairly thick, but tender, roughed with considerable rusting. Dull green or yellowish in color. Flesh fairly fine except for grit at center. Buttery, moderately juicy, spicy, rich flavor. Rates well as a dessert variety where small size can be desirable. Tree is fairly vigorous, willowy and spreading in habit, reasonably productive, moderately susceptible to blight.

witches milk. Secretion of the mammary gland of the newborn of both sexes; due to the presence of the hormone prolactin that travels from the blood of the mother into the fetus. Also known as sorcerers' milk.

witch hazel. A North American shrub which is of economic importance as the source of a healing lotion obtained by distilling the leaves in alcohol. The plant has branches of a very peculiar appearance, for they twist and curve in all directions. In olden times the witch hazel was believed to have supernatural power, and the forked twigs were used as divining rods. The plant does not bloom until late in the fall, and the fruits ripen the following year. The yellow flowers grow in showy clusters. A small, woody capsule encloses the seeds.

withania cheese. A kind of cheese so named because the rennet used in making it comes from withania berries (*W. coagulans,* a member of *Solanaceae family*). Cheese made fro withania rennet is said to have a good flavour if ania rennet is said to have a good flavour if ripened to the right degree, but with age it develops an acrid flavour. It is made in East Indies where religion and prejudice make the use of animal rennet impracticable.

woad. A group of plants of the mustard family, chiefly natives of the Mediterranean region. Dyer's woad, a species yielding a blue dye, was formerly much cultivated. This has been superseded by indigo; but a fine blue is still obtained by mixing the two. The leaves when gathered are reduced to a paste, fermented for two weeks, made into balls, sun-dried, and subjected to further fermentation.

wood alcohol. CH_3OH. Classical name for methyl alcohol, it is highly toxic. Its presence in methylated spirits accounts for the toxicity of the latter.

woolgreen B. Food green S. Food Green S is triarymethane dye having a structural formula closely similar to that of Fast Green. It is the monosodium salt of 4,4-bis-(dimethy-lamino)-diphenyl-methylene-2-naphthol-3,6-disulphonic acid. It is a dull bluish-green powder, soluble in water (8% at 25°C) but only slightly soluble in glycerol and ethanol (95%). It has poor light-stability, but is quite stable in acid media and in the presence of sulphur dioxide. This colour is not normally used alone, but is a useful component of green shades.

Worcester sauce. A special kind of sauce, characterized by spicy flavour, sediment and thin supernatant liquid. Recipes usually secret but basically soya, tamarinds, anchovies, garlic and spices, plus sugar, salt and vinegar, maturated six months in oak casks.

wormwood. *Artemisia absinthium.* Wormwood is a shrubby perennial herb with greyish-white stems covered with fine silky hairs. The leaves are silky, hair and glandular with small, resinous particles are yellowish green in colour. The plant emits an aromatic odour and yields a spicy, somewhat bitter taste. It's native to Europe, northern Africa and western Asia, but now extensively cultivated. Parts used are the leaves and flowering tops (fresh and dried), harvested just before or during flowering. Wormwood has been used in the manufacture of vermouth. Sweet wormwood, another species (*A. annua*) is often grown as an ornamental, but contains an essential oil that has strong antifungal and antibacterial activities.

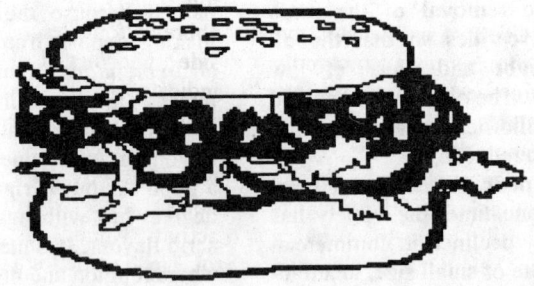

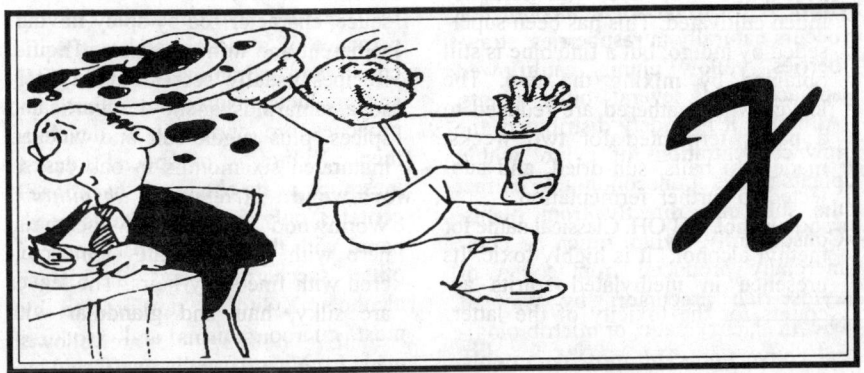

xanthine. A purine that is an intermediate compound in the oxidative degradation of adenine and guanine to uric acid.

xanthine oxidase. An enzyme of purine catabolism that catalyzes the oxidation of xanthine to uric acid and the oxidation of hypoxanthine to xanthine; a molybdenum-containing flavoprotein that also catalyzes the oxidation of aldehydes. It is present in milk and in liver; specific for the two purines, xanthine and hypoxanthine (which it oxidizes to uric acid), and will also oxidize a range of aldehydes to the corresponding acids. It is identical with Schardinger's enzyme of milk.

xanthophylls. Class of oxygenated hydrocarbon compounds structurally related to carotene. Xanthophylls are yellow pigments, some of which function as photosynthetic accessory pigments in plants. However, in the brown algae the xanthophylls fucoxanthin and peridinin are the primary light-absorbing pigments.

The yellow pigment of milk fat is a xanthophyll. These carotenoid fat-soluble pigments are synthesized by plants. Their colour range from deep yellow to greenish yellow. The Xan-thophylls are not absorbed by dairy cattle in quantities proportionate to their occurrence in the food. The xanthophylls are principal oxygen-containing carotenoid in green plants, in many seeds, and the one occurring in greatest amount in eggs yolk. This pigment has also been called lutein.

xanthoproteic test. For proteins (actually for the benzene nucleus of tyrosine and tryptophan which occur in nearly all proteins). Yellow colour on boiling with nitric acid, turns orange on adding ammonia.

xanthosine. The ribonucleoside of xan-thine. Xanthosine mono-, di-, and triphosphate are abbreviated, respectively, as XMP, XDP, and XTP. The abbreviations refer to the 5'-nucleoside phosphates unless otherwise indicated.

xerophilic microorganisms. Microorganisms that grow best under low water activity conditions, and may not be able to grow at high water activity values.

Xtol. Trade name for a distilled grade tall oil; used in the preparation of surfactants, soaps, asphalt, alkyds, and as a chemical intermediate.

xylan. A homopolysaccharide of xylose that occurs in plants.

xylitol. A 5-carbon sugar alcohol that occurs naturally in raspberries, strawberries, yellow plums, cauliflower, spinach, and several other plants. Although it is widely distributed, the low concentrations of xylitol within plants makes it uneconomic to extract the substance directly from plants. Consequently, xylitol much be commercially produced from xylan or xylose-rich precursors by way of chemical, enzymatic, or microbiological conversion. The most commonly used and highest yield xylan sources as of the early 1980s are birch tree chips.

Other appropriate starting materials include beech and other hardwood chips, almond and pecan shells, cotton-seed hulls, straw, cornstalks (maize), and corn cobs. These xylan sources are routinely converted to xylitol by hydrolysis of xylan to D-xylose. Reduction of xylose to xylitol by pressure hydrogenation in the presence of a nickel catalyst; Purification and crystallization of xylitol end-products. Numerous other approaches are currently in development. Xylitol is of special interest inasmuch as its chemical "backbone" contains only 5 carbon atoms compared with the 6-carbon backbone of other saccharides and the sugar alcohols. Xylitol is not utilized by most microorganisms and products made from it are usually unaffected by microbial attack. Xylitol is a normal intermediate product of carbohydrate metabolism in humans and animals, and it occurs naturally in plants as previously mentioned. The use of xylitol in various food substances is being investigated by regulatory agencies in a number of countries.

xylose. Pentose sugar found in plant tissues as complex polysaccharide; it is 40% as sweet as sucrose.

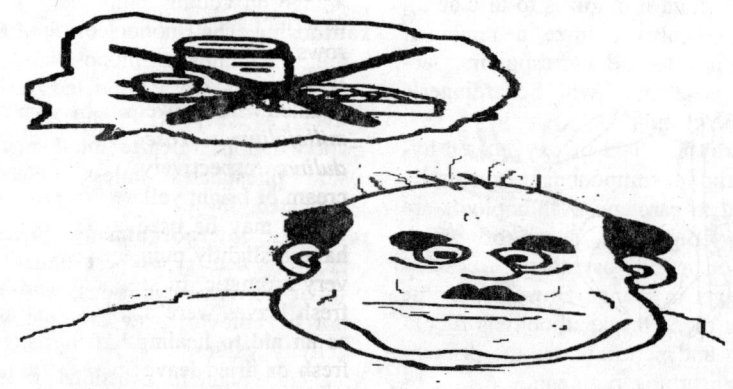

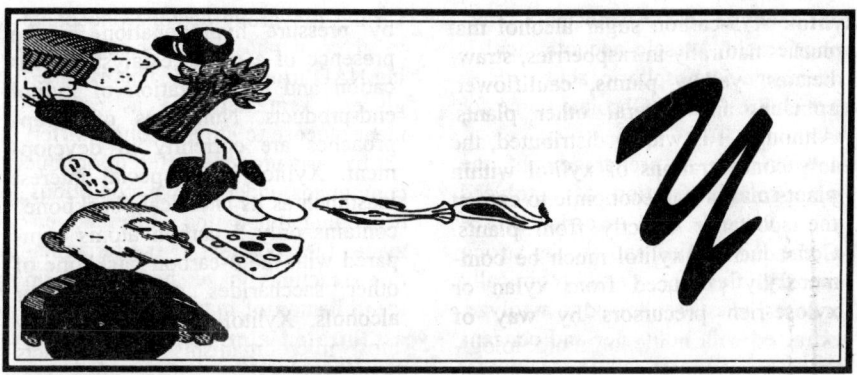

yam. A plant having edible roots much like the sweet potato. It is found in the temperate and subtropical parts of America, in China and in the islands of the Southern Pacific. In Australia and China a species known as winged yam produces edible tubers from one and a half to three feet long which sometimes weigh thirty pounds. The skin is dark brown and the reddish flesh is sweet and juicy and very palatable when baked. A large yam is also found in India, though there the small white yam is more in demand for foot.

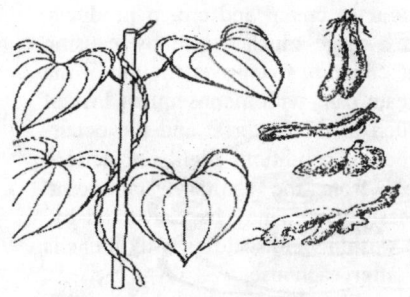

The yam has become an important vegetable in the US. While it contains less starch than the Irish potato, it contains more nitrogen and a high percentage of sugar. The wild species contain toxins (saponins and alkaloids) and these can appear in cultivated varieties under poor conditions of growth. The average composition per 100 g is: carbohydrate 25%; 2% protein; iron 1 mg; vitamin B_1 0.04 mg; vitamin B_2 0.05 mg; nicotinic acid 0.5 mg; and vitamin C 20 mg.

. . mor. Trade name for refined pine oil which is used to increase the detergency of soaps, for dyes, and as a solvent for oils and greases.

yarrow. *Achillea millefolium.* A hardy perennial and native to Europe, grows as a rampant weed in fields and hedge rows, where it can vary from a low. It has flat heads of minute five-petalled white flowers. Other forms (*A. millefolium v. rosea* and *A. filipendulina,* respectively) have pink-and-cream or bright yellow flowers. Fresh leaves may be used in salads. They have a slightly pungent taste and are very aromatic. In self-help medicine, fresh leaves were applied to wounds as an aid to healing. An infusion of fresh or dried leaves may be used to apply to minor cuts and grazes, and a decoction may be used to wash the hair; it was thought to prevent baldness. It can also be helpful as an astringent for greasy skin.

yeast adenylic acid. Adenosine-3-phosphoric acid. Muscle adenolic acid is adenosine-5-phosphoric acid.

yeast eluate factor. Obsolete name for vitamin B_6.

yeast extract. A preparation of the water-soluble fraction of autolyzed yeast, valuable both as a rich source of the B vitamins and for its strong savoury flavour. Yeast (comically brewers' yeast) is allowed to autolyze, extracted with hot water and concentrated by evaporation. The commercial preparations are Marmite and Yeastrel.

yeast fermentation, bottom. Fermentation during the manufacture of beer with a yeast that sinks to the bottom of the tank. Most beers are produced this way; ale, porter and stout being the principal beers produced by top fermentation.

yeast fermentation. The yeast cells tissue can metabolize glucose both under anaerobic as well as aerobic conditions. In muscle tissue, under anaerobic condition, lactic acid formation helps to regenerate NAD^+ from NADH, for the flow of glycolytic reactions. The yeast cells also need a similar mechanism but lack the enzyme lactate dehydrogenase. These cells, however, possess pyruvate decarboxylase and alcohol dehydrogenase to achieves the same purpose. Acetaldehyde formed in this way, is next reduced to ethyl alcohol, by the enzyme alcohol dehydrogenase. In this reaction NAD^+ is regenerated from NADH needed by glyceraldehyde-3-phosphate dehydrogenase enzyme in the glycolytic reactions. If sodium bisulphite is added to the fermenting medium it reacts with acetaldehyde and blocks the final reaction regenerating NAD^+. The yeast under these circumstances start converting dihydroxy acetone-phosphate to glycerol phosphate for regenerating NAD^+ from NADH. This is called glycerol fermentation. Yeast can ferment glucose to ethyl alcohol, different bacteria produce different organic compounds under similar conditions, depending upon the different enzymes they possess. These fermentation reactions have been used in identification of many bacteria.

yeast filtrate factor. Obsolete name for pantothenic acid.

Yeastrel. Trade name for a yeast extract; the average composition per 100 g is: 4.2 mg vitamin B_2 and 40 mg nicotinic acid.

yeasty cream. Cream which has under gone a gassy fermentation by the presence of lactose fermenting yeast. The taste is yeasty and the cream foams. *Torula cremoris* is the most common species of yeast causing this defect in cream. Yeasty cream in its first stages is of a pleasantly aromatic "nutty" flavour and odour, which gradually changes into a disagreeable bitterness. The yeasts, while usually present in most cream, develop only under favourable temperature conditions. Besides spoiling flavour and odour of cream and cream products, they cause much waste by causing the cream to foam over the top of the cream cans with a consequent loss of much of the butterfat and the occurrence of conditions highly objectionable from the sanitary standpoint. Yeasty cream may be prevented by:
(a) washing and scalding milk utensils after each use,
(b) cooling the cream to below 5°C, and keeping it cool.

yeast. Fungi; consist of cell wall enclosing cytoplasm and nucleus, some can spore (true yeasts), others reproduce only by cell division (false yeasts). In general, the term yeast is used to describe a relatively small number of *Ascomycetes* fungi (a few hundred), as compared with the vast number of other fungi (several thousand) that have been identified. The term mold does not have a specific mycological definition. While the yeasts have a preponderantly positive value to the food field, the molds make some positive contributions (some cheeses, etc.), but participate in many more negative ways (leaf molds on plants; blue-green molds on fruits; machinery mold; related food-borne diseases). Some authorities identify all or most molds as saprophytes, that is, plants that obtain their nourishment from nonliving substances.

Large quantities of bakers' yeast are used in the production of bread, rolls, sweet doughs, pretzels, pizzas, crackers, doughnuts, bagels, Danish pastry, and the like. The chief advantages of yeast leavening, as compared to chemical leavening, are that it contributes characteristic tastes and aromas and that the evolution of carbon dioxide can be made to continue over a much longer period of time. The main disadvantage is that it is somewhat more difficult to control. Also, in some food, fermentation flavors can be undesirable, certain cookies, for example. The yeast leavening process is generally more costly than chemical aeration, not only because yeast can be more expensive than chemical leaveners, but because the yeast cells consume other materials (sugars) as a result of their activity. Gas is generated during fermentation as part of the metabolic activity of yeast. Many microorganisms can ferment sugars with the production of carbon dioxide, but the organism that seems to function best

in doughs is *Saccharomyces cerevisiae,* or bakers' yeast.

The importance of the economically useful yeasts can be attributed to two main factors:

(a) Fermentation- the transformation of simple sugars and other organic chemicals to other desirable chemicals; and

(b) Respiratory (Oxidative) metabolism-the great capacity of some yeasts for a protein synthesis during growth in richly aerated media containing a wide variety of carbonaceous and nitrogenous nutrients.

Thus, yeasts have been found to be useful in several ways:

1. As dried, nonfermentative whole cells or hydrolyzed cell matter, yeasts contribute nutrition and flavor to human diets and animal rations.

2. As living cells, they are biocatalysts in the production of bread, wine, beer, distilled, beverages, among many other important food products.

3. As producers of vitamins and other biochemicals, yeasts are a rich source of enzymes, coenzymes, nucleic acids, nucleotides, sterols, and metabolic intermediates.

4. As a versatile biochemical tool, yeasts aid research studies in nutrition, enzymology, and molecular biology. The destruction of numerous substances by molds has both positive and negative connotations.

Molds can play an important role in the biodegradation of unwanted substances. *Saccharomyces cerevisiae* is used in brewing and baking; *S. cerevisiae* var. *ellipsoideus* is used in wind making (occurs on grapes). Other species of this genus used in production of fermented milk liquors, like Koumiss, Kefir, etc. Sub-genus

Zygosaccharomyces can ferment highly concentrated sugar products like jam, honey and sugar confectionery, and therefore important to the food technologist. Also in the Tribe Saccharomyceteae are *Pichia* and *Hansenula*, contaminants in brewing that form esters instead of alcohol from sugar. Also grow as films on pickle brines, film yeasts. Varieties such as *Candida utilis* called Food yeast (formerly *Torula utilis*) are grown on waste carbohydrate sources and petroleum residues, as a potential supplement to animal feed. The composition varies with growing conditions, approximately 50% protein of NPU about 50, and relatively high concentrations of most of the B vitamins, 5% fat (*Rhodotorula gracilis* can produce 50% fat.).

Brewer's yeast contains an extremely rich concentration of nutrients. It comes closer than anything else to being a 'super food'. It contains 16 of the 20 amino acids and the complete B-complex range; it is especially rich in B_1 and B_2 but also contains niacinamide, pantothenic acid, biotin, cholin, pyridoxine, folic acid, vitamin B_{12} and inositol. It also has large amounts of phosphorus, iron and calcium and two of the vital trace elements, chromium and selenium, Yeast varies according to the medium on which it is grown and not all brewer's yeast contains B_{12}. The torula (nutritional or 'candida') yeast was developed with a de-bittered taste. It is usually grown on waste sulphite liquor from wood pulp. It is advised not to take baker's yeast or any other live yeast as a food supplement. The live yeast goes on working in the gut and actually eats up the vitamin B in the body. This includes yeast used for brewing. If you are a home brewer and you want to make use of spent yeast you should rinse it in fresh water, dry it and then deactivate the yeast by heating it in the oven for 30 minutes.

yeast, compressed. In making compressed yeast, the washed yeast suspension is filtered and extruded to form a firm cake containing about 69% to 70% water. On a dry weight basis, extruded material will contain 50% to 60% protein, 4% to 5% fat, 2.8% to 3.0% phosphorus, and 6% to 8% ash. Fractional percentages of additives such as emulsifiers may be present. Compressed yeast stored at refrigerator temperatures of -10°C will lose about 10% of its activity in four weeks. At higher storage temperatures, the yeast rapidly loses its leavening power and develops unpleasant odors, and the cakes turn brown at the edges. Of course, compressed yeast should never be stored at room temperature. Many baking problems can be traced to the use of compressed yeast that has deteriorate in storage. Compressed yeast with a higher content of carbohydrate and a lower protein content is said to be more resistant to storage deterioration.

yeast, deteriorated. A number of methods have been suggested for improving the storage stability of yeasts. Patents have been granted for coating yeast cells with fats and oils. A process for preserving active dry yeast by applying polyethylene glycol having a molecular weight in the range of 3,350-4,600 to the surface of the yeast. The coating is applied in a fluid bed dryer by spraying the molten glycol on to the surface of the particles. Glutathione, a reducing agent, is one of the substances released from dried yeast when the yeast is rehydrated. The physical properties of doughs may be adversely affected by this substance-they may become softer, sticker, and less retentive of gas. Glutathione is present in all yeast, including compressed yeast, but semi-permeable membranes in the cell prevent it from leaking out if the cells are fully hydrated. The membrane's control of permeation is lost (or greatly reduced) when it is dehydrated, however, and soluble substances inside the cell can be dissolved and eluted before permeability is completely re-established after the cell contracts liquid water. Published data indicate that the amount of glutathione released from instant ADY is considerably less than that extracted from regular ADY, when the rehydration conditions are similar. It might be thought that addition of oxidizing agents would counteract the reducing action of glutathione, but there does not seem to be any practical way of balancing these reactions. Compressed yeast cells that have been killed, as by high temperature storage, will also release glutathione when they are mixed with water. The effects on dough properties are similar to those described above. Of course, the loss of organized metabolic activity in heat damage cells will eliminate any significant gas formation by these cells. Dead yeast cells autolyze, i.e., they break down completely, producing compounds having unpleasant flavors that carry through to the baked loaf.

yeast, instant active dry. This product differs from regular dried yeast in that the instant version does not require a separate rehydration step. That is, the instant product can be added directly from its container to the dough mixer. The difference results

both from the yeasts's genetic constitution and the method used for processing it. A method of preparing instant active dry yeast is as follows: Fresh compressed yeast (special strain of S. cerevisiae) containing 1-3% of methyl cellulose and about the same amount of a wetting agent is divided into a mass of particles having a particle size of 0.2-2.0 mm. The particles are dried by passing through them a drying gas (e.g., air) as a temperature of not more than 160°C. In not more than 120 minutes, a dry matter content of 85% or more is achieved without raising the temperature of the particles above 50°C. Because instant ADY is dried to a moisture content lower than 5%, it will absorb water from air at normal ranges of relative humidity. This partial rehydration can lead to rapid deterioration with loss of gassing power. Oxygen uptake is also determental to the shelf life of ADY. Consequently, the package is designed to have low gas transmission rates. It usually is a pouch of four-ply construction including layers of aluminium foil and polyester. Pouch and contents are vacuumed before heat sealing.

yeast, regular active dry. There are several types of active dry yeast (ADY). Most, if not all, of these products are manufactured from strains selected to be resistant to dehydration damage. Yeast cream is the raw material. Free water is removed by vacuum filters or filter presses. If a vacuum filter is used, the yeast cream is first treated with an aqueous solution of a salt such as sodium chloride to extract some internal water from the cells through osmotic action. The most common type of ADY has been dehydrated at low temperatures until it reaches a moisture content of about 7.5-8.5%. Otherwise, its composition is very similar to that of compressed yeast. It can be produced as short thin strands, small pellets, salt granules, or powder, and it is normally packed in polyethylene-lined fiber drums or in flexible pouches. About 1% of its activity will be lost per month of room temperature storage if the yeast has been packed in nitrogen or carbon dioxide, while up to 8% per month may be lost if it has not been packed in one of these inert gases. The regular ADY must be rehydrated with water having a temperature of 40° to 45°C if maximum fermentative activity is to be obtained. It should never been rehydrated with either chilled water or hot water. Rehydration of the individual cells is very rapid, but it may take a few minutes for water to penetrate to the center of the granules. After rehydration is complete, the yeast may be chilled, or even heated to slightly above the rehydration range, without causing significant damage to its fermentation ability. When substituting ADY for compressed yeast in a formula which has been designed for the latter, multiply the compressed yeast weight by 0.6-0.75, and add enough water to make up the difference. All active dry yeasts must be clearly distinguished from inactive dry yeast, which is manufactured as a nutritional additive or as a raw material for preparing flavors and other greatly modified products. It has no fermentative ability at all, and is probably never used in bakery products. Some inactive dried yeasts are made from species other than S. cerevisiae.

Yeatex. Trade name for yeast extract, autolyzed Brewers' yeast; used as a flavouring ingredient. The average composition per 100 g is: 40% protein; 11% carbohydrate; 1 mg thiamin; 2 mg riboflavin; 42 mg nicotinic acid; 5 mg pantothenic acid; 2.2 mg pyridoxine; and 1 mg folic acid.

yellow clover. *Trifolium agrarium.* A variety of true clover and an annual with yellow flowers and a low-growing profile. It is frequently found along highways and is not of agricultural importance. It should not to confused with yellow sweet clover.

yellow colours. Oil yellow GG - mixture of 4-phenylazoresorcinol and 4,6 - (phenylazo resorcinol. Yellow 2 G - disodium salt of 1-(2,5-dichloro-4-sulphophenyl)-5-hydroxy-3-methyl-4-p-sulpho-phenylazopyrazole. Yellow RFS - disodium salt of 4-sulpho-4-(sulphomethylamino)-azobenzene. Yellow RY - disodium salt of 6-p-sulphophenylazoresorcinol-4-sulphonic acid. Sunset yellow FCF - disodium salt of 1-p-sulphophenylazo-2-naphthol-6-sulphonic acid; yellow-orange colour used to simulate the colour of eggs or orange, called Yellow No. 6 in US Oil yellow XP-3-methyl-1-phenyl-4-(2,4-xylazo)-5-pyrazolone. Naphthol yellow S-disodium or potassium salt of 2,4-dinitro-1-naphthol-7-sulphonic acid.

yellow dock. *Rumex crispus.* Yellow dock is a perennial plant considered by some to be a troublesome weed in many fields and waste places throughout Europe, the US and southern Canada. Its spindle-shaped, yellow taproot sends up a smooth, rather slender stem. Lanceolate to oblong lanceolate in shape, the pointed light green leaves have predominantly wavy margins. The lower leaves are larger and longer-petioled than the upper are. The numerous pale green, drooping flowers are loosely whirled in panicled racemes. The seed is a pointed, three-angled and heart-shaped kind of nut.

yellow enzyme. One of a group of flavoprotein dehydrogenases that contain a yellow flavin prosthetic group.

yellow milk. Milk which has acquired a yellow colour due to an organism described a yellow colour due to an organism described as *Bacillus synxanthus* which redissolves the cure to form a yellow liquid. There are probably several organisms which produce a yellow colour; all seem to have proteolytic functions. Yellow milk is very rare, though it is very common to see dirty vessels which have contained milk become quite yellow.

yerba mate. *See* mate.

Yersinia enterocolitica. A Gram-negative, nonspore-forming bacillus that is a frequent cause of gastroenteritis in humans. The organism is transmitted to humans by contact with infected domestic animals or by ingestion of faecal contaminated food or water.

Yersinia pestis. The small, oval, pleomorphic, nonmotile, Gram-negative rods that grow best at 27°C. Masses of the *Y. pestis* partially obstruct the digestive tract of infected rat fleas. Important changes occur in *Y. pestis* when they grow in the human host:

(a) The organism produces an antiphagocytic capsule when it grows at 310K, the temperature of human body.

(b) The organism produces a plasmid-dependent cytotoxic factor at 30°C, that kills macrophages.

(c) Plasmid-dependent synthesis of a cytoplasmic protein, V antigen, it occurs in response to low intracellular calcium concentration of macrophages. It is thought to be an important virulence factor because antibody to it protects experimental animals from plague.

Yersinia ruckeri. The pathogenic yersinia that causes disease in fish and other aquatic life. It causes red-mouth disease in rainbow-trout.

Yestamin. Trade name for a variety of preparations of dried Saccharomyces yeast (debittered brewers' yeast) used to enrich foods. The average composition per 100 g is: 44% protein; 1-2% fat; 36% carbohydrate; 5-27 mg thiamin; 3-7 mg riboflavin; 20-60 mg nicotinic acid; 2-6 mg panthothenic acid; 2-3 mg pyridoxine; and 2 mg folic acid.

yield. For the isolation of an enzyme; the total activity at a given step in the isolation divided by the total activity at a reference step.

yield coefficient. The weight of bacteria obtained from a culture divided by the weight of a limiting material that was utilized by the bacteria during their growth.

Ymer. trade name for a sour milk drink which is becoming popular in Denmark and to a large extent replacing Yoghurt. It is made from skim milk, soured as ordinary lactic acid starters most of the curd by separating out the whey, artier which cream is added. Then this mixture is homogenized and bottled, the mixture filled into bottles at a temperature of about 5°C. The bottles are held at ice temperatures until consumed.

yogurt. The product obtained by inoculating pasteurized milk with a mixed culture of *Streptococcus thermophilus* and *Lactobacillus bulgaricus*, and incubating the mixture at 30°C until the lactose is fermented. In commercial production, nonfat or low-fat milk is pasteurized, cooled, inoculated with *streptococcus thermophilus* and *Lactobacillus bulgaricus. S. thermophilus* grows more quickly at first and renders the milk anaerobic and weakly acidic. *L. bulgaricus* then acidifies the milk even more. Acting together, the two species, ferment almost all the lactose to lactic acid and flavour the yoghurt with diacetyl and acetaldehyde. Fruits or the fruit flavour to be added are pasteurized separately and then combined with yoghurt. Yoghurt has the same food value as milk except that it has a lower sugar level and is more acidic. It is a good source of protein and calcium and contains as few calories, so it is good for dieters (but beware of the commercially flavoured yoghurts). It is an excellent whole protein in itself and contains significant amounts of carbohydrate and vitamins B_2 and B_3. Many manufacturers also add vitamins A, C and D. The yoghurt breaks down milk to lactic acid and the bacteria which cause putrefaction in the form of gas cannot live in this lactic acid. Yoghurt bacteria are also capable of manufacturing the entire range of B-complex vitamins in the intestine. This is very important because many modern drugs kill intestinal flora. Another advantage of yoghurt is that people who are allergic to milk can generally eat it safely. The bacterial culturing agent consumes most of the lactose, which is one of the main reasons for intolerance to milk, particularly in adults. The bacteria also acts on the milk protein so that it becomes in effect predigested. The changes to the lactose and protein of milk in yoghurt render it easily digestible, even by chronic invalids.

yohimbine. *Corynanthe yohimbe.* Schizandra fruit. *Schizandra chenensis.* Ginkgo. *Ginkgo biloba.* These three are included together because of their remarkable sexual rejuvenating properties, particularly when used in conjunction with each other. Yohimbine is the popularized name of a real tongue-twisting chemical known officially as 17 α-hydroxyyohimban-16-α-carboxylic acid methylester. The flowers adorning it may be either pink or white. The nourishing fruit is a collection of berry-like, ripened carpels in a short, spike-like, drooping head that's fleshy but not splitting open when ripened. Gingko happens to be the only living representative left of a once vast order of tall, resinous trees widely distributed throughout the Mesozoic. Era. The drupe-like fruit yields yellow seeds when it matures and acquires a rather foul-smelling odour to it. The outer fleshy portion of the fruit provokes a very warm sensation to the skin when brought in contact with it. The leaves also are used as well. Both schizandra and ginko are very popular in Chinese folk medicine for a *wide variety* of health complaints, especially sexual frigidity.

yolk index. Index of freshness of an egg; the ratio of height to diameter of yolk under defined conditions. As the egg deteriorates the yolk index decreases.

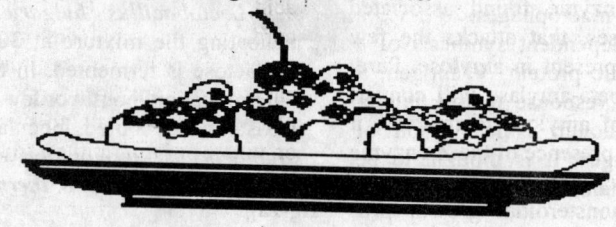

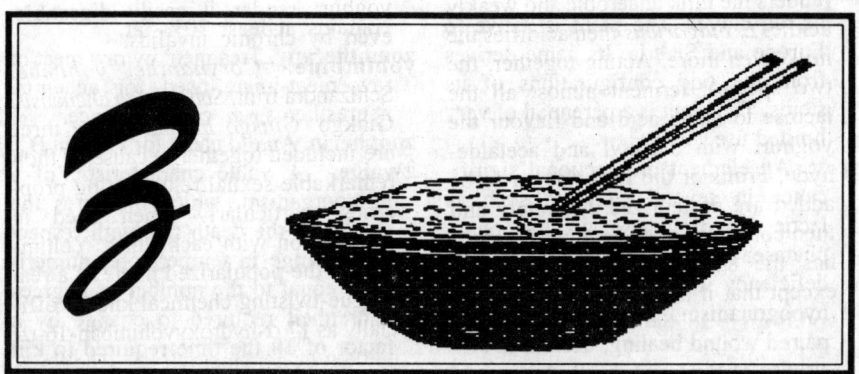

zedoary root. The roots of *Curcuma zedoaria*, an Indian plant of the ginger family; used in the manufacture of flavours and bitters.

zein. Protein obtained from maize (*Zea mais*), soluble in alcohol but not water or dilute alkali. It is of poor nutritive value as it completely lacks lysine and is poor in tryptophan. It is present in corn gluten and is separated from the gluten by solvent extraction and precipitation. Zein is used as a binder in tablet making and for gloss and protection in tablet coatings used in the pharmaceutical industry. It is used as a functional ingredient in some food products. It is also used as a protective coating for confections and grains, as well as a coating on nut meats, where protection against moisture penetration is required for long periods, and for the vitamin enrichment coating of rice.

Z-enzyme. Enzyme found associated with amylases, that attacks the few 1,3-β-links present in amylose. Pure, crystalline beta-amylase will convert only 70% of amylose to maltose, it requires the presence of the Z-enzyme for complete conversion.

zeranol. A nonsteroidal growth promoter used in cattle to improve feed conversion efficiency. It has mild oestrogenic properties, and is thought to act as an anabolic by stimulating the pituitary to increase production of somatotrophin (growth hormone). It causes increased nitrogen retention, increased muscle and bone growth, mobilization of fat, elevated blood cose and insulin, and an increase in the size of the adrenal glands.

zest. Outer skin of citrus fruits.

zexanthin. One of the carotenoid pigments in maize, egg yolk and *Physalis*; has no vitamin A activity; used as a colouring.

Ziegel cheese. A kind of cheese made in Austria from either whole milk or whole milk to which 15% of cream has been added. It is ready for market after about 8 weeks.

Ziger-Schottenziger-albumin. A German whey-protein cheese made by coagulating the albumin with heat and acid, then skimming it off the hot curd, cooling and draining tit on cheesecloth and pressing it in a Swiss cheese press for 24 hours. Then it is placed in a salt bath to which cider or vinegar is sometimes added. Also known as ricotta.

zig-zag clover. *Trifolium medium*. A variety of true clover and an offshoot of red clover. The plant is native to Europe and Siberia. Its name derives from the odd configurations of its stems. The plant is a perennial of very limited use.

zinc. An element of functional significance in several enzymes such as lactic dehydrogenase, alkaline phosphatase, and carbonic anhydrase. The deficiency of zinc in diet causes hypogonadism, growth failure, impaired wound healing, decreased sensitivity of taste and smell. At least 15 mg/day of zinc is required by adults, while pregnant and lactating women require more zinc. It is essential for plant growth, and a dietary essential for man and animals. Its deficiency results in hypogonadism. Present as part of enzymes carbonic anhydrase and uricase, and in crystalline insulin. Found in traces in most foods. Oysters concentrate zinc from seawater and can contain up to 0.3%.

Zinfandel grape. An extensively planted red wine grape which is quite productive. The exact origin of this grape has not been successfully traced. The wine yielded is of good quality and with a characteristic flavor of its own, identified as a "bramble" flavor (suggestive of wild blackberries or dewberries) by some tasters.

Zomma cheese. A variety of Turkish, plastic-curd Caviocavallo-type cheese, which is similar to Katschkawalj; it contains at least 30% fat.

zomotherapy. Treatment by raw meat or raw meat-juice; used for anaemia, neurasthenia, in convalescence.

zoopherin. An old name for vitamin B_{12}.

z-value. A value characteristic of a microorganism, which measures the change in the death rate with respect to a change in temperature; numerically equal to the number of degrees Fahrenheit required to change by a factor of 10 the time required to kill an organism at a specified temperature; dimension of temperature degrees. (i.e., °F). The z-value is a basic parameter in the heat process evaluation scheme.

zwieback. German term for twice-baked bread. Ordinary dough plus eggs and butter, baked, sliced, baked again to a rusk and sometimes sugar coated.

zymase. Name given to the mixture of enzymes in yeast that is responsible for fermentation.

zymogen. Any inactive enzyme precursor that, following secretion, is chemically altered to the active form of the enzyme. Trypsin is secreted by the pancreas as zymogen trypsinogen, this is changed in the small intestine by the action of another enzyme, enterokinase, to the active form. Zymogens are often packaged in the cell, especially in secretory cells of pancreas, for example, such packages are termed zymogen granules.